Essentials
of Psychiatric
Mental Health
Nursing SECOND EDITION

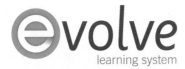
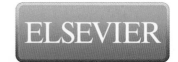
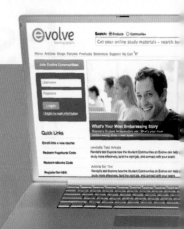

Essentials *of* Psychiatric Mental Health Nursing

SECOND EDITION

A Communication Approach to Evidence-Based Care

Elizabeth M. Varcarolis, RN, MA
Professor Emeritus
Formerly Deputy Chairperson, Department of Nursing
Borough of Manhattan Community College;
Associate Fellow
Albert Ellis Institute for Rational Emotional Behavioral Therapy (REBT)
New York, New York

ELSEVIER
SAUNDERS

3251 Riverport Drive
St. Louis, Missouri 63043

Notice

Knowledge and best practice in this field are constantly changing. As new research and experience broaden our knowledge, changes in practice, treatment, and drug therapy may become necessary or appropriate. Readers are advised to check the most current information provided (i) on procedures featured or (ii) by the manufacturer of each product to be administered, to verify the recommended dose or formula, the method and duration of administration, and contraindications. It is the responsibility of the practitioner, relying on their own experience and knowledge of the patient, to make diagnoses, to determine dosages and the best treatment for each individual patient, and to take all appropriate safety precautions. To the fullest extent of the law, neither the Publisher nor the Authors assume any liability for any injury and/or damage to persons or property arising out of or related to any use of the material contained in this book.

The Publisher

Library of Congress Cataloging-in-Publication Data
Varcarolis, Elizabeth M.
  Essentials of psychiatric mental health nursing: a communication approach to evidence-based care/ Elizabeth M. Varcarolis. — 2nd ed.
      p. ; cm.
  Includes bibliographical references.
  ISBN 978-1-4557-0661-7 (pbk. : alk. paper)
  I. Title.
  [DNLM: 1. Mental Disorders—nursing. 2. Evidence-Based Nursing. 3. Nurse-Patient Relations. 4. Nursing Process. 5. Psychiatric Nursing—ethics. 6. Psychiatric Nursing—methods. WY 160]
  616.89'0231—dc23   2012022983

Senior Content Strategist: Yvonne Alexopoulos
Senior Content Developmental Specialist: Lisa P. Newton
Publishing Services Manager: Jeff Patterson
Project Manager: Jeanne Genz
Designer: Ashley Eberts

Printed in China

Last digit is the print number: 9   8   7   6   5   4   3   2   1

To the memory of Josiah and Ruth Merrill, who
gave me life and opportunity and who I miss every day.

And especially to my husband Paul, whose love
and devotion become more and more evident as time
passes. Thanks for the wonderful years.

To the memory of Ruth Matheney
and Suzanne Lego, who as mentors made such
a difference in my professional career.

Betsy Varcarolis

ACKNOWLEDGMENTS

As is always the case, I owe a huge debt of gratitude to many for their contributions and support.

I thank Dr. Margaret (Peggy) Jordan Halter for her generous and outstanding contributions to the first edition of *Essentials*. Peggy brings multiple talents and expertise to any project she undertakes. Thank you Peggy for your hard work on the first edition. She has since taken over as the sole editor/author of the popular ***Foundations of Psychiatric Mental Health Nursing: A Clinical Approach***, a huge undertaking. She was the sole editor/author of the sixth edition and will continue through future editions. She is launching this well-regarded text into the 21st century.

The two unique and creative features that are the "gems" of this text continue in this edition. They are enticing, interesting, and great learning tools for our students. The first of these features is "Examining the Evidence" boxes. I am grateful to Lois Angelo, MSN, APRN, for her contributions to all but three of the "Examining the Evidence" boxes and for her diligence in introducing pressing issues within the practice of psychiatric nursing as well as the latest evidence to help guide nurses in their care and understanding of current issues. I thank Dr. Margaret Halter for her "Examining the Evidence" box in Chapter 1, which was used in the first edition of this text.

I have been fortunate enough to have Dr. Dolly C. Sadow and Marie Ryder, CPRP, CNS-BC, submit "Examining the Evidence" boxes on "stigma" and "peer supervision in consumer providers" in Chapters 2 and 3, respectively.

The second gem is the "Applying the Art" boxes, all contributed by Dawn Scheick; they are found in all of the clinical chapters (Chapters 10-19). Dawn offers excellent examples of how a nurse can incorporate effective and insightful communication while working with patients possessing a variety of needs and displaying a wide range of behaviors.

Communication is one of the arts taught to all nursing students, and effective communication strategies are the cornerstone of psychiatric mental health nursing. The text offers many pedagogical features that will benefit both the cognitive as well as the visual learner. It is hoped that the reader will gain fresh insights, attain a broader understanding, and learn effective tools in their interactions with vulnerable individuals during their treatment toward a more mentally healthy quality of life.

I want to offer special thanks to the amazing authors who have contributed to this edition of *Essentials of Psychiatric Mental Health Nursing* and for their expertise and hard work. Sincere and profound thanks go to Peggy Halter, Dorothy Varchol, Penny Brooke, Kathleen Ibrahim, Kathy Kramer-Howe, and Ed Herzog in order of the appearance of their chapters.

A very special thanks to Teresa Burckhalter and Mary Gilkey for their creative work on the instructor and student ancillaries to accompany this book.

I have been fortunate to be part of a patient and hard-working team. The people working behind the scenes are always pivotal to the production of any successful text. These are the people who have provided support, kept the project on track, and solved a myriad of problems that are inherent in any production:

- Yvonne Alexopoulos, Senior Content Strategist, always supported and provided everything needed to make the second edition of *Essentials* a success.
- Lisa P. Newton, Senior Content Developmental Specialist, pulled together resources, provided support, and untangled dilemmas during the publication process.
- Kit Blanke, Editorial Assistant, handled multiple details for the book.
- Jeanne Genz, Project Manager, managed consistency to the minutest detail and has made me look good through the process. Thanks Jeanne.
- Ashley Eberts, Book Designer, created a vivid, exciting, and reader-friendly design.

CONTRIBUTORS

Lois Angelo, MSN, APRN, BC
Assistant Professor of Nursing
University of New Hampshire
Durham, New Hampshire

Ann Wolbert Burgess, DNSc, APRN, BC, FAAN
Professor of Psychiatric Nursing
William F. Connell School of Nursing
Boston College
Chestnut Hill, Massachusetts

Margaret Jordan Halter, PhD, APRN
Associate Dean
Ashland University College of Nursing
Ashland, Ohio

Edward A. Herzog, MSN, APRN
Faculty
Kent State University
Kent, Ohio

Kathleen Ibrahim, MA, APRN, BC
Assistant to the Director of Nursing
New York State Psychiatric Institute
New York, New York

Kathy Kramer-Howe, MSW, LCSW
Hospice of the Valley
Phoenix, Arizona

Dolly C. Sadow, PhD, ABPP
Med Options of Massachusetts
Bedford, Massachusetts

Dawn M. Scheick, EdD RN, PMHCNS, BC
Chair and Professor of Nursing
Alderson-Broaddus College;
Therapist
Barbour County Health Department
Philippi, West Virginia

Sheila Rouslin Welt, MS, APN
Private Practice, Psychotherapy
Morristown, New Jersey;
Educational Consultation
The Pingry School
Short Hills, New Jersey

Marie K. Ryder, CPRP, CNS-BC
Professor of Nursing
Middlesex Community College
Bedford, Massachusetts

Penny Simpson Brooke, APRN, MS, JD
University of Utah
College of Nursing
Salt Lake City, Utah

Shirley A. Smoyak, RN, PhD, FAAN
Professor II (distinguished)
Rutgers University
New Brunswick, New Jersey

Dorothy A. Varchol, RNBC, MA, MSN
Nursing Faculty in Health and Public Safety
Cincinnati State Technical and Community College
Cincinnati, Ohio

Teresa S. Burckhalter, MSN, RN, BC
Nursing Faculty
Technical College of the Lowcountry
Beaufort, South Carolina
Test Bank

Mary Blessing Gilkey, APRN, BC, MS
Assistant Professor
Hampton University
Hampton, Virginia
Student Resources

Marie Messier, MSN, RN
Associate Professor of Nursing
Germanna Community College
Locust Grove, Virginia
Student Resources

REVIEWERS

Janet Flynn, RN, MSN
Associate Professor of Nursing
Elgin Community College
Elgin, Illinois

Phyllis Jacobs, BSN, MSN
Assistant Professor/Director
Undergraduate Nursing Program
Wichita State University
Wichita, Kansas

Loyce A. Kennedy, MSN, RN
Assistant Professor of Nursing
Arkansas Tech University—Fort Smith
Sparks Hospital
Fort Smith, Arkansas

Cindy Parsons, DNP, PMHNP-BC, FAANP
Assistant Professor of Nursing
University of Tampa
Tampa, Florida

Marie K. Ryder, CPRP, CNS-BC
Professor of Nursing
Middlesex Community College
Bedford, Massachusetts

Kathleen Slyh, RN, MSN
Nursing Instructor
Technical College of the Lowcountry
Beaufort, South Carolina

Donna Webb, RN, BSN, MSN
Nursing Instructor
Texas State Technical College
Brownwood, Texas

Essentials of Psychiatric Mental Health Nursing: A Communication Approach to Evidence-Based Care, ed 2, presents the essential content for a shorter course without sacrificing either the current research or the nursing and psychotherapeutic interventions necessary to sound practice. In fact, all efforts have been taken to ensure research and psychotherapeutic interventions reflect current knowledge.

This *Essentials,* ed 2, continues to provide a comprehensive but concise review of the prominent theorists and all therapeutic modalities in use today, including milieu, group, and family therapies, in Chapter 3, "Theories and Therapies." Within each of the clinical chapters (Chapters 10 through 19), chapters that examine various psychiatric emergencies (Chapters 20-25), and chapters that address discrete patient populations across the life span (Chapters 26 through 28), specific therapeutic modalities that have proven effective for each topic are thoroughly covered.

In addition to the overview of medication groups in Chapter 4, "Biological Basis for Understanding Psychopharmacology," specific medications are covered in full for each of the discrete clinical disorders, including patient and family teaching guidelines. Integrative therapies are also included in each of the clinical chapters where they have proven effective.

In order to present the most essential base of knowledge for a shorter course, the pertinent information on some topics has been incorporated into the clinical chapters where applicable, rather than included in a separate chapter. For example, rather than include a general chapter on culture, each of the clinical chapters incorporates relevant information on cultural aspects of the various clinical disorders, which can also help give the reader a broader cultural perspective.

Forensic issues related to the nursing care of patients are included in specific chapters, especially "Child, Partner, and Elder Violence" (Chapter 21) and "Sexual Violence" (Chapter 22). This is in addition to Chapter 6, "Legal and Ethical Basis for Practice."

THE SCIENCE AND ART OF PSYCHIATRIC MENTAL HEALTH NURSING

The American Nurses Association's *Psychiatric Mental Health Nursing: Scope and Standards of Practice* begins with the following statement that stresses the importance of both the art and the science employed by nurses caring for patients with mental health problems and psychiatric disorders:

"Psychiatric–mental health nursing, a core mental health profession, employs a purposeful use of self as its art and a wide range of nursing, psychosocial, and neurobiological theories and research evidence as its science."

In *Essentials of Psychiatric Mental Health Nursing: A Communication Approach to Evidence-Based Care,* ed 2, there is an effort to integrate and balance these two aspects of nursing care and present all of the essential information on each so that students will be prepared to offer the best possible care when they enter practice.

The Science

Over the past couple decades we have seen remarkable scientific progress in our understanding of the workings of the brain and how abnormalities in the function of the brain are related to mental illness. As confidence in this research grew, the focus on scientific research expanded and led to more scientifically based treatment approaches, and the concept of *evidence-based practice* became a dominant focus of mental health treatment.

While writing this text a great effort was made to provide the most current evidence-based information in the field while at the same time keeping the material comprehensible and reader-friendly. Relevant information drawn from science is woven throughout the book.

Chapter 1, "Practicing the Science and Art of Psychiatric Nursing," introduces the student to the evolution of evidence-based practice (EBP) and the mechanics of the practice and gives the reader guidelines for where and how to gather information for applying EBP in psychiatric nursing practice.

Perhaps one of the two most unique features of this book is the **Examining the Evidence** feature, which is introduced in Chapter 1 and runs throughout the clinical chapters. Each box poses a question, walks the readers through the process of gathering evidence-based data from a variety of sources, and presents the evidence from different points of view.

The Art

In comparison with the medical model, the *recovery model* is a more social, relationship-based model of care. The focus of the recovery model is more of a nurse/physician partner relationship. The recovery model began in the addiction field, in which the goal was for individuals to recover from substance abuse and addictions. Today the recovery model is gaining momentum in the larger mental health community. Its focus is on empowering patients by supporting hope, strengthening social ties, developing more effective coping skills, and fostering the use of spiritual strength, and more.

By definition, nurses are primed to incorporate the biopsychosocial and cultural/spiritual approaches to care. Some nursing leaders express concern that the "art" of nursing is becoming marginalized by the emphasis on evidence-based practice. Chapter 1 covers some of these often minimized and uncharted interventions such as the art of caring, the skill of attending, and patient advocacy. However, what also might be minimized and deemphasized are the tools that make nurses unique. Some of these tools include possessing effective communication skills, forming therapeutic relationships, and understanding ways of interviewing and assessing our patients' needs. These areas are stressed in Chapter 8, "Communication Skills: Medium for All Nursing Practice," and Chapter 9, "Therapeutic Relationships and the Clinical Interview." There is also a section in each of the clinical chapters on useful communications techniques for a specific disorder or situation.

The second of the unique features that are also included in the clinical chapters are the **Applying the Art** boxes, which depict a clinical scenario demonstrating the interactions between a student and a patient (both therapeutic and non-therapeutic), the student's perception of the interaction, and the identification of the mental health nursing concepts in play.

ORGANIZATION

Organized into five units, the chapters in the book have been grouped to emphasize the clinical perspective and to facilitate locating information. All clinical chapters are organized in a clear, logical, and consistent format with the nursing process as the strong, visible framework. The basic outline for clinical chapters is:

- Prevalence and Comorbidity
  Knowing the comorbid disorders that are often part of the clinical picture of specific disorders helps students as well as clinicians understand how to better assess and treat their patients.
- Theory
- Cultural Considerations
- Clinical Picture
- ***Application of the Nursing Process***
  - Assessment
    Presents appropriate assessment for a specific disorder, including assessment tools and rating scales. The rating scales included help highlight important areas in the assessment of a variety of behaviors or mental conditions. Because many of the answers are subjective, experienced clinicians use these tools as a guide when planning care, in addition to their knowledge of their patients.
  - Diagnosis
    Includes the latest NANDA-I (2012-2014) terminology.
  - Outcomes Identification
  - Planning
  - Implementation
    Interventions follow the categories set by the ANA Psychiatric–Mental Health Nursing: Scope and Standards of Practice (2007). Various interventions for each of the clinical disorders are chosen based on which of them most fit specific patient needs, including communication guidelines, health teaching and health promotion, milieu therapy, psychotherapy, and pharmacological, biological, and integrative therapies.
  - Evaluation

FEATURES

In addition to boxes **Examining the Evidence** boxes and **Applying the Art** tables described above, the following features are included in the book to inform, heighten understanding, and engage the reader:

- Chapters open with **Objectives** and **Key Terms and Concepts** to orient the reader.
- Numerous **Vignettes** describing psychiatric patients and their disorders attract and hold the readers' interest.
- **Assessment Guidelines** are included in clinical chapters to familiarize readers with methods of assessing patients; also for use in the clinical setting.
- **Potential Nursing Diagnoses** tables list several possible nursing diagnoses for a particular disorder along with the associated signs and symptoms.
- **Nursing Interventions** tables list interventions for a given disorder or clinical situation, along with rationales for each intervention.
- **Key Points to Remember** present the main concepts of each chapter in an easy to comprehend and concise bulleted list.
- **Critical Thinking** questions at the end of all chapters introduce clinical situations in psychiatric nursing and encourage critical thinking processes essential for nursing practice.
- **Chapter Review** questions at the end of each chapter reinforce key concepts. Answers are listed on the Evolve website.
- Appendixes provide the ***DSM-IV-TR*** and a list of the latest **NANDA-I diagnoses**.

LEARNING AND TEACHING AIDS

For Students

The Evolve Student Resources for this book include the following:

- *Chapter Review Answers*, including rationales and page references
- *Case Studies* and *Nursing Care Plans* for clinical disorders
- *Concept Supplements* for additional help
- *Nurse, Patient, and Family Resources*, which include web addresses, association information, and additional resources for patient teaching material, medication information, and support groups

For Instructors

The Evolve Instructor Resources for this book include the following:

- ***TEACH for Nurses* Lesson Plans**, based on textbook chapter Learning Objectives, serve as ready-made, modifiable lesson plans and a complete roadmap to link all parts of the educational package. These concise and straightforward lesson plans can be modified or combined to meet your particular scheduling and teaching needs.
- ***Test Bank*** in ExamView formats, featuring approximately 800 test items, complete with correct answer, rationale, cognitive level, nursing process step, appropriate NCLEX© label, and corresponding textbook page references. The

ExamView program allows instructors to create new tests; edit, add, and delete test questions; sort questions by NCLEX category, cognitive level, and nursing process step; and administer and grade tests online.

- *PowerPoint Presentations* with more than 600 customizable lecture slides.
- *Audience Response Questions* for i>clicker and other systems with 2 to 5 multiple-answer questions per chapter to stimulate class discussion and assess student understanding of key concepts.

I hope you all find that *Essentials of Psychiatric Mental Health Nursing: A Communication Approach to Evidence-Based Care,* ed 2, provides you with the information you need to be successful in your practice of nursing... Good luck to you all.

Betsy Merrill Varcarolis

CONTENTS

UNIT 5   AGE-RELATED MENTAL HEALTH DISORDERS

Essential Theoretical Concepts for Practice

Hildegard E. Peplau (1909-1999)
"Mother of Psychiatric Nursing"

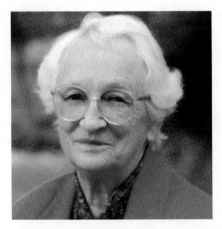

Hildegard Peplau has had the most profound effect on the practice of nursing since Florence Nightingale. Peplau's interpersonal theory of nursing was strongly influenced by Harry Stack Sullivan's Interpersonal Relationship Theory, as well as Maslow, Freud and others. Peplau was the first nursing theorist to bring in theory from other scientific fields and integrate them into a nursing theory. Her interpersonal theories lead to a paradigm shift in the nature of the nurse-patient relationship (now often referred to in medicine as the patient-centered relationship). Peplau was the first to theorize that the nurse's therapeutic use of self during the nurse-patient interactions had a direct bearing on the outcome of the patient's well-being.

Hildegard Peplau received a master's and doctorate degree from Teachers College, Columbia University and it was there that she developed the first graduate program specific to psychiatric nursing. At Rutgers University, New Jersey (1954 to 1974) she created a Master's program for the preparation of clinical specialists in psychiatric nursing, the first of its kind for any nursing discipline.

As you read through this text you will learn about the different levels of anxiety, the phases of the nurse-patient relationship, and the importance of observing your own thoughts and feelings within the context of the nurse-patient interaction. These are all indispensible tools used by competent nurses today, all contributions from Hildegard Peplau. Peplau's model and contributions have served as a springboard for later nurse theorists and clinicians in developing more sophisticated and therapeutic nursing interventions.

Peplau's contribution goes way beyond psychiatric nursing. She promoted the idea of advanced practice nursing which lead to professional standards and regulation through credentialing. Even nurses who never heard of Hildegard Peplau are profoundly affected by the art and the science she brought to nursing, and are fundamental to nursing as well as the practice of psychiatric nursing.

1

Practicing the Science and the Art of Psychiatric Nursing

Elizabeth M. Varcarolis

evolve WEBSITE

http://evolve.elsevier.com/Varcarolis/essentials

KEY TERMS AND CONCEPTS

5 A's, p. 4
attending, p. 8
caring, p. 6
clinical algorithms, p. 5
clinical/critical pathways, p. 6
clinical practice guidelines, p. 5

evidence-based practice (EBP), p. 3
nurse-patient partnership, p. 3
patient advocate, p. 8
psychiatric mental health
   nursing, p. 3
recovery model, p. 3

SELECTED CONCEPT: Patient Advocacy

Three fundamental elements of patient advocacy include:

- To ensure that patients are informed of their rights in a particular situation, including the right to refuse treatment.
- To support patients and decisions they make.
- To protect patients, which includes reporting threats to their well-being.

Inherent in the responsibilities of advocating for patients include the following protections:

- Privacy
- Confidentiality
- Protection in participation in research
- Standards and review mechanisms
- Acting on questionable practices
- Addressing impaired practice

(Marcus, 2011; ANA, 2001)

OBJECTIVES

1. Contrast and compare the focus and approach of the mental health recovery model to the evidence-based practice (EBP) model.
2. Identify the "5 A's" in the simple multistep process of evidence-based practice and describe what is inherent in each step of this process.
3. Discuss at least three current dilemmas nurses face when they seek the best evidence for their interventions.
4. Identify four resources that nurses can use as guidelines for best-evidence interventions.
5. Defend why the concept of "caring" should be a basic ingredient to the practice of nursing and how it is expressed by nurses in the clinical setting.
6. Discuss what is meant by being a patient advocate.

Psychiatric nursing is a specialized area of nursing practice. Its focus is the treatment of human responses to mental health problems and psychiatric disorders. "Psychiatric–mental health nursing, a core mental health profession, employs a purposeful use of self as its art and a wide range of nursing, psychosocial, and neurobiological theories and research evidence as its science" (ANA, 2007, p. 1).

Starting around the 1990s (the "Decade of the Brain") more funding for brain research became available and remarkable progress was made in our understanding of how to treat illnesses caused by brain dysfunction. The method for using treatment approaches to medical illness and mental health illness that are scientifically grounded or evidence based became known as evidence-based practice (EBP). In psychiatry the evidence-based focus extends to treatment approaches in which there is scientific evidence for psychological and sociological treatment methodologies, as well as evidence related to the neurobiology of psychiatric disorders and psychopharmacology. Therefore evidence-based practice strives to decrease the gap between research and practice (Dorn, 2005). This model is consistent with the familiar traditional medical model.

The mental health recovery model, on the other hand, is more of a social model of disability than a medical model of disability. Therefore the focus shifts from one of illness and disease to an emphasis on rehabilitation and recovery (Caldwell et al., 2010). The recovery model originated from the 12-step program of Alcoholics Anonymous and was advanced by a grassroots advocacy initiative called the Consumer/Survivor/Ex-patient Movement during the 1980s and early 1990s. The concept of recovery refers primarily to managing symptoms, reducing psychosocial disability, and improving role performance (Pratt et al., 2006). Holistic interventions are designed to increase recovery as evidenced by engagement in work and engagement in community/social life, as well as a reduction of symptoms (Beebe, 2010). Recovering from a mental illness is viewed as a personal journey of healing.

The goal of recovery is to empower those with mental illness to find meaning and satisfaction in their lives, realize personal potential, and function at their optimal level of independence. It has been found that supportive relationships, social inclusion, acquisition of needed coping skills, recovery-oriented services, and sense of hope for the future can lead to a sustainable belief in oneself; to a sense of empowerment and self-determination, meaning, and satisfaction; and to the highest quality of life within the limitations of the illness. The principles of the recovery model have been adopted by a number of countries and states. The focus of the recovery model has the following mandates (Caldwell et al., 2010, p. 43):

- Mental health care is to be consumer and family driven.
- Care must focus on increasing consumer's ability to be successful in coping with life's challenges, facilitating recovery, and building resilience—not just managing symptoms.
- An individualized plan of care is to be at the core of consumer-centered recovery—recovery-oriented services that allow consumers to realize improved mental health and quality of life.
- Consumers must be partners in decision making in all aspects of care.

Therefore the concept of the **nurse-patient relationship,** or physician-patient relationship originating from the medical model, suggests an unequal status with the nurse/health care worker as the person in authority. The emphasis today is much more on the nurse-patient partnership, which is more in line with the emphasis on "relationships" in the recovery model (Stuart, 2011).

Forchuk (2001), Benner (2004), and other psychiatric nursing leaders stress the importance of psychiatric nursing taking a leadership role in creating patient-centered care that demonstrates how to establish a relationship within a recovery-based model and at the same time understand and incorporate the evidence related to the neurobiology of psychiatric disorders and psychotropic medications.

THE SCIENCE OF NURSING: FINDING THE EVIDENCE FOR THE PRACTICE

Basing nursing and medical practice on a systematic approach to care is not new. In the past century, nursing began with a strong emphasis on practice. McDonald (2001) states that Florence Nightingale (1820 to 1910), the founder of modern nursing, had a philosophy reflecting an evidence-based framework. Nightingale advocated for the "best possible research, access the best available governmental statistics and expertise…" (p. 2). During the 1860 International Statistical Congress held in London, Nightingale made a proposal that was to result in "the first model for systemic collection of hospital data using a uniform classification of diseases and operations and was to form the basis of the *International Statistical Classification of Diseases and Related Health Problems* (ICD) used today worldwide" (Keith, 1988). Mental health professionals in the United States substitute the *Diagnostic and Statistical Manual of Mental Disorders (DSM)* for the mental health section of the *ICD*. The *DSM* is discussed in more detail in Chapter 2.

Hildegard Peplau (1909 to 1999), considered the mother of psychiatric nursing, had a passion for clarifying and developing the art and science of professional nursing practice and believed that a scientific approach was essential to the practice of psychiatric nursing (Haber, 2000). Her contributions went far beyond what she brought to the field of psychiatric nursing. She introduced the concept of advanced nursing practice and promoted professional standards and regulation through credentialing among a multitude of other contributions to nursing (Tomey, 2006).

It should be noted that psychiatry was one of the first medical specialties to extensively use randomized controlled trials. One of the founding principles of clinical psychology in the 1950s was that practice should be based on the results of experimental comparisons of treatment methods (Geddes et al., 2004). However, without scientific evidence for practice, much of nursing care has been based on tradition, personal experience, unsystematic trial and error, and the earlier experiences of nurses and others in the health care profession (Wilson, 2004; Zauszniewski & Suresky, 2003).

The emergence of evidence-based nursing practice in the United States originated from the evidence-based practice movement in the medical community in England and Canada during the 1980s and 1990s (Mick, 2005). During that time there was an increase in research-related journals, the most relevant of which for nurses was the development of the *Evidence-Based Nursing* journal in 1998.

The University of Minnesota defines EBP as "the process by which the best available research evidence (from well-designed studies), clinical expertise, and patient preferences are used for making clinical decisions." Melnyk (2004) states there is no magic bullet that provides a formula describing the weight of evidence that patient values and preferences and clinical expertise should take in making clinical decisions. Mantzoukas (2007) warns that although EBP is equated with effective decision making, avoidance of habitual practice, and enhanced clinical performance, there is a tendency to overlook certain types of knowledge that through reflection can provide useful information for individualized and effective practice.

Numerous definitions delineate the multistep process of integrating EBP into clinical practice. One that is simply stated and apt is used at the Children's Mercy Hospital in Kansas City, Missouri (Mick, 2005), referred to as the 5 A's:

1. *Ask a question.* Identify a problem or need for change for a specific patient or situation.
2. *Acquire literature.* Search the literature for scientific studies and articles that address the issue(s) of concern.
3. *Appraise the literature.* Evaluate and synthesize the research evidence regarding its validity, relevance, and applicability using criteria of scientific merit.
4. *Apply the evidence.* Choose interventions that are based on the best available evidence with the understanding of the patient's preference and needs.
5. *Assess the performance.* Evaluate the outcomes, using clearly defined criteria and reports, and document results.

Evaluating the evidence is done through a hierarchical rating system. Randomized controlled studies and evidence-based clinical practice guidelines provide the strongest evidence on which to base clinical practice. In a randomized controlled trial (RCT) patients are chosen at random (by chance) to receive one of several clinical interventions. One intervention would be the intervention under study and another might be the standard intervention or a placebo. The weakest level is from expert committee reports, opinions, clinical experience, or descriptive studies. Table 1-1 presents a hierarchy of evidence and grading for each level.

The first Surgeon General's report published on the topic of mental health was in 1999 (U.S. Department of Health and Human Services [USDHHS], 1999). This landmark document was based on an extensive review of the scientific literature and in consultation with mental health providers and consumers (Zauszniewski & Suresky, 2003). The document concluded that there are numerous effective psychopharmacological and psychosocial treatments for most mental disorders. However, it raised some questions for psychiatric nurses, including the following (Stuart, 2001):

• Are psychiatric nurses aware of the efficacy of the treatment and interventions they provide?
• Are they truly practicing evidence-based care?
• Is there documentation of the nature and outcomes of the care they provide?

There is no question that emphasis on evidence-based practice in medicine and mental health is expanding. Interventions based on the best research evidence combined with clinical expertise seem an ideal approach. However, this approach will not provide easy answers, and much discussion and questions are raised regarding the practice of evidence-based mental health nursing. First, who interprets "best evidence"?

Second, not all nursing problems are able to be reduced to a clear issue solvable by scientific experiments (White, 1997). White continues to stress that many problems are addressed by using "artistry" to find solutions.

Third, relatively few studies backed by rigorous quantitative research are available from which to select nursing interventions and to guide psychiatric nursing care practices. Of 227 data-based studies published between 2000 and 2003, only 52 (23%) included nurses, student nurses, or other mental health care professionals. Of these 52 studies, only 11 (21%) involved examining psychiatric nursing interventions. Promoting EBP in psychiatric nursing will require increasing the number of studies by researchers who possess clinical knowledge and research expertise (Zauszniewski & Suresky, 2003).

Fourth, there is the question: How do nurses who are practicing in an environment of reduced staffing, increased

TABLE 1-1   HIERARCHY OF EVIDENCE AND GRADING OF RECOMMENDATIONS

Each recommendation has been allocated a grading that directly reflects the hierarchy of evidence on which it has been based. Please note that the hierarchy of evidence and the recommendation gradings relate to the strength of the literature, not to clinical importance.

HIERARCHY OF EVIDENCE		GRADING OF RECOMMENDATIONS	
Level	Type of Evidence	Level	Type of Evidence
Ia	Evidence from systematic reviews or meta-analyses of randomized controlled trials	A	Based on hierarchy I evidence
Ib	Evidence from at least one randomized controlled trial		
IIa	Evidence from at least one controlled study without randomization	B	Based on hierarchy II evidence or extrapolated from hierarchy I evidence
IIb	Evidence from at least one other type of quasi-experimental study		
III	Evidence from nonexperimental descriptive studies, such as comparative studies, correlation studies, and case control studies	C	Based on hierarchy III evidence or extrapolated from hierarchy I or II evidence
IV	Evidence from expert committee reports or opinions and/or clinical experience of respected authorities	D	Directly based on hierarchy IV evidence or extrapolated from hierarchy I, II, or III evidence

From Hierarchy of evidence and grading of recommendations. (2004). *Thorax, 59*(3), 181-272.

complexity, and stress on issues of cost-effectiveness find time to research the literature, evaluate numerous studies (if indeed they are available), and make decisions on "best evidence?" This question still needs a definitive answer; however, some of the following provide valuable guidelines for current practice:

1. *Internet mental health resources.* A number of sites provide mental health resources online for information, treatment provisions, and the results of recent clinical studies. There are self-tests for people to see if they may be experiencing, at least in part, a specific syndrome or disorder (e.g., depression, elation, attention deficit/hyperactivity disorder [ADHD]). There are also resources for acquiring support and treatment. Box 1-1 provides a short list of popular mental health sites. It is best to focus on sites that are maintained by professional societies, professional librarians, or other organizations whose quality is evidence based in order to reduce the amount of uncensored information of low quality.

2. *Clinical practice guidelines.* Clinical practice guidelines are systematically developed statements that identify, appraise, and summarize the best evidence about prevention, diagnosis, prognosis, therapy, and other knowledge necessary to make informed decisions about specific health problems. They are based on literature review (scientific research in the form of randomized controlled clinical trials; reports of series, or case studies; or "expert clinical experience" [AAPMR, 2006]). The development and use of practice guidelines can increase quality and consistency of care and facilitate outcome research. Essentially, they (1) identify practice questions and explicitly identify all the decision options and outcomes; (2) identify the "best evidence" about prevention, diagnosis, prognosis, therapy, harm, and cost-effectiveness; and (3) identify the decision points

BOX 1-1   MENTAL HEALTH WEB RESOURCES

- American Association of Pastoral Counselors: www.aapc.org
- American Psychiatric Association: www.psych.org
- American Psychological Association: www.apa.org
- American Psychiatric Nurses Association: www.apna.org
- Brain Technologies: www.braintechnologies.com
- Centre for Addiction and Mental Health: www.camh.net
- National Institute of Mental Health: www.nimh.nih.gov
- National Institute of Nursing Research: www.ninr.nih.gov
- U.S. Department of Health and Human Services, National Guideline Clearinghouse: www.guidelines.gov

at which this "best evidence" needs to be integrated with individual clinical experience and patients' needs and goals in deciding on a course of action. The American Psychiatric Association's (APA) *Clinical Practice Guidelines* and the National Quality Measures Clearinghouse offer such guidelines. The U.S. Department of Health and Human Services sponsors a National Guidelines Clearinghouse of evidence-based guidelines pertaining to a wide range of medical and mental health conditions (www.guidelines.gov).

3. *Clinical algorithms.* Clinical algorithms are step-by-step guidelines prepared in a flowchart format. Alternative diagnostic and treatment approaches are described based on decisional points using a large database relevant for the symptoms, diagnosis, or treatment modalities. Algorithms are especially helpful in deciding what medication

to use considering a wide variety of variables related to the patient's personal situation (e.g., age, gender, current medications, ethnic origin, allergies). Figure 1-1 depicts a clinical algorithm for the suspicion of suicide risk.

4. *Clinical/critical pathways.* Clinical/critical pathways are usually specific to the institution using them. They are most often used in relation to hospitalized patients and target a specific population (e.g., suicidal patient, bipolar patient–manic, a depressed patient, an individual with schizophrenia). These clinical pathways serve as a "map" for specified treatments and interventions to occur within a specific time frame, often days. For example, the clinical guide may state for the day of admission certain goals are to be reached and specific interventions are to be carried out by different members of the health team (e.g., physicians, nurses, social workers, dietitians). The interventions include preadmission workup, tests, diet and health teaching, medication, and observation of effectiveness or adverse effects, through discharge plans and follow-up care. Each pathway lists the expected outcomes using a measurable, time-limited format, and documentation is ongoing. Some institutions computerize these clinical pathways within the patient's chart. Clinical/critical pathways and maps offer a great opportunity for the integration of research into clinical practice when the interventions are evidence based.

The Research-Practice Gap

Unfortunately, there is a wide gap between the best evidence treatments and their effective delivery into practice. The need for continued research on how best to apply the findings of clinically relevant issues and their delivery into clinical practice has been the emphasis of the Institute of Medicine (IOM) (2006):

> "…research that has identified the efficacy of specific treatments under rigorously controlled conditions has been accompanied by almost no research identifying how to make these same treatments effective when delivered in usual settings of care…when administered by service providers without specialized education in the therapy" (p. 350).

Effective research is reported in language that is understandable and free of statistical and research jargon (Zauszniewski & Suresky, 2003), and appropriate dissemination of findings needs to reach nursing practitioners. Despite the complexities and concerns that demand to be addressed, evidence-based nursing is becoming a foundation for nursing practice. Eventually the use of scientific evidence-based practice will reduce the use of unwarranted nursing practices and alleviate the severity of nursing errors. Furthermore, the use of evidence-based practice optimizes the process of evaluation and facilitates the nurse's development and professional advancement (Jasmine, 2009).

To help the reader understand how best evidence is identified and applied to nursing interventions, this textbook contains a feature titled Examining the Evidence. It is hoped that this feature, presented in each of the clinical chapters, will underscore the importance of sound scientific inquiry and ignite the reader's interest in research.

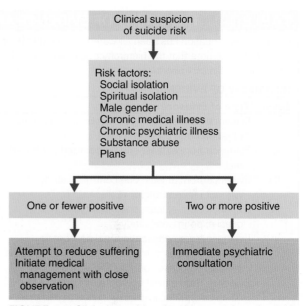

FIGURE 1-1 Clinical algorithm for the suspicion of suicide risk. (Modified from Goldman, L., & Ausiello, D. [2008]. *Cecil medicine* [23rd ed.]. Philadelphia: Saunders.)

THE ART OF NURSING: DEVELOPING THE SKILLS FOR THE PRACTICE

Contemporary nursing relies on a high level of scientific thought in its theories, research, and knowledge base. However, there is an "art" to nursing as well. Even the best evidence-based guidelines may not be sufficient for the patient who stands in front of you with a very individualized set of problems and capacities. Such individuality is complex, demanding that nurses use intuition, interpersonal skills, and the therapeutic use of self. These "arts" complement nursing's scientific base and are indispensable for treating any patient effectively. As Williams and Garner (2002, p. 8) conclude, "Too great an emphasis on evidence-based medicine oversimplifies the complex and interpersonal nature of clinical care."

What components are integral to nursing as an art as well as a science? Benner (2004) suggests that many of the attributes of nursing that fall under the "art of nursing" are invisible, intangible, rarely charted, and almost never suggested in a nursing care plan. Consequently, these attributes are often marginalized, undervalued, and demeaned. Three areas inherent in the "art" of nursing addressed here are (1) caring, (2) attending, and (3) patient advocacy.

Caring

Kari Martinsen (born 1943), a psychiatric nurse and philosopher from Norway, believed that "caring involves how we relate to each other, how we show concern for each other in our daily life. Caring is the most natural and the most fundamental aspect of human existence" (Alvsvåg, 2006, p. 173). A survey by Schoenhofer and colleagues (1998) used a group process method (13 groups of 3 to 5 people each) to synthesize what

EXAMINING THE EVIDENCE
The Importance of Evidence-Based Research in Practice

***Nursing Mental Diseases* is a textbook that was written in 1934 by a registered nurse, Harriet Bailey (Bailey, 1934). It is fascinating, informative, and well written, yet clearly dated. Let us try to answer a hypothetical question based on information presented in this textbook of common nursing measures used during this period.**

Nursing measures to improve a patient's mood include all of the following *except:*

1. Hosing them down alternately with hot and cold water
2. Providing a diet that consists exclusively of milk for several days
3. Encouraging social support and family involvement
4. Putting the patient to bed for 4 to 10 weeks

Incorrect answers: 1. Hydrotherapy was commonly used as a "nerve stimulant" to improve mood. 2. A milk diet was followed by a sudden introduction of a full diet (no rationale given; your guess is as good as mine). 4. Bed rest was seen as a treatment for mental illness.

Correct answer: 3. The patient was removed from family and friends who may have sympathized or criticized too much; after 4 to 10 weeks patients were permitted to receive a letter from home on a test basis.

Psychiatric nurses today do not hose down patients, provide milk diets, or enforce prolonged bed rest. They do encourage patients to interact with others and promote family involvement when possible. Although sophistication in psychiatric nursing interventions has improved drastically in the past century, it is certain that some currently accepted treatments and nursing interventions will one day be abandoned and replaced with interventions that are more effective.

Formal decisions to adopt practice protocols or guidelines (innovation) or abandon old ones (exnovation) are not typically based on a single study, but are made after a comprehensive review of information. Evidence-based practice includes not only evaluating research but also integrating it with input from experts and patients (Polit & Beck, 2006).

Although the vast majority of nurses—professionals charged with decisions about lives and even life and death issues—do not conduct extensive literature reviews, it is essential to consider your education a continual endeavor. Reading professional journals and keeping abreast of current research play an essential role in this education.

In each of this text's clinical chapters, an interesting question (which is how *any* research project initially starts—with a question) about mental health, psychiatric disorders, and treatment that you might actually ask yourself is presented. Literature and expert opinions are provided that explore possible responses and opposing positions to the question. You are encouraged to read these boxes and evaluate the evidence. What is your opinion? What other information would you need to draw a conclusion? How can researchers best approach this question?

We hope that these boxes will not only make you think but also increase your appreciation for research and explain why it is necessary.

Bailey, H. (1934). *Mental health nursing* (2nd ed.). New York: Macmillan.
Polit, D. F., & Beck, C. T. (2006). *Essentials of nursing research: method, appraisal, and utilization* (6th ed.). Philadelphia: Lippincott.
Margaret J. Halter (Taken from first edition of Essentials of Psychiatric Mental Health Nursing).

was meant by caring to the participants. The following three themes emerged from the shared narratives:

1. Caring is evidenced by empathic understanding, actions, and patience on another's behalf.
2. Caring for one another by actions, words, and being there leads to happiness and touches the heart.
3. Caring is giving of self while preserving the importance of self.

Dr. Jean Watson's caring theory incorporates humanistic-altruistic values, creative problem solving, faith-hope, existential and spiritual forces, and more.

The caring nurse is first and foremost a competent nurse (Cooper & Powell, 1998). Indeed, Locsin (1995) expanded the concept of caring in the theory of technological competence as caring in critical care nursing. Without knowledge and competence, the demonstration of compassion and caring alone is powerless to help those under our care. Without a base of knowledge and skills, care alone cannot eliminate another person's confusion, grief, or pain, but a response of care can transform fear, pain, and suffering into a tolerable, shared experience (Cooper, 2001).

However, a nurse may be at a level of competence but unable to demonstrate caring. The absence of caring can leave memorable scars and make patients feel distrustful, disconnected, uneasy, and discouraged (Halldorsdottir & Hamrin, 1997). Using communications that are destructive or devalue a patient's worth can have lasting negative effects. Examples of uncaring behaviors include denying patients' feelings, responding with indifference to patients' concerns, and failing to check to see if medications given to relieve discomfort or distress are working. These are examples of behaviors that violate a patient's integrity and dignity and are never justified (Cooper, 2001).

Comforting can also be assumed under the mantle of caring. Benner (2004) states that comforting includes providing social, emotional, physical, and spiritual support for a patient that is consistent with the holistic approach to nursing care. The provision of comfort measures can even be lifesaving in fragile patients, and is a basic component to good care. Caring as practiced from a caring perspective/theory applies to all settings, all populations (including cultural/ethnic/minority groups), and all age groups (Jasmine, 2009). Unfortunately, there are many impediments to practicing "caring" in our present health care system that are driven by economic considerations. We continue to be in a period of nursing shortage in institutions (e.g., hospitals, community centers, emergency departments) with many graduating nurses not being hired at this time because of budgetary factors. This low staffing puts a greater burden on nurses while working with greater workloads and sicker patients. However, as Cooper aptly points out, caring is both an attitude that one communicates, a way of being with a patient, as well as a set of skills that can be learned and developed. Both require nurturing and practice. Cooper goes on to say that while it does take time to listen to patients, "in time you will be able to do the tasks of nursing while attending to the patient, and get to know the patient as you are doing an assessment or intervention" (p. 95).

Attending

Attending refers to an *intensity of presence,* being there for and in tune with the patient. The experience of emotional or physical suffering can be isolating. When patients perceive that the nurse is there for them, a human connection is made and the patient's sense of isolation is minimized or eliminated (Cooper, 2001). Being present requires entering the patient's experience. Attending behaviors may include listening, touching, or giving attentive physical care (Cooper, 2001). It is through active listening skills and the use of effective communication skills that we can fully understand another person's immediate experience and distressing fears, perceptions, and concerns. Attending behaviors are learned and are inherent in a true therapeutic relationship. Chapter 9 discusses attending behaviors in more detail within the context of the nurse-patient relationship.

Patient Advocacy

Essentially, a patient advocate is one who speaks up for another's cause, who helps others by defending and comforting them, especially when the other person lacks the knowledge, skills, ability, or status to speak for himself/herself. Lawyers are often viewed as advocates for their clients; however, in nursing,

being a patient advocate is not a legal role but rather an ethical one. Ethics is an integral part of the foundation of nursing. You, no doubt, have had a class that includes the ethical code for nurses. However, the role of patient advocate bears mentioning here. The term *patient advocate* was first placed in the 1976 American Nurses Association (ANA) *Code of Ethics for Nurses,* revision, and remains essentially unchanged up to the present. It reads:

> The nurse must be alert to and take appropriate action regarding any instances of incompetent, unethical, illegal, or impaired practices(s) by any member of the health team or the health care system itself, or any action on the part of others that places the rights or best interest of the patient in jeopardy (ANA, 2001, 3.5).

And, yes, sometimes it takes a great deal of courage to advocate for our patients when we witness behaviors or actions of other health care professionals that could have serious consequences for the patient.

Advocacy in nursing includes a commitment to patients' health, well-being, and safety across the life span, and the alleviation of suffering and promoting a peaceful, comfortable, and dignified death (ANA, 2001). Nurses advocate for patients when they advise patients of their rights (including the right to refuse treatment), provide accurate and current information so patients can make informed decisions, and support those decisions (Mallik, 1997). Advocating for the patient demonstrates respect for human life (the patient's as well as our own) and validates the belief in the value of human life, whether it is to save a life or to bring comfort to those who are dying. Psychiatric mental health nurses function as advocates when they engage in public speaking, write articles for the popular press, and lobby congressional representatives to help improve and expand mental health care for everyone (ANA, 2007).

Throughout the text a special feature titled Applying the Art gives the reader a glimpse of a nurse-patient interaction and the nurse's thought processes while attending to the patient's immediate concern.

KEY POINTS TO REMEMBER

- Evidence-based practice (EBP) is a process by which the best available research evidence, clinical expertise, and patient preferences are used for making clinical decisions.
- The "5 A's" process to delineate the multistep process of integrating best evidence into clinical practice includes (1) asking, (2) acquiring, (3) appraising, (4) applying, and (5) assessing.
- The mental health recovery model is one of helping people with psychiatric disabilities effectively manage their symptoms, reduce psychosocial disability, and find a meaningful life in a community of their choosing.
- Some sources for obtaining research findings are (1) Internet mental health resources, (2) clinical practice guidelines, (3) clinical algorithms, and (4) clinical/critical pathways.

- A sound body of knowledge of effective psychiatric nursing interventions is available and in use today. However, a great deal more observations and studies need to be done to ascertain whether we are using best-evidence interventions in our clinical practice.
- Best evidence for appropriate medication and therapies for use in patients with specific mental health conditions has been more readily studied and documented.
- Three specific areas are inherent within the art of nursing: (1) caring, (2) attending, and (3) patient advocacy.

APPLYING CRITICAL JUDGMENT

1. A friend of yours has recently returned from the war in Afghanistan. You are startled when you see him on the street in a disheveled state. He appears frightened, seems to be talking to himself, and jumps a mile when a car backfires nearby. You are astounded because he was always so smart and well liked, thought of as kind and personable, and had a good career ahead of him as a computer programmer. When you approach him he backs away in a protective manner.
   A. How would the contribution of evidence-based practice (EBP) be helpful to his recovery? Give examples.
   B. What might be some specific needs that could be met under the recovery model?
   C. Discuss how nurses can incorporate both EBP and the recovery model in their practice.
   D. Explain which model might be the most useful during the acute phase of his recovery, and which model might be more effective in the continuation period of his recovery.
2. A friend of yours says that he heard about a new practitioner in the area that is going to teach alcoholics how to safely drink in moderation. You are thinking of two of your friends who are now in recovery, one of whom nearly died from an alcoholic event. You state that from all you have read, and from your friends' experience, that "controlled drinking isn't thought to be an acceptable practice." Your friend says, sure there is good evidence, "This professional has lots of stories and affidavits from people who are alcoholics whom he has treated with success to drink in a controlled manner." You tell him that that is not good evidence for such a claim.
   A. How would you, as a nurse, evaluate this claim? Explain the five steps you would take to find the strength of this claim.
   B. Using Table 1-1, what would you say about the quality of the evidence given above?
   C. If your friend were in recovery and thinking of trying this treatment, what would you say to him that would make a strong argument against such a decision?
3. You are a new nursing student and a friend of yours says, "What the devil is the 'art of nursing'? Isn't that from the middle ages?"
   A. Discuss three components that might be considered under the art of nursing.
   B. Give your friend an example of how nurses demonstrate "caring" in the clinical area.
   C. Explain why patients need to have nurses act as their advocate. Can you think of an example from your clinical experience?
4. Go to the Centre for Evidence-Based Mental Health at www.cebmh.com and check out at least one available clinical trial.

CHAPTER REVIEW QUESTIONS

Choose the most appropriate answer(s).
1. The "art" of psychiatric mental health nursing, according to Benner, includes: (select all that apply)
   1. caring.
   2. attending.
   3. patient advocacy.
   4. ethics.
2. The "science" of psychiatric mental health nursing includes: (select all that apply)
   1. a sense of tradition.
   2. nursing theory.
   3. psychosocial theory.
   4. neurobiological theory.
3. Caring is: (select all that apply)
   1. an attitude that one communicate.
   2. a way of being with the patient.
   3. intensity of presence.
   4. giving of self.
4. Patient advocacy:
   1. is a legal role.
   2. requires courage.
   3. is an optional aspect of nursing.
   4. was developed in 2007.
5. When an experienced psychiatric nurse listens carefully to a patient's detailed recounting of a traumatic emotional experience, the nurse is:
   1. acting as a patient advocate.
   2. using an attending behavior.
   3. interpreting "best evidence."
   4. using a systematic approach to care.

REFERENCES

Alvsvåg, H. (2006). Philosophy of caring. In A. M. Tomey, & M. R. Alligood (Eds.), *Nursing theorists and their work.* St Louis: Mosby.

American Academy of Physical Medicine and Rehabilitation (AAPMR). (2006). *Practice guidelines committee develops definitions of term.* Retrieved August 24, 2006, from www.aapmr.org/hpl/pracguide/terms.htm.

American Nurses Association (ANA). (2007). *Psychiatric–mental health nursing: scope and standards of practice.* Silver Spring, MD: The Association.

American Nurses Association (ANA). (2001). *Code of ethics with interpretive statements.* Silver Spring, MD: The Association.

Beebe, L. H. (2010). Adjunctive psychiatric treatments and recovery-focused care. *Journal of Psychosocial Nursing Mental Health Services, 48*(11), 4–5.

Benner, P. (2004). Relational ethics of comfort, touch, and solace endangered arts? *American Journal of Critical Care, 13,* 346–349.

Caldwell, B. A., Sclasani, M., Swarbrick, M., & Piren, K. (2010). Psychiatric nursing practice & the recovery model of care. *Journal of PSN, 48*(7), 42–48.

Cooper, C. (2001). *The art of nursing: a practical introduction.* Philadelphia: Saunders.

Cooper, C., & Powell, E. (1998). Technology and care in a bone marrow transplant unit: creating and assuaging vulnerability. *Holistic Nursing Practice, 12,* 57–68.

Dorn, K. (2005). Topics in advanced practice nursing. *E Journal, 4*(4). Medscape.

Forchuk, C. (2001). Evidence-based psychiatric/mental health nursing. *Evidence-Based Mental Health, 4*(2), 39–40.

Geddes, J., Reynolds, S., Streiner, D., & Szatmari, P. (2004). *Evidence based practice in mental health.* Centre for Evidence-Based Medicine. Retrieved from www.cebm.utoronto.ca/syllabi/men/intro.htm.

Haber, J. (2000). Hildegard Peplau: the psychiatric nursing legacy of a legend. *Journal of the American Psychiatric Nurses Association, 6*(2), 56–62.

Halldorsdottir, S., & Hamrin, E. (1997). Caring and uncaring encounters in nursing and health care from the cancer patient's perspective. *Cancer Nursing, 20,* 120–128.

Institute of Medicine (IOM). (2006). *Improving the quality of health care for mental and substance-use conditions.* Institute of Medicine of the National Academies. Washington, DC: National Academies Press.

Jasmine, T. (2009). Art, science, or both? Keeping the care in nursing. *Nursing Clinics of North America, 44,* 415–421.

Keith, J. M. (1988). Florence Nightingale: statistician and consultant epidemiologist. *International Nursing Review, 35,* 147–150.

Locsin, R. C. (1995). Machine technologies and caring in nursing. *Image: Journal of Nursing Scholarship, 27*(3), 201–203.

Mallik, M. (1997). Advocacy in nursing: a review of the literature. *Journal of Advanced Nursing, 23,* 130–138.

Mantzoukas, S. (2007). A review of evidence-based practice, nursing research and reflection: leveling the hierarchy. *Journal of Clinical Nursing, 17*(2), 214–223.

Marcus, K. (2011). The nurse as patient advocate: is there a conflict of interest? In P. S. Cowen, & S. Moorehead (Eds.), *Current issues in nursing* (8th ed., pp. 609–674). St Louis: Mosby/Elsevier.

McDonald, L. (2001). Florence Nightingale and the early origins of evidence-based nursing. *Evidence-Based Nursing, 4,* 68–69.

Melnyk, B. M. (2004). Integrating levels of evidence into clinical decision making. *Pediatric Nursing, 30*(4), 323–324.

Mick, K. (2005). *Evidence-based nursing practice: putting the pieces together.* Retrieved July 18, 2006, fromwww.apon.org.

Pratt, C., Gill, K., Barrett, N., & Roberts, M. (2006). *Psychiatric rehabilitation* (2nd ed.). San Diego: Academic Press.

Schoenhofer, S., Bingham, V., & Hutchins, G. (1998). Giving of oneself on another's behalf: the phenomenology of everyday caring. *International Journal of Human Caring, 2*(2). 32–29.

Stuart, G. W. (2001). Evidence-based psychiatric nursing practice: rhetoric or reality? *Journal of the American Psychiatric Nurses Association, 7*(4), 103–114.

Stuart, G. W. (2011). Psychiatric mental health nursing: recent changes in current issues. In P. S. Cowen, & S. Moorehead (Eds.), *Current issues in nursing.* St Louis: Mosby/Elsevier.

Tomey, A. M. (2006). Nursing theorists of historical significance. In A. M. Tomey, & M. R. Alligood (Eds.), *Nursing theorists and their work* (6th ed.). St Louis: Mosby.

U.S. Department of Health and Human Services (USDHHS). (1999). *Mental health: a report from the surgeon general.* Rockville, MD: National Institute of Mental Health.

White, S. I. (1997). Evidence-based practice and nursing: the new panacea? *British Journal of Nursing, 6*(3), 175–178.

Williams, D. D. R., & Garner, J. (2002). The case against "the evidence": a different perspective on evidence-based medicine. *British Journal of Psychiatry, 180,* 8–12.

Wilson, H. S. (2004). Evidence-based practice in psychiatric-mental health nursing. In C. R. Kneisl, H. S. Wilson, & E. Trigoboff (Eds.), *Contemporary psychiatric-mental health nursing.* Upper Saddle River, NJ: Pearson Prentice-Hall.

Zauszniewski, J. A., & Suresky, J. (2003). Evidence for psychiatric nursing practice: an analysis of three years of published research. *Online Journal of Issues in Nursing, 9*(1). Retrieved July 18, 2006, from http://nursingworld.org/ojin/hirsh/topic4/tpc4_1.htm.

Mental Health and Mental Illness

Elizabeth M. Varcarolis

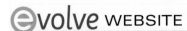

http:evolve.elsevier.com/Varcarolis/essentials

KEY TERMS AND CONCEPTS

biologically based mental
    illness, p. 16
culture-related syndromes, p. 22
*Diagnostic and Statistical
    Manual of Mental Disorders
    (DSM),* p. 13
epidemiology, p. 14
mental disorders, p. 13
mental health, p. 13

mental illness, p. 13
myths and misconceptions, p. 14
prevalence rate, p. 14
psychiatry's definition of normal
    mental health, p. 14
psychobiological disorder, p. 17
resiliency, p. 14
stigma/stigmatizing, p. 18

**SELECTED CONCEPT: Stigma and
Mental Health**
False beliefs, myths, and lack of understanding of mental illness can cause tremendous pain and negative consequences
for individuals or groups who develop mental health problems. Stigma may be obvious and direct, or expressed in more subtle
behaviors.

Some of the harmful effects of stigma
toward those with mental health issues
include:

- Discrimination at work or school
- Difficulty finding housing
- Bullying, physical violence or
  harassment
- Health insurance that doesn't adequately cover a person's mental
  health dysfunction/disorder
- Instilling self-doubt regarding ability
  to succeed in certain challenges and
  perceiving that there is nothing that
  can help
- Further isolation from friends, family,
  and colleagues.

(Mayo Clinic, 2011)

OBJECTIVES

1. Assess mental health using the seven signs of mental health identified in this chapter (Table 2-1 and Figure 2-1).
2. Summarize factors that can affect the mental health of an individual and the ways that these factors influence conducting a holistic nursing assessment.
3. Discuss some dynamic factors (including social climate, politics, cultural beliefs, myths, and biases) that contribute to making a clear-cut definition of mental health elusive.
4. Identify the processes leading up to stigmatizing, and some of the effects stigma can have on the medical and psychological well-being of an individual, group, and/or culture.
5. Demonstrate how the *DSM* multiaxial system can influence a clinician to consider a broad range of information before making a *DSM* diagnosis.
6. Compare and contrast a *DSM* diagnosis with a nursing diagnosis.
7. Give examples of how consideration of norms and other cultural influences can affect making an accurate *DSM* diagnosis.

TABLE 2-1   MENTAL HEALTH VERSUS MENTAL ILLNESS

SIGNS OF MENTAL HEALTH	SIGNS OF MENTAL ILLNESS
Happiness	**Major Depressive Episode**
Finds life enjoyable	Loses interest or pleasure in all or almost all usual activities and pastimes
Can see in objects, people, and activities the possibilities for meeting his or her needs	Describes mood as depressed, sad, hopeless, discouraged, "down in the dumps"
Control Over Behavior	**Control Disorder: Undersocialized, Aggressive**
Can recognize and act on cues to existing limits	Shows repetitive and persistent pattern of aggressive conduct in which basic rights of others are violated
Can respond to rules, routines, and customs of any group to which he or she belongs	
Appraisal of Reality	**Schizophrenic and Other Disorders**
Accurate picture of what is happening around the individual	Shows bizarre delusions, such as delusions of being controlled
Good sense of consequences, both good and bad, that will follow his or her acts	Has auditory hallucinations
Can see difference between "as if" and "for real" in situations	Manifests delusions with persecutory or jealous content
Effectiveness in Work	**Adjustment Disorder With Work (or Academic) Inhibition**
Within limits set by abilities, can do well in tasks attempted	Shows inhibition in work or academic functioning in which previously there was adequate performance
When meeting mild failure, persists until determines whether he or she can do the job	
Healthy Self-Concept	**Dependent Personality Disorder**
Sees self as approaching individual ideals, as capable of meeting demands	Passively allows others to assume responsibility for major areas of life because of inability to function independently
Has reasonable degree of self-confidence that helps in being resourceful under stress	Lacks self-confidence (i.e., sees self as helpless, stupid)
Satisfying Relationships	**Borderline Personality Disorder**
Experiences satisfaction and stability in relationships	Shows pattern of unstable and intense interpersonal relationships
Socially integrated and can rely on social supports	Has chronic feelings of emptiness
Effective Coping Strategies	**Substance Dependencies**
Uses stress reduction strategies that address the problem, issue, threat (e.g., problem solving, cognitive restructuring)	Repeatedly self-administers substances despite significant substance-related problems (e.g., threat to job, family, social relationships)
Uses coping strategies in a healthy way that does not cause harm to self or others	

Modified from Redl, F., & Wattenberg, W. (1959). *Mental hygiene in teaching* (pp. 198-201). New York: Harcourt, Brace & World; American Psychiatric Association. (2000). *Diagnostic and statistical manual of mental disorders* (4th ed., text rev.). Washington, DC: Author; Farber, E.W., & Kaslow, F.W. (2003). Social psychology: theory, research, and mental health implications. In A. Tasman, J. Kay, & J.A. Lieberman (Eds.), *Psychiatry* (2nd ed.). West Sussex, England: Wiley.

Mental health and mental illness are not specific entities but rather they exist on a continuum. The mental health continuum is dynamic and ever-shifting, ranging from mild to moderate to severe to psychosis (see Figure 2-1).

The groundbreaking *Report of the Surgeon General* (USDHHS, 1999) defines mental health as successful performance of mental functions, resulting in the ability to engage in productive activities, enjoy fulfilling relationships, and adapt to change and cope with adversity. Mental health is from early childhood until death "the springboard of thinking and communication skills, learning, emotional growth, resilience, and self-esteem" (USDHHS, 1999). It is a state of well-being in which individuals are able to realize their abilities within the normal stresses of life and function productively within their personal lives as well as contribute to their community (WHO, 2010).

According to the National Alliance on Mental Illness (NAMI, 2011) mental illnesses are medical conditions that affect a person's thinking, feeling, mood, ability to relate to others, and daily functioning. Basically, mental illness can be seen as the result of a chain of events that include flawed biological, psychological, social, and cultural processes. However, mental illnesses are treatable, and individuals can experience relief from their symptoms with treatment and support. Although there may not be a cure, recovery is possible (NAMI, 2011).

This chapter discusses concepts of mental health and mental illness. The reader will be introduced to the concept of mental disorders as medical diseases. You will come to understand how mental disorders are categorized using the Diagnostic and Statistical Manual of Mental Disorders (DSM). The *DSM* is the manual that classifies mental disorders and is considered the "bible" for mental health workers (e.g., psychiatrists, psychiatric nurses, psychologists, and others who plan care for people experiencing mental distress/dysfunction). The *DSM* focuses on research and clinical observation when constructing diagnostic categories

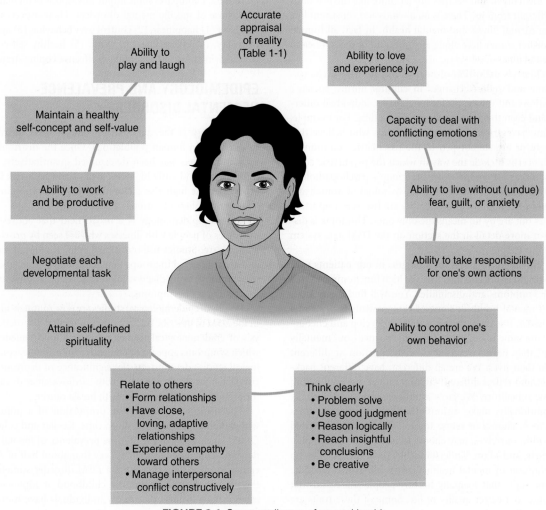

FIGURE 2-1 Some attributes of mental health.

for a discrete mental disorder. This chapter describes how nursing diagnoses can be used to ensure appropriate care. This chapter also addresses the importance of assessing a person's ethnic background, culture, and minority group before making a valid diagnosis and executing an effective treatment plan.

CONCEPTS OF MENTAL HEALTH AND ILLNESS

The World Health Organization declared that 4 of the 10 leading causes of disability in the United States and other developed countries are mental health disorders (NAMI, 2011). Unfortunately our understanding of mental illness is plagued by a host of myths and misconceptions. One myth is that to be mentally ill is to be different and odd. Another misconception is that to be mentally healthy, a person must be logical and rational. All of us dream "irrational" dreams at night, and "irrational" emotions not only are universal human experiences but also are essential to a fulfilling life. There are people who show extremely abnormal behavior and are characterized as mentally ill and yet they are far more like the rest of us than different from us. There is no obvious and consistent line between mental illness and mental health. In fact, all human behavior lies somewhere along a continuum of mental health and mental illness.

Psychiatry's definition of normal mental health changes over time and reflects changes in cultural norms, society's expectations and values, professional biases, individual differences, and even the political climate of the time. For example, criticisms have arisen from various groups who believe that they were or are stereotyped in the psychiatric community. Their concerns include the way in which the psychiatric community places an emphasis on the group's psychopathology rather than on health attributes. The psychology of women and the issues surrounding homosexuality are two very important examples but are by no means the only ones. This topic is discussed in more detail in the section on the DSM axis system later in this chapter.

We are taught to assess the strengths in our patients with mental health issues and their areas of high functioning, as well as their symptoms and disabilities. You will find many attributes of mental health in some of your patients with mental health issues. It is these strengths that we develop and encourage. By the same token, those who are "normal" or "mentally healthy" may have several areas of dysfunction at different times in their lives. We are all different, have different backgrounds, and reflect different cultural influences, even within the same subculture. We grow at different rates intellectually and emotionally, make various decisions at different times in our lives, choose or refuse to evaluate our behaviors and grow within ourselves, may choose to have deep-seated spiritual beliefs, and so on. Understandably, then, there can be no one definition of mental health that fits all. However, there are some traits that mentally healthy people share and that contribute to a better quality of life. Some of these traits are depicted in Figure 2-1.

A characteristic of mental health that is increasingly being promoted is the concept of resiliency. Resiliency is the ability to recover from or adjust easily to misfortune and change. Resiliency is closely associated with the process of adapting and helps people facing tragedy, loss, trauma, and severe stress (American Psychological Association, 2004). Research has demonstrated that this ability to recover from painful experiences and difficult events is not an unusual quality, but is a trait possessed by many people and can be developed in almost everyone. Disasters occur all too frequently, such as terrorist attacks (World Trade Towers), the devastation of hurricanes (Katrina), senseless shootings (Columbine, Tuscon, Ohio) and crippling floodings (Haiti, Australia, Japan). These are just a few of the many disasters in which people united to help one another and continue their lives despite horrendous loss, illustrating resilience. Being resilient does not mean that people are unaffected by stressors. It means that rather than falling victim to the negative emotions, resilient people recognize the feelings, readily deal with them, and learn from the experience given time.

Table 2-1 compares some important aspects of mental health with those of specific mental disorders. These aspects include degree of (1) happiness, (2) control over behavior, (3) appraisal of reality, (4) effectiveness in work, (5) healthy self-concept, (6) satisfying relationships, and (7) effective coping strategies.

EPIDEMIOLOGY AND PREVALENCE OF MENTAL DISORDERS

Epidemiology is the quantitative study of the distribution of disorders in human populations. Once the distribution of mental disorders has been determined quantitatively, epidemiologists can identify high-risk groups and high-risk factors. Study of these high-risk factors may lead to important clues about the etiology of various mental disorders.

Clinical epidemiology is a broad field that addresses the outcomes of people with illnesses who are seen by providers of clinical care. Studies use traditional epidemiological methods and are conducted in groups that are usually defined by illness or symptoms, or by diagnostic procedures or treatments given for the illness or symptoms.

Results of epidemiological studies are now routinely included in the *DSM* to describe the frequency of mental disorders. Analysis of epidemiological studies can assess the frequency with which symptoms appear concurrently. For example, epidemiological studies demonstrate the significance of depression as a risk factor for death in people with cardiovascular disease and for premature death in people with breast cancer.

The prevalence rate is the proportion of a population with a mental disorder at a given time. Kessler and colleagues (2005) latest study of the lifetime prevalence of mental disorders and concluded in their survey that about half of Americans will meet the criteria for a *DSM* disorder sometime in their life, with the first onset in childhood or adolescence. It is important to note that many individuals have more than one mental disorder at a time. For example, some people diagnosed with a depressive disorder may also have a coexisting anxiety disorder. Therefore some people have dual diagnoses (coexisting disorders).

Table 2-2 shows the prevalence rates and includes the epidemiology of some psychiatric disorders in the United States.

MENTAL ILLNESS AND POLICY ISSUES

Many factors can affect the severity and progress of a mental illness, biologically based or otherwise, and these same factors can affect a "normal" person's mental health as well. Some of

TABLE 2-2	PREVALENCE AND EPIDEMIOLOGY OF PSYCHIATRIC DISORDERS IN THE UNITED STATES		
DISORDER	PREVALENCE OVER 12 MONTHS (%)	ESTIMATED NUMBER OF PEOPLE AFFECTED BY DISORDER IN THE UNITED STATES	EPIDEMIOLOGY
Schizophrenia	1.1	2.2 million	Affects men and women equally; may appear earlier in men than in women
Any affective (mood) disorder; includes major depression, dysthymic disorder, and bipolar disorder	9.5	18.8 million	Women affected twice as much as men (12.4 million women; 6.4 million men); depressive disorders may appear earlier in life in those born in recent decades compared with past; often co-occurs with anxiety and substance abuse
Major depressive disorder	5	9.9 million	Leading cause of disability in the United States and established economies worldwide; nearly twice as many women (6.5%) as men (3.3%) suffer from a major depressive disorder every year
Bipolar affective disorder	1.2	2.3 million	Affects men and women equally
Anxiety disorders; includes panic disorder, obsessive-compulsive disorder, posttraumatic stress disorder (PTSD), generalized anxiety disorder, and phobias	13.3	19.1 million	Anxiety disorders frequently co-occur with depressive disorders, eating disorders, and/or substance abuse
Panic disorder	1.7	2.4 million	Typically develops in adolescence or early adulthood; about one in three people with panic disorder develops agoraphobia
Obsessive-compulsive disorder	2.3	3.3 million	First symptoms begin in childhood or adolescence
PTSD	3.6	5.2 million	Can develop at any time; approximately 30% of Vietnam veterans experienced PTSD after the war; percentage high among first responders to 9/11/01 terrorist attacks
Generalized anxiety disorder	2.8	4 million	Can begin across life cycle; risk is highest between childhood and middle age
Social phobia	3.7	5.3 million	Typically begins in childhood or adolescence
Agoraphobia	2.2	3.2 million	
Specific phobia	4.4	6.3 million	
Any substance abuse	11.3		
Alcohol dependence	7.2		

Data from National Institute of Mental Health. (2004). *The numbers count: mental disorders in America* (NIH Pub. No. 01-4584). Retrieved August 1, 2004, from www.nimh.nih.gov/publicat/numbers.cfm.

these factors include available support systems, family influences, developmental events, cultural or subcultural beliefs and values, health practices, and negative influences impinging on an individual's life. If possible, these influences need to be evaluated and factored into an individual's plan of care. Figure 2-2 identifies some influences that can have an effect on a person's mental health. In 1996 the Mental Health Parity Act was passed by Congress. This legislation required insurers that provide mental health coverage to offer benefits at the same level provided for medical and surgical coverage. In 2000 the Government Accounting Office found that although 86% of health plans complied with the 1996 law, 87% of health plans that complied with the law imposed new limits on mental health coverage.

The 1999 USDHHS report entitled *Mental Health: A Report of the Surgeon General* stated the following:

- Mental health is fundamental to health.
- Mental disorders are real health conditions that have an immense impact on individuals and families.

- The efficacy of mental health treatment is well documented.
- A range of treatments exists for most mental disorders.

On April 29, 2002, President George W. Bush endorsed parity and established a new mental health commission. In February 2003, the Senator Paul Wellstone Mental Health Equitable Treatment Act was introduced into the Senate and the House of Representatives. In July 2003, the President's New Freedom Commission on Mental Health also endorsed parity.

Since 1996 the limited federal law has been kept in place through a series of 1-year extensions, and stronger bills have repeatedly been introduced and vetoed (National Mental Health Association [NMHA], 2004). State bills were proposed to close the federal loopholes, and as of 2006, 34 states had adopted laws. However, many require full insurance parity for only a limited number of psychiatric diagnoses. One method many states use to determine coverage is by making a distinction of whether the problem is a biologically based mental illness, that is, a mental disorder caused by neurotransmitter dysfunction, abnormal brain structure, inherited genetic

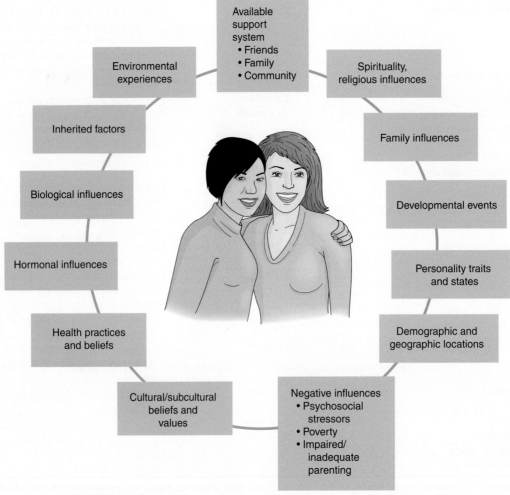

FIGURE 2-2 Influences that can have an effect on an individual's mental health.

factors, or other biological causes. Another term for such an illness is psychobiological disorder. These biologically influenced illnesses include the following:

- Schizophrenia
- Bipolar disorder
- Major depression
- Obsessive-compulsive and panic disorders
- Posttraumatic stress disorder
- Autism

Other severe and disabling mental disorders include the following:

- Anorexia nervosa
- Attention deficit/hyperactivity disorder
- Many of the most prevalent and disabling mental disorders have been found to have strong biological influences; therefore we can look at these disorders as "diseases."

The *DSM* cautions that the emphasis on the term *mental disorder* implies a distinction between "mental" disorder and "physical" disorder, which is an outdated concept, and stresses mind-body dualism: "There is much 'physical' in 'mental' disorders and much 'mental' in 'physical' disorders" (American Psychiatric Association, 2000).

MEDICAL DIAGNOSIS AND NURSING DIAGNOSIS OF MENTAL ILLNESS

To perform their professional responsibilities, clinicians and researchers need clear and accurate guidelines for identifying and categorizing mental illness. Such guidelines help clinicians plan and evaluate treatment for their patients. A necessary element for categorization includes agreement regarding which behaviors constitute a mental illness.

Medical Diagnoses and the *DSM*

In the *DSM* each of the mental disorders is conceptualized as a clinically significant behavioral or psychological syndrome or pattern that occurs in an individual and is associated with present **distress** (e.g., a painful symptom) or **disability** (i.e., impairment in one or more important areas of functioning) or with a significantly increased risk of suffering death, pain, disability, or an important loss of freedom. This syndrome or pattern must not be merely an expected and culturally sanctioned response to a particular event, such as the death of a loved one. Whatever the original cause, it must currently be considered a manifestation of a behavioral, psychological, or biological dysfunction in the individual within the individual's cultural boundaries. Deviant behavior (e.g., political, religious, or sexual) and conflicts between the individual and society are not considered mental disorders unless the deviance or conflict is a symptom of a dysfunction in the individual.

It is important to stress that the *DSM* classifies disorders that people have, and not the person. For this reason, the text of the *DSM* avoids the use of expressions such as "a schizophrenic" or "an alcoholic" and instead uses the more accurate terms "an individual with schizophrenia" or "an individual

with alcohol dependence." Since the third edition of the *DSM* appeared in 1980, the criteria for classification of mental disorders have been sufficiently detailed for clinical, teaching, and research purposes.

The *DSM* in Culturally Diverse Populations

Special efforts have been made in the *DSM* to incorporate an awareness that the manual is used in culturally diverse populations in the United States and internationally. It is true that culture is an inclusive term and there are many definitions for culture; most anthropologists agree that "culture includes traditions of thought and behavior, such as language and history that can be socially acquired, shared, and passed on to new generations" (Hays, 2008). However, evaluations of an individual's cultural background should also include minority groups. Minorities need to include not only different ethnicities but also older adults; people who have disabilities; lesbian, gay, bisexual, and transgender (LGBT) individuals; and women, for example (Hays, 2008). Therefore clinicians are urged to evaluate individuals from numerous ethnic groups/cultural backgrounds and minority backgrounds. Assessment can be especially challenging when a clinician from one ethnic/cultural or minority group uses the *DSM* classification to evaluate an individual from a different ethnic/cultural or minority group.

PSYCHIATRY AND SPIRITUALITY

An important part of a culture is spirituality, which for a long time played a secondary role in the medical holistic assessment of people with mental health distress and/or disorders. However, be aware there have been many leaders in nursing who have advanced the importance of the concept of spirituality in health care and healing, and have made significant contributions in research and writings to the nursing literature. Finally, psychiatry is beginning to comprehend the importance of spiritual belief. Spirituality is a much broader concept than just religion alone; spirituality "provides an essential core, enriching experience, and a reason to live for many people" (Favazza, 2009, p. 2633). There are many ways to achieve a spiritual moment and lead a spiritual life. For example, among certain cultural groups, particular religious practices or beliefs (e.g., hearing or seeing a deceased relative during bereavement) may be misdiagnosed as manifestations of a psychotic disorder; furthermore, a syndrome often manifests in different superficial forms in different cultures. Also, people from minority or migrant populations may have good reason to be distrustful, and it should not be assumed that these patients are suffering from paranoia or paranoid schizophrenia. There are many ways that people can induce or enhance spirituality. Favazza (2009) cites the following examples of how people obtain an altered state of consciousness, which is spiritually enriching and brings peace and serenity into people's lives. Mysticism, meditation (e.g., Dhyana, a form of concentrated meditation taught by Buddha; Zen Buddhism, a Japanese practice in which a spiritual master instructs students in meditation, used throughout the United States; and transcendental meditation, a Hindu meditative process), and mindfulness meditation (derived from Buddhist practice) are just a few examples. Mindfulness meditation is used today and has many health benefits; it is a valuable tool for dealing with chronic pain and stress. It is actively employed with dialectic behavioral therapy (DBT), stress reduction programs, and some forms of cognitive therapy (Favazza, 2009). Prayer is most widely used in the United States; it is used for many reasons and is also tied to many different cultures. For example, some people pray by singing; others pray by dancing, spinning, or reciting the rosary; some people pray at certain times of the day and/or facing a specific direction; and still other people only pray in private or only in public. In all cases prayer represents a way to connect with a supreme spiritual being and to activate spiritual energy, which can reveal itself in everyday life (Favazza, 2009).

The *DSM* Multiaxial System

The *DSM* axis system forces the diagnostician to consider a broad range of information by requiring judgments to be made on each of five axes.

Axis I refers to the collection of signs and symptoms that together constitute a particular disorder (for example, schizophrenia) or a condition that may be a focus of treatment. (Refer to Appendix A for a list of all the mental disorders catalogued in the current *DSM*.) Axis II refers to the personality disorders and mental retardation. Thus Axes I and II constitute the classification of abnormal behavior. Axes I and II were separated to ensure that the possible presence of long-term disturbance is considered when attention is directed to the current disorder. For example, a heroin addict would be diagnosed on Axis I as having a substance-related disorder; this patient might also have a long-standing antisocial personality disorder, which would be noted on Axis II. This is another example of a person having more than one mental disorder at the same time. This phenomenon of coexisting disorders is often termed *co-occurring* or *dual diagnosis.*

Although the remaining three axes are not needed to make the actual diagnosis, their inclusion in the *DSM* indicates the recognition that factors other than a person's symptoms should be considered in an assessment. On Axis III the clinician indicates any general medical conditions believed to be relevant to the mental disorder in question. In some individuals a physical disorder (e.g., a neurological dysfunction) may be the cause of the abnormal behavior, whereas in others it may be an important factor in the individual's overall condition (e.g., diabetes in a child with a conduct disorder).

Axis IV is for reporting psychosocial and environmental problems that may affect the diagnosis, treatment, and prognosis of a mental disorder. These may include occupational problems, educational problems, economic problems, interpersonal difficulties with family members, and a variety of problems in other life areas. Often a psychosocial assessment will uncover these (see Chapter 7).

Finally, Axis V, called Global Assessment of Functioning (GAF), gives an indication of the person's best level of psychological, social, and occupational functioning during the preceding year, rated on a scale of 1 to 100 (1 indicates persistent danger of severely hurting oneself or others, and 100 indicates superior functioning in a variety of activities at the time of the evaluation, as well as the highest level of functioning for at least a few months during the past year). Box 2-1 presents the GAF scale.

Caution must be exercised to avoid labeling or stereotyping when a medical diagnosis or a nursing diagnosis is being formulated. Anthropologists, historians, and students of cross-cultural society have long observed that every society has its own view of health and illness and its own classification of diseases.

Over the last 13 to 14 years, stigma has been acknowledged to be a major barrier to mental health treatment and recovery to people with mental health disorders (Pinto-Foltz et al., 2009). Stigma is a "collection of negative attitudes, beliefs, thoughts, and behaviors that influence the individual, or the general public, fear, reject, or avoid, be prejudiced, and discriminate people" (Gary, 2005, p. 980). Goffman's classic definition of stigma is "an attribute that is deeply discrediting where a person is reduced from a whole unusual person to a tainted, discounted one" (Goffman, 1963). Stereotyping, labeling, separating, status, loss, and discrimination in a context of power imbalance are many of the psychosocial processes that lead to stigmatization. Stigmatizing attitudes toward the mentally ill can have harmful effects on an individual and family, especially if the diagnosis is made on the basis of insufficient evidence and proves faulty. These attitudes result in social isolation and reduced opportunities. For example, stigmatizing interferes with the person establishing and maintaining friendships, employment, and housing. It also impacts the person's ability to obtain psychological treatment and general medical treatment (Sadow & Ryder, 2008). Stigmatizing a group or an individual results in painful feelings of shame, and a negative sense of self, which can directly impact recovery. Stigmatization erodes an individual's or a group's confidence in the fact that mental illnesses "are treatable health conditions" (NAMI, 2011).

An example of the influence of cultural and social stigmatizing when making a bias on psychiatric diagnosis is the inclusion of homosexuality as a psychiatric disease in both the first and second editions of the *DSM*. All research consistently failed to demonstrate that people with a homosexual orientation were any more maladjusted than heterosexuals, but despite the research data, change occurred in the medical community only when gay rights' activists advocated an end to discrimination against lesbians and gay men. No longer is homosexuality classified as a mental disorder.

Instances of stigma and prejudicial bias toward minority groups encompass a wide range of circumstances, such as people with different sexual orientations, African Americans, the mentally ill, the disabled, and cognitively impaired older adults, children, and women. Biases are often reflected in our

BOX 2-1 GLOBAL ASSESSMENT OF FUNCTIONING (GAF) SCALE*

Consider psychological, social, and occupational functioning on a hypothetical continuum of mental health to mental illness. Do not include impairment in functioning that is a result of physical (or environmental) limitations. *Note:* Use intermediate codes when appropriate (e.g., 45, 68, 72).

Code

100 **Superior functioning in a wide range of activities, life's problems never seem to get out of hand, is**
↓ **sought out by others because of his or her many positive qualities. No symptoms.**
91

90 **Absent or minimal symptoms** (e.g., mild anxiety before an exam), **good functioning in all areas, interest-**
↓ **ed and involved in a wide range of activities, socially effective, generally satisfied with life, no more**
81 **than everyday problems or concerns** (e.g., an occasional argument with family members).

80 **If symptoms are present, they are transient and expected reactions to psychosocial stressors** (e.g.,
↓ difficulty concentrating after family argument); **no more than slight impairment in social, occupational,**
71 **or school functioning** (e.g., temporarily falling behind in schoolwork).

70 **Some mild symptoms** (e.g., depressed mood and mild insomnia) **OR some difficulty in social, occu-**
↓ **pational, or school functioning** (e.g., occasional truancy, or theft within the household), **but generally**
61 **functioning pretty well, has some meaningful interpersonal relationships.**

60 **Moderate symptoms** (e.g., flat affect and circumstantial speech, occasional panic attacks) **OR moderate dif-**
↓ **ficulty in social, occupational, or school functioning** (e.g., few friends, conflicts with peers or coworkers).
51

50 **Serious symptoms** (e.g., suicidal ideation, severe obsessional rituals, frequent shoplifting) **OR any serious**
↓ **impairment in social, occupational, or school functioning** (e.g., no friends, unable to keep a job).
41

40 **Some impairment in reality testing or communication** (e.g., speech is at times illogical, obscure, or
↓ irrelevant) **OR major impairment in several areas, such as work or school, family relations, judg-**
31 **ment, thinking, or mood** (e.g., depressed man avoids friends, neglects family, and is unable to work; child frequently beats up younger children, is defiant at home, and is failing at school).

30 **Behavior is considerably influenced by delusions or hallucinations OR serious impairment in commu-**
↓ **nication or judgment** (e.g., sometimes incoherent, acts grossly inappropriately, suicidal preoccupation) **OR**
21 **inability to function in almost all areas** (e.g., stays in bed all day; no job, home, or friends).

20 **Some danger of hurting self or others** (e.g., suicide attempts without clear expectation of death; frequently
↓ violent; manic excitement) **OR occasionally fails to maintain minimal personal hygiene** (e.g., smears
11 feces) **OR gross impairment in communication** (e.g., largely incoherent or mute).

10 **Persistent danger of severely hurting self or others** (e.g., recurrent violence) **OR persistent inability to**
↓ **maintain minimal personal hygiene OR serious suicidal act with clear expectation of death.**
1

0 **Inadequate information.**

*The rating of overall psychological functioning on a scale of 0 to 100 was operationalized by Luborsky (1962) in the Health-Sickness Rating Scale. Spitzer and colleagues developed a revision of the Health-Sickness Rating Scale called the Global Assessment Scale (GAS) (Endicott, J., et al., 1976). A modified version of the GAS was included in the *Diagnostic and Statistical Manual of Mental Disorders,* third edition, revised (American Psychiatric Association, 1987), as the Global Assessment of Functioning scale. This rating scale highlights important areas in the assessment of functioning. Because many of the judgments are subjective, experienced clinicians use this tool as a guide when planning care, and draw on their knowledge of their patients.
From American Psychiatric Association. (2000). *Diagnostic and statistical manual of mental disorders (DSM-IV-TR)* (4th ed., text rev.). Washington, DC: Author.

power structures and political systems. Awareness of the cultural bias and dangers in stereotyping and holding stigmatizing attitudes has enormous implications for nursing practice, especially in the field of mental health, because nurses often take their cues from the medical structure. "Increasing awareness about the pervasive nature of stigma as well as special

educational interventions can help nurses and other health professionals in training to avoid this pitfall" (Sadow, 2011).

Nursing Diagnoses and NANDA International

Psychiatric mental health nursing includes the diagnosis and treatment of human responses to actual or potential mental health problems. NANDA International (NANDA-I) describes a nursing diagnosis as a clinical judgment about individual, family, or community responses to actual or potential health problems and life processes. Therefore the *DSM* is used to diagnose a psychiatric disorder, whereas a well-defined nursing diagnosis provides the framework for identifying appropriate nursing interventions for dealing with the phenomena a patient with a mental health disorder is experiencing (e.g., hallucinations, self-esteem issues, impaired ability to function). See Chapter 7 for more on the formulation of nursing diagnoses in psychiatric nursing.

Appendix B lists NANDA-I–approved nursing diagnoses. The individual clinical chapters offer suggestions for potential nursing diagnoses for the behaviors and phenomena often encountered in association with specific disorders.

INTRODUCTION TO CULTURE AND MENTAL ILLNESS

The *DSM* includes information specifically related to culture in three areas:
1. A discussion of cultural variations for each of the clinical disorders
2. A description of culture-bound syndromes
3. An outline designed to assist the clinician in evaluating and reporting the impact of the individual's cultural context

Health care providers must consider the norms and influence of culture in determining the mental health or mental illness of the individual. Throughout history, people have interpreted health or sickness according to their own cultural views. People in the Middle Ages, for example, regarded bizarre behavior as a sign that the disturbed person was possessed by a demon. To exorcise the demon, priests resorted to prescribed religious rituals. During the 1880s, when the "germ theory" of illness was popular, physicians interpreted bizarre behavior as stemming from attacks by biological agents.

Cultures differ not only in the way they view mental illness but also in the types of behavior categorized as mental illness. For example, the content of a person's delusions, hallucinations, obsessional thoughts, and phobias often reflects what is important in the person's culture.

A number of culture-related syndromes appear to be more influenced by culture alone and are not seen in all areas of the world. For example, one form of mental illness recognized in parts of Southeast Asia is **running amok,** in which someone (usually a male) runs around engaging in furious, almost indiscriminate violent behavior. **Pibloktoq** is an uncontrollable desire to tear off one's clothing and expose oneself to severe winter weather; it is a recognized form of psychological disorder in parts of Greenland, Alaska, and the Arctic regions of Canada. In our own society, we recognize **anorexia nervosa** as a psychobiological disorder that entails voluntary starvation. This disorder is well-known in Europe, North America, and Australia, but unheard of in many other parts of the world.

What is to be made of the fact that certain disorders occur in some cultures but are absent in others? One interpretation is that the conditions necessary for causing a particular disorder occur in some places but are absent in other places. Another interpretation is that people learn certain kinds of abnormal behavior by imitation. However, the fact that some disorders may be culturally determined does not prove that all mental illnesses are so determined. The best evidence suggests that schizophrenia and bipolar affective disorders are found throughout the world. The symptom patterns of schizophrenia have been observed among indigenous Greenlanders and West African villagers, as well as in our own Western culture.

Many believe that the helpers of choice for many people from minority cultures are their traditional helpers/therapists. This is particularly true for problems that have psychological or psychosocial aspects. One example would be people of Central and Latin American cultures. Many people from this area of the world may prefer *curanderos* (male healers) or *curanderas* (female healers), who would be sought for healing a number of symptoms that are perceived to originate from psychological components, such as *susto* (fright) and *mal de ojo* (evil eye) (Falicop, 1998, p. 173; Hays, 2008). Another example is that of the Mexican and Mexican Americans who primarily prefer female healers. The practices employed by these healers are a mixture of Catholicism, ancient Mayan and Aztec cultures, and herbology (Hays, 2008; Novas, 1994).

A traditional helping strategy that we use in American mainstream therapies, especially with children, is that of storytelling. It is also one that is common to many indigenous cultures. The "therapist" uses a metaphor in the form of a "story" that offers a social message, but does not directly give advice or tell the person what to do. The listeners are then left to draw their own conclusions and make changes if they are ready to do so (Swinomish Tribal Community, 1991).

Indeed, psychotherapy would be considered the treatment of last resort in many cultures because (1) it is unavailable, (2) shame is attached to using therapies in the dominant culture, or (3) there are more effective or preferred treatments in their own culture (Hays, 2008; Yeh et al., 2006). The most effective therapists will be those who are eclectic in their knowledge, come from a background of working with different cultures, have a broad knowledge of coping strategies, and are flexible in their approach (Hays, 2008).

EXAMINING THE EVIDENCE

What is stigma?

The American Heritage Dictionary (1991) defines stigma as "a mark of infamy, disgrace or reproach." People often feel that stigma disqualifies one from full social acceptance. Many groups are stigmatized in our society, but we will focus on the stigma of mental illness to illustrate the effects of stigma.

What are the effects of stigma?

Stigma and discrimination against people with mental illness are often major barriers to success in relationships, employment, and treatment programs (Gill, 2008). Even worse, efforts to achieve rehabilitation and recovery from mental illness can be sabotaged by prejudice and negative assumptions (Hinshaw & Stier, 2008). The availability of health care in general is also affected by the stigma of mental illness. People with mental illness receive fewer medical services than those not labeled in this manner (Thornicroft et al., 2007).

Well, do they at least receive the best psychiatric treatment?

Not always. There are several mechanisms by which stigma affects mental health care including avoiding treatment, abandoning treatment, and harming one's sense of self (Corrigan et al., 2010).

Well, stigma sounds not only unpleasant, but is also dangerous to one's health. The mentally ill, though, work with health and mental health professionals, and they are not like that.

Health care providers are not immune. A proportion of providers hold negative and unfounded views of people with mental illness today (Rao et al., 2009). Negative attitudes and discrimination towards mental illness within the nursing profession have also been studied (Ross & Goldner, 2009).

Is there anything we can do to reduce stigma?

There are multiple methods that can be employed to reduce stigma; unfortunately, they are efficacious only some of the time with some populations (Lyons et al., 2009). Some campaigns in the media have focused on changing the presentation of people with mental illness. Others have educated the general public or targeted populations about the treatability of mental illness. Other efforts have focused on exposing the public to real people with mental illness in an effort to reduce stigma (Lyons et al., 2009). Stigma then might be reduced by education, by contact or personal acquaintance, and by offering different ways of perceiving people and situations.

This all sounds complicated. Is there a cost-effective, simple intervention that can be used in a classroom and that will make some difference?

Yes. Sadow and Ryder (2008) found that exposure to a person living with mental illness, but being in recovery, significantly reduces stigmatizing attitudes held by nursing students. It is important to have a person in recovery speak to the class and be available to answer questions. This personal exposure was found to be more effective than using books or movies to change the perception of mental illness. Health professionals are often exposed to people whose mental illness is in its most acute phase, when they do not function well. Professional do not often have an opportunity to see patients when they are well and are leading normal lives. Thus professionals erroneously conclude that no recovery is possible. Cohen and Cohen (1984), in a classic paper, call this "the clinician's illusion." This illusion is not factual. A seminal long-term (3 decades) study in Maine and Vermont (DeSisto et al., 1995) found that many people coping with serious mental illness improved over time, even if they did not receive treatment.

Where can someone find an "appropriate" person in recovery to speak to a class?

Contact NAMI.org (National Alliance on Mental Illness) or call 1-800-950-NAMI (6269) and ask for 'In Our Own Voice' (IOOV). This program (IOOV) will connect you with people who are trained speakers who generously share personal testimonies about living with and overcoming the challenges posed by mental illness. You and your class will be assisted in arranging a free presentation in your area.

Why bother?

There are two very important reasons. First, preliminary research indicates that people who attend an IOOV presentation experience a promising reduction in stigmatizing attitudes (Corrigan & O'Shaughnessy, 2007). Second, research (Sadow & Ryder, 2008) indicates that student nurses, after completing their psychiatric clinical experience, have an increase in stigmatizing attitudes. Consequently, it is imperative that student nurses experience programs such as IOOV in order to be exposed to people who had previously been hospitalized with mental illness and are now recovered and focused on living/building full lives. This may encourage us, as healers, to embrace the concepts of hope and recovery, and begin to eliminate the stigma of mental illness.

References

Cohen, P., & Cohen, J. (1984). The clinician's illusion. *Archives of General Psychiatry, 41*(12), 1178–1182. Retrieved from EBSCOhost.

Corrigan, P. W., Morris, S., Larson, J., Rafacz, J., Wassel, A., et al. (2010). Self-stigma and coming out about one's mental illness. *Journal of Community Psychology, 38*(3), 259–275. Retrieved from EBSCOhost.

Corrigan, P. W., & O'Shaughnessy, J. R. (2007). Changing mental illness stigma as it exists in the real world. *Australian Psychologist, 42*(2), 90–97. doi:10.1080/00050060701280573.

Continued

EXAMINING THE EVIDENCE—cont'd

DeSisto, M., Harding, C., McCormick, R., Ashikaga, T., & Brooks, G. (1995). The Maine and Vermont three decade studies of serious mental illness. I. Matched comparison of cross-sectional outcome. *British Journal of Psychiatry: Journal of Mental Science, 167*(3), 331–338. Retrieved from EBSCOhost.

Gill, K. J. (2008, Winter). The persistence of stigma and discrimination. *Psychiatric Rehabilitation Journal,* 183–184. doi:10.2975/31.3.2008.183.184.

Hinshaw, S. P., & Stier, A. (2008, April). Stigma as related to mental disorders. *Annual Review of Clinical Psychology, 4,* 367–393. Retrieved from www.annualreviews.org///.1146 /.clinpsy.4.022007.141245.

Lyons, C. C., Hopley, P. P., & Horrocks, J. J. (2009). A decade of stigma and discrimination in mental health: plus ça change, plus c'est la même chose (the more things change, the more they stay the same). *Journal of Psychiatric and Mental Health Nursing, 16*(6), 501–507. doi:10.1111/j.1365-2850.2009.01390.x.

NAMI: *In our own voice.* (n.d.). Retrieved March 17, 2011, from National Alliance on Mental Illness website: www.nami.org/ template.cfm?section=In_Our_Own_Voice.

Rao, H. H., Mahadevappa, H. H., Pillay, P. P., Sessay, M. M., Abraham, A. A., et al. (2009). A study of stigmatized attitudes towards people with mental health problems among health professionals. *Journal of Psychiatric and Mental Health Nursing, 16*(3), 279–284. doi:10.1111/j.1365-2850.2008.01369.x.

Ross, C. A., & Goldner, E. M. (2009). Stigma, negative attitudes and discrimination towards mental illness within the nursing profession: a review of the literature. *Journal of Psychiatric and Mental Health Nursing, 16*(6), 558–567. doi:10.1111/j.1365-2850.2009.01399.x.

Sadow, D., & Ryder, M. (2008, November). Reducing stigmatizing attitudes held by future health professionals: the person is the message. *Psychological Services, 5*(4), 362–372. doi:10.1037/.5.4.362.

Thornicroft, G., Rose, D., & Kassam, A. (2007). Discrimination in health care against people with mental illness. *International Review of Psychiatry, 19*(2), 113–122. doi:10.1080/09540260701278937.

Contributed by Dolly Sadow and Marie Ryder.

KEY POINTS TO REMEMBER

- Mental illness is difficult to define, and people have many myths regarding mental illness.
- Mental health can be conceptualized along a continuum, from mild to moderate to severe to psychosis.
- There are many important aspects of mental health (e.g., happiness, control over behavior, appraisal of reality, effectiveness in work, a healthy self-concept, presence of satisfying relationships, and effective coping strategies). Some components of mental health are identified in Figure 2-1.
- The processes that lead to stigmatization (labeling, stereotyping, status, loss, and discrimination in a context of power imbalance) can lead to an increase in social isolation, an enhanced struggle to recover, poor social functioning, significant barriers to obtaining psychiatric and medical services, and more. The mental anguish and excruciating pain caused by stigmatization effect tremendous damage to individuals and their families, groups, and/or cultures.
- The study of epidemiology can help identify high-risk groups and behaviors. In turn, this can lead to a better understanding of the causes of some disorders. Prevalence rates help us identify the proportion of a population with a mental disorder at a given time.
- With the current recognition that many common mental disorders are biologically based, it is easier to see how these biologically based disorders can be classified as medical diseases as well.

- Clinicians use the five axes of the *DSM* and the GAF scale as a guide for diagnosing and categorizing mental disorders, allowing for a more holistic approach to the assessment. Medical condition, psychosocial and environmental influences, and present and past levels of functioning are considered.
- Factors that may influence the intensity or cause of a mental illness are illustrated in Figure 2-2.
- Using well-conceived nursing diagnoses helps target the symptoms and needs of patients so that ideally they may achieve a higher level of functioning and a better quality of life.
- The influence of culture on behavior and the way in which symptoms present may reflect a person's cultural patterns. Symptoms need to be understood in terms of a person's cultural background.
- Caution is recommended for all health care professionals concerning the damage and disservice that stigmatizing/stereotyping can cause for medical and mental health patients. Stigmatizing is acknowledged to be a barrier to proper or appropriate mental health/recovery and medical services as well. Indeed, it may even prevent a person from accessing or receiving help. Stigmatizing/stereotyping causes shame and pain for the individual and their families, or the groups being stigmatized, and greatly impacts the quality of life or ability to lead a healthy life.

APPLYING CRITICAL JUDGMENT

1. Timothy Harris is a college sophomore with a grade point average of 3.4. He was brought to the emergency department after a suicide attempt. He has been extremely depressed since the death of his girlfriend 5 months previously when the car he was driving careened out of control and crashed. Timothy's parents have been very distraught since the accident. To compound things, the parents' religious beliefs include the conviction that taking one's own life will prevent a person from going to heaven. Timothy has epilepsy and has developed increased seizures since the accident; he refuses help because he says he should be punished for his carelessness and does not care what happens to him. He has not been to school and has not shown up for his part-time job of tutoring younger children in reading.
   A. Questions regarding Timothy and the use of the *DSM* multiaxial system:
      (1) What might be a possible *DSM* diagnosis for Axis I?
      (2) What information should be included on Axis III?
      (3) What should be included on Axis IV?
      (4) What score (range) might you give to Timothy on the GAF scale?
   B. Questions regarding mental health and mental illness:
      (1) What are some factors that you would like to assess regarding aspects of Timothy's overall mental health and other influences that can affect mental health before you plan your care?
      (2) If an antidepressant medication could help him with his depression, explain why this alone would not meet his multiple needs. What issues do you think have to be addressed if Timothy is to receive a holistic approach to care?
      (3) Formulate at least two potential nursing diagnoses for Timothy.
      (4) Would the religious beliefs of Timothy's parents affect your plan of care? If so, how?

2. Using Table 2-1, evaluate yourself and one of your patients in terms of mental health.

3. In a small study group, share experiences you have had with others from unfamiliar cultural, ethnic, or racial backgrounds and identify two positive learning experiences from these encounters.

4. Before your first day of clinical experience write what you honestly think about people who have for one reason or another developed a mental health disorder.
   A. After your clinical rotation, write what you now honestly think about individuals who have developed a mental health disorder.
   B. If your impressions are different after your experience, clarify what is different.
   C. Explore with your classmates how the clinical rotation and what you have learned from your readings and your instructors influenced the changes in your thinking, if there are changes.

CHAPTER REVIEW QUESTIONS

Choose the most appropriate answer(s).

1. Which statement about mental illness is true?
   1. Mental illness is a matter of individual nonconformity with societal norms.
   2. Mental illness is present when individual irrational and illogical behavior occurs.
   3. Mental illness is defined in relation to the culture, time in history, political system, and group in which it occurs.
   4. Mental illness is evaluated solely by considering individual control over behavior and appraisal of reality.

2. Axis V of the *DSM* multiaxial system:
   1. refers to medical illnesses.
   2. reports psychosocial and environmental problems.
   3. indicates a need for substance abuse treatment.
   4. describes a person's level of functioning.

3. Why is it important for a nurse to be aware of the multiple factors that can influence an individual's mental health?
   1. Rates of illness differ among various groups.
   2. The *DSM* cannot be used without information on multiple factors.
   3. The nurse diagnoses and treats human responses, which are influenced by many factors.
   4. The nurse must contribute these data for epidemiological research.

4. Factors that affect a person's mental health are: (select all that apply)
   1. support systems.
   2. developmental events.
   3. socioeconomic status.
   4. cultural beliefs.

5. Which statement best describes a major difference between a *DSM-IV-TR* diagnosis and a nursing diagnosis?
   1. There is no functional difference between the two. Both serve to identify a human deviance.
   2. The *DSM-IV-TR* diagnosis disregards culture, whereas the nursing diagnosis takes culture into account.
   3. The *DSM-IV-TR* is associated with present distress or disability, whereas a nursing diagnosis considers past and present responses to actual mental health problems.
   4. The *DSM-IV-TR* diagnosis distinguishes a person's specific psychiatric disorder, whereas a nursing diagnosis offers a framework for identifying interventions for phenomena a patient is experiencing.

REFERENCES

Altrocchi, J. (1980). *Abnormal behavior.* New York: Harcourt Brace Jovanovich.

American Psychiatric Association. (2000). *Diagnostic and statistical manual of mental disorders (DSM-IV-TR)* (4th ed., text rev.). Washington, DC: Author.

American Psychological Association. (2004). *The road to resilience.* Washington, DC: Author.

Endicott, J., Spitzer, R. L., Fleiss, J. L., et al. (1976). The global assessment scale: a procedure for measuring overall severity of psychiatric disturbance. *Archives of General Psychiatry, 33,* 766–771.

Falicop, C. J. (1998). *Latino families in therapy.* New York: Guilford Press.

Favazza, A. (2009). Psychiatry and spirituality. In B. J. Sadock, V. A. Sadock, & P. Ruiz (Eds.), *Kaplan and Sadock's comprehensive textbook of psychiatry* (9th ed., Vol. 11, pp. 2033–2049). Philadelphia: Williams & Wilkins.

Gary, F. A. (2005). Stigma: barrier to mental health care among ethnic minorities. *Issues in Mental Health Nursing, 26,* 979–999.

Goffman, E. (1963). *Stigma: notes on the management of spoiled identity.* Upper Saddle River, NJ: Prentice Hall.

Hays, P. A. (2008). *Addressing cultural complexities in practice: assessment, diagnosis, and therapy* (2nd ed.). Washington, DC: American Psychological Association.

Kessler, R. C., Berglund, P., Demler, O. L., et al. (2005). Lifetime prevalence and age-of-onset distribution of *DSM-IV* disorders in the national comorbidity survey replication. *Archives of General Psychiatry, 62,* 593–602.

Luborsky, L. (1962). Clinician's judgments of mental health. *Archives of General Psychiatry, 7,* 407–417.

Mayo Clinic Staff. (2011). *Mental health: overcoming the stigma of mental health.* Retrieved July 10, 2011, from www.mayoclinic.com/health/mental-health/MH00076/Method= print.

National Alliance on Mental Illness (NAMI). (2011). *What is mental illness: mental illness facts.* Retrieved July 9, 2011, from www.nami.org/PrinterTemplate.cfm?section= about_mental_illness.

National Institute of Mental Health. (2004). *The numbers count: mental disorders in America* (NIH Pub. No. 01–4584). Retrieved August 1, 2004, from www.nimh.nih.gov/publicat/numbers.cfm.

National Mental Health Association. (2004). *Congress must pass mental health parity now.* Retrieved July 31, 2004, from www.nmha.org/federal/parity/parityfactsheet.cfm.

Novas, H. (1994). *Everything you need to know about Latino history.* New York: Plume/Penguin.

Pinto-Foltz, M., Space, D., & Logsdon, M. C. (2009). Reducing stigma related to mental disorders: initiatives, interventions, and recommendations for nursing. *Archives of Psychiatric Nursing, 23*(1), 32–40.

Sadock, B. J., & Sadock, V. A. (2007). *Kaplan and Sadock's synopsis of psychiatry* (10th ed.). Philadelphia: Lippincott Williams & Wilkins.

Sadow, D. (personal communication). January 30, 2011.

Sadow, D., & Ryder, M. (2008). Reducing stigmatizing attitudes held by future health professionals: the person is the message. *Psychological Services, 5*(4), 362–372.

Swinomish Tribal Community. (1991). *A gathering of wisdom: tribal mental health: a cultural perspective.* LaConnor, WA: Author.

U.S. Department of Health and Human Services (USDHHS). (1999). *Mental health: a report of the Surgeon General.* Rockville, MD: USDHHS, Center for Mental Health Services, National Institutes of Health.

World Health Organization (WHO). (2010). *Mental health: strengthening our response.* Retrieved July 9, 2011, from www.who.int/mediacenter.

Yeh, C. J., Innan, A. G., Kim, A. B., & Okubo, Y. (2006). Asian American families collective coping strategies in response to 9/11. *Cultural Diversity and Ethnic Minority Psychology, 12,* 134–148.

Theories and Therapies

Margaret Jordan Halter

KEY TERMS AND CONCEPTS

automatic thoughts, p. 33
boundaries, p. 42
cognitive distortions, p. 33
conscious, p. 26
conservation, p. 35
countertransference, p. 27
curative factors, p. 40
ego, p. 26
group content, p. 39
group process, p. 39

id, p. 26
object permanence, p. 35
operations, p. 35
preconscious, p. 26
recovery model, p. 34
schemata, p. 34
self-actualization, p. 31
superego, p. 26
transference, p. 27
unconscious, p. 26

SELECTED CONCEPT: Recovery Model of Care

The Mental Health Recovery Model is not a focus on a cure, but instead emphasizes living adaptively with chronic mental illness. It is viewed as both an overarching philosophy of life for people with mental illness and as an approach to care for use by those who treat, finance, and support mental health care.

The recovery model switches the focus from nurse-patient relationship to nurse-partner relationship and had its initial success with those struggling with substances of abuse.

(Halter, the Text)

OBJECTIVES

1. Discuss the contributions of theories and therapies from a variety of disciplines and areas of expertise.
2. Choose two of the major theories that you believe are among the most relevant to psychiatric and mental health nursing care and defend your choice, giving examples.
3. Identify the origins and progression of dominant theories and treatment modalities.
4. Discuss the relevance of these theories and treatments to the provision of psychiatric and mental health care.

5. Demonstrate comprehensive understanding of Peplau's theoretical base for practice that is beneficial to all settings.
6. Identify three different theoretical models of mental health care and demonstrate how each could be used in specific circumstances.
7. Distinguish models of care used in clinical settings, and cite benefits and limitations of these models.

We expect ourselves and others to behave in certain ways, and we seek explanations for behavior that deviates from what we believe to be normal. What causes excessive sadness or extreme happiness? How do we explain mistrust, anxiety, confusion, or apathy—degrees of which may range from mildly disturbing to incapacitating? It is by understanding a problem that we can begin to devise solutions to treat or eradicate it. Mental illness has long defied explanation, even as other so-called physical illnesses were being quantified and often controlled.

It was not until the late 1800s that psychological models and theories were conceived, developed, and disseminated into mainstream thinking. They provided structure for considering developmental processes and possible explanations about how we think, feel, and behave. The theorists believed if complex workings of the mind could be understood they also could be treated, and from these models and theories therapies evolved.

Early practitioners used various forms of talk therapy, or **psychotherapy,** focusing on the complexity and inner workings of the mind and emphasizing environmental influences on its development and its stability. Beginning in the early twentieth century, biological explanations for mental alterations began to gain acceptance. Currently the dominant and common belief is that mental health and mental illness are on a continuum and comprised of both psychological and biological factors and that there is a dynamic interplay between the two.

Mental health professionals continue to rely on theoretical models as a basis for understanding and treating psychiatric alterations and mental health issues. No single model fully explains psychiatric illness and pathology. This chapter provides an overview of developmental theories, psychotherapeutic models, and related treatments and discusses the potential connection between them and the provision of psychiatric nursing care. Table 3-1 provides a brief overview of the major theories.

PROMINENT THEORIES AND THERAPEUTIC MODELS

Psychoanalytic Theory

Sigmund Freud (1856 to 1939), an Austrian neurologist, is considered the "father of psychiatry." His work was based on psychoanalytic theory, in which Freud claims that most psychological disturbances are the result of early trauma or incidents that are often not remembered or recognized.

Freud (1961) identified three layers of mental activity: the conscious, the preconscious, and the unconscious mind. The conscious mind is your current awareness—thoughts, beliefs, and feelings. However, most of the mind's activity occurs outside of this conscious awareness, like an iceberg with its bulk hidden underwater. The preconscious mind contains what is lying immediately below the surface, not currently the subject of our attention, but accessible. The biggest chunk of the iceberg is the unconscious mind; it is here where our primitive feelings, drives, and memories reside, especially those that are unbearable and traumatic. The conscious mind is then influenced by the preconscious and unconscious mind (Figure 3-1).

One of Freud's later and widely known constructs concerns the intrapsychic struggle that occurs within the brain among the id, the ego, and the superego. The id is the primitive, pleasure-seeking part (particularly sexual pleasure) of our personalities that lurks in the unconscious mind.

The ego is our sense of self and acts as an intermediary between the id and the world by using ego defense mechanisms, such as repression, denial, and rationalization (see Chapter 11).

The superego is our conscience and is greatly influenced by our parents' or caregivers' moral and ethical stances. In healthy individuals, the ego is able to realistically evaluate situations, limit the id's primitive impulses, and keep the superego from becoming too rigid and obsessive.

TABLE 3-1   MAJOR THEORIES OF PSYCHIATRIC CARE

THEORY	THEORIST	TENETS	THERAPEUTIC MODEL
Psychoanalytic	Freud	Unconscious thoughts; psychosexual development	Psychoanalysis to learn unconscious thoughts; therapist is nondirective and interprets meaning
Interpersonal	Sullivan	Relationships as basis for mental health or illness	Therapy focuses on here and now and emphasizes relationships; therapist is an active participant
Behavioral	Pavlov, Watson-Skinner	Behavior is learned through conditioning	Behavioral modification addresses maladaptive behaviors by rewarding adaptive behavior
Cognitive	Beck	Negative and self-critical thinking causes depression	Cognitive behavioral therapists assist in identifying negative thoughts patterns and replacing them with rational ones
Biological	Many	Psychiatric disorders are the result of physical (brain) alterations	Neurochemical imbalances are corrected through medication and talk therapy

Freud's theory of development focused on sexual urges and has been criticized for being sexist; perhaps his harshest criticism stems from the notion of "penis envy"—in which girls suffer from feelings of inferiority for not having male genitalia. Freud describes each developmental stage in terms of the id's focus on an erogenous zone of the body. Fixation, typically as the result of childhood sexual abuse, at any given point results in pathologic conditions and personality disorders. Table 3-2 provides a comparison of Freud's, Sullivan's, and Erikson's developmental stages.

Therapeutic Model

Psychoanalytic therapy was Freud's answer for a scientific method to relieve emotional disturbances by knowing the unconscious mind. An often time-consuming (sometimes daily), expensive, and emotionally painful process, the goal of this therapy is to know and understand what is happening at the unconscious level in order to uncover the truth. The analyst uses *free association* to search for forgotten and repressed memories by encouraging the patient to say anything that comes to mind. For example, "What do you think of when I say 'water'?" A patient may respond, "Warm…June…darkness …can't breathe," revealing a long-forgotten, but traumatic near-drowning incident.

The analyst is nondirective, but does make interpretations of symbols, thoughts, and dreams. **Psychodynamic therapy** is theoretically related to psychoanalytic therapy and views the mind in essentially the same way. It tends to be shorter, about 10 to 12 sessions (Sadock & Sadock, 2008), and the therapist takes a more active role because the therapeutic relationship is part of the healing process. Transference occurs as the patient projects intense feelings onto the therapist related to unfinished work from previous relationships; safe expression of these feelings is crucial to successful therapy. Psychodynamic therapists recognize that they, too, have unconscious emotional responses to the patient, or countertransference, which must be scrutinized in order to prevent damage to the therapeutic relationship.

Interpersonal Theory

Interpersonal theory focuses on what occurs between people, as opposed to psychoanalytic theory that is rooted in what occurs in the mind. Harry Stack Sullivan (1892 to 1949), an American psychiatrist, believed that personality dynamics and disorders

were caused primarily by social forces and interpersonal situations. Human beings are driven by the need for interaction; indeed, Sullivan (1953) viewed loneliness as the most painful human experience. He emphasized the early relationship with the *significant other* (primary parenting figure) as crucial for personality development, and believed that healthy relationships were necessary for a healthy personality. Anxiety is an interpersonal phenomenon that is transmitted empathically from the significant other to the child, and also by perceived degrees of approval or disapproval felt by the child. According to Sullivan, all behavior is aimed at avoiding anxiety and threats to self-esteem.

One of the ways that we avoid anxiety is by focusing on our positive attributes, or the *good me* ("I'm a good skier"), and by hiding the negative aspects, or the *bad me* ("I failed an exam"), of ourselves from others and maybe even from ourselves. The *not me* is used to separate us from parts of ourselves that we cannot imagine being part of us and is pushed deeply into the unconscious. An example is an adolescent in a strict and conservative family who begins to have stirrings of attraction, yet firmly maintains (and believes) that she does not have feelings for boys.

Sullivan's theory of development echoes that of Freud's in that personalities are influenced by the social environment as children, particularly as adolescents. He believed that personality is most influenced by the mother, but that personality could be molded even as adults. Stages occur in a stepwise fashion that is environmentally influenced (see Table 3-2).

Therapeutic Model

Interpersonal therapy (IPT) is a hands-on system in which therapists actively guide and challenge maladaptive behaviors and distorted views. The focus is on the "here and now" with an emphasis on the patient's life and relationships at home, at work, and in the social realm. The therapist becomes a "participant observer" and reflects the patient's interpersonal behavior, including responses to the therapist. The premise for this work is that if people are aware of their dysfunctional patterns and unrealistic expectations, they can modify them.

Behavioral Theories

As the psychoanalytic movement was developing in the twentieth century, so too was the behaviorist school of thought. Ivan Pavlov (1927) is famous for investigating *classical conditioning,* in which involuntary behavior or reflexes could be conditioned to respond to neutral stimuli. Pavlov's experimental dogs became accustomed to receiving food after a bell was rung; later these dogs salivated in response to the ring alone. For human beings, classical conditioning can occur under such circumstances as when a baby's crying induces a milk let-down reflex or when a rape victim begins to hyperventilate and sweat when she hears footsteps behind her.

John B. Watson (1930) rejected psychoanalysis and was seeking an objective therapy that did not focus on

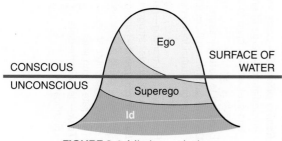

FIGURE 3-1 Mind as an iceberg.

TABLE 3-2 DEVELOPMENT OF PERSONALITY ACCORDING TO FREUD, SULLIVAN, AND ERIKSON*

FREUD	SULLIVAN	ERIKSON
Oral—birth to 1½ years ***Pleasure-pain principle*** ***Id,*** the instinctive and primitive mind, is dominant Demanding, impulsive, irrational, asocial, selfish, trustful, omnipotent, and dependent Primary thought processes Unconscious instincts—source-energy-aim-object Mouth—primary source of pleasure Immediate release of tension/anxiety and immediate gratification through oral gratification ***Task***—develop a sense of trust that needs will be met	**Infancy**—birth to 1½ years Mothering object relieves tension through empathic intervention and tenderness, leading to decreased anxiety and increased satisfaction and security; mother becomes symbolized "good mother" Goal is biological satisfaction and psychological security Denial of tension relief creates anxiety, and mother becomes symbolized as "bad mother" Anxiety in mother yields anxiety and fear in child via empathy These states are experienced by the child in diffuse-undifferentiated manner ***Task***—learn to count on others for satisfaction and security to trust	**Infancy**—birth to 1½ years ***Trust vs. mistrust*** Egocentric ***Danger***—during second half of first year, an abrupt and prolonged separation may intensify the natural sense of loss and may lead to a sense of mistrust that may last throughout life ***Task***—develop a basic sense of trust that leads to hope Trust requires a feeling of physical comfort and a minimal experience of fear or uncertainty; if this occurs, the child will extend trust to the world and self
Anal—1½ to 3 years ***Reality principle***—postpone immediate discharge of energy and seek actual object to satisfy needs Learning to defer pleasure Gaining satisfaction from tolerating some tension-mastering impulses Focus on toilet training—retaining/letting go; power struggle ***Ego development***—functions of the ego include problem-solving skills, perception, ability to mediate id impulses ***Task***—delay immediate gratification	**Childhood**—1½ to 6 years Muscular maturation and learning to communicate verbally Learning social skills through consensual validation Beginning to develop self-esteem via reflected appraisals: Good me Bad me Not me Levels of awareness Awareness Selective inattention Dissociation ***Task***—learn to delay satisfaction of wishes with relative comfort	**Early childhood**—1½ to 3 years ***Autonomy vs. shame/doubt*** Develop confidence in physical and mental abilities that leads to the development of an autonomous will ***Danger***—development of a deep sense of shame/doubt if child is deprived of the opportunity to rebel; learns to expect defeat in any battle of wills with those who are bigger and stronger ***Task***—gain self-control of and independence within the environment

Phallic—3 to 7 years
Superego develops via incorporating moral values, ideals, and judgments of right and wrong that are held by parents; superego is primarily unconscious and functions on the **reward and punishment principle** (sexual identity attained via resolving oedipal conflict)
Conflict differs for boy and girl
Task—develop sexual identity through identification with same-sex parent

Latency—7 to 12 years
De-sexualization; libido diffused
Involved in learning social skills, exploring, building, collecting, accomplishing, and hero worship
Peer group loyalty begins
Gang and scout behavior
Growing independence from family
Task—sexuality is repressed during this time; learn to form close relationship(s) with same-sex peers

Play—3 to 6 years
Initiative vs. guilt
Interest in socially appropriate goals leads to a sense of purpose
Imagination is greatly expanded because of increased ability to move around freely and increased ability to communicate
Intrusive activity and curiosity and consuming fantasies, which lead to feelings of guilt and anxiety
Establishment of conscience
Danger—may develop a deep-seated conviction that he or she is essentially bad, with a resultant stifling of initiative or a conversion of moralism to vindictiveness
Task—achieve a sense of purpose and develop a sense of mastery over tasks

Juvenile—6 to 9 years
Absorbed in learning to deal with ever-widening outside world, peers, and other adults
Reflections and revisions of self-image and parental images
Task—develop satisfying interpersonal relationships with peers that involve competition and compromise

Preadolescence—9 to 12 years
Develops intimate interpersonal relationship with person of same sex who is perceived to be much like oneself in interests, feelings, and mutual collaboration
Task—learn to care for others of same sex who are outside the family; Sullivan called this the "normal homosexual phase"

School age—6 to 12 years
Industry vs. inferiority
Develops a healthy competitive drive that leads to confidence
In learning to accept instruction and to win recognition by producing "things," the child opens the way for the capacity of work enjoyment
Danger—the development of a sense of inadequacy and inferiority in a child who does not receive recognition
Task—gain a sense of self-confidence and recognition through learning, competing, and performing successfully

Continued

TABLE 3-2   DEVELOPMENT OF PERSONALITY ACCORDING TO FREUD, SULLIVAN, AND ERIKSON*—cont'd

FREUD	SULLIVAN	ERIKSON
Genital phase (adolescence)— 13 to 20 years Fluctuation regarding emotion stability and physical maturation Very ambivalent and labile, seeking life goals and emancipation from parents Dependence vs. independence Reappraisal of parents and self; intense peer loyalty **Task**—form close relationships with members of the opposite sex based on genuine caring and pleasure in the interaction	**Adolescence**—12 to 20 years *Early adolescence*—*12 to 14 years* Establishing satisfying relationships with opposite sex *Late adolescence*—*14 to 20 years* Interdependent and establishing durable sexual relations with a select member of the opposite sex **Task**—form intimate and long-lasting relationships with the opposite sex and develop a sense of identity	**Adolescence**—12 to 20 years **Identity vs. role confusion** Diffusion Differentiation from parents leads to fidelity (sense of self) Physiological revolution that accompanies puberty (rapid body growth and sexual maturity) forces the young person to question beliefs and to refight many of the earlier battles **Danger**—temporary identity diffusion (instability) may result in a permanent inability to integrate a personal identity **Task**—integrate all the tasks previously mastered into a secure sense of self **Young adulthood**—20 to 30 years **Intimacy and solidarity vs. isolation** Maturity and social responsibility results in the ability to love and be loved As people feel more secure in their identity, they are able to establish intimacy with themselves (their inner life) and with others, eventually in a love-based satisfying sexual relationship with a member of the opposite sex **Danger**—fear of losing identity may prevent intimate relationship and result in a deep sense of isolation **Task**—form intense long-term relationships and commit to another person, cause, institution, or creative effort **Adulthood**—30 to 65 years **Generativity vs. self-absorption** Interest in nurturing subsequent generations creates a sense of caring, contributing, and generativity **Danger**—lack of generativity results in self-absorption and stagnation **Task**—achieve life goals and obtain concern and awareness of future generations **Senescence**—65 years to death **Integrity vs. despair** Acceptance of mortality and satisfaction with life leads to wisdom Satisfying intimacy with other human beings and adaptive response to triumphs and disappointments Marked by a sense of what life is, was, and its place in the flow of history **Danger**—without this "accrued ego integration," there is despair, usually marked by a display of displeasure and distrust **Task**—derive meaning from one's whole life and obtain/maintain a sense of self-worth

*Developed from original sources by Freud, Sullivan, and Erikson.

unconscious motivations. He contended that personality traits and responses, adaptive and maladaptive, were learned. In a famous (but terrible) experiment, Watson conditioned Little Albert, a 9-month-old child, to be terrified at the sight of white fur or hair. He concluded that through behavioral techniques anyone could be trained to be anything, from a beggar to a merchant.

B.F. Skinner (1938) conducted research on operant conditioning in which voluntary behaviors are learned through consequences of positive reinforcement (a consequence that causes the behavior to occur more frequently) or negative reinforcement or punishment (a consequence that causes the behavior to occur less frequently). Studying hard results in good grades and increases the chances that studying will continue to occur; driving too fast may result in a speeding ticket and in mature and healthy individuals can decrease the chances that speeding will recur.

Therapeutic Models

Behavioral therapy, or **behavior modification,** uses basic tenets from each of the behaviorists described previously. It attempts to correct or eliminate maladaptive behaviors or responses by rewarding and reinforcing adaptive behavior.

Systematic desensitization is based on classical conditioning. The premise is that learned responses can be reversed by first promoting relaxation and then gradually facing a particular anxiety-provoking stimulus. This method has been particularly successful in extinguishing phobias. Agoraphobia, the fear of open places, can be treated initially by visualizing trips outdoors while using relaxation techniques. Later, the individual can practice more challenging excursions, which should result in eliminating or reducing agoraphobia.

Aversion therapy is based on both classical and operant conditioning and is used to eradicate unwanted habits by associating unpleasant consequences with them. A pharmacologically based aversion therapy is a regimen of disulfiram (Antabuse); people who take this medication and then ingest alcohol become extremely ill. Aversion therapy also has been used with sex offenders who may, for example, receive electric shocks in response to arousal from child pornography.

Biofeedback is a technique in which individuals learn to control physiological responses such as breathing rates, heart rates, blood pressure, brain waves, and skin temperature. This control is achieved by providing visual or auditory biofeedback of the physiological response and then using relaxation techniques such as slow, deep breathing or meditation.

Humanistic Theory

Humanistic psychologists rejected the psychoanalysts' focus on unconscious conflicts, which they considered overpessimistic. They also rejected the behaviorists' focus on learning, which they considered overscientific. They sought a psychological science concerned with the human potential for development, knowledge attainment, motivation, and understanding.

Maslow's hierarchy of needs theory was developed in 1954 by Abraham Maslow (1970). Needs are placed conceptually on a pyramid, with the most basic and important needs on the lower level (Figure 3-2). The higher levels, the more distinctly human needs, occupy the top sections of the pyramid. According to Maslow, when lower level needs are met, higher level needs are able to emerge.

- *Physiological needs.* The most basic needs are the physiological drives, including the need for food, oxygen, water, sleep, sex, and a constant body temperature. If all the needs were deprived, this level would take priority.
- *Safety needs.* Once physiological needs are met, the safety needs emerge. They include security, protection, freedom from fear/anxiety/chaos, and the need for law, order, and limits.
- *Belongingness and love needs.* People have a need for an intimate relationship, love, affection, and belonging and will seek to overcome feelings of loneliness and alienation. Maslow stresses the importance of having a family and a home and being part of identifiable groups.
- *Esteem needs.* People need to have a high self-regard and have it reflected to them from others. If self-esteem needs are met, we feel confident, valued, and valuable. When self-esteem is compromised, we feel inferior, worthless, and helpless.
- *Self-actualization.* We are preset to strive to be everything that we are capable of becoming. Maslow said, "What a man *can* be, he *must* be." What we are capable of becoming is highly individual—an artist must paint, a writer must write, and a healer must heal. The drive to satisfy this need is felt as a sort of restlessness, a sense that something is missing. It is up to each person to choose a path that will result in inner peace and fulfillment.

Although Maslow's early work included only five levels of needs, he later took into account two additional factors: (1) cognitive needs (the desire to know and understand) and (2) aesthetic needs (Maslow, 1970). He describes the acquisition of knowledge (first) and the need to understand (second) as being hard-wired and essential. Furthermore, he identified aesthetic needs as a craving for beauty and symmetry, a universal need.

Rogers' Person-Centered Theory

Carl Rogers, an American psychologist, popularized person-centered theory in the 1940s. Rogers, unlike Freud, saw people as basically healthy and good. He identified people and all living organisms as having innate self-actualizing tendencies to grow, to develop, and to realize their full potential (Rogers, 1986). He believed that clients (he did not call them patients) were in the best position to explore, understand, and identify solutions to their own problems. He uses the analogy of teaching a child

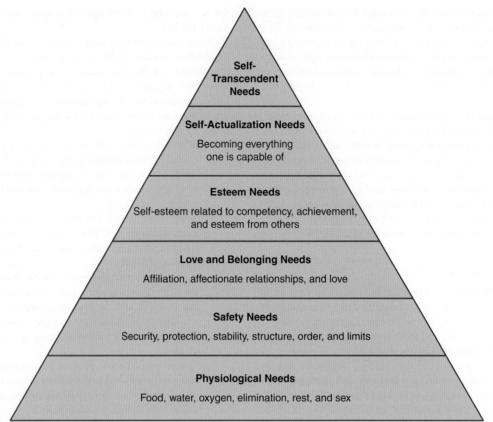

FIGURE 3-2 Maslow's hierarchy of needs. (Adapted from Maslow, A. H. [1972]. *The farther reaches of human nature.* New York: Viking.)

to ride a bicycle. It is not enough to tell the child how to ride, but is imperative that the child tries to ride the bike. (Refer to Chapter 9 for further discussion on Rogers' use of therapeutic relationships.)

Therapeutic Models

Patient-centered therapy is an existentially based therapy; the emphasis is on self-awareness and on the present, because the past has already occurred and the future has not yet occurred (Boeree, 2006). The role of the therapist is that of a nondirective facilitator who seeks clarification and provides encouragement in this process. Three essential qualities in the therapist are congruence (genuineness), empathy, and respect. If these three qualities are present, the patient will improve; without them, there is little chance that the therapy will be successful.

Cognitive Theory

Aaron T. Beck was convinced that depressed people generally had standard patterns of negative and self-critical thinking (Beck, 1963). Cognitive appraisals of events therefore lead to emotional responses—it is not the stimulus itself that causes the response, but instead one's evaluation of the stimulus. An example of the stimulus-appraisal-response relationship would

be a woman whose sister had been depressed since their tumultuous and unsteady childhoods. In response to a question about how she and her sibling handled their parents' divorce and subsequent move to a small apartment, one of the siblings observed: "My sister fell apart. She retreated, barely talked. Mom asked me how I was doing. I told her I was excited to get a new bedroom and make new friends. And I was telling the truth."

Therapeutic Model

Cognitive behavioral therapy (CBT) is a popular and commonly used effective and well-researched therapeutic tool. It is based on both cognitive and behavioral theory and seeks to modify negative thoughts that lead to dysfunctional emotions and actions. Several concepts underlie this therapy. One is that we all have *schemata*, or unique assumptions about ourselves, others, and the world around us. For example, if someone has a schema that no one can be trusted but themselves, this person will question everyone else's motives and expect deception and eventual pain from relationships with others. Other negative schemata include incompetence, abandonment, evilness, and vulnerability.

Typically, people are unaware of their basic assumptions; however, their beliefs and attitudes will make them apparent.

TABLE 3-3   EXAMPLES OF COGNITIVE DISTORTIONS

DISTORTION	DEFINITION	EXAMPLE
All-or-nothing thinking	Thinking in black and white, reducing complex outcomes into absolutes	Cheryl got second-highest score in the cheerleading competition. She considers herself a loser.
Overgeneralization	Using a bad outcome (or a few bad outcomes) as evidence that nothing will ever go right again	Marty had a traffic accident. She refuses to drive and says, "I shouldn't be allowed on the road."
Labeling	A form of generalization where a characteristic or event becomes definitive and results in an overly harsh label for self or others	"Because I failed the advanced statistics exam, I am a failure. I might as well give up."
Mental filter	Focusing on a negative detail or bad event and allowing it to taint everything else	Anne's boss evaluated her work as exemplary and gave her a few suggestions for improvement. She obsessed about the suggestions and ignored the rest.
Disqualifying the positive	Maintaining a negative view by rejecting information that supports a positive view as being irrelevant, inaccurate, or accidental	"I've just been offered the job I've always wanted. No one else must have applied."
Jumping to conclusions	Making a negative interpretation despite the fact that there is little or no supporting evidence	"My fiancé, Mike, didn't call me for 3 hours; therefore, he doesn't love me."
a. Mind reading	Inferring negative thoughts, responses, and motives of others	The grocery store clerk was grouchy and barely made eye contact. "I must have done something wrong."
b. Fortune-telling error	Anticipating that things will turn out badly as an established fact	"I'll ask her out, but I know she won't have a good time."
Magnification or minimization	Exaggerating the importance of something (such as a personal failure or the success of others) or reducing the importance of something (such as a personal success or the failure of others)	"I'm alone on a Saturday night because no one likes me. When other people are alone, it's because they want to be."
a. Catastrophizing	An extreme form of magnification in which the very worst is assumed to be a probable outcome	"If I don't make a good impression on the boss at the company picnic, she will fire me."
Emotional reasoning	Drawing a conclusion based on an emotional state	"I'm nervous about the exam. I must not be prepared. If I were, I wouldn't be afraid."
"Should" and "must" statements	Rigid self-directives that presume an unrealistic amount of control over external events	"My patient is worse today. I should give better care so that she will get better."
Personalization	Assuming responsibility for an external event or situation that was likely out of personal control	"I'm sorry that your party wasn't more fun. It's probably because I was there."

Adapted from Burns, D. D. (1980). *Feeling good: the new mood therapy*. New York: William Morrow.

Rapid, unthinking responses based on these schemata are known as **automatic thoughts.** These responses are particularly intense and frequent in psychiatric disorders such as depression and anxiety. Often these automatic thoughts, or **cognitive distortions,** are irrational because people make false assumptions and misinterpretations. Common cognitive distortions are listed in Table 3-3.

The goal of CBT is to identify the negative patterns of thought that lead to negative emotions. Once the maladaptive patterns are identified, they can be replaced with rational thoughts. A particularly useful technique in CBT is to use a four-column format to record the precipitating event or situation, the resulting automatic thought, the ensuing feeling(s) and behavior(s), and, finally, a challenge to the negative

thoughts based on rational evidence and thoughts. This is sometimes referred to as the ABCs of irrational beliefs and is a good exercise for nursing students to try for themselves (Box 3-1).

A Note on How Psychotherapy Changes the Brain

Numerous studies have indicated that all mental processes are derived from the brain. Therefore psychotherapeutic outcomes such as changes in symptoms, psychological abilities, personality, or social functioning, are generally accepted to be attributed to brain changes brought about either by medication or psychotherapy (Karisson, 2011). Numerous studies compiled by Karisson (2011) substantiate positive treatment responses with various psychotherapies resulting

---

BOX 3-1 EXAMPLE OF ABCs OF IRRATIONAL BELIEFS

Activating Event
Edward has been in counseling for depression. His therapist's secretary called and canceled this week's appointment.

Belief
My therapist is disgusted with me and wants to avoid me.

Consequence
Sadness, rejection, and hopelessness. Decides to call off work and return to bed.

Reframing
There is no evidence to believe that I disgust my therapist. Why would he have rescheduled if he really didn't want to see me?

---

in brain changes for the following disorders: major depressive disorder (MDD), anxiety disorders (panic disorder, social anxiety disorder, specific phobias), posttraumatic stress disorder (PTSD), borderline personality disorder, and obsessive-compulsive disorder (OCD). These studies suggest that at present the most effective therapies that result in brain changes are cognitive behavioral therapy (CBT), dialectic behavior therapy (DBT), psychodynamic psychotherapy, and interpersonal psychotherapy (IP) are effective for treating the aforementioned disorders (Karisson, 2011).

Mental Health Recovery Model

Although we tend think of recovery as regaining health or being cured from an episode of illness, the term recovery in this model has a different meaning. The mental health recovery model is not a focus on a cure, but instead emphasizes living adaptively with chronic mental illness. It is viewed both as an overarching philosophy of life for people with mental illness and as an approach to care for use by those who treat, finance, and support mental health care. It is also an effective approach to dealing with substance abuse.

A diagnosis of mental illness once meant that you listened to health care professionals and relied upon them to chart your course in life. This medical model approach often results in apathy and discouragement: "They want me to take medication for the rest of my life; I don't like it and won't take it." The recovery model shifts the responsibility for care from the provider to the individual: "I will discuss the medication side effects with my friends who have similar problems and then talk to my nurse practitioner about my options and preferences."

This model emphasizes hope, social connection, empowerment, coping strategies, and meaning in life. A recovery approach to care has been embraced by the American Psychiatric Association from a service perspective. The U.S. Department of Health and Human Services uses recovery concepts to guide federal and state initiatives, particularly as they relate to empowering mental health consumers (people with mental illness) and in campaigns to reduce mental illness stigma.

The Recovery Model in Psychiatric Nursing

The use of the recovery model in psychiatric nursing is a natural extension of what we have traditionally done. Peplau (1952) set the standard by urging nurses to develop therapeutic interpersonal relationships; the recovery model moves this relationship from nurse-patient to nurse-partner. According to Hanrahan and colleagues (2011), it is crucial to increase individual and family roles in recovery. Caldwell and colleagues (2010) assert that psychiatric nurses should educate other health care professionals about recovery concepts and suggest methods to empower consumers and promote recovery:

- Advocate for self-administration of medications when possible, with appropriate supports in the community.
- Encourage the development of medication records to schedule dosing and to share with other health care providers.
- Develop a personal relapse prevention program by knowing the symptoms of relapse, by realizing the effects of environmental and internal triggers on emotional well-being, and by enlisting others for support.
- Recommend supported employment in regular community settings to reduce isolation and improve confidence.
- Utilize psychiatric advance directives to enable consumers to plan for mental health treatment in the event of a crisis should they become incompetent.

OTHER MAJOR THEORIES

Cognitive Development

Jean Piaget (1896 to 1980) was a Swiss psychologist and researcher (Smith, 1997). While working at a boys' school run by Alfred Binet, developer of the Binet Intelligence Test, Piaget helped to score these tests. He became fascinated by the fact that young children consistently gave wrong answers on intelligence tests, wrong answers that revealed a discernible pattern of cognitive processing that was different from that of older children and adults. He concluded that cognitive development was a dynamic progression from primitive awareness and simple reflexes to complex thought and responses (Piaget & Inhelder, 1969). Our mental representations of the world, or schemata, depend on the cognitive stage we have reached.

An understanding of cognitive development can assist nurses to tailor their care to suit the cognitive level of the patient. For example, the concept of dying is difficult to grasp for the 5-year-old child who has lost a parent; support for this child will require different skills than those required for a 10-year-old child, who can understand the permanence of death. Whereas each of the cognitive stages describes a child, Piaget's theory can be useful in understanding cognitive ability in people with problems such as developmental delay and mental retardation:

- *Sensorimotor stage (birth to 2 years).* Begins with basic reflexes and culminates with purposeful movement, spatial abilities, and hand-eye coordination. Physical interaction with the environment provides the child with a basic understanding of the world. By about 9 months, object permanence is achieved and the child can conceptualize objects that are no longer visible. The delight of the game of peek-a-boo can be explained by this emerging skill as the child begins to anticipate the face hidden behind the hands.
- *Preoperational stage (2 to 7 years).* Operations is a term used to describe thinking about objects. Children are not yet able to think abstractly or generalize qualities in the absence of specific objects, but rather think in a concrete fashion. Egocentric thinking is demonstrated through a tendency to expect others to view the world as they do. They are also unable to conserve mass, volume, or number. An example of this is thinking that a tall, thin glass holds more liquid than a short, wide glass.
- *Concrete operational stage (7 to 11 years).* Logical thought appears and abstract problem solving is possible. The child is able to see a situation from another's point of view and can take into account a variety of solutions to a problem. Conservation is possible; for example, 2 small cups of liquid can be seen to equal a tall glass. They are able to classify based on discrete characteristics, order objects in a pattern, and understand the concept of reversibility.
- *Formal operational stage (11 years to adulthood).* Conceptual reasoning commences at approximately the same time as does puberty. At this stage the child's basic abilities to think abstractly and problem solve mirror those of an adult.

Theory of Psychosocial Development

The German-born American Erik Erikson (1902 to 1994) was a child psychoanalyst. Erikson (1963) described development as occurring in eight predetermined life stages, stages whose levels of success are related to the preceding stage (see Table 3-2). These stages are characterized by developmental tasks that ideally result in a successful resolution. One of the stages, for example, occurs from the ages of 7 to 12. During that time, the child's task is to gain a sense of his or her own abilities and competence, and expand relationships beyond the immediate family to include peers. The attainment of this task *(industry)* brings with it the virtue of confidence. If children are unable to gain a mastery of age-appropriate tasks, and cannot make a connection with their peers, they will feel like failures *(inferiority)*.

It is important to note that the resolution of each stage does not depend completely on integrating the positive characteristic and completing eschewing the negative. Ideally, harmony is achieved between the two characteristics. For example, we would not want a child to be 100% trusting—a child who trusted everyone would be totally vulnerable; a degree of mistrust is essential to survival. Additionally, Erikson did not states that developmental tasks had to be mastered within the prescribed time period, but he did believe that some tasks are naturally easier at certain junctures. For example, a child had inconsistent and abusive parenting; he may grow into a mistrustful adult. However, by experiencing corrective, dependable, and positive relationships later in life, he could become an appropriately trusting adult.

Theory of Object Relations

The theory of object relations was developed by interpersonal theorists, who emphasize past relationships in influencing a person's sense of self as well as the nature and quality of relationships in the present. The term *object* refers to another person, particularly a significant person.

Margaret Mahler (1895 to 1985) was a Hungarian-born child psychologist who worked with emotionally disturbed children. She developed a framework for studying how an infant transitions from complete self-absorption, with an inability to separate from its mother, to a physically and psychologically differentiated toddler. Mahler believed that psychological problems were largely the result of a disruption of this separation (Mahler et al., 1975).

During the first 3 years, the significant other (e.g., the mother) provides a secure base of support that promotes enough confidence for the child to separate. This is achieved by a balance of holding (emotionally and physically) a child enough for the child to feel safe, while encouraging independence and natural exploration.

Problems may arise in this process. If a toddler leaves his or her mother on the park bench and wanders off to the sandbox, the child should be encouraged with smiles and reassurance, "Go on honey; it's safe to go away a little." Then the mother needs to be reliably present when the toddler returns, thereby rewarding his or her efforts. Mahler notes that raising healthy children does not require that parents never make mistakes, and that "good enough parenting" will promote successful separation-individuation.

Theories of Moral Development
Stages of Moral Development

Lawrence Kohlberg (1927 to 1987) was an American psychologist whose work reflected and expanded on Piaget's by applying his theory to moral development, a development that coincided with cognitive development (Crain, 1985). While visiting Israel, Kohlberg became convinced that children living in a kibbutz had advanced moral development, and he believed that the atmosphere of trust, respect, and self-governance nurtured this development. In the United States, he created schools or "just communities" that were based on these concepts. Based on interviews with youths, Kohlberg developed a theory of how people progressively develop a sense of morality (Kohlberg & Turiel, 1971).

His theory provides a framework for understanding the progression from black-and-white thinking about right and wrong to a complex, variable, and context-dependent decision-making process regarding the rightness or wrongness of action.

Pre-conventional level

Stage 1: Obedience and punishment. The hallmarks of this stage are a focus on rules and on listening to authority. People at this stage believe that obedience is the method to avoid punishment.

Stage 2: Individualism and exchange. Individuals become aware that not everyone thinks the way that they do, and that rules are seen differently by different people. If they or others decide to break the rules, they are risking punishment.

Conventional level

Stage 3: Good interpersonal relationships. Children begin to view rightness or wrongness as related to motivations, personality, or the goodness or badness of the person. Generally speaking, people should get along and have similar values.

Stage 4: Maintaining the social order. A "rules are rules" mindset returns. However, the reasoning behind it is not simply to avoid punishment; it is because the person has begun to adopt a broader view of society. Listening to authority maintains the social order; bureaucracies and big government agencies often seem to operate with this tenet.

Post-conventional level

Stage 5: Social contract and individual rights. People in stage 5 still believe that the social order is important, but the social order must be *good*. For example, if the social order is corrupt, then rules should be changed and it is a duty to protect the rights of others.

Stage 6: Universal ethical principles. Actions should create justice for everyone involved. We are obliged to break unjust laws.

Ethics of Care Theory

Carol Gilligan (born 1936) is an American psychologist, ethicist, and feminist who inspired the normative ethics of care theory. She worked with Kohlberg as he developed his theory of moral development and later criticized his work for being based on a sample of boys and men. Additionally, she believed that he used a scoring method that favored males' methods of reasoning, resulting in lower moral development scores for girls as compared to boys. Based on Gilligan's critique, Kohlberg later revised his scoring methods, which resulted in greater similarity between girls' and boys' scores.

Gilligan's 1982 book, *In a Different Voice: Psychological Theory and Women's Development,* suggests that a morality of care should replace Kohlberg's "justice view" of morality, which maintains that we should do what is right no matter the personal cost or the cost to those we love. Gilligan's "care view" emphasizes the importance of forming relationships, banding together, and putting the needs of those for whom we care above the needs of strangers. Gilligan asserts that a female approach to ethics has always been in existence but has been trivialized. Like Kohlberg, Gilligan asserts that moral development progresses through three major divisions: pre-conventional, conventional, and post-conventional. These transitions are not dictated by cognitive ability, but rather through personal development and changes in a sense of self (Table 3-4).

MODELS, THEORIES, AND THERAPIES IN CURRENT PRACTICE

Biological Model

Psychiatric care is dominated by the biological model, in which mental disorders are believed to have physical causes; therefore

TABLE 3-4	GILLIGAN'S STAGES OF MORAL DEVELOPMENT	
STAGE	**GOAL**	**ACTION**
Pre-conventional	Goal is individual survival—selfishness	Caring for self
Conventional	Self-sacrifice is goodness—responsibility to others	Caring for others
Post-conventional	Principle of nonviolence—do not hurt others or self	Balancing caring for self with caring for others

mental disorders will respond to physical treatment. Sigmund Freud himself researched neurological causes for mental illness and considered cocaine a possible treatment.

In the 1950s a surgeon noticed that surgical patients were calmed by the administration of chlorpromazine (Thorazine); it soon became widely used for the treatment of schizophrenia and dramatically reduced the use of restraint and seclusion. This discovery spurred the development of other drug-based treatments and the adoption of a chemical imbalance theory of mental disorders.

If chemical imbalances exist, how do they develop? Twin studies have been useful to support the genetic transmission of certain disorders. Whereas only 1% of the population has schizophrenia, among identical twins the concordance rate (the percent of the time that both twins will be affected) is about 50% (Sadock & Sadock, 2008). Although this indicates genetic involvement, it cannot be the whole story. If it were, the concordance rate of schizophrenia in identical twins would be 100%. It is likely that the environment exerts an influence on the developing embryo or child. Research has shown that toxins, viruses, hostile environments, and brain traumas have been proposed as catalysts for the development of psychiatric disorders (see Chapter 4).

Biological Therapy

Psychopharmacology is the primary biological treatment for mental disorders. (Refer to Chapter 4 for a full discussion of the biological basis for understanding psychopharmacology.) Major classifications of medications are antidepressants, antipsychotics, antianxiety agents, mood stabilizers, and psychostimulants. Clinicians recognize the importance of optimizing other biological variables, such as correcting hormone levels (as in hypothyroidism), regulating nutritionally deficient diets, and balancing inadequate sleep patterns. (Refer to Chapters 10 through 19 for relevant uses of psychopharmacology.)

Electroconvulsive therapy (ECT) has proven to be an effective treatment for severe depression and other psychiatric conditions. ECT is a procedure that uses electrical current

TABLE 3-5   NURSING THEORETICAL WORKS RELEVANT TO PSYCHIATRIC NURSING

THEORIST	MODEL/THEORY	FOCUS OF NURSING	EXAMPLE
Dorothy Johnson	Behavioral system	Helping a patient return to a state of equilibrium when exposed to stressors by reducing or removing them and by supporting adaptive processes (Johnson, 1980)	Providing prn antianxiety medication and encouraging slow, deep breathing for a patient who is experiencing panic attacks
Imogene King	Goal attainment	Developing an interpersonal relationship and helping the patient to achieve his/her goals based on the patient's roles and social contexts (King, 1981)	Sitting with a new mother who is experiencing depression and developing a discharge plan in the context of childcare and financial deficits
Madeleine Leininger*	Culture care	Promoting health and helping people to cope with illness while recognizing cultural issues and their importance to health (Leininger, 1995)	Including the family in the plan of care for an Amish man who has recently attempted suicide
Betty Neuman*	System model	Developing a nurse-patient relationship; assessing and intervening with the person's response to stress (Neuman, 1982)	Considering the impact of shingles and graduate school stressors on a person diagnosed with generalized anxiety disorder
Dorothea Orem	Self-care deficit	Addressing self-care deficits and encouraging patients to be actively involved in their own care (Orem, 2001)	Temporarily helping a person with an exacerbation of paranoia to meet his/her hygiene needs
Ida Orlando*	Dynamic nurse-patient relationship	Addressing the patient's immediate need for help; the longer the unmet need, the more stress will be experienced (Orlando, 1990)	Asking, "Would you like to talk?" to a man who has begun pacing in the hallway and shaking his head
Hildegard Peplau*	Interpersonal relations	Using the interpersonal environment as a therapeutic tool for healing and in reduction of anxiety (Peplau, 1992)	Sitting quietly beside a new father who has recently lost his job and attempted suicide and does not want to talk
Jean Watson*	Transpersonal caring	Caring is as important as procedures and tasks; developing a nurse-patient relationship that results in a therapeutic outcome (Watson, 2007)	Taking time from a busy assignment to meet a patient's husband

*Psychiatric nursing background.

to induce a seizure, and is thought to work by affecting neurotransmitters and neuroreceptors (see Chapter 15 for more discussion regarding ECT).

Most mental health professionals combine biological approaches with talk therapy. Research indicates that using medication and cognitive behavioral therapy is an extremely effective treatment for many psychiatric disorders, especially major depression (Black & Andreasen, 2011; Sadock & Sadock, 2008). If a hostile environment can trigger negative brain chemistry or transmission, then a positive environment may reverse and improve the process.

Nursing Models

We have been examining theories and therapies developed by professionals from a variety of disciplines that date back to the late 1800s. It was not until the 1950s that the profession of nursing began to develop, record, and test theories (Alligood & Tomey, 2010). The drive to create these theories began as a result of nursing education being moved from hospital-based programs to college- and university-based programs where nurses became involved in research. This research became the impetus for nurses to develop theories and a strong scientific body of knowledge.

Hildegard Peplau's work in the early 1950s is most often associated with psychiatric nursing, and her work will be presented in the following section. However, most nursing theories are applicable and of value to psychiatric nursing because interpersonal relations, caring, and communication are keys to the foundation of nursing. A summary of selected nursing theorists, the focus of their theoretical works, and examples of how their contributions could be utilized in psychiatric nursing is provided in Table 3-5. It is worth noting that among nurse theorists, psychiatric nurses are well-represented.

Interpersonal Relations in Nursing

Hildegard Peplau's (1909 to 1999) seminal work, *Interpersonal Relations in Nursing,* was first published in 1952 and has served as a foundation for understanding and conducting therapeutic nursing relationships ever since. Peplau based her work on Sullivan's interpersonal theory and emphasized that the nature of the nurse-patient relationship strongly influenced the outcome for the patient.

Peplau made an extremely useful contribution to understanding anxiety by conceptualizing the four levels still in use today:

1. Mild anxiety is day-to-day, "I'm awake and taking care of business" alertness. Stimuli in the environment are perceived and understood, and learning can easily take place.
2. Moderate anxiety is felt as a heightened sense of awareness, such as when you are about to take an exam. The perceptual field is narrowed and an individual hears, sees, and understands less. Learning can still take place, although it may require more direction.
3. Severe anxiety interferes with clear thinking and the perceptual field is greatly diminished. Nearly all behavior is directed at reducing the anxiety. An example of this is your response to skidding your car on wet pavement.
4. Panic anxiety is overwhelming and results in either paralysis or dangerous hyperactivity. An individual cannot communicate, function, or follow direction. This is the sort of anxiety that is associated with the terror of panic attacks.

Refer to Chapter 11 for application of these levels to the nursing process.

One of the most useful constructs of Peplau's theory is in providing structure for how we view the therapeutic relationship, which she divided into four phases. Each of these overlapping and interlocking phases includes tasks, the expression of needs by the patient, and the interventions facilitated by the nurse. Refer to Chapter 9 for more information on the phases of the nurse-patient relationship.

Influence of Theories and Therapies on Nursing Care

Other theories and therapies presented earlier in this chapter also are relevant to nursing care. Nurses constantly borrow concepts and carry out interventions that are supported by these models. Some examples of how they may be used are as follows:

- **Behavioral:** Promoting adaptive behaviors through reinforcement can be valuable and important in working with patients, especially when working with a pediatric population. These patients look forward to positive reinforcement for good behavior and will work hard for gold stars or other privileges.
- **Cognitive:** Helping patients identify negative thought patterns is a worthwhile intervention in promoting healthy functioning and improving neurochemistry. Workbooks are available to aid in the process of identifying these cognitive distortions.
- **Psychosocial development:** Erikson's theory provides structure for understanding critical junctures in development. The older adult gentleman who has suffered a stroke may be depressed and despairing because he can no longer take care of his house. In this case the nurse and patient could explore ways of optimizing the patient's remaining strengths and talents, such as by nurturing and tutoring young people or by developing attainable and progressive goals such as getting the mail, taking out the trash, and so forth.
- **Hierarchy of needs:** Maslow's work is useful in prioritizing nursing care. When working with an actively suicidal patient, students sometimes think it is rude to ask if the patients are thinking about killing themselves. However, safety supersedes this potential threat to self-esteem. Although the "must do's" in nursing begin with physical care (such as providing medication and hydration through IV fluids), the goal should also include higher level needs, which can be obtained by listening, observing, and collaborating with the patient in the development of the plan of care.

EXAMINING THE EVIDENCE

Let's give a warm welcome to the Consumer Providers (CPs) who are now joining the Mental Health Team!!!

OK...But who *are* consumer providers?

The Rand Corporation, a nonprofit research organization, has identified the following important information about Consumer Providers:

"Consumer Providers (CPs) are individuals with serious mental illness who are trained to use their experiences to provide recovery–oriented services and to support others with mental illness in a mental health delivery setting" (Chinman et al., 2008, p. v). The CP receives specialized training in mental health concepts with a focus on hope and recovery. After completing this intensive training, some CPs take a rigorous national exam, and if they successfully pass, they become Certified Peer Specialists. In order to maintain their certification, they must be involved in continuing education programs and, like all mental health professionals, need supervision in the clinical setting (Chinman et al., 2008).

So, what is the role of CPs in the clinical setting?

CPs serve as role models to encourage people who are struggling with mental health issues. When appropriate, they share their personal recovery story to show that recovery from mental illness is possible.

CPs teach goal setting, problem solving, symptom management skills, and a variety of recovery tools.

CPs facilitate or lead groups to provide peer support for clients (Chinman et al., 2008).

EXAMINING THE EVIDENCE—cont'd

What are the advantages of having CPs on the mental health team?

It must be noted that, although reasonable evidence supports the efficacy of structured self-management programs for physical conditions such as diabetes, there is far less research to evaluate outcomes for mental disorders (Cook et al., 2009). That point being noted, Cook and colleagues examined changes in measures of recovery and psychosocial outcomes of participants involved in a peer-led intervention called Wellness Recovery Action Planning (WRAP). The results of this research concluded that "the efficacy and effectiveness of peer-led self-management has the potential to enhance self-determination and promote recovery for people with psychiatric disabilities" (Cook et al., 2009, p. 1). Additionally, many investigators are presently engaged in research that will definitively answer the questions regarding the efficacy of having CPs provide peer-led services. Still, "overall the results suggest that peer support services have a positive impact in the lives of those that receive this care, and help foster recovery and promote resiliency" (Daniels et al., 2009, p. 10).

Since "money makes the world go round," how are the services of CPs billed?

More frequently, state mental health systems are allowing CP services to be reimbursed under Medicaid (Salzer et al., 2010.) Additionally, it is noteworthy that the Veterans Administration has created job codes for CPs and allows billing of their services (Chinman et al., 2008).

So, having CPs on the mental health team sounds like a sweeping movement that is transforming the mental health system!

Yes! Now that the idea of "recovery" is the focus of mental health treatment, CPs provide an important strategy for making mental health care more oriented to the goal of leading people to paths of resiliency and recovery (Chinman et al., 2008).

EXCELLENT!!! So, as nurses, we will be sure to give a resounding welcome to consumer providers, who bring the essential elements of hope and recovery to the Mental Health Team!

References

Chinman, M., Hamilton, A., Butler, B., Knight, E., Murray, S., et al. (2008). *Mental health consumer providers: a guide for clinical staff*. Retrieved from Rand Health website: www.rand.org/////_reports//_TR584.html.

Cook, J., Copeland, M. E., Hamilton, M., et al. (2009). Initial outcomes of mental illness self-management program based on Wellness Recovery Action Planning. *Psychiatric Services*, *60*, 246–249.

Daniels, A. S., Grant, E. A., Filson, B., Powell, I. G., Fricks, L., et al. (2009, November 17). Pillars of peer support: transforming mental health systems of care through peer support services. In *Pillars of peer support services summit*. Atlanta, GA: Symposium conducted at The Carter Center. Retrieved from www.parecovery.org/documents/Pillars_of_Peer_Support.pdf.

Salzer, M., Schwenk, E., & Brusilovskity, E. (2010). Certified peer specialists roles and activities: results from a national survey. *Psychiatric Services*, *61*(5), 520–523.

Submitted by Marie Ryder & Dolly Sadow.

Therapies for Specific Populations

Group Therapy

This therapeutic method is commonly derived from interpersonal theory and operates under the assumption that interaction among participants can provide support or bring about desired change among individual participants.

A **group** is defined as (a) "a gathering of two or more individuals (b) who share a common purpose and (c) meet over a substantial time period (d) in face-to-face interaction (e) to achieve an identifiable goal" (Arnold & Boggs, 2011, p. 525). Experts disagree on the ideal size of the group, but it is usually somewhere from 6 to 10 members. A group that is too small will limit diversity of opinion and put pressure on members to participate. Overly large groups reduce the members' ability to share, especially if some members dominate the group.

Setting. Settings for groups are important. The room should be private, and the seating should be comfortable and arranged so that people can see one another. Using tables is discouraged because they can be psychological barriers between group members. One of the worst arrangements for discussion is the traditional "classroom seating" with everyone facing a central speaker, thereby limiting free interaction among participants.

Groups possess both content and process dimensions. Group content refers to the actual dialogue between members or the type of information that can be transcribed (written or recorded) in minutes of meetings. Group process includes all the other elements of human interaction, such as nonverbal communication, adaptive and maladaptive roles, energy flow, power plays, conflict, hidden agendas, and silences. Although the content is essential to the group's work, it is the process that becomes the real challenge for leaders as well as participants.

Group development tends to follow a sequential pattern of growth and requires less leadership with time. Understanding this pattern is especially helpful to the leader in order to anticipate distinct phases and provide guidance and interventions that are most effective. Tuckman's (1965) model of group development has four stages: forming, storming, norming, and performing. A fifth stage, adjourning (mourning), was later added (Tuckman & Jensen, 1977). These stages are comparable to human development from infancy into old age, accompanied by varying levels of maturity, confidence, and need for direction (Table 3-6).

TABLE 3-6   TUCKMAN'S STAGES OF GROUP DEVELOPMENT AND COMPARABLE LIFE PHASE

STAGE	COMPARABLE LIFE PHASE	DESCRIPTION
Forming	Infancy	The task and/or purpose of the group is defined. Connecting with others, desiring acceptance, and avoiding conflict define early groups. Members gather commonalities and differences as they attempt to know one another. The leader is the main connection and necessary for direction.
Storming	Adolescence	Important issues are being addressed, and conflict begins to surface. Personal relations may interfere with the task at hand. Some members will dominate, and some will be silent. Rules and structure are helpful. Members may challenge the role of the leader, who has the opportunity to model adaptive behavior.
Norming	Early adulthood	Members know one another, and rules of engagement (norms) are evident. There is a sense of group identity and cohesion. Members resist change, which could lead to a group breakup or a return to the discomfort of storming. Leadership is shared.
Performing	Mature adulthood	Groups who reach this stage are characterized by loyalty, flexibility, interdependence, and productivity. There is a balance between focus on work and focus on the welfare of group members.
Adjourning (mourning)	Older adult years	Groups in this stage are ready to disband, tasks are terminated, and relationships are disengaged. Accomplishments are recognized and members are pleased to have been part of the group. A sense of loss is an inevitable consequence.

From Tuckman, B. W., & Jensen, M. A. (1977). Stages of small-group development revisited. *Group & Organization Management, 2,* 419-427.

Roles of group members. Studies of group dynamics have identified informal roles of members that are necessary to develop a successful group. The most common descriptive categories for these roles are task, maintenance, and individual roles (Benne & Sheats, 1948). Task roles serve to keep the group focused and attend to the business at hand. Maintenance roles function to keep the group together and provide interpersonal support. There are also individual roles that can interfere with the group's functioning because they are not related to the group goals, but rather to specific personalities. Table 3-7 describes roles of group members.

Roles of the group leader. The group leader has multiple responsibilities in starting, maintaining, and terminating a group. In the initial forming phase, the leader defines the structure, size, composition, purpose, and timing for the group. The leader facilitates communication and ensures that meetings start and end on time. In the adjourning phase, the leader ensures that each member summarizes individual accomplishments and gives positive and negative feedback regarding the group experience.

Leadership style depends on group type (Jacobs et al., 2012). A leader selects the style that is best suited to the therapeutic needs of a particular group. The **autocratic leader** exerts control over the group and does not encourage much interaction among members. In contrast, the **democratic leader** supports extensive group interaction in the process of problem solving. A **laissez-faire leader** allows the group members to behave in any way that they choose and does not attempt to control the direction of the group. For example, staff leading a community meeting with a fixed, time-limited agenda may tend to be more autocratic. In a psychoeducational group, the leader may be more democratic to encourage members to share their experiences. In a creative group such as an art or horticulture group, the leader may choose a laissez-faire style, giving minimal direction to allow for a variety of responses.

Types of groups. Education groups form for the purpose of imparting information and require active expert leadership and careful planning. Task groups are typically time limited and have a common goal, and the role of the leader is to facilitate team building and cooperation. Support groups bring together people with common concerns and may be facilitated by a supportive leader or by group members. Therapy groups are led by professional group therapists whose styles may range from a directive and confrontational approach to a more hands-off, let the group members learn from each other, approach.

Benefits of Group Therapy

One of the commonly cited benefits of group therapy is that it is more efficient, both pragmatically and financially, because many people can engage in therapy at once. However, it is the nature of the interaction between people with common concerns and frames of references that seems to provide the greatest benefit. Yalom (1985) identified 11 benefits, or curative factors, of group membership (Table 3-8).

Roles of Nurses

Psychiatric–mental health nurses are involved in a variety of therapeutic groups in acute care and long-term treatment settings. For all group leaders, a clear theoretical framework is necessary to provide a structure to understand the group interaction. Co-leadership of groups is a common practice and has several benefits: it provides training for less experienced

TABLE 3-7   ROLES OF GROUP MEMBERS

ROLE	FUNCTION
Task Roles	
Coordinator	Connects various ideas and suggestions
Initiator-contributor	Offers new ideas or a new outlook on an issue
Elaborator	Gives examples and follows up meaning of ideas
Energizer	Encourages group to make decisions or take action
Evaluator	Measures group's work against a standard
Information/opinion giver	Shares opinions, especially to influence group values
Orienter	Notes progress of the group toward goals
Maintenance Roles	
Compromiser	In a conflict, yields to preserve group harmony
Encourager	Praises and seeks input from others; warm and accepting
Follower	Attentive listener and integral to the group
Gatekeeper	Ensures participation, encourages participation, points out commonality of thought
Harmonizer	Mediates conflicts constructively among members
Standard setter	Assesses explicit and implicit standards for group
Individual Roles	
Aggressor	Criticizes and attacks others' ideas and feelings
Blocker	Disagrees with group issues, opposes others, stalls the process
Help seeker	Asks for sympathy of group excessively, self-deprecating
Playboy/playgirl	Distracts others from the task; jokes, introduces irrelevant topics
Recognition seeker	Seeks attention by boasting and discussing achievements
Monopolizer	Dominates conversation, thereby preventing equal input
Special interest pleader	Advocates for a special group, usually with own prejudice or bias

Data from Benne, K. D., & Sheats, F. (1948). Functional roles of group members. *Journal of Social Issues, 4*(2), 41.

TABLE 3-8   YALOM'S CURATIVE FACTORS OF GROUP MEMBERSHIP

CURATIVE FACTOR	DEFINITION	EXAMPLE
Altruism	Giving appropriate help to other members	"We've spent all this time talking about me. Lou needs to talk about his visit with his dad. Let's focus on him."
Cohesiveness	Feeling connected to other members and belonging to the group	"People in our group always listen to each other. We've been polite since the first day."
Interpersonal learning	Learning from other members	"Sammi said it takes 2 weeks for Prozac to really work. I should give it more time."
Guidance	Receiving help and advice	"I've also had that feeling where I just had to have a drink, Don. Just pick up the phone and call me next time it happens."
Catharsis	Releasing feelings and emotions	A new mother of twins begins to cry and says, "It sounds terrible, but sometimes I wish I'd never had children."
Identification	Modeling after member or leader	David notices that the leader projects confidence by speaking clearly, making good eye contact, and sitting up straight. David does the same.
Family reenactment	Testing new behaviors in a safe environment	"I learned to always smile and agree so Dad wouldn't go off on me. I don't have to be cheery and I can speak my mind here."
Self-understanding	Gaining personal insights	Dale realizes that his negativity has kept him from getting the friends he wants.
Instillation of hope	Feeling hopeful about one's life	"Sue has managed to stay sober for 2 years. I think I can do this."
Universality	Feeling that one is not alone	Aaron, a quiet group member finally comments, "My son has schizophrenia, too, and it helps to hear that other people have the same worries I do."
Existential factors	Coming to understand what life is about	"I guess I've been obsessing about being a perfect housekeeper and haven't noticed that my children are growing up without me."

From Yalom, I. D. (1985). *The theory and practice of group psychotherapy.* New York: Basic Books.

staff; it allows for immediate feedback between the leaders after each session; and it gives two role models for teaching communication skills to members.

Basic level registered nurses have biopsychosocial educational backgrounds and are ideally suited to teach a variety of health subjects. *Psychoeducational groups* are established to teach about subjects. These groups may be time limited or may be supportive for long-term treatment. Generally, written handouts or audiovisual aids are used to focus on specific teaching points. The following psychoeducational groups are commonly led by nurses:

- **Medication education groups** allow patients to hear the experiences of others who have taken medication and have an opportunity to ask questions without the fear of being judged and learning to take the medications correctly.
- **Dual-diagnosis groups** focus on co-occurring psychiatric illness and substance abuse. The registered nurse (RN) may co-lead this group with a dual-diagnosis specialist (master's level clinician).
- **Multifamily groups** have evidence-based support as an effective method within the severely mentally ill population (Lemmens et al., 2009). The focus is on education about the mental illness and strategies for the family to cope with long-term disability.
- **Symptom management groups** are designed for patients to share coping skills regarding a common problem, such as anger or psychosis. Self-control is improved and relapse is reduced by helping patients to develop a plan for action.
- **Stress management groups** teach members about various relaxation techniques, including deep breathing, exercise, music, and spirituality.
- **Self-care groups** focus on basic hygiene issues such as bathing and grooming.

Advanced practice registered nurses (APRNs) may lead any of the groups described earlier as well as psychotherapy groups. Psychotherapy groups require specialized training in techniques that allow for deep disclosure, sharing, confrontation, and healing among participants.

Therapeutic Milieu

A therapeutic milieu, or healthy environment, combined with a healthy social structure within an inpatient setting or structured outpatient clinic is essential to supporting and treating those with mental illness. Within these small versions of society, people are safe to test new behaviors and increase their ability to interact adaptively within the outside community.

Community meetings usually include all patients and the treatment team. Functions include orienting new members to the unit, encouraging patients to engage in treatment, and evaluating the treatment program. Nursing staff are the largest group of providers and give valuable feedback to the team about group interactions. Goal-setting meetings may be conducted in inpatient settings and partial hospitalization programs to plan daily goals for each patient.

Other therapeutic milieu groups aim to help increase patients' self-esteem, decrease social isolation, encourage appropriate social behaviors, and educate patients in basic living skills. These groups are often led by occupational or recreational therapists, although nurses frequently co-lead them. Examples of therapeutic milieu groups are recreational groups, physical activity groups, creative arts groups, and storytelling groups.

Family Therapy

Family therapy developed around the mid-twentieth century as an adjunct to individual treatment and refers to the treatment of the family as a whole. Family therapists use a variety of theoretical philosophies to effect change in dysfunctional patterns of behavior and interaction. Some therapists may focus on the present, whereas others may rely more heavily on the family's history and reports of interactions between sessions. Terms related to family therapy are listed in Box 3-2.

BOX 3-2   CENTRAL CONCEPTS TO FAMILY THERAPY

- **Boundaries:** *Clear boundaries* maintain distinctions between individuals within the family and between the family and the outside world. Clear boundaries allow for balanced flow of energy between members. *Diffuse* or *enmeshed boundaries* are those in which there is a blending of the roles, thoughts, and feelings of the individuals so that clear distinctions among family members fail to emerge. *Rigid* or *disengaged boundaries* are those in which the rules and roles are followed in spite of the consequences.
- **Triangulation:** The tendency, when two-person relationships are stressful and unstable, to engage a third person to stabilize the system through formation of a coalition in which two members are pitted against the third.
- **Scapegoating:** A form of displacement in which a family member (usually the least powerful) is blamed for another family member's distress. The purpose is to keep the focus off the painful issues and the problems of the blamers.
- **Double bind:** A double bind is a no-win situation in which you are "darned if you do, darned if you don't."
- **Hierarchy:** The function of power and its structures in families, differentiating parental and sibling roles and generational boundaries.
- **Differentiation:** The ability to develop a strong identity and sense of self while maintaining an emotional connectedness with one's family of origin.
- **Sociocultural context:** The framework for viewing the family in terms of the influence of gender, race, ethnicity, religion, economic class, and sexual orientation.
- **Multigenerational issues:** The continuation and persistence from generation to generation of certain emotional interactive family patterns (e.g., reenactment of fairly predictable patterns; repetition of themes or toxic issues; and repetition of reciprocal patterns such as those of overfunctioner and underfunctioner).

Although different therapists may adhere to different theories and use a wide variety of methods, the goals of family therapy are basically the same. These goals include the following (Nichols, 2009):

- To reduce dysfunctional behavior of individual family members
- To resolve or reduce intrafamily relationship conflicts
- To mobilize family resources and encourage adaptive family problem-solving behaviors
- To improve family communication skills

- To heighten awareness and sensitivity to other family members' emotional needs and help family members meet their needs
- To strengthen the family's ability to cope with major life stressors and traumatic events, including chronic physical or psychiatric illness
- To improve integration of the family system into the societal system (e.g., school, medical facilities, workplace, and especially the extended family)

■ KEY POINTS TO REMEMBER

- Theoretical models and therapeutic strategies provide a useful framework for the delivery of psychiatric nursing care.
- The psychoanalytic model is based on unconscious motivations and the dynamic interplay between the primitive brain (id), the sense of self (ego), and the conscience (superego). The focus of psychoanalytic theory is on understanding the unconscious mind.
- The interpersonal model maintains that the personality and disorders are created by social forces and interpersonal experiences. Interpersonal therapy aims to provide positive and repairing interpersonal experiences.
- The behavioral model suggests that because behavior is learned, behavioral therapy should improve behavior through rewards and reinforcement of adaptive behavior.
- The humanist model is based on human potential, and therapy is aimed at maximizing this potential. Maslow developed a theory of personality that is based on the hierarchical satisfaction of needs. Rogers' person-centered theory uses self-actualizing tendencies to promote growth and healing.
- The cognitive model posits that disorders, especially depression, are the result of faulty thinking. Cognitive behavioral therapy is empirically supported and focuses on the recognition of distorted thinking and the replacement with more accurate and positive thoughts.

- The biological model is currently the dominant model and focuses on physical causation for personality problems and psychiatric disorders. Medication is the primary biological therapy.
- Developmental theories provide general guidelines for expected progression throughout the life span. Theories focus on stage-specific tasks, the attainment of a separate sense of self, cognitive maturation, and moral maturity.
- A variety of nursing theories are useful to psychiatric nursing. Hildegard Peplau developed an important interpersonal theory for the provision of psychiatric nursing care.
- Group therapy offers the patient significant interpersonal feedback from multiple people.
- Groups transition through predictable stages, benefit from therapeutic factors, and are characterized by members filling specific roles.
- Family therapy is based on various theoretical models and aims to decrease emotional reactivity among family members and encourage differentiation among individual family members.

■ APPLYING CRITICAL JUDGMENT

1. How could the theorists discussed in this chapter impact your nursing care? Specifically:
   A. How do Freud's concepts of the conscious, preconscious, and unconscious affect your understanding of patients' behaviors?
   B. Can you remember a young patient whose development was impacted by illness? How can Erikson's psychosocial stages be applied to this patient?
   C. What are the implications of Sullivan's focus on the importance of interpersonal relationships for your interactions with patients?

   D. Can you think of anyone who seems to be self-actualized? What is your reason for this conclusion?
   E. How do you utilize Maslow's hierarchy of needs in your nursing practice?
   F. What do you think about the behaviorist point of view that to change behaviors is to change personality?
2. Which of the therapies described here do you think can be the most helpful to you in your nursing practice? What are your reasons for this choice?

CHAPTER REVIEW QUESTIONS

Choose the most appropriate answer(s).

1. Which of the following contributions to modern psychiatric nursing practice was made by Freud?
   1. The theory of personality structure and levels of awareness
   2. The concept of a "self-actualized personality"
   3. The thesis that culture and society exert significant influence on personality
   4. Provision of a developmental model that includes the entire life span

2. The theory of interpersonal relationships developed by Hildegard Peplau is based on the foundation provided by which of the following early theorists?
   1. Freud
   2. Piaget
   3. Sullivan
   4. Maslow

3. According to Maslow's Hierarchy of Needs, the most basic needs for psychiatric mental health nursing are:
   1. physiological.
   2. safety.
   3. love and belonging.
   4. self-actualization.

4. The premise that an individual's behavior and affect are largely determined by the attitudes and assumptions the person has developed about the world underlies:
   1. modeling.
   2. milieu therapy.
   3. cognitive behavioral therapy.
   4. psychoanalytic psychotherapy.

5. Providing a safe environment for patients with impaired cognition, referring an abused spouse to a "safe house," and conducting a community meeting are nursing interventions that address aspects of:
   1. milieu therapy.
   2. cognitive therapy.
   3. behavioral therapy.
   4. interpersonal psychotherapy.

REFERENCES

Alligood, M. R., & Tomey, A. M. (2010). *Nursing theorists and their work*. Maryland Heights, MO: Mosby/Elsevier.

Arnold, E., & Boggs, K. U. (2011). *Interpersonal relationships: professional communication skills for nurses* (6th ed.). St Louis: Saunders.

Beck, A. T. (1963). Thinking and depression. *Archives of General Psychiatry, 9*, 324–333.

Benne, K. D., & Sheats, F. (1948). Functional roles of group members. *Journal of Social Issues, 4*(2), 41–49.

Black, D. W., & Andreasen, N. C. (2011). *Introductory textbook of psychiatry* (5th ed.). Washington, DC: American Psychiatric Publishing, Inc.

Boeree, C. G. (2006). *Personality theories: Carl Rogers*. Retrieved April 11, 2011 from http://webspace.ship.edu/cgboer/rogers.html.

Caldwell, B. A., Sclafani, M., Swarbrick, M., & Piren, K. (2010). Psychiatric nursing practice and the recovery model of care. *Journal of Psychosocial Nursing, 48*(7), 42–48.

Crain, W. C. (1985). *Theories of development* (2nd ed.). Englewood Cliffs, NJ: Prentice Hall.

Erikson, E. (1963). *Childhood and society*. New York: Norton.

Freud, S. (1961). The ego and id. In J. Strachey (Ed. and Trans.), *The standard edition of the complete psychological works of Sigmund Freud* (vol. 19, pp. 3–66). London: Hogarth Press. (Original work published 1923.).

Gilligan, C. (1982). *In a different voice: psychological theory and women's development*. Cambridge: Harvard University Press.

Hanrahan, N. P., Delaney, K. R., & Stuart, G. W. (2011). Blueprint for the development of the psychiatric nurse workforce. *Nursing Outlook*. doi:10.1016/j.outlook.2011.04.007.

Jacobs, E. E., Masson, R. L., Harvill, R. L., & Schimmel, C. J. (2012). *Group counseling: strategies and skills* (7th ed.). Pacific Grove, CA: Brooks/Cole.

Johnson, D. E. (1980). The behavioral system model for nursing. In J. P. Riehl, & C. Roy (Eds.), *Conceptual models for nursing practice* (2nd ed). New York: Appleton-Century-Crofts.

Karisson, H. (2011). *How psychotherapy changes the brain*. Retrieved January 6, 2012 from http://www.psychiatrictimes.com/print/article/10168/192-6705?printable= true.

King, I. M. (1981). *A theory for nursing: systems, concepts, process*. New York: Wiley.

Kohlberg, L., & Turiel, E. (1971). Moral development and moral education. In G. S. Lesser (Ed.), *Psychology and educational practice*. Glenview, IL: Scott Foresman.

Leininger, M. (1995). Culture care theory, research, and practice. *Nursing Science Quarterly, 9*(2), 71–78.

Lemmens, G., Eisler, E., Lietaer, G., & Demyttenaere, K. (2009). Therapeutic factors in a systemic multi-family group treatment for major depression: patients' and partners' perspectives. *Journal of Family Therapy, 31*(3), 250–269.

Mahler, M. S., Pine, F., & Bergman, A. (1975). *The psychological birth of the human infant*. New York: Basic Books.

Maslow, A. H. (1970). *Motivation and personality* (2nd ed.). New York: Harper and Row.

Nichols, M. P. (2009). *Family therapy: concepts and methods* (9th ed.). Upper Saddle River, NJ: Prentice Hall.

Orem, D. E. (2001). *Nursing: concepts of practice* (6th ed.). St Louis: Mosby.

Orlando, I. J. (1990). *The dynamic nurse-patient relationship: function, process, and principles*. (Pub. No. 15–2341), New York: National League for Nursing.

Pavlov, I. P. (1927). *Conditioned reflexes*. London: Routledge and Kegan Paul.

Peplau, H. E. (1992). *Interpersonal relations in nursing*. New York: Putnam.

Peplau, H. E. (1952). *Interpersonal relations in nursing: a conceptual frame of reference for psychodynamic nursing*. New York: Putnam.

Piaget, J., & Inhelder, B. (1969). *The psychology of a child*. New York: Basic Books.

Rogers, C. R. (1986). Carl Rogers on the development of the person-centered approach. *Person-Centered Review, 1*(3), 257–259.

Sadock, B. J., & Sadock, V. A. (2008). *Concise textbook of clinical psychiatry* (3rd ed.). Philadelphia: Lippincott.

Skinner, B. F. (1938). *The behavior of organisms.* New York: Appleton-Century-Crofts.

Smith, L. (1997). Jean Piaget. In N. Sheehy, A. Chapman, & W. Conroy (Eds.), *Biographical dictionary of psychology.* London: Routledge.

Sullivan, H. S. (1953). *The interpersonal theory of psychiatry.* New York: Norton.

Tuckman, B. W. (1965). Developmental sequence in small groups. *Psychological Bulletin, 63,* 384–399.

Tuckman, B. W., & Jensen, M. A. (1977). Stages of small-group development revisited. *Group & Organization Management, 2,* 419–427.

Watson, J. (2007). *Watson Caring Science Institute.* Retrieved April 13, 2011, from www.watsoncaringscience.org/caring_science/index.html.

Watson, J. B. (1930). *Behaviorism* (rev. ed.). Chicago: University of Chicago Press.

Yalom, I. D. (1985). *The theory and practice of group psychotherapy.* New York: Basic Books.

CHAPTER

4

Biological Basis for Understanding Psychopharmacology

Dorothy A. Varchol

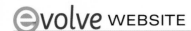 WEBSITE

http://evolve.elsevier.com/Varcarolis/essentials

KEY TERMS AND CONCEPTS

acetylcholine, p. 51
agonist, p. 52
agranulocytosis, p. 63
antagonist, p. 52
antianxiety or anxiolytic drugs, p. 48
basal ganglia, p. 48
circadian rhythms, p. 50
conventional antipsychotic
    drugs, p. 62
extrapyramidal symptoms
    (EPS), p. 49
γ-aminobutyric acid (GABA), p. 51
hypnotic, p. 61
limbic system, p. 48
lithium, p. 61
monoamines, p. 58
monoamine oxidase (MAO), p. 58
monoamine oxidase inhibitors
    (MAOIs), p. 58
mood stabilizing drugs, p. 62
neuroimaging, p. 50

neurons, p. 47
neurotransmission, p. 50
neurotransmitter, p. 51
pharmacodynamic
    interactions, p. 58
pharmacokinetic
    interactions, p. 57
plasticity, p. 47
psychoneuroimmunology
    (PNI), p. 64
psychotropic, p. 47
receptors, p. 51
reticular activating system
    (RAS), p. 49
reuptake, p. 51
second-generation antipsychotics
    or atypical antipsychotics, p. 63
selective serotonin reuptake
    inhibitors (SSRIs), p. 58
synapse, p. 51
therapeutic index, p. 61

SELECTED CONCEPT:
Pharmacogenetics
Pharmacology and genetics have merged into a new field called pharmacogenetics.
    Genetic factors play a role in how individuals respond to drugs (if it works on them or not) and the side effects experienced (toxicity or tolerates well). How a drug is used in the body is determined by genetically mediated patterns of protein structures, receptor sensitivities, enzyme activity, and drug metabolism. These differences are present not just through individual genetic factors, but are greatly determined by ethnic associations as well.
    Psychogenetics may one day lead to personalized medications, safer drugs, and targeted pharmacological therapies determined by genetically inherited factors.
(Preston et al., 2010)

OBJECTIVES

1. Identify at least three major brain structures and eight major brain functions that can be altered by mental illness and psychotropic medications.
2. Describe how neuroimaging techniques can be helpful in understanding mental illness.
3. Explain the basic process of neurotransmission and synaptic transmission using Figures 4-5, 4-6, and 4-7.
4. Identify the main neurotransmitters affected by the following psychotropic drugs and their subgroups:
   a. Antidepressants
   b. Antianxiety agents
   c. Sedative-hypnotics
   d. Mood stabilizers
   e. Antipsychotic agents
   f. Anticholinesterase drugs
5. Explain the relevance of psychodynamic and psychokinetic drug interactions in the delivery of safe, effective nursing care.
6. Discuss the rationale for special dietary and drug restrictions with monoamine oxidase inhibitors (MAOIs).
7. Compare and contrast the side effect profiles of conventional antipsychotic drugs with the side effect profiles of atypical antipsychotic drugs.
8. Discuss the relationship between the immune system and the nervous system in mental health and mental illness.
9. Describe how genes and culture affect an individual's response to psychotropic medication.

Whether conscious or unconscious, all mental activity has its locus in the brain. A primary goal of psychiatric mental health nursing is to understand the biological basis of both normal and abnormal brain function and apply this understanding to the care of individuals treated with drugs referred to as psychotropic. Because all brain functions are carried out by similar mechanisms (interactions of neurons), often in similar locations, it is not surprising that mental disturbances are frequently associated with alterations in other brain functions and that the drugs used to treat mental disturbances can also interfere with other activities of the brain. Box 4-1 summarizes some of the major brain functions.

BRAIN STRUCTURES AND FUNCTIONS

For the brain to perform its many and varied activities, each part must act both independently and in concert with other regions.

BOX 4-1   FUNCTIONS OF THE BRAIN

- Monitor changes in the external world.
- Monitor the composition of body fluids.
- Regulate the contractions of the skeletal muscles.
- Regulate the internal organs.
- Initiate and regulate the basic drives: hunger, thirst, sex, aggressive self-protection.
- Mediate conscious sensation.
- Store and retrieve memories.
- Regulate mood (affect) and emotions.
- Think and perform intellectual functions.
- Regulate the sleep cycle.
- Produce and interpret language.
- Process visual and auditory data.

Cerebrum

The cerebrum consists of surface and deep areas of integrating gray matter (the cerebral cortex and basal ganglia) as well as connecting tracts of white matter that link these areas with each other and the rest of the nervous system. The gray matter consists predominantly of neuronal cell bodies, dendrites, and glial cells whereas the white matter is composed of myelinated nerve fibers (axons).

Progressive loss of both gray and white matter has been associated with schizophrenia as well as use of antipsychotic medication (Ho et al., 2011), but it is not known whether volume loss is necessarily harmful because eliminating dysfunctional or transformed cells may actually contribute to preserving brain function. Plasticity is evident throughout life as gray matter shrinks or thickens and synaptic connections are pruned or forged, especially in areas where learning and memory occur.

Each hemisphere of the cerebral cortex is divided into four lobes (Figure 4-1) that control sensory and motor function as well as higher mental activities (e.g., language, decision making, problem solving, and a conscious sense of being). Sensory areas are responsible for specific sensations: the **parietal** for touch, **temporal** for sound, and **occipital** for vision. Motor areas in the **frontal** lobes control voluntary movement. The **prefrontal cortex (PFC)** coordinates complex cognitive functions and enables us to plan and execute goals (Fuster, 2008). When circuitry in the PFC is impaired by a mental disorder (e.g., schizophrenia, major depression, or alcohol intoxication), there is a decrease in executive function, attention, impulse control, socialization, regulation of drives (such as libido), and emotions. Drugs targeting specific molecules within PFC circuits are being developed to normalize disrupted PFC activity.

In addition to the gray matter forming the cortex, there are pockets of integrating gray matter lying deep within the cerebrum: the hippocampus, the amygdala, and the basal ganglia. The **hippocampus** interacts with the PFC in making new memories. The **amygdala** plays a major role in processing fear

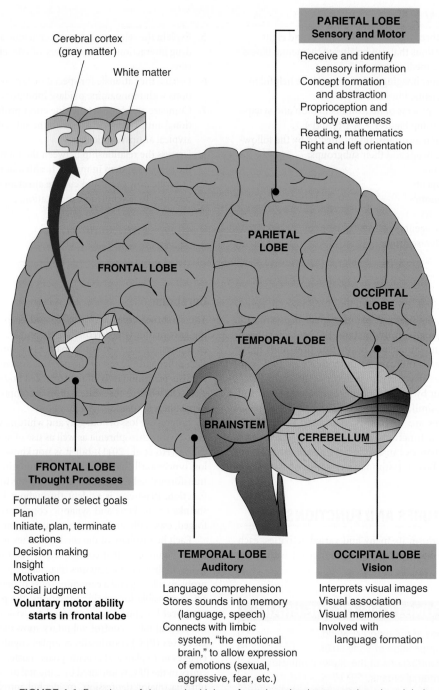

FIGURE 4-1 Functions of the cerebral lobes: frontal, parietal, temporal, and occipital.

and anxiety. The hippocampus and amygdala, along with the hypothalamus and thalamus, are part of a circle of structures called the limbic system or "emotional brain." Linking the frontal cortex, basal ganglia, and upper brainstem, the limbic system mediates thought and feeling through complex, bidirectional connections. Antianxiety drugs (anxiolytics) slow the limbic system.

Subcortical Structures
Basal Ganglia

The four subcortical basal ganglia that lie deep within the cerebrum are the striatum, the pallidum, the substantia nigra, and the subthalamic nucleus. This group of gray matter nuclei plays a major role in motor responses via the extrapyramidal motor system, which relies on the neurotransmitter dopamine to

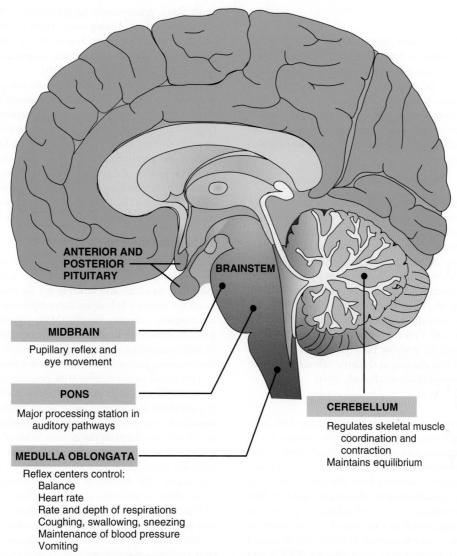

ANTERIOR AND POSTERIOR PITUITARY

BRAINSTEM

MIDBRAIN

Pupillary reflex and eye movement

PONS

Major processing station in auditory pathways

MEDULLA OBLONGATA

Reflex centers control:
Balance
Heart rate
Rate and depth of respirations
Coughing, swallowing, sneezing
Maintenance of blood pressure
Vomiting

CEREBELLUM

Regulates skeletal muscle coordination and contraction
Maintains equilibrium

FIGURE 4-2 Functions of the brainstem and cerebellum.

maintain proper muscle tone and motor stability. Neuroimaging has recently shown that the antipsychotic agent haloperidol can reduce striatal volume within hours, temporarily changing brain structure and predicting abnormal involuntary motor symptoms **(extrapyramidal symptoms [EPS])** with high precision (Tost et al., 2010). In the basal ganglia, two types of movement disturbances may occur: (1) acute extrapyramidal symptoms, which develop early in treatment; and (2) tardive dyskinesia, which usually occurs much later. Conventional antipsychotics (the first generation of antipsychotic medications) and high doses of the atypical agent (second generation of antipsychotic medications) risperidone (Risperdal) are most likely to cause extrapyramidal side effects.

It is important to remember that movement is regulated by the basal ganglia, including the diaphragm—essential for

breathing—and the muscles of the throat, tongue, and mouth—essential for speech. Thus drugs that affect brain function can stimulate or depress respiration or affect speech patterns (e.g., slurred speech).

Brainstem

Basic vital life functions occur through the brainstem, composed of the midbrain, pons, and medulla (Figure 4-2).

Through projections called the **reticular activating system (RAS),** the brainstem sets the level of consciousness and regulates the cycle of sleep and wakefulness. Unfortunately, drugs used to treat psychiatric problems may interfere with the regulation of sleep and alertness, thus the warning to take sedating drugs at bedtime and to use caution while driving.

Cerebellum

Located behind the brainstem, the cerebellum (see Figure 4-2) is mainly a coordinator of motor function. However, it also interacts with the cerebrum in higher cognitive functions such as speech memory, facial recognition, visual attention, and awareness (Andreasen & Pierson, 2008; Baier et al., 2010). Cerebellar hypoactivation affecting posture and equilibrium is well-documented as occurring in some people with schizophrenia, but the role of the cerebellum in cognition is still under investigation (Picard et al., 2008).

Thalamus

Located above the brainstem, the thalamus serves as a major relay station for sensory impulses on their way to the cerebral cortex. Dopamine reduces the thalamic sensory filter, allowing more sensory input to escape from the thalamus to the cortex (Stahl & Muntner, 2008). Corticostriatal-thalamic pathways are disrupted in schizophrenia, obsessive-compulsive disorder (OCD), and attention deficit/hyperactivity disorder (ADHD). The thalamus also plays a role in complex reflex movements, body-alerting mechanisms, and even emotions by associating sensory impulses with various feelings (Patton et al., 2012). Current researchers are studying the role of the thalamus in bipolar I disorder and changes in thalamic volume that occur with lithium treatment (Radenbach et al., 2010).

Hypothalamus

The **hypothalamus** maintains homeostasis. It regulates temperature, blood pressure, perspiration, libido, hunger, thirst, and circadian rhythms, such as sleep and wakefulness. Hypothalamic **neurohormones,** often called releasing hormones, direct the secretion of hormones from the anterior pituitary gland. For example, **corticotropin-releasing hormone (CRH)** is involved in the stress response. It stimulates the pituitary to release corticotropin, which in turn stimulates the cortex of each adrenal gland to secrete cortisol. This system is disrupted in mood disorders, posttraumatic stress disorder (PTSD), and Alzheimer's dementia, but abnormalities in the system may someday be reversed by CRH antagonists (Beyer & Stahl, 2010).

The hypothalamic-pituitary-thyroid axis is involved in the regulation of nearly every organ system because all major hormones and catecholamines (e.g., cortisol, gonadal hormones, insulin) depend on thyroid status. Release of thyrotropin-releasing hormone (TRH) results in pituitary secretion of thyrotropin (thyroid-stimulating hormone or TSH), which in turn stimulates the thyroid gland to release the thyroid hormones—thyroxine (T_4) and triiodothyronine (T_3). Thyroid hormones are used to treat people with depression or rapid-cycling bipolar I disorder. They are also used as replacement therapy for people who develop a hypothyroid state from lithium treatment (Sadock & Sadock, 2007).

The hypothalamic neurohormone dopamine inhibits the release of prolactin. When excess dopamine is blocked by conventional antipsychotic drugs, blood prolactin levels increase (hyperprolactinemia) with subsequent amenorrhea, galactorrhea (milk flow), gynecomastia (development of breast tissue), or sexual dysfunction. Among antipsychotics, conventional agents and the atypical drug risperidone are the most frequent and serious offenders whereas most atypical antipsychotics are prolactin sparing (Madhusoodanan et al., 2010).

In addition to working with the endocrine system, the hypothalamus sends instructions to the **autonomic nervous system,** divided into the **sympathetic and parasympathetic systems** (Figure 4-3). The sympathetic system usually increases heart rate, respirations, and blood pressure to prepare for fight or flight, whereas the parasympathetic system slows the heart rate and begins the process of digestion. The sympathetic system is highly activated by sympathomimetic drugs, such as amphetamine and cocaine, as well as by withdrawal from sedating drugs, such as alcohol, benzodiazepines, and opioids (Sadock & Sadock, 2007).

Visualizing the Brain

Neuroimaging visualizes a brain that is structurally and functionally interconnected. Some common brain imaging techniques measuring structure and function are identified in Table 4-1. Structural imaging techniques are computed tomography (CT) and magnetic resonance imaging (MRI). CT scans use a series of x-rays to view brain structure and have been largely supplanted by MRI scans, which use a strong magnetic field and radio waves, distinguishing gray and white matter better than CT scans.

Functional neuroimaging with positron emission tomography (PET) and single photon emission computed tomography (SPECT) use ionizing radiation to localize brain regions associated with perceptual, cognitive, emotional, and behavioral functions. Based on the increase in blood flow to the local vasculature that accompanies neural activity, PET scans have provided evidence of decreased metabolism in unmedicated individuals with depression or schizophrenia and increased metabolism in obsessive-compulsive disorder (Figure 4-4). PET and SPECT have also shown dopamine system dysregulation in schizophrenia and loss of monoamines in depression.

Functional magnetic resonance imaging (fMRI) demonstrates cognitive function without contrast injections or invasive tests. It is the major method used by cognitive neuroscientists to observe changes that occur in various parts of the brain while subjects perform tasks involving higher intellectual processes such as memory or attention. In addition, fMRI maps the modulatory effects of psychotropic medication, illustrating how a therapeutic response can be achieved at minimal doses. Antipsychotic medications are now prescribed at a fraction of the dosages that were once considered standard, in large part because of imaging studies.

CELLULAR COMPOSITION OF THE BRAIN

Neurons

The brain is composed of a vast network of more than 100 billion interconnected nerve cells (neurons) and the supporting cells that surround these neurons. An essential feature of neurons is their ability to initiate signals and conduct an electrical impulse from one end of the cell to the other called neurotransmission

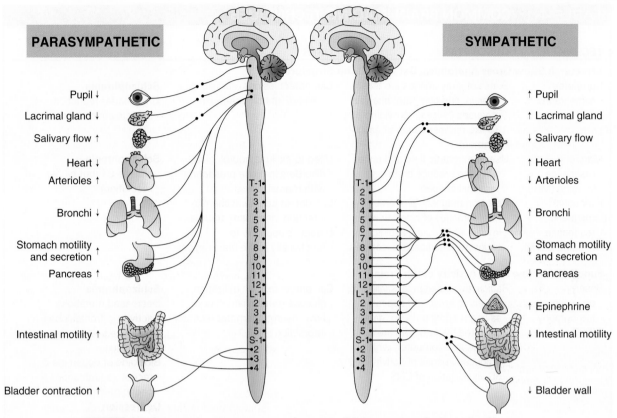

FIGURE 4-3 Autonomic nervous system has two divisions: sympathetic and parasympathetic. The sympathetic division is dominant in stress situations, such as fear and anger—known as the fight-or-flight response.

(Figure 4-5). Electrical signals within neurons are then converted at synapses into chemical signals through the release of molecules called **neurotransmitters,** which then elicit electrical signals on the other side of the synapse. Together, these two signaling mechanisms (action potentials and synaptic signals) enable information processing in the brain.

Synaptic Transmission

Once an electrical impulse reaches the end of a neuron, the neurotransmitter is released from the axon terminal at the presynaptic neuron. This transmitter then diffuses across a narrow space, or **synapse,** to an adjacent postsynaptic neuron, where it attaches to specialized **receptors** on the cell surface and either inhibits or excites the postsynaptic neuron. It is the interaction between neurotransmitter and receptor that is a major target of psychotropic drugs. Figure 4-6 shows how an insufficient degree of transmission may be caused by a deficient release of neurotransmitters from the presynaptic cell or by a decrease in receptors. Figure 4-7 illustrates how excessive transmission may be due to excessive release of a transmitter or to increased receptor responsiveness, as occurs in schizophrenia.

After attaching to a receptor and exerting its influence on the postsynaptic cell, the transmitter separates from the receptor

and is destroyed. Some transmitters (e.g., acetylcholine) are destroyed by specific enzymes (e.g., acetylcholinesterase) at the postsynaptic cell. In the case of monoamine transmitters (e.g., norepinephrine, dopamine, serotonin), the destructive enzyme is monoamine oxidase (MAO).

Other transmitters (e.g., norepinephrine) are taken back into the cell from which they were originally released by a process called cellular **reuptake.** On return to these cells, the transmitters are either reused or destroyed by intracellular enzymes. The two basic mechanisms of destruction are described in Box 4-2.

Neurotransmitters

A **neurotransmitter** is a chemical messenger between neurons by which one neuron triggers another. Four major groups of neurotransmitters in the brain are monoamines (biogenic amines), amino acids, peptides, and cholinergics (e.g., acetylcholine). Monoamine neurotransmitters (**dopamine, norepinephrine, serotonin**) and **acetylcholine** are implicated in a variety of neuropsychiatric disorders.

Amino acid neurotransmitters, such as the inhibitory γ-aminobutyric acid (GABA) and the excitatory **glutamate,** balance brain activity. Peptide neurotransmitters such as hypothalamic CRH can be thought of as modulating or adjusting general

TABLE 4-1 COMMON BRAIN IMAGING TECHNIQUES

TECHNIQUE	DESCRIPTION	USES	CLINICAL RESEARCH EXAMPLES
Structural: Show Gross Anatomical Details of Brain Structures			
Computed tomography (CT)	Series of x-ray images are taken of brain, and computer analysis produces "slices," providing a 3D-like reconstruction of each segment	Can detect lesions, abrasions, areas of infarct, aneurysm	**Schizophrenia** Gray matter reduction Ventricle abnormalities
Magnetic resonance imaging (MRI)	Uses a magnetic field and radio waves to produce cross-sectional images	Used to exclude neurological disorders in those presenting with mental illness	**Schizophrenia** Same as CT (but higher resolution)
Functional magnetic resonance imaging (fMRI)	Relies on magnetic properties to see images of blood flow in brain as it occurs; avoids exposure to radioactive isotopes	Can detect edema, ischemia, infection, neoplasm, trauma Detects blood flow to functionally active brain regions	
Functional: Show Some Activity of the Brain			
Positron emission tomography (PET)	Radioactive substance is injected, travels to brain, and appears as bright spots on scan; data collected by detectors are relayed to a computer, which produces images of activity and 3D visualization of CNS	Can detect oxygen utilization, glucose metabolism, blood flow, neurotransmitter receptor interaction	**Schizophrenia** Decreased metabolic activity in frontal lobes Dopamine system dysregulation Blockade of dopamine receptors with antipsychotic medications **Depression** Blockade of serotonin transporter receptors with antidepressant medications **Alzheimer's disease** Reduction in nicotinic receptor subtype
Single photon emission computed tomography (SPECT)	Similar to PET but uses γ-radiation (photons) SPECT is less costly, but resolution is poorer	Similar to PET	See PET

brain function. Table 4-2 lists important neurotransmitters, types of receptors to which they attach, and mental disorders that are associated with an increase or decrease in neurotransmitters.

Interaction of Neurons, Neurotransmitters, and Receptors

Most psychotropic drugs produce effects through alteration of synaptic concentrations of dopamine, acetylcholine, norepinephrine, serotonin, histamine, GABA, or glutamate. These changes are thought to result from activation of receptor antagonists (blocking activity of a neurotransmitter) or agonists (promoting activity of a neurotransmitter), interference with neurotransmitter reuptake, enhancement of neurotransmitter release, or inhibition of enzymes (Sadock & Sadock, 2007).

Dopamine

The monoamine **dopamine** is an important neurotransmitter that is involved in cognition, motivation, and movement. It controls emotional responses and the brain's reward and pleasure centers, stimulates the heart, and increases blood flow to vital organs.

Drugs such as cocaine interfere with the reuptake of dopamine, thereby allowing more of the neurotransmitter to stay active in the synapse for a longer time. The dopamine hypothesis of schizophrenia originated from the observation that drugs (e.g., amphetamines) that stimulate dopamine activity can induce psychotic symptoms whereas drugs that block dopamine receptors (e.g., haloperidol) have antipsychotic activity (Sadock & Sadock, 2007).

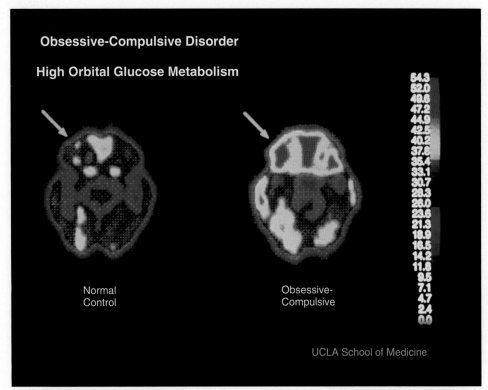

FIGURE 4-4 Positron emission tomographic scans show increased brain metabolism *(brighter colors)*, particularly in the frontal cortex, in a patient with obsessive-compulsive disorder (OCD), compared with a normal control. This suggests altered brain function in OCD. (From Lewis Baxter, MD, University of Alabama, courtesy National Institute of Mental Health.)

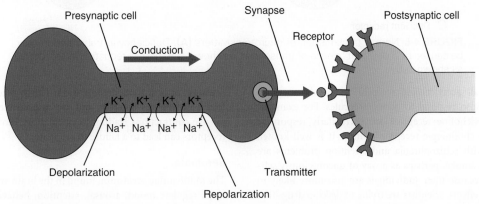

FIGURE 4-5 Activities of neurons. Conduction along a neuron involves the inward movement of sodium ions (Na+) followed by the outward movement of potassium ions (K+). When the current reaches the end of the cell, a neurotransmitter is released. The transmitter crosses the synapse and attaches to a receptor on the postsynaptic cell. The attachment of transmitter to receptor either stimulates or inhibits the postsynaptic cell.

Acetylcholine

Dopamine is balanced by the neurotransmitter acetylcholine. Neurons that release acetylcholine are said to be cholinergic and are thought to be involved in cognitive functions, especially memory. Because acetylcholine is deficient in Alzheimer's disease, attempts have been made to enhance the function of neurons that secrete acetylcholine by use of drugs that inhibit the enzyme that degrades acetylcholine (i.e., acetylcholinesterase). Therefore **acetylcholinesterase (AChE) inhibitors** such as donepezil (Aricept), galantamine (Razadyne), and rivastigmine (Exelon) are prescribed to delay cognitive decline in Alzheimer's disease.

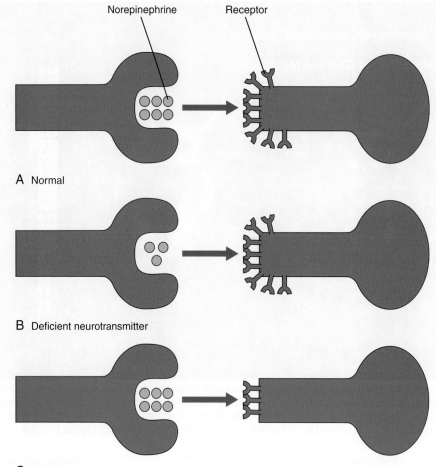

FIGURE 4-6 Normal transmission of neurotransmitters **(A).** Deficiency in transmission may be caused by a deficient release of transmitter, as shown in **B,** or by a reduction in receptors, as shown in **C.**

Although all acetylcholine receptors respond to acetylcholine, they also respond to other molecules. For example, nicotinic acetylcholine receptors are particularly responsive to nicotine, a cholinergic receptor agonist. It is well-known that people with schizophrenia and attention problems are more likely to smoke, perhaps as a way of unconsciously self-medicating. Because these individuals are also more likely to suffer adverse effects, scientists are trying to develop drugs that target the nicotine receptors without the carcinogenic, cardiovascular, and addictive effects.

Norepinephrine

Neurons that release the monoamine **norepinephrine (NE)** are called noradrenergic. NE and serotonin play a major role in regulating mood. A deficiency of one or both of these monoamines within the limbic system is thought to underlie depression, whereas an excess has been associated with mania. Many of the standard first-generation antipsychotic drugs act as antagonists at the α_1 receptors for NE. Blockage of these receptors can cause vasodilation and a consequent drop in blood

pressure, or orthostatic hypotension. The α_1 receptors are also found on the vas deferens and are responsible for the propulsive contractions leading to ejaculation. Blockage of these receptors can lead to a failure to ejaculate.

Serotonin

The monoamine **serotonin,** found in the brain and spinal cord, helps regulate mood, arousal, attention, behavior, and body temperature. When some antidepressants are combined with other drugs or supplements that increase serotonin production (e.g., St. John's wort or over-the-counter cough and cold medications containing dextromethorphan), the serotonin syndrome may occur. Symptoms of high levels of serotonin range from mild (restlessness, shivering, and diarrhea) to severe (muscle rigidity, fever, and seizures). These symptoms can be alleviated by muscle relaxants and drugs that block serotonin production. Current research focuses on serotonin dysfunction in impulsive aggression and suicide (Cardish, 2007).

Serotonin release by platelets plays an important role in hemostasis. Drugs with the highest degree of serotonin reuptake

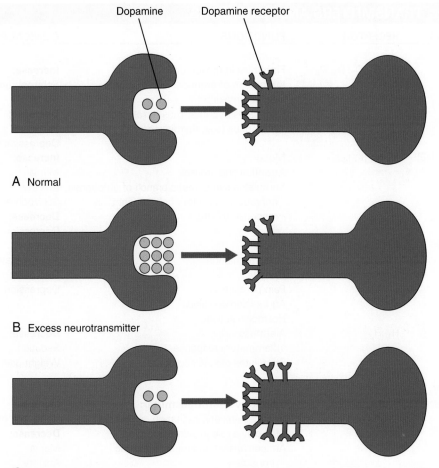

A   Normal

B   Excess neurotransmitter

C   Excess receptors

FIGURE 4-7 Causes of excess transmission of neurotransmitters. Excess transmission may be caused by excess release of transmitter, as shown in **B,** or excess responsiveness of receptors, as shown in **C.**

BOX 4-2   DESTRUCTION OF NEUROTRANSMITTERS

A full explanation of the various ways in which psychotropic drugs alter neuronal activity requires a brief review of the manner in which neurotransmitters are destroyed after attaching to the receptors. To avoid continuous and prolonged action on the postsynaptic cell, the neurotransmitter is released shortly after attaching to the postsynaptic receptor. Once released, the transmitter is destroyed in one of two ways.

One way is the immediate inactivation of the transmitter at the postsynaptic membrane. An example of this method of destruction is the action of the enzyme acetylcholinesterase on the neurotransmitter acetylcholine. Acetylcholinesterase is present at the postsynaptic membrane and destroys acetylcholine shortly after it attaches to nicotinic or muscarinic receptors on the postsynaptic cell.

A *second* method of neurotransmitter inactivation is a little more complex. After interacting with the postsynaptic receptor, the transmitter is released and taken back into the presynaptic cell, the cell from which it was released. This process, referred to as the reuptake of neurotransmitter, is a common target for drug action. Once inside the presynaptic cell, the transmitter is either recycled or inactivated by an enzyme within the cell. The monoamine neurotransmitters norepinephrine, dopamine, and serotonin are all inactivated in this manner by the enzyme monoamine oxidase.

In looking at this second method, one might naturally ask what prevents the enzyme from destroying the transmitter before its release. The answer is that before release the transmitter is stored within a membrane and is thus protected from the degradative enzyme. After release and reuptake, the transmitter is either destroyed by the enzyme or reenters the membrane to be reused.

TABLE 4-2   TRANSMITTERS AND RECEPTORS

TRANSMITTERS	RECEPTORS	FUNCTIONS	CLINICAL RELEVANCE
Monoamines			
Dopamine (DA)	D_1, D_2, D_3, D_4, D_5	Fine muscle movement Integration of emotions and thoughts Decision making Stimulates hypothalamus to release hormones (sex, thyroid, adrenal)	**Increase:** Schizophrenia Mania **Decrease:** Parkinson's disease Depression

Norepinephrine (NE)
(noradrenaline)
	α_1, α_2, β_1, β_2	Mood
		Attention and arousal
		Stimulates sympathetic branch of autonomic
		  nervous system for "fight or flight" in
		  response to stress
			Increase:
			Mania
			Anxiety
			Schizophrenia
			Decrease:
			Depression

Serotonin (5-HT)	5-HT, 5-HT_2, 5-HT_3, 5-HT_4	Mood Sleep regulation Hunger Pain perception Aggression and libido Hormonal activity	**Increase:** Anxiety states **Decrease:** Depression
Histamine	H_1, H_2	Alertness Inflammatory response Stimulates gastric secretion	**Decrease:** Sedation Weight gain
Amino Acids			

γ-Aminobutyric acid
(GABA)
	GABA_A, GABA_B	**Inhibitory neurotransmitter:**
		Reduces anxiety, excitation, aggression
		May play a role in pain perception
		Anticonvulsant and muscle-relaxing
		  properties
		May impair cognition and psychomotor
		  functioning
			Increase:
			Reduction of anxiety
			Decrease:
			Mania
			Anxiety
			Schizophrenia

Glutamate	NMDA, AMPA	**Excitatory neurotransmitter:**
		AMPA plays a role in learning
		  and memory
			Increase NMDA:
			Prolonged increase can kill
			  neurons (neurotoxicity)
			Neurodegeneration in
			  Alzheimer's disease
			Decrease NMDA:
			Psychosis
			Increase AMPA:
			Improvement of cognitive
			  performance in
			  behavioral tasks

Cholinergics			
Acetylcholine (ACh)	Nicotinic, muscarinic (M_1, M_2, M_3)	Plays a role in learning, memory Regulates mood: mania, sexual aggression Affects sexual and aggressive behavior Stimulates parasympathetic nervous system	**Decrease:** Alzheimer's disease Huntington's chorea Parkinson's disease **Increase:** Depression

TABLE 4-2 TRANSMITTERS AND RECEPTORS—cont'd

TRANSMITTERS	RECEPTORS	FUNCTIONS	CLINICAL RELEVANCE
Peptides (Neuromodulators)			
Substance P (SP)	SP	Centrally active SP antagonist has antidepressant and antianxiety effects in depression Promotes and reinforces memory Enhances sensitivity to pain receptors to activate	Involved in regulation of mood and anxiety Role in pain management
Somatostatin (SRIF)	SRIF	Altered levels associated with cognitive disease	**Decrease:** Alzheimer's disease Decreased levels of SRIF in spinal fluid of some depressed patients **Increase:** Huntington's chorea
Neurotensin (NT)	NT	Endogenous antipsychotic-like properties	Decreased levels in spinal fluid of schizophrenic patients

AMPA, α-Amino-3-hydroxy-5-methyl-4-isoxazolepropionic acid; *NMDA,* N-methyl-D-aspartate; *SRIF,* somatotropin release-inhibiting factor.

inhibition—fluoxetine, paroxetine, and sertraline—are more frequently associated with altered anticoagulant effects; thus concomitant use of nonsteroidal anti-inflammatory drugs (NSAIDs), aspirin, warfarin, or other drugs that affect coagulation potentiates the risk of bleeding (Halperin & Reber, 2007).

Histamine

Many standard antipsychotic agents, as well as a variety of other psychiatric drugs, block the H_1 receptors for **histamine.** Two significant side effects of blocking these receptors are sedation and substantial weight gain. Sedation may be beneficial in severely agitated patients, but weight gain can lead to disturbances in glucose and lipid metabolism and insulin resistance.

γ-Aminobutyric Acid (GABA)

The major inhibitory neurotransmitter γ-aminobutyric acid (GABA) modulates neuronal excitability and is associated with the regulation of anxiety. Most antianxiety (anxiolytic) drugs act by increasing the effectiveness of this transmitter, primarily by increasing receptor responsiveness. Combining selective serotonin reuptake inhibitors (SSRIs) and antipsychotics produces changes in $GABA_A$ receptors and related signaling systems that differ from the effects of either drug administered alone. This synergism significantly improves negative symptoms in patients unresponsive to antipsychotic treatment (Danovich et al., 2011). Researchers are examining an antipsychotic drug to simultaneously target dopamine hyperactivity and GABA hypoactivity, thereby reducing anxiety and improving cognitive function in schizophrenic individuals (Davidson, 2007).

Glutamate

Glutamate is a potent excitability neurotransmitter that activates N-methyl-D-aspartate (NMDA) receptors. High concentrations of glutamate or overly sensitive receptors can lead to overstimulation and cell death, as occurs in neurodegenerative conditions such as Alzheimer's disease. As a corollary, NMDA receptor antagonists, such as the drug memantine, decrease excitability and neurotoxicity. In schizophrenia it is theorized that glutamate excitotoxicity may occur early in the illness and NMDA receptor hypoactivation later, resulting in psychotic symptoms comparable to those seen with NMDA antagonists, phencyclidine (PCP), and ketamine. Both NMDA and α-amino-3-hydroxy-5-methyl-4-isoxazolepropionic acid (AMPA) receptors are binding sites for glutamate, and the interplay of the two receptors is being explored in developing ketamine-like drugs to rapidly reverse depressive symptoms (Li et al., 2010).

PSYCHOTROPIC DRUGS AND INTERACTIONS

Psychotropic drugs work by mechanisms not yet fully understood, and understanding their action has become more challenging when drug interactions alter or modify their effects.

Pharmacokinetic interactions are the effects of drugs on the plasma concentrations of each other. These interactions involve four basic processes: absorption, distribution, metabolism, or elimination. Most pharmacokinetic interactions are a result of inhibition or induction of cytochrome P450 (CYP450) enzymes. When a potent CYP450 enzyme inhibitor or inducer is added to drugs metabolized by one or more CYP450 enzymes, the patient experiences an adverse drug effect or therapeutic failure.

Pharmacodynamic interactions are the combined effects of drugs. For example, when two agents that produce the same or similar end result are coadministered, there is an additive or synergistic effect. This is most evident in the enhanced sedation (central nervous system [CNS] depression) that occurs when alcohol is taken with psychotropic medications. Drugs with opposing effects would reduce the response to one or both drugs. An example would be the antagonistic effect of a benzodiazepine with concurrent use of theophylline. Older adults with chronic illnesses, such as major depressive disorder, are likely to experience more pharmacodynamic interactions because of multiple comorbidities requiring other medications (Ereshefsky, 2009).

ANTIDEPRESSANT DRUGS

Several hypotheses of depression have been proposed for the action of antidepressants:

1. The monoamine hypothesis suggests a lack of three monoamines (dopamine, norepinephrine, or serotonin) in various brain regions. However, there is no clear evidence that monoamine deficiency accounts for depression.
2. The monoamine receptor hypothesis suggests that low levels of neurotransmitters cause increased receptor sensitivity (up-regulation) over time; thus it may take several weeks for patients to feel better when they are taking antidepressants.
3. More recent hypotheses focus on "downstream molecular events" that the receptors trigger, including the regulation of genes. For example, one hypothesis is that the gene for brain-derived neurotrophic factor (BDNF) is repressed in depression and may be activated by antidepressants. Neurotrophic factors such as BDNF are critical for the survival of neurons and enhance the sprouting of axons to form new synaptic connections (Stahl & Muntner, 2008).

Monoamine Oxidase Inhibitors (MAOIs)

To understand the action of these drugs, keep in mind the following definitions:

- **Monoamines:** a type of organic compound, including the neurotransmitters that are further divided into subgroups called catecholamines (e.g., norepinephrine, epinephrine, dopamine) and indolamines (e.g., serotonin) and many different drugs and food substances
- **Monoamine oxidase (MAO):** an enzyme that destroys monoamines
- **Monoamine oxidase inhibitors (MAOIs):** drugs that increase concentrations of monoamines by inhibiting the action of MAO (Figure 4-8)

Because MAOIs block the enzyme that metabolizes monoamines, they may occasionally be used to increase the levels of serotonin and norepinephrine in intractable depression. However, selective serotonin reuptake inhibitors (SSRIs) and serotonin-norepinephrine reuptake inhibitors (SNRIs) are more commonly used antidepressants because of the vasopressor effects that occur when MAOIs are combined with other sympathomimetics (amines that stimulate the sympathetic nervous system). The most feared vasopressor effect is the **hypertensive crisis** that can result if a patient takes over-the-counter medications with pseudoephedrine or consumes the adrenergic monoamine tyramine, commonly found in aged foods and beverages. Dietary restriction of tyramine must be maintained for 2 weeks after stopping MAOIs to allow the body to resynthesize the MAO enzyme. The EMSAM patch delivers the MAOI selegiline through the skin, and has diminished hypertensive effects compared to the oral preparations phenelzine (Nardil) and tranylcypromine (Parnate). However, dietary precautions are still required. Chapter 15 contains a list of foods and beverages to avoid while taking MAOIs, and gives nursing measures and instructions for teaching patients who are taking MAOIs. For a more detailed description of how MAOIs work, visit the Evolve website at http://evolve.elsevier.com/Varcarolis/essentials.

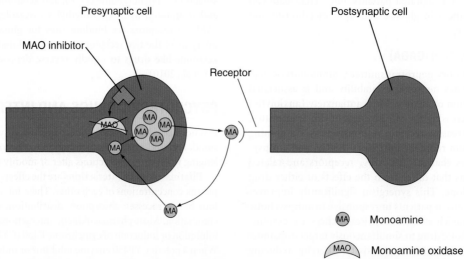

FIGURE 4-8 Blocking of monoamine oxidase (MAO) by inhibiting agents (MAOIs), which prevents the breakdown of monoamine by MAO.

Tricyclic Antidepressants (TCAs)

Originally termed tricyclic antidepressants (TCAs), these agents are more accurately called cyclic antidepressants (CAs) because newer members of this class have a four-ring structure. TCAs, such as amitriptyline (Elavil) and nortriptyline (Pamelor), act primarily by blocking the presynaptic transporter protein receptors for norepinephrine and, to a lesser degree, serotonin (Figure 4-9). This blocking prevents norepinephrine from coming into contact with its degrading enzyme, MAO, and thus increases the level of norepinephrine at the synapse.

Multiple pharmacological mechanisms of TCAs have proven beneficial in treating difficult cases of depression and chronic pain. However, multiple actions on several receptors also earned TCAs the name "dirty drugs" because of their many side effects. For example, to varying degrees TCAs block muscarinic receptors that normally bind acetylcholine, leading to anticholinergic effects. Again to varying degrees, TCAs block H_1 receptors, causing sedation and weight gain. Strong binding at adrenergic receptors causes dizziness and hypotension, thereby increasing the risk for falls. Pharmacokinetics must be considered in TCA overdose fatalities because TCAs are highly lipid soluble and rapidly absorbed. This may result in cardiotoxicity and death

before the patient can reach a hospital, especially if the patient is an older adult with a slower rate of drug elimination. For a more detailed description of how TCAs work, visit the Evolve website at http://evolve.elsevier.com/Varcarolis/essentials.

Selective Serotonin Reuptake Inhibitors (SSRIs)

As the name implies, SSRIs such as fluoxetine (Prozac), sertraline (Zoloft), paroxetine (Paxil), citalopram (Celexa), and escitalopram (Lexapro), preferentially block the reuptake and thus the destruction of serotonin. Vilazodone (Viibryd) (see *Viibryd Medication Guide,* 2011) is a new dual-action antidepressant that shows a significant effect as early as the first week of administration. It is an SSRI and partial agonist at serotonin 5-hydroxytryptamine 1A (5-HT$_{1A}$) receptors. The idea behind a partial agonist is that it will effectively block the negative feedback caused by higher levels of serotonin and increase serotonin release even more. Refer to Figure 4-10 for an explanation of the mechanism of action of SSRIs. For a more detailed description of how SSRIs work, visit the Evolve website at http://evolve.elsevier.com/Varcarolis/essentials.

Selectivity results in fewer side effects because SSRIs do not inhibit receptors for other neurotransmitters (e.g., acetylcholine, histamine, norepinephrine). However, too much

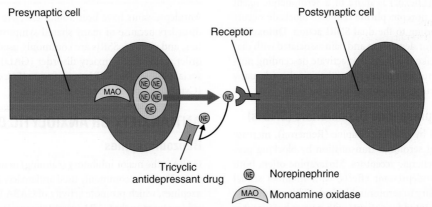

FIGURE 4-9 Mechanism by which tricyclic antidepressant drugs block the reuptake of norepinephrine.

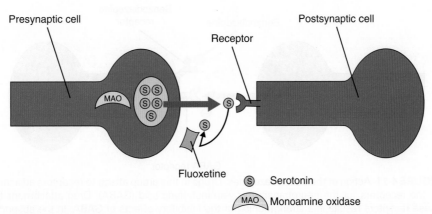

FIGURE 4-10 Mechanism of action of selective serotonin reuptake inhibitors (SSRIs).

serotonergic activity can result in *anxiety, insomnia, sexual dysfunction,* and *gastrointestinal disturbances.* Serotonin toxicity may occur with coadministration of other serotonergic drugs (e.g., MAOIs, SSRIs, SNRIs, lithium, triptan, buspirone, tramadol, over-the-counter cough and cold medications containing dextromethorphan) or antidopaminergic drugs. Similarly, the risk of serotonin toxicity may be increased by pharmacokinetic interactions because serotonergic antidepressants are metabolized by cytochrome P450 (CYP450) enzymes, and any drug that inhibits a CYP450 enzyme increases serotonin levels. For example, metabolism by CYP3A4 is a major elimination pathway for SSRIs, so doses should be reduced with coadministered CYP3A4 inhibitors (e.g., ketoconazole). On the other hand, CYP34A inducers (e.g., rifampin) can result in inadequate plasma concentrations and diminished effectiveness.

Adverse events can occur upon discontinuation of serotonergic antidepressants, particularly when discontinuation is abrupt. The discontinuation syndrome is most likely to occur with SSRIs or SNRIs having a short half-life. Thus it is more common with paroxetine (Paxil) than with fluoxetine (Prozac).

Serotonin-Norepinephrine Reuptake Inhibitors (SNRIs)

SNRIs increase the levels of both serotonin and norepinephrine. **Venlafaxine** (Effexor) is more of a serotonergic agent at lower doses, but norepinephrine reuptake blockade occurs at higher doses, leading to the dual SNRI action. **Duloxetine** (Cymbalta) is used for depression and pain associated with diabetic neuropathy. Like the TCAs that activate descending norepinephrine and serotonin pathways to the spinal cord, many SNRIs have therapeutic effects on neuropathic pain.

Serotonin-Norepinephrine Disinhibitors (SNDIs)

SNDIs, represented by only mirtazapine (Remeron), increase norepinephrine and serotonin transmission by blocking presynaptic α_2-noradrenergic receptors. Mirtazapine offers both antianxiety and antidepressant effects, with minimal sexual dysfunction secondary to serotonin blockade. This antidepressant is particularly suited for patients with nausea because it is an antiemetic via serotonin blockade.

OTHER ANTIDEPRESSANTS

Norepinephrine-Dopamine Reuptake Inhibitors (NDRIs)

Unlike other currently used antidepressants, **bupropion** (Wellbutrin) does not act on the serotonin system. It inhibits dopamine-norepinephrine reuptake, and it also inhibits nicotinic acetylcholine receptors to reduce the addictive action of nicotine. Thus the bupropion preparation Zyban is also prescribed for smoking cessation.

Trazodone (Desyrel) is not a first choice for antidepressant treatment, but it is often given along with another agent because sedation, one of its side effects, helps with insomnia. Trazodone's sedative effect is from potent histamine-1 blockade. The trazodone extended-release formulation claims to maintain blood levels within a therapeutic range for 24 hours, potentially reducing side effects while maintaining efficacy. Potent α-adrenergic blocking properties can cause priapism (painful prolonged penile erections). Refer to Chapter 15 for more information on the antidepressant medications, nursing considerations, and patient and family teaching.

TREATING ANXIETY DISORDERS WITH ANTIDEPRESSANTS

Antidepressants have been found effective in treating anxiety disorders because of many shared symptoms, neurotransmitters, and circuits. SSRIs are commonly used to treat panic disorder, generalized anxiety disorder (GAD), OCD, PTSD, and social phobia. The SNRIs venlafaxine (Effexor) and duloxetine (Cymbalta) are also used to treat GAD.

ANTIANXIETY OR ANXIOLYTIC DRUGS

Benzodiazepines

GABA is the major inhibitory (calming) neurotransmitter in the CNS. The most commonly used antianxiety agents are **benzodiazepines,** which promote activity of GABA by binding to a specific receptor on the $GABA_A$ receptor complex. Figure 4-11 shows that benzodiazepines such as diazepam (Valium), clonazepam

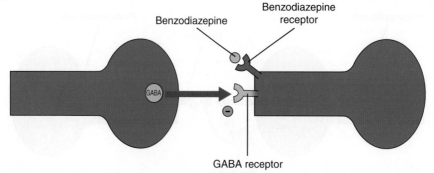

FIGURE 4-11 Action of the benzodiazepines. Drugs in this group attach to receptors adjacent to the receptors for the neurotransmitter γ-aminobutyric acid (GABA). Drug attachment to these receptors results in a strengthening of the inhibitory effects of GABA. In the absence of GABA, there is no inhibitory effect of benzodiazepines.

(Klonopin), and alprazolam (Xanax) bind to GABA$_A$ receptors with different α subunits. α$_2$ subunits may be the most important for decreasing anxiety.

The fact that benzodiazepines do not inhibit neurons in the absence of GABA limits the potential toxicity of these drugs. However, patients taking benzodiazepines have the potential to develop tolerance and withdrawal reactions. Some of the various benzodiazepines, such as flurazepam (Dalmane) and triazolam (Halcion), have a predominantly hypnotic (sleep-inducing) effect, whereas others, such as lorazepam (Ativan) and alprazolam (Xanax), reduce anxiety without being as **soporific** (sleep producing).

The ability of benzodiazepines to potentiate GABA could account for their ability to reduce neuronal excitement in seizures and alcohol withdrawal. When used alone, even at high dosages, benzodiazepines rarely inhibit the brain to the degree that respiratory depression, coma, and death result. However, when combined with other central nervous system (CNS) depressants, such as alcohol, opiates, or TCAs, the inhibitory actions of the benzodiazepines can lead to life-threatening respiratory depression.

Any drug that inhibits electrical activity in the brain can interfere with motor ability and judgment. Therefore, patients must be cautioned about engaging in activities that could be dangerous if reflexes and attention are impaired (e.g., driving). Ataxia is a common side effect secondary to the abundance of GABA receptors in the cerebellum.

Non-Benzodiazepines
Buspirone
Buspirone (BuSpar) is a drug that reduces anxiety without having strong sedative-hypnotic properties. Its mechanism of action is unknown, but it has a high affinity for serotonin receptors, acting as a serotonin 1A partial agonist. It is not a CNS depressant and thus does not have as great a danger of interaction with other CNS depressants, such as alcohol. Also, the potential for addiction that exists with benzodiazepines does not exist for buspirone.

Short-Acting Sedative-Hypnotic Sleep Agents
Non-benzodiazepine hypnotic agents, such as zolpidem (Ambien), zaleplon (Sonata), and eszopiclone (Lunesta), demonstrate selectivity for GABA$_A$ receptors containing α$_1$ subunits. Termed the "Z-hypnotics," they have sedative effects without the antianxiety, anticonvulsant, or muscle relaxant effects of benzodiazepines.

Melatonin Receptor Agonists
Ramelteon (Rozerem), a hypnotic, acts much the same way as endogenous melatonin. It has a high selectivity at the melatonin-1 receptor site—thought to regulate sleepiness—and at the melatonin-2 receptor site—thought to regulate circadian rhythms.

MOOD STABILIZERS
Lithium
Although the efficacy of lithium (Eskalith, Lithobid) as a mood stabilizer in bipolar disorder is well established, its mechanism

of action is not well understood. Theories include interaction with sodium and potassium at the cell membrane to stabilize electric activity, reduction in the levels of the excitatory neurotransmitter glutamate, and inhibition of the second messenger enzyme inositol monophosphatase. As a positively charged ion, similar to sodium, it may act by stabilizing electrical activity in neurons. If the alteration of electrical currents is not responsible for its beneficial effects, it certainly explains some adverse effects such as cardiac dysrhythmias, seizures, or tremors.

Primarily because of its effects on electrical conductivity, lithium has a low therapeutic index (the ratio of the lethal dose to the effective dose); therefore it is important to monitor blood lithium levels, which are dependent on kidney function. Lithium is particularly sensitive to interactions during excretion, and even minor changes in serum sodium or hydration levels can cause lithium to accumulate. Lithium doses are difficult to titrate if interacting medications (e.g., thiazide diuretics or sodium-containing antacids) are taken intermittently. Long-term use of lithium increases the risk of both kidney and thyroid disease. Chapter 16 considers lithium treatment in more detail.

Anticonvulsant Mood Stabilizers
Valproate, available as **divalproex sodium** (Depakote) and **valproic acid** (Depakene), is recommended in bipolar disorder for mixed episodes and rapid cycling. It is very effective in managing impulsive aggression. When lithium is not tolerated, divalproex may be used for long-term maintenance therapy. Its action in bipolar illness is unknown, but it may be related to increased bioavailability of the inhibitory neurotransmitter GABA. Baseline lab work includes liver function tests and complete blood count (CBC). Once the patient is stable, valproate levels are measured every 6 months and generally range from 50 to 100 mcg/mL.

Carbamazepine (Tegretol), in a controlled-release formula, is used to treat acute mania. A CBC must be done periodically because of rare but serious blood dyscrasias (e.g., aplastic anemia and agranulocytosis).

Lamotrigine (Lamictal), approved for maintenance treatment of bipolar disorder, modulates the release of glutamate and aspartate and is effective in decreasing the time between episodes of bipolar depression. The most common adverse effects are usually mild, but about 8% of patients who begin lamotrigine will develop a rash during the first 4 months of treatment. If this occurs, the drug should be discontinued. Although the rash is usually benign, there is a concern that it is an early manifestation of a toxic epidermal necrolysis called Stevens-Johnson syndrome (Sadock & Sadock, 2007). Another rare but serious side effect of lamotrigine is aseptic meningitis.

Other Agents
Off-label mood stabilizers include oxcarbazepine (Trileptal), gabapentin (Neurontin), and topiramate (Topamax). Benzodiazepines may be used for their calming effects during mania, and sometimes antipsychotics and antidepressants are used

along with a mood stabilizer. Refer to Chapter 16 for nursing considerations and patient and family teaching for the mood stabilizing drugs.

ANTIPSYCHOTIC DRUGS

Conventional Antipsychotics

The conventional antipsychotic drugs (i.e., typical, traditional, standard antipsychotics) were once called **neuroleptics** because they caused significant neurological effects. They are also referred to as **dopamine receptor agonists** (**DRAs**) because they bind to dopamine type 2 (D_2) receptors and reduce dopamine transmission as illustrated in Figure 4-12.

D_2 blockade achieves the therapeutic effect of decreasing positive symptoms in schizophrenia, but it also can lead to extrapyramidal side effects such as dystonia (muscle stiffness), akathisia (restlessness), tardive dyskinesia (TD), and drug-induced parkinsonism. D_2 blockade also may lead to a rare but life-threatening complication called neuroleptic malignant syndrome (NMS) involving autonomic, motor, and behavioral symptoms. The antipsychotic agent should be stopped immediately if the patient develops signs of NMS such as severe muscle rigidity, confusion, agitation, and increased temperature, pulse, and blood pressure.

In addition to adverse effects occurring with D_2 blockade, unpleasant effects also result from antipsychotics blocking other receptors, such as those identified in Figure 4-13. For

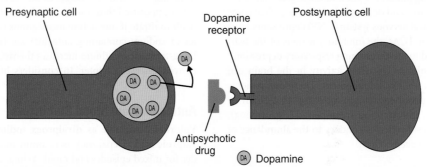

FIGURE 4-12 Mechanism by which antipsychotics block dopamine receptors.

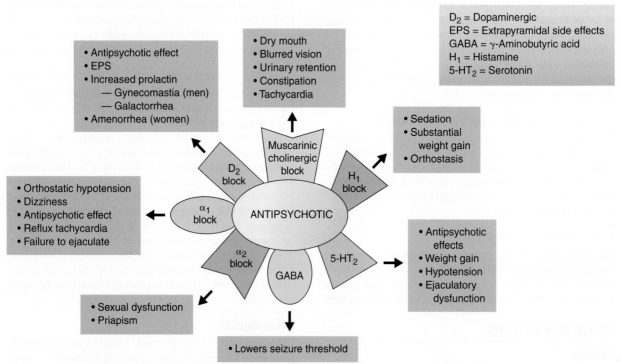

FIGURE 4-13 Adverse effects of receptor blockage of antipsychotic agents. (From Varcarolis, E. [2011]. *Manual of psychiatric nursing care plans* [4th ed.]. St Louis: Saunders Elsevier.)

example, blocking **muscarinic cholinergic** receptors can result in blurred vision, dry mouth, constipation, and urinary hesitancy. Antagonism of the **histamine$_1$** receptors causes sedation and weight gain. Blockage at the α_1 **receptors for norepinephrine** can affect vasodilation and a consequent drop in blood pressure, or orthostatic hypotension. Antagonism of either α_1 receptors or **5-HT$_2$** receptors may result in ejaculatory dysfunction. For a more detailed description of how the antipsychotic drugs block specific receptors, visit the Evolve website at http://evolve.elsevier.comVarcarolis/essentials.

Conventional antipsychotics have been divided into two groups: high potency and low potency. Low-potency neuroleptics such as **chlorpromazine** (Thorazine) are used less frequently than high-potency neuroleptic medications because of problems with orthostatic hypotension. Their sedative effect was seen as advantageous in controlling aggression in violent patients, but this calming effect can also be obtained by combining lorazepam (Ativan) with a high-potency drug such as **haloperidol** (Haldol).

Although high-potency haloperidol and **fluphenazine** (Prolixin) have less sedation and fewer anticholinergic effects, they cause more extrapyramidal symptoms (EPS) than low-potency agents. An acute dystonic reaction (ADR) is more likely to occur early in treatment with a high-potency neuroleptic, especially if the patient uses cocaine.

In a large government-sponsored trial called "The CATIE Project," the moderate-potency conventional antipsychotic perphenazine (Trilafon) was found to be comparable in efficacy to newer atypical agents. This finding, as well as the cost-effectiveness of conventional antipsychotics, has renewed interest in their use.

Atypical Antipsychotics

Second-generation antipsychotics or atypical antipsychotics are prescribed more frequently because their different receptor-binding profile accounts for fewer EPS, and they have a greater ability to target negative symptoms of schizophrenia. All antipsychotics, regardless of class, have the ability to improve cognitive function (Goff et al., 2010), but there is controversy regarding whether the atypicals are superior in this function. Their tolerability may facilitate treatment adherence, which in turn may result in greater cognitive improvement (Selva-Vera et al., 2010). Also, the higher incidence of EPS with conventional antipsychotics may necessitate treatment with anticholinergic medication, such as benztropine (Cogentin). Anticholinergics themselves can produce sedation, inattention, and memory disturbance, illustrating how both mental illness and pharmacotherapy disrupt cognition.

Atypicals are known as serotonin-dopamine antagonists (SDAs) because they have a higher ratio of serotonin (5-HT$_2$) to dopamine D$_2$-receptor blockade than conventional dopamine receptor antagonists (DRAs) (Sadock & Sadock, 2007). In addition to being potent serotonin type 2A (5-HT$_{2a}$) receptor antagonists, some SDAs have significant anticholinergic and antihistaminic activity.

Clozapine

Clozapine (Clozaril), the first of the atypicals, is several times more potent in blocking serotonin 5-HT$_2$ receptors than dopamine D$_2$ receptors. Preferential blocking of dopamine receptors in the limbic system, rather than those in striatal areas, is thought to account for a low prevalence of movement disorders (Rothschild, 2009).

Clozapine also has binding activity at a variety of other receptors, which may account for its advantages in treating patients who respond poorly to other antipsychotics, both typical and atypical (Joober & Boksa, 2010). Clozapine is not used as a first-line treatment because it may suppress bone marrow, resulting in a rare but serious decrease in the level of granulated white blood cells (WBCs) called agranulocytosis. The risk of neutropenia and agranulocytosis is highest in the first few months of treatment.

Clozapine has the potential for inducing seizures, a dose-related side effect, in 3.5% of patients. Caution should be used with coadministration of SSRIs because these drugs increase the risk of seizures by elevating clozapine concentrations. When clozapine-treated patients are partial responders, topiramate may be used for augmentation. This drug combination has been associated with weight loss and metabolic benefit (Hahn et al., 2010).

Olanzapine

Olanzapine (Zyprexa), a derivative of clozapine, has comparable receptor occupancies and similar metabolic side effects, such as weight gain. Metabolic monitoring for all patients being administered atypical antipsychotics is recommended, although risperidone (Risperdal) and quetiapine (Seroquel) have a lower weight gain and ziprasidone (Geodon) and aripiprazole (Abilify) are considered weight neutral.

Metabolic monitoring usually includes measurements of body weight, body mass index (BMI), waist circumference, fasting plasma glucose level, and fasting lipid profile.

In addition, metformin—a medication used to regulate blood glucose level—has been shown to halt weight gain, decrease measures of insulin resistance, and possibly increase medication adherence. Although weight gain and metabolic effects are unhealthy, these adverse effects are often more tolerable than the neurological adverse effects of conventional antipsychotics.

Olanzapine is sedating because of its antagonism of H$_1$ receptors, so it is common practice to administer the medication at bedtime. Olanzapine was the first antipsychotic available as orally disintegrating tablets for patients who are unable or unwilling to swallow.

Risperidone

Risperidone (Risperdal) exhibits high levels of D$_2$-receptor blockade and a very high affinity for 5-HT$_2$ receptors. EPS may occur if the dosage is only slightly higher than the effective dose. The patient should be carefully monitored for motor difficulties if the dosage exceeds 4 to 6 mg/day. Because risperidone blocks α_1 and H$_1$ receptors, it can cause orthostatic hypotension and sedation, which can lead to falls—a serious problem for older adults. Weight gain, sedation, and sexual dysfunction also are adverse effects that may affect adherence with the medication regimen.

Risperidone (Risperdal Consta), the first atypical antipsychotic available as a long-acting injectable, was hypothesized to result in greater improvement, increased stability, and lower rates of relapse in unstable patients with schizophrenia because of its ability to achieve "steady state" concentrations (Schatzberg & Nemeroff, 2009). However, recent evidence shows that long-acting risperidone is not superior to oral risperidone, and has the added burden of adverse effects at the injection site and more EPS (Rosenheck et al., 2011). Long-acting injectables still have their place with nonadherent patients when it is necessary to keep the dosage regimen constant, particularly in patients with schizophrenia incarcerated for violent acts (Nasrallah, 2011). Further research is needed to compare the atypical injectable Risperdal Consta with the conventional long-acting injectables haloperidol and fluphenazine decanoate.

Paliperidone is the principal active metabolite of risperidone in INVEGA extended-release tablets. Unlike risperidone, paliperidone is eliminated almost independently of the CYP2D6 pathway and is cleared through the kidneys. The Osmotic Release Oral System (OROS) provides consistent 24-hour release of medication, leading to minimal peaks and troughs in plasma concentration.

Quetiapine

Quetiapine (Seroquel) has a broad receptor-binding profile. Its strong blockage of histamine-1 receptors accounts for high sedation. The combination of histamine-1 and serotonin receptor blockage leads to weight gain and moderate risk for metabolic syndrome. Orthostatic hypotension is explained by antagonism of adrenergic α_1 receptors. Quetiapine has a low risk for EPS or prolactin level elevation from low D_2 dopamine binding because of rapid dissociation at these receptors. Once-daily Seroquel XR tablets is expected to increase adherence by simplifying the dosing routine.

Ziprasidone

Ziprasidone (Geodon) is a serotonin-norepinephrine reuptake inhibitor. The main side effects are dizziness and sedation. One major safety concern with ziprasidone, as well as the atypicals listed earlier, is prolongation of the QT_c interval, which can be fatal if the patient has a history of cardiac dysrhythmias. Thus a baseline electrocardiogram is recommended before treatment. Food increases its absorption up to twofold; therefore ziprasidone is always taken with food. It is unlikely to cause significant interactions with drugs metabolized by cytochrome P450. Ziprasidone may be given intramuscularly for acute agitation, but it is important to note that it is not a long-acting preparation.

Aripiprazole

Aripiprazole (Abilify) is a unique atypical known as a *dopamine system stabilizer*. In areas of the brain with excess dopamine, it lowers the dopamine level by acting as a receptor antagonist; however, in regions with low dopamine concentration, it stimulates receptors to raise the dopamine level, acting as a dopamine agonist. It is also an antagonist at serotonin $5-HT_2$ receptors and a partial agonist at $5-HT_1$ receptors. It has little sedation and weight gain. Although it is not common, aripiprazole does cause akathisia, described as restlessness or agitation. Headache, insomnia, and nausea are other adverse effects reported. Aripiprazole is available in a ready-to-use vial for intramuscular injection and control of agitation in schizophrenia or bipolar disorder.

Iloperidone

Iloperidone (Fanapt) functions as an antagonist at the dopamine D_2 and D_3, serotonin $5-HT_{1A}$, and norepinephrine α_1/α_{2c} receptors. The dose might be reduced in patients coadministered a strong CYP2D6 inhibitor (fluoxetine) or CYP34A inhibitor or in those who are poor metabolizers. Approximately 7% to 10% of Caucasians and 3% to 8% of Black/African Americans lack the capacity to metabolize CYP2D6 substrates. Iloperidone can be administered without regard to meals.

Lurasidone Hydrochloride

Lurasidone HCl (Latuda) is similar to other atypicals in having high binding affinity for dopamine D_2 and serotonin $5-HT_{2A}$ receptors, and its efficacy for treatment of acute schizophrenia is established. Available in a once-daily dose, it also targets selected other serotonin receptors that may play a role in cognition (Terry et al., 2008). Lurasidone should not be used with strong inhibitors or inducers of the enzyme CYP3A4. It is absorbed in the gastrointestinal tract, and reaches maximum concentration (C_{max}) in 1 to 3 hours. The C_{max} doubles when lurasidone is administered with food (Lincoln & Tripathi, 2011). Refer to Chapter 17 for more information on adverse and toxic effects, nursing considerations, and patient and family teaching of the antipsychotics.

Psychoneuroimmunology (PNI)

Psychoneuroimmunology (PNI) is a research field that focuses on the relationship between the immune system and the nervous system. Studies investigate molecular, cellular, and neuronal events to determine their role in psychiatric disorders. For example, scientists are identifying the neural circuits involved in cytokine-induced depression (Loftis et al., 2010) and in stress-related disorders. Neuroinflammatory processes related to cytokines, the signaling molecules of the immune system, are also being studied as biological mechanisms underlying cognitive deficits in Alzheimer's disease and in tetrahydrocannabinol (THC) use. Activation of innate immune inflammatory responses and their regulation by neuroendocrine pathways in patients with cancer are known to result in changes in neurotransmitter metabolism, neuropeptide function, sleep-wake cycles, regional brain activity, and ultimately behavior (Miller et al., 2008). Neuroimmunopharmacology focuses on drugs modulating neuroimmune processes, and is beginning to explore highly advanced technologies such as nanotechnology to develop approved nano-drugs.

CONSIDERING CULTURE

Cultural and ethnic beliefs surrounding mental illness and pharmacotherapy affect a person's perception of the need for treatment, adherence, reporting of adverse events, and the preference for alternative or complementary therapies.

Cross-cultural psychopharmacology explores different effects or responses that exist among ethnic groups and the reasons for these effects. To predict patients' responses, scientists search for variants in genes that code for drug metabolizing enzymes in the liver. **Pharmacogenetics** studies how genes influence drug metabolism and response, with much attention focusing on drug metabolism via the CYP450 enzyme systems. Variation in drug response is particularly important in nonresponders and adverse responders who require adjusted doses or alternate medications. Although the genetic underpinnings of mental illness have yet to be determined, genetic profiles may someday explain why some patients respond to certain drugs and which patients are poor or ultrarapid metabolizers. At present, medications treat "target symptoms" of mental disorders so that people can function. In the future, genetic research might personalize treatment by targeting genetic flaws or underlying causes of these disorders, thereby leading to a cure for mental illness.

KEY POINTS TO REMEMBER

- All actions of the brain—sensory, motor, intellectual—are carried out physiologically through the interactions of nerve cells. These interactions involve impulse conduction, transmitter release, and receptor response. Alterations in these basic processes can lead to mental disturbances and physical manifestations.
- In particular, it seems that excess activity of dopamine, among other factors, is involved in the thought disturbances of schizophrenia, and deficiencies of norepinephrine, serotonin, or both underlie depression and anxiety. Insufficient activity of GABA also plays a role in anxiety.
- Pharmacological treatment of mental disturbances is directed at the suspected transmitter-receptor problem. Antipsychotic drugs decrease dopamine levels, antidepressant drugs increase synaptic levels of norepinephrine and/or serotonin, and antianxiety drugs increase the effectiveness of GABA or increase 5-HT and/or norepinephrine levels.
- Because the immediate target activity of a drug can result in many downstream alterations in neuronal activity, drugs with a variety of chemical actions may show efficacy in treating the same clinical condition. Thus, newer drugs with novel mechanisms of action are being used in the treatment of schizophrenia, depression, and anxiety.
- Unfortunately, agents used to treat mental disease can cause various undesired effects. Prominent among these can be sedation or excitement, motor disturbances, muscarinic blockage, α-adrenergic antagonism, sexual dysfunction, and weight gain. There is a continuing effort to develop new drugs that are effective, safe, and well tolerated.

APPLYING CRITICAL JUDGMENT

1. No matter where you practice nursing, individuals under your care will be taking psychotropic drugs. Consider the importance of understanding normal brain structure and function as they relate to mental disturbances and psychotropic drugs by addressing the following questions:
   A. How can you use your knowledge of normal brain function (control of peripheral nerves, skeletal muscles, the autonomic nervous system, hormones, and circadian rhythms) to better understand how a patient can be affected by psychotropic drugs or psychiatric illness?
   B. What information from the various brain imaging techniques can you use to understand and treat patients with mental disorders and provide support to their families? How might you use that information for patient and family teaching?
2. Based on your understanding of symptoms that may occur when the following neurotransmitters are altered, what specific information would you include in medication teaching?
   A. Dopamine D_2 (as with use of antipsychotic drugs)
   B. Blockage of muscarinic receptors (as with use of phenothiazines and other drugs)
   C. α_1 receptors (as with use of phenothiazines and other drugs)
   D. Histamine (as with use of phenothiazines and other drugs)
   E. Monoamine oxidase (MAO) (as with use of a monoamine oxidase inhibitor [MAOI])
   F. γ-Aminobutyric acid (GABA) (as with the use of benzodiazepines)
   G. Serotonin (as with the use of selective serotonin reuptake inhibitors [SSRIs] and other drugs)
   H. Norepinephrine (as with the use of serotonin-norepinephrine reuptake inhibitors [SNRIs])

CHAPTER REVIEW QUESTIONS

Choose the most appropriate answer(s).

1. All mental activity has its locus in the:
   1. environmental stimuli of the patient.
   2. brain.
   3. personality structure.
   4. emotions.
2. Standard anti-psychotic drugs: (select all that apply)
   1. lower the seizure threshold.
   2. increase blood pressure.
   3. can cause extrapyramidal symptoms (EPS).
   4. may lead to neuroleptic malignant syndrome.
3. A psychiatric nurse routinely administers the following drugs to patients in the community mental health center. The patients who should be most carefully assessed for untoward cardiac side effects are those receiving:
   1. lithium.
   2. clozapine.
   3. diazepam.
   4. sertraline.
4. Clozaril: (select all that apply)
   1. is an atypical anti-psychotic drug.
   2. may cause agranulocytosis.
   3. is indicated for severely ill schizophrenics.
   4. is used for first-line treatment of psychosis.
5. Pharmacological agents:
   1. are equally effective with all cultural groups.
   2. rarely cause side effects.
   3. may have undesired effects in some cultural groups.
   4. Are best if they are naturally processed.

REFERENCES

Andreasen, N. C., & Pierson, R. (2008). The role of the cerebellum in schizophrenia. *Biological Psychiatry, 64*(2), 81–88. EpubApr8.

Baier, B., Dieterich, M., Stoeter, P., Birklein, F., & Muller, N. G. (2010). Anatomical correlate of impaired covert visual attentional processes in patients with cerebellar lesions. *Journal of Neuroscience, 30*(10), 3770–3776.

Beyer, C. E., & Stahl, S. M. (2010). *Next generation antidepressants: moving beyond monoamines to discover novel treatment strategies for mood disorders.* London: Cambridge University Press.

Brunton, L., Chabner, B., & Knollman, B. (2011). *Goodman & Gilman's the pharmacological basis of therapeutics* (12th ed.). New York: McGraw Hill Medical.

Cardish, R. J. (2007). Psychopharmacologic management of suicidality in personality disorders. *Canadian Journal of Psychiatry, 52* (6 Suppl. 1), S115–S127.

Danovich, L., Weinreb, O., Youdim, M. B. H., & Silver, H. (2011). The involvement of $GABA_A$ receptor in the molecular mechanisms of combined selective serotonin reuptake inhibitor-antipsychotic treatment. *International Journal of Neuropsychopharmacology, 14*, 143–155.

Davidson, M. (2007). *First antipsychotic targeting GABA to enter phase II trials.* Schizophrenia.com. Retrieved February 14, 2007, from www.schizophrenia.com/sznews/archives/004647.html.

Ereshefsky, L. (2009). Drug-drug interactions with the use of psychotropic medications. *CNS Spectrums Supplement, 14*(8).

Fuster, J. M. (2008). *The prefrontal cortex* (4th ed.). St Louis: Elsevier.

Goff, D. C., Hill, M., & Barch, D. (2010). The treatment of cognitive impairment in schizophrenia. *Pharmacology Biochemistry & Behavior.* Accessed online April 14, 2011.

Hahn, M. K., Remington, G., Bois, D., & Cohn, T. (2010). Topiramate augmentation in clozapine-treated patients with schizophrenia: clinical and metabolic effects. *Journal of Clinical Psychopharmacology, 30*(6), 706–710.

Halperin, D., & Reber, G. (2007). Influence of antidepressants on hemostasis. *Dialogues Clinical Neuroscience, 9*(1), 47–59.

Ho, B. -C., Andreasen, N. C., Ziebell, S., Pierson, R., & Magnotta, V. (2011). Long-term antipsychotic treatment and brain volumes: a longitudinal study of first-episode schizophrenia. *Archives of General Psychiatry, 68*(2), 128–137.

Joober, R., & Boksa, P. (2010). Clozapine: a distinct, poorly understood and under-used molecule. *Journal of Psychiatry and Neuroscience, 35*(3), 147–149.

Li, N., Boyoung, L., Liu, R., Banasr, M., Dwyer, J. M., et al. (2010). mTOR-dependent synapse formation underlies the rapid antidepressant effects of NMDA antagonists. *Science, 329*(5994), 959–964.

Lincoln, J., & Tripathi, A. (2011). Lurasidone for schizophrenia. *Current Psychiatry Online, 10*(1). Accessed April 14, 2011.

Loftis, J. M., Huckans, M., & Morasco, B. J. (2010). Neuroimmune mechanisms of cytokine-induced depression: current theories and novel treatment strategies. *Neurobiological Disorders, 37*(3), 519–533.

Madhusoodanan, S., Parida, S., & Jimenez, C. (2010). Hyperprolactinemia associated with psychotropics: a review. *Human Psychopharmacology: Clinical and Experimental, 25*(4), 281–297.

Miller, A. H., Ancoli-Israel, S., Bower, J. E., Capuron, L., & Irwin, M. R. (2008). Neuroendocrine-immune mechanisms of behavioral comorbidities in patients with cancer. *Journal of Clinical Oncology*, 971–982.

Nasrallah, H. A. (February 2011). Two vastly underutilized interventions can improve schizophrenia outcomes. *Current Psychiatry Online, 10*(2).

Patton, K. T., Thibodeau, G. A., & Douglas, M. M. (2012). *Essentials of anatomy & physiology.* St Louis: Elsevier Mosby.

Picard, H., Amado, I., Mouchet-Mages, I., et al. (2008). The role of the cerebellum in schizophrenia: an update of clinical, cognitive, and functional evidence. *Schizophrenia Bulletin, 34*(1), 155–172.

Preston, J. D., O'Neal, J. H., & Talaga, M. C. (2010). *Handbook of clinical psychopharmacology for therapists* (6th ed.). Oakland, CA: New Harbinger.

Radenbach, K., Flaig, V., Schneider-Axmann, T., Usher, J., Reith, W., et al. (2010). Thalamic volumes in patients with bipolar disorder. *European Archives of Psychiatry, 260*(8), 601–607.

Rosenheck, R. R., Krystal, J. H., Lew, R., Barnett, P. G., Fiore, L., et al. (2011). Long-acting risperidone and oral antipsychotics in unstable schizophrenia. *New England Journal of Medicine, 364,* 842–851.

Rothschild, A. J. (Ed.). (2009). *The evidence-based guide to antipsychotic medications.* Arlington, VA: American Psychiatric Publishing.

Sadock, B. J., & Sadock, V. A. (2007). *Kaplan & Sadock's synopsis of psychiatry: behavioral sciences/clinical psychiatry* (10th ed.). Philadelphia: Lippincott Williams & Wilkins.

Schatzberg, A. F., & Nemeroff, C. B. (2009). *The American Psychiatric Association Publishing textbook of psychopharmacology* (4th ed.). Arlington, VA: American Psychiatric Publishing.

Selva-Vera, G., Balanza-Martinez, V., Salazar-Fraile, J., Sanchez-Moreno, J., Martinez-Aran, A., et al. (2010). The switch from conventional to atypical antipsychotic treatment should not be based exclusively on the presence of cognitive deficits. A pilot study in individuals with schizophrenia. *BMC Psychiatry.* Posted 8/04/2010. Accessed April 14, 2011, on Medscape.

Stahl, S. M., & Muntner, N. (2008). *Stahl's essential pharmacology* (3rd ed.). New York: Cambridge University Press.

Terry, A. V., Buccafusco, J. J., & Wilson, C. (2008). Cognitive dysfunction in neuropsychiatric disorders: selected serotonin receptor subtypes as therapeutic targets. *Behavioral Brain Research, 195*(1), 30–38.

Tost, H., Braus, D. F., Hakimi, S., Ruf, M., Vollmert, C., et al. (2010). Acute D(2) receptor blockade induces rapid, reversible remodeling in human cortical-striatal circuits. *Nature Neuroscience.* Jun 6.

Viibryd Medication Guide. Accessed April 14, 2011, at www.fda.gov/downloads/Drugs/DrugSafety/UCM241524.pdf.

5

Settings for Psychiatric Care

Margaret Jordan Halter

ⓔvolve WEBSITE

KEY TERMS AND CONCEPTS

comorbid conditions
  (co-occurring), p. 74
elopement, p. 72
least restrictive environment, p. 69

mental health parity, p. 76
primary care providers (PCPs), p. 70
stigma, p. 69
therapeutic milieu, p. 72

SELECTED CONCEPT
Patient-Centered Medical Homes (PCMH) received strong support from the Affordable Care Act of 2010. These health homes were developed in response to fragmented care that resulted in some services never being delivered while others were duplicated. The focus of care is patient-centered and provides access to physical health, behavioral health, and supportive community and social services.

Electronic communication (e.g., follow-up emails and reminders) and record keeping are viewed as essential to this process.
(Halter, text)

OBJECTIVES

1. Describe the evolution of treatment settings for psychiatric care.
2. Compare and contrast inpatient and outpatient treatment environments in which psychiatric care is provided.
3. Discuss the role of mental health professionals in assisting people with mental illness symptoms or mental illnesses.
4. Explain methods for financing psychiatric care.

Obtaining traditional health care is fairly straightforward. For example, if you wake up with a sore throat, you know what to do and basically what will happen. It is likely that if you feel bad enough, you will see your primary care provider (PCP), be examined, and maybe get a throat culture to diagnose the problem. If the cause is bacterial, you will probably be prescribed an antibiotic. If you do not improve in a certain length of time, your PCP may order more tests or recommend that you see an ear, nose, and throat specialist.

Compared to obtaining treatment for physical disorders, entry into the health care system for the treatment of psychiatric problems can be a mystery. In fact, although 46% of the population will have a diagnosable mental disorder over the course of a lifetime, and 80% of that population will eventually seek treatment, the delay in treatment is often years or decades (Kessler et al., 2005).

Challenges in accessing and navigating this care system exist for several reasons. One reason is that we just do not have much of a frame of reference. We are unlikely to benefit from the experience of others because having a psychiatric illness is often hidden as a result of embarrassment or concern over the stigma, or a sense of responsibility, shame, and being flawed associated with these disorders (refer to Chapter 2 for more on stigma). You may know that when your grandmother had heart disease, she saw a cardiac specialist and had a coronary artery bypass, but you may be unaware that she was also treated for depression by a psychiatrist.

Seeking treatment for mental health problems is also complicated by the very nature of mental illness. At the most extreme, disorders with a psychotic component may disorganize thoughts and impede a person's ability to recognize the need for care. Even major depression, a common psychiatric disorder, may interfere with motivation to seek care because the illness often causes feelings of apathy, hopelessness, and anergia (lack of energy).

Mental health symptoms are also confused with other problems. For example, anxiety disorders often manifest in somatic symptoms such as racing heartbeat, sweaty palms, and dizziness, which could be symptoms of cardiac problems. Prudence would dictate ruling out other causes, such as physical illness, particularly because diagnosing psychiatric illness is largely based on symptoms and not on objective measurements such as electrocardiograms (ECGs) and blood counts. This necessary process of ruling out other illnesses often results in an often-troublesome treatment delay.

Further complicating treatment for mental illness is the unique nature of the system of care, which is rooted in the public as well as private sectors. The purpose of this chapter is to provide an overview of this system, briefly examine the evolution of mental health care, and explore different venues by which people receive treatment for mental health problems. Treatment options are presented in order of acuteness, beginning with those in the least restrictive environment—the setting that provides the necessary care while allowing the greatest personal freedom. This chapter also explores how mental health care is funded and the challenges in securing adequate funding.

BACKGROUND

Although people with financial resources have a variety of psychiatric treatment options, state or county governments coordinate a separate care system for uninsured individuals, often for those with the most serious and persistent illnesses. This separate system of care has its roots in asylums that were created in most existing states before the Civil War. These asylums were created with good intentions in an environment of optimism about recovery and belief that states had a special responsibility to care for the "insane." Effective treatments were not yet developed and community care was virtually nonexistent. By the early 1950s, there were only two real options for psychiatric care—a private psychiatrist's office or a mental hospital. At that time, there were 550,000 patients in state hospitals. A majority were individuals with disabling conditions who had become "stuck" in the asylums.

The number of people in state-managed psychiatric hospitals began to decrease with the creation of Medicare and Medicaid during the 1960s Great Society reform period. Medicaid had an especially potent effect because it paid for short-term hospitalization in general hospitals and medical centers, and for long-term care in nursing homes; however, it did not cover care for most patients in psychiatric hospitals. These incentives stimulated development of general hospital psychiatric units, and also led states to transfer geriatric patients from 100% state-paid psychiatric hospitals to Medicaid-reimbursed nursing facilities.

In the 1999 Olmstead decision, the Supreme Court decreed that keeping people in psychiatric hospitals was "unjustified isolation." The opinion of the court was that mental illness is a disability and institutionalization is in violation of the Americans With Disabilities Act, and that all people with disabilities have a right to live in the community.

These forces combined to lead to the gradual and incomplete creation of state- and county-financed community care systems to complement, and largely replace, functions of the state hospitals. The number of state psychiatric hospitals continues to be cut and has been reduced to about 220 facilities (National Association of State Mental Health Program Directors, 2011). Figure 5-1 illustrates the current structure of one state mental health and substance abuse system. In Ohio, two state agencies—the Ohio Department of Mental Health and the Ohio Department of Alcohol and Drug Addiction Services—certify, monitor, and fund agencies that provide services. These agencies may be for profit or nonprofit. County board(s) (depending on whether the alcohol or substance abuse and mental health boards are combined) provide(s) more local oversight and management of these agencies.

Related to the shift from hospital to community care were the pharmacological breakthroughs in the latter half of the

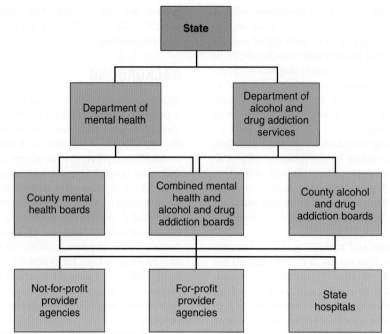

FIGURE 5-1 An example of a state system of mental health and substance abuse care.

twentieth century that led to dramatic changes in the provision of psychiatric care. The introduction of chlorpromazine (Thorazine), the first antipsychotic medication, in the early 1950s contributed to hospital discharges. Gradually, more psychopharmacological agents were added to treat psychosis, depression, anxiety, and other disorders, and treatment could be provided not only from specialists in psychiatry but also from general practitioners.

Our current system of psychiatric care includes inpatient and outpatient settings. Decisions for level of care tend to be based on the condition being treated and the acuteness of the problem. However, these are not the only criteria. Levels of care may be influenced by such factors as a concurrent psychiatric or substance abuse problem, medical problems, acceptance of treatment, social supports, and disease chronicity or potential for relapse.

OUTPATIENT CARE SETTINGS

Primary care providers (PCPs) are the first choice for most people when they are ill, but what about mental disorders? Imagine that you are feeling depressed, so depressed, in fact, that you are miserable and cannot carry out your normal activities. You recall that a friend who was depressed saw a psychiatrist (or was that a psychologist?), but that seems too drastic. You do not feel *that* bad. Perhaps you are coming down with something. After all, you have been tired and you are not eating very well. You decide to visit your PCP, a general health care provider who may be a physician, advanced practice nurse, or physician's assistant in an office, hospital, or clinic.

This is not an unusual choice. Seeking help for mental health problems from PCPs rather than from mental health specialists is common and similar to seeking help for other medical disorders. This is especially true because most psychiatric disorders are accompanied by unexplained physical symptoms. Most people treated for psychiatric disorders will not go beyond this level of care and may feel more comfortable being treated in a familiar setting. Furthermore, being treated in primary care rather than in the mental health system may lessen the degree of stigma, self-perceived or societally, attached to getting psychiatric care.

Disadvantages to being treated by PCPs include time constraints, because a 15-minute appointment is usually inadequate for a mental and physical assessment. Because PCPs typically have limited training in psychiatry, they may lack the expertise in the diagnosis and treatment of psychiatric disorders (Boscarino et al., 2010). Whereas this may be the only source many people use for receiving mental health services, sometimes PCPs refer people into specialty mental health care.

Patient-centered medical homes (PCMHs) or **primary care medical homes** received strong support from the Affordable Care Act of 2010 under President Obama. These health homes were developed in response to fragmented care that resulted in some services never being delivered while others were duplicated. The focus of care is patient centered and provides access to physical health, behavioral health, and supportive community and social services. Services range from preventive care and acute medical problems to chronic conditions and end-of-life issues. According to the Agency for

Healthcare Research and Quality (2011), these homes have five key characteristics:

1. Patient centered—Care is relationship based with the patient (family) and takes into account the unique needs of the whole person. The patient is a core member of the team who manages and organizes the care.
2. Comprehensive care—All levels (preventive, acute, and chronic) of mental and physical care are addressed. Physicians or advanced practice nurses lead teams that include nurses, physician assistants, pharmacists, nutritionists, social workers, educators, and care coordinators.
3. Coordination of care—Care is coordinated with the broader health system such as hospitals, specialty care, and home health.
4. Improved access—Patients do not wait until Monday through Friday from 9 AM to 5 PM to get the care they need. In addition to extended hours of service, these homes provide e-mail and phone support.
5. Systems approach—Evidence-based care is provided with a continuous feedback loop of evaluation and quality improvement.

The treatment of psychiatric disorders and mental health alterations can be addressed as part of a comprehensive approach to care. Electronic communication (e.g., follow-up e-mails and reminders) and record keeping are viewed as essential to this process.

Community mental health centers (CMHCs) developed from President Kennedy's Community Mental Health Centers Act of 1963, signaling a new policy preference for community care as opposed to institutionalization. Although only about 700 of the anticipated 2800 CMHCs were funded, the legislation marked a change in direction and led to state laws and budgets favoring community care. CMHCs are regulated through state mental health departments and funded by the state. Some areas may provide local funding. Because of this limited government funding, financial support services may be restricted to those whose income and medical expenses make them eligible. Typically, fees are determined using a sliding scale based on income and ability to pay.

Community-based facilities provide comprehensive services to prevent and treat mental illness. These services include assessment, diagnosis, individual and group counseling, case management, medication management, education, rehabilitation, and vocational or employment services. Some centers may provide an array of services across the life span, whereas others may be population specific, such as adult, geriatric, or children.

People with serious mental illness may benefit from **psychiatric rehabilitation** in the community. This is a social model that emphasizes and supports recovery and integration into society rather than a medical model of dysfunction. Serious disorders can result in isolation, poverty, and regression. These services focus on the development of social skills, the ability to access resources, and the acquisition of optimal social, working, living, and learning environments (United States Psychiatric Rehabilitation Services, 2011).

Psychiatric home care can be provided by any mental health professional, but it is typically nurses with inpatient experience who are able to provide biologically based and psychotherapeutic care while working through agencies such as visiting nurses. Home care may reduce the need for costly and disruptive hospitalizations and may provide a more comfortable and safe alternative to clinical settings. To qualify for reimbursement, patients must have a psychiatric diagnosis, be under the care of a PCP, and be homebound. The designation of homebound generally is given when patients cannot safely leave home, if leaving home causes undue stress, if the nature of the illness results in a refusal to leave home, or if they cannot leave home unaided. However, Medicare reimbursement does allow for the person to leave home once a week for religious services and once a week for hair care.

Intensive outpatient programs (IOPs) provide structured programs to bridge the gap between inpatient and outpatient treatment for people who require more than outpatient care or who may need a transition from an intensive setting. Treatment includes individual and group therapy and psychosocial education for at least 4 hours per week.

Partial hospitalization programs (PHPs) have been around since the 1960s, and like IOPs, function as an intermediate step between outpatient and inpatient care. They are the most intensive of outpatient options and tend to be 4 to 8 hours per day for up to 5 days a week. Structured programs are provided with nursing and medical supervision, intervention, and treatment. They are located within general hospitals, in psychiatric hospitals, and as part of community mental health programs. Patients whose symptoms are under control spend a certain number of hours at the facility each day and at night return to their homes, where family and friends can support them. Additionally, coping strategies that are learned during the program can be applied and practiced in the outside world, and then later explored and discussed. A multidisciplinary team facilitates group therapy, individual therapy, other therapies (e.g., art and occupational), and pharmacological management. Patients who are admitted to PHPs are closely monitored in case of need for readmission to inpatient care.

Role of Nurses in Outpatient Care Settings

Registered nurses who work in outpatient settings provide nursing care for individuals with mental illness, alcoholism, substance abuse problems, mental retardation, or developmental disabilities, as well as their families or caretakers. Community mental health nurses work to develop and implement a plan of care along with the multidisciplinary treatment team. They may choose to be certified in psychiatric mental health nursing or hold advanced practice degrees.

Community mental health nurses need to be very knowledgeable about community resources such as shelters for

TABLE 5-1	NUMBER AND RATE OF 24-HOUR HOSPITAL AND RESIDENTIAL TREATMENT BEDS BY TYPE OF MENTAL HEALTH ORGANIZATION			
TYPE OF ORGANIZATION	**1980**	**1990**	**2000**	**2004**
Number of 24-Hour Hospital and Residential Treatment Beds				
All organizations	274,713	325,529	214,186	212,231
State and county mental hospitals	156,482	102,307	61,833	57,034
Private psychiatric hospitals	17,157	45,952	26,402	28,422
Nonfederal general hospitals with separate psychiatric services	29,384	53,576	40,410	41,403
Veterans Administration (VA) medical centers*	33,796	24,799	8,989	—
Residential treatment centers for emotionally disturbed children	20,197	35,170	33,508	33,835
All other organizations†	1,433	63,745	43,044	53,536
24-Hour Hospital and Residential Treatment Beds per 100,000 Civilian Population				
All organizations	124.3	128.5	74.8	71.2
State and county mental hospitals	70.2	40.4	21.6	19.1
Private psychiatric hospitals	7.7	18.1	9.2	9.5
Nonfederal general hospitals with separate psychiatric services	13.7	21.2	14.1	13.9
VA medical centers	15.7	9.9	3.1	—
Residential treatment centers for emotionally disturbed children	9.1	13.9	11.7	11.4
All other organizations†	0.6	25.2	15.0	17.3

*Department of Veterans Affairs medical centers (VA general hospital psychiatric services and VA psychiatric outpatient clinics) were dropped from the survey as of 2004.
†Includes free-standing psychiatric outpatient clinics, partial care organizations, and multiservice mental health organizations.
Data from Center for Mental Health Services. (2006). In R. W. Manderscheid & J. T. Berry (Eds.), *Mental health, United States, 2004.* USDHHS Pub. No. (SMA)-06-4195, Rockville, MD: Substance Abuse and Mental Health Services Administration.

abused women, food banks for people with severe financial limitations, and agencies that provide employment options for people with mental illness. Nurses may also assess the patient and living arrangements in the home, provide teaching, refer to community supports, and supervise unlicensed care staff. An important concept for community mental health nurses is viewing the entire community as a patient. This perspective promotes community interventions such as conducting stress reduction classes and facilitating grief support groups.

INPATIENT CARE SETTINGS

Inpatient care has undergone significant change over the past 25 years. During the 1980s, inpatient stays were at their peak as private and nonfederal general hospital psychiatric units proliferated. During the mid-1990s, the number of patient days, psychiatric beds, and psychiatric facilities dipped sharply (Table 5-1). This decline was caused by improvements instigated by managed care, tougher limitations of covered days by insurance plans, and alternatives to inpatient hospitalization such as partial hospitalization programs and residential facilities.

Inpatient facilities provide 24-hour nursing care in a safe and structured setting for people who are in need of this most restrictive environment. Such a setting is essential to caring for those who are in need of protection from suicidal ideation, aggressive impulses, medication adjustment and monitoring, crisis stabilization, substance abuse detoxification, and behavior modification. Referrals for inpatient treatment may come from a PCP or mental health provider, agencies, another hospital unit, emergency facilities, or nursing homes. Hospital admissions are made under the services of a psychiatrist, although a PCP also may have admitting privileges.

Patients may be admitted voluntarily or involuntarily (see Chapter 6). Units may be unlocked or locked. Locked units provide privacy and prevent elopement—leaving before being discharged (also referred to as being "away without leave" or AWOL). There may also be psychiatric intensive care units (PICUs) within the general psychiatric units to provide better monitoring of those who display an increased risk for danger to self or others.

The therapeutic milieu is essential to successful inpatient treatment. Milieu refers to the environment in which holistic treatment occurs and includes all members of the treatment team (Box 5-1), a positive physical setting, interactions

BOX 5-1   MEMBERS OF THE TREATMENT TEAM

- **Psychiatric nurse generalists** are licensed registered nurses whose focus is on mental health and illness. They may or may not have certification in psychiatric mental health nursing.
- **Advanced practice psychiatric nurses** have post–baccalaureate degrees and work as either clinical nurse specialists (CNSs) or nurse practitioners (NPs) and have state certification. Both assess health and psychiatric disorders, provide psychotherapy, and prescribe medications. CNSs tend to focus more on leadership, program development, education, and psychotherapy, whereas NPs focus on differential diagnoses, treatment, medication management, and psychotherapy.
- **Psychiatrists** are medical doctors who have additional specialized training in diagnosing and treating psychiatric disorders. Medication is the dominant treatment used by psychiatrists, although psychotherapy and other psychosocial interventions continue to be used.
- **Psychologists** practice under state regulations and hold doctor of philosophy in psychology degrees (which differ from doctor of medicine). Their expertise lies in evaluation, psychological testing, psychotherapy, and counseling. Some states may allow prescriptive authority for psychologists.
- **Social workers** are licensed by the state and enter general practice with a bachelor's degree in social work, or pursue advanced practice with a master's degree in social work. They may provide counseling and plan for supportive services such as housing, health care, and treatment after the patient is returned to the community.
- **Counselors** possess a master's degree in psychology, counseling, or a related field and are licensed by the state. They are trained to diagnose and provide individual and group counseling.
- **Occupational therapists** are usually state regulated and are prepared at the bachelor's, master's, or doctoral level. They assist individuals to develop or regain independent living skills, activities of daily living, and role performance that have been affected by mental disorders.
- **Physical therapists** possess master's or doctoral degrees and are accredited by the state. Their role is to rehabilitate individuals with physical disabilities that may be present concurrent with psychiatric disabilities.
- **Art therapists** are prepared at the master's level in art therapy and registered through a professional association. They use art to help people understand their problems, enhance healthy development, and reduce the effects of their illnesses.
- **Recreation therapists** are typically bachelor's prepared and may be licensed by the state or be nationally certified. Recreational activities are used to improve emotional, physical, cognitive, and social well-being.
- **Pharmacists** are state licensed and are prepared through 6 years of secondary education for a Doctor of Pharmacy (PharmD) degree. They provide distribution and centralized monitoring of drug regimens.
- **Medical personnel** are physicians whose focus is the provision of nonpsychiatric care for comorbid conditions.
- **Mental health workers** or psychiatric aides are nonprofessional staff who may be state certified. They have extensive contact with patients while assisting with hygiene and meals and participating in unit activities. Mental health workers communicate important information concerning the patient's condition to professional staff.
- **Pastoral counselors** are clergy who have clinical pastoral education and are certified through the American Association of Pastoral Counselors. They provide individual and group counseling.
- **Consumer providers.** "Consumer Providers (CPs) are individuals with serious mental illness who are trained to use their experiences to provide recovery–oriented services and to support others with mental illness in a mental health delivery setting" (Chinman et al., 2008, p. v).

Chinman, M., Hamilton, A., Butler, B., Knight, E., Murray, S., et al. (2008). *Mental health consumer providers: a guide for clinical staff.* Retrieved from Rand Health website: www.rand.org/////_reports//_TR584.pdf.

---

between those who are hospitalized, and activities that promote recovery. Inpatient care provides structure in which patients eat meals, receive medication (if necessary), attend activities, and participate in individual and group therapies on a schedule. For those younger than the age of 18, school attendance is required. Patients are active participants in their plans of care and have the right to refuse treatments as long as they have not been declared incompetent. Advocates are usually available to provide advice and counsel for people who have doubts, and most facilities distribute a patient's bill of rights on admission or have it clearly posted. Box 5-2 provides a sample list of patient's rights.

Inpatient rooms are usually less institutional looking than other hospital rooms and tend to resemble hotel rooms. Showers may be in the individual rooms or dorm-style, with one or two per hallway. Rooms are private, semiprivate, or, occasionally, wards. Units may be made up solely of males or of females, or may be coed. Rooms are designed with safety in mind. Hanging is the most common method of inpatient suicide; therefore strict measures are taken to prevent it. Closet rods and hooks, towel bars, and shower rods are constructed to break if subjected to more than a minimal amount of weight. Sprinkler and shower heads tend to be flush mounted, and utility pipes are enclosed. Other safety

---

BOX 5-2   TYPICAL ITEMS INCLUDED IN HOSPITAL STATEMENTS OF A PATIENT'S RIGHTS

- Right to be treated with dignity
- Right to be involved in treatment planning and decisions
- Right to refuse treatment, including medications
- Right to request to leave the hospital, even against medical advice
- Right to be protected against the possible impulse to harm oneself or others that might occur as a result of a mental disorder
- Right to the benefit of the legally prescribed process of an evaluation occurring within a limited period (in most states, 72 hours) in the event of a request for discharge against medical advice that may lead to harm to self or others
- Right to legal counsel
- Right to vote
- Right to communicate privately by telephone and in person

- Right to informed consent
- Right to confidentiality regarding one's disorder and treatment
- Right to choose or refuse visitors
- Right to be informed of research and to refuse to participate
- Right to the least restrictive means of treatment
- Right to send and receive mail and to be present during any inspection of packages received
- Right to keep personal belongings unless they are dangerous
- Right to lodge a complaint through a plainly publicized procedure
- Right to participate in religious worship

---

measures include locked windows, platform beds rather than mechanical hospital beds to prevent possible crushing, and furniture with rounded corners to reduce intentional injury. Furniture for inpatient rooms tends to be heavy and durable so that it cannot be thrown or dismantled and used as a weapon.

Inpatient care begins with a medical assessment to rule out or consider co-occurring/comorbid conditions. Comprehensive assessments are conducted by a multidisciplinary team, and a plan of care is developed, monitored, evaluated, and refined. Crisis intervention and stabilization and patient safety are goals of inpatient care. Psychotropic medication evaluation, prescription, and management are usually part of the plan of care, as is individual therapy. Electroconvulsive therapy (ECT) may be ordered for certain conditions, particularly for patients with depression who have been unresponsive to antidepressants.

Group therapy is an important facet of inpatient care. Coping skills are taught and enhanced through cognitive behavioral groups that focus on symptom management. Occupational therapy provides an opportunity to practice life skills that have been delayed, hampered, or eroded. Psychoeducational groups focus on specific psychiatric disorders, medication, goal setting, life planning, and recovery.

Length of stay varies depending on the severity of the illness and symptoms. Nationwide, the mental health average length of stay is 8 days, and for substance abuse the average length of stay is 4.8 days (Piper Report, 2011). At the state level these averages may vary significantly. Therapeutic passes may be helpful so that the patient may go home for limited periods. In some cases, especially with children and people with severe mental illness, privileges and rewards, such as recreational outings, walks on the hospital grounds, and tokens to buy items from a unit "store," may be earned in order to reinforce adaptive behaviors.

Discharge planning begins on the first day of admission based on the patient's unique needs. Case management and collaboration with the patient's outpatient clinician, PCP, family, and community agencies such as the visiting nurse agency facilitate an integrated approach and establish comprehensive transition plans from inpatient to the community setting. This allows the patient to live effectively and safely in the community. Effective case management and collaboration also reduce recidivism.

At discharge, patients should be stabilized. Discharge instructions include follow-up appointments, medication directions, education and prescriptions, and, if necessary, assistance with living arrangements that may include a private residence, shelter, halfway house, or group home.

Crisis care is provided in emergency departments of general hospitals or in community-based *crisis intervention centers*. Crisis care may be initiated by the individual, friends, family, health care provider, or law enforcement personnel. Some patients are involuntarily committed. Psychiatric emergencies may include suicidal (or homicidal) ideation, acute psychosis, or behavioral responses to drugs. The stay in such facilities tends to be short, usually less than 24 hours. At that point the patient may be discharged to home, referred for inpatient care, or transferred to another community facility such as a shelter.

Residential treatment programs are structured short- or long-term living environments in which individuals are provided with varying levels of supervision and support. The residents also learn to access community support as an alternative to hospitalization and are encouraged to achieve maximal independence.

State Acute Care System

Today's state-operated psychiatric hospitals are an extension of what remains of the old system, although the quality of care in state hospitals has improved dramatically. The clinical role of state hospitals is to serve the most seriously ill patients, but this role varies widely, depending on available levels of community care and on payments by state Medicaid programs. In some states, state hospitals primarily provide intermediate treatment for patients unable to be stabilized in short-term general hospital units, and long-term care for individuals judged too ill for community care. In other states the emphasis is on acute care that is reflective of gaps in the private sector, especially for the uninsured or for those who have exhausted limited insurance benefits.

In most states the state hospitals provide forensic (court-related) care and monitoring as part of their function for those found not guilty by reason of insanity (NGRI). The state or county system also advises the courts as to defendants' sanity who may be judged to have been so ill when they committed the criminal act that they cannot be held responsible, but require treatment instead. One tragic example is that of Andrea Yates, the Texas woman who in 2001 drowned her five young children under the delusional belief she was saving them from their sinfulness. She was found NGRI and was committed to a Texas state psychiatric facility.

General Hospital Psychiatric Units and Private Psychiatric Hospital Acute Care

Acute care general hospital psychiatric units tend to be housed on a floor or floors of a general hospital. Private psychiatric hospitals are free-standing facilities. As noted, the dramatic growth of acute care psychiatric hospitals and hospital units is the result of a shift away from institutionalization in state-managed hospitals. Since that time, reduced reimbursement, increased managed care, enhanced outpatient options, and expanded availability of outpatient and partial hospitalization programs have resulted in the steady decline of these facilities. Average length of stay was declining, but has stabilized at about 9 days among the general population, 12 days for children's programs, and approximately 15 days for older adults (National Association of Psychiatric Health Systems, 2009).

Role of Psychiatric Nurses in Inpatient Care Settings

As professional care providers available around the clock every day of the week, nurses are at the center of any acute care inpatient facility. Management of these units, ideally, is by nurses with backgrounds in psychiatric mental health nursing, preferably with advanced practice degrees. Staff nurses tend to be nurse generalists, that is, nurses who have basic training as registered nurses. Some registered nurses obtain national certification in psychiatric mental health nursing through the American Nurses Credentialing Center. The staff psychiatric registered nurse carries out the following nursing responsibilities:

- Completing comprehensive data collection that includes the patient, family, and other health care workers
- Developing, implementing, and evaluating plans of care
- Assisting or supervising mental health care workers (e.g., nursing assistants with or without additional training in working with people who have mental illnesses)
- Maintaining a safe and therapeutic environment
- Facilitating health promotion through teaching
- Monitoring behavior, affect, and mood
- Maintaining oversight of restraint and seclusion

- Coordinating care by the treatment team

Medication management is an essential skill for psychiatric nurses. In this specialty area nurses often exert a strong influence on medication decisions because continual observation of the expected, interactive effects and adverse effects of medications provides the data necessary for medication adjustment. For example, feedback about a patient's excessive sedation or increased agitation will lead to a decision to decrease or increase the dosage of an antipsychotic medication.

A common misperception regarding psychiatric nurses in acute care settings is that because they "just talk" they lose their skills, including physical tasks such as starting and maintaining intravenous (IV) lines and changing dressings. First, therapeutic communication itself is a skill that people are not born with and must learn. Second, patients on the psychiatric unit are not limited to *DSM-IV-TR* diagnoses and often have complex health care needs. For example, an older adult male with brittle diabetes and a recent foot amputation may become actively suicidal. In this case, it is likely he will be transferred to the psychiatric unit, where his blood glucose level will be monitored and wound care completed.

SPECIALTY TREATMENT SETTINGS

Treatment options are available that provide specialized care for specific groups of people. These options include inpatient, outpatient, and residential care.

Pediatric Psychiatric Care

Children with mental illnesses have the same range of treatment options as do adults but receive them apart from adults in pediatric settings. Inpatient care may be necessary if the child's symptoms become severe. Parental or guardian—including Department of Children and Families—involvement in the plan of care is integral so that they understand the illness, treatment, and the family's role in supporting the child. Additionally, hospitalized children, if able, attend school several hours a day.

Geriatric Psychiatric Care

The older adult population may be treated in specialized mental health settings that take into account the effects of aging on psychiatric symptoms. Physical illness and loss of independence can be strong precipitants in the development of depression and anxiety. Dementia is a particularly common problem encountered in geriatric psychiatry. Treatment is aimed at careful evaluation of the interaction of mind and body and provision of care that optimizes strengths, promotes independence, and focuses on safety.

Veterans Administration Centers

Active military personnel and veterans who were not dishonorably discharged may receive federally funded inpatient or outpatient care and medication for psychiatric and alcohol or substance abuse. One of the greatest challenges veterans face is dealing with the aftereffects of the traumas of active combat. During Civil

War times these late effects were termed "soldiers heart." After World War I, soldiers had "shell shock" and after World War II it was termed "battle fatigue." Currently mental health services are inundated by people suffering from posttraumatic stress disorder (PTSD). There is a prevalence of PTSD in the general population of about 7% and nearly 14% for veterans of the wars in Iraq and Afghanistan. This creates a tremendous need for strong psychiatric services for this population (Gradus, 2010).

Forensic Psychiatric Care

Incarcerated populations, both adult and juvenile, have higher than average incidences of mental disorders or substance abuse. Researchers estimate that there are more people with mental illness in prisons than in hospitals (Torrey et al., 2010). Treatment may be provided within the prison system, where inmates are often separated from the general prison population. State hospitals also treat forensic patients. Most facilities provide psychotherapy, group counseling, medication management, and assistance with transition to the community.

Alcohol and Drug Abuse Treatment

All the mental health settings that were previously described may provide treatment for alcohol and substance abuse, although specialized treatment centers exist apart from the mental health care system. More than 4 million people aged 12 or older (nearly 2% of the population) received treatment for alcohol or illicit drug use in 2009 (Substance Abuse and Mental Health Services Administration [SAMHSA], 2010). This treatment is typically outpatient and includes counseling, education, medication management, and 12-step programs. Because alcohol detoxification can be life-threatening, inpatient care may be required for medical management. Drug rehabilitation facilities provide inpatient care for detoxification of drugs, including opiates and chemicals, and offer all levels of outpatient care.

Self-Help Options

Obtaining sufficient sleep, meditating, eating right, exercising, abstaining from smoking, and limiting the use of alcohol are healthy responses to a variety of illnesses such as diabetes and hypertension. As with other medical conditions, lifestyle choices and self-help responses can have a profound influence on the quality of life and the course, progression, and outcome of psychiatric disorders. If we accept the notion that psychiatric disorders are usually a combination of biochemical interactions, genetics, and environment, then it stands to reason that by providing a healthy living situation, we are likely to fare better. If, for example, a person has a family history of anxiety and has demonstrated symptoms of anxiety, then a good first step (or an adjunct to psychiatric treatment) could be to learn yoga and balance the amounts of life's obligations with relaxation.

A voluntary network of self-help groups operates outside the formal mental health care system to provide education, contacts, and support. Since the introduction of Alcoholics Anonymous in the early twentieth century, self-help groups have multiplied and have proven to be effective in the treatment and support of psychiatric problems. Groups specific to anxiety, depression, loss, caretakers' issues, bipolar disorder, posttraumatic stress disorder, and almost every other psychiatric issue are widely available in most communities.

Consumers, people who use mental health services, and their family members have successfully united to shape the delivery of mental health care. Nonprofit organizations such as the National Alliance on Mental Illness (NAMI) encourage self-help and promote the concept of **recovery,** or the self-management of mental illness. Introduced in Chapter 1 and discussed further in Chapters 3 and 19, these grassroots' groups also confront social stigma, influence policies, and support the rights of people experiencing mental illness.

PAYING FOR MENTAL HEALTH CARE

Most Americans are covered by private insurance that pays varying amounts for mental health care. Standard policies not only allow people to choose their providers and seek treatment but also provide some portion of reimbursement. Managed care plans stipulate the providers members may visit and then may cover the entire costs or require copays from the members. Low-income Medicaid and Medicare recipients may also be enrolled in managed care plans. Both standard policies and managed care plans provide coverage for mental health care, although it is often not at the same rate as is coverage for physical care.

Limits in health insurance are problematic in terms of coverage for mental illnesses. Because most health insurance is employer based and because serious mental illness can lead to job loss, many individuals with serious mental illness have no coverage. State systems exist, in part, as a "safety net" for the limits in health insurance. Furthermore, most private insurance plans (along with Medicare) have enacted coverage limits that are more restrictive for treatment of mental illness than other illnesses with annual or lifetime caps on days of care or on total expenses.

In 1996 the federal government enacted a mental health parity law that made it illegal for companies with more than 50 employees to limit annual or lifetime mental health benefits unless they also limited benefits for physical illnesses. Although this federal legislation was a good start, problems remained. One problem is that reimbursement does not include substance abuse or chemical dependency treatment. The Paul Wellstone and Pete Domenici Mental Health Parity and Addiction Equity Act of 2008 expanded the 1996 legislation by adding addictions to the mental health benefits list; this act became effective in early 2010 (SAMHSA, 2010). It is important to note that both legislators had relatives with severe mental illness—Wellstone's brother had a severe mental illness and Domenici's daughter has schizophrenia.

This latest federal legislation protects state parity laws that may actually be stronger, but preempts (takes the place of) weaker state parity laws. Coverage varies by state. For example, Arkansas provides coverage for all mental illness. Other states limit the coverage to a specific list of biologically based—a term with several definitions—mental illnesses. In Ohio this list includes schizophrenia, schizoaffective disorder, major depressive disorder, bipolar disorder, paranoia and other psychotic disorders, obsessive-compulsive disorder, and panic disorder (Ohio Laws, 2007). As of February 2010, 30 states were designated as offering full parity for mental illness insurance coverage (National Conference of State Legislatures, 2010).

In addition to the state systems of care, public assistance is available for mental health care and costs of living. Four assistance programs are Medicare, Medicaid, Social Security, and the Veterans Administration (VA). Medicare is a national program that provides benefits to those who are 65 years of age or older and to those who have become totally disabled. In the case of mental illness, benefits are limited and coverage may be 50% for outpatient care compared with 80% for non–mental health outpatient care. Medicaid operates under federal guidelines and state regulations and pays mental health care costs for people who have extreme financial need.

States vary widely in how they fund mental health care, but all states must provide benefits for inpatient care, PCP services, and treatment for those younger than age 21. Social Security has two federal programs designed to help people with disabilities. Social Security Disability Insurance (SSDI) may be awarded to individuals who have worked a required length of time, have paid into Social Security, and are disabled for 12 months or more. Supplemental Security Income (SSI) provides benefits based on economic need (Social Security Administration, 2011). Among people receiving Social Security disability income, psychiatric disorders are the largest and fastest growing subgroup (Drake et al., 2009).

A VISION FOR MENTAL HEALTH CARE IN AMERICA

Despite the availability and variety of community psychiatric treatments in the United States, many patients in this country in need of services are not receiving them. In addition to stigma, there are geographic, financial, and systems factors that impede access to psychiatric care. For example, mental health services are scarce in some rural areas, and many American families cannot afford health insurance even if they are working. The President's New Freedom Commission on Mental Health was charged with studying the mental health system and issuing recommendations for its transformation (2003). It is likely that their recommendations will influence the direction of mental health care for the next 2 decades. Their final report identifies that in a transformed mental health care system:
- Americans understand that mental health is essential to overall health.
- Mental health care is consumer and family driven.
- Disparities in mental health services are eliminated.
- Early mental health screening, assessment, and referral to services are common practice.

- Excellent mental health care is delivered and research is accelerated.
- Technology is used to access mental health care and information.

Psychiatric registered nurses are uniquely qualified to address each of the aforementioned goals by virtue of an integrated educational background that includes biology, psychology, and the social sciences. Nurses specializing in this area will increasingly be in demand. As the population ages, more geropsychiatric nurses will be needed to work with older adult psychiatric patients with complex health problems. Advanced practice psychiatric nurses may collaborate more with primary health care practitioners or in independent practice to fill the gap in existing community services. Psychiatric nurses can help make the vision statement from the President's New Freedom Commission on Mental Health (2003) a reality:

> We envision a future when everyone with a mental illness will recover, a future when mental illnesses can be prevented or cured, a future when mental illnesses are detected early, and a future when everyone with a mental illness at any stage of life has access to effective treatment supports— essentials for living, working, learning, and participating fully in the community.

On March 23, 2010, President Obama, signed into law the **Affordable Care Act**. This groundbreaking piece of legislation will help insure millions of people who could not previously afford healthcare insurance. This will include millions of children and adults with mental health conditions who will no longer be denied healthcare because of pre-existing conditions. Some other provisions under this law include:
- Insurance companies can no longer deny a person because of pre-existing conditions or for resending or taking away insurance for health/mental health related reasons
- Expansion of coverage for young adults up to the age of 26 under the parents' family policy
- A provision for people over 65 on Medicare — a 50% discount for name brand drugs who reach the Medicare "doughnut-hole"
- Provides small business tax credits
- Provides affordable coverage to millions of Americans who aren't able to afford care
- People with existing healthcare coverage are able to keep or choose their doctors

Parts of this law have already gone into effect, and the complete Affordable Care Act is due to go into effect in 2014.

KEY POINTS TO REMEMBER

- Compared to seeking care for physical disorders, finding care for psychiatric disorders can be complicated by a two-tiered system of care provided in the private and public sectors.
- Nonspecialist primary care providers treat a significant portion of psychiatric disorders.
- Psychiatric care providers are specialists who are licensed to prescribe medication and conduct therapy. They include psychiatrists, advanced practice psychiatric nurses, physicians' assistants, and, in some states, psychologists.
- Community mental health centers are state-regulated and state-funded facilities that are staffed by a variety of mental health care professionals.
- Other outpatient settings include psychiatric home care, intensive outpatient programs, and partial hospitalization programs.
- Inpatient care is used when less restrictive outpatient options are insufficient in dealing with symptoms. It can be provided in general medical centers, private psychiatric centers, crisis units, and state hospitals.
- Nurses provide the basis for inpatient care and are part of the overall unit milieu that emphasizes the role of the total environment in providing support and treatment.
- Specific populations such as children, veterans, geriatrics, and forensics benefit from treatment geared to their unique needs.
- Financing psychiatric care has been complicated by lack of parity, or equal payment for physical as compared to psychiatric disorders. Legislation has been proposed and passed to improve mental health parity.

APPLYING CRITICAL JUDGMENT

1. You are a community psychiatric mental health nurse working at a local mental health center. You are conducting an assessment interview with a single male patient who is 45 years old. He reports that he has not been sleeping and that his thoughts seem to be "all tangled up." He informs you that he hopes you can help him today because he does not know how much longer he can go on. He does not make any direct reference to suicidal intent. He is disheveled and has been sleeping at shelters. He has little contact with his family and starts to become agitated when you suggest that it might be helpful for you to contact them. He refuses to sign any release of information forms. He admits to recent hospitalization at the local veterans' hospital and reports previous treatment at a dual-diagnosis facility even though he denies substance abuse. In addition to his mental health problems, he says that he has tested positive for human immunodeficiency virus and takes multiple medications that he cannot name.

   A. What are your biopsychosocial and spiritual concerns about this patient?
   B. What is the highest priority problem to address before he leaves the clinic today?
   C. Do you feel that you need to consult with any other members of the multidisciplinary team today about this patient?
   D. In your role as case manager, what systems of care will you need to coordinate to provide quality care for this patient?
   E. How will you start to develop trust with the patient to gain his cooperation with the treatment plan?

CHAPTER REVIEW QUESTIONS

Choose the most appropriate answer(s).

1. A 24-year-old female is diagnosed with alcohol dependence and requires acute detoxification. The most appropriate setting is:
   1. partial hospitalization.
   2. residential setting.
   3. rehab unit.
   4. acute inpatient care.
2. A significant influence allowing psychiatric treatment to move from the hospital to the community was:
   1. television.
   2. the development of psychotropic medications.
   3. identification of external causes of mental illness.
   4. the use of a collaborative approach by patients and staff focusing on rehabilitation.
3. Which of the following is a benefit for patients being treated for mental health problems by a primary care physician rather than a psychiatrist?
   1. A high level of expertise in the diagnosis of psychiatric disorders
   2. Extended time in the physician's office for a thorough psychiatric assessment
   3. Feeling that there is less stigma attached to treatment
   4. A high level of expertise in the management of psychopharmacological medications for psychiatric illnesses
4. A 45-year-old patient experiencing increased symptoms of anxiety lives in a rural community over 100 miles from the nearest psychiatrist. Other health team members are located closer to his residence. Which of the following health care

professionals could provide an initial screening and treatment plan for this patient? (Select all that apply.)

1. Social worker
2. Psychologist
3. Primary care provider
4. Advanced practice psychiatric nurse

5. A community mental health student nurse is asked by her supervisor to develop a stress reduction class for the residents in the surrounding community. The student nurse resists, saying that her responsibilities are to her patient caseload.

The supervisor explains to the student why this assignment is appropriate for her role. Which is the most suitable rationale that the supervisor can provide to the student nurse?

1. Stress reduction is important to a patient's mental health.
2. Funding sources will support the class only if it is developed by a nurse.
3. An important concept for community health nursing is to view the entire community as a patient.
4. Research has demonstrated that stress reduction reduces hypertension in mental health patients.

REFERENCES

Agency for Healthcare Research and Quality. (2011). *What is PCMH?* Retrieved 12/29/2011 from http://ahrq.gov/portal/server.pt/community/pcmh__home/1483/what_is_pcmh.

Boscarino, J. A., Larson, S., Ladd, I., Hill, E., & Paolucci, S. J. (2010). Mental health experiences and needs among primary care providers treating OEF/OIF veterans: preliminary findings from the Geisinger Veterans Initiative. *International Journal of Emergency Mental Health, 12*(3), 161–170.

Drake, R. E., Skinner, J. S., Bond, G. R., & Goldman, H. H. (2009). Social security and mental illness: reducing disability with supported employment. *Health Affairs, 28*(3), 761–770.

Gradus, J. L. (2010). Epidemiology of PTSD. In *United States Department of Veterans Affairs.* Retrieved April 16, 2011, from www.ptsd.va.gov/professional/pages/epidemiological-facts-ptsd.asp.

Kessler, R. C., Berglund, P., Demler, O., et al. (2005). Lifetime prevalence and age-of-onset distributions of *DSM-IV* disorders in the national comorbidity survey replication. *Archives of General Psychiatry, 62*, 593–602.

National Association of Psychiatric Health Systems. (2009). *2008 NAPHS Annual Survey.* Washington, DC: Author.

National Association of State Mental Health Program Directors. (2011). *State psychiatric hospitals.* Retrieved April 14, 2011, from www.nasmhpd.org/state_hospitals.cfm.

National Conference of State Legislatures. (2010). *State laws mandating or regulating mental health benefits.* Retrieved April 20, 2011, from www.ncsl.org/default.aspx?tabid=14352.

Ohio Laws. (2007). Health coverage plans—biologically based mental illness. Ohio Revised Code. Retrieved April 20, 2011, from http://codes.ohio.gov/orc/3923.282.

Piper Report. (2011). *Hospitalizations for mental health and substance abuse disorders: costs, length of stay, patient mix, and payor mix.* Retrieved June 1, 2012, from http://www.pipperreport.com/blog/2011/06/25/hospitalizations-for-mental-health-and-substance-abuse-disorders.

President's New Freedom Commission on Mental Health. (2003). *Achieving the promise: transforming mental health care in America.* Retrieved February 18, 2008, from www.mentalhealthcommission.gov/reports/FinalReport/toc.html.

Social Security Administration. (2011). *Understanding supplemental security income.* Retrieved April 20, 2011, from www.ssa.gov/ssi/text-eligibility-ussi.htm.

Substance Abuse and Mental Health Services Administration. (2010). *Results from the 2009 national survey on drug use and health.* Retrieved April 16, 2011, from http://oas.samhsa.gov/NSDUH/2k9NSDUH/2k9Results.htm#Ch3.

Torrey, E. F., Kennard, A. D., Eslinger, D., Lamb, R., & Pavle, J. (2010). *More mentally ill persons are in jails and prisons than hospitals: a survey of the states.* Retrieved April 16, 2011, from http://74.125.155.132/scholar?q=cache:_ulTyMxYGAsJ:scholar.google.com/+percent+of+prison+population+with+a+mental+disorder&hl=en&as_sdt=0,36&as_ylo=2009.

United States Psychiatric Rehabilitation Services. (2011). *About the US Psychiatric Rehabilitation Association.* Retrieved April 19, 2011, from https://netforum.avectra.com/eweb/DynamicPage.aspx?Site=USPRA&WebCode=about.

Legal and Ethical Basis for Practice

Penny Simpson Brooke

evolve WEBSITE

http://evolve.elsevier.com/Varcarolis/essentials

KEY TERMS AND CONCEPTS

SELECTED CONCEPT: Right to Treatment

With the enactment of the Hospitalization of the Mentally Ill Act in 1964, the federal statutory right to psychiatric treatment in public hospitals was created. The statute requires that medical and psychiatric care and treatment be provided to everyone admitted to a public hospital.

Based on the decisions of a number of early court cases, treatment must meet the following criteria:

- The environment must be humane.
- Staff must be qualified and sufficient to provide adequate treatment.
- The plan of care must be individualized.

OBJECTIVES

1. Compare and contrast the different admissions procedures including admission criteria.
2. Summarize patients' rights as they pertain to the patient's (a) right to treatment, (b) right to refuse treatment, and (c) right to informed consent.
3. Delineate the steps nurses are advised to take if they suspect negligence or illegal activity on the part of a professional colleague or peer.
4. Discuss the legal considerations of patient privilege (a) after a patient has died, (b) if the patient tests positive for human immunodeficiency virus, or (c) if the patient's employer states a "need to know."
5. Summarize situations in which health care professionals have a duty to break patient confidentiality.
6. Discuss a patient's civil rights and describe how they pertain to restraint and seclusion.
7. Discuss in detail the balance between the patient's rights and the rights of society with respect to the following legal concepts relevant in nursing and psychiatric nursing: (a) duty to intervene, (b) documentation and charting, and (c) confidentiality.

This chapter introduces you to current legal and ethical issues that may be encountered in the practice of psychiatric nursing. A fundamental goal of psychiatric care is to strike a balance between the rights of the individual patient and the rights of society at large. This chapter is designed to assist you in understanding the implications of ethical or legal issues on the provision of care in a psychiatric setting.

An **ethical dilemma** results when there is a conflict between two or more courses of action, each carrying with them favorable and unfavorable consequences. How we respond to these dilemmas is based partly on our own morals (beliefs of right or wrong) and values. Suppose you are caring for a pregnant woman with schizophrenia who wants to carry the baby to term, but whose family insists she get an abortion. In order to promote fetal safety, her antipsychotic medication will need to be reduced, putting her at risk of exacerbation of the illness. Furthermore, there is a question as to whether she can safely care for the child. If you relied on the ethical principle of autonomy, you may conclude that she has the right to decide. Would other ethical principles be in conflict with autonomy in this case?

At times your values may be in conflict with the value system of the institution. This situation further complicates the decision-making process and necessitates careful consideration of the patient's desires. For example, you may experience a conflict in a setting where older adult patients are routinely tranquilized to a degree that you find excessive. Whenever one's value system is challenged, increased stress results.

LEGAL AND ETHICAL CONCEPTS

Ethics is the study of philosophical beliefs about what is considered right or wrong in a society. **Bioethics** is a more specific term that refers to the ethical questions that arise in health care. The five basic principles of bioethics are as follows:

1. **Beneficence:** The duty to act so as to benefit or promote the good of others. Spending extra time to help calm an extremely anxious patient is a beneficent act.
2. **Autonomy:** Respecting the rights of others to make their own decisions. Acknowledging the patient's right to refuse medication is an example of promoting autonomy.
3. **Justice:** The duty to distribute resources or care equally, regardless of personal attributes. An example of justice is when an intensive care unit (ICU) nurse devotes equal attention both to a patient who has attempted suicide and to another patient who suffered a brain aneurysm.
4. **Fidelity** (nonmaleficence): Maintaining loyalty and commitment to the patient and doing no wrong to the patient. Maintaining expertise in nursing skill through nursing education demonstrates fidelity to patient care.
5. **Veracity:** One's duty to communicate truthfully. Describing the purpose and side effects of psychotropic medications in a truthful and nonmisleading way is an example of veracity.

Law and ethics are closely related because law tends to reflect the ethical values of society. It should be noted that although you may feel obligated to follow ethical guidelines, these guidelines should not override laws. For example, if you are aware of a statute or a specific rule or regulation created by the state board of nursing that prohibits a certain action (e.g., restraining patients against their will) and you feel you have an ethical obligation to protect the patient by engaging in such an action (e.g., using restraints), you would be wise to follow the law.

MENTAL HEALTH LAWS

Laws have been enacted to regulate the care and treatment of the mentally ill. Mental health laws, or statutes, vary from state to state; in order to understand the legal climate of your specific state, you are encouraged to review its code. This can be accomplished by visiting the webpage of your state mental health department or by doing an Internet search using the following key words: 'mental + health + statutes + (your state).'

Many of these laws have undergone major revision since 1963, which reflects a shift in emphasis from state or institutional care of the mentally ill to community-based care. This was heralded by the enactment of the Community Mental Health Center Act of 1963 under President John F. Kennedy.

Along with this shift in emphasis has come the more wide-spread use of psychotropic drugs in the treatment of mental illness—which has enabled many people to integrate more readily into the larger community—and an increasing awareness of the need to provide the mentally ill with humane care that respects their civil rights. Parity in health insurance coverage for mental health treatment was addressed in 2010 by two separate laws. The Paul Wellstone and Pete Domenici Mental Health Parity and Addiction Equity Act states that if mental health or substance abuse care is covered by a private insurance plan, then these conditions must receive coverage equitable to other physical medical conditions. The 2010 Health Insurance Exchanges program requires that each state offers mental health care and substance abuse services equal to other medical services (Bazelon, 2010).

Civil Rights

People with mental illness are guaranteed the same rights under federal and state laws as any other citizen. Most states specifically prohibit any person from depriving an individual receiving mental health services of his or her civil rights, including the right to vote; the right to civil service ranking; the rights related to granting, forfeit, or denial of a driver's license; the right to make purchases and to enter contractual relationships (unless the patient has lost legal capacity by being incompetent); and the right to press charges against another person. The psychiatric patient's rights include the right to humane care and treatment. The medical, dental, and psychiatric needs of the patient must be met in accordance with the prevailing standards accepted in these professions. The mentally ill in prisons and jails are afforded the same protections. The right to religious freedom and practice, the right to social interaction, and the right to exercise and recreational opportunities are also protected.

In recent years many states have established Mental Health Courts to process criminal cases involving defendants with mental illnesses. These courts attempt to direct the offender to treatment and services in the community (Bazelon, 2011).

ADMISSION AND DISCHARGE PROCEDURES

Due Process in Civil Commitment

The courts have recognized that involuntary civil commitment to a mental hospital is a "massive curtailment of liberty" (*Humphrey v. Cady*, 1972) requiring due process protections in the civil commitment procedure. This right derives from the Fifth Amendment of the U.S. Constitution, which states that "no person shall…be deprived of life, liberty, or property without due process of law." The Fourteenth Amendment explicitly prohibits states from depriving citizens of life, liberty, and property without due process of law. State civil commitment statutes, if challenged in the courts on constitutional grounds, must afford minimal due process protections to pass the court's scrutiny (*Zinermon v. Burch*, 1990). In most states, a patient can challenge commitments through a writ of habeas corpus, which means a "formal written order"

to "free the person." The writ of habeas corpus is the procedural mechanism used to challenge unlawful detention by the government.

The writ of habeas corpus and the least restrictive alternative doctrine are two of the most important concepts applicable to civic commitment cases. The least restrictive alternative doctrine mandates that the least drastic means be taken to achieve a specific purpose. For example, if someone can safely be treated for depression on an outpatient basis, hospitalization would be too restrictive and unnecessarily disruptive.

Admission to the Hospital

All students are encouraged to become familiar with the important provisions of the laws in their own states regarding admissions, discharges, patient's rights, and informed consent.

A medical standard or justification for admission should exist. A well-defined psychiatric problem must be established, based on current illness classifications in the current *Diagnostic and Statistical Manual of Mental Disorders (DSM)* authored by the American Psychiatric Association. The presenting illness should also be of such a nature that it causes an immediate crisis situation or that other less restrictive alternatives are inadequate or unavailable. There should also be a reasonable expectation that the hospitalization and treatment will improve the presenting problems.

In the case of *Olmstead v. L.C.* (1999) the Supreme Court of the United States ruled that states are required to place patients with mental health illness in less restrictive community settings, rather than institutions, when the treatment profession has determined that a community setting is appropriate and the patient is not opposed to the decision to transfer from an institution to a community facility.

Voluntary Admission

Generally, voluntary admission is sought by the patient or the patient's guardian through a written application to the facility. Voluntarily admitted patients have the right to demand and obtain release. However, few states require voluntarily admitted patients to be notified of the rights associated with their status. In addition, many states require that a patient submit a written release notice to the facility staff, who reevaluate the patient's condition for possible conversion to involuntary status according to criteria established by state law.

Involuntary Admission (Commitment)

Involuntary admission is made without the patient's consent. Generally, involuntary admission is necessary when a person is in need of psychiatric treatment, presents a danger to self or others, or is unable to meet his or her own basic needs. Involuntary commitment requires that the patient retain freedom from unreasonable bodily restraints as well as the right to informed consent and the right to refuse medications, including psychotropic or antipsychotic medications.

Three different commitment procedures are commonly available: **judicial determination, administrative determination,** and **agency determination.** In addition, a specified number of physicians must certify that a person's mental health status justifies detention and treatment. Involuntary hospitalization can be further categorized by the nature and purpose of the involuntary admission: emergency hospitalization; observational or temporary hospitalization; long-term or formal commitment; or outpatient commitment.

Emergency involuntary hospitalization. Most states provide for emergency involuntary hospitalization or civil **commitment** for a specified period (1 to 10 days on average) to prevent dangerous behavior that is likely to cause harm to self or others. Police officers, physicians, and mental health professionals may be designated by law to authorize the detention of mentally ill individuals who are a danger to themselves or others.

Observational or temporary involuntary hospitalization. Civil commitment for observational or temporary involuntary hospitalization is of longer duration than emergency hospitalization. The primary purpose of this type of hospitalization is observation, diagnosis, and treatment for those who have mental illness or pose a danger to themselves or others. The length of time and procedures vary markedly from state to state. A guardian, family member, physician, or other public health officer may apply for this type of admission. Certification by two or more physicians, a judicial review, or administrative review and order is often required for involuntary admission.

Long-term or formal commitment. Long-term commitment for involuntary hospitalization has as its primary purpose extended care and treatment of the mentally ill. Those who undergo extended involuntary hospitalization are committed through medical certification, judicial, or administrative action. Some states do not require a judicial hearing before commitment, but often provide the patient with an opportunity for a judicial review after commitment procedures. This type of involuntary hospitalization generally lasts 60 to 180 days, but may be for an indeterminate period.

Involuntary outpatient commitment. Beginning in the 1990s, states began to pass legislation that permitted outpatient commitment as an alternative to forced inpatient treatment. Recently states are using **involuntary outpatient commitment** as a preventive measure, allowing a court order before the onset of a psychiatric crisis that would result in an inpatient commitment. The order for involuntary outpatient commitment is usually tied to receipt of goods and services provided by social welfare agencies, including disability benefits and housing. To access these goods and services the patient is mandated to participate in treatment and may face inpatient admission if he or she fails to participate in treatment (Chan, 2003; Monahan et al., 2003; Rainey, 2001). Forced treatment raises ethical dilemmas regarding autonomy versus paternalism, privacy rights, duty to protect, and right to treatment; and has been challenged on constitutional grounds.

Discharge from the Hospital

Release from hospitalization depends on the patient's admission status. Patients who sought informal or voluntary admission, as previously discussed, have the right to request and receive release. Some states, however, do provide for conditional release of voluntary patients, which enables the treating physician or administrator to order continued treatment on an outpatient basis if the clinical needs of the patient warrant further care.

Conditional Release

Conditional release usually requires outpatient treatment for a specified period to determine the patient's adherence with medication protocols, ability to meet basic needs, and ability to reintegrate into the community. Generally a voluntarily hospitalized patient who is conditionally released can only be committed through the usual methods for involuntary hospitalization. However, an involuntarily hospitalized patient who is conditionally released may be reinstitutionalized while the commitment is still in effect without recommencement of formal admission procedures.

Unconditional Release

Unconditional release, or **discharge**, is the termination of a patient-institution relationship. This release may be court ordered or administratively ordered by the institution's officials. Generally, the administrative officer of an institution has the discretion to discharge patients.

Release Against Medical Advice (AMA)

In some cases there is a disagreement between mental health care providers and patients as to whether continued hospitalization is necessary. When treatment seems beneficial, but there is no compelling reason (e.g., danger to self or others) to seek an involuntary continuance of stay, patients may be released against medical advice.

PATIENTS' RIGHTS UNDER THE LAW

Psychiatric facilities usually provide patients with a written list of basic patient rights. These rights are derived from a variety of sources, especially legislation that developed during the 1960s. Since then, they have been modified to some degree, but most lists share commonalities in the following text.

Right to Treatment

With the enactment of the Hospitalization of the Mentally Ill Act in 1964, the federal statutory right to psychiatric treatment in public hospitals was created. The statute requires that medical and psychiatric care and treatment be provided to everyone admitted to a public hospital.

Although state courts and lower federal courts have decided that there may be a federal constitutional right to treatment, the U.S. Supreme Court has never firmly defined the **right to treatment** in a constitutional principle. The evolution of these cases in the courts provides an interesting history of the development and shortcomings of our mental health delivery system. Based on the decisions of a number of early court cases, treatment must meet the following criteria:

- The environment must be humane.
- Staff must be qualified and sufficient to provide adequate treatment.
- The plan of care must be individualized.

The initial cases presenting the psychiatric patient's right to treatment arose in the criminal justice system. An interesting case regarding a person's right to treatment is *O'Connor v. Donaldson* (1975). The Court held that a "state cannot constitutionally confine a nondangerous individual who is capable of surviving safely in freedom by himself or with the help of willing and responsible family members or friends."

Right to Refuse Treatment

A companion to the right to consent to treatment is the right to withhold consent. A patient may also withdraw consent at any time. Retraction of consent previously given must be honored, whether it is verbal or written. However, the mentally ill patient's right to refuse treatment with psychotropic drugs has been debated in the courts, based partly on the issue of mental patients' competency to give or withhold consent to treatment and their status under the civil commitment statutes. These early cases, initiated by state hospital patients, considered medical, legal, and ethical considerations, such as basic treatment problems, the doctrine of informed consent, and the bioethical principle of autonomy. For a summary of the evolution of one landmark set of cases regarding the patient's right to refuse treatment, see Table 6-1.

The notion of refusing treatment becomes especially important if we consider medication to be a "chemical restraint." If it is, then the infringement on a person's liberty is at least equal to that with involuntary commitment. In this circumstance, the noninstitutionalized, competent, mentally ill patient has the right, through substituted judgment, to determine whether to be involuntarily committed or to be medicated.

Cases involving the right to refuse psychotropic drug treatment are still evolving. Without clear direction from the Supreme Court, there will be different case outcomes in different jurisdictions.

The numerous cases involving the right to refuse medication have illustrated the complex and difficult task of translating social policy concerns into a clearly articulated legal standard.

Right to Informed Consent

The principle of informed consent is based on a person's right to self-determination, as enunciated in the landmark case of *Canterbury v. Spence* (1972):

> The root premise is the concept, fundamental in American jurisprudence, that every human being of adult years and sound mind has a right to determine what shall be done with his own body.... True consent to what happens to one's self is the informed exercise of choice, and that entails an opportunity to evaluate knowledgeably the options available and the risks attendant on each.

Proper orders for specific therapies and treatments are required and must be documented in the patient's chart. Consent for surgery, electroconvulsive treatment, or the use of experimental drugs or procedures must be obtained. In some state institutions, consent is required for every medication addition or change. Patients have the right to refuse participation in experimental treatments or research and the right to voice grievances and recommend changes in policies or services offered by the facility, without fear of punishment or reprisal.

TABLE 6-1	RIGHT TO REFUSE TREATMENT: EVOLUTION OF MASSACHUSETTS CASE LAW TO PRESENT LAW	
CASE	**COURT**	**DECISION**
Rogers v. Okin, 478 F. Supp. 1342 (D. Mass. 1979)	Federal district court	Ruled that involuntarily hospitalized patients with mental illness are competent and have the right to make treatment decisions. Forcible administration of medication is justified in an emergency if needed to prevent violence and if other alternatives have been ruled out. A guardian may make treatment decisions for an incompetent patient.
Rogers v. Okin, 634 F. 2nd 650 (1st Cir. 1980)	Federal court of appeals	Affirmed that involuntarily hospitalized patients with mental illness are competent and have the right to make treatment decisions. The staff has substantial discretion in an emergency. Forcible medication is also justified to prevent the patient's deterioration. A patient's rights must be protected by judicial determination of competency or incompetency.
Mills v. Rogers, 457 U.S. 291 (1982)	U.S. Supreme Court	Set aside the judgment of the court of appeals with instructions to consider the effect of an intervening state court case.
Rogers v. Commissioner of the Department of Mental Health, 458 N.E.2d 308 (Mass. 1983)	Massachusetts Supreme Judicial Court answering questions certified by federal court of appeals	Ruled that involuntarily hospitalized patients are competent and have the right to make treatment decisions unless they are judicially determined to be incompetent.

For consent to be effective legally, it must be informed. Generally, the informed consent of the patient must be obtained by the physician or other health professional who will perform the treatment or procedure. Patients must be informed of the nature of their problem or condition, the nature and purpose of a proposed treatment, the risks and benefits of that treatment, the alternative treatment options available, the probability that the proposed treatment will be successful, and the risks of not consenting to treatment. It is important for psychiatric nurses to know that the presence of psychotic thinking does not mean that the patient is incompetent or incapable of understanding.

Neither voluntary nor involuntary admission to a mental facility determines whether patients are capable of making informed decisions about the health care they may need. Patients must be considered legally competent until they have been declared incompetent through a legal proceeding. Competency is related to the capacity to understand the consequences of one's decisions. The determination of legal competency is made by the courts. If found incompetent, the court may appoint a legal guardian or representative who is legally responsible for giving or refusing consent for a person the court has found to be incompetent. A court-appointed guardian must always consider the patient's wishes. Guardians are usually selected from among family members. The order of selection is usually (1) spouse, (2) adult children or grandchildren, (3) parents, (4) adult brothers and sisters, and (5) nieces and nephews. In the event that a family member is either unavailable or unwilling to serve as guardian, the court may also appoint a court-trained and court-approved social worker representing the county or state or a member of the community.

Many procedures that nurses perform have an element of implied consent attached. For example, if you approach the patient with a medication in hand and the patient indicates a willingness to receive the medication, implied consent has occurred. It should be noted that many institutions, particularly state psychiatric hospitals, have a requirement to obtain informed consent for every medication given. A general rule for you to follow is that the more intrusive or risky the procedure, the higher the likelihood that informed consent must be obtained. The fact that you may not have a legal duty to be the person to inform patients of the associated risks and benefits of a particular medical procedure does not excuse you from clarifying the procedure to patients and ensuring their expressed or implied consent.

Rights Surrounding Involuntary Commitment and Psychiatric Advance Directives

Patients concerned that they may be subject to involuntary psychiatric commitment can prepare an advance psychiatric directive document that will express their treatment choices. The advance directive for mental health decision making should be followed by health care providers when patients are not competent to make informed decisions for themselves. This document can clarify the patient's choice of a surrogate decision maker and instructions about hospital choices, medications, treatment options, and emergency interventions. Identification of individuals who are to be notified of the patient's hospitalization and who may have visitation rights is especially helpful given the privacy demands of the Health Insurance Portability and Accountability Act (HIPAA) (Bazelon, 2003).

Rights Regarding Restraint and Seclusion

As mentioned, the use of the least restrictive means of restraint for the shortest duration is always the general rule. Verbal interventions or enlisting the cooperation of patients are examples of first-line interventions. Typically, medication is considered if verbal interventions fail. Chemical interventions are usually considered less restrictive than mechanical, but can have a greater effect on the patient's ability to relate to the environment. When used judiciously, psychopharmacology is extremely effective and helpful as an alternative to other physical methods of restraint.

The history of mechanical restraint and seclusion is one that is marked by abuses and overuse, and even a tendency to use restraint as punishment. This was especially true before the 1950s, when there were no effective chemical treatments. Legislation has dramatically reduced this problem by mandating strict guidelines. Behavioral restraint and seclusion are authorized as an intervention under the following circumstances:

- When the particular behavior is physically harmful to the patient or a third party
- When alternative or less restrictive measures are insufficient in protecting the patient or others from harm
- When a decrease in sensory overstimulation (seclusion only) is needed
- When the patient anticipates that a controlled environment would be helpful and requests seclusion

As indicated, most state laws prohibit the use of unnecessary physical restraint or isolation. The use of seclusion and restraint is permitted only under the following circumstances (Simon, 1999):

- On the written order of a physician
- When orders are confined to specific time-limited periods (e.g., 2 to 4 hours)
- When the patient's condition is reviewed and documented regularly (e.g., every 15 minutes)
- When the original order is extended after review and reauthorization (e.g., every 24 hours) and specifies the type of restraint

In an emergency, the nurse may place a patient in seclusion or restraint and obtain a written or verbal order as soon as possible thereafter. With the exception of a patient-initiated request to be placed in seclusion, federal laws require an emergency situation to exist in which an immediate risk of harm to the patient or others can be documented. While in restraints the patient must be protected from all sources of harm. The behavior leading to restraint or seclusion and the time the patient is placed in and released from the restraint must be documented; the patient in restraint must be assessed at regular and frequent intervals (e.g., every 15 to 30 minutes) for physical needs (e.g., food, hydration, toileting), safety, and comfort, and these observations also must be documented (every 15 to 30 minutes). The patient must be removed from restraints when safer and quieter behavior is observed.

Recent changes in the law regarding the use of restraints and seclusion have prompted agencies to revise their policies and procedures, further limiting these practices. Despite deeply held beliefs among practitioners who have used restraints, most agencies have found no negative effect associated with the reduced use of restraints and seclusion. Alternative methods of therapy and cooperation with the patient have been successful. Nurses also need to know under which circumstances the use of seclusion and restraints is contraindicated (Box 6-1).

BOX 6-1 CONTRAINDICATIONS TO SECLUSION AND RESTRAINT

- Extremely unstable medical and psychiatric conditions*
- Delirium or dementia leading to inability to tolerate decreased stimulation*
- Severe suicidal tendencies*
- Severe drug reactions or overdoses or need for close monitoring of drug dosages*
- Desire for punishment of patient or convenience of staff

*Unless close supervision and direct observation are provided.
From Simon, R.I. (2001). *Concise guide to psychiatry and law for clinicians* (3rd ed., p. 117). Washington, DC: American Psychiatric Press.

MAINTENANCE OF PATIENT CONFIDENTIALITY

Ethical Considerations

Confidentiality of care and treatment is also an important right for all patients, particularly psychiatric patients. Any discussion or consultation involving a patient should be conducted discreetly and only with individuals who have a need and a right to know this privileged information. The American Nurses Association (ANA) *Code of Ethics for Nurses with Interpretive Statements* (2001) asserts the duty of the nurse to protect confidential patient information (Box 6-2). Failure to provide this protection may harm the nurse-patient relationship, as well as the patient's well-being. However, the code clarifies that this duty is not absolute. In some situations disclosure may be mandated to protect the patient, other people, or the public health.

Legal Considerations
Health Insurance Portability and Accountability Act

The psychiatric patient's right to receive treatment and to have confidential medical records is legally protected. The fundamental principle underlying the ANA *Code of Ethics for Nurses* on confidentiality is a person's constitutional right to privacy. Generally, your legal duty to maintain confidentiality is to protect the patient's right to privacy. The Health Insurance Portability and Accountability Act (HIPAA) became effective on April 14, 2003. Therefore, you may not, without the patient's consent, disclose information obtained from the patient or information in the medical record to anyone except those individuals for whom it is necessary for implementation

---

BOX 6-2 CODE OF ETHICS FOR NURSES

The House of Delegates of the American Nurses Association approved these nine provisions at its June 30, 2001, meeting in Washington, D.C. In July 2001, the Congress of Nursing Practice and Economics voted to accept the new language of the interpretive statements, resulting in a fully approved revised *Code of Ethics for Nurses with Interpretive Statements*.

1. The nurse, in all professional relationships, practices with compassion and respect for the inherent dignity, worth, and uniqueness of every individual, unrestricted by considerations of social or economic status, personal attributes, or the nature of health problems.
2. The nurse's primary commitment is to the patient, whether an individual, family, group, or community.
3. The nurse promotes, advocates for, and strives to protect the health, safety, and rights of the patient.
4. The nurse is responsible and accountable for individual nursing practice and determines the appropriate delegation of tasks consistent with the nurse's obligation to provide optimum patient care.

5. The nurse owes the same duties to self as to others, including the responsibility to preserve integrity and safety, to maintain competence, and to continue personal and professional growth.
6. The nurse participates in establishing, maintaining, and improving health care environments and conditions of employment conducive to the provision of quality health care and consistent with the values of the profession through individual and collective action.
7. The nurse participates in the advancement of the profession through contributions to practice, education, administration, and knowledge development.
8. The nurse collaborates with other health professionals and the public in promoting community, national, and international efforts to meet health needs.
9. The profession of nursing, as represented by associations and their members, is responsible for articulating nursing values, for maintaining the integrity of the profession and its practice, and for shaping social policy.

From American Nurses Association. (2001). *Code of ethics for nurses with interpretive statements.* Washington, DC: Nursesbooks.org.

of the patient's treatment plan. Special protection of notes used in psychotherapy that are kept separate from the patient's health information was created by this HIPAA rule (2003). Discussions about a patient in public places such as elevators and the cafeteria, even when the patient's name is not mentioned, can lead to disclosures of confidential information and liabilities for you and the hospital.

Patients' Employers

Your release of information to the patient's employer about the patient's condition, without the patient's consent, is a breach of confidentiality that subjects you to liability for the tort of invasion of privacy as well as a HIPAA violation. On the other hand, discussion of a patient's history with other staff members to determine a consistent treatment approach is not a breach of confidentiality.

Generally, for a situation to be created in which information is privileged, a patient–health professional relationship must exist and the information must concern the care and treatment of the patient. The health professional may refuse to disclose information to protect the patient's privacy. However, the right to privacy is the patient's right, and health professionals cannot invoke confidentiality for their own defense or benefit.

Rights After Death

A person's reputation can be damaged even after death. It is therefore important not to divulge information after a person's death that could not have been legally shared before the death. The Dead Man's Statute protects confidential information about people when they are not alive to speak for themselves.

A legal privilege of confidentiality is enacted legislatively and in some states exists to protect the confidentiality of professional communications (e.g., nurse-patient, physician-patient, attorney-patient). The theory behind such privileged communications is that patients will not be comfortable or willing to disclose personal information about themselves if they fear that nurses will repeat their confidential conversations.

In some states in which the legal privilege of confidentiality has not been legislated for nurses, you must respond to a court's inquiries regarding the patient's disclosures even if this information implicates the patient in a crime. In these states the confidentiality of communications cannot be guaranteed. If a duty to report exists, you may be required to divulge private information shared by the patient.

Patient Privilege and Human Immunodeficiency Virus Status

Some states have enacted mandatory or permissive statutes that direct health care providers to warn a spouse if a partner tests positive for human immunodeficiency virus (HIV). Nurses must understand the laws in their jurisdiction of practice regarding privileged communications and warnings of infectious disease exposure.

Exceptions to the Rule

Duty to warn and protect third parties. The California Supreme Court, in its 1974 landmark decision *Tarasoff v. Regents of University of California,* ruled that a psychotherapist has a **duty to warn** a patient's potential victim of potential harm. A university student who was in counseling at a California university was despondent over being rejected by Tatiana Tarasoff. The psychologist notified police verbally and in writing that the young man may be dangerous to Tarasoff. The police questioned the student, found him to be rational, and secured his promise to stay away from his love interest. The student killed Tarasoff 2 months later. This case created much controversy and confusion in the psychiatric and medical communities over breach of patient confidentiality and its effect on the therapeutic relationship in psychiatric care and over the ability of the psychotherapist to predict when a patient is truly dangerous. This trend continues as other jurisdictions have adopted or modified the California rule despite the objections of the psychiatric community. These jurisdictions view public safety to be more important than privacy in narrowly defined circumstances.

The *Tarasoff* case acknowledged that generally there is no common law duty to aid third parties. An exception is when special relationships exist, and the court found the patient-therapist relationship sufficient to create a duty of the therapist to aid Ms. Tarasoff, the victim. The duty to protect the intended victim from danger arises when the therapist determines—or, pursuant to professional standards, should have determined—that the patient presents a serious danger to another. Any action reasonably necessary under the circumstances, including notification of the potential victim, the victim's family, and the police, discharges the therapist's duty to the potential victim.

In 1976, the California Supreme Court issued a second ruling in the case of *Tarasoff v. Regents of University of California* (now known as *Tarasoff II*). This ruling broadened the earlier ruling, the duty to warn, to include the **duty to protect.**

Most states have similar laws regarding the duty to warn third parties of potential life threats. The duty to warn usually includes the following:

- Assessing and predicting the patient's danger of violence toward another
- Identifying the specific individual(s) being threatened
- Taking appropriate action to protect the identified victims

Nursing implications. As this trend toward making it the therapist's duty to warn third parties of potential harm continues to gain wider acceptance, it is important for students and nurses to understand its implications for nursing practice. Although none of these cases has dealt with nurses, it is fair to assume that in jurisdictions that have adopted the Tarasoff doctrine, the duty to warn third parties will be applied to advanced practice psychiatric mental health nurses in private practice who engage in individual therapy.

If, however, a staff nurse who is a member of a team of psychiatrists, psychologists, psychiatric social workers, and other psychiatric nurses does not report patient threats of harm against specified victims or classes of victims to the team of the patient's management psychotherapist for assessment and evaluation, this failure is likely to be considered substandard nursing care.

So, too, the failure to communicate and record relevant information from police, relatives, or the patient's old records might also be deemed negligent. Breach of patient-nurse confidentiality should not pose ethical or legal dilemmas for nurses in these situations, because a team approach to the delivery of psychiatric care presumes communication of pertinent information to other staff members to develop a treatment plan in the patient's best interest.

Child and Elder Abuse Reporting Statutes

Because of their interest in protecting children, all 50 states and the District of Columbia have enacted child abuse reporting statutes. Although these statutes differ from state to state, they generally include a definition of child abuse, a list of individuals required or encouraged to report abuse, and the governmental agency designated to receive and investigate the reports. Most statutes include civil penalties for failure to report. Many states specifically require nurses to report cases of suspected abuse.

There is a conflict between federal and state laws with respect to child abuse reporting when the health care professional discovers child abuse or neglect during the suspected abuser's alcohol or drug treatment. Federal laws and regulations governing confidentiality of patient records, which apply to almost all drug abuse and alcohol treatment providers, prohibit any disclosure without a court order. In this case, federal law supersedes state reporting laws, although compliance with the state law may be maintained under the following circumstances:

- If a court order is obtained, pursuant to the regulations
- If a report can be made without identifying the abuser as a patient in an alcohol or drug treatment program
- If the report is made anonymously (some states, to protect the rights of the accused, do not allow anonymous reporting)

As reported incidents of abuse to other persons in society surface, states may require health professionals to report other kinds of abuse. A growing number of states are enacting elder abuse reporting statutes, which require registered nurses (RNs) and others to report cases of abuse of older adults. Agencies who receive federal funding (i.e., Medicare or Medicaid) must follow strict guidelines for reporting and preventing elder abuse. Older adults are defined as adults 65 years of age and older. These laws also apply to dependent adults—that is, adults between 18 and 64 years of age whose physical or mental limitations restrict their ability to carry out normal activities or to protect themselves—when the RN has actual knowledge that the person has been the victim of physical abuse.

Under most state laws, a person who is required to report suspected abuse, neglect, or exploitation of a disabled adult and who willfully does not do so is guilty of a misdemeanor crime. Most state statutes declare that anyone who makes a report in good faith is immune from civil liability in connection with the report.

You may also report knowledge of, or reasonable suspicion of, mental abuse or suffering. Dependent adults as well as older adults are protected by the law from purposeful physical or fiduciary neglect or abandonment. **Because state laws vary, students are encouraged to become familiar with the requirements of their states.**

TORT LAW APPLIED TO PSYCHIATRIC SETTINGS

Torts are a category of civil law that commonly applies to health care practice. A tort is a civil wrong for which money damages may be collected by the injured party (the plaintiff) from the wrongdoer (the defendant). The injury can be to person, property, or reputation. Because tort law has general applicability to nursing practice, this section may contain a review of material previously covered elsewhere in your nursing curriculum.

Bullying has become a recognized form of violence in our society. Nurses may encounter bullying behaviors from nursing supervisors, peers, patients, and even family members of patients. The root of this controlling type of behavior can be anxiety, stress, fear, or possibly even guilt felt by the bully (Boudreaux, 2010).

When nurses in psychiatric settings encounter provocative, threatening, or violent behavior from patients, the use of restraint or seclusion might be required until a patient demonstrates quieter and safer behavior. Accordingly, the nurse in the psychiatric setting should understand the intentional torts of battery, assault, and false imprisonment (described in Box 6-3). More on the use of restraints and seclusion is found in Chapters 16 and 24.

Common Liability Issues
Protection of Patients

Legal issues common in psychiatric nursing relate to the failure to protect the safety of patients. If a suicidal patient is left alone with the means to harm himself or herself, the nurse who has a duty to protect the patient will be held responsible for the resultant injuries. Leaving a suicidal patient alone in a room on the sixth floor with an open window is an example of unreasonable judgment on the part of the nurse. Precautions to prevent harm must be taken whenever a patient is restrained. Miscommunications and medication errors are common in all areas of nursing, including psychiatric care. A common area of liability in psychiatry is abuse of the therapist-patient relationship. Issues of sexual misconduct during the therapeutic relationship have become a source of concern in the psychiatric community. Misdiagnosis is also frequently charged in legal suits. See Table 6-2 for common liability issues.

Violence

Violent behavior is not acceptable in our society. The incidence of violence and violent acts appears to be escalating in our society. Therefore we see nurses confronting increasing amounts of violence in the workplace. Nurses must protect themselves in both institutional and community settings. Employers are

BOX 6-3 FALSE IMPRISONMENT AND NEGLIGENCE: PLUMADORE V. STATE OF NEW YORK (1980)

Mrs. Plumadore was admitted to Saranac Lake General Hospital for a gallbladder condition. Her medical workup revealed emotional problems stemming from marital difficulties, which had resulted in suicide attempts several years before her admission. After a series of consultations and tests, she was advised by the attending surgeon that she was scheduled to have gallbladder surgery later that day. After the surgeon's visit, a consulting psychiatrist who examined Mrs. Plumadore directed her to dress and pack her belongings because he had arranged to have her admitted to a state hospital at Ogdensburg.

Subsequently, two uniformed state troopers handcuffed Mrs. Plumadore and strapped her into the backseat of a patrol car. She was also accompanied by a female hospital employee and was transported to the state hospital. On arrival, the admitting psychiatrist recognized that the referring psychiatrist lacked the requisite authority to order her involuntary commitment. He therefore requested that she sign a voluntary admission form, which she refused to do. Despite Mrs. Plumadore's protests regarding her admission to the state hospital, the psychiatrist assigned her to a ward without physical or psychiatric examination and without the opportunity to contact her family or her medical physician. The record of her admission to the state hospital noted an "informed admission," which is patient-initiated voluntary admission in New York.

The court awarded $40,000 to Mrs. Plumadore for false imprisonment, negligence, and malpractice.

TABLE 6-2 COMMON LIABILITY ISSUES

ISSUE	EXAMPLES
Patient safety	Suicide risks
	Restraints
	Miscommunication
	Medication errors
	Boundary violations (e.g., sexual misconduct)
	Misdiagnosis
Defamation of character	Harms patient's reputation
• Slander (spoken)	Confidential information divulged
• Libel (written)	Truth is a defense
Supervisory liability (vicarious liability)	Inappropriate delegation of duties
	Lack of supervision of those supervising
Intentional torts	Voluntary acts intended to bring a physical or mental consequence
• May carry criminal penalties	Purposeful acts
• Punitive damages may be awarded	Carelessness or recklessness
• Not covered by malpractice insurance	No patient consent
	Self-defense or protection of others may serve as a defense to charges of an intentional tort
Negligence or malpractice	Carelessness
	Foreseeability of harm
Assault and battery	Person apprehensive (assault) of harmful or offensive touching (battery)
	Threat to use force (words not enough) with opportunity and ability
	Treatment without patient's consent
False imprisonment	Intent to confine to a specific area
	Indefensible use of seclusion or restraints
	Detain voluntarily admitted patient with no agency or legal policies to support detaining

not typically held responsible for employee injuries caused by violent patient behavior. Nurses have placed themselves knowingly in the range of danger by agreeing to care for unpredictable patients. It is therefore important for nurses to protect themselves by participating in setting policies that create a safe environment. Good judgment means not placing oneself in a potentially violent situation. Nurses, as citizens, have the same rights as patients—that is, to be free from being threatened or harmed. Appropriate security support should be readily available to the nurse practicing in an institution. When you work in community settings, you must avoid placing yourself unnecessarily in dangerous environments, especially when alone at night. You should use common sense and enlist the support of local law enforcement officers when needed. A violent patient is not being abandoned if placed safely in the hands of the authorities.

The psychiatric mental health nurse must also be aware of the potential for violence in the community when a patient is discharged following a short-term stay. The duty of the nurse to protect the patient as well as others who may be threatened by the violent patient is discussed in the preceding section in this chapter titled Duty to Warn and Protect Third Parties. The nurse's assessment of the patient's potential for violence must be documented and monitored if there is legitimate concern regarding discharge of a patient who is discussing or exhibiting potentially violent behavior. The psychiatric mental health nurse must communicate his or her observations to the medical staff when discharge decisions are being considered.

Negligence/Malpractice

Negligence or **malpractice** is an act or an omission to act that breaches the duty of due care and results in or is responsible for a person's injuries. The five elements required to prove negligence are (1) duty, (2) breach of duty, (3) cause in fact, (4) proximate cause, and (5) damages. Foreseeability or likelihood of harm is also evaluated.

Duty is measured by a standard of care. When nurses represent themselves as being capable of caring for psychiatric patients and accept employment, a duty of care has been assumed. The duty is owed to psychiatric patients to understand the theory and medications used in the specialty care of these patients. People who represent themselves as possessing superior knowledge and skill, such as psychiatric nurse specialists, are held to a higher standard of care in the practice of their profession. The staff nurse who is assigned to a psychiatric unit must be knowledgeable enough to assume a reasonable or safe duty of care for the patients.

If you are not capable of providing the standard of care that other nurses would be expected to provide under similar circumstances, you have breached the duty of care. **Breach of duty** is the conduct that exposes the patient to an unreasonable risk of harm, through either commission or omission of acts by the nurse. If you do not have the required education and experience to provide certain interventions, you have breached the duty by neglecting or omitting to provide necessary care. You can also act in such a way that the patient is harmed and can thus be guilty of negligence through acts of commission.

Cause in fact may be evaluated by asking the question, "Except for what the nurse did, would this injury have occurred?" **Proximate cause,** or legal cause, may be evaluated by determining whether there were any intervening actions or individuals that were, in fact, the causes of harm to the patient. **Damages** include actual damages (e.g., loss of earnings, medical expenses, and property damage) as well as pain and suffering. Foreseeability of harm evaluates the likelihood of the outcome under the circumstances.

DETERMINATION OF A STANDARD OF CARE

Professional standards of practice determined by professional associations differ from the standards embodied in the minimal qualifications established by state licensure for entry into the profession of nursing. The ANA has established standards for psychiatric mental health nursing practice and credentialing for the psychiatric mental health RN and the advanced practice RN in psychiatric mental health nursing (ANA, 2007).

Standards for psychiatric mental health nursing practice differ markedly from minimal state requirements because the primary purposes for setting these two types of standards are different. The state's qualifications for practice provide consumer protection by ensuring that all practicing nurses have successfully completed an approved nursing program and passed the national licensing examination. The professional association's primary focus is to elevate the practice of its members by setting standards of excellence.

Nurses are held to the standard of care provided by other nurses possessing the same degree of skill or knowledge in the same or similar circumstances. In the past, community standards existed for urban and rural agencies. However, with greater mobility and expanded means of communication, national standards have evolved. Psychiatric patients have the right to the standard of care recognized by professional bodies governing nursing, whether they are in a rural or an urban facility. Nurses must participate in continuing education courses to stay current with existing standards of care.

Hospital policies and procedures establish institutional criteria for care, and these criteria, such as the frequency of rounds for patients in seclusion, may be introduced to prove a standard that the nurse met or failed to meet. The shortcoming of this method is that the hospital's policy may be substandard. For example, the state licensing laws for institutions might set a minimal requirement for staffing or frequency of rounds for certain patients, and the hospital policy might fall below that minimum. **Substandard institutional policies do not absolve the individual nurse of responsibility to practice on the basis of professional standards of nursing care.**

Like hospital policy and procedures, customs can be used as evidence of a standard of care. For example, in the absence of a written policy on the use of restraint, testimony might be offered regarding the customary use of restraint in emergency situations in which the combative, violent, or confused patient poses a threat of harm to self or others. Using traditions to establish a standard of care may result in the same defect as in using hospital policies and procedures: customs may not comply with the laws, recommendations of the accrediting body, or other recognized standards of care. Customs must be carefully and regularly evaluated to ensure that substandard routines have not developed. Substandard customs do not protect you when a psychiatric patient charges that a right has been violated or that harm has been caused by the staff's common practices.

Guidelines for Nurses Who Suspect Negligence

It is not unusual for a student or practicing nurse to suspect negligence on the part of a peer. In most states, as a nurse you have a legal duty to report such risks of harm to the patient. It is also important that you document the evidence clearly and accurately before making serious accusations against a peer. If you question a physician's orders or actions, or those of a fellow nurse, it is wise to communicate these concerns directly to the person involved. If the risky behavior continues, you have an obligation to communicate these concerns to a supervisor, who should then intervene to ensure that the patient's rights and well-being are protected.

If you suspect a peer of being chemically impaired or of practicing irresponsibly, you have an obligation to protect not only the rights of the peer but also the rights of all patients who could be harmed by this impaired peer. If, after you have reported suspected behavior of concern to a supervisor, the danger persists, you have a duty to report the concern to someone at the next level of authority. It is important to follow the channels of communication in an organization, but it is also important to protect the safety of the patients. If the supervisor's actions or inactions do not rectify the dangerous situation, you have a continuing duty to report the behavior of concern to the appropriate authority, such as the state board of nursing.

A useful reference for nurses is the ANA's *Guidelines on Reporting Incompetent, Unethical, or Illegal Practices* (1994), and the ANA's *Code of Ethics for Nurses with Interpretive Statements* (2001, p. 154, 2010 reissue).

> *Reporting unethical, illegal, and in incompetent, or impaired nurse practices, even when done appropriately, may present substantial risk to the nurse; nevertheless such risks do not eliminate the obligation to address serious threats to patient safety.*

Duty to Intervene and Duty to Report

The psychiatric mental health nurse has a duty to intervene when the safety or well-being of the patient or another person is obviously at risk. A nurse who follows an order that is known to be incorrect or that the nurse believes will harm the patient is responsible for the harm that results to the patient. **If you have information that leads you to believe that the physician's orders need to be clarified or changed, it is your duty to intervene and protect the patient.** It is important that you communicate with the physician who has ordered the treatment to explain the concern. If the treating physician does not appear willing to consider your concerns, you should carry out the duty to intervene through other appropriate channels.

It is important for you to express your concerns to the supervisor to allow the supervisor to communicate with the appropriate medical staff for intervention in the physician's treatment plan. As the patient's advocate, you have a duty to intervene to protect the patient; at the same time, you do not have the right to interfere with the physician-patient relationship.

It is also important to follow agency policies and procedures for communicating differences of opinion. If you fail to intervene and the patient is injured, you may be partly liable for the injuries that result because of failure to use safe nursing practice and good professional judgment.

The legal concept of **abandonment** may also arise when a nurse does not leave a patient safely reassigned to another health professional before discontinuing treatment. When the nurse is given an assignment to care for a patient, the nurse must provide the care or ensure that the patient is safely reassigned to another nurse. Abandonment issues arise when accurate, timely, and thorough reporting has not occurred or when follow-through of patient care, on which the patient is relying, has not occurred. The same principles apply for the psychiatric mental health nurse who is working in a community setting. For example, if a suicidal patient refuses to come to the hospital for treatment, you cannot abandon the patient but must take the necessary steps to ensure the patient's safety. These actions may include enlisting the assistance of the legal system in temporarily involuntarily committing the patient.

The duty to intervene on the patient's behalf poses many legal and ethical dilemmas for nurses in the workplace. Institutions that have a chain-of-command policy or other reporting mechanisms offer some assurance that the proper authorities in the administration are notified. Most patient care issues regarding physicians' orders or treatments can be settled fairly early in the process by the nurse's discussion of the concerns with the physician. If further intervention by the nurse is required to protect the patient, the next step in the chain of command can be followed. Generally, the nurse then notifies the immediate nursing supervisor; the supervisor thereupon discusses the problem with the physician, and then with the chief of staff of a particular service, until a resolution is reached. If there is no time to resolve the issue through the normal process because of the life-threatening nature of the situation, the nurse must act to protect the patient's life.

Unethical or Illegal Practices

The issues become more complex when a professional colleague's conduct, including that of a student nurse, is criminally unlawful. Specific examples include the diversion of drugs from the hospital and sexual misconduct with patients. Increasing media attention and the recognition of substance abuse as an occupational hazard for health professionals have led to the establishment of substance abuse programs for health care workers in many states. These programs provide appropriate treatment for impaired professionals to protect the public from harm and to rehabilitate the professional.

The problem previously discussed—of reporting impaired colleagues—becomes a difficult one, particularly when no direct harm has occurred to the patient. Concern for professional reputations, damaged careers, and personal privacy rather than public protection has generated a code of silence regarding substance abuse among health professionals.

Several states now require reporting of impaired or incompetent colleagues to the professional licensing boards. In the absence of such a legal mandate, the questions of whether to report and to whom to report become ethical ones. You are again urged to use the ANA's *Guidelines on Reporting Incompetent,*

Unethical, or Illegal Practices (1994). Chapter 19 deals more fully with issues related to the chemically impaired nurse.

The duty to intervene includes the duty to report known abusive behavior. Most states have enacted statutes to protect children and older adults from abuse and neglect. Psychiatric mental health nurses working in the community may be required by law to report unsafe relationships they discover.

DOCUMENTATION OF CARE

Purpose of Medical Records

The purpose of the medical record is to provide accurate and complete information about the care and treatment of patients and to give health care personnel responsible for that care a means of communicating with each other. The medical record allows for continuity of care. A record's usefulness is determined by evaluating, when the record is read later, how accurately and completely it portrays the patient's behavioral status at the time it was written. The patient has the right to see the chart, but the chart belongs to the institution. The patient must follow appropriate protocol to view his or her records.

For example, if a psychiatric patient describes to a nurse a plan to harm himself or herself or another person and that nurse fails to document the information, including the need to protect the patient or the identified victim, the information will be lost when the nurse leaves work, and the patient's plan may be executed. The harm caused could be linked directly to the nurse's failure to communicate this important information. Even though documentation takes time away from the patient, the importance of communicating and preserving the nurse's memory through the medical record cannot be overemphasized.

Facility Use of Medical Records

The medical record has many other uses aside from providing information on the course of the patient's care and treatment to health care professionals. A retrospective chart review can provide valuable information to the facility on the quality of care provided and on ways to improve that care. A facility may conduct reviews for risk management purposes to determine areas of potential liability for the facility and to evaluate methods used to reduce the facility's exposure to liability. For example, documentation of the use of restraints and seclusion for psychiatric patients may be reviewed by risk managers. Accordingly, the chart may be used to evaluate care for quality assurance or peer review. Utilization review analysts review the chart to determine appropriate use of hospital and staff resources consistent with reimbursement schedules. Insurance companies and other reimbursement agencies rely on the medical record in determining what payments they will make on the patient's behalf.

Medical Records as Evidence

From a legal perspective, the chart is a recording of data and opinions made in the normal course of the patient's hospital care. It is deemed to be good evidence because it is presumed to be true, honest, and untainted by memory lapses. Accordingly, the medical record finds its way into legal cases for a variety of reasons. Some examples of its use include determining (1) the extent of the patient's damages and pain and suffering in personal injury cases, such as when a psychiatric patient attempts suicide while under the protective care of a hospital; (2) the nature and extent of injuries in child abuse or elder abuse cases; (3) the nature and extent of physical or mental disability in disability cases; and (4) the nature and extent of injury and rehabilitative potential in workers' compensation cases.

Medical records may also be used in police investigations, civil conservatorship proceedings, competency hearings, and commitment procedures. In states that mandate mental health legal services or a patients' rights advocacy program, audits may be performed to determine the facility's compliance with state laws or violation of patients' rights. Finally, medical records may be used in professional and hospital negligence cases.

During the discovery phase of litigation, the medical record is a pivotal source of information for attorneys in determining whether a cause of action exists in a professional negligence or hospital negligence case. Evidence of the nursing care rendered will be found in the notes charted by the nurse.

Nursing Guidelines for Computerized Charting

Accurate, descriptive, and legible nursing notes serve the best interests of the patient, the nurse, and the institution. As computerized charting becomes more widely available, it will also be important for psychiatric mental health nurses to understand how to protect the confidentiality of these records. Institutions must also protect against intrusions into the privacy of the patient record systems.

Concerns for the privacy of the legitimate patient's records have been addressed legally by federal laws that provide guidelines for agencies that use computerized charting. These guidelines include the recommendation that staff be assigned a password for entering patients' records in order to identify staff who have accessed patients' confidential information. There are penalties, including grounds for firing the staff, if staff enter a record for which they are not authorized to have access. Only those staff who have a legitimate need to know about the patient are authorized to access a patient's computerized chart.

It is important for you to keep your password private and never to allow someone else to access a record under your password. You are responsible for all entries into records using your password. The various systems used allow specific timeframes within which the nurse must make any necessary corrections if a charting error is made.

Any charting method that improves communication between care providers should be encouraged. Courts assume that nurses and physicians read each other's notes on patient progress. Many courts take the attitude that if care is not documented, it did not occur. Your charting also serves as a valuable memory refresher if the patient sues years after the care is rendered. In providing complete and timely information on the care and treatment of patients, the medical record enhances communication among health professionals. Internal institutional audits of the record can improve the quality of care rendered. Nurses' charting is improved by following the guidelines in Box 5-6. Chapter 7 describes common charting forms and gives examples as well as the pros and cons of each.

FORENSIC NURSING

Forensic nursing is the application of psychiatric nursing or any medical specialty principles of practice when used in a court of law to assist the court to utilize this knowledge to reach a decision on a contested issue. The nurse acts as an advocate, educating the court about the science of nursing in this courtroom-based practice of forensic nursing. Examples of psychiatric forensic nursing may include cases related to patient competency, fitness to stand trial, and commitment or responsibility for a crime. The relevance of nursing facts is presented and applied to the legal facts. Forensic cases also pertain to personal injury and murder proceedings. A dentist may serve as a forensic dentist in identifying a tooth as it relates to a corpse.

KEY POINTS TO REMEMBER

- States' power to enact laws for public health and safety and for the care of those unable to care for themselves often pits the rights of society against the rights of the individual.
- Psychiatric nurses frequently encounter problems requiring ethical choices.
- The nurse's privilege to practice nursing carries with it the responsibility to practice safely, competently, and in a manner consistent with state and federal laws.

- Knowledge of the law, the ANA's *Code of Ethics for Nurses with Interpretive Statements,* and the ANA's standards of care from *Psychiatric–Mental Health Nursing: Scope and Standards of Practice* is essential to provide safe, effective psychiatric nursing care and will serve as a framework for decision making when the nurse is presented with complex problems involving competing interests.

APPLYING CRITICAL JUDGMENT

1. Two nurses, Joe and Beth, have worked on the psychiatric unit for 2 years. During the past 6 months, Beth has confided to Joe that she has been experiencing a particularly difficult marital situation. Joe has observed that over the 6 months Beth has become increasingly irritable and difficult to work with. He notices that minor tranquilizers are frequently missing from the unit dose cart on the evening shift. He complains to the pharmacy and is informed that the drugs were stocked as ordered. Several patients state that they have not been receiving their usual drugs. Joe finds that Beth has recorded that the drugs have been given as ordered. He also notices that Beth is diverting the drugs.
   A. What action, if any, should Joe take?
   B. Should Joe confront Beth with his suspicions?
   C. If Beth admits that she has been diverting the drugs, should Joe's next step be to report Beth to the supervisor or to the board of nursing?
   D. Should Joe make his concern known to the nursing supervisor directly by identifying Beth, or should he state his concerns in general terms?
   E. Legally, must Joe report his suspicions to the board of nursing?
   F. Does the fact that harm to the patients is limited to increased agitation affect your responses?

2. A 40-year-old man who is admitted to the emergency department for a severe nosebleed has both nares packed. Because of his history of alcoholism and the probability of ensuing delirium tremens, the patient is transferred to the psychiatric unit. He is admitted to a private room, placed in restraints, and checked by a nurse every hour per physician's orders. While unattended, the patient suffocates, apparently by inhaling the nasal packing, which had become dislodged from the nares. On the next 1-hour check, the nurse finds the patient without pulse or respiration. A state statute requires that a restrained patient on a psychiatric unit be assessed by a nurse every hour for safety, comfort, and physical needs.
   A. If standards are not otherwise specified, do statutory requirements set forth minimal or maximal standards?
   B. Does the nurse's compliance with the state statute relieve him or her of liability in the patient's death?
   C. Does the nurse's compliance with the physician's orders relieve him or her of liability in the patient's death?
   D. Was the order for the restraint appropriate for this type of patient?
   E. What factors did you consider in making your determination?
   F. Was the frequency of rounds for assessment of patient needs appropriate in this situation?
   G. Did the nurse's conduct meet the standard of care for psychiatric nurses? Why or why not?
   H. What nursing action should the nurse have taken to protect the patient from harm?

3. Assume that there are no mandatory reporting laws for impaired or incompetent colleagues in the following clinical situation. In a private psychiatric unit in California, a 15-year-old boy is admitted voluntarily at the request of his parents because of violent, explosive behavior that seems to stem from his father's recent remarriage after his parents' divorce. A few days after admission, while in group therapy, he has an explosive reaction to a discussion about

APPLYING CRITICAL JUDGMENT—cont'd

weekend passes for Mother's Day. He screams that he has been abandoned and that nobody cares about him. Several weeks later, on the day before his discharge, he elicits from the nurse a promise to keep his plan to kill his mother confidential. Consider the ANA's *Code of Ethics for Nurses* on patient confidentiality, the principles of psychiatric nursing, the statutes on privileged communications, and the duty to warn third parties in answering the following questions:

A. Did the nurse use appropriate judgment in promising confidentiality?

B. Does the nurse have a legal duty to warn the patient's mother of her son's threat?

C. Is the duty owed to the patient's father and stepmother?

D. Would a change in the admission status from voluntary to involuntary protect the patient's mother without violating the patient's confidentiality?

E. Would your response be different depending on the state in which the incident occurred? Why or why not?

F. What nursing action, if any, should the nurse take after the disclosure by the patient?

CHAPTER REVIEW QUESTIONS

Choose the most appropriate answer(s).

1. A researcher tells the nurse that she would like to include one of her patients in a medication study. The nurse is responsible for:
   1. instructing the patient in the details of the study.
   2. encouraging the patient to participate.
   3. directing the client in appropriate study behaviors.
   4. assessment of the client's ability to give informed consent.

2. The single most important action nurses can take to protect the rights of a psychiatric patient is to:
   1. be aware of that state's laws regarding care and treatment of the mentally ill.
   2. refuse to participate in imposing restraint or seclusion.
   3. document concerns about unit short staffing.
   4. practice the five principles of bioethics.

3. To provide appropriate care for a patient who has been admitted involuntarily to a psychiatric unit, the nurse must be aware of the fact that the patient has the right to:
   1. refuse psychotropic medications.
   2. be treated by unit staff of his or her choice.
   3. be released within 24 hours of making a written request.

   4. have a consultation with other mental health professionals at the hospital's expense.

4. A client, covered in mud and grime, has refused to wash himself upon admission to the inpatient unit. Despite his protests, 2 male staff force him into the shower and wash him down with soap and water. What statement is correct regarding patient rights?
   1. No violation as his was a threat to self
   2. Violation due to forcing him against his will
   3. No violation due to need for appropriate hygiene
   4. Violation due to mandate for least restrictive alternative

5. Observing the patient's right to privacy permits the psychiatric mental health nurse to:
   1. freely disclose information in the medical record to the patient's employer.
   2. use information about the patient when preparing a journal article.
   3. discuss observations about the patient with the treatment team.
   4. disclose confidential information after the patient's death.

REFERENCES

American Nurses Association (ANA). (2001, 2010 reissue). *Code of ethics for nurses with interpretive statements.* Washington, DC: Nursesbooks.org.

American Nurses Association (ANA). (1994). *Guidelines on reporting incompetent, unethical, or illegal practices.* Kansas City, MO: Author.

American Nurses Association (ANA), American Psychiatric Nursing Association, and International Society of Psychiatric Mental Health Nurses. (2007). *Psychiatric–mental health nursing: scope and standards of practice.* Silver Springs, MD: Nursesbooks.org.

American Psychiatric Association (APA). (2000). *Diagnostic and statistical manual of mental disorders (DSM-IV-TR)* (4th ed., text rev.). Washington, DC: Author.

Bazelon, D. L. (2011). *Diversion from incarceration.* Retrieved March 4, 2011, from http://bazelon.org/where-we-stand/access-to-services/-diversion-from incarceration.

Bazelon, D. L. (2010). *Mental health parity.* Washington, DC: Bazelon Center for Mental Health Law. Retrieved March 4, 2011, from http://bazelon.org/where-we-stand/accesstoservices//mental-health parity.aspx.

Bazelon, D. L. (2003). *Advance psychiatric directives.* Washington, DC: Bazelon Center for Mental Health Law.

Boudreaux, A. (2010). Keeping your cool with difficult family members. *Nursing, 40*(12), 50.

Canterbury v. Spence, 464 F.2d 772 (D.C. Cir. 1972), quoting *Schloendorff v. Society of N.Y. Hosp.,* 211 N.Y. 125, 105 N.E. 92, 93 (1914).

Chan, C. (2003). *Mandatory outpatient treatment: issues to consider.* Chicago: Paper presented at the 153rd Annual Meeting of the American Psychiatric Association.

Health Insurance Portability and Accountability Act (HIPAA). U.S.C. 45 C.F.R § 164.501 (2003).

Humphrey v. Cady, 405 U.S. 504 (1972).

Monahan, J., Swartz, M., & Bonnie, R. J. (2003). Mandated treatment in the community for people with mental disorders. *Health Affairs, 22*(5), 28–38.

O'Connor v. Donaldson, 422 U.S. 563 (1975).

Olmstead v. L.C. (98–536), 527 U.S. 581 (1999).

Plumadore v. State of New York, 427 N.Y.S.2d 90 (1980).

Rainey, C. J. (2001). *Mandated outpatient treatment resources and data.* Orlando, FL: Presented at the American Psychiatric Association 53rd Institute on Psychiatric Services.

Simon, R. I. (1999). The law and psychiatry. In R. E. Hales, S. C. Yudofsky, & J. A. Talbott (Eds.), *The American Psychiatric Press textbook of psychiatry* (3rd ed.). Washington, DC: American Psychiatric Press.

Tarasoff v. Regents of University of California, 551 P.2d 334, 131 Cal Rptr 14 (1976).

Tarasoff v. Regents of University of California, 529 P.2d 553, 118 Cal Rptr 129 (1974).

Zinermon v. Burch, 494 U.S. 113, 108 L.Ed.2d 100, 110 S. Ct. 975 (1990).

UNIT 2

Tools for Practice of the Art

Madeleine Leininger, PhD, RN, LhD, FAAN (1925-Present)
Founder of Transcultural Nursing

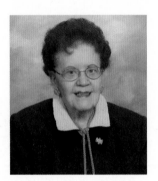

Madeleine Leininger is a nurse pioneer, scientist, anthropologist, researcher, theorist, leader, certified transcultural nurse specialist, and author/editor of more than 27 books. Leininger developed her Theory of Cultural Care and Universality based on her observations in the 1950s and 1960s of the people of New Guinea, where she lived for 2 years. She recognized the need for nurses to deliver care that combined both humanism and scientific knowledge that would be meaningful to people from culturally diverse backgrounds.

She was the first graduate-prepared nurse to earn a PhD in cultural and social anthropology. In 1954 Leininger later obtained a master's degree in psychiatric nursing from The Catholic University of America in Washington, DC. Soon afterwards, she developed the first master's level clinical specialist program in child psychiatric nursing at the University of Cincinnati. She subsequently developed the first graduate transcultural nursing program in psychiatric nursing also at the University of Cincinnati.

Simply stated, transcultural nursing is the practice of nursing that provides culturally congruent, competent, and equitable care practices in a world that has become increasingly multicultural in nature.

Leininger (1998) states that when nurses do not take into account a patient's spiritual/religious beliefs, family ties, and economic and educational factors, the nurse is at risk for demonstrating a noncaring attitude that may result in nonbeneficial outcomes. Human care/caring is defined within the context of culture. Leininger's transcultural nursing theory has at its focus "caring." She stated that "...*a caring focus must become the dominant focus of all areas of nursing. It is the holistic and most complete and creative way to help people*" (Leininger, 1981).

Leininger, M.M. (1998). *What is transcultural nursing?* Livonia, MI: Transcultural Nursing Society.
Leininger, M.M. (1981). *Caring: an essential human need.* Thorofare, NJ: Charles B. Slack.

Nursing Process and QSEN: The Foundation for Safe and Effective Care

Elizabeth M. Varcarolis

evolve WEBSITE

http://evolve.elsevier.com/Varcarolis/essentials

KEY TERMS AND CONCEPTS

evidence-based practice (EBP), p. 108
health teaching, p. 109
mental status examination (MSE), p. 101
milieu therapy, p. 109
Nursing Interventions Classification (NIC), p. 108
Nursing Outcomes Classification (NOC), p. 105

outcomes criteria, p. 105
Psychiatric Mental Health Nursing Standards of Practice, p. 98
psychosocial assessment, p. 101
Quality and Safety Education for Nurses (QSEN), p. 98
self-care activities, p. 109

SELECTED CONCEPT: Quality and Safety Education for Nurses (QSEN) Pre-Licensure Competencies
The primary goal of QSEN is to prepare future nurses with the knowledge, skills, and attitudes (KSAs) to increase the quality, care, and safety in the healthcare setting.
1. Patient-centered care
2. Teamwork and collaboration
3. Quality improvement (QI)
4. Evidence-based practice
5. Safety
6. Informatics

OBJECTIVES

1. Conduct a mental status examination.
2. Perform a psychosocial assessment including cultural and spiritual components.
3. Explain three principles a nurse follows in planning actions to reach approved outcome criteria.
4. Construct a plan of care for a patient with a mental or emotional health problem.
5. Identify three advanced practice psychiatric nursing interventions.
6. Demonstrate basic nursing interventions and evaluation of care using the Standards of Practice (ANA, 2007).
7. Compare and contrast the Nursing Interventions Classification, Nursing Outcomes Classification, and evidence-based nursing practice.
8. Access www.qsen.org and read the prelicensure quality and safety competencies for knowledge, skills, and attitudes (KSAs) needed to prepare nurses for employment in the health care system.

The nursing process continues to be the basic framework for all significant action taken by nurses in providing developmentally and culturally relevant psychiatric mental health care to all patients. The nursing process is integral to *Psychiatric Mental Health Nursing: Scope and Standards of Practice* as defined by the American Nurses Association (ANA, 2007). The **Psychiatric Mental Health Nursing Standards of Practice** are the bases for the following:

- Criteria for certification
- Legal definition of nursing, as reflected in many states' nurse practice acts
- National Council of State Boards of Nursing Licensure Examination (NCLEX-RN®)
- The Six Standards of Practice defining the critical thinking model known as the nursing process.

By this time, you are most likely familiar with the nursing process—the six-step problem-solving approach to holistic nursing care. A patient may be an individual, a family, a group, or a community. Psychiatric mental health nursing practice bases nursing judgments and behaviors on an accepted theoretical framework. Whenever possible, interventions are supported by evidence-based research. The importance of a theoretical framework has been supported by *Psychiatric–Mental Health Nursing: Scope and Standards of Practice* (ANA, 2007). Figure 7-1 depicts the nursing process in psychiatric mental health nursing. This process is intended to facilitate and identify safe and quality care for patients

Safety and quality care for patients has become the new standard for nursing education. As of the late 1990s, the Institute of Medicine (IOM; based on their *Quality Chasm* reports) and other organizations found a need to improve the quality and safety outcomes of health care delivery. As nursing practice focused more on quality and safety issues, it became evident that graduating nursing students were missing critical competencies for safety and quality of care. The context and approach of nursing education is changing, and new models of education are needed (Valiga & Champagne, 2011). The competencies mandated by the IOM require changes throughout health professionals' education to better prepare students with the responsibilities and realities in the health care setting. There is now "a major national initiative centered on patient safety and quality" known as **Quality and Safety Education for Nurses (QSEN)** (Sullivan, 2010). The primary goal of QSEN is to prepare future nurses with the knowledge, skills, and attitudes (KSAs) required to enhance quality, care, and safety in the health care settings in which they are employed (Cronenwett et al., 2007). QSEN bases their work on six competencies (Box 7-1).

The Pilot Schools Collaborative, supported by a QSEN grant, chose 15 schools to partner with clinical experts to develop teaching strategies that included the 6 QSEN competencies in their nursing programs. The Collaborative included schools in which the following degrees were offered: BSN, APN, and diploma programs. Findings reflected the need to increase knowledge about patient safety practices, the benefits of faculty development, and the value of redesigning student learning experiences (Sherwood & Hicks, 2011). There is a definite need to offer students more experience in interactive learning that would incorporate both knowledge and skills with real-world examples (Durham & Sherwood, 2008). For example, simulation programs are popular and effective. These programs portray virtual clinical settings, such as the use of avatars, and offer students a chance to implement their knowledge, skills, and attitudes without the potential for patient harm (Durham & Sherwood, 2008). Nurse educators have described how to incorporate QSEN's six competencies into curricula and proposed guidelines explaining how educators can incorporate these six competencies into their own curricula (Valiga & Champagne, 2011). This new trend in education is often referred to as performance-based learning.

Performance-based learning is a trend that is fundamentally changing nursing education. Performance skills are learned more effectively through interactive strategies, which require changes in the traditional roles of teachers and students. There is less emphasis on lecturing and more on participation with the student in collaborative and simulated hands-on strategies to achieve actual practice competencies (Lasater & Nielsen, 2009; Lenburg, 2011). The influence of concept-based learning activities and students' clinical judgment development is part of a new revolution (Lasater & Nielson, 2009).

Suggestions for the use of QSEN competencies in the discussion of Standards of Practice can be found in 'Competency Knowledge, Skills, Attitudes (Pre-Licensure)' at the website www.qsen/ksas_pre-licensure.php.

STANDARD 1: ASSESSMENT

A view of the individual as a complex blend of many parts is consistent with nurses' **holistic approach to care.** Nurses who care for people with physical illnesses ideally maintain a holistic view that involves an awareness of psychological, social, cultural, and spiritual issues as well as ethnicity, sexual orientation, and age (e.g., child, teenager, older woman). Likewise, nurses who work in the mental health field need to assess, or have access to, past and present medical history, a recent physical examination, and any physical complaints the patient is experiencing, as well as document any observable physical conditions or behaviors (e.g., unsteady gait, abnormal breathing pattern, facial grimacing, or changing position to relieve discomfort).

Assessments are conducted by a variety of professionals including nurses, psychiatrists, social workers, dietitians, and other therapists. Every patient should have a thorough and formal nursing assessment on entering treatment to develop a basis for the plan of care in preparation for discharge. Subsequent to the formal assessment, data are collected continually and systematically as the patient's condition changes and hopefully improves. Perhaps the patient entered treatment actively suicidal, and the initial focus of care was on protection from injury; through regular assessment it may be determined that although suicidal ideation has diminished, negative self-evaluation is still certainly a problem.

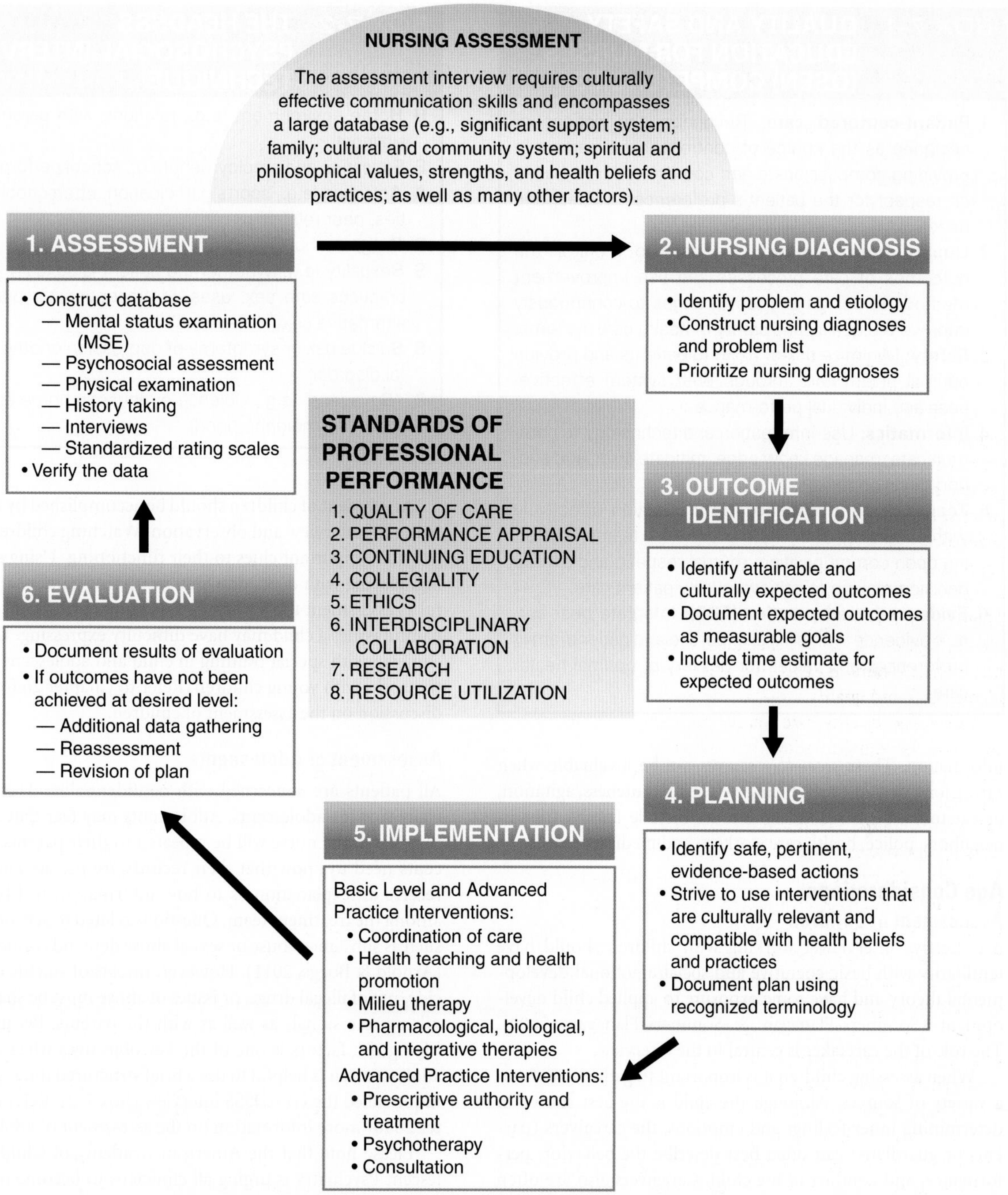

NURSING ASSESSMENT

The assessment interview requires culturally effective communication skills and encompasses a large database (e.g., significant support system; family; cultural and community system; spiritual and philosophical values, strengths, and health beliefs and practices; as well as many other factors).

1. ASSESSMENT

- Construct database
  — Mental status examination (MSE)
  — Psychosocial assessment
  — Physical examination
  — History taking
  — Interviews
  — Standardized rating scales
- Verify the data

2. NURSING DIAGNOSIS

- Identify problem and etiology
- Construct nursing diagnoses and problem list
- Prioritize nursing diagnoses

STANDARDS OF PROFESSIONAL PERFORMANCE

1. QUALITY OF CARE
2. PERFORMANCE APPRAISAL
3. CONTINUING EDUCATION
4. COLLEGIALITY
5. ETHICS
6. INTERDISCIPLINARY COLLABORATION
7. RESEARCH
8. RESOURCE UTILIZATION

3. OUTCOME IDENTIFICATION

- Identify attainable and culturally expected outcomes
- Document expected outcomes as measurable goals
- Include time estimate for expected outcomes

6. EVALUATION

- Document results of evaluation
- If outcomes have not been achieved at desired level:
  — Additional data gathering
  — Reassessment
  — Revision of plan

4. PLANNING

- Identify safe, pertinent, evidence-based actions
- Strive to use interventions that are culturally relevant and compatible with health beliefs and practices
- Document plan using recognized terminology

5. IMPLEMENTATION

Basic Level and Advanced Practice Interventions:
- Coordination of care
- Health teaching and health promotion
- Milieu therapy
- Pharmacological, biological, and integrative therapies

Advanced Practice Interventions:
- Prescriptive authority and treatment
- Psychotherapy
- Consultation

FIGURE 7-1 The nursing process in psychiatric mental health nursing.

Virtually all facilities have standardized nursing assessment forms to aid in organization and consistency among reviewers. These forms may be hardcopy or computerized, according to the resources and preferences of the institution. The time required for the nursing interview varies, depending on the assessment form and on the patient's response pattern (e.g., a lengthy or rambling historian, a patient prone to tangential thought, or a patient having memory disturbances or markedly slowed responses). In emergency situations, immediate intervention is often based on a minimal amount of data. Refer to Chapter 9 for sound guidelines for setting up and conducting a clinical interview.

The nurse's *primary source* for data collection is the patient; however, there may be times when it is necessary to supplement or rely completely on another source for the assessment

---

BOX 7-1 QUALITY AND SAFETY EDUCATION FOR NURSES (QSEN) COMPETENCIES

1. **Patient-centered care:** Recognize the patient or designee as the source of control and full partner in providing compassionate and coordinated care based on respect for the patient's preferences, values, and needs.
2. **Quality improvement:** Use data to monitor the outcomes of care processes and use improvement methods to design and test changes to continuously improve the quality and safety of health care systems.
3. **Safety:** Minimize risk of harm to patients and provide optimal health care through both system effectiveness and individual performance.
4. **Informatics:** Use information and technology to communicate, manage knowledge, mitigate error, and support decision making.
5. **Teamwork and collaboration:** Function effectively within nursing and interprofessional teams, fostering open communication, mutual respect, and shared decision making to achieve quality patient care.
6. **Evidence-based practice (EBP):** Integrate best current evidence with clinical expertise and patient/family preferences and values for delivery of optimal health care.

BOX 7-2 THE HEADSSS PSYCHOSOCIAL INTERVIEW TECHNIQUE

H **H**ome environment (e.g., relations with parents and siblings)
E **E**ducation and employment (e.g., school performance)
A **A**ctivities (e.g., sports participation, afterschool activities, peer relations)
D **D**rug, alcohol, or tobacco use
S **S**exuality (e.g., whether the patient is sexually active, practices safe sex, uses contraception, or practices alternative sexual lifestyles)
S **S**uicide risk or symptoms of depression or other mental disorder
S "**S**avagery" (e.g., violence or abuse in home environment or in neighborhood)

---

information. These *secondary sources* can be invaluable when caring for a patient experiencing psychosis, muteness, agitation, or catatonia. Such secondary sources include family, friends, neighbors, police, health care workers, and medical records.

Age Considerations

Assessment of Children

An effective interviewer working with children should have familiarity with basic cognitive and social/emotional developmental theory and have some exposure to applied child development (Sommers-Flanagan & Sommers-Flanagan, 2009). The role of the caretaker is central in the interview.

When assessing children it is important to gather data from a variety of sources. Although the child is the best source in determining inner feelings and emotions, the caregivers (parents or guardians) can often best describe the behavior, performance, and conduct of the child. Caregivers also are often helpful in interpreting the child's words and responses. However, a separate interview is advisable when an older child is reluctant to share information, especially in cases of suspected abuse (Arnold & Boggs, 2011).

As mentioned, developmental levels should be considered in the evaluation of children. One of the hallmarks of psychiatric disorders in children is the tendency to regress—that is, to return to a previous level of development. Although it is developmentally appropriate for toddlers to suck their thumbs, such a gesture is unusual in an older child.

Assessment of children should be accomplished by a combination of interview and observation. Watching children at play provides important clues to their functioning. Using storytelling, playing with dolls, drawing, or playing games can be useful as assessment tools when determining critical concerns and painful issues a child may have difficulty expressing. Usually, a clinician with special training in child and adolescent psychiatry works with young children. Refer to Chapter 26 for further discussion on the assessment of children.

Assessment of Adolescents

All patients are concerned with confidentiality. This is especially true for adolescents. Adolescents may fear that anything they say to the nurse will be repeated to their parents. Adolescents need to know that their records are private and should receive an explanation as to how information will be shared among the treatment team. Questions related to sensitive issues such as substance abuse or sexual abuse demand confidentiality (Arnold & Boggs, 2011). However, threats of suicide or homicide, use of illegal drugs, or issues of abuse must be shared with other professionals as well as with the parents. Because identifying risk factors is one of the key objectives when assessing adolescents, it is helpful to use a brief structured interview technique called the HEADSSS interview (Box 7-2). Refer to Chapter 26 for more information on the assessment of adolescents.

Please note that the American Academy of Child & Adolescent Psychiatry is urging all clinicians to become more culturally sensitive and develop greater cultural competency, and they have developed a model curriculum to address this need (Mian et al., 2010).

Assessment of the Older Adult

Older adults often need special attention. The nurse needs to be aware of any physical limitations—any sensory condition (vision or hearing deficits), motor condition (difficulty walking or maintaining balance), or medical condition (cardiac condition)—that could cause increased anxiety, stress, or physical discomfort for the patient while attempting to assess mental and emotional needs.

It is wise to identify any physical deficits the patient may have at the onset of the assessment and make accommodations for them. For example, if the patient is hard of hearing, speak a little more slowly and in clear, louder tones (but not too loud) and seat the patient close to you without invading his or her personal space. Refer to Chapter 28 for more on communicating with the older adult.

Psychiatric Nursing Assessment

The psychiatric nursing assessment has many goals, including the following:

- Establish rapport.
- Obtain an understanding of the current problem or chief complaint.
- Review physical status and obtain baseline vital signs.
- Assess for risk factors affecting the safety of the patient or others.
- Perform a mental status examination (MSE).
- Assess psychosocial status.
- Identify mutual goals for treatment.
- Formulate a plan of care.

Gathering Data

Review of systems. The mind-body connection is significant in the understanding and treatment of psychiatric disorders. Many patients who are admitted for treatment of psychiatric conditions also are given a thorough physical examination by a primary care provider. Likewise, most nursing assessments include a physical component, such as obtaining a baseline set of vital statistics, a historical and current review of body systems, and a documentation of allergic responses.

People with certain physical conditions may be more prone to psychiatric disorders such as depression. It is generally believed that the disease process of multiple sclerosis itself may actually cause depression. Other medical diseases that are typically associated with depression are coronary artery disease, diabetes, and stroke. In fact, a recent study demonstrated that women with both depression and diabetes have a significantly higher risk for mortality and cardiovascular disease than do women with either depression or diabetes alone (Brauser & Barclay, 2011). Individuals need to be evaluated for any medical origins of their depression or anxiety.

There are many medical conditions that can mimic psychiatric illnesses (Box 7-3). By the same token, often when depression is secondary to a known medical condition, it remains unrecognized and thus untreated. Conversely, psychiatric disorders can result in physical or somatic symptoms such as abdominal pain, headaches, lethargy, insomnia, and intense fatigue. Therefore all patients presenting to the health care system need to have both a medical and a psychological health evaluation to ensure a correct diagnosis and appropriate care.

Laboratory data. Disorders such as hypothyroidism may have the clinical appearance of depression, and hyperthyroidism may appear to be a manic phase of bipolar disorder; a simple blood test can usually differentiate between depression and

thyroid disorders. Abnormal liver enzyme levels can explain irritability, depression, and lethargy. People who have chronic renal disease often suffer from the same symptoms when their blood urea nitrogen and electrolyte levels are abnormal. Results of a toxicology screen for the presence of either prescription or illegal drugs also may provide useful information.

Mental status examination. Fundamental to the assessment is a mental status examination (MSE). In fact, an MSE is part of the assessment in all areas of medicine. The MSE in psychiatry is analogous to the physical examination in general medicine. The purpose of the MSE is to evaluate an individual's current cognitive processes. For acutely disturbed patients it is typical for the mental health clinician to administer MSEs every day. Sommers-Flanagan and Sommers-Flanagan (2009) advise anyone seeking employment in the medical–mental health field to be competent in communicating with other professionals via MSE reports. Box 7-4 lists the elements of a basic MSE. An example of a mental status examination is printed on the inside back cover of this text.

Generally the mental status exam aids in collecting and organizing *objective data*. The nurse observes the patient's physical behavior, nonverbal communication, appearance, speech patterns, mood and affect, thought content, perceptions, cognitive ability, and insight and judgment. Box 7-4 is an example of a standardized MSE.

Psychosocial assessment. A psychosocial assessment provides additional information from which to develop a plan of care beyond the MSE. It includes obtaining the following information about the patient:

- Central or chief complaint (in the patient's own words)
- History of violent, suicidal, or self-mutilating behaviors
- Alcohol and/or substance abuse
- Family psychiatric history
- Personal psychiatric treatment including medications and complementary therapies
- Stressors and coping methods
- Quality of activities of daily living
- Personal background
- Social background including support system
- Weaknesses, strengths, and goals for treatment
- Racial, ethnic, and cultural beliefs and practices
- Spiritual beliefs or religious practices

The patient's psychosocial history is most often the *subjective* part of the assessment. The focus of the history is the patient's perceptions and recollections of current lifestyle, and life in general (e.g., family, friends, education, work experience, coping styles, and spiritual and cultural beliefs).

Spiritual and/or religious assessment. The importance of spirituality and religious beliefs is an often overlooked element of patient care, although numerous empirical studies have suggested that being part of a spiritual community is helpful to people coping with illness and recovering from surgery (Kling, 2011). Spirituality and religious beliefs have the potential to exert an influence on how people understand meaning and purpose in their lives and how they use critical judgment to solve problems (e.g., crises of illness).

BOX 7-3   SOME MEDICAL CONDITIONS THAT MAY MIMIC PSYCHIATRIC ILLNESS

Depression

Neurological disorders:
- Cerebrovascular accident (stroke)
- Alzheimer's disease
- Brain tumor
- Huntington's disease
- Epilepsy (seizure disorder)
- Multiple sclerosis
- Parkinson's disease
- Cancer

Infections:
- Mononucleosis
- Encephalitis
- Hepatitis
- Tertiary syphilis
- Human immunodeficiency virus (HIV) infection

Endocrine disorders:
- Hypothyroidism and hyperthyroidism
- Cushing's syndrome
- Addison's disease
- Parathyroid disease

Gastrointestinal disorders:
- Liver cirrhosis
- Pancreatitis

Cardiovascular disorders:
- Hypoxia
- Congestive heart failure

Respiratory disorders:
- Sleep apnea

Nutritional disorders:
- Thiamine deficiency
- Protein deficiency
- B_{12} deficiency
- B_6 deficiency
- Folate deficiency

Collagen vascular diseases:
- Lupus erythematosus
- Rheumatoid arthritis

Anxiety

Neurological disorders:
- Alzheimer's disease
- Brain tumor
- Stroke
- Huntington's disease

Infections:
- Encephalitis
- Meningitis
- Neurosyphilis
- Septicemia

Endocrine disorders:
- Hypothyroidism and hyperthyroidism
- Hypoparathyroidism
- Hypoglycemia
- Pheochromocytoma
- Carcinoid

Metabolic disorders:
- Low calcium level
- Low potassium level
- Acute intermittent porphyria
- Liver failure

Cardiovascular disorders:
- Angina
- Congestive heart failure
- Pulmonary embolus

Respiratory disorders:
- Pneumothorax
- Acute asthma
- Emphysema

Drug effects:
- Stimulants
- Sedatives (withdrawal)

Lead, mercury poisoning

Psychosis

Medical conditions:
- Temporal lobe epilepsy
- Migraine headaches
- Temporal arteritis
- Occipital tumors
- Narcolepsy
- Encephalitis
- Hypothyroidism
- Addison's disease
- HIV infection

Drug effects:
- Hallucinogens (e.g., LSD)
- Phencyclidine
- Alcohol withdrawal
- Stimulants
- Cocaine
- Corticosteroids

The terms spirituality and religion are different although not mutually exclusive. Spirituality refers to how we find meaning, hope, purpose, and a sense of peace in our lives. Spirituality is more of an internal phenomenon centering on universal personal questions and needs. It is the part of us that seeks to understand life. The term spirituality is more about the believer's faith being more personal, less dogmatic, and more inclusive considering that there are many spiritual paths and no one "real path." A person's spiritual beliefs may or may not be connected with the community or with religious rituals.

Religion is an external system that includes beliefs, patterns of worship, and symbols. Religious affiliation is a choice to

BOX 7-4   CONTENT OF A MENTAL STATUS EXAMINATION

Personal Information
- Age
- Gender
- Marital status
- Religious preference
- Race
- Ethnic background
- Employment
- Living arrangements

Appearance
- Grooming and dress
- Level of hygiene
- Pupil dilation or constriction
- Facial expression
- Height, weight, nutritional status
- Presence of body piercing or tattoos, scars, other
- Relationship between appearance and age

Behavior
- Excessive or reduced body movements
- Peculiar body movements (e.g., scanning of the environment, odd or repetitive gestures, level of consciousness, balance and gait)
- Abnormal movements (e.g., tardive dyskinesia, tremors)
- Level of eye contact (keep cultural differences in mind)

Speech
- Rate: slow, rapid, normal
- Volume: loud, soft, normal

- Disturbances (e.g., articulation problems, slurring, stuttering, mumbling)
- Cluttering (e.g., rapid, disorganized, tongue-tied speech)

Affect and Mood
- Affect: flat, bland, animated, angry, withdrawn, appropriate to context
- Mood: sad, labile, euphoric

Thought
- Thought process (e.g., disorganized, coherent, flight of ideas, neologisms, thought blocking, circumstantiality)
- Thought content (e.g., delusions, obsessions, suicidal thought)

Perceptual Disturbances
- Hallucinations (e.g., auditory, visual)
- Illusions

Cognition*
- Orientation: time, place, person
- Level of consciousness (e.g., alert, confused, clouded, stuporous, unconscious, comatose)
- Memory: remote, recent, immediate
- Fund of knowledge
- Attention: performance on serial sevens, digit span tests
- Abstraction: performance on tests involving similarities, proverbs
- Insight
- Judgment

*Refer to the inside back cover for the Saint Louis University Mental Status (SLUMS) exam.

connect personal spiritual beliefs with a larger organized group or institution and typically involves rituals. Belonging to a religious community can provide support during difficult times. For many individuals, prayer is a source of hope, comfort, and support in healing. (Refer to Chapter 2 for examples of the culturally different forms of prayer.)

Spiritual and religious practices have been determined to enhance healthy behaviors, social support, and a sense of meaning in people's lives, all of which are linked to decreased overall mental and physical stress, which in turn relate to a decreased incidence of illness in many people. (Refer to Chapter 10 for the effect of stress on health and illness.)

O'Rioran (2010) in an interview with Dr. Donald Lloyd-Jones (Northwestern University Fienberg School of Medicine, Chicago, IL) quoted him as saying:

In general, from the perspective of overall health, healthcare utilization, and outcomes, the suggestion has been from some of the studies that greater religiosity, in terms of participation or spirituality, is typically associated with better health outcomes.

Cultural and social assessment. Because nurses are increasingly faced with caring for culturally diverse populations, there is a growing need for nursing assessment, nursing diagnoses, and subsequent care to be planned around unique cultural health care beliefs, values, and practices. It is becoming more evident that all mental health professionals, and perhaps especially nurses, have a thorough understanding of the complexity of the cultural and social factors that influence health and illness. Awareness of individual cultural beliefs and health care practices can help all health care workers from stereotyping, stigmatizing, and labeling patients.

For patients who have difficulty using and understanding the English language, federal law maintains the use of a trained interpreter (Arnold & Boggs, 2011). Refer to Box 7-5 for an example of a psychosocial assessment.

After the assessment, it is useful to summarize pertinent data with the patient. This summary provides patients with reassurance that the health care provider understands their message, and it gives the patient an opportunity to clarify any misinformation. The patient should be told what will happen next. For example, if the initial assessment takes

BOX 7-5 PSYCHOSOCIAL ASSESSMENT

A. Previous hospitalizations

B. Educational background

C. Occupational background
1. Employed? Where? What length of time?
2. Special skills

D. Social patterns
1. Describe family.
2. Describe friends.
3. With whom does the patient live?
4. To whom does the patient go in time of crisis?
5. Who makes the decisions in your family?
6. Describe a typical day.

E. Sexual patterns
1. Sexually active? Practices safe sex? Practices birth control?
2. Sexual orientation
3. Sexual difficulties

F. Interests and abilities
1. What does the patient do in his or her spare time?
2. In which sport, hobby, or leisure activity does the patient participate?
3. Does the patient excel in any particular activity or hobby?
4. What gives the patient pleasure?

G. Substance use and abuse
1. What medications does the patient take? How often? How much?
2. What herbal or over-the-counter drugs does the patient take? How often? How much?
3. What psychotropic drugs does the patient take? How often? How much?
4. How many drinks of alcohol does the patient take per day? Per week?
5. What recreational drugs does the patient take? How often? How much?
6. Does the patient identify the use of drugs as a problem?

H. Coping abilities
1. What does the patient do when he or she gets upset?
2. To whom can the patient talk?
3. What usually helps to relieve stress?
4. What did the patient try this time?

I. Spiritual assessment
1. Does the patient have a spiritual or religious affiliation?
2. What gives the patient strength and hope?
3. Does the patient participate in any spiritual/religious activities?
4. What role does religion/spiritual practice play in the patient's life?
5. Do the patient's spiritual or religious beliefs help him or her in stressful situations?
6. Are there any restrictions on diet or medical interventions within the patient's religious, spiritual, or cultural beliefs?

J. Cultural assessment
1. Does the patient need an interpreter?
2. What is the first thing the patient does when he or she becomes ill to address the illness?
3. How has the patient been treating this illness?
4. How is this condition (medical or mental) viewed in the patient's culture?
5. Are there special health care practices within the patient's culture that address his or her medical/mental problem?
6. What are the attitudes toward mental illness in the patient's culture?
7. Does the patient have culture-specific beliefs that help him or her cope (with racism, prejudice, or discrimination)?
8. Does the patient's diet consist of culture-specific foods? If so, what foods should not be part of the patient's diet?

place in the hospital, you should tell the patient who he or she will be seeing next. If the initial assessment was conducted by a psychiatric nurse in a mental health clinic, the patient should be told when and how often he or she will meet with the nurse to work on the patient's problems. If you believe a referral is necessary, this should be discussed with the patient.

Self-awareness assessment. Self-awareness is a positive trait and a competent and effective interviewer needs to possess a high degree of psychological, emotional, and social/cultural self-awareness to perform optimally (Sommers-Flanagan & Sommers-Flanagan, 2009).

We all have personal biases and "off days" (i.e., days we feel sad or upset, for example), and we all hold our own expectations of the outcome of the interview. In addition, we all come from a specific culture/subculture with inherent expectations, traditions, and well-ingrained social beliefs. Being consciously aware of our personal biases and emotional states can help us become cognizant of how these traits can influence and distort our understanding of the patient (Sommers-Flanagan & Sommers-Flanagan, 2009) as well as our patient's experience of us as a safe and empathetic health care provider.

It is a good idea to be aware of cultural and social beliefs that may influence your interactions with a person from another background with inherently different cultural, social, and spiritual/religious beliefs. Also examine how you are feeling at the moment before an interview. We are not always aware of personal feelings or how they are affecting us when we first begin an interview, with the exceptions of students who will always feel anxious in the beginning, a very healthy sign. How do we obtain a good picture of ourselves in relationship to our interviewing skills? One way is clinical supervision from a seasoned and effective psychiatric nurse or clinician. Another effective way is by the use of videotapes of ourselves during an interview (usually a very painful experience, initially). Even seasoned interviewers can be shocked and surprised by their videotapes. With a confident colleague or supervisor, although these insights may be painful they are enormously helpful in becoming more self-aware and they increase our awareness of our patient as well. Taking notes shortly after an interview of what the patient said and what you said (**process recordings**) is a useful exercise because these "verbatim" notes provides an overall evaluation of your interaction, which may help you reevaluate and review not only what you missed but also what you could has done differently to be more effective. Process recordings are also useful for reviewing alternatives to what the patient has meant. Although these assessment methods are not as popular as they were in the past in nursing education, they offer the opportunity for important learning experiences in improving communication skills (refer to Applying the Art features throughout the clinical chapters).

Validating the Assessment

To gain an even clearer picture of your patient, it is helpful to look to outside sources. Emergency department records can be a valuable resource in understanding an individual's presenting behavior and problems. Police reports may be available in cases in which hostility and legal altercations occurred. Using informatics is a way of checking previous admissions, validating current information, or adding new information to your database. If the patient was admitted to a psychiatric unit in the past, information about the patient's previous level of functioning and behavior gives you a baseline for making clinical judgments. Occasionally consent forms may need to be signed by the patient or other appropriate relative, in order to obtain access to records.

Using Rating Scales

A number of standardized rating scales are useful for psychiatric evaluation and monitoring. Rating scales are often administered by a clinician, but many are self-administered. Table 7-1 lists some of the common scales in use today. Many of the clinical chapters in this book include a rating scale.

> ### ⚡ QUALITY AND SAFETY ALERT
>
> Some possible QSEN competencies inherent when assessing patients include the following:
> - **Patient-centered care:** Elicit patient values, preferences, and expressed needs as part of the clinical interview.
> - **Informatics:** Navigate the electronic health record.
> - **Teamwork and collaboration:** Identify the need for an interpreter; recognize contributions of other individuals or groups to help patient/family achieve health goals (not directly from QSEN).

STANDARD 2: DIAGNOSIS

Formulating a Nursing Diagnosis

A nursing diagnosis is a clinical judgment about a patient's response, needs, actual and potential psychiatric disorders, mental health problems, and potential comorbid (co-occurring) physical illnesses. A well-chosen and well-stated nursing diagnosis is the basis for selecting therapeutic outcomes and interventions (NANDA-I, 2012-2014). Refer to Appendix B for list of NANDA-I–approved nursing diagnoses.

A nursing diagnosis has three structural components:
1. Problem (unmet need)
2. Etiology (probable cause)
3. Supporting data (signs and symptoms)

The *problem,* or unmet need, describes the state of the patient at present. Problems that are within the nurse's domain to prescribe for and treat are termed *nursing diagnoses.* The nursing diagnostic title states what should change—for example: *Hopelessness.*

Etiology, or probable cause, is linked to the diagnostic title with the words "related to." Stating the etiology or probable cause tells what needs to be addressed to effect the change and identifies causes that the nurse can treat through nursing interventions—for example: *Hopelessness related to multiple losses.*

Supporting data, or signs and symptoms, state what the condition is like at present. It may be linked to the diagnosis and etiology with the words "as evidenced by." Supporting data (defining characteristics) that validate the diagnosis include the following:
- Patient's statement (e.g., "It's no use; nothing will change.")
- Lack of involvement with family and friends
- Lack of motivation to care for self or environment

The complete nursing diagnosis might be *Hopelessness* related to multiple losses as evidenced by lack of motivation to care for self and the statement, "It's no use, nothing will change."

> ### ⚡ QUALITY AND SAFETY ALERT
>
> Suggested QSEN competencies inherent when planning nursing diagnoses include the following:
> - **Patient-centered care:** Integrate understanding of multiple dimensions of patient-centered care, including patient's needs, preferences, and values within their cultural parameters.

STANDARD 3: OUTCOMES IDENTIFICATION

Determining Outcomes

Outcomes criteria are the optimal goal outcomes that reflect the maximal level of patient health that can realistically be achieved through nursing interventions. Whereas nursing diagnoses identify nursing problems, outcomes reflect the desired change. The expected outcomes provide direction for continuity of care (ANA, 2007). Outcomes need to take into account the patient's culture, values, and ethical beliefs. *Specifically, outcomes are stated in attainable and measurable terms and include a time estimate for attainment* (ANA, 2007). Therefore outcomes criteria are patient centered, geared to each individual, and documented as obtainable goals.

Moorhead and colleagues (2008) have compiled a standardized list of nursing outcomes in Nursing Outcomes Classification (NOC). NOC includes a total of 385 standardized outcomes that provide a mechanism for communicating the effect of

TABLE 7-1	STANDARDIZED RATING SCALES*
USE	**SCALE**
Depression	Beck Inventory
	Geriatric Depression Scale (GDS)
	Hamilton Depression Scale
	Zung Self-Report Inventory
	Patient Health Questionnaire (PHQ-9)
Anxiety	Modified Spielberger State Anxiety Scale
	Hamilton Anxiety Scale
Substance use disorders	Addiction Severity Index (ASI)
	Recovery Attitude and Treatment Evaluator (RAATE)
	Brief Drug Abuse Screen Test (B-DAST)
Obsessive-compulsive behavior	Yale-Brown Obsessive-Compulsive Scale (Y-BOCS)
Mania	Mania Rating Scale
Schizophrenia	Scale for Assessment of Negative Symptoms (SANS)
	Brief Psychiatric Rating Scale (BPRS)
Abnormal movements	Abnormal Involuntary Movement Scale (AIMS)
	Simpson Neurological Rating Scale
General psychiatric assessment	Brief Psychiatric Rating Scale (BPRS)
	Global Assessment of Functioning Scale (GAF)
Cognitive function	Mini-Mental State Examination (MMSE)
	Cognitive Capacity Screening Examination (CCSE)
	Alzheimer's Disease Rating Scale (ADRS)
	Memory and Behavior Problem Checklist
	Functional Assessment Screening Tool (FAST)
	Global Deterioration Scale (GDS)
Family assessment	McMaster Family Assessment Device
Eating disorders	Eating Disorders Inventory (EDI)
	Body Attitude Test
	Diagnostic Survey for Eating Disorders

*These rating scales highlight important areas in psychiatric assessment. Because many of the answers are subjective, experienced clinicians use these tools as a guide when planning care and also rely on their knowledge of their patients.

nursing interventions on the well-being of patients, families, and communities. Each outcome has an associated group of indicators that is used to determine patient status in relation to the outcome. Table 7-2 provides suggested NOC indicators for the outcome of Suicide Self-Restraint along with the Likert scale that quantifies the achievement on each indicator from 1 (never demonstrated) to 5 (consistently demonstrated).

However, NOC does not distinguish between short- and long-term outcomes. It is helpful when assessing the effectiveness of nursing interventions to use long- and short-term outcomes, often stated as goals. The use of long- and short-term outcomes or goals is particularly helpful for teaching and learning purposes. It is also valuable for providing guidelines for appropriate interventions. The use of goals guides nurses in building incremental steps toward meeting the desired outcome. All outcomes (goals) are written in positive terms following the criteria established by the Standards of Practice. Table 7-3 shows how a specific outcome criterion might be stated for a suicidal individual with a nursing diagnosis of *Risk for Suicide* related to depression and suicide attempt.

> ⚡ **QUALITY AND SAFETY ALERT**
>
> **Patient-Centered Care**
> - Integrate understanding of multiple dimensions of patient-centered care.
> - Engage patients or designated surrogates (e.g., family members) and active partnerships that promote health, safety and well-being, and self-remanagement.
> - Plan goals that are congruent with the patient/family and are realistic and meet patient's needs (not directly from QSEN).

STANDARD 4: PLANNING

More inpatient and community-based facilities are using standardized tools (e.g., care plans, flowcharts, clinical pathways) for patients with specific diagnoses. Standard tools allow for inclusion of evidence-based practice and newly tested interventions as they become available. They are more time-efficient, although less focused on the specific individual patient needs. Whatever the care planning procedures in a specific institution, the nurse considers the following specific principles when planning care:

- *Safe.* They must be safe for the patient as well as for other patients, staff, and family.
- *Appropriate.* They must be compatible with other therapies and with the patient's personal goals and cultural values, as well as with institutional rules.
- *Individualized.* They should be realistic (1) within the patient's capabilities given the patient's age, physical strength, condition, and willingness to change; (2) based on the number of staff available; (3) reflective of the actual available community resources; and (4) within the student's or nurse's capabilities.
- *Evidence based.* They should be based on scientific principles when available.

TABLE 7-2 SUICIDE SELF-RESTRAINT (NOC)

Definition:
Personal actions to refrain from gestures and attempts at killing self

Outcome Target Rating:
Maintain at _____. Increase to _____.

SUICIDE SELF-RESTRAINT OVERALL RATING	NEVER DEMONSTRATED 1	RARELY DEMONSTRATED 2	SOMETIMES DEMONSTRATED 3	OFTEN DEMONSTRATED 4	CONSISTENTLY DEMONSTRATED 5	
Indicators						
Expresses feelings	1	2	3	4	5	NA
Expresses sense of hope	1	2	3	4	5	NA
Maintains connectedness in relationship	1	2	3	4	5	NA
Obtains assistance as needed	1	2	3	4	5	NA
Seeks help when feeling self-destructive	1	2	3	4	5	NA
Verbalizes suicidal ideas	1	2	3	4	5	NA
Controls impulses	1	2	3	4	5	NA
Refrains from gathering means for suicide	1	2	3	4	5	NA
Refrains from giving away possessions	1	2	3	4	5	NA
Refrains from inflicting serious injury	1	2	3	4	5	NA
Refrains from using nonprescribed mood-altering substance(s)	1	2	3	4	5	NA
Discloses plan for suicide if present	1	2	3	4	5	NA
Upholds suicide contract	1	2	3	4	5	NA
Maintains self-control without supervision	1	2	3	4	5	NA
Refrains from attempting suicide	1	2	3	4	5	NA
Obtains treatment for depression	1	2	3	4	5	NA
Obtains treatment for substance abuse	1	2	3	4	5	NA
Reports adequate pain control for chronic pain	1	2	3	4	5	NA
Uses suicide prevention resources	1	2	3	4	5	NA
Uses social support group	1	2	3	4	5	NA
Uses available mental health services	1	2	3	4	5	NA
Plans for future	1	2	3	4	5	NA

From Moorhead, S., Johnson, M., Maas, M.L., & Swanson, E. (2008). *Nursing outcomes classification (NOC)* (4th ed.). St Louis: Mosby.

TABLE 7-3	EXAMPLES OF LONG- AND SHORT-TERM GOALS FOR A SUICIDAL PATIENT	
LONG-TERM GOALS OR OUTCOME	**SHORT-TERM GOALS OR OUTCOMES**
1. Patient will remain free from injury throughout the hospital stay.	a. Patient will state he or she understands the rationale and procedure of unit's protocol for suicide precautions.
	b. Patient will find staff and/or friend or family member when feeling overwhelmed or self-destructive during hospitalization.
2. By discharge, patient will state he or she no longer wishes to die and has at least two people to contact if suicidal thoughts arise.	a. Patient will meet with the nurse twice a day for 15 minutes to problem solve alternatives to the situation throughout the hospital stay.
	b. Patient will meet with social worker to find supportive resources in his or her community on discharge.
	c. By discharge, patient will state the purpose of medication, time and dose, adverse effects, and who to call for questions or concerns.

Using best-evidence interventions and treatments as they become available is being stressed in all areas of medical and mental health care (as discussed in detail in Chapter 1). David Sackett, one of the founders of evidence-based medicine, had the quintessential definition of evidence-based practice: "the conscientious, explicit, and judicious use of current best evidence in making decisions about the care of individual patients" (Sackett et al., 2000). **Evidence-based practice (EBP)** for nurses is a combination of clinical skills and the use of clinically relevant research in the delivery of effective patient-centered care. Therefore, the use of best available research coupled with patient preferences and sound clinical judgment and skills makes an optimal patient-centered nurse-patient relationship (Sackett et al., 2000). Box 7-6 lists several websites available for nurses to use as resources on evidence-based practice. Keep in mind that any interventions that are chosen to be used need to be acceptable and appropriate to the individual patient.

Interventions Planning

The **Nursing Interventions Classification (NIC)** (Bulechek et al., 2008) is a research-based standardized listing of 542 interventions that the nurse can use to plan care, and reflects current clinical practice. Nurses in all settings can use NIC to support quality patient care and incorporate evidence-based nursing actions. Although many safe and appropriate interventions may not be included in NIC, it is a useful guide for standardized care, but individualizing interventions to meet a patient's special needs should always be part of the planning.

When choosing nursing interventions from NIC or other sources, the nurse uses not just those that fit the nursing diagnosis (e.g., *Risk for Suicide*) but also those that match the defining data. Although the outcome criteria (NOC) might be similar or the same (e.g., Suicide Self-Restraint), the safe and appropriate interventions may be totally different because of the defining data. For example, consider the nursing diagnosis *Risk for Suicide* related to feelings of despair as evidenced by two recent suicide attempts and repeated statements that "I want to die."

BOX 7-6 USEFUL EVIDENCE-BASED PRACTICE WEBSITES

- Academic Center for Evidence-Based Nursing (ACE): www.acestar.uthscsa.edu
- Center for Research and Evidence-Based Practice (CREP): www.son.rochester.edu/son/research/centers/research-evidenced-based-practice
- Centre for Evidence-Based Mental Health: www.cebmh.com
- The Cochrane Collaboration: www.cochrane.org
- The Joanna Briggs Institute: www.joannabriggs.edu.au
- The Sarah Cole Hirsch Institute for Best Nursing Practice Based on Evidence: http://fpb.case.edu/HirshInstitute/index.shtm
- University of Iowa, Evidence-Based Practice Guidelines: www.nursing.uiowa.edu/products_services/evidence_based.htm
- University of Minnesota Evidence-Based Health Care Project: http://evidence.ahc.umn.edu/ebn.htm

The planning of appropriate nursing interventions might include the following:

- Initiate suicide precautions (e.g., ongoing observations and monitoring of the patient, provision of a protective environment) for the person who is at serious risk for suicide.
- Search the newly hospitalized patient and personal belongings for weapons or potential weapons during the inpatient admission procedure, as appropriate.
- Use protective interventions (e.g., area restriction seclusion, physical restraints) if the patient lacks the restraint to refrain from harming self, as needed.
- Assign hospitalized patient to a room located near the nursing station for ease in observations, as appropriate.

However, if the defining data are different, so will be the appropriate interventions. For example: *Risk for Suicide* related to loss of spouse as evidenced by lack of self-care and statements evidencing loneliness.

The nurse might choose the following interventions for this patient's plan of care:

- Determine the presence and degree of suicidal risk.
- Facilitate support of the patient by family and friends.
- Consider strategies to decrease isolation and opportunities to act on harmful thoughts.
- Assist the patient in identifying a network of supportive personnel and resources within the community (e.g., support groups, clergy, care providers).
- Provide information about available community resources and outreach programs.
- Chapter 23 addresses assessment of and intervention for the suicidal patient in more depth.

⚡ QUALITY AND SAFETY ALERT

Some possible QSEN competencies inherent in planning care include the following:

- **Patient-centered care:** Respect patient preferences for degree of active engagement in care process toward helping the patient meet his or her needs and goals.
- **Evidence-based practice:** Base individualized care plan on patient's values, clinical expertise, and evidence.
- **Informatics:** Document and plan patient care in an electronic health record.

STANDARD 5: IMPLEMENTATION

Psychiatric–Mental Health Nursing: Scope and Standards of Practice (ANA, 2007) identifies seven areas for intervention. Recent graduates and practitioners new to the psychiatric setting will participate in many of these activities with the guidance and support of more experienced health care professionals. The following four interventions identified in psychiatric mental health nurse (PMHN) practice guidelines (ANA, 2007) are performed both by the psychiatric mental health nurse (basic education) as well as by the advanced practice psychiatric mental health nurse (master's prepared).

The basic level for the psychiatric mental health registered nurse is accomplished through the nurse-patient relationship and therapeutic intervention skills. The nurse implements the plan using evidence-based interventions whenever possible, utilizing community resources, and collaborating with nursing colleagues.

Basic Level and Advanced Practice Interventions
Coordination of Care
The psychiatric mental health nurse coordinates the implementation of the plan and provides documentation.

Health Teaching and Health Promotion
Psychiatric mental health nurses use a variety of health teaching methods adaptive to the patient's needs (e.g., age, culture, ability to learn, readiness), integrating current knowledge and research and seeking opportunities for feedback and effectiveness of care. Health teaching includes identifying the health education needs of the patient and teaching basic principles of physical and mental health, such as giving information about coping, interpersonal relationships, social skills, mental disorders, the treatments for such illnesses and their effects on daily living, relapse prevention, problem-solving skills, stress management, crisis intervention, and self-care activities. The last of these, self-care activities, assists the patient in assuming personal responsibility for activities of daily living (ADLs) and is aimed at improving the patient's mental and physical well-being.

Milieu Therapy
Milieu therapy is an extremely important consideration for the nurse working with a patient who should feel comfortable and safe. Milieu management includes orienting patients to their rights and responsibilities, selecting specific activities that meet patients' physical and mental health needs, and ensuring that patients are maintained in the least restrictive environment. Among other things, it also includes that patients are informed in a culturally competent manner about the need for limits and the conditions necessary to remove them.

Pharmacological, Biological, and Integrative Therapies
Nurses need to know the intended action, therapeutic dosage, adverse reactions, and safe blood levels of medications being administered. The nurse also must monitor these values when appropriate (e.g., blood levels for lithium). The nurse is expected to discuss and provide medication teaching tools to the patient and family regarding drug action, adverse side effects, dietary restrictions, and drug interactions, and to provide time for questions. The nurse's assessment of the patient's response to psychobiological interventions is communicated to other members of the mental health team. Interventions are also aimed at alleviating untoward effects of medication.

Advanced Practice Interventions Only
The following three interventions are carried out by the advanced practice registered nurse in psychiatric mental health (APRN-PMH).

Prescriptive Authority and Treatment
The APRN-PMH is educated and clinically prepared to prescribe psychopharmacological agents for patients with mental health or psychiatric disorders in accordance with state and federal laws and regulations. Such prescriptions take into account the individual variables such as culture, ethnicity, gender, religious beliefs, age, and physical health.

Psychotherapy
The APRN-PMH is educationally and clinically prepared to conduct individual, couples, group, and family psychotherapy using evidence-based psychotherapeutic frameworks and nurse-patient therapeutic relationships (ANA, 2007).

Consultation

The APRN-PMH works with other clinicians to provide consultation, influence the identified plan, enhance the ability of other clinicians, provide services for patients, and effect change.

⚡ QUALITY AND SAFETY ALERT

Some possible QSEN competencies for implementing patient-centered care include the following:

Patient-Centered Care
- Provide patient-centered care with sensitivity and respect for the diversity of human experience.
- Recognize the boundaries of therapeutic relationships.
- Participate in building consensus or resolving conflict in the context of patient care.

Safety
- Do the interventions based on your care plan minimize the risk of harm to patients and providers through both system effectiveness and individual performance?

Teamwork and Collaboration
- Initiate request for help when appropriate to the situation.
- Integrate the contributions of others who play a role in helping patient/family achieve health goals in order to achieve quality patient care.

STANDARD 6: EVALUATION

Unfortunately, evaluation of patient outcomes is often the most neglected part of the nursing process. Evaluation of the individual's response to treatment should be systematic, ongoing, and criterion-based. Supporting data are included to clarify the evaluation. Ongoing assessment of data allows for revisions of nursing diagnoses, changes to more realistic outcomes, or identification of more appropriate interventions when outcomes are not met.

⚡ QUALITY AND SAFETY ALERT

Suggested QSEN competencies inherent when evaluating care include the following:

Quality Improvement (QI)
- Seek information about outcomes of care populations served in care setting.
- Evaluate and monitor the patient's outcomes (long- and short-term goals) and make changes to improve and increase the quality and safety of patient care (not directly from QSEN).

⚡ QUALITY AND SAFETY ALERT

Suggested QSEN competencies inherent in the documentation of care include the following:
- **Informatics:** Communicates information to the rest of the team on the patient's progress and employs communication technologies to coordinate care for patients.

DOCUMENTATION

Documentation could be considered the seventh step in the nursing process. Keep in mind that patient records are legal documents and may be used in a court of law (see Chapter 6). Besides the evaluation of stated outcomes, the chart should record changes in patient condition, record of informed consents (for medications and treatments), reaction to medication, documentation of symptoms (verbatim when appropriate), concerns of the patient, and any untoward incidents in the health care setting. Documentation of patient progress is the responsibility of the entire mental health team.

Although communication among team members and coordination of services are the primary goals when choosing a system for charting, practitioners in all settings must also consider professional standards, legal issues, requirements for reimbursement by insurers, and accreditation by regulatory agencies.

Information also must be in a format that is retrievable for quality assurance monitoring, utilization management, peer review, and research. Documentation, using the nursing process as a guide, is reflected in many of the different formats that are commonly used in health care settings (Table 7-4). Computerized clinical documentation is used increasingly in today's medical settings. Nurses need to be trained to use these technologies and the medical setting should be prepared to provide further training for nurses in the use of terminology, progress notes relating to needs assessment, nursing interventions, and nursing diagnoses (Hayrinen, 2010). Any documentation format used by a health care facility must be focused, organized, and pertinent and must conform to certain legal and other generally accepted principles (Box 7-7).

TABLE 7-4 NARRATIVE VERSUS PROBLEM-ORIENTED CHARTING*

NARRATIVE CHARTING	PROBLEM-ORIENTED CHARTING: SOAPIE
Characteristics	
A descriptive statement of patient status written in chronological order throughout a shift. Used to support assessment finding from a flow sheet. In charting by exception, narrative notes are used to indicate significant symptoms, behaviors, or events that are exceptions to norms identified on assessment flow sheet.	Developed in the 1960s for physicians to reduce inefficient documentation. Intended to be accompanied by a problem list. Originally SOAP, with IE added later. Emphasis is on problem identification, process, and outcome. **S:** Subjective data (patient statement) **O:** Objective data (nurse observations) **A:** Assessment (nurse interprets S and O and describes either a problem or a nursing diagnosis) **P:** Plan (proposed intervention) **I:** Interventions (nurse's response to problem) **E:** Evaluation (patient outcome)
Example	
Date/time/discipline Patient was agitated in the morning and pacing in the hallway. Blinked eyes, muttered to self, and looked off to the side. Stated heard voices. Verbally hostile to another patient. Offered 2 mg of haloperidol (Haldol) prn and sat with staff in quiet area for 20 minutes. Patient returned to community lounge and was able to sit and watch television.	Date/time/discipline **S:** "I'm so stupid. Get away, get away." "I hear the devil telling me bad things." **O:** Patient paced the hall, mumbling to self and looking off to the side. Shouted derogatory comments when approached by another patient. Watched walls and ceiling closely. **A:** Patient was having auditory hallucinations and increased agitation. **P:** Offered patient haloperidol prn. Redirected patient to less stimulating environment. **I:** Patient received 2 mg of haloperidol PO prn. Sat with patient in quiet room for 20 minutes. **E:** Patient calmer. Returned to community lounge, sat, and watched television.
Advantages	
Uses a common form of expression (narrative writing). Can address any event or behavior. Explains flow sheet findings. Provides multidisciplinary ease of use.	Structured. Provides consistent organization of data. Facilitates retrieval of data for quality assurance and utilization management. Contains all elements of the nursing process. Minimizes inclusion of unnecessary data. Provides multidisciplinary ease of use.
Disadvantages	
Unstructured. May result in different organization of information from note to note. Makes it difficult to retrieve quality assurance and utilization management data. Frequently leads to omission of elements of the nursing process. Commonly results in inclusion of unnecessary and subjective information.	Requires time and effort to structure the information. Limits entries to problems. May result in loss of data about progress. Not chronological. Carries negative connotation.

*Today most charting is computerized, and each institution has its own system.

BOX 7-7 LEGAL CONSIDERATIONS FOR DOCUMENTATION OF CARE

Do's

- Chart in a timely manner all pertinent and factual information.
- Be familiar with the nursing documentation policy in your facility and make your charting conform to this standard. The policy generally states the method, frequency, and pertinent assessments, interventions, and outcomes to be recorded. If your agency's policies and procedures do not encourage or allow for quality documentation, bring the need for change to the administration's attention.
- Chart legibly in ink.
- Chart facts fully, descriptively, and accurately.
- Chart what you see, hear, feel, and smell.
- Chart pertinent observations: psychosocial observations, physical symptoms pertinent to the medical diagnosis, and behaviors pertinent to the nursing diagnosis.
- Chart follow-up care provided when a problem has been identified in earlier documentation. For example, if a patient has fallen and injured a leg, describe how the wound is healing.
- Chart fully the facts surrounding unusual occurrences and incidents.
- Chart all nursing interventions, treatments, and outcomes (including teaching efforts and patient responses), and safety and patient protection interventions.
- Chart the patient's expressed subjective feelings.
- Chart each time you notify a physician and record the reason for notification, the information that was communicated, the accurate time, the physician's instructions or orders, and the follow-up activity.

- Chart physicians' visits and treatments.
- Chart discharge medications and instructions given for use, as well as all discharge teaching performed, and note which family members were included in the process.

Don'ts

- Do *not* chart opinions that are not supported by the facts.
- Do *not* defame patients by calling them names or by making derogatory statements about them (e.g., "an unlikable patient who is demanding unnecessary attention").
- Do *not* chart before an event occurs.
- Do *not* chart generalizations, suppositions, or pat phrases (e.g., "patient in good spirits").
- Do *not* obliterate, erase, alter, or destroy a record. If an error is made, draw one line through the error, write "mistaken entry" or "error," and initial. Follow your agency's guidelines closely.
- Do *not* leave blank spaces for chronological notes. If you must chart out of sequence, chart "late entry." Identify the time and date of the entry and the time and date of the occurrence.
- If an incident report is filed, *do not note in the chart that one was filed.* This form is generally a privileged communication between the hospital and the hospital's attorney. Describing it in the chart may destroy the privileged nature of the communication.

▌ KEY POINTS TO REMEMBER

- The nursing process is a six-step problem-solving approach to patient care to help secure safety and quality care for patients.
- The Institute of Medicine (IOM) and QSEN faculty have established mandates to prepare future nurses with the knowledge, skills, and attitudes (KSAs) necessary for achieving quality and safety as they engage in the six competencies of nursing: patient-centered care, teamwork and collaboration, evidence-based practice (EBP), quality improvement (QI), safety, and informatics.
- The *primary source* of assessment is the patient. *Secondary sources* of information include the family, neighbors, friends, police, and other members of the health team.
- The assessment interview includes gathering objective data (mental or emotional status) and subjective data (psychosocial assessment). A number of tools are provided in this textbook for the evaluation of cultural, spiritual/religious, and mental status.
- Medical examination, history, and systems review complete a comprehensive assessment.

- An important part of planning patient-centered care is to understand how spiritual/religious beliefs play in a person's life and how they deal with stress.
- Caregivers should also have an awareness of the person's cultural background and social attachments, and how these issues affect the way a person experiences healing in his or her culture.
- Assessment tools and standardized rating scales may be used to evaluate and monitor a patient's progress. Emphasis needs to be placed on further evaluation of progress and sharing of this information with other members of the health care team.
- Self-assessment is an important part of the assessment process. There are a number of ways that novice interviewers can gain valuable feedback, support, and supervision.
- Determination of the nursing diagnosis (NANDA-I) defines the practice of nursing, improves communication between staff members, and assists in accountability for care.
- A nursing diagnosis consists of (1) an unmet need or problem, (2) an etiology or probable cause, and (3) supporting data.

KEY POINTS TO REMEMBER—cont'd

- Outcomes are variable, measurable, and stated in terms that reflect a patient's actual state. NOC provides 330 standardized outcomes. Planning involves determining desired outcomes.
- Behavioral goals support outcomes. Goals are measurable, indicate the desired patient behavior(s), include a set time for achievement, and are short and specific.
- Planning nursing actions (NIC or other sources) to achieve the outcomes includes the use of the following specific principles: the plan should be (1) safe, (2) evidence based whenever possible, (3) realistic, and (4) compatible with other therapies. NIC provides nurses with standardized nursing interventions that are applicable for use in all settings.
- Practice in psychiatric nursing encompasses four basic-level interventions: coordination of care; health teaching and health promotion; milieu therapy; and pharmacological, biological, and integrative therapies.

- Advanced practice interventions are carried out by a nurse who is educated at the master's level or higher. Nurses certified for advanced practice psychiatric mental health nursing can practice psychotherapy, prescribe certain medications, and perform consulting work.
- The evaluation of care is a continual process of determining to what extent the outcome criteria have been achieved. The plan of care may be revised on the basis of the evaluation.
- Documentation of patient progress through evaluation of outcome criteria is crucial. The chart is a legal document and should accurately reflect the patient's condition, medications, treatment, tests, responses, and any untoward incidents.

APPLYING CLINICAL JUDGMENT

1. Pedro Gonzales, a 37-year-old Hispanic man, arrived by ambulance from a supermarket, where he had fallen. He remains lethargic. On his arrival to the emergency department (ED), his breath smelled "fruity." He appears confused and anxious, saying that "they put the 'evil eye' on me, they want me to die, they are drying out my body… it's draining me dry…they are yelling, they are yelling… no, no I'm not bad…oh God don't let them get me." When his mother arrives in the ED, she tells the staff, through the use of an interpreter, that Pedro is a severe diabetic and has a diagnosis of paranoid schizophrenia, and this happens when he does not take his medications. In a group or in collaboration with a classmate respond to the following:
   A. A number of nursing diagnoses are possible in this scenario. Formulate in writing at least two nursing diagnoses (problems) given the preceding information, and include "related to" and "as evidenced by."
   B. For each of your nursing diagnoses, list one long-term outcome (e.g., the problem, what should change). Include a timeframe, desired change, and three criteria that will help you evaluate if the outcome has been met, not met, or partially met.
   C. For each long-term outcome, list two short-term outcomes (goals) (the steps that need to be taken in order for the goal to be accomplished), including timeframe, desired outcomes, and evaluation criteria.
   D. What are the four basic principles for planning nursing interventions?
   E. What specific needs might you take into account when planning nursing care for Mr. Gonzales?
   F. Using informatics, evaluate optimal outcomes for Mr. Gonzalez at your current health care setting, or use the charting method employed by the institution.
   G. Give an example of the QSEN competencies you might stress when planning care for Mr. Gonzalez.

CHAPTER REVIEW QUESTIONS

Choose the most appropriate answer(s).
1. Which statement by a nurse suggests an undesirable outcome of a psychiatric assessment interview conducted by the psychiatric nurse?
   1. "I think I was able to establish good rapport with the patient."
   2. "I believe the patient understands that my values differ from his."
   3. "I was able to obtain a good understanding of the patient's current problem."
   4. "I was able to perform a complete assessment of the patient's level of psychological functioning."

2. Assessment of an older adult patient will be facilitated if the nurse:
   1. identifies and accommodates patient physical needs early.
   2. pledges complete confidentiality of all topics to the patient.
   3. adheres strictly to the order of questions on the standardized assessment tool.
   4. interprets data without regard to the patient's spiritual and cultural beliefs and practices.
3. Outcome criteria includes the: (select all that apply)
   1. time estimated for attainment.
   2. measurable terms.
   3. initial assessment.
   4. identifying data.

CHAPTER REVIEW QUESTIONS — cont'd

4. Which statement about a nursing diagnosis is correct?
   1. A nursing diagnosis has three structural components: a problem, the etiology of the problem, and supporting data that validate the diagnosis.
   2. A nursing diagnosis is complete when the problem statement reflects an unmet need and the etiology given reflects a probable cause.
   3. An accurate nursing diagnosis requires a problem statement that identifies causes the nurse can treat via nursing interventions.
   4. A nursing diagnosis always must be based on objective data measured by the nurse; subjective data may be used only as supporting data to validate the diagnosis.

5. The purpose of the psychiatric nursing assessment is to: (select all that apply)
   1. establish rapport.
   2. review physical status.
   3. determine risk factors.
   4. evaluate the care plan.

REFERENCES

American Nurses Association (ANA), American Psychiatric Nurses Association, & International Society of Psychiatric–Mental Health Nurses. (2007). *Psychiatric–mental health nursing: scope and standards of practice*. Washington, DC: Nursesbooks.org.

Arnold, E. C., & Boggs, K. U. (2011). *Interpersonal relationships: professional communication skills for nurses* (5th ed.). St Louis: Saunders.

Brauser, D. (2011). *Deadly combination of depression and diabetes doubles mortality risk*. Retrieved from www.Medscape.org/viewarticle/735714?SRE=cmemp.

Bulechek, G. M., Butcher, H. K., & Dochterman, J. M. (2008). *Nursing interventions classification (NIC)* (5th ed.). St Louis: Mosby.

Cronenwett, L., Sherwood, G., Bronsteiner, J., Disch, J., Johnson, J., Mitchell, P., Sullivan, D., & Water and, J. (2007). Quality and safety education for nurses. *Nursing Outlook, 55*(3), 122–131.

Durham, C. F., & Sherwood, G. D. (2008). Education to bridge the quality gap: a case to study approach. *Urologic Nursing, 28*(6), 431–438.

Hayrinen, K. (2010). Evaluation of electronic nursing documentation—nursing process model and standardized terminologies as key to visible and transparent nursing. *International Journal of Medical Informatics, 79*(8), 554–564.

Kling, J. (2011). *Spirituality an important component of patient care*. Retrieved July 23, 2011, from www.medscape.com/viewarticle/738237.

Lasater, K., & Nielsen, A. (2009). The influence of concept-based learning activities on students' clinical judgment development. *Journal of Nursing Education, 48*(8), 441–446.

Lenburg, C. E. (2011). The influence of contemporary trends and issues in nursing education. In B. Cherry, & S. R. Jacob (Eds.), *Contemporary nursing: issues, trends, & management* (5th ed.). St Louis: Elsevier.

Mian, A. I., Al-Mateen, C. S., & Cerda, G. (2010). Training child and adolescent psychiatrists to be culturally competent. *Child and Adolescent Psychiatric Clinics of North America, 19*(4), 7–31.

Moorhead, S., Johnson, M., Maas, M. L., & Swanson, E. (2008). *Nursing outcomes classification (NOC)* (4th ed.). St Louis: Mosby.

North American Nursing Diagnosis Association International (NANDA-I). (2012-2014). *Nursing diagnoses—definitions and classification 2012-2014*. Copyright © 2012, 1994–2012 by NANDA International, Philadelphia: Author. Used by arrangement with Blackwell Publishing Limited, a company of John Wiley and Sons, Inc.

O'Riordan, M. (2000). *Religion, spirituality not associated with better cardiovascular health*. Retrieved March 16, 2012 from http://www.theheart.org/article/104-5327.do.

Sackett, D. L., Straus, S., Richardson, W., et al. (2000). *Evidence-based medicine: how to practice and teach EBM*. London: Churchill Livingstone.

Sherwood, G., & Hicks, R. W. (2011). Quality and safety education in nursing (QSEN). In B. Cherry, & S. R. Jacob (Eds.), *Contemporary nursing: issues, trends, & management* (5th ed.). St Louis: Elsevier.

Sommers-Flanagan, J., & Sommers-Flanagan, R. (2009). *Clinical interviewing* (4th ed.). Hoboken, NJ: John Wiley & Sons.

Sullivan, D. T. (2010). Connecting nursing education and practice: a focus on shared goals for all of me and safety. *Creative Nursing, 16*(1), 37–43.

Valiga, T. M., & Champagne, M. (2011). Creating the future of nursing education: challenges and opportunities. In P. Slavik Cowen, & S. Moorhead (Eds.), *Current issues in nursing* (8th ed.). St Louis: Mosby/Elsevier.

Communication Skills: Medium for All Nursing Practice

Elizabeth M. Varcarolis

evolve WEBSITE

http://evolve.elsevier.com/Varcarolis/essentials

KEY TERMS AND CONCEPTS

cultural filters, p. 128
double messages, p. 119
double-bind messages, p. 119
e-health/e-medicine, telehealth,
    p. 128
feedback, p. 117

nontherapeutic techniques, p. 120
nonverbal communication, p. 118
therapeutic communication, p. 116
therapeutic techniques, p. 120
verbal communication, p. 118

SELECTED CONCEPT: Telehealth Technologies

"Telehealth is the use of electronic information and telecommunication technologies to support long-distance clinical healthcare, patient and professional health-related education, public health and health administration. Technologies include videoconferencing, the Internet, store-and-forward imaging, streaming media, and terrestrial and wireless communications." *(HRSA Rural Health)*

Since the whole area of psychiatry, psychology, counseling and nursing is based on human interaction, there still remains a need for "human to human sensitivity, acknowledgment, and respect for the patient care experience" with the use of any of the information communication technologies (ICT).
(Malloch, 2010, p. 1) (Arnold & Boggs, 2011).

OBJECTIVES

1. Identify three personal and two environmental factors that can impede accurate communication.
2. Discuss the differences between verbal and nonverbal communication and demonstrate at least five areas of nonverbal communication.
3. Identify two attending behaviors that you will work on to increase your communication skills.
4. Relate problems that can arise when nurses are insensitive to cultural differences in patients' communication styles.
5. Compare and contrast the range of verbal and nonverbal communication of your cultural groups with two other cultural groups in the areas of (a) communication style, (b) eye contact, and (c) touch. Give examples.
6. Demonstrate with a classmate the use of four techniques that can enhance communication, highlighting what makes them effective.
7. Demonstrate with a classmate the use of four techniques that can obstruct communication, highlighting what makes them ineffective.
8. Role play with a classmate the techniques of "What if" and the "Miracle Question" and then switch roles. Identify what new information you might have learned about your classmate, and what new insight you might have about yourself.
9. What are some advantages of telemedicine and telepsychiatry in the community in which you live?

Humans have a fundamental need to relate to others, and our advanced ability to communicate gives our life sustenance and meaning. We also share a need to be understood and form satisfying relationships with others. This is usually accomplished through the use of effective communication skills. On the other hand, when stress or negative feelings occur within the relationship, effective communication usually fails. Our ability to communicate is a fundamental aspect of being human; in fact, all of our actions, words, and expressions convey meaning to others. It is even said that we cannot *not* communicate. Silence, for example, can communicate acceptance, anger, or thoughtfulness. In the provision of nursing care, however, communication has a new emphasis. Just as social relationships are different from therapeutic relationships, basic communication is different from the professional, goal-directed, and scientifically based communication we call therapeutic communication.

COMMUNICATION

Therapeutic communication is crucial to forming a patient-centered nurse-patient relationship and is based on human interaction. Therapeutic communication is essential in nursing care regardless of the setting. Developing the skill to determine levels of pain in the postoperative patient, to listen as parents express feelings of fear concerning their child's diagnosis, or to understand, without hearing the words, the needs of the intubated voiceless patient in the intensive care unit is essential to the provision of quality nursing care. In psychiatric nursing communication skills assume a different and new emphasis because psychiatric disorders cause not only physical symptoms (such as fatigue, loss of appetite, and insomnia) but also emotional symptoms (such as sadness, anger, hopelessness, and euphoria) that affect a person's very ability to relate to others.

It is often in the psychiatric rotation that students discover the utility of therapeutic communication and begin to rely on techniques they once considered artificial. With continued practice, you will develop your own style and rhythm, and eventually these techniques will become a part of the way you communicate with others.

Novice psychiatric practitioners are often concerned that they may say the wrong thing, especially when learning to apply therapeutic techniques. Will you say the wrong thing? The answer is, yes, you probably will. That is how we all learn to find more useful and effective ways of helping individuals reach their goals. The challenge is to recover from your mistakes and use them for learning and growth (Sommers-Flanagan & Sommers-Flanagan, 2009).

Will saying the wrong thing be harmful to the patient? This is doubtful, especially if your intent is honest, your approach is respectful, and you have a genuine concern for the patient. Communication is up to 90% nonverbal, and individuals pay attention to the intent, as discussed in greater detail later in this chapter. Scientific investigations have identified special skills and methods that can aid people in becoming more effective helpers. However, knowledge of skills and techniques is not enough. Being an effective communicator, whether in nursing or in any other area of life, is not just a matter of knowing what techniques to use. Genuine respect for the individual, the ability to listen and to understand the person's concerns, and a desire to work with the individuals to help their situation are also key factors.

The Communication Process

Communication is the process of sending and receiving messages. One way of thinking about the process of communication is to use Berlo's classic communication model (1960), which has the following basic premises:

1. One person has a need to communicate with another (**stimulus**). For example, the stimulus for communication can be a need for information, comfort, or advice.
2. The person sending the message (**sender**) initiates interpersonal contact.
3. The **message** is the information sent or expressed to another. The clearest messages are those that are well organized and expressed in a manner familiar to the receiver.

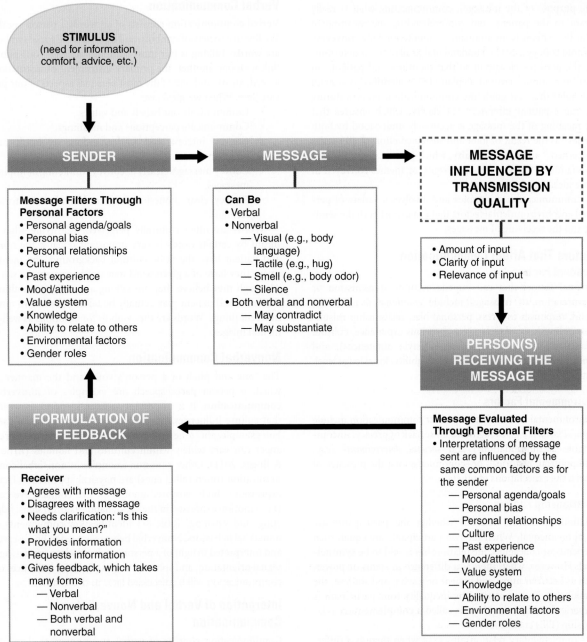

FIGURE 8-1 Operational definition of communication. (Adapted from Ellis, R.B., Gates, B., & Kenworthy, N. [2003]. *Interpersonal communication in nursing: theory and practice.* London: Churchill Livingstone Elsevier.)

4. The message can be sent through a variety of **media,** including auditory (hearing), visual (seeing), tactile (touch), olfactory (smell), or any combination of these.

5. The person receiving the message (**receiver**) then interprets the message and responds to the sender by providing feedback. The nature of the feedback often indicates whether the meaning of the message sent has been correctly interpreted by the receiver. Validating the accuracy of the sender's message is extremely important. An accuracy check may be obtained by simply asking the sender, "Is this what you mean?" or "I notice you turn away when we talk about your going back to college. Is there a conflict there?"

Figure 8-1 shows this simple model of communication along with some of the many factors that affect communication.

Effective communication in helping relationships depends on the nurse understanding what he or she is trying to convey (the purpose of the message), communicating what is really meant to the patient, and comprehending the meaning of what the patient is intentionally or unintentionally conveying (Arnold & Boggs, 2011). Fundamental to all of this is determining the person's viewpoint so that the nurse and patient can start on common ground. Peplau (1952) identified two main principles that can guide the communication process during the nurse-patient interview: (1) **clarity,** which ensures that the meaning of the message is accurately understood by both parties "as the result of joint and sustained effort of all parties concerned," and (2) **continuity,** which promotes connections among ideas "and the feelings, events, or themes conveyed in those ideas" (p. 290).

Communication is complex and involves a variety of personal and environmental factors that can distort both the sending and the receiving of messages.

Factors That Affect Communication
Personal Factors
Personal factors that can impede accurate transmission or interpretation of messages include *emotional factors* (e.g., mood, responses to stress, personal bias, relationship misunderstandings), *social factors* (e.g., previous experience, cultural differences, language differences, lifestyle differences), and *cognitive factors* (e.g., problem-solving ability, knowledge level, language use).

Environmental Factors
Environmental factors that may affect communication include *physical factors* (e.g., background noise, lack of privacy, uncomfortable accommodations) and *societal determinants* (e.g., sociopolitical, historical, or economic factors; the presence of others; the expectations of others).

Relationship Factors
Relationship factors refer to whether the participants are equal or unequal. When the two participants are equal, such as friends or colleagues, the relationship is said to be **symmetrical.** However, when there is a difference in status or power, such as between nurse and patient or teacher and student, the relationship is characterized by inequality (one participant is "superior" to the other) and is called a **complementary** relationship (Ellis et al., 2007).

Complementary relationships exist when there is a difference in status between the participants. For example, in all cultures social status, age or developmental differences, gender differences, and educational differences can be influential in the communication process.

In the United States, capitalism intimately ties systems of privilege (high-power groups) with systems of oppression (low-power groups) through economic control. Because high-status groups hold more power, they have more control over lower status groups. One way that power groups retain control (unequal) is through stereotypes, prejudice, and bias. In other words, stigma plays a big part in keeping relationship factors unbalanced (Hays, 2008).

Verbal Communication
Verbal communication consists of all words a person speaks. We live in a society of symbols, and our supreme social symbols are words. Talking is our most common activity—our public link with one another, the primary instrument of instruction, a need, an art, and one of the most personal aspects of our private lives. When we speak, we:
- Communicate our beliefs and values.
- Communicate perceptions and meanings.
- Convey interest and understanding *or* insult and judgment.
- Convey messages clearly *or* convey conflicting or implied messages.
- Convey clear, honest feelings *or* disguised, distorted feelings.

Words are often culturally perceived. Clarifying what is meant by certain words is very important. Even if the nurse and patient have the same cultural background, the mental image they have of a given word may not be exactly the same. Although they believe they are talking about the same thing, the nurse and patient may actually be talking about two quite different things. Words are the symbols for emotions as well as mental images.

Nonverbal Communication
The tone and pitch of a person's voice and the manner in which a person paces speech are examples of nonverbal communication. It is important to keep in mind, however, that culture influences the pitch and the tone a person uses. For example, the tone and pitch of a voice used to express anger can vary widely within cultures and families (Arnold & Boggs, 2011). Other common examples of nonverbal communication (often called **cues**) are physical appearance, facial expressions, body posture, amount of eye contact, eye cast (i.e., emotion expressed in the eyes), hand gestures, sighs, fidgeting, and yawning. Table 8-1 identifies key components of nonverbal behaviors. Nonverbal behaviors need to be observed and interpreted in light of a person's culture, class, gender, age, sexual orientation, and spiritual norms. Cultural influences on communication will be discussed later in this chapter.

Interaction of Verbal and Nonverbal Communication
Communication consists of verbal and nonverbal elements. Although we tend to think of communication primarily in terms of what is said, Shea (1998), a nationally renowned psychiatrist and communication workshop leader, indicates that communication is roughly 10% verbal and 90% nonverbal. Others believe that nonverbal behaviors comprise from 65% to 95% of a sent message. Both sets of statistics point to the surprising degree to which nonverbal behaviors and cues influence communication. Effective communicators pay attention to verbal as well as nonverbal cues.

Communication thus involves two radically different but interdependent kinds of symbols. The first type is the **spoken word,** which represents our public selves. Verbal assertions

TABLE 8-1	NONVERBAL BEHAVIORS	
BEHAVIOR	**POSSIBLE NONVERBAL CUES**	**EXAMPLE**
Body behaviors	Posture, body movements, gestures, gait	The patient is slumped in a chair, puts her face in her hands, and occasionally taps her right foot.
Facial expressions	Frowns, smiles, grimaces, raised eyebrows, pursed lips, licking of lips, tongue movements	The patient grimaces when speaking to the nurse; when alone, he smiles and giggles to himself.
Eye cast	Angry, suspicious, and accusatory looks	The patient's eyes harden with suspicion.
Voice-related behaviors	Tone, pitch, level, intensity, inflection, stuttering, pauses, silences, fluency	The patient talks in a loud sing-song voice.
Observable autonomic physiological responses	Increase in respirations, diaphoresis, pupil dilation, blushing, paleness	When the patient mentions discharge, she becomes pale, her respirations increase, and her face becomes diaphoretic.
Personal appearance	Grooming, dress, hygiene	The patient is dressed in a wrinkled shirt and his pants are stained; his socks are dirty and he is unshaven.
Physical characteristics	Height, weight, physique, complexion	The patient appears grossly overweight and his muscles appear flabby.

can be straightforward comments or skillfully can be used to distort, conceal, deny, and generally disguise true feelings. The second type, **nonverbal behaviors,** covers a wide range of human activities, from body movements to responses to the messages of others. How a person listens and uses silence and sense of touch may also convey important information about the private self that is not available from conversation alone, especially when viewed from a cultural perspective.

Some elements of nonverbal communication, such as facial expressions, seem to be inborn and are similar across cultures. Matsumoto (1992) and Matsumoto & Sung Hwang (2011) cited studies that found a high degree of agreement in spontaneous facial expressions or emotions across 10 different cultures. In public, however, some cultural groups (e.g., Japanese) may control their facial expressions when observers are present. Other types of nonverbal behaviors, such as how close people stand to each other when speaking, depend on cultural conventions. Some nonverbal communication is formalized and has specific meanings (e.g., the military salute, the Japanese bow).

Messages are not always simple and can appear to be one thing when in fact they are another. An interaction consists of verbal and nonverbal messages. Often, people have more conscious awareness of their verbal messages and less awareness of their nonverbal behaviors. The verbal message is sometimes referred to as the **content** of the message, and the nonverbal behavior is called the **process** of the message.

When the content is congruent with the process, the communication is more clearly understood and is considered healthy. For example, if a student says, "It's important that I get good grades in this class," that is *content*. If the student has purchased the books for the class, takes good notes, and has a study buddy, that is *process*. Therefore the content and process are congruent and straightforward, and there is a "healthy" message. If, however, the verbal message is not reinforced or is in fact contradicted by the nonverbal behavior, the message is confusing. For example, if the student does not have the books, skips several classes, and does not study, that is *process*. Here the student is conveying two different messages.

Conflicting messages are known as double messages or *mixed messages.* One way a nurse can respond to verbal and nonverbal incongruity is to reflect and validate the patient's feelings. "You say you are upset that you did not pass this semester, but I notice that you look more relaxed and less conflicted than you have all term. What do you see as some of the pros and cons of not passing the course this semester?"

Pioneers in the field of family therapy, Bateson and colleagues (1956) coined the term double-bind messages. Messages are sent to create meaning but also can be used defensively to hide what is actually occurring, create confusion, and attack relatedness (Ellis et al., 2007). A double-bind message is a mix of content (what is said) and process (what is transmitted nonverbally) that has both a neutral/nurturing aspect, as in what is said, and a hurtful/negative aspect, which is often implied. For example:

> **VIGNETTE**
> A 17-year-old female who lives at home with her mother wants to go out for an evening with her friends. She is told by her chronically ill but not helpless mother: "Oh, that's okay, go ahead, have fun. I'll just sit here by myself, and I can always call 911 if I don't feel well, but you go ahead and have fun." The mother says this while looking sad, eyes cast down, slumped in her chair, and letting her cane drop to the floor.

The recipient of this double-bind message is caught between contradictory statements so that she cannot do the right thing. If she goes out for the evening, the implication is that she is being selfish by leaving her sick mother alone, but if she stays, the mother could say, "I told you to go have fun." If she does go out, the chances are she will not have much fun. No matter what the daughter does, she just cannot win.

With experience, nurses become increasingly aware of a patient's verbal and nonverbal communication. Nurses can compare patients' dialogue with their nonverbal communication to gain important clues about the real message. What individuals do either may express and reinforce or may contradict what they say. As in the saying "Actions speak louder than words," actions often reveal the true meaning of a person's intent, whether it is conscious or unconscious.

EFFECTIVE COMMUNICATION SKILLS FOR NURSES

The art of communication was emphasized by Peplau to highlight the importance of nursing interventions in facilitating achievement of quality patient care and quality of life (Haber, 2000). Therefore, as stated, the goals of the nurse in the mental health setting are to help the patient:

- Feel understood and comfortable.
- Identify and explore problems relating to others.
- Discover healthy ways of meeting emotional needs.
- Experience satisfying interpersonal relationships.

The goal for the nurse is to establish and maintain a relationship in which the patient will feel safe and hopeful that positive change is possible.

Once specific needs and problems have been identified, the nurse can work with the patient on increasing critical thinking skills, learning new coping behaviors, and experiencing more appropriate and satisfying ways of relating to others. To do this the nurse needs to have a sound knowledge of communication skills. Therefore nurses must become more aware of their own interpersonal methods, eliminating obstructive nontherapeutic techniques and developing additional responses that maximize nurse-patient interactions and increase the use of helpful therapeutic techniques.

Useful tools for nurses when communicating with their patients are (1) silence, (2) active listening, and (3) clarifying techniques.

Use of Silence

Silence can frighten interviewers as well as patients (Sommers-Flanagan & Sommers-Flanagan, 2009). In our society, and in nursing, there is an emphasis on action. In communication we tend to expect a high level of verbal activity. Many students and practicing nurses find that when the flow of words stops, they become uncomfortable. **Silence** is not the absence of communication; it is a specific channel for transmitting and receiving messages. The practitioner needs to understand that silence is a significant means of influencing and being influenced by others, and if used judiciously, it can be a powerful listening response.

In the initial interview the patient may be reluctant to speak because of the newness of the situation, the fact that the nurse is a stranger, self-consciousness, embarrassment, or shyness.

Talking is highly individualized; some find the telephone a nuisance, but others talk/text on their cell phones almost constantly (e.g., while driving, shopping, in a restaurant with friends, and, yes, sitting in a classroom or meeting). The nurse must recognize and respect individual differences in styles and tempos of responding. People who are quiet, those who have a language barrier or speech impediment, older adults, and those who lack confidence in their ability to express themselves may communicate a need for support and encouragement through their silence.

Although there is no universal rule concerning how much silence is too much, silence has been said to be worthwhile only as long as it is serving some function and not frightening the patient. Knowing when to speak during the interview largely depends on the nurse's perception about what is being conveyed through the silence. Icy silence may be an expression of anger and hostility. Being ignored or given the silent treatment is recognized as an insult and is a particularly hurtful form of communication. Silence among some African-American patients may relate to anger, insulted feelings, or acknowledgment of a nurse's lack of cultural sensitivity (Smedley et al., 2002).

Silence may provide meaningful moments of reflection for both participants. It gives each an opportunity to contemplate thoughtfully what has been said and felt, weigh alternatives, formulate new ideas, and gain a new perspective on the matter under discussion. If the nurse waits to speak and allows the patient to break the silence, the patient may share thoughts and feelings that would otherwise have been withheld. Nurses who feel compelled to fill every void with words often do so because of their own anxiety, self-consciousness, and embarrassment. When this occurs, the nurse's need for comfort tends to take priority over the needs of the patient.

Conversely, prolonged and frequent silences by the nurse may hinder an interview that requires verbal articulation. Although the untalkative nurse may be comfortable with silence, this mode of communication may make the patient feel like a fountain of information to be drained dry. Moreover, without feedback, patients have no way of knowing whether what they said was understood.

Active Listening

People want more than just physical presence in human communication. Most people want the other person to be there for them psychologically, socially, and emotionally. **Active listening** includes the following:

- Observing the patient's nonverbal behaviors
- Listening to and understanding the patient's verbal message
- Listening to and understanding the person in the context of the social setting of his or her life
- Listening for "false notes" (i.e., inconsistencies or things the patient says that need more clarification)
- Providing the patient with feedback about himself or herself of which the patient might be unaware

Sommers-Flanagan and Sommers-Flanagan (2009) advise students, as well as experienced clinicians, to learn to quiet themselves: "They need to rein in any natural urges to help, personal needs, and anxieties" (p. 5). Relaxation techniques may help some before an interview with the patient (e.g., closing one's eyes and breathing slowly for a few minutes or using mindfulness training/meditation). This usually results in more concentration on the patient, and less distraction by personal worries or personal thoughts of what to say next.

Effective interviewers must become accustomed to silence, but it is just as important for effective interviewers to learn to become active listeners when the patient is talking, as well as when the patient becomes silent. During active listening nurses carefully note what the patient is saying verbally and nonverbally, as well as monitor their own nonverbal responses. Using silence effectively and learning to listen on a deeper, more significant level—to the patient as well as to your own thoughts and reaction—are both key ingredients in effective communication. Both skills take time to develop but can be learned; you will become more proficient with guidance and practice.

Some principles important to active listening are always relevant, such as the following (Mohl, 2003):
- The answer is always inside the patient.
- Objective truth is never as simple as it seems.
- Everything you hear is modified by the patient's filters.
- Everything you hear is modified by your own filters.
- It is okay to feel confused and uncertain.
- Listen to yourself, too.

Active listening helps strengthen the patient's ability to use critical thinking in order to solve problems. By giving the patient undivided attention, the nurse communicates that the patient is not alone. This kind of intervention enhances self-esteem and encourages the patient to direct energy toward finding ways to deal with problems. Serving as a sounding board, the nurse listens as the patient tests thoughts by voicing them aloud. This form of interpersonal interaction often enables the patient to clarify thinking, link ideas, and tentatively decide what should be done and how best to do it. Active listening is an art that develops with practice over time.

Clarifying Techniques

Understanding depends on clear communication, which is aided by verifying with the patient the nurse's interpretation of the patient's messages. The nurse must request feedback on the accuracy of the message received from verbal as well as nonverbal cues. The use of **clarifying techniques** helps both participants identify major differences in their frame of reference, giving them the opportunity to correct misperceptions before these cause any serious misunderstandings. The patient who is asked to elaborate on or to clarify vague or ambiguous messages needs to know that the purpose is to promote mutual understanding.

Paraphrasing

For clarity, the nurse might use **paraphrasing,** which means restating in different (often fewer) words the basic content of a patient's message. Using simple, precise, and culturally relevant terms, the nurse may readily confirm interpretation of

the patient's previous message before the interview proceeds. By prefacing statements with a phrase such as, "I'm not sure I understand" or "In other words, you seem to be saying…," the nurse helps the patient form a clearer perception of what may be a bewildering mass of details. After paraphrasing, the nurse must validate the accuracy of the restatement and its helpfulness to the discussion. The patient may confirm or deny the perceptions through nonverbal cues or by direct response to a question such as, "Was I correct in saying…?" As a result, the patient is made aware that the interviewer is actively involved in the search for understanding.

Restating

In **restating,** the nurse mirrors the patient's overt and covert messages; thus this technique may be used to echo feeling as well as content. Restating differs from paraphrasing in that it involves repeating the same key words the patient has just spoken. If a patient remarks, "My life is empty…it has no meaning," additional information may be gained by restating, "Your life has no meaning?" The purpose of this technique is to explore more thoroughly subjects that may be significant. However, too frequent and indiscriminate use of restating might be interpreted by patients as inattention, disinterest, or worse.

It is easy to overuse this tool so that its application becomes mechanical. Parroting or mimicking what another has said may be perceived as poking fun at the person, so that use of this nondirective approach can become a definite barrier to communication. To avoid overuse of restating, the nurse can combine restatements with direct questions that encourage descriptions: "What does your life lack?" "What kind of meaning is missing?" "Describe one day in your life that appears empty to you."

Reflecting

Reflection is a means of assisting people to better understand their own thoughts and feelings. **Reflecting** may take the form of a question or a simple statement that conveys the nurse's observations of the patient when sensitive issues are being discussed. The nurse might then describe briefly to the patient the apparent meaning of the emotional tone of the patient's verbal and nonverbal behavior. For example, to reflect a patient's feelings about his or her life, a good beginning might be, "You sound as if you have had many disappointments."

Sharing observations with a patient shows acceptance. The nurse helps make the patient aware of inner feelings and encourages the patient to own them. For example, the nurse may tell a patient, "You look sad." Perceiving the nurse's concern may allow a patient spontaneously to share feelings. The use of a question in response to the patient's question is another reflective technique (Arnold & Boggs, 2011). For example:

Patient: "Nurse, do you think I really need to be hospitalized?"
Nurse: "What do you think, Jane?"
Patient: "I don't know; that's why I'm asking you."

Nurse: "I'll be willing to share my impression with you at the end of this first session. However, you've probably thought about hospitalization and have some feelings about it. I wonder what they are."

Exploring

A technique that enables the nurse to examine important ideas, experiences, or relationships more fully is **exploring.** For example, if a patient tells the nurse that he does not get along well with his wife, the nurse will want to further explore this area. Possible openers include the following:

- *"Tell me* more about your relationship with your wife."
- *"Describe* your relationship with your wife."
- *"Give me an example* of how you and your wife don't get along."

Asking for an example can greatly clarify a vague or generic statement made by a patient.

Patient: "No one likes me."

Nurse: "Give me an example of one person who doesn't like you."

or

Patient: "Everything I do is wrong."

Nurse: "Give me an example of one thing you do that you think is wrong."

Table 8-2 lists more examples of techniques that enhance communication.

Projective Questions: The *"What If"* Question

Projective questions usually start with a *"what if"* to help people articulate, explore, and identify thoughts and feelings. Projective questions can also help people imagine thoughts, feelings, and behaviors they might have in certain situations (Sommers-Flanagan & Sommers-Flanagan, 2009, p. 87):

- If you had three wishes what would you wish for?
- What if you could go back and change how you acted in (X situation/significant life event); what would you do differently now?
- What would you do if you were given $1 million, no strings attached?

Presupposition Questions: The *"Miracle Question"*

- Suppose you woke up in the morning and a miracle happened and this problem had gone away. What would be different? How would it change your life?

These two questions can reveal a lot about a person that can be used in identifying goals that the patient may be motivated to pursue, and often get to the crux of what might be the most important issues in a person's thinking/life.

NONTHERAPEUTIC TECHNIQUES

Although people may use nontherapeutic techniques in their daily lives, they can become problematic when one is working with patients. Table 8-3 offers samples of nontherapeutic techniques and suggestions for more helpful responses.

Asking Excessive Questions

Excessive questioning, or asking multiple questions at the same time, especially closed-ended questions, casts the nurse in the role of interrogator, raising a demand for information without respect for the patient's willingness or readiness to respond. This approach conveys lack of respect for and sensitivity to the patient's needs. Excessive questioning or asking multiple questions at the same time controls the range and nature of the response and can easily result in a therapeutic stall or shut down an interview. It is a controlling tactic and may reflect the interviewer's lack of security in letting the patient tell his or her own story. It is better to ask more open-ended questions and follow the patient's lead. For example:

Excessive questioning: "Why did you leave your wife? Did you feel angry at her? What did she do to you? Are you going back to her?"

More therapeutic approach: "Tell me about the situation between you and your wife."

Keep in mind that knowing a lot of facts about a person is not synonymous with helping. You might end up with a lot of facts, but miss the person entirely (Egan, 2010).

Giving Approval or Disapproval

"You look great in that dress." "I'm proud of the way you controlled your temper at lunch." "That's a great quilt you made." What could be bad about giving someone a pat on the back once in a while? Nothing, if it is done without carrying a judgment (positive or negative) by the nurse. We often give our friends and family approval when they do something well. However, in a nurse-patient situation, **giving approval** often becomes much more complex. A patient may be feeling overwhelmed, experiencing low self-esteem, feeling unsure of where his or her life is going, and very needy for recognition, approval, and attention. Yet, when people are feeling vulnerable, a value comment might be misinterpreted. For example:

Giving approval: "You did a great job in group telling John just what you thought about how rudely he treated you."

Implied in this message is that the nurse was pleased by the manner in which the patient talked to John. The patient then sees such a response as a way to please the nurse by doing the right thing. To continue to please the nurse (and get approval), the patient may continue the behavior. The behavior might be useful for the patient, but when a behavior is being done to please another person, it is not coming from the individual's own volition or conviction.

Also when the other person whom the patient needs to please is not present, the motivation for the new behavior might not be there either. Thus the new response really is not a change in behavior as much as a ploy to win approval and acceptance from another person. Giving approval also stops further communication. It is a statement of the observer's (nurse's) judgment about another person's (patient's) behavior. A more useful comment would be the following:

More therapeutic approach: "I noticed that you spoke up to John in group yesterday about his rude behavior. How did it feel to be more assertive?"

TABLE 8-2 TECHNIQUES THAT ENHANCE COMMUNICATION

TECHNIQUE	DISCUSSION	EXAMPLES
Using silence	Gives the person time to collect thoughts or think through a point.	Encourage a person to talk by waiting for the answers.
Accepting	Indicates that the person has been understood. The statement does not necessarily indicate agreement but is nonjudgmental. However, nurses should not imply that they understand when they do not understand.	"Yes." "Uh-huh." "I follow what you say."
Giving recognition	Indicates awareness of change and personal efforts. Does not imply good or bad, or right or wrong.	"Good morning, Mr. James." "You've combed your hair today." "I notice that you shaved today."
Offering self	Offers presence, interest, and a desire to understand. Is not offered to get the person to talk or behave in a specific way.	"I would like to spend time with you." "I'll stay here and sit with you awhile."
Offering general leads	Allows the other person to take direction in the discussion. Indicates that the nurse is interested in what comes next.	"Go on." "And then?" "Tell me about it."
Giving broad openings	Clarifies that the lead is to be taken by the patient. However, the nurse discourages pleasantries and small talk.	"Where would you like to begin?" "What are you thinking about?" "What would you like to discuss?"
Placing the events in time or sequence	Puts events and actions in better perspective. Notes cause-and-effect relationships and identifies patterns of interpersonal difficulties.	"What happened before?" "When did this happen?"
Making observations	Calls attention to the person's behavior (e.g., trembling, nail biting, restless mannerisms). Encourages the person to notice the behavior to describe thoughts and feelings for mutual understanding. Helpful with mute and withdrawn people.	"You appear tense." "I notice you're biting your lips." "You appear nervous whenever John enters the room."
Encouraging description of perception	Increases the nurse's understanding of the patient's perceptions. Talking about feelings and difficulties can lessen the need to act them out inappropriately.	"What do these voices seem to be saying?" "What is happening now?" "Tell me when you feel anxious."
Encouraging comparison	Reveals recurring themes in experiences or interpersonal relationships. Helps the person clarify similarities and differences.	"Has this ever happened before?" "Is this how you felt when...?" "Was it something like...?"
Restating	Repeats the main idea expressed. Gives the patient an idea of what has been communicated. If the message has been misunderstood, the patient can clarify it.	*Patient:* "I can't sleep. I stay awake all night." *Nurse:* "You have difficulty sleeping?" *Patient:* "I don't know...he always has some excuse for not coming over or keeping our appointments." *Nurse:* "You think he no longer wants to see you?"
Reflecting	Directs questions, feelings, and ideas back to the patient. Encourages the patient to accept his or her own ideas and feelings. Acknowledges the patient's right to have opinions and make decisions and encourages the patient to think of self as a capable person.	*Patient:* "What should I do about my husband's affair?" *Nurse:* "What do you think you should do?" *Patient:* "My brother spends all of my money and then has the nerve to ask for more." *Nurse:* "You feel angry when this happens?"
Focusing	Concentrates attention on a single point. It is especially useful when the patient jumps from topic to topic. If a person is experiencing a severe or panic level of anxiety, the nurse should not persist until the anxiety lessens.	"This point you are making about leaving school seems worth looking at more closely." "You've mentioned many things. Let's go back to your thinking of 'ending it all'."

Continued

TABLE 8-2 TECHNIQUES THAT ENHANCE COMMUNICATION—cont'd

TECHNIQUE	DISCUSSION	EXAMPLES
Exploring	Examines certain ideas, experiences, or relationships more fully. If the patient chooses not to elaborate by answering no, the nurse does not probe or pry. In such a case, the nurse respects the patient's wishes.	"Tell me more about that." "Would you describe it more fully?" "Could you talk about how it was that you learned your mom was dying of cancer?"
Giving information	Makes available facts the person needs. Supplies knowledge from which decisions can be made or conclusions drawn. For example, the patient needs to know the role of the nurse; the purpose of the nurse-patient relationship; and the time, place, and duration of the meetings.	"My purpose for being here is…" "This medication is for…" "The test will determine…"
Seeking clarification	Helps patients clarify their own thoughts and maximize mutual understanding between nurse and patient.	"I am not sure I follow you." "What would you say is the main point of what you just said?" "Give an example of a time you thought everyone hated you."
Presenting reality	Indicates what is real. The nurse does not argue or try to convince the patient, just describes personal perceptions or facts in the situation.	"That was Dr. Todd, not a terrorist stalking and trying to harm you." "That was the sound of a car backfiring." "Your mother is not here; I am a nurse."
Voicing doubt	Undermines the patient's beliefs by not reinforcing the exaggerated or false perceptions.	"Isn't that unusual?" "Really?" "That's hard to believe."
Seeking consensual validation	Clarifies that both the nurse and the patient share mutual understanding of communications. Helps the patient become clearer about what he or she is thinking.	"Tell me whether my understanding agrees with yours."
Verbalizing the implied	Puts into concrete terms what the patient implies, making the patient's communication more explicit.	*Patient:* "I can't talk to you or anyone else. It's a waste of time." *Nurse:* "Do you feel that no one understands?"
Encouraging evaluation	Aids the patient in considering people and events from the perspective of the patient's own set of values.	"How do you feel about…?" "What did it mean to you when he said he couldn't stay?"
Attempting to translate into feelings	Responds to the feelings expressed, not just the content. Often termed *decoding*.	*Patient:* "I am dead inside." *Nurse:* "Are you saying that you feel lifeless? Does life seem meaningless to you?"
Suggesting collaboration	Emphasizes working with the patient, not doing things for the patient. Encourages the view that change is possible through collaboration.	"Perhaps you and I can discover what produces your anxiety." "Perhaps by working together we can come up with some ideas that might improve your communications with your spouse."
Summarizing	Combines the important points of the discussion to enhance understanding. Also allows the opportunity to clarify communications so that both nurse and patient leave the interview with the same ideas in mind.	"Have I got this straight?" "You said that…" "During the past hour, you and I have discussed…"
Encouraging formulation of a plan of action	Allows the patient to identify alternative actions for interpersonal situations the patient finds disturbing (e.g., when anger or anxiety is provoked).	"What could you do to let anger out harmlessly?" "The next time this comes up, what might you do to handle it?" "What are some other ways you can approach your boss?"

Adapted from Hays, J.S., & Larson, K. (1963). *Interacting with patients*. New York: Macmillan. Copyright ©1963 Macmillan Publishing.

TABLE 8-3 NONTHERAPEUTIC COMMUNICATION

NONTHERAPEUTIC TECHNIQUE	EXAMPLES	DISCUSSION	MORE HELPFUL RESPONSE
Giving premature advice	"Get out of this situation immediately."	Assumes the nurse knows best and the patient cannot think for self. Inhibits problem solving and fosters dependency.	*Encouraging problem solving:* "What are the pros and cons of your situation?" "What were some of the actions you thought you might take?" "What are some of the ways you have thought of to meet your goals?"
Minimizing feelings	*Patient:* "I wish I were dead." *Nurse:* "Everyone gets down in the dumps." "I know what you mean." "You should feel happy you're getting better." "Things get worse before they get better."	Indicates that the nurse is unable to understand or empathize with the patient. The patient's feelings or experiences are being belittled, which can cause the patient to feel small or insignificant.	*Empathizing and exploring:* "You must be feeling very upset. Are you thinking of hurting yourself?"
Falsely reassuring	"I wouldn't worry about that." "Everything will be all right." "You will do just fine; you'll see."	Underrates the patient's feelings and belittles the patient's concerns. May cause the patient to stop sharing feelings if the patient thinks he or she will be ridiculed or not taken seriously.	*Clarifying the patient's message:* "What specifically are you worried about?" "What do you think could go wrong?" "What are you concerned might happen?"
Making value judgments	"How come you still smoke when your wife has lung cancer?"	Prevents problem solving. Can make the patient feel guilty, angry, misunderstood, not supported, or anxious to leave.	*Making observations:* "I notice you are still smoking even though your wife has lung cancer. Is this a problem?"
Asking "why" questions	"Why did you stop taking your medication?"	Implies criticism; often has the effect of making the patient feel defensive.	*Asking open-ended questions; giving a broad opening:* "Tell me some of the reasons that led up to your not taking your medications."
Asking excessive questions	*Nurse:* "How's your appetite? Are you losing weight? Are you eating enough?" *Patient:* "No."	Results in the patient's not knowing which question to answer and possibly being confused about what is being asked.	*Clarifying:* "Tell me about your eating habits since you've been depressed."
Giving approval; agreeing	"I'm proud of you for applying for that job." "I agree with your decision."	Implies that the patient is doing the *right* thing—and that not doing it is wrong. May lead the patient to focus on pleasing the nurse or clinician; denies the patient the opportunity to change his or her mind or decision.	*Making observations:* "I noticed that you applied for that job. What factors led you to change your mind about applying for that job?" *Asking open-ended questions; giving a broad opening:* "What led to that decision?"

Continued

TABLE 8-3 NONTHERAPEUTIC COMMUNICATION—cont'd			
NONTHERAPEUTIC TECHNIQUE	EXAMPLES	DISCUSSION	MORE HELPFUL RESPONSE
Disapproving; disagreeing	"You really should have shown up for the medication group." "I disagree with that."	Can make a person defensive.	*Exploring:* "What was going through your mind when you decided not to come to your medication group?" "That's one point of view. How did you arrive at that conclusion?"
Changing the subject	*Patient:* "I'd like to die." *Nurse:* "Did you go to Alcoholics Anonymous like we discussed?"	May invalidate the patient's feelings and needs. Can leave the patient feeling alienated and isolated and increase feelings of hopelessness.	*Validating and exploring:* *Patient:* "I'd like to die." *Nurse:* "This sounds serious. Have you thought of harming yourself?"

Adapted from Hays, J.S., & Larson, K. (1963). *Interacting with patients.* New York: Macmillan. Copyright ©1963 Macmillan Publishing.

This opens the way for finding out if the patient was scared or comfortable, wants to work more on assertiveness, or has other issues to discuss. It also suggests that this was a self-choice the patient made. The patient is given recognition for the change in behavior, and the topic is also opened for further discussion.

Disapproving is moralizing and implies that the nurse has the right to judge the patient's thoughts or feelings. Again, an observation should be made instead.

> *Disapproving:* "You really should not cheat, even if you think everyone else is doing it."
>
> *More therapeutic approach:* "Can you give me two examples of how cheating could negatively affect your goal of graduating?"

Advising

Although we ask for and give advice all the time in daily life, **giving advice** to a patient is rarely helpful. Often when we ask for advice, our real motive is to discover if we are thinking along the same lines as someone else or if they would agree with us. When the nurse gives advice to a patient who is having trouble assessing and finding solutions to conflicted areas in his or her life, the nurse is interfering with the patient's ability to make personal decisions. Giving a person a solution robs the patient of self-responsibility (Egan, 2010). When the nurse offers the patient solutions, the patient eventually begins to think that the nurse does not view the patient as capable of making effective decisions.

People often feel inadequate when they are given no choices over decisions in their lives. Giving advice to patients can foster dependency ("I'll have to ask the nurse what to do about....") and can undermine their sense of competence and adequacy. However, people do need information to make informed decisions. Often the nurse can help the patient define a problem

and identify what information might be needed to attain an informed decision. A more useful approach would be, "What do you see as some possible actions you can take?" It is much more constructive to encourage critical thinking by the patient. At times the nurse can suggest several alternatives that a patient might consider (e.g., "Have you ever thought of telling your friend about the incident?"). The patient is then free to say yes or no and make a decision from among the suggestions.

Asking "Why" Questions

"Why did you come late?" "Why didn't you go to the funeral?" "Why didn't you study for the exam?" Very often **"why" questions** imply criticism. We may ask our friends or family such questions, and in the context of a solid relationship the "why?" may be understood more as "what happened?" With people we do not know—especially an anxious person who may be feeling overwhelmed—a "why" question from a person in authority (nurse, physician, teacher) can be experienced as intrusive and judgmental, which serves only to make the person defensive.

It is much more useful to ask *what* is happening rather than *why* it is happening. Questions that focus on who, what, where, and when often elicit important information that can facilitate problem solving and further the communication process.

CULTURAL CONSIDERATIONS: NEGOTIATING BARRIERS

Ethnically diverse populations are a rapidly growing segment of the American population. Health care professionals are gradually becoming aware of the need to become more familiar with the verbal and nonverbal communication characteristics of the diverse multicultural populations now using the health care system. The nurse's awareness of the cultural meaning of certain verbal and nonverbal communications in initial face-to-face encounters with a patient can lead to the formation of positive therapeutic alliances with members of culturally diverse populations (Kavanaugh, 2008) or lead to frustration and misunderstanding by both the nurse and the patient. Always assess the patient's ability to speak and understand English well, and provide an interpreter when needed.

Unrecognized differences between aspects of the cultural identities of patient and nurse can result in assessment and interventions that are not optimally respectful of the patient and can be inadvertently biased or prejudiced (Lu and Mezzich, 1995). Lu and colleagues further emphasized that health care workers need to have not only knowledge of various patients' cultures but also awareness of their own cultural identities. Especially important are nurses' attitudes and beliefs toward those from ethnically diverse populations and subcultures (e.g., alternate lifestyles, the elderly), because these will affect their relationships with their patients. Four areas that may prove problematic for the nurse interpreting specific verbal and nonverbal messages of the patient include the following:

1. Communication styles
2. Use of eye contact
3. Perception of touch
4. Cultural filters

Communication Styles

People from some ethnic backgrounds may communicate in an intense and highly emotional manner. For example, from the perspective of a non-Hispanic person, Hispanic Americans may appear to use dramatic body language when describing their emotional problems. Such behavior may be perceived as out of control and thus viewed as having a degree of pathology that is not actually present. Within the Hispanic culture, however, intensely emotional styles of communication often are culturally appropriate and are to be expected (Kavanaugh, 2008). French and Italian Americans also show animated facial expressions and expressive hand gestures during communication that can be mistakenly interpreted by others.

Conversely, in other cultures, a calm facade may mask severe distress. For example, in Asian cultures, expression of either positive or negative emotions is a private affair, and open expression of emotions is considered to be in bad taste and possibly to be a weakness. A quiet smile by an Asian American may express joy, an apology, stoicism in the face of difficulty, or even anger (USDHHS, 2001). In general, Asian individuals exercise emotional restating communication and interpersonal conflicts are not directly addressed or even allowed (Arnold & Boggs, 2011). German and British Americans also value highly the concept of self-control and may show little facial emotion in the presence of great distress or emotional turmoil.

It is important to understand an ethnic minority in light of the historical context in which it evolved and its relationship to the dominant culture. For example, African Americans, whose historical background in the United States is one of slavery and oppression, are likely to be aware of a basic need for survival. As a result of their experiences, many African Americans have become highly selective and guarded in their communication

with those outside their cultural group, which may explain the distrust that many African Americans have about the American health care system (Eiser & Ellis, 2007). Therefore, a tendency toward guarded and selective communication among African-American patients may represent a healthy cultural adaptation (Smedley et al., 2002; USDHHS, 2001).

Eye Contact

Fontes (2008) warns that the presence or absence of eye contact should not be used to assess attentiveness, to judge truthfulness, or to make assumptions on the degree of engagement one has with the patient. Culture dictates a person's comfort or lack of comfort with direct eye contact. Some cultures consider direct eye contact disrespectful and improper. For example, Hispanic individuals have traditionally been taught to avoid eye contact with authority figures such as nurses, physicians, and other health care professionals. Avoidance of direct eye contact is seen as a sign of respect to those in authority. To nurses or other health care workers from non-Hispanic backgrounds, however, this lack of eye contact may be wrongly interpreted by the interviewer as disinterest in the interview or even as a lack of respect. Conversely, the nurse is expected to look directly at the patient when conducting the interview (Kavanaugh, 2008).

Similarly, in Asian cultures respect is shown by avoiding eye contact. For example, in Japan direct eye contact is considered to show lack of respect, and to be a personal affront; preference is for shifting or downcast eyes or focus on the speaker's neck. Among many Chinese, gazing around and looking to one side when listening to another is considered polite. However, when speaking to an older adult, direct eye contact is used (Kavanaugh, 2008). Philippine Americans may try to avoid eye contact; however, once it is established, it is important to return and maintain eye contact.

Many Native Americans also believe it is disrespectful or even a sign of aggression to engage in direct eye contact, especially if the speaker is younger. Direct eye contact by members of the dominant culture in the health care system can and does cause discomfort for some patients and is considered a sign of disrespect, while listening is considered a sign of respect and essential to learning about the other individual (Kalbfleisch, 2009; Kavanaugh, 2008).

On the other hand, among German Americans, direct and sustained eye contact indicates that the person listens or trusts, is somewhat aggressive, or, in some situations, is sexually interested. Russians also find direct, sustained eye contact the norm for social interactions (Giger & Davidhizar, 2007). In Haiti, it is customary to hold eye contact with everyone but the poor (Kavanaugh, 2008; USDHHS, 2001). French, British, and many African Americans maintain eye contact during conversation; avoidance of eye contact by another person may be interpreted as being disinterested, not telling the truth, or avoiding the sharing of important information. In some Arab cultures, for a woman to make direct eye contact with a man may imply a sexual interest or even promiscuity. In Greece, staring in public is acceptable (Kavanaugh, 2008).

Touch

The therapeutic use of touch is a basic aspect of the nurse-patient relationship, and touch is normally perceived as a gesture of warmth and friendship. However, in some cultures touch can be perceived as an invasion of privacy or an invitation to intimacy by some patients. The response to touch is often culturally defined. For example, many Hispanic Americans are accustomed to frequent physical contact. Holding the patient's hand in response to a distressing situation or giving the patient a reassuring pat on the shoulder may be experienced as supportive and thus help facilitate openness early in the therapeutic relationship (Kavanaugh, 2008).

When the nurse is working with a Mexican American, for example, often the touch of the nurse is welcome because in the minds of some Mexican Americans, this action can both prevent and treat illness (Giger & Davidhizar, 2007). People of Italian and French backgrounds may also be accustomed to frequent touching during conversation (USDHHS, 2001). In the Soviet Union, touch is often an important part of nonverbal communication used freely with intimate and close friends (Giger & Davidhizar, 2007). However, the degree of comfort conveyed by touch in the nurse-patient relationship depends on the country of origin.

Within the context of an interview, touch might easily be experienced as patronizing, intrusive, aggressive, or sexually inviting. For example, among German, Swedish, and British Americans, touch practices are infrequent, although a handshake may be common at the beginning and end of an interaction. In India, men may shake hands with other men but not with women; an Asian Indian man may greet a woman by nodding and holding the palms of his hands together but not touching the woman. In Japan, handshakes are acceptable; however, a pat on the back is not. Chinese Americans may not like to be touched by strangers. Some Native Americans extend their hand and lightly touch the hand of the person they are greeting rather than shake hands (Kavanaugh, 2008).

Even among people of the same culture, the use of touch has different interpretations and rules when the touch is between individuals of different genders and classes. Students are urged to check the policy manual of their facility because some facilities have a "no touch" policy, particularly with adolescents and children who may have experienced inappropriate touch and would not know how to interpret the touch of the health care worker.

Cultural Filters

It is important to recognize that it is impossible to listen to people in an unbiased way. In the process of socialization we develop cultural filters through which we listen to ourselves, others, and the world around us. Cultural filters are a form of cultural bias or cultural prejudice that determines what we notice and what we ignore (Egan, 2010).

We need these cultural filters to provide structure for ourselves and to help us interpret and interact with the world.

However, unavoidably, these cultural filters also introduce various forms of bias into our listening because they are bound to influence our personal, professional, familial, and sociological values and interpretations. If the cultural filters are strong, the likelihood for bias is increased (Egan, 2010). Bias builds a distorted understanding, and a tendency to pigeonhole a person because of such factors as race, sexual orientation, nationality, social status, religious persuasion, or lifestyle (Egan, 2010).

We all need a frame of reference to help us function in our world. The trick is to understand that other people use many other frames of reference to help them function in their worlds. Acknowledging that others view the world quite differently and trying to understand other people's ways of experiencing and living in the world can go a long way toward minimizing our personal distortions in listening. Building acceptance and understanding of those culturally different from ourselves is a skill, too.

TELEHEALTH THROUGH INFORMATION COMMUNICATION TECHNOLOGIES (ICTs)

E-health/e-medicine, telehealth technology has found widespread uses within the United States, and is still evolving. However, it has only recently been adopted for behavioral health and mental health care (Ryan, 2011). Telehealth is used as a live interactive mechanism, as a way to track clinical data and provide access to people who otherwise might not receive good medical or psychosocial help. It is a valuable tool for consumers as well as practitioners to access current psychiatric and medical breakthroughs, diagnoses, and treatment options (Arnold & Boggs, 2011). As ICTs advance, it is possible that electronic house calls, Internet support groups, and virtual health examination may well be the wave of the future, eliminating office visits altogether (Arnold & Boggs, 2011; Kinsella, 2003).

Castelli (2010) states that besides providing better health care for those in rural areas or for those who cannot travel, telehealth helps relieve the impending nursing shortage. Nursing schools are having a difficult time meeting the nursing shortage because of a decrease in financial resources and retiring faculty (Castelli, 2010). The use of telehealth/tele–home care technologies allows nurses to monitor patients' vital signs, including lung sounds, and identify changes in patients' physiological states. Clinicians can conduct remote physical assessment and consults, which are especially helpful in facilities that have limited nursing resources, including schools, prisons, health clinics, or rural hospitals (Castelli, 2010).

Essentially, "Telehealth is the use of electronic information and telecommunication technologies to support long-distance clinical health care, patient and professional health-related education, public health and health administration. Technologies include videoconferencing, the Internet, store-and-forward imaging, streaming media, and terrestrial and wireless communications" (USDHHS-HRSA, 2011). Ryan (2011) states that one in four adults could be diagnosed with a mental health issue. It could be anxiety, stress, marital issues, depression, or substance abuse. Most of these mental health issues are not addressed because of the fear of stigma, the scarcity of health care providers in remote areas, or problems with transportation (e.g., because of anxiety, physical limitations, or lack of transportation). The consequences of not seeking help can be significant. For example, consequences can range from problems at work to domestic violence, increased depression, and suicide—consequences that can result in a host of other ramifications (Joch, 2008).

The U.S. Department of Defense is particularly interested in implementing and expanding the use of these technologies because, according to Weckerlein (2011), up to 25% of service members screened positive for mental health concerns. These technologies can be used for telepsychiatric appointments ranging from treating posttraumatic stress disorder and depression to providing wellness and resiliency interventions, especially in rural areas (Weckerlein, 2011).

Because the practices of psychiatry, psychology, counseling, and nursing are based on human interaction, there still remains a need for "human to human sensitivity, acknowledgment, and respect for the patient care experience" (Arnold & Boggs, 2011; Malloch, 2010, p. 1). (See the Examining the Evidence box.)

EXAMINING THE EVIDENCE

Telehealth—The Long-Distance Patient-Centered Relationship

What exactly is "telehealth" and can it help a person deal with the problems of mental illness? If so, are insurance companies willing to pay for it?

This is a fast-moving trend in today's information communication technology (ICT). This new type of innovative communication is transforming the frontlines of health care. Telehealth can deliver therapy and manage and monitor disease (GSM, 2011). "Tele" is a prefix meaning "at a distance." With the use of telehealth, services can be delivered via telecommunications that may involve optical, sound, or visual media technologies (Glasper, 2011). Telehealth has already shown that it can maximize health and improve patient disease management skills and confidence with the disease process (Suter, 2011).

For those with mental health issues, Intel has developed a mobile phone application that mirrors cognitive behavioral techniques for people to use who cannot or do not want to see a therapist or as an adjunct to weekly face-to-face therapy sessions. The Touchscreen Mood Map aimed for Android and iPhone invites people to plot their mood throughout the day and view trends to investigate what circumstances spark a drop or rise in mood. Based on their emotional state, individuals can select from a variety of self-directed therapeutic applications involving cognitive restructuring and relaxation exercises. The Mind Scan exercise encourages cognitive reappraisal of thoughts that can lead to anger and depression. One prompt asks, "May I be exaggerating the urgency of a situation?" In a breathing exercise of the application a blue circle expands and contracts slowly to encourage deliberate and slower breathing to reduce anxiety. Participants described greater self-awareness of their emotional patterns (GSM, 2011).

Also, the University of Colorado Hospital is working with children/families with autism spectrum disorder and anxiety utilizing videoconferencing and Skype. Many rural parents had felt disconnected from services because expert interventions were not available to them in rural areas. Parents are now provided with webinars on specific topics and/or small group discussions via videoconferencing (Kaiser, 2011).

Although telehealth's improved health outcomes regularly show cost savings for patient payers and the nation as a whole, one significant barrier to broad-scale telehealth delivery is the current lack of reimbursement for remote patient monitoring by third-party payers. A telemonitoring visit is not counted as a visit by payers (Suter, 2011). In the future, however, Medicare will be looking at formulas that reward quality. Utilizing electronic media to routinely check on recently discharged patients to ensure their recovery is on track enhances quality and, thus, rewards (payments). Studies have shown that patients greatly appreciate the added contact after discharge (Augustine, 2011).

As the health care sector is increasing its use of information technology, health care professionals need to maintain appropriate skills, in particular communication techniques to enhance delivery of care to patients (Warm, 2011). Nurses must continue to utilize therapeutic techniques—those pertaining to both verbal and nonverbal communication. Whether in person or at a distance, it is essential that trust is developed with each patient, that professional boundaries are maintained, and that the therapeutic relationship continues to be a major tool of the nurse.

Augustine, J. (2011). With patient satisfaction under increasing scrutiny, consider patient callbacks, *ED Management, 23*(7), 81-83.

Glasper, A. (2011). Telehealth care—where is it going? *British Journal of Nursing, 20*(12), 714.

Kaiser, K. (2011). Telehealth: families finding ways to connect in rural Colorado, *EP Magazine,* April.

Research Activities Newsletter (GSM). (2011). *Social media use is one of many innovations in care delivery transforming the frontlines of care,* Agency for Healthcare Research and Quality, No. 11, pp. 2-5.

Suter, P. (2011). Theory-based telehealth and patient empowerment. *Population Health Management, 14*(2), 87-92.

Warm, T. (2011). A review of the effectiveness of the clinical informaticist role. *Nursing Standards, 25*(44), 35-38.

Contributed by Lois Angelo.

FACILITATIVE SKILLS CHECKLIST

Instructions: Periodically during your clinical experience, use this checklist to identify areas where growth is needed and progress has been made. Think of your clinical client experiences. Indicate the extent of your agreement with each of the following statements by marking the scale: *SA,* strongly agree; *A,* agree; *NS,* not sure; *D,* disagree; *SD,* strongly disagree.

1. I maintain good eye contact.	SA	A	NS	D	SD
2. Most of my verbal comments follow the lead of the other person.	SA	A	NS	D	SD
3. I encourage others to talk about feelings.	SA	A	NS	D	SD
4. I am able to ask open-ended questions.	SA	A	NS	D	SD
5. I can restate and clarify a person's ideas.	SA	A	NS	D	SD
6. I can summarize in a few words the basic ideas of a long statement made by a person.	SA	A	NS	D	SD
7. I can make statements that reflect the person's feelings.	SA	A	NS	D	SD
8. I can share my feelings relevant to the discussion when appropriate to do so.	SA	A	NS	D	SD
9. I am able to give feedback.	SA	A	NS	D	SD
10. At least 75% or more of my responses help enhance and facilitate communication.	SA	A	NS	D	SD
11. I can assist the person to list some alternatives available.	SA	A	NS	D	SD
12. I can assist the person to identify some goals that are specific and observable.	SA	A	NS	D	SD
13. I can assist the person to specify at least one next step that might be taken toward the goal.	SA	A	NS	D	SD

FIGURE 8-2 Facilitative skills checklist. (Adapted from Myrick, D., & Erney, T. [2000]. *Caring and sharing* [2nd ed., p. 168]. Copyright © 2000 by Educational Media Corp., Minneapolis, MN.)

EVALUATION OF CLINICAL SKILLS

After you have had some introductory clinical experience, you may find the facilitative skills checklist in Figure 8-2 useful for evaluating your progress in developing interviewing skills. Note that some of the items might not be relevant for some of your patients (e.g., numbers 11 through 13 may not be possible when a patient is highly psychotic). Self-evaluation of clinical skills is a way to focus on therapeutic improvement. Role playing can be a useful tool for preparation for the clinical experience as well as a practice in acquiring more effective and professional communication skills.

KEY POINTS TO REMEMBER

- Knowledge of communication and interviewing techniques is the foundation for development of any patient-centered relationship. Goal-directed professional communication is referred to as therapeutic communication.
- Communication is a complex process. Berlo's communication model has five parts: stimulus, sender, message, medium, and receiver. Feedback is a vital component of the communication process for validating the accuracy of the sender's message.
- A number of factors can minimize or enhance the communication process. For example, differences in culture, language, and knowledge levels; noise; lack of privacy; the presence of others; and expectations can all influence communication.
- There are verbal and nonverbal elements in communication; the nonverbal elements often play the larger role in conveying a person's message. Verbal communication consists of all words a person speaks. Nonverbal communication consists of the behaviors displayed by an individual, in addition to the actual content of speech.
- Communication has two levels: the content level (verbal) and the process level (nonverbal behavior). When content is congruent with process, the communication is said to be healthy. When the verbal message is not reinforced by the communicator's actions, the message is ambiguous; we call this a double-bind (or mixed) message.
- Cultural background (as well as individual differences) has a great deal to do with what nonverbal behavior means to different individuals. The degree of eye contact and the use of touch are two nonverbal aspects that can be misunderstood by individuals of different cultures.
- There are a number of communication techniques that nurses can use to enhance their nursing practices. Many widely used communication enhancers are cited in Table 8-2.

KEY POINTS TO REMEMBER—cont'd

- There are also a number of nontherapeutic techniques that nurses can learn to avoid to enhance their effectiveness with people. Some are cited in Table 8-3 along with suggestions for more helpful responses.
- Most nurses are most effective when they use nonthreatening and open-ended communication techniques.
- Effective communication is a skill that develops over time and is integral to the establishment and maintenance of a therapeutic alliance.

- The application of telehealth in the psychosocial sciences is relatively new, but viewed as an invaluable tool for helping people with mental health and issues in behavioral medicine. It is particularly well suited for individuals in rural areas and for those to whom assessing health care/mental health clinics is not possible either physically or financially.

APPLYING CRITICAL JUDGMENT

1. Keep a log for 30 minutes a day of your communication pattern (a tape recorder is ideal). Name four effective techniques that you notice you use frequently. Identify two techniques that are obstructive. In your log, rewrite these nontherapeutic communications and replace them with statements that would better facilitate discussion of thoughts and feelings. Share your log and discuss the changes you are working on with one classmate.

2. Role play with a classmate at least five nonverbal communications and have your partner identify the message he or she was receiving.

3. Using touch and use of eye contact, act out how the nurse would use the nonverbal messages in three different cultural groups.

4. When interviewing Tom shortly after his return from Afghanistan, he makes the following statement to you. For each of the following techniques, reply using the technique indicated.

I am so afraid to go to sleep at night since I came back from Afghanistan. The nightmares are so real, I can hear the screams of the wounded, and the visions in my mind are terrifying.	Restating Rephrasing Giving information Reflecting feelings	Your responses using these techniques

5. Answer the following questions as honestly as you can to a good friend/partner (Sommers-Flanagan & Sommers-Flanagan, 2009, p. 403):
   A. Has there ever been a time in your life when you experienced racism or discrimination? What were your thoughts and feelings related to this experience?
   B. Can you relate a time when your own thoughts about people who are different from you affected how you treated them? Would you do anything differently now?
   C. How would you describe the "American culture"? What part of this culture do you embrace? What parts do you reject? How does your internalization of the "American culture" impact what you think constitutes a "mentally healthy individual"?

6. How would information communication technologies (ICTs) be best used in your community? Specifically, which ICTs would you choose if you were opening a telehealth communication center in your community?

CHAPTER REVIEW QUESTIONS

Choose the most appropriate answer(s).

1. Paraphrasing, restating, reflecting, and exploring are techniques used for the purpose of:
   1. clarifying.
   2. summarizing.
   3. encouraging comparison.
   4. placing events in time and sequence.

2. Which communication technique would yield positive results within the context of a therapeutic relationship?
   1. Advising
   2. Giving approval
   3. Listening actively
   4. Asking "why" questions

3. Which nontherapeutic communication technique is used in the following example?
   Patient: I am really upset about being discharged.
   Nurse: Where do you live?
   1. False reassurance
   2. Excessive questioning
   3. Changing the subject
   4. Presenting reality

4. Which statement by the nurse to a patient would be considered nontherapeutic?
   1. "I know exactly how you feel."
   2. "I'm not sure I understand what you mean."
   3. "Tell me more about what happened when you resigned."
   4. "I see that you are wringing your hands as we talk about the job interview."

5. When the patient says, "I have no idea what to do about my job," and the nurse responds, "Can you describe a specific concern you have about your job?," the nurse is using the communication technique of:
   1. exploring.
   2. reflecting.
   3. focusing.
   4. paraphrasing.

REFERENCES

Arnold, E. C., & Boggs, K. U. (2011). *Interpersonal relationships: professional communication skills for nurses* (6th ed.). St Louis: Elsevier Saunders.

Bateson, G., Jackson, D., & Haley, J. (1956). Toward a theory of schizophrenia. *Behavioral Sciences, 1*(4), 251–264.

Berlo, D. K. (1960). *The process of communication.* San Francisco: Reinhart Press.

Castelli, D. (2010). *Telehealth technologies addressing the global impending nursing shortage.* Retrieved August 31, 2011, from www.nursingcenter.com/CareerCenter/static.asp?pageid=800469.

Egan, G. (2010). *The skilled helper: a problem-management approach and opportunity-development approach to helping* (9th ed.). Belmont, CA: Brooks/Cole, Cengage Learning.

Eiser, A., & Ellis, G. (2007). Cultural competence and the African-American experience with healthcare: the case for specific content and cross-cultural education. *Academic Medicine, 82,* 176–183.

Ellis, R. B., Gates, B., & Kenworthy, N. (2007). *Interpersonal communicating in nursing* (2nd ed.). London: Churchill Livingstone.

Fontes, L. A. (2008). *Interviewing clients across cultures: a practitioners guide.* New York: The Guilford Press.

Giger, J. N., & Davidhizar, R. E. (2007). *Transcultural nursing: assessment and intervention* (5th ed.). St Louis: Mosby Elsevier.

Haber, J. (2000). Hildegard E. Peplau: the psychiatric nursing legacy of a legend. *Journal of the American Psychiatric Nursing Association, 6*(2), 58–62.

Hays, P. A. (2008). *Addressing cultural complexities in practice.* Washington, DC: American Psychological Association.

Joch, A. (2008). *Tele-therapy.* Retrieved August 28, 2011, from http://govhealthit.com/news/tele-therapy.

Kalbfleisch, P. (2009). Effective health communication in native populations in North America. *Journal of Language and Social Psychology, 28*(two), 158–173.

Kavanaugh, K. H. (2008). Transcultural perspectives in mental health nursing. In M. Andrews, & J. Boyle (Eds.), *Transcultural concepts in nursing care* (5th ed.). Philadelphia: Lippincott Williams & Wilkins.

Kinsella, A. (2003). Telemedicine connection. *Advance for Providers of Post-Acute Care (May-June),* 24–26.

Lu, F. G., & Mezzich, J. E. (1995). Issues in the assessment and diagnosis of culturally diverse individuals. In J. M. Oldham, & M. B. Riba (Eds.), *Review of psychiatry* (Vol. 14, pp. 477–510). Washington, DC: American Psychiatric Press.

Mallach, E. G. (2010). Information systems conversion in SMEs. In M. Cruiz-Cunho (Ed.), *Enterprise information systems for business integration and SMEs: technological, organizational, and social dimensions* (pp. 15–23). doi:10.4018/978-1-60566-892-5-.

Matsumoto, D. (1992). American-Japanese cultural differences in name recognition of universal facial expressions. *Journal of Cross Cultural Psychology, 23*(one), 72–84.

Matsumoto, D., & Sung Hwang, H. (2011). *Reading facial expressions of emotion.* Retrieved January 2, 2012 from http://www.apa.org/science/about/psa/2011/05/facial-expressions.aspx.

Mohl, P. C. (2003). Listening to the patient. In A. Tasman, J. Kay, & J. A. Lieberman (Eds.), *Psychiatry* (2nd ed.). West Sussex, England: Wiley.

Peplau, H.E. (1952). *Interpersonal relations in nursing: a conceptual frame of reference for psychodynamic nursing.* New York: Putnam.

Ryan, A. (2011). *Technology's new role in mental health care.* Retrieved August 28, 2011, from www.newstrib.com/articles/print-articles/?id= 595FE9FD494635CF72C0B4444C01DFA.

Shea, S. C. (1998). *Psychiatric interviewing: the art of understanding* (2nd ed.). Philadelphia: Saunders.

Smedley, B., Stith, A., & Nelson, A. (2002). *Unequal treatment: confronting racial and ethnic disparities in healthcare* (Institute of Medicine Report). Washington, DC: National Academies Press.

Sommers-Flanagan, J., & Sommers-Flanagan, R. (2009). *Clinical interviewing* (4th ed.). Hoboken, NJ: Wiley.

U.S. Department of Health and Human Services. (2001). *Mental health: culture, race, and ethnicity: supplement to mental health: a report of the Surgeon General*. Rockville, MD: USDHHS, Substance Abuse and Mental Health Services Administration, Center for Mental Health Services.

U.S. Department of Health and Human Services, Health Resources and Services Administration (USDHHS-HRSA). *Rural health*. Retrieved August 28, 2011, from www.hrsa.gov/ruralhealth/about/Telehealth/.

Weckerlein, J. (2011). *Technology to aid DoD mental health services*. Retrieved August 28, 2011, from http://science.dodlive.mil/2011/08/05/8089/.

Therapeutic Relationships and the Clinical Interview

Elizabeth M. Varcarolis

evolve WEBSITE

http://evolve.elsevier.com/Varcarolis/essentials

KEY TERMS AND CONCEPTS

clinical supervision, p. 148
confidentiality, p. 142
contract, p. 142
countertransference, p. 138
empathy, p. 144
genuineness, p. 144
intimate distance, p. 147
orientation phase, p. 139
personal distance, p. 147
process recordings, p. 148
public distance, p. 147

rapport, p. 142
social distance, p. 147
social relationship, p. 136
termination phase, p. 143
therapeutic encounter, p. 137
therapeutic relationship/
    partnership, p. 136
transference, p. 137
values, p. 148
working phase, p. 142

SELECTED CONCEPT:
Cultural Self-awareness
"Whether two people can understand each other depends not so much on racial or cultural backgrounds, but how strongly each of them believed in their correctness and or even the superiority of what is personally familiar.

Truly understanding someone from another culture begins with acceptance of differences as normal, interesting, and even desirable aspects of being human."
(Sommers-Flanagan & Sommers-Flanagan, 2009, p. 29)

OBJECTIVES

1. Compare and contrast the three phases of the nurse-patient relationship.
2. Compare and contrast a social relationship and a therapeutic relationship regarding purpose, focus, communications style, and goals.
3. Identify at least four patient behaviors a nurse may encounter in the clinical setting.
4. Explore aspects that foster a therapeutic nurse-patient relationship and those that are inherent in a nontherapeutic nursing interactive process.
5. Define and discuss the role of empathy, genuineness, and positive regard on the part of the nurse in a nurse-patient relationship.

Psychiatric mental health nursing is based on principles of *science*. A background in anatomy, physiology, and chemistry is the basis for the safe and effective provision of biological treatments. For example, it is assumed the nurse has knowledge of how medications work, indications for use, and adverse effects based on best-evidence studies and trials. However, it is the caring relationship and the development of the skills needed to enhance and maintain these relationships that make up the *art* of psychiatric nursing. Quinlan (1996) states that "the development of that very human relationship allows a place for caring and healing to occur. This use of the essential humanness of the nurse as a person is the most critical part of the way nurses make themselves available to both patients and colleagues" (p. 7). Quinlan goes on to say that how this is achieved remains within the domain of the individual nurse.

NURSE-PATIENT RELATIONSHIPS

The term "patient-centered care" is being rapidly advanced by the medical community. In the medical field these terms are an "innovative approach to the planning, delivery, and evaluation of healthcare that is grounded in mutually beneficial partnerships among healthcare patients, families and providers" (Gordon et al., 2010; Public Broadcasting Service [PBS], 2006). The core concepts of patient- and family-centered care consist of (a) dignity and respect, (b) information sharing, (c) patient and family participation, and (d) collaboration in policy and program development. These tenants have long been subsumed in the nursing profession as what is known as the nurse-patient relationship, so for our purposes we will continue to use the term nurse-patient relationship throughout this text. What is becoming new within the term "nurse-patient relationship," however, is a shift to the term "nurse-patient partnership," which has been introduced in Chapters 1, 3, and 19, and elsewhere.

The therapeutic nurse-patient relationship is the basis of all psychiatric nursing treatment approaches regardless of the specific aim. The very first connections between nurse and patient are to establish an understanding that the nurse is safe, confidential, reliable, and consistent, and that the relationship is conducted within appropriate and clear boundaries.

It is true that many disorders, such as schizophrenia and major affective disorders, have strong biochemical and genetic components. However, many accompanying emotional problems such as poor self-image, low self-esteem, and difficulties

with adherence to treatment regimen can be significantly improved through a therapeutic patient-centered alliance or relationship (LaRowe, 2004). All too commonly, those entering treatment have taxed or exhausted their familial and social resources and have found themselves in a position of isolation from people who will listen for more than a few minutes.

The nurse-patient relationship is a creative process and unique to each nurse. Each person brings his or her own uniqueness to the nurse-patient relationship. Each of us has unique gifts that we can learn to use creatively to form positive bonds with others. Historically this has been referred to as the "therapeutic use of self." Therapeutic use of self is an example of the practice of the "art of nursing." *Important to remember,* the efficacy of this therapeutic use of self has been scientifically substantiated as an evidence-based intervention. Randomized clinical trials have repeatedly found that development of a positive alliance (therapeutic relationship) is one of the best predictors of positive outcomes in therapy (Gordon et al., 2010; Kopta et al., 1999). On the other hand, noncompliance with treatment and poor outcomes in therapy are related to a patient feeling unheard, disrespected, or otherwise unconnected with the clinician/health care worker (Gordon et al., 2010). Research suggests that therapeutic success is a result of the personal characteristics of the clinician and the patient, not necessarily a result of the particular process employed. Furthermore, there is evidence that psychotherapy (talk therapy) and a therapeutic alliance actually change brain chemistry in much the same way as medication, thus resulting in the adage that the best treatment for most psychiatric problems (less so with psychotic disorders) is a combination of medication and psychotherapy. Cognitive behavioral therapy, in particular, has met with great success in the treatment of depression, phobias, obsessive-compulsive disorders, and others.

Establishing a therapeutic alliance or relationship with a patient takes time. Skills in this area gradually improve with guidance from those with more skill and experience. When patients do not engage in a therapeutic alliance, chances are that no matter what plans of care or planned interventions are made, nothing significant will happen except mutual frustration and mutual withdrawal.

Therapeutic Versus Other Types of Relationships

The nurse-patient relationship is often loosely defined, but a therapeutic relationship incorporating principles of mental health nursing is more clearly defined and differs from other relationships. A therapeutic nurse-patient relationship has specific goals and functions. Goals in a therapeutic relationship include the following:

- **Facilitating** communication of distressing thoughts and feelings
- **Assisting** patients with problem solving to help facilitate activities of daily living
- **Helping** patients examine self-defeating behaviors and test alternatives
- **Promoting** self-care and independence

A relationship is an interpersonal process that involves two or more people. Throughout life we meet people in a variety of settings and share a variety of experiences. With some individuals we develop long-term relationships; with others the relationship lasts only a short time. Naturally the kinds of relationships we enter vary from person to person and from situation to situation. Generally, relationships can be defined as (1) social or (2) therapeutic.

Social Relationships

A social relationship can be defined as a relationship that is primarily initiated for the purpose of friendship, socialization, enjoyment, or accomplishment of a task. Mutual needs are met during social interaction (e.g., participants share ideas, feelings, and experiences). Communication skills used in social relationships may include giving advice and (sometimes) meeting basic dependency needs, such as lending money and helping with jobs. Often the content of the communication remains superficial. During social interactions, roles may shift. Within a social relationship there is little emphasis on the evaluation of the interaction:

Patient: "Oh, gosh, I just hate to be alone. It is getting me down and sometimes it hurts so much."

Nurse: "I know just how you feel. I don't like it either. What I do is get a friend and go to a movie or something. Do you have someone to hang with?" *(In this response the nurse is minimizing the patient's feelings and giving advice prematurely.)*

Patient: "No, not really, but often I don't even feel like going out. I just sit at home feeling scared and lonely."

Nurse: "Most of us feel like that at one time or another. Maybe if you took a class or joined a group you could meet more people. I know of some great groups you could join. It's not good to be stuck in by yourself all of the time." *(Again, the nurse is not "hearing" the patient's distress, and in so doing, is minimizing again her pain and isolation. The nurse goes on to give the patient banal advice, thus closing off the patient's feelings and experience.)*

Therapeutic Relationships

The therapeutic relationship between nurse and patient differs from both a social and an intimate relationship in that the nurse maximizes his or her communication skills, understanding of human behaviors, and personal strengths to enhance the patient's growth. Patients more easily engage in the relationship when the clinician's interactions address their concerns, respect the patient as a partner in decision making,

and use language that is straightforward (Gordon et al., 2010). That suggests the focus of the relationship needs to be on the patient's ideas, experiences, and feelings. Inherent in a therapeutic relationship is the nurse's focus on significant personal issues introduced by the patient during the clinical interview. The nurse and the patient identify areas that need exploration and periodically evaluate the degree of change in the patient.

Although the nurse may assume a variety of roles as mentioned (e.g., teacher, counselor, socializing agent, liaison), **the relationship is consistently focused on the patient's problem and needs.** Nurses must meet their own needs outside of the therapeutic relationship. When nurses begin to want the patient to "like them," "do as they suggest," "be nice to them," or "give them recognition," the needs of the patient cannot be adequately met, and the interaction could be detrimental (nontherapeutic) to the patient.

Working under supervision is an excellent way to keep the focus and boundaries clear. Communication skills and knowledge of the stages of and phenomena occurring in a therapeutic relationship are crucial tools in the formation and maintenance of that relationship. Within the context of a helping relationship, the following occur:

- The needs of the patient are identified and explored.
- Alternate problem-solving approaches are taken.
- New coping skills may develop.
- Behavioral change is encouraged.

Staff nurses as well as students may struggle with the boundaries between social and therapeutic relationships. There is a fine line. In fact, students often feel more comfortable "being a friend" because it is a more familiar role, especially with people close to their own age. However, when this occurs, the nurse or student needs to make it clear (to themselves and the patient) that the relationship is a therapeutic one. This does *not* mean that the nurse is not friendly toward the patient, and it does *not* mean that talking about innocuous topics (e.g., television, weather, children's pictures) is forbidden. It does mean, however, that the nurse follows the prior stated guidelines regarding a therapeutic relationship; essentially, the focus is on the patient, and the relationship is not designed to meet the nurse's needs. The patient's problems and concerns are explored, potential solutions are discussed by both patient and nurse, and solutions are implemented by the patient:

Patient: "Oh, gosh, I just hate to be alone. It is getting me down and sometimes it hurts so much."

Nurse: "Loneliness can be painful. What is going on now that you are feeling so alone?"

Patient: "Well, my mom died 2 years ago, and last month, my—oh, I am so scared." *(Patient takes a deep breath, looks down, and looks like she might cry.)*

Nurse: *(Sits in silence while the patient recovers.)* "Go on…"

Patient: "My boyfriend left for Afghanistan. I haven't heard from him, and they say he is missing. He was my best friend and we were going to get married, and if he dies I don't want to live."

Nurse: "Have you thought of harming yourself?"

Patient: "Well, if he dies I will. I can't live without him."

Nurse: "Have you ever felt like this before?"

Patient: Yes, when my mom died. I was depressed for about a year until I met my boyfriend."

Nurse: "It sounds like you are going through a very painful and scary time. Perhaps you and I can talk some more and come up with some ways for you to feel less anxious, scared, and overwhelmed. Would you be willing to work on this together?"

The ability of the nurse to engage in interpersonal interactions in a goal-directed manner for the purpose of assisting patients with their emotional or physical health needs is the foundation of the nurse-patient relationship. The nurse-patient relationship is synonymous with a professional helping relationship. Behaviors that have relevance to health care workers, including nurses, are as follows:

- **Accountability:** Nurses assume responsibility for their conduct and the consequences of their actions.
- **Focus on patient needs:** The interest of the patient rather than the nurse, other health care workers, or the institution is given first consideration. The nurse's role is that of patient advocate.
- **Clinical competence:** The criteria on which the nurse bases his or her conduct are principles of knowledge and those that are appropriate to the specific situation. This involves awareness and incorporation of the latest knowledge made available from research (evidence-based practice).
- **Delaying judgment:** Ideally, nurses refrain from judging patients and avoid transferring their own values and beliefs to others.
- **Supervision** by a more experienced clinician or team is essential to developing one's competence in this area.

Nurses interact with patients in a variety of settings, such as emergency departments, medical-surgical units, obstetric and pediatric units, clinics, community settings, schools, and patients' homes. Nurses who are sensitive to patients' needs and have effective assessment and communication skills can significantly help patients confront current problems and anticipate future choices.

The type of relationship that occurs may be informal and not extensive, such as when the nurse and patient meet for only a few sessions. However, even though it is brief, the relationship may be substantial, useful, and important for the patient. This limited relationship is often referred to as a therapeutic encounter. When the nurse shows true concern for another's circumstances (has positive regard, empathy), even a short encounter with the individual can have a powerful effect on that individual's life.

At other times, the encounters may be longer and more formal, such as in inpatient settings, mental health units, crisis centers, and mental health facilities, as well as in private practice. This longer time span allows greater development of an effective therapeutic nurse-patient relationship.

Establishing Relationship Boundaries

A well-defined therapeutic relationship allows the establishment of clear patient boundaries that provide a safe space through which the patient can explore feelings and treatment issues. The nurse's role in the therapeutic relationship is theoretically rather well-defined. The patient's needs are separated from the nurse's needs, and the patient's role is different from that of the nurse. Therefore the boundaries of the relationship seem to be well stated. In reality, boundaries are at risk of blurring, and a shift in the nurse-patient relationship may lead to nontherapeutic dynamics. Examples of circumstances that can produce blurring of boundaries include the following:

- When the relationship slips into a social context
- When the nurse's needs are met at the expense of the patient's needs

There are warning signals that indicate a nurse may be blurring boundaries.

- **Overhelping:** Doing for patients what they are able to do themselves or going beyond the wishes or needs of patients
- **Controlling:** Asserting authority and assuming control of patients "for their own good"
- **Narcissism:** Having to find weakness, helplessness, and/or disease in patients to feel helpful, at the expense of recognizing and supporting patients' healthier, stronger, and more competent features

When situations such as these arise, the relationship has ceased to be a helpful one and the phenomenon of control becomes an issue. Role blurring is often a result of unrecognized transference or countertransference.

Transference

Transference is a phenomenon originally identified by Sigmund Freud when he used psychoanalysis to treat patients. Transference is the process whereby a person unconsciously and inappropriately displaces (transfers) onto individuals in his or her current life those patterns of behavior and emotional reactions that originated in relation to significant figures in childhood. The patient may even say, "You remind me of my _____" (e.g., mother, sister, father, brother). See the following example:

Patient: "Oh, you are so high and mighty. Did anyone ever tell you that you are a cold, unfeeling machine, just like others I know?"

Nurse: "Tell me about one person who is cold and unfeeling toward you." (*In this example, the patient is experiencing the nurse in the same way she did with significant other[s] during her formative years. In this case, the patient's mother was very aloof, leaving her with feelings of isolation, worthlessness, and anger.*)

Although the transference phenomenon occurs in all relationships, transference seems to be intensified in relationships of authority. Because the process of transference is accelerated toward a person in authority, physicians, nurses, and social workers are all potential objects of transference. It is important to realize that the patient may experience thoughts, feelings, and reactions toward a health care worker that are realistic and appropriate; these are *not* transference phenomena.

Common forms of transference include the desire for affection or respect and the gratification of dependency needs.

Other transferential feelings the patient might experience are hostility, jealousy, competitiveness, and love. Requests for special favors (e.g., cigarettes, water, extra time in the session) are concrete examples of transference phenomena.

Countertransference

Countertransference refers to the tendency of the nurse to displace onto the patient feelings related to people in his or her past. Frequently, the patient's transference to the nurse evokes countertransference feelings in the nurse. For example, it is normal to feel angry when attacked persistently, annoyed when frustrated unreasonably, or flattered when idealized. A nurse might feel extremely important when depended on exclusively by a patient. If the nurse does not recognize his or her own omnipotent feelings as countertransference, encouragement of independent growth in the patient might be minimized at best. Recognizing our countertransference reactions maximizes our ability to *empower* our patients. When we fail to recognize our countertransferences toward our patients, the therapeutic relationship stalls, and essentially we *disempower* our patients by experiencing them not as individuals but rather as inner projections. See the following examples:

> *Patient:* "Yeah, well I decided not to go to that dumb group. 'Hi, I'm so and so, and I'm an alcoholic.' Who cares?" *(Patient sits slumped in a chair chewing gum, nonchalantly looking around.)*
>
> *Nurse: (in a very impassioned tone)* "You always sabotage your chances. You need AA to get in control of your life. Last week you were going to go and now you have disappointed everyone." *(Here the nurse is reminded of her mother who was an alcoholic. The nurse had tried everything to get her mother into treatment and took it as a personal failure and deep disappointment that her mother never sought recovery. After the nurse sorts out her thoughts and feelings, she realizes the frustration and feelings of disappointment and failure come from feelings toward her mother and not the patient. The nurse starts out the next session with the following approach.)*
>
> *Nurse:* "Look, I was thinking about last week and I realize the decision to go to AA or find other help is solely up to you. It is true that I would like you to live a fuller and more satisfying life, but it is your decision. I am wondering, however, what happened to change your mind to not go to AA."

If the nurse feels either a strongly positive or a strongly negative reaction to a patient, the feeling most often signals countertransference in the nurse. One common sign of countertransference in the nurse is overidentification with the patient. In this situation the nurse may have difficulty recognizing or understanding problems the patient has that are similar to the nurse's own. For example, a nurse who is struggling with an alcoholic family member may feel disinterested, cold, or disgusted toward an alcoholic patient. Other indications of countertransference occur when the nurse becomes involved in power struggles, competition, or arguments with the patient.

Identifying and working through various transference and countertransference issues is crucial if the nurse is to achieve professional and clinical growth and allow for positive change in the patient. These issues are best handled through the use of supervision by either the peer group or the therapeutic team. Regularly scheduled supervision sessions provide the nurse with the opportunity to increase self-awareness, clinical skills, and growth, as well as allow for continued growth of the patient.

Self-Check on Boundary Issues

It is helpful for all of us to take time out to be reflective and to try to be aware of our thoughts and actions with patients, as well as with colleagues, friends, and family. Figure 9-1 is a helpful self-test you can use throughout your career, no matter what area of nursing you choose.

Phases of the Nurse-Patient Relationship

Hildegard Peplau introduced the concept of the nurse-patient relationship in 1952 in her ground-breaking book *Interpersonal Relations in Nursing*. This model of the nurse-patient relationship is well accepted in the United States and Canada and has become an important tool for all nursing practice. Peplau (1952) proposed that the nurse-patient relationship "facilitates forward movement" for both the nurse and the patient (p. 12). Peplau's interactive nurse-patient process is designed to facilitate the patient's boundary management, independent problem solving, and decision making that promotes autonomy (Haber, 2000).

It is most likely that in the brief period you have for your psychiatric nursing rotation, all the phases of the nurse-patient relationship will not have time to develop. However, it is important for you to be aware of these phases because you must be able to recognize and use them later. It is also important to remember that any contact that is caring and respectful and demonstrates concern for the situation of another person can have an enormous positive impact on that person.

Peplau (1952, 1999) described the nurse-patient relationship as evolving through interlocking, overlapping phases. The distinctive phases of the nurse-patient relationship are generally recognized as follows:

- Orientation phase
- Working phase
- Termination phase

Although various phenomena and goals are identified for each phase, they often overlap. Even before the first meeting, the nurse may have many thoughts and feelings related to the first clinical session. This is sometimes referred to as the *preorientation phase*.

Preorientation Phase

Novice health care professionals usually have many concerns and experience a mild to moderate degree of anxiety on their first clinical day. Commonly, nursing instructors will encourage students to identify concerns about working with psychiatric patients in preconference on the first clinical day. These concerns focus on being afraid of people with psychiatric problems, saying "the wrong thing," and being unaware of the proper responses to certain patient behaviors. There really are no magic words. Talking with the instructor and supervised

NURSING BOUNDARY INDEX SELF-CHECK

Please rate yourself according to the frequency with which the following statements reflect your behavior, thoughts, or feelings within the past 2 years while providing patient care.*

1. Have you ever received any feedback about your behavior being overly intrusive with patients and their families?	Never ____	Rarely ____	Sometimes ____	Often ____
2. Do you ever have difficulty setting limits with patients?	Never ____	Rarely ____	Sometimes ____	Often ____
3. Do you ever arrive early or stay late to be with your patient for a longer period?	Never ____	Rarely ____	Sometimes ____	Often ____
4. Do you ever find yourself relating to patients or peers as you might to a family member?	Never ____	Rarely ____	Sometimes ____	Often ____
5. Have you ever acted on sexual feelings you have for a patient?	Never ____	Rarely ____	Sometimes ____	Often ____
6. Do you feel that you are the only one who understands the patient?	Never ____	Rarely ____	Sometimes ____	Often ____
7. Have you ever received feedback that you get "too involved" with patients or families?	Never ____	Rarely ____	Sometimes ____	Often ____
8. Do you derive conscious satisfaction from patients' praise, appreciation, or affection?	Never ____	Rarely ____	Sometimes ____	Often ____
9. Do you ever feel that other staff members are too critical of "your" patient?	Never ____	Rarely ____	Sometimes ____	Often ____
10. Do you ever feel that other staff members are jealous of your relationship with your patient?	Never ____	Rarely ____	Sometimes ____	Often ____
11. Have you ever tried to "match-make" a patient with one of your friends?	Never ____	Rarely ____	Sometimes ____	Often ____
12. Do you find it difficult to handle patients' unreasonable requests for assistance, verbal abuse, or sexual language?	Never ____	Rarely ____	Sometimes ____	Often ____

* Any item that is responded to with "Sometimes" or "Often" should alert the nurse to a possible area of vulnerability. If the item is responded to with "Rarely," the nurse should determine whether it is an isolated event or a possible pattern of behavior.

FIGURE 9-1 Nursing boundary index self-check. (From Pilette, P.C., Berck, C.B., & Achber, L.C. [1995]. Therapeutic management of helping boundaries. *Journal of Psychosocial Nursing and Mental Health Services, 33*[1], 45.)

peer group discussion will add confidence, feedback, and suggestions. Chapter 8 discusses the use of communication strategies in clinical practice.

Often, students new to the mental health setting are concerned about being in situations that they may not know how to handle. These concerns are universal and often arise in the clinical setting. Table 9-1 identifies common patient behaviors (e.g., crying, asking the nurse to keep a secret, threatening to commit suicide, giving a gift) and gives examples of an appropriate response, the rationale for the response, and a possible verbal statement. The exact words depend on the situation, but understanding the rationale will aid you in applying the information in future interactions.

Most experienced psychiatric nursing faculty and staff monitor the unit atmosphere and have a sixth sense as it pertains to behaviors that indicate escalating tension. They are trained in crisis interventions, and formal security is often available onsite to give the staff support. Your instructor will set the ground rules for safety during the first clinical day. For example, do not enter a patient's room alone, know if there are any patients who should not be engaged, stay in open areas that have other health care personnel, and recognize the signs and symptoms of escalating anxiety. There are certain rules of thumb regarding actions a nurse can take if a patient's anger begins to escalate (see Chapter 24). You should always trust your own instincts. If you feel uncomfortable for any reason, excuse yourself for a moment and discuss your feelings with your instructor or a staff member. In addition to obtaining reassurance and support, students can often provide valuable information about the patient's condition by sharing these perceptions.

Orientation Phase

The orientation phase can last for a few meetings or can extend over a longer period. It is the first time the nurse and the patient meet, and they are strangers to each other. When strangers meet, they interact according to their own backgrounds, standards, values, and experiences. This fact—that each person has a unique frame of reference—underlies the need for

TABLE 9-1 COMMON PATIENT BEHAVIORS AND NURSE RESPONSES

POSSIBLE REACTIONS BY NURSE	USEFUL RESPONSES BY NURSE
What to Do If the Patient Says He or She Wants to Kill Himself or Herself	
The nurse may feel overwhelmed or responsible for "talking the patient out of it." The nurse may pick up some of the patient's feelings of hopelessness.	The nurse assesses whether the patient has a plan and the lethality of the plan. The nurse tells the patient that this is serious, that the nurse does not want harm to come to the patient, and that this information needs to be shared with other staff. "This is very serious, Mr. Lamb. I do not want any harm to come to you. I will have to share this with the other staff." The nurse can then discuss with the patient the feelings and circumstances that led up to this decision. (Refer to Chapter 23 for strategies in suicide intervention.)
What to Do If the Patient Asks the Nurse to Keep a Secret	
The nurse may feel conflict because the nurse wants the patient to share important information but is unsure about making such a promise.	The nurse *cannot* make such a promise. The information may be important to the health or safety of the patient or others. "I cannot make that promise. It might be important for me to share it with other staff." The patient then decides whether to share the information.
What to Do If the Patient Asks the Nurse a Personal Question	
The nurse may think that it is rude not to answer the patient's question. A new nurse might feel relieved to delay the start of the interview. The nurse may feel uneasy and want to leave the situation. New nurses are often manipulated by a patient into changing roles. This keeps the focus off the patient and prevents the creation of a relationship.	The nurse may or may not answer the patient's query. If the nurse decides to answer a natural question, he or she answers in a word or two, then refocuses back on the patient. *Patient:* Are you married? *Nurse:* Yes. Do you have a spouse? *Patient:* Do you have any children? *Nurse:* This time is for you—tell me about yourself. *Patient:* You can just tell me if you have any children. *Nurse:* This is your time to focus on your concerns. Tell me something about your family.
What to Do If the Patient Makes Sexual Advances	
The nurse feels uncomfortable but may feel conflicted about "rejecting" the patient or making him or her feel "unattractive" or "not good enough."	The nurse needs to set clear limits on expected behavior. "I am not comfortable having you touch (kiss) me. This time is for you to focus on your problems and concerns." Frequently restating the nurse's role throughout the relationship can help maintain boundaries. If the patient does not stop the inappropriate behavior, the nurse might say, "If you can't stop this behavior, I'll have to leave. I'll be back at [time] to spend time with you then." Leaving gives the patient time to gain control. The nurse returns at the stated time.
What to Do If the Patient Cries	
The nurse may feel uncomfortable and experience increased anxiety or feel somehow responsible for making the person cry.	The nurse should stay with the patient and reinforce that it is all right to cry. Often it is at that time that feelings are closest to the surface and can be best identified. "You seem ready to cry." "You are still upset about your brother's death." "What are you thinking right now?" The nurse offers tissues when appropriate.

TABLE 9-1 COMMON PATIENT BEHAVIORS AND NURSE RESPONSES—cont'd	
POSSIBLE REACTIONS BY NURSE	**USEFUL RESPONSES BY NURSE**

What to Do If the Patient Leaves Before the Session Is Over

The nurse may feel rejected, thinking it was something that he or she did. The nurse may experience increased anxiety or feel abandoned by the patient.	Some patients are not able to relate for long periods without experiencing an increase in anxiety. On the other hand, the patient may be testing the nurse. "I will wait for you here for 15 minutes, until our time is up." During this time, the nurse does not engage in conversation with any other patient or even with the staff. When the time is up, the nurse approaches the patient, says the time is up, and restates the day and time the nurse will see the patient again.

What to Do If the Patient Says He or She Does Not Want to Talk

The nurse new to this situation may feel rejected or ineffectual.	At first, the nurse might say something to this effect: "It's all right. I would like to spend time with you. We don't have to talk." The nurse might spend short, frequent periods (e.g., 5 minutes) with the patient throughout the day. "Our 5 minutes is up. I'll be back at 10 AM and stay with you 5 more minutes." This gives the patient the opportunity to understand that the nurse means what he or she says and is back on time consistently. It also gives the patient time between visits to assess how he or she feels and what he or she thinks about the nurse, and perhaps to feel less threatened.

What to Do If the Patient Gives the Nurse a Present

The nurse may feel uncomfortable when offered a gift. The meaning needs to be examined. Is the gift (1) a way of getting better care, (2) a way to maintain self-esteem, (3) a way of making the nurse feel guilty, (4) a sincere expression of thanks, or (5) a cultural expectation?	Possible guidelines: If the gift is expensive, the only policy is to graciously refuse. If it is inexpensive, then (1) if it is given at the end of hospitalization when a relationship has developed, graciously accept; (2) if it is given at the beginning of the relationship, graciously refuse and explore the meaning behind the present. "Thank you, but it is our job to care for our patients. Are you concerned that some aspect of your care will be overlooked?" If the gift is money, it is always graciously refused.

What to Do If Another Patient Interrupts During Time With Your Selected Patient

The nurse may feel a conflict. The nurse does not want to appear rude. Sometimes the nurse tries to engage both patients in conversation.	The time the nurse had contracted with a selected patient is that patient's time. By keeping his or her part of the contract, the nurse demonstrates that the nurse means what he or she says and views the sessions as important. "I am with Mr. Rob for the next 20 minutes. At 10 AM, after our time is up, I can talk to you for 5 minutes."

self-awareness on the part of the nurse. The initial interview includes the following:

- An atmosphere is established in which rapport can grow.
- The nurse's role is clarified, and the responsibilities of both the patient and the nurse are defined.
- The contract containing the time, place, date, and duration of the meetings is discussed.
- Confidentiality is discussed and assumed.

- The terms of termination are introduced (these are also discussed throughout the orientation phase and beyond).
- The nurse becomes aware of transference and countertransference issues.
- Patient problems are articulated, and mutually agreed goals are established.

Establishing rapport. A major emphasis during the first few encounters with the patient is on providing an atmosphere in which trust and understanding, or **rapport,** can grow. As in any relationship, rapport can be nurtured by demonstrating genuineness and empathy, developing positive regard, showing consistency, and offering assistance in problem solving and in providing support. It is important for the nurse to first identify how the patient wants to be addressed. In some countries, it is very important that people are addressed by their professional title if they have one. To some people, calling them by their first name, such as a young person addressing an older person by "John" or "Phoebe," would be insulting and likely stall the process. The health care workers simply asks, "What do people call you?" or "How should I address you?"

Parameters of the relationship. The patient needs to know about the nurse (who the nurse is and the nurse's background) and the purpose of the meetings. For example, a student might furnish the following information:

> *Student:* "Hello, Mrs. Rodriquez. I am Jim Thompson from Scottsdale Community College. I am in my psychiatric rotation and will be coming here for the next six Thursdays. I would like to spend time with you each Thursday if you are still here. I'm here to be a support person for you as you work on your treatment goals."

Formal or informal contract. A contract emphasizes the patient's participation and responsibility because it shows that the nurse does something *with* the patient rather than *for* the patient. The **contract,** either stated or written, contains the place, time, date, and duration of the meetings. During the orientation phase, the patient may begin to express thoughts and feelings, identify problems, and discuss realistic goals. Therefore the mutual agreement on goals is also part of the contract.

> *Student:* "Mrs. Rodriquez, we will meet at 10 AM each Thursday in the consultation room at the clinic for 45 minutes from September 15 to October 27. We can use that time for further discussion of your feelings of loneliness and anger and explore some things you could do to make the situation better for yourself."

Confidentiality. The patient has a right to know who else will be given the information shared with the nurse and that the information may be shared with specific people, such as a clinical supervisor, the physician, the staff, or other students in conference. The patient also needs to know that the information will *not* be shared with relatives, friends, or others outside the treatment team, except in extreme situations. Safeguarding the privacy and confidentiality of individuals not only is the nurse's ethical obligation but also is a legal responsibility as well.

Extreme situations include (1) child or elder abuse, (2) threats of self-harm or harm to others, or (3) intention not to follow through with the treatment plan. If information must be given to others, this is usually done by the physician, according to legal guidelines (refer to Chapter 6). The nurse must be aware of the patient's right to **confidentiality** and must not violate that right.

> *Student:* "Mrs. Rodriquez, I will be sharing some of what we discuss with my nursing instructor, and at times I may discuss certain concerns with my peers in conference or with the staff. However, I will *not* be sharing this information with your husband or any other members of your family or anyone outside the hospital without your permission."

Termination. Termination begins in the orientation phase. It also may be mentioned when appropriate during the working phase if the nature of the relationship is time limited (e.g., six or nine sessions). The date of the termination phase should be clear from the beginning. In some situations the nurse-patient contract may be renegotiated when the termination date has been reached. In other situations, when the therapeutic nurse-patient relationship is an open-ended one, the termination date is not known.

> *Student:* "Mrs. Rodriquez, as I mentioned earlier, our last meeting will be on October 27. We will have three more meetings after today."

Working Phase

The development of a strong working relationship can allow the patient to experience increased levels of anxiety and demonstrate dysfunctional behaviors in a safe setting while trying out new and more adaptive coping behaviors. Moore and Hartman (1988) identified specific tasks of the **working phase** of the nurse-patient relationship that remain relevant today in current clinical practice:

- Maintain the relationship.
- Gather further data.
- Promote the patient's problem-solving skills, self-esteem, and use of language.
- Facilitate behavioral change.
- Overcome resistance behaviors.
- Evaluate problems and goals, and redefine them as necessary.
- Promote practice and expression of alternative adaptive behaviors.

During the working phase, the nurse and patient together identify and explore areas in the patient's life that are causing problems. Often, the patient's present ways of handling situations stem from earlier means of coping devised to survive in a chaotic and dysfunctional family environment. Although certain coping methods may have worked for the patient at an earlier age, they now interfere with the patient's interpersonal relationships and prevent him or her from attaining current goals. The patient's dysfunctional behaviors and basic assumptions about the world are often defensive, and the patient is usually unable to change the dysfunctional behavior at will. Therefore, most of the problem behaviors or thoughts continue because of unconscious motivations and needs that are beyond the patient's awareness.

The nurse can work with the patient to identify these unconscious motivations and assumptions that keep the patient from finding satisfaction and reaching potential. Describing, and often reexperiencing, old conflicts generally awakens high levels of anxiety in the patient. Patients may use various defenses against anxiety and displace their feelings onto the nurse. Therefore during the working phase, intense emotions such as anxiety, anger, self-hatred, hopelessness, and helplessness may surface. Defense mechanisms, such as acting out anger inappropriately, withdrawing, intellectualizing, manipulating, and denying, are to be expected.

During the working phase, the patient may unconsciously transfer strong feelings into the present and onto the nurse that belong to significant others from the past (transference). The emotional responses and behaviors in the patient may also awaken strong countertransference feelings in the nurse. **The nurse's awareness of personal feelings and reactions to the patient are vital for effective interaction with the patient.**

Termination Phase

The termination phase is the final, integral phase of the nurse-patient relationship. Termination is discussed during the first interview, and again during the working stage at appropriate times. Termination may occur when the patient is discharged or when the student's clinical rotation ends. Basically, the tasks of termination are as follows:

- Summarizing the goals and objectives achieved in the relationship
- Discussing ways for the patient to incorporate into daily life any new coping strategies learned during the time spent with the nurse
- Reviewing situations that occurred during the time spent together
- Exchanging memories, which can help validate the experience for both nurse and patient and facilitate closure of that relationship

Termination often awakens strong feelings in both nurse and patient. Termination of the relationship signifies a loss for both, although the intensity and meaning of termination may be different for each. If a patient has unresolved feelings of abandonment, loneliness, or rejection, these feelings may be reawakened during the termination process. This process can be an opportunity for the patient to express these feelings, perhaps for the first time.

Important reasons for the student or nurse to address the termination phase are as follows:

- Feelings are aroused in both the patient and the nurse with regard to the experience they have shared; when these feelings are recognized and shared, patients learn that it is acceptable to feel sadness and loss when someone they care about leaves.
- Termination can be a learning experience; patients can learn that they are important to at least one person.
- By sharing the termination experience with the patient, the nurse demonstrates caring for the patient.
- This may be the first successful termination experience for the patient.

If a nurse has been working with a patient for a while, it is important for her to help the patient acknowledge any feelings and reactions he or she may be experiencing related to separations. If a patient denies that the termination is having an effect (assuming the nurse-patient relationship was strong), the nurse may say something like, "Goodbyes are difficult for people. Often they remind us of other goodbyes. Tell me about another separation in the past." If the patient appears to

be displacing anger, either by withdrawing or by being overtly angry at the nurse, the nurse may use generalized statements such as, "People may experience anger when saying goodbye. Sometimes they are angry with the person who is leaving. Tell me how you feel about my leaving." New practitioners as well as students in the psychiatric setting need to consider their last clinical experience with their patient and work with their supervisor or instructor to facilitate communication during this time.

A common response of beginning practitioners, especially students, is feeling guilty about terminating the relationship. These feelings may, in rare cases, be manifested by the student's giving the patient his or her telephone number, making plans to get together for coffee after the patient is discharged, continuing to see the patient afterward, or exchanging letters. Maintaining contact after discharge is not acceptable and is in opposition to the goals of a therapeutic relationship. Often this is in response to the student's need to (1) feel less guilty for "using the patient for learning needs," (2) maintain feelings of being "important" to the patient, or (3) sustain the illusion that the student is the only one who "understands" the patient, among other student-centered rationales.

Indeed, part of the termination process may be to explore, after discussion with the patient's case manager, the patient's plans for the future: where the patient can go for help, which agencies to contact, and which people may best help the patient find appropriate and helpful resources.

What Hinders and What Helps

Not all nurse-patient relationships follow the classic phases as outlined by Peplau. Some nurse-patient relationships start in the orientation phase but move to a mutually frustrating phase and finally to mutual withdrawal (Figure 9-2).

Forchuk and associates (2000) conducted a qualitative study of the nurse-patient relationship that remains relevant today. They examined the phases of both the therapeutic and the nontherapeutic relationship. From this study they identified certain behaviors that were beneficial to the progression of the nurse-patient relationship as well as those that hampered the development of this relationship. The study emphasized the

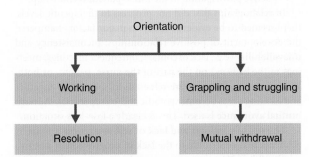

FIGURE 9-2 Phases of therapeutic and nontherapeutic relationships. (From Forchuk, C., Westwell, J., Martin, M., et al. [2000]. The developing nurse-client relationship: nurses' perspectives. *Journal of the American Psychiatric Nurses Association, 6*[1], 3-10.)

importance of consistent, regular, and private interactions with patients as essential to the development of a therapeutic alliance. Nurses in this study stressed the importance of listening, pacing, and consistency.

Specifically, Forchuk and associates (2000) found evidence that the following factors enhanced the nurse-patient relationship, allowing it to progress in a mutually satisfying manner:

- **Consistency** includes ensuring that a nurse is always assigned to the same patient and that the patient has a regular routine for activities. Interactions are facilitated when they are frequent and regular in duration, format, and location. Consistency also refers to the nurse being honest and consistent (congruent) in what is said to the patient.
- **Pacing** includes letting the patient set the pace and letting the pace be adjusted to fit the patient's moods. A slow approach helps reduce pressure, and at times it is necessary to step back and realize that developing a strong relationship may take a long time.
- **Listening** includes letting the patient talk when needed. The nurse becomes a sounding board for the patient's concerns and issues. Listening is perhaps the most important skill for nurses to master. Truly listening to another person, attending to what is behind the words, is a learned skill.
- **Initial impressions,** especially positive initial attitudes and preconceptions, are significant considerations in how the relationship will progress. Preconceived negative impressions and feelings toward the patient usually bode poorly for the positive growth of the relationship. In contrast, the nurse's feeling that the patient is "interesting" or "a challenge" and a positive attitude about the relationship are usually favorable signs for the developing therapeutic alliance.
- **Comfort and control,** that is, promoting patient comfort and balancing control, usually reflect caring behaviors. Control refers to keeping a balance in the relationship: not too strict and not too lenient.
- **Patient factors** that seem to enhance the relationship include trust on the part of the patient and the patient's active participation in the nurse-patient relationship.

In relationships that did not progress to therapeutic levels, there seemed to be evidence that two major factors hampered the development of positive relationships: **inconsistency** and **unavailability** (e.g., lack of contact, infrequent meetings, meetings in the hallway) on the part of the nurse, patient, or both. When nurse and patient are reluctant to spend time together and meeting times become sporadic and/or superficial, the term **mutual avoidance** is used. This is clearly a lose-lose situation.

The nurse's feelings and lack of self-awareness are major elements that contribute to the lack of progression of positive relationships. Negative preconceived ideas about the patient and negative feelings (e.g., discomfort, dislike, fear, and avoidance) seem to be a constant in relationships that end in frustration and mutual withdrawal. Sometimes these feelings are known, and sometimes the nurse is only vaguely aware of them.

Factors That Enhance Growth

Rogers and Truax (1967) identified three personal characteristics that help promote change and growth in patients, which are classic guidelines that are vital components for establishing a therapeutic alliance or relationship: (1) genuineness, (2) empathy, and (3) positive regard. These are some of the intangibles that are at the heart of the art of nursing.

Genuineness

Genuineness, or self-awareness of one's feelings as they arise within the relationship and the ability to communicate them when appropriate, is a key ingredient in building trust. When a person is genuine, one gets the sense that what is displayed on the outside of the person is congruent with the internal processes. It is conveyed by listening to and communicating with others without distorting their messages, and being clear and concrete in communications with patients. Being genuine in a therapeutic relationship implies the ability to use therapeutic communication tools in an appropriately spontaneous manner, rather than rigidly or in a parrot-like fashion.

Empathy

Empathy is a complex multidimensional concept that has moral, cognitive, emotional, and behavioral components (Mercer & Reynolds, 2002). Perhaps Carl Rogers (1980) explained empathy most clearly:

> It means entering the private perceptual world of the other and becoming thoroughly at home with it. It involves being sensitive, moment by moment, to the changing felt meanings which flow in this other person, to the fear or rage or tenderness or confusion or whatever that he or she is experiencing. It means temporarily living in the other's life, moving about in it delicately without making judgments (p. 142).

Therefore, empathy signifies a central focus and feeling with and in the patient's world. According to Mercer and Reynolds (2002) it involves the following:

- Accurately perceiving the patient's situation, perspective, and feelings
- Communicating one's understanding to the patient and checking with the patient for accuracy
- Acting on this understanding in a helpful (therapeutic) way toward the patient

Empathy versus sympathy. There is much confusion regarding empathy versus sympathy. A simple way to distinguish them is that in empathy we *understand* the feelings of others. In sympathy we *feel* the feelings of others. When a helping person is feeling sympathy for another, objectivity is lost, and the ability to assist the patient in solving a personal problem ceases. Furthermore, sympathy is associated with feelings of pity and commiseration. Although these are considered nurturing human traits, they may not be particularly useful in a therapeutic relationship. When people express sympathy, they express agreement with another, which in some situations may discourage further exploration of a person's thoughts and feelings.

The following examples are given to clarify the distinction between empathy and sympathy. A friend tells you that her mother was just diagnosed with inoperable cancer. Your friend then begins to cry and pounds the table with her fist.

> *Sympathetic response:* "I know exactly how you feel. My mother was hospitalized last year and it was awful. I was so depressed. I still get upset just thinking about it." *(You go on to tell your friend about the incident.)*

Sometimes when nurses try to be sympathetic, they are apt to project their own feelings onto those of the patient, which thus limits the patient's range of responses. A more useful response might be as follows:

> *Empathic response:* "How upsetting this must be for you. Something similar happened to my mother last year and I had so many mixed emotions. What thoughts and feelings are you having?" *(You continue to stay with your friend and listen to his or her thoughts and feelings.)*

In the practice of psychotherapy or counseling, empathy is an essential ingredient in a therapeutic relationship both for the better-functioning patient and for the patient who functions at a more primitive level.

Positive Regard

Positive regard implies respect. It is the ability to view another person as being worthy of caring about and as someone who has strengths and achievement potential. Positive regard is usually communicated indirectly by the following actions rather than directly by words.

Attitudes. One attitude through which a nurse might convey respect is willingness to work with the patient. That is, the nurse takes the patient and the relationship seriously. The experience is viewed not as "a job," "part of a course," or "time spent talking," but as an opportunity to work with patients to help them develop personal resources and actualize more of their potential in living.

Actions. Some actions that manifest an attitude of respect are attending, suspending value judgments, and helping patients develop their own resources.

Attending. Attending behavior is a crucial element in a successful interview. To succeed, nurses must pay attention to their patients in culturally and individually appropriate ways (Sommers-Flanagan & Sommers-Flanagan, 2009). *Attending* is a special kind of listening that refers to an intensity of presence, or being with the patient. At times, simply being with another person during a painful time can make a difference.

Body posture, eye contact, and body language are nonverbal behaviors that reflect the degree of attending and are highly culturally influenced. The cultural components of body posture, eye contact, and body language are covered in more depth in The Clinical Interview section of this chapter.

Suspending value judgments. Although we will always have personal opinions, nurses are more effective when they guard against using their own value systems to judge patients' thoughts, feelings, or behaviors. For example, if a patient is taking drugs or is involved in sexually risky behavior, you might recognize that these behaviors are hindering the patient from living a more satisfying life, posing a potential health threat, or preventing the patient from developing satisfying relationships. However, labeling these activities as bad or good is not useful. Rather, focus on exploring the behavior of the patient and work toward identifying the thoughts and feelings that influence this behavior. Judgmental behavior on the part of the nurse will most likely interfere with further exploration.

The first steps in eliminating judgmental thinking and behaviors are to (1) recognize their presence, (2) identify how or where you learned these responses to the patient's behavior, and (3) construct alternative ways to view the patient's thinking and behavior.

Denying judgmental thinking will only compound the problem.

> *Patient:* "I am really sexually promiscuous and I love to gamble when I have money. I have sex whenever I can find a partner and spend most of my time in the casino. This has been going on for at least 3 years."

A judgmental response would be the following:

> *Nurse A:* "So your promiscuous sexual and compulsive gambling behaviors really haven't brought you much happiness, have they? You are running away from your problems and could end up with AIDS and broke."

A more helpful response would be the following:

> *Nurse B:* "So, your sexual and gambling activities are part of the picture also. You sound as if these activities are not making you happy."

In this example, Nurse B focuses on the patient's behaviors and the possible meaning they might have to the patient. Nurse B does not introduce personal value statements or prejudices regarding promiscuous behavior, as does Nurse A. Empathy and positive regard are essential qualities in a successful nurse-patient relationship.

Helping patients develop resources. The nurse becomes aware of patients' strengths and encourages patients to work at their optimal level of functioning. The nurse does not act for patients unless absolutely necessary, and then only as a step toward helping them act on their own. It is important that patients remain as independent as possible to develop new resources for problem solving.

> *Patient:* "This medication makes my mouth so dry. Could you get me something to drink?"
>
> *Nurse:* "There is juice in the refrigerator. I'll wait here for you until you get back."

or

> *Nurse:* "I'll walk with you while you get some juice from the refrigerator."

or

> *Patient:* "Could you ask the doctor to let me have a pass for the weekend?"
>
> *Nurse:* "Your doctor will be on the unit this afternoon. I'll let her know that you want to speak with her."

Consistently encouraging patients to use their own resources helps minimize the patients' feelings of helplessness and dependency and validates their potential for change.

THE CLINICAL INTERVIEW

The content and direction of the clinical interview are decided by the patient. The patient leads. The nurse employs communication skills and active listening to better understand the patient's situation. During the clinical interview, the nurse provides the opportunity for the patient to reach specific goals, including the following:

- To feel understood and comfortable
- To identify and explore problems relating to others
- To discuss healthy ways of meeting emotional needs
- To experience a satisfying interpersonal relationship

Preparing for the Interview

Helping a person with an emotional or medical problem is rarely a straightforward task. The goal of assisting a patient to regain psychological or physiological stability can be difficult to achieve. Extremely important to any kind of counseling is permitting the patient to set the pace of the interview, no matter how slow the progress may be (Arnold & Boggs, 2011).

Setting

Effective communication can take place almost anywhere. However, because the quality of the interaction—whether in a clinic, a clinical unit, an office, or the patient's home—depends on the degree to which the nurse and patient feel safe, establishing a setting that enhances feelings of security can be important to the helping relationship. A health care setting, a conference room, or a quiet part of the unit that has relative privacy but is within view of others is ideal. When the interview takes place in the home, it offers the nurse a valuable opportunity to assess the person in the context of everyday life.

Seating

In all settings, chairs need to be arranged so that conversation can take place in normal tones of voice and eye contact can be comfortably maintained or avoided. For example, a non-threatening physical environment for nurse and patient would involve the following:

- Assuming the same height, either both sitting or both standing.
- Avoiding a face-to-face stance when possible; a 90- to 120-degree angle or side-by-side position may be less intense and the patient and nurse can look away from each other without discomfort.
- Providing safety and psychological comfort in terms of exiting the room. The patient should not be positioned between the nurse and the door, nor should the nurse be positioned in such a way that the patient feels trapped in the room.
- Avoiding a desk barrier between the nurse and the patient.

Introductions

In the orientation phase, students tell the patient who they are, what the purpose of the meeting is, and how long and at what time they will be meeting with the patient. The issue of confidentiality is addressed during the initial interview. Please remember that all health care professionals must respect the private, personal, and confidential nature of the patient's communication except in specific situations as outlined earlier (e.g., harm to self or others, child abuse, elder abuse). What is discussed with staff and your clinical group in conference should not be discussed outside with others, no matter who they are (e.g., patient's relatives, news media, friends). The patient needs to know that whatever is discussed will stay confidential unless permission is given for it to be disclosed.

The nurse can then ask the patient how he or she would like to be addressed. This question accomplishes a number of tasks (Arnold & Boggs, 2011). For example:

- It conveys respect.
- It gives the patient direct control over an important ego issue. (Some patients like to be called by their last names; others prefer being on a first-name basis with the nurse.)

Initiating the Interview

Once introductions have been made, the nurse can turn the interview over to the patient by using one of a number of open-ended statements such as the following:

- "Where should we start?"
- "Tell me a little about what has been going on with you."
- "What are some of the stresses you have been coping with recently?"
- "Tell me a little about what has been happening in the past couple of weeks."
- "Perhaps you can begin by letting me know what some of your concerns have been recently."
- "Tell me about your difficulties."

Communication can be facilitated by appropriately **offering leads** (e.g., "Go on"), making **statements of acceptance** (e.g., "Uh-huh"), or otherwise conveying interest.

Tactics to Avoid

The nurse needs to avoid certain behaviors as outlined by Moscato in 1988; they still serve as important guidelines today. For example:

Do Not:	Try To:
Argue with, minimize, or challenge the patient.	Keep focus on facts and the patient's perceptions.
Give false reassurance.	Make observations of the patient's behavior. "Change is always possible."
Interpret to the patient or speculate on the dynamics.	Listen attentively, use silence, and try to clarify the patient's problem.

Do Not:	Try To:
Question or probe patients about sensitive areas that they do not wish to discuss.	Pay attention to nonverbal communication. Strive to keep the patient's anxiety decreased.
Try to sell the patient on accepting treatment.	Encourage the patient to look at pros and cons.
Join in attacks patients launch on their mates, parents, friends, or associates.	Focus on facts and the patient's perceptions. Be aware of nonverbal communication.
Participate in criticism of another nurse or any other staff member.	Focus on facts and the patient's perceptions. Check out serious accusations with the other nurse or staff member. Have the patient meet with the nurse or staff member in question and senior staff or clinician and clarify perceptions.

Helpful Guidelines

Some classic guidelines for conducting the initial interviews are offered by Meier and Davis (2001):

- Speak briefly.
- When you do not know what to say, say nothing.
- When in doubt, focus on feelings.
- Avoid advice.
- Avoid relying on questions.
- Pay attention to nonverbal cues.
- Keep the focus on the patient.

Attending Behaviors: The Foundation of Interviewing

Engaging in attending behaviors and listening well are two key principles of counseling on which just about everyone agrees (Sommers-Flanagan & Sommers-Flanagan, 2009). Attending behaviors were addressed earlier but are covered more thoroughly here as they relate to the clinical interview. Ivey and Ivey (1999) define attending behaviors as "culturally and individually appropriate...eye contact, body language, vocal qualities, and verbal tracking" (p. 15). Sommers-Flanagan and Sommers-Flanagan (2009) state that positive attending behaviors can open up communication and encourage free expression. However, negative attending behaviors are more likely to inhibit expression. These behaviors need to be evaluated in terms of cultural patterns and past experiences of both the interviewer and the interviewee. There are no universals; however, there are guidelines that students can follow.

Eye Contact

Even among people from similar cultural backgrounds there may be variation in what an individual is personally comfortable with in terms of eye contact. For some patients and interviewers, sustained eye contact is normal and comfortable, whereas for other patients and interviewers it may be more comfortable and natural to make brief eye contact but look away or down much of the time. Sommers-Flanagan and Sommers-Flanagan (2009) state that it is appropriate for most nurse clinicians to maintain more eye contact when the patient speaks and less constant eye contact when the nurse speaks. However, in general, white patients are more comfortable with more sustained eye contact much of the time, whereas Native Americans, African Americans, and Asian patients often prefer less eye contact.

Body Language

Body language involves two elements: kinesics and proxemics. *Kinesics* is associated with physical characteristics such as body movements and postures. The way someone holds the head, legs, and shoulders; facial expressions; eye contact or lack thereof; and so on convey a multitude of messages. For example, a person who slumps in a chair, rolls the eyes, and sits with arms crossed in front of the chest can be perceived as resistant and unreceptive to what another wants to communicate.

On the other hand, positive body language may include leaning in slightly toward the speaker, maintaining a relaxed and attentive posture, making direct eye contact, making hand gestures that are unobtrusive and smooth while minimizing the number of other movements, and matching one's facial expressions to one's feelings or to the patient's feelings.

Proxemics refers to personal space and what distance between oneself and others is comfortable for an individual. Proxemics takes into account that these distances may be different for different cultural groups. **Intimate distance** in the United States is 0 to 18 inches and is reserved for those we trust most and with whom we feel most safe. **Personal distance** (18 to 40 inches) is for personal communications such as those with friends or colleagues. **Social distance** (4 to 12 feet) is applied to strangers or acquaintances, often in public places or formal social gatherings. **Public distance** (12 feet or more) relates to public space (e.g., public speaking). In public space one may hail another, and the parties may move about while communicating with one another.

Vocal Qualities

Vocal quality, or **paralinguistics,** encompasses voice loudness, pitch, rate, and fluency. Sommers-Flanagan and Sommers-Flanagan (2009) state that "effective interviewers use vocal qualities to enhance rapport, communicate interest and empathy and to emphasize special issues or conflicts" (p. 56). This supports the old adage, "It's not *what* you say, but *how* you say it." Speaking in soft and gentle tones is apt to encourage a person to share thoughts and feelings, whereas speaking in a rapid, high-pitched tone may convey anxiety and create it in the patient. Consider, for example, how tonal quality can affect communication in a simple sentence like "I will see you tonight."

1. "*I* will see you tonight." (I will be the one who sees you tonight.)
2. "I *will* see you tonight." (No matter what happens, or whether you like it or not, I will see you tonight.)
3. "I will see *you* tonight." (Even though others are present, it is you I want to see.)
4. "I will see you *tonight*." (It is definite, tonight is the night we will meet.)

Verbal Tracking

Verbal tracking is just that: tracking what the patient is saying. Individuals cannot know if you are hearing or understanding what they are saying unless you provide them with cues. Verbal tracking is giving neutral feedback in the form of restating or summarizing what the patient has already said. It does not include personal or professional opinions of what the patient has said (Sommers-Flanagan & Sommers-Flanagan, 2009). For example:

Patient: "I don't know what the fuss is about. I smoke marijuana to relax and everyone makes a fuss."

Nurse: "Do you see this as a problem for you?"

Patient: "No, I don't. It doesn't affect my work…well, most of the time, anyway. I mean, of course, if I have to think things out and make important decisions, then obviously it can get in the way. But most of the time I'm cool."

Nurse: "So when important decisions have to be made, then it interferes; otherwise, you don't see it affecting your functioning."

Patient: "Yeah, well, most of the time I'm cool."

Meier and Davis (2001) state that verbal tracking involves pacing the interview with the patient by sticking closely with the patient's speech content (as well as speech volume and tone as discussed earlier). It can be difficult to know which leads to follow if the patient introduces many topics at once.

Clinical Supervision and Process Recordings

Communication and interviewing techniques are acquired skills. Nurses learn to increase their ability to use communication and interviewing skills through practice and clinical supervision. In clinical supervision, the focus is on the nurse's behavior in the nurse-patient relationship. The nurse and the supervisor examine and analyze the nurse's feelings and reactions to the patient and the way they affect the relationship.

• "And I would emphasize that, no matter how good we become at being our own inner supervisor, professional help and support from experienced (external) supervisor is essential to good practice"(Fox, 2008, p. 21).

• Farkas-Cameron (1995) observed that clinical supervision can be a therapeutic process for the nurse. During the process, feelings and concerns are ventilated as they relate to the developing nurse-patient relationship. The opportunity to examine interactions, obtain insights, and devise alternative strategies for dealing with various clinical issues enhances clinical growth and minimizes frustration and burnout. Clinical supervision is a necessary professional activity that fosters professional growth and helps minimize the development of nontherapeutic nurse-patient relationships.

The best way to increase communication and interviewing skills is to review clinical interactions exactly as they occur. This process offers students the opportunity to identify themes and patterns in their own, as well as their patients', communications. Students also learn to deal with the variety of situations that arise in the clinical interview.

If taping or videotaping the interaction is not available, the use of process recordings is a good mechanism to identify patterns in the student's and the patient's communication. Process recordings are written records of a segment of the nurse-patient session that reflect as closely as possible the verbal and nonverbal behaviors of both patient and nurse. have some disadvantages because they rely on memory and are subject to distortions. However, they can be a useful tool for identifying communication patterns. It is usually best if the student can write notes verbatim (word for word) in a private area immediately after the interaction has taken place. Although the use of process recordings is decreasing in many schools of nursing, they remain a useful tool for students, as well as new clinicians, to reflect on the interview, examine the process, and consider more appropriate responses, thereby improving communication skills.

VALUES AND CULTURAL INFLUENCES WITHIN A RELATIONSHIP

Relationships are complex. We bring into our relationships a multitude of thoughts, feelings, beliefs, and attitudes—some rational and some irrational. We form these from families or culture, our spiritual beliefs and experiences, and our "heroes." It is helpful, even crucial, that we have an understanding of our own values and attitudes so that we may become aware of the beliefs or attitudes we hold that may interfere with the establishment of positive relationships with those under our care.

Increasingly we are working with, living with, and caring for people from diverse cultures and subcultures whose life experiences and life values may be quite different from our own. Values are abstract standards and represent an ideal, either positive or negative. For example, in the United States, to create a social order in which people can live peaceably together and feel secure in their person and property, society has adopted the two values of respecting one another's liberty and working cooperatively for a common goal. Not all the nation's people live up to these ideals all the time.

You may have noticed that there may be a dichotomy between theory and practice in the lives of some. For example, some people may pay lip service to the values of authority, but their behavior contradicts these values. They may stress honesty and respect for the law, yet cheat on their taxes and in their business practices. They may love their neighbors on Sunday and preach the love of God but demean or downgrade others around them for the rest of the week. They may declare themselves patriots, but label others traitors or even deny freedom of speech to any dissenters whose concept of patriotism differs from theirs.

A person's value system greatly influences both daily and long-range choices. Values and beliefs provide a framework for the life goals people develop and for what they want their life to include. Our values are usually culturally oriented and influenced in a variety of ways through our parents, teachers, religious institutions, workplaces, peers, and political leaders as well as through Hollywood and the media. All these influences attempt to instill their values and to form and influence ours (Simon et al., 1995).

We also form our values through the example of others. **Modeling** is perhaps one of the most potent means of value education because it presents a vivid example of values in action. We all need role models to guide us in negotiating life's many choices. Young people in particular are hungry for role models and will find them among peers as well as adults. As nurses, parents, bosses, coworkers, friends, lovers, teachers, spouses, and singles, we are constantly (in either a positive or a negative manner) providing a role model to others.

Our culture, and more precisely our subculture, defines the guidelines that provide structure to our lives. It is through this that our beliefs, thoughts, behaviors, and feelings are interpreted (Korn, 2001; Sommers-Flanagan & Sommers-Flanagan, 2009). Culture provides meaning to our lives and our environment in the form of an operating system or interpretive system. How we view the world and how we are supposed to behave, think, believe, and live are influenced by this interpretive system. Problems arise when the interpretive system of the clinician and that of the individual seeking guidance are glaringly different. When the nurse is working with an individual from a culturally distinct environment, the interpretive system between them might be so distinct at times that it is difficult for the patient and clinician to connect in a clinically meaningful way (Hays, 2008). "Developing cultural self-awareness begins with acceptance of differences as normal, interesting, and even desirable aspects of being human" (Sommers-Flanagan & Sommers-Flanagan, 2009, p. 29).

There are many ways this can be problematic. Although we emphasize that the patient and the nurse identify outcomes together, what happens when the nurse's beliefs, values, and interpretive system are very different from those of a patient? For example, the patient wants an abortion, which is against the nurse's values (or vice versa). The patient engages in irresponsible sex with multiple partners, and that is against the nurse's values. The patient puts material gain and objects far ahead of loyalty to friends and family, in direct contrast with the nurse's values (or vice versa). The patient's lifestyle includes taking illicit drugs, and substance abuse is against the nurse's values. The patient is deeply religious, and the nurse is a nonbeliever who shuns organized religion. Can nurses develop a working relationship and help patients solve a problem when the values, goals, and interpretive systems of the patients are so different from their own?

As nurses, it is useful for us to understand that our values and beliefs are not necessarily right and certainly not right for everyone. It is helpful to realize that our values and beliefs (1) reflect our own culture, (2) are derived from a whole range of choices, and (3) are those we have *chosen* for ourselves from a variety of influences and role models. These chosen values guide us in making decisions and taking the actions we hope will make our lives meaningful, rewarding, and full.

Personal values may change over time; indeed, they may change many times over the course of a lifetime. The values you held as a child are different from those you held as an adolescent and so forth. Self-awareness requires that we understand what we value and those beliefs that guide our behavior. It is critical that as nurses we not only understand and accept our own values and beliefs but also are sensitive to and accepting of the unique and different values and beliefs of others.

KEY POINTS TO REMEMBER

- The nurse-patient relationship (patient-centered, nurse-patient partnership) is well-defined, and the roles of the nurse and the patient must be clearly stated.
- It is important that the nurse be aware of the differences between a therapeutic relationship and a social or intimate relationship. In a therapeutic nurse-patient relationship, the focus is on the patient's needs, thoughts, feelings, and goals. The nurse is expected to meet personal needs outside this relationship in other professional, social, or intimate arenas.
- Genuineness, positive regard, and empathy are personal strengths in the helping person that foster growth and change in others.
- Although the boundaries of the nurse-patient relationship generally are clearly defined, they can become blurred; this blurring can be insidious and may occur on an unconscious level. Usually, transference and countertransference phenomena are operating when boundaries are blurred.
- It is important to have a grasp of common countertransferential feelings and behaviors and of the nursing actions to counteract these phenomena.
- Supervision aids in promoting the professional growth of the nurse as well as in the nurse-patient relationship, allowing the patient's goals to be worked on and met.
- The phases of the nurse-patient relationship include the orientation, working, and termination phases.

KEY POINTS TO REMEMBER — cont'd

- The clinical interview is a key component of psychiatric mental health nursing. Presented are considerations needed for establishing a safe setting and planning for appropriate seating, introduction, and initiation of the interview.
- Attending behaviors (e.g., eye contact, body language, vocal qualities, and verbal tracking) are a key element in effective communication.

- Cultural background (as well as individual values and beliefs) has a great deal to do with what nonverbal behavior means to different individuals. The degree of eye contact and the use of touch are two nonverbal aspects that can be misunderstood by individuals of different cultures.
- A meaningful therapeutic relationship is facilitated when values and cultural influences are considered. It is the nurse's responsibility to seek to understand the patient's perceptions.

APPLYING CRITICAL JUDGMENT

1. On your first clinical day you spend time with an older woman, Mrs. Schneider, who is very depressed. Your first impression is "Oh, my, she looks like my mean Aunt Helen. She even sits like her." Mrs. Schneider asks you, "Who are you and how can you help me?" She tells you that "a student" could never understand what she is going through. She then says, "If you really wanted to help me you could get me a good job after I leave here."

   A. Identify transference and countertransference issues in this situation. What is your most important course of action? What in the classic study of Forchuk and associates (2000) indicates that this is a time for you to exercise self-awareness and self-insight to establish the potential for a therapeutic encounter or relationship?

   B. How could you best respond to Mrs. Schneider's question about who you are? What other information will you give her during this first clinical encounter? Be specific.

   C. What are some useful responses you could give her regarding her legitimate questions about ways you could be of help to her?

   D. Analyze Mrs. Schneider's request that you find her a job. How does this request relate to boundary issues, and how can this be an opportunity for you to help Mrs. Schneider develop resources? Keeping in mind the aim of Peplau's interactive nurse-patient process, describe some useful ways you could respond to this request.

2. You are attempting to conduct a clinical interview with a very withdrawn patient. You have tried silence and open-ended statements, but all you get is one-word answers. What other actions could you take at this time?

CHAPTER REVIEW QUESTIONS

Choose the most appropriate answer(s).

1. Which of the following is an accurate statement about transference?
   1. Transference occurs when the patient attributes thoughts and feelings toward the therapist that pertain to a person in the patient's past.
   2. Transference occurs when the therapist attributes thoughts and feelings toward the patient that pertain to a person in the patient's past.
   3. Transference occurs when the therapist understands and builds a value system consistent with the patient's value system.
   4. Transference occurs when the therapist recalls circumstances in his or her life similar to those the patient is experiencing and shares this with the patient.

2. A basic tool the nurse uses when establishing a relationship with a patient with a psychiatric disorder is:
   1. narcissism.
   2. role blurring.
   3. consistency.
   4. formation of value judgments.

3. Which nurse behavior jeopardizes the boundaries of the nurse-patient relationship?
   1. Focusing on patient needs
   2. Suspending value judgments

   3. Recognizing the value of supervision
   4. Allowing the relationship to become social

4. Which nurse behavior would not be considered a boundary violation?
   1. Narcissism
   2. Controlling
   3. Genuineness
   4. Keeping secrets about the relationship

5. Which statement describes an event that would occur during the working phase of the nurse-patient relationship?
   1. The nurse summarizes the objectives achieved in the relationship.
   2. The nurse assesses the patient's level of psychological functioning, and mutual identification of problems and goals occurs.
   3. Some regression and mourning occur about the nurse-patient relationship, although the patient demonstrates satisfaction and competence.
   4. The patient strives for congruence among actions, thoughts, and feelings and engages in problem solving and testing of alternative behaviors.

REFERENCES

Arnold, E. C., & Boggs, K. U. (2011). *Interpersonal relationships: professional communication skills for nurses* (5th ed.). St Louis: Saunders.

Farkas-Cameron, M. M. (1995). Clinical supervision in psychiatric nursing. *Journal of Psychosocial Nursing and Mental Health Services, 33*(2), 40–47.

Forchuk, C., Westwell, J., Martin, M., et al. (2000). The developing nurse-client relationship: nurse's perspectives. *Journal of the American Psychiatric Nurses Association, 6*(1), 3–10.

Fox, S. (2008). *Relating to clients: the therapeutic relationship for complementary therapists.* London and Philadelphia: Jessica Kingsley Publishers.

Gordon, C., Phillips, M., & Bereson, E. V. (2010). The doctor-patient relationship. In T. A. Stern, G. L. Fricchione, N. H. Cassen, M. S. Jellinek, & J. F. Rosenbaum (Eds.), *Massachusetts General Hospital: handbook of general hospital psychiatry* (6th ed.). Philadelphia: Saunders/Elsevier.

Haber, J. (2000). Hildegard E. Peplau: the psychiatric nursing legacy of a legend. *Journal of the American Psychiatric Nurses Association, 6*(2), 56–62.

Hays, P. (2008). *Addressing cultural complexities in practice* (2nd ed.). Washington, DC: American Psychological Association.

Ivey, A. E., & Ivey, M. (1999). *Intentional interviewing and counseling* (4th ed.). Pacific Grove, CA: Brooks/Cole.

Kopta, S. M., Saunders, S. M., Lueger, R. L., & Howard, K. I. (1999). Individual psychotherapy outcome and process research: challenge leading to great turmoil or positive transition? *Annual Review of Psychology, 50,* 441–469.

Korn, M. L. (2001). *Cultural aspects of the psychotherapeutic process.* Retrieved June 20, 2006, from http://doctor.medscape.com/viewarticle/418608.

LaRowe, K. (2004). *The therapeutic relationship.* Retrieved February 3, 2005, from http://compassion-fatigue.com/Index.asp?PG=89.

Meier, S. T., & Davis, S. R. (2001). *The elements of counseling* (4th ed.). Pacific Grove, CA: Brooks/Cole.

Mercer, S. W., & Reynolds, W. (2002). Empathy and quality of care. *British Journal of General Practice, 52*(Suppl), S9–S12.

Moore, J. C., & Hartman, C. R. (1988). Developing a therapeutic relationship. In C. K. Beck, R. P. Rawlins, & S. R. Williams (Eds.), *Mental health–psychiatric nursing.* St Louis: Mosby.

Moscato, B. (1988). The one-to-one relationship. In H. S. Wilson, & C. S. Kneisel (Eds.), *Psychiatric nursing* (3rd ed.). Menlo Park, CA: Addison-Wesley.

Peplau, H. E. (1999). *Interpersonal relations in nursing: a conceptual frame of reference for psychodynamic nursing.* New York: Springer.

Peplau, H.E. (1952). *Interpersonal relations in nursing: a conceptual frame of reference for psychodynamic nursing.* New York: Putnam.

Pilette, P. C., Berck, C. B., & Achber, L. C. (1995). Therapeutic management of helping boundaries. *Journal of Psychosocial Nursing and Mental Health Services, 33*(1), 40–47.

Public Broadcasting Service (PBS). (2006). *Receiving patient-centered care.* Retrieved July 24, 2011, from www. pbs.org/remaking American medicine/care.html.

Quinlan, J. C.F. (1996). *Co-creating personal and professional knowledge through peer support and peer approval in nursing.* Submitted for degree of PhD of the University of Bath, England, 1996. Retrieved July 17, 2006, from www.bath.ac.uk/carpp/jquinlan/titlepage.htm.

Rogers, C. R. (1980). *A way of being.* Boston: Houghton Mifflin.

Rogers, C. R., & Truax, C. B. (1967). The therapeutic conditions antecedent to change: a theoretical view. In C. R. Rogers (Ed.), *The therapeutic relationship and its impact.* Madison: University of Wisconsin Press.

Simon, S. B., Howe, L. W., & Kirschenbaum, H. (1995). *Values clarification.* New York: Warner Books.

Sommers-Flanagan, J., & Sommers-Flanagan, R. (2009). *Clinical interviewing* (3rd ed.). Hoboken, NJ: Wiley.

Caring for Patients With Psychobiological Disorders

Pioneering the Process of Certification in Psychiatric Mental Health Nursing

Sheila Rouslin Welt, MS, APN

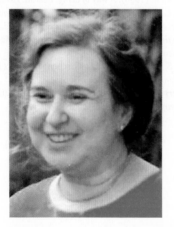

Sheila Rouslin Welt is a Clinical Specialist in Psychiatric Nursing; she established the first position for clinical specialists in community mental health centers in the state of New Jersey and was one of the first private practice nurses in psychotherapy. A long-time editor of *Perspectives in Psychiatric Care,* Ms. Rouslin Welt was the first nurse to coauthor a book on group psychotherapy (the first of 6 books) and has authored more than 15 articles and book chapters. For 12 years she taught in the graduate psychiatric nursing program at Rutgers University. A national and international lecturer, for the past 30 years Ms. Rouslin Welt has maintained a private psychotherapy, supervision, and consultation practice in New Jersey.

Ms. Rouslin Welt was part of the movement to gain certification for the practice of Clinical Specialists in Psychiatric Nursing. The following is her story.

The credentialing process began in the early 1970s. Marcia Stachyra, a fellow graduate of Peplau's program, spearheaded the process. Although graduate education at the time permitted a nurse to attain the title of Clinical Specialist in Psychiatric Nursing and act as a psychotherapist, the practice of nurse psychotherapy was unprotected by existing Nurse Practice Acts or specialty certification. Therefore, the need for credentialing criteria arose. Indeed, changes or advances in clinical practice typically precede laws that protect and govern the professionals or the public. For example, in the state of New York anyone could practice as a psychotherapist. In New Jersey, however, the Psychology Practice Act specified psychotherapy as within the purview of some disciplines, but not nursing.

With the help of psychologist Allan Williams, the New York State Psychological Association's Executive Director and a member of their legal team, several of us began the process of certification that would legitimize our practice. We worked with the New York State Nurses Association in a process that included revising the Nurse Practice Act in a way that, through regulations guiding practice, psychotherapy by a properly prepared nurse could be included as a legitimate treatment process. This led to the development of postdegree certification through a designated process of clinical supervision and testing. Not only did the process become a model for New Jersey, the next battleground, but also it became the prototype for national certification, demonstrating growth of the profession.

The New Jersey process was more complex and difficult, however. Although we formed The Society of Certified Clinical Specialists in Psychiatric Nursing, we were vulnerable because psychologists "owned" psychotherapy through their Act; therefore if we practiced psychotherapy, we would be labeled as practicing psychology. We were not one of the "exempt" professions. The medical doctors, though, even nonpsychiatrists, could practice anything considered in the scope of medical practice. Meanwhile, a group of mainly social workers evolved into a credentialing body called Marriage and Family Counselors. In the process of surveying helping professionals such as physicians, nurses, social workers, and clergy in order to "exempt" them from the need for the new credential or to attain legacy status, they advanced the question to a prominent nursing educator whether any nurses were prepared for psychotherapeutic work, and she said, "No." Obviously, this was not so, and it led to difficult times ahead, including a member of the fledgling Society being sued for practice for which she was deemed educationally unprepared and uncredentialed. Somehow, we faced the hurdles and survived those years, again with the need for revision of the New Jersey Nurse Practice Act in order to broaden the scope of practice.

CHAPTER

10

Stress and Stress-Related Disorders

Elizabeth M. Varcarolis

evolve WEBSITE

http://evolve.elsevier.com/Varcarolis/essentials

KEY TERMS AND CONCEPTS

acute stress disorder, p. 159
compassion fatigue/secondary
    stress trauma, 161
distress, p. 155
eustress, p. 155

flashbacks, p. 159
posttraumatic stress disorder
    (PTSD), p. 156
stress response, p. 155

SELECTED CONCEPT: Compassion Fatigue/Secondary Stress Trauma
Secondary stress trauma and *compassion fatigue* are synonymous terms. Compassion fatigue/secondary stress trauma is the term used when health care workers are indirectly traumatized when they cannot help the patient going through a devastating illness or severe trauma. As a result, nurses/health care workers are left with profound feelings such as depression, isolation, high levels of anxiety, nightmares, somatic symptoms, and more.
(Yoder, 2010)

OBJECTIVES

1. Discuss four examples of how *eustress* has helped you in your life and two examples of how *distress* has affected you in your life.
2. Describe some of the common symptoms people experience when they are stressed.
3. Describe the physiological manifestations of the fight-or-flight response of the autonomic nervous system when triggered by a stressor.
4. Describe the physiological manifestations of the hypothalamus-pituitary-adrenal cortex axis in the role of chronic stress in terms of the fight-or-flight response.

OBJECTIVES—cont'd

5. Teach a classmate about posttraumatic stress disorder (PTSD), including (a) the symptoms, (b) the way it could affect our veterans returning from the wars in Iraq and Afghanistan, (c) possible sequelae (results) of untreated PTSD, (d) potential treatments, and (e) the potential role of PTSD in first responders.

6. Explain how assessing for traumatic brain injury (TBI) would fit into *evidence-based practice* when working with returning war veterans, as well as other members of the population who are involved in traumatic injury (e.g., head injuries, sports injuries, physical abuse).

7. Compare and contrast the differences between PTSD and acute stress disorder.

8. Describe what is meant by secondary traumatic stress/compassion fatigue in terms of (a) symptoms and (b) health care workers who might be the most vulnerable.

We are all familiar with stress. The annual stress survey commissioned by the American Psychological Association has found that for the last 2 years nearly 25% of Americans are experiencing high levels of stress, which is measured by a score of 8 or higher on a 10-point scale. Another 50% reported moderate stress levels (a score of 4 to 7) (American Psychological Association, 2010; Harvard Health Publications, 2011).

Actually, some stress is termed "good" stress, or eustress. Eustress is beneficial stress; it motivates people to develop the skills they need to solve problems and meet personal goals. However, it is the distress that causes problems. **Distress** is a negative experience that can drain our energy. Increased stress and anxiety can trigger depression, cause confusion, and instill helplessness/hopelessness, causing fatigue. When individuals feel "stressed-out" they may have trouble sleeping or eating, experience headaches or back pain, lose interest in favorite activities, feel tense and become irritable, and often feel powerless. Long-term chronic stress can cause us physiological harm and emotional difficulties.

A stressor—that which triggers stress—can be real or perceived. Stress can be psychological (e.g., anxiety, guilt, or joy) or physical (e.g., stressful environment, such as loud noises, extreme heat or cold, or other disturbing physical condition). Stress can be psychosocial (e.g., threat to self-esteem, acceptance in a group, social status, and respect). Stress can also be spiritual (such as an existential crisis): What should I be doing with my life? Where am I going in life? Who am I really? Is there a God? What does God want of me? We all have individual thresholds for stress, but stress is a part of everyday life for everyone. Response to stress can be operationally defined (Figure 10-1).

PHYSIOLOGICAL AND PSYCHOLOGICAL RESPONSES TO STRESS

The Autonomic Nervous System—Fight-or-Flight Response

The stress response is also referred to as the "fight-or-flight response." The fight or flight response is a survival mechanism by which our body and mind become immediately ready to meet a threat or stress.

When a threat appears imminent the hypothalamus receives information from almost all parts of the brain including the limbic system (considered the emotional brain), particularly the amygdala (the component of the limbic system that contributes to emotional processing). The hypothalamus functions as the command-and-control center when receiving stressful signals. The hypothalamus responds to signals of stress by engaging the autonomic nervous system. The autonomic nervous system is comprised of the sympathetic (fight-or-flight response) and parasympathetic nervous systems (relaxation response).

In times of stress the sympathetic nervous system assumes control (fight-or-flight response) and sends signals to the adrenal glands, releasing epinephrine (or adrenaline). The circulating adrenaline increases heart rate, elevates blood pressure, increases blood flow to the skeletal muscles, and increases muscle tension. Respirations also increase, bringing more oxygen to the lungs, which is then sent to the brain, increasing alertness.

As the initial rush of epinephrine subsides, the hypothalamus stimulates the HPA axis (hypothalamus, pituitary gland, and adrenal glands). If the stress is prolonged, the hypothalamus releases corticotropin-releasing hormone (CRH), which in turn travels to the pituitary gland and triggers the release of adrenocorticotropic hormone (ACTH) (Harvard Mental Health Letter, 2011). ACTH then travels to the adrenal glands, stimulating release of cortisol. Cortisol is the primary stress hormone. Cortisol helps to supply cells with amino acids and fatty acids for energy, as well as diverts glucose from muscles for use by the brain to maintain vigilance.

As the threat passes, the parasympathetic branch of the autonomic nervous system, the part that helps maintain homeostasis and relaxation, takes over. Cortisol levels drop as the body returns to a more normal and healthier state that allows individuals to function as they did before the threat.

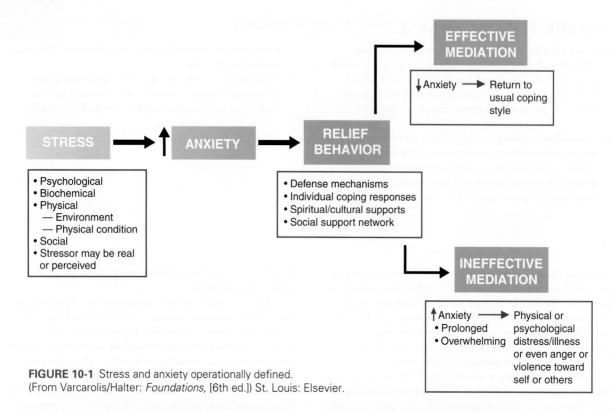

FIGURE 10-1 Stress and anxiety operationally defined. (From Varcarolis/Halter: *Foundations*, [6th ed.]) St. Louis: Elsevier.

However, when stress is prolonged or people are not able to relax, they remain in chronic low levels of stress. The body stays alert for a prolonged period of time. The chemicals produced by the stress response (cortisol, adrenaline, and other catecholamines) can have damaging effects on the body, causing physical diseases including a substantial negative effect on the immune system, leaving individuals vulnerable to autoimmune diseases. According to the Centers for Disease Control and Prevention, up to 90% of diseases are stress-related (The New Wellness, 2009). Stress alone does not cause disease, but it does contribute to it.

The stress response is pictorially presented in Figure 10-2.

STRESS REDUCTION TECHNIQUES

Perhaps some of the most common techniques that people use to combat stress include the following:
- Elicit the relaxation response (e.g., meditation, prayer, mindfulness).
- Perform physical activity, which deepens breathing, relieves muscle tension, and can elevate levels of the body's own endorphins, which induces a sense of well-being (e.g., yoga, tai chi, running, walking briskly).
- Seek social support (e.g., close family ties, acquaintances, spouses, friends). Studies have shown that social interactions provide great buffers for stress and help people cope better with stress.

For more on selected stress reduction techniques, refer to Box 10-1.

STRESS-RELATED DISORDERS

Posttraumatic Stress Disorder

The symptoms of posttraumatic stress disorder are terrifying and often disrupt a person's ability to carry out his or her daily activities. Actually, it is hard for many people to just get through the day (WebMD, 2011). Posttraumatic stress disorder (PTSD) occurs in people who have experienced a highly traumatic event, witnessed a traumatic event (e.g., watching a friend die an atrocious death), or been repeatedly exposed to stories about a traumatic event. Events instigating PTSD often involve threats of death or serious injury to self and others, inducing feelings of intense fear, helplessness, or horror (Black & Andreasen, 2011). PTSD usually occurs after a traumatic event that is outside the range of usual experience. Examples are childhood physical abuse, torture/kidnap, military combat, sexual assault, and natural disasters such as floods, tornados, earthquakes, and tsunamis; human disasters such as plane and train accidents; crime-related events such as bombing, terrorist attacks, assault, mugging, rape, incest, or being taken hostage; or diagnosis of a life-threatening illness. The common element in all these experiences is the individual's extraordinary helplessness or powerlessness in the face of such stressors (Preston et al., 2010). Gilbertson and colleagues (2008) quoted statistics that suggested approximately 94% of rape victims met the full PTSD symptom criteria 1 week following the traumatic event.

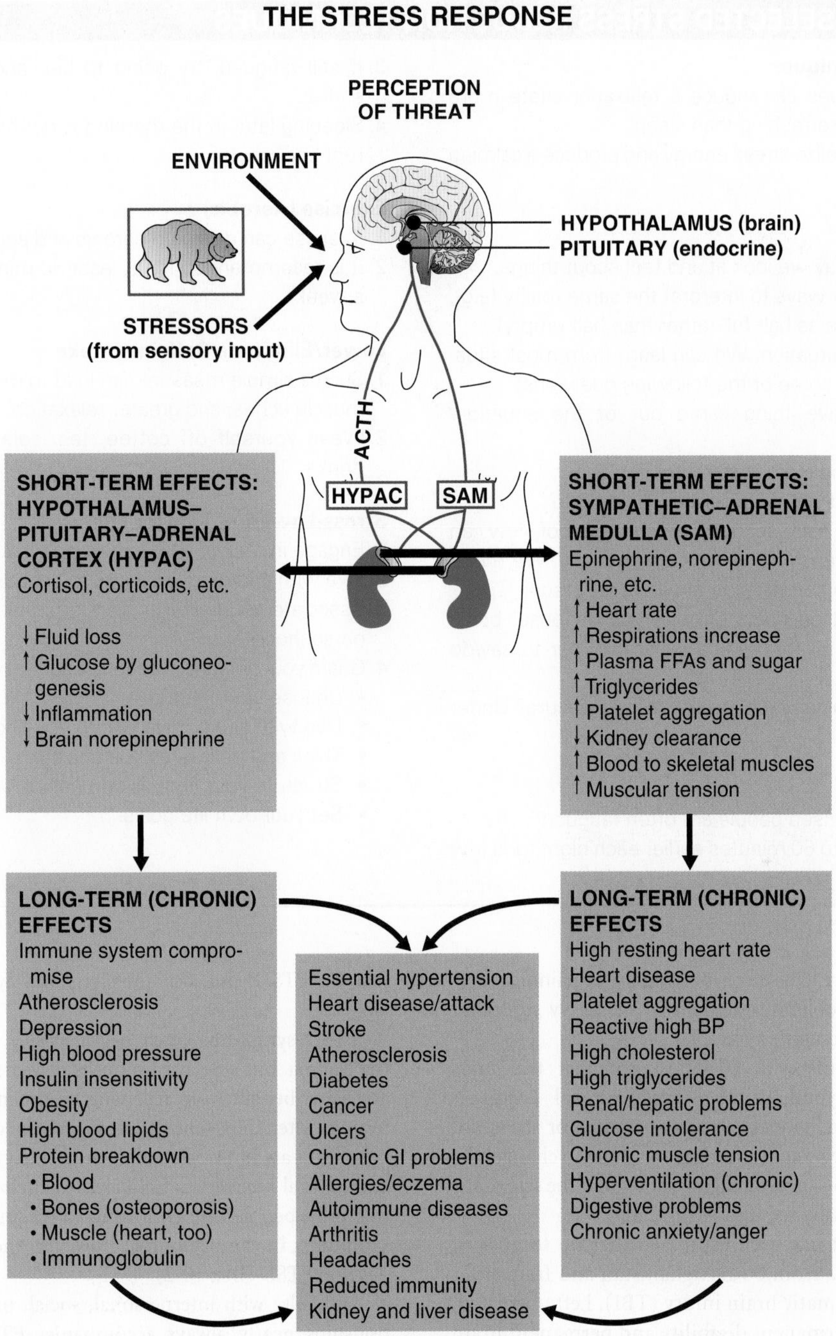

THE STRESS RESPONSE

FIGURE 10-2 The Stress Response. (Brigham, D.D. [1994]. *Imagery for getting well: clinical applications of behavioral medicine*. New York: WW Norton.)

Although the prevalence of PTSD is about 7% in the general population (Black & Andreasen, 2011) the incidence of PTSD in Afghanistan and Iraq war veterans is 19% to 20% (RAND Corp., 2008; Ritchie & Cavazos, 2005). War veterans of Iraq and Afghanistan who have screened positive for PTSD were four times more likely to endorse suicidal ideation then non-PTSD veterans (Jakupcak, 2009) and have dangerous levels of alcohol use (Tull, 2010). Major depression frequently co-occurs with PTSD. The RAND Report (2008) researchers also found that when PTSD and a major depressive disorder (MDD) are

BOX 10-1   SELECTED STRESS REDUCTION TECHNIQUES

Relaxation Techniques
1. These techniques can induce a relaxation state more physiologically refreshing than sleep.
2. They help neutralize stress energy and produce a calming effect.

Reframing
1. Changes the way we look at and feel about things.
2. There are many ways to interpret the same reality (e.g., seeing the glass as half full rather than half empty).
3. Reassess the situation. We can learn from most situations by asking some of the following questions:
   - "What positive thing came out of the situation/experience?"
   - "What did you learn in this situation?"
   - "What would you do differently next time?"
4. Considering life from another person's point of view can help dissipate tension and develop empathy. We might even feel some compassion toward the person.
   - "What might be going on with your (spouse, boss, teacher, friend) that would cause him/her to say/do that?"
   - "Is he/she having problems? Feeling insecure? Under pressure"?

Sleep
1. Chronically stressed people are often fatigued.
2. Go to sleep 30 to 60 minutes earlier each night for a few weeks.

3. If still fatigued, try going to bed another 30 minutes earlier.
4. Sleeping later in the morning is not helpful and can disrupt body rhythms.

Exercise (Aerobic)
1. Exercise can dissipate chronic and acute stress.
2. It is recommended for at least 30 minutes, three times a week.

Lower/Eliminate Caffeine Intake
1. Such a simple measure can lead to more energy, fewer muscle aches, and greater relaxation.
2. Wean yourself off coffee, tea, colas, and chocolate drinks.

Stress-Lowering Tips for Life
1. Engage in meaningful, satisfying work.
2. Live with and/or love whom you choose.
3. Associate yourself with gentle people who affirm your personhood.
4. Guard your personal freedom, especially your freedom to:
   - Choose your friends.
   - Live with and/or love whom you choose.
   - Think and believe as you choose.
   - Structure your time as you desire.
   - Set your own life goals.

untreated or undertreated, there is a long list of painful repercussions: marital problems, unemployment, heavy substance abuse, and suicide, to name a few.

Studies of patients with PTSD suggest that the stress response of the hypothalamus-pituitary-adrenal cortex is abnormal in these individuals. Repeated trauma or stress not only alters the release of neurotransmitters but also changes the anatomy of the brain—neuroimaging shows that the size of the hippocampus is actually reduced (Krill, 2009).

Besides PTSD, it has been estimated that up to 20% of our combat veterans from both Afghanistan and Iraq suffer some degree of traumatic brain injury (TBI). Left untreated, TBI can result in permanent disability and permanent brain damage. A new blood test is under study in an effort to win FDA approval to test for biomarkers in the blood indicative of mild traumatic brain damage. Apparently, unique proteins can be found in the bloodstream from damaged brain cells (Zoroya, 2010). This blood test not only will help medical professionals treat our soldiers more effectively but also could be used in the civilian population to help identify TBI in people involved in contact sports, accidents, falls, shaken baby syndrome, or Alzheimer's disease, for example. Therefore returning veterans of war should be closely assessed not

just for PTSD, but also for signs and symptoms of TBI as well.

PTSD symptoms often begin within a few months after the trauma, but a delay of months or years is not uncommon. Survivors benefit from receiving treatments for PTSD within months after the event. If left for a year or more, and severe symptoms are not treated, they most likely will become chronic and natural recovery is unlikely. It is helpful to keep in mind that most people who go through a traumatic event may have symptoms in the beginning; however, they do not go on to develop PTSD (Box 10-2).

Difficulty with interpersonal, social, or occupational relationships nearly always accompanies PTSD, and trust is a common issue of concern. Child and spousal abuse may be associated with hypervigilance and irritability. Chemical abuse (alcohol or other mind-altering substances) may begin as an attempt to self-medicate to relieve anxiety.

It is important for health care workers to realize that exposure to stimuli reminiscent of those associated with the original trauma may cause an exacerbation of the trauma. For example, one nurse therapist observed that the attack on the World Trade Center on September 11, 2001, caused an exacerbation of PTSD symptoms in veterans of World War II (Kaiman, 2003).

BOX 10-2   POTENTIAL SYMPTOMS OF PTSD

Adaptations of the typical symptoms experienced in a person with PTSD according to the *ICD-10* (WHO, 1992) and Preston and colleagues (2010) are as follows:
- Episodes of repeated reliving of the event
  - Intrusive memories of the traumatic event are experienced with the same fear and horror that occurred with the actual event, as if the person is reliving the actual event. One type of reliving of the event is in the form of dissociated and unbidden memories and feelings that are called **flashbacks**. Flashbacks are dissociative reactions in which the individual feels or acts as if the traumatic event were recurring. Often there is a trigger—such as a car backfiring, which could be a trigger for a war veteran, or hearing or reading about a rape, which could be a trigger for a person re-experiencing the horror and helplessness associated with a brutal sexual assault.
  - Dreams/nightmares that re-enact the horror of the event are also common in people with PTSD.
- Avoidance of people or situations that could trigger memories of the event.
- Persistent emotional blunting, unresponsiveness to surroundings. Numbing of feelings, such as feeling detached or estranged from others or feeling empty inside. Activities that used to be pleasurable no longer hold any value.
- Increased autonomic hyperarousal with hypervigilance. Increased hypervigilance may take the form of becoming exceedingly alert and constantly on the lookout for danger, suddenly becoming angry or irritable, having trouble sleeping or concentrating, or having an exaggerated startle response. Often the person may exhibit reckless or self-destructive behavior.
- Transient psychotic symptoms such as realization, delusions, and hallucinations.
- Associated features may include major depression. Panic attacks, substance abuse, and suicidal ideation are often present.

From Preston, J.D., O'Neal, J.H., & Talaga, M.C. (2010). *Handbook of clinical psychopharmacology for therapists* (6th ed., p. 196, Fig. 11-1) Oakland, CA: New Harbinger Publications.

GOALS OF TREATMENT

The following are the optimal outcomes for the PTSD patient:
- Patient and others (e.g., family, friends) will remain safe.
- Patient will receive treatment for co-occurring conditions, which is always part of active treatment (e.g., alcohol/drug addiction, depression, anxiety disorders, specifically panic attacks).
- Patient will attend support group meetings.
- Patient will expand social support network.
- Patient will exhibit an increase in restful sleep periods.
- Patient will have fewer nightmares and flashbacks.
- Patient will express decreased irritability.
- Patient will be able to demonstrate effective anxiety reduction techniques (cognitive or behavioral).

(Refer to Chapters 20 and 22 for more information about PTSD.)

PSYCHOTHERAPEUTIC TREATMENT STRATEGIES

Cognitive behavioral therapy (CBT) typically is included in the treatment regimen of PTSD patients (refer to Chapter 3). Both CBT and selective serotonin reuptake inhibitors (SSRIs) have become first-line treatment options for many people suffering from PTSD (Pollack et al., 2010). Group therapy with others who have experienced similar experiences (e.g., victims of sexual violence or child abuse, war veterans) has proven beneficial for many. Family therapy is an important therapeutic modality as well. As mentioned previously, early treatment of any comorbid condition needs to be addressed concurrently. A multimodal approach is always encouraged. Refer to Table 10-1 for a review of therapeutic approaches.

PSYCHOPHARMACOLOGY

The treatment of choice for individuals with posttraumatic stress disorder is psychotherapy, and the most successful psychotherapy is exposure-based cognitive therapy. However, when target symptoms arise and become serious, medications can be used and may serve to help the patient achieve emotional control (Preston et al., 2010). Target symptoms are included in Table 10-2.

Acute Stress Disorder

Acute stress disorder can occur after the same kind of triggers that exist in posttraumatic stress disorder, which include experiencing a violent event or repeatedly witnessing a violent or traumatic event (e.g., first responders at the scene of a mass casualty incident, police officers repeatedly exposed to details of child abuse). Possible precipitating traumatic events are the same as those listed under Posttraumatic Stress Disorder. However, in an acute stress disorder, the resolution of the symptoms resolves within 1 month.

CRITICAL INCIDENT DEBRIEFING

Critical incident stress debriefing may be valuable for ameliorating symptoms in people with an acute stress response. Benzodiazepines may be used to treat daytime anxiety, and

EXAMINING THE EVIDENCE

PTSD—A Holistic View

I just completed a clinical rotation at the Veterans Administration and it was so sad to see young veterans from Iraq and Afghanistan suffering with PTSD. Are there any new approaches to treatment?

This is a very timely and critical quetion. Since 2001 more than 1.5 million U.S. troops have been deployed to Iraq or Afghanistan. A recent study indicated that 10% to 20% of military personnel met the criteria for PTSD (Tuerk et al., 2009). In addition, those diagnosed with PTSD are more likely to have comorbid conditions, including osteoarthritis, diabetes, heart disease, depression, obesity, and elevated lipid levels (Weiss & Skelton, 2011); suffer from chronic pain; and self-medicate with alcohol and nonprescribed medications (Hoge, 2011). Symptoms and complications of PTSD are not time limited, but often present many decades after the traumatic experience (Durai & Chopra, 2011).

As many veterans return home from a difficult tour in a war zone, there is great concern that appropriate services be provided to facilitate their readjustment and address the physical and emotional toll. Recent literature documents that from 1997 to 2005 there was a steady and constant growth in the number of veterans using mental health services (Harpaz-Rotem & Rosenheck, 2011). The U.S. Department of Defense and Veterans' Affairs has implemented numerous programs in the area of screening, education, stigma reduction, and clinical care. However, veterans with PTSD are reluctant to seek care, with only 50% of those diagnosed utilizing mental health services. New research among veterans found negative perceptions of mental health care, which included distrust of mental health professionals and consideration of treatment as "unhealthy" or a "last resort." This may be due to the belief that the roles of military personnel are similar to those of police and other first responders—they are trained to deal with multiple traumatic events. They do not normally perceive themselves as victims, nor do they see their reactions as pathological. The paradox of war-related PTSD is that reactions labeled "symptoms" upon return home can be highly effective in combat—hypervigilance and the ability to deny emotions (Hoge, 2011).

Presently, according to the Institute of Medicine (IOM), the most effective treatment for PTSD is cognitive behavioral therapy (CBT) that focuses on awareness of current thoughts/feelings; utilization of psychoeducation and learning skills to challenge thoughts; insight about common changes in beliefs following trauma and prolonged exposure (PE), which stresses talking through the trauma to obtain control of thoughts and feelings; and adoption of real-world practices to reduce distress in situations that have been previously avoided. Medications, such as selective serotonin reuptake inhibitors (SSRIs), are often used, but not considered a first-line intervention (Forbes et al., 2010). The IOM is actively involved in the study of "innovative" treatments for PTSD such as acupuncture, yoga, and the therapeutic use of animals (IOM, 2011). Other successful strategies are eye movement desensitization reprocessing (EMDR)—focusing on mental images and muscular tension and adopting positive thoughts/images while performing particular eye movements and using creative narration—imagining different scenarios to the reality of the actual traumatic event (Lahad et al., 2010).

Significant improvement in the care of war veterans requires a holistic approach with attention to both mental and physical concerns; collaboration with primary care and mental health practitioners is essential concomitant with greater understanding from therapists regarding specifics of the military role and sensitivity and knowledge regarding grief and survivor's guilt. In addition, there is a need for reinforcement of social connections through peer programs as well as support services for family members of those suffering from PTSD (Hoge, 2011).

Durai, B., & Chopra, M. (2011). Exposure to trauma and PTSD in older veterans attending primary care: comorbid conditions and self-rated health status. *Journal of the American Geriatrics Society*, *59*(6), 1087–1092.

Forbes, D., Creamer, M., et al. (2010). A guide to guidelines for treatment of PTSD and related conditions. *Journal of Traumatic Stress*, *23*(5), 537–552.

Harpaz-Rotem, I., & Rosenheck, R. (2011). Serving those who served: retention of newly returning veterans from Iraq and Afghanistan in mental health treatment. *Psychiatric Services*, *62*(1), 22–27.

Hoge, C. (2011). Interventions for war-related PTSD: meeting veterans where they are. *Journal of the American Medical Association*, *306*(5), 549–551.

Institute of Medicine. (2011). Assessment of ongoing efforts in treatment of PTSD. *IOM Newsletter*. July 11, 2011.

Lahad, M., et al. (2010). Preliminary study of a new integrative approach in treating PTSD. *Arts in Psychotherapy*, *37*, 391–399.

Tuerk, P., Anouk, L., et al. (2009). Diagnosis and treatment of PTSD-related compulsive checking behaviors in veterans of the Iraq war: the influence of military context on the expression of PTSD symptoms. *American Journal of Psychiatry*, *166*, 762–767.

Weiss, T., & Skelton, K. (2011). PTSD is a risk factor for metabolic syndrome in an impoverished urban population. *General Hospital Psychiatry*, *33*, 135–142.

Contributed by Lois Angelo.

TABLE 10-1 THERAPEUTIC APPROACH

DISORDER	THERAPEUTIC MODALITY	COMMENTS
Posttraumatic stress disorder	Psychotherapy (e.g., exposure-based cognitive behavioral therapy) Family therapy Vocational rehabilitation Group therapy with others who have shared similar experiences (e.g., veterans, partner abuse, sexual violence) Relaxation techniques	More than one treatment modality should be used: a. Establish support b. Focus on abreaction, survivor guilt or shame, anger, and helplessness

TABLE 10-2 PHARMACOLOGY FOR TARGET SYMPTOMS FOR PTSD PATIENTS

TARGET SYMPTOMS	POTENTIAL TREATMENT
Depression	1. Antidepressants
Intrusive experiences (flashbacks, avoidance, and numbing)	2. SSRI antidepressants, second-generation antipsychotics
Treatment-resistant PTSD	Second-generation antipsychotics, anticonvulsants
Panic attacks	Antidepressants, monoamine oxidase inhibitors, high-potency benzodiazepines
Hyperarousal	Antidepressants, benzodiazepines, anticonvulsants
Nightmares	Minipress (Prazosin)

From Preston, J.D., O'Neal, J.H., & Talaga, M.C. (2010). *Handbook of clinical psychopharmacology for therapists* (6th ed., p. 139, Fig. 11-B). Oakland, CA: New Harbinger Publications.

sedative-hypnotics may be used for sleep. However, these medications are prescribed short term and are used in conjunction with crisis intervention and other psychological treatments (Preston et al., 2010). Refer to Chapter 24 for more information on critical incident debriefing.

SELF-CARE FOR NURSES

Nurses should be alert to secondary traumatic stress, also known as compassion fatigue. These terms are used interchangeably and describe the emotional effect that nurses and other health care workers may experience by being indirectly traumatized when helping or trying to help a person who has experienced primary traumatic stress (Beck, 2011; Yoder, 2010). Beck (2011) summarizes secondary traumatic stress/compassion fatigue as:

- Increased negative arousal
- Intrusive thoughts/images of another's critical experience
- Difficulty separating work from personal life
- Lowered frustration tolerance
- Increased outbursts of anger or rage
- Dread of working with certain individuals
- Depression
- Ineffective and/or destructive self-soothing behaviors
- Hypervigilance
- Decreased feelings of work competence
- Diminished sense of purpose/enjoyment with career
- Lowered self-esteem in nonprofessional situations
- Loss of hope

Nurses who work with patients with posttraumatic stress disorder and hear their stories as well as nurses who are constantly exposed to patients who describe traumatic events in their lives may be vulnerable to compassion fatigue/secondary traumatic stress. Yoder (2010) sites specific patient care situations in which compassion fatigue is often triggered:

- When nurses who believe that their actions would "not make a difference" or "never seem to be enough" experience problems with the system (high patient census, heavy patient assignments, overtime, and extra weekends)
- When nurses have personal issues, such as inexperience or inadequate energy
- When nurses identified with the patient
- When nurses overlooked serious patient symptoms

Examples of nurses who are at high risk for compassion fatigue/secondary trauma stress are those who work in hospice care, pediatrics, emergency departments (EDs), oncology, and forensic nursing, and certainly psychiatric nurses who work closely with individual patients. Also, the emotional character of the nurse can potentiate compassion fatigue; for example, if the nurse has unrealistic self-expectations, is overinvolved with the patient, is inexperienced, or is having a personal crisis (Beck, 2011; Yoder, 2010). Studies show that psychiatrists, in particular, are prone to high levels of stress as evidenced by high rates of suicide, severe depression, and secondary general compassion fatigue (Yoder, 2010). However, there have been no studies as yet that include the incidence of compassion fatigue/secondary traumatic stress in psychiatric mental health nurses.

- Some stress is useful in our lives; *eustress* is stress that makes us strive to reach our goals, repair important relationships, improve our work, and stimulate creative problem-solving processes and improve critical thinking.
- Stress is common in our lives, but when stress is prolonged and increased it may be experienced more as *distress*, which is a negative experience. When stress becomes chronic it can cause physiological harm and emotional difficulties.
- When we are confronted with a serious stressor, our autonomic nervous system reacts with the fight-or-flight response. This response involves a complex network of nerve pathways, brain structures, and glands to help our bodies and mind deal with the stressor.
- The second part of the fight-or-flight response is caused by the hypothalamus-pituitary-adrenal (HPA) cortex, which activates the response.
- When the stress response is prolonged and becomes chronic, it can have damaging effects on the body by lowering the resistance of the immune system and contributing to both physical illness and mental trauma (e.g., depression, hopelessness, helplessness, increased sustained anxiety).
- Some suggestions for stress reduction are given in Box 10-1.

- Posttraumatic stress disorder (PTSD) usually occurs after a severe traumatic event (e.g., childhood abuse, torture/kidnap, military combat, sexual assault, incest, natural disasters, life-threatening illness). It is estimated that up to 20% of our combat veterans returning from Afghanistan and Iraq have PTSD.
- If PTSD is not treated, serious consequences often result, including severe depression, alcohol/substance abuse, suicide, inability to trust, and social and occupational disruptions, as well as a host of mentally damaging symptoms and/or disorders.
- The major symptoms of PTSD and acute stress disorder have been addressed in this chapter.
- Pharmacological and therapeutic interventions that have proven successful with PTSD have been identified.
- Nurses are cautioned to be alert for secondary traumatic stress, also known as compassion fatigue, when trying to help a patient who has experienced a primary traumatic event. Symptoms a health care worker might experience are included in this chapter. Health care workers who might be vulnerable to compassion fatigue have been identified; however, this is not an exclusive list.

■ **APPLYING CRITICAL JUDGMENT**

1. A friend of yours, Juan, arrives to class breathing hard and looking pale and shaken. He tells you that he just missed getting run over by a car and that his heart keeps pounding.
   A. Once Juan becomes calm, how would you explain to him about his body's physiological response to the fight-or-flight response?
2. Another friend of yours, Teresa, tells you that after failing the midterm exam she just cannot stop thinking about her failure. She feels preoccupied and stressed all the time.
   A. If Teresa is experiencing chronic stress, describe what is happening physiologically.
   B. If this response continues for a long time, what might be some of the sequelae (results)?
   C. Depending on the situation, what are some suggestions you could offer both Juan and Teresa that might help reduce stress?

3. After witnessing a brutal murder of four bank guards 3 months ago, Laura continues to have nightmares and jumps at any loud noise. At the health clinic where you work, she tells you that she does not sleep well at night and cannot stop thinking about the traumatic event.
   A. If Laura is diagnosed with PTSD, identify and define other signs and symptoms you might notice.
   B. Besides her symptoms, what would you include in your assessment in order to plan effective interventions for Laura?
   C. If Laura tells you she has flashbacks and cannot function at school and work, what medication might alleviate her symptoms?
   D. List three interventions that have been found to help patients with PTSD, naming the most important intervention first.

CHAPTER REVIEW QUESTIONS

Choose the most appropriate answer(s).

1. Your patient, a student highly stressed from school, has been attending yoga sessions for relaxation. Which response would indicate that this physical activity has been successful?
   1. Decreased energy
   2. Decreased blood pressure
   3. Increased heart rate
   4. Increased respiratory rate

2. A young woman, recently divorced, is learning to cope with some additional stressors. The most appropriate interventions are to: (select all that apply)
   1. alter her general lifestyle by moving to another area.
   2. arrange to increase her job hours, to avoid home life.
   3. control stress by increased physical activity.
   4. change her reactions to stress with cognitive behavioral therapy.

3. The patient you are assigned unexpectedly has a respiratory arrest. During this emergency situation, your body under stress will secrete a large amount of:
   1. carbon dioxide.
   2. growth hormone.
   3. epinephrine.
   4. aldosterone.

4. You are helping your elderly patient to develop stress reduction techniques. Which interventions are most appropriate? (select all that apply)
   1. Limit visits to friends and family.
   2. Schedule a daily walk.
   3. Run 4-5 miles per day.
   4. Continue the use of daily prayer.

5. Two days ago, a client was admitted to the inpatient psychiatric unit with a diagnosis of PTSD and a history of violence. Currently, he continues to have sleep problems, trouble with concentration, and has been feeling increased anger toward another patient who reminds him of a former colleague. Select the priority nursing diagnosis.
   1. Risk for violence
   2. Ineffective individual coping
   3. Sleep deprivation
   4. Decisional conflict

REFERENCES

American Psychological Association (2010). *Stress in America findings: mind/body/health: for a healthy mind and body, talk to a psychologist.* Retrieved November 9, 2010, from www.apa.org/news/press/releases/stress/indexaspx.

Beck, C. T. (2011). Secondary traumatic stress in nurses: a systemic review. *Archives of Psychiatric Nursing, 25*(1), 1–10.

Black, D. W., & Andreasen, N. A. (2011). *Introductory textbook of psychology* (5th ed.). Washington, DC: American Psychiatric Publishing.

Gilbertson, M. W., Orr, S. P., Rauch, S. L., & Pigman, R. K. (2008). Trauma and posttraumatic stress disorder. In T. A. Stern, J. F. Rosenbaum, M. Fava, J. Biedermann, & S. L. Rauch (Eds.), *Massachusetts General Hospital, comprehensive clinical psychology* (pp. 465–480). Philadelphia: Mosby/Elsevier.

Harvard Health Publications. (2011). *Understanding the stress response.* Retrieved July 27, 2011, from www.health.harvard.edu/newsletters/Harvard_Mental_Health.

Jakupcak, M. (2009). Posttraumatic stress disorder as a risk factor for suicidal ideation in Iraq and Afghanistan war veterans. *Journal of Traumatic Stress, 22*(4), 303–306.

Kaiman, C. (2003). PTSD in the World War II combat veterans. *American Journal of Nursing, 103*(11), 32–40.

Krill, W. E. (2009). *The brain, brain chemistry, and PTSD.* Retrieved January 3, 2011, from http://krillco.hubpages.com/hub/The-Brain-Brain-Chemistry-And-PTSD-.

Preston, J. D., O'Neal, J. H., & Talaga, M. C. (2010). *Handbook of clinical psychopharmacology for therapists* (6th ed.). Oakland, CA: New Harbinger Publications.

RAND Corporation. (2008). *One in five Iraq and Afghanistan veterans suffer from PTSD or major depression.* Retrieved February 14, 2011, from rand.org/news/press/2008/04/17. html.

Ritchie, E. C., & Cavazos (2005). Meeting the mental health needs of veterans of wars in Iraq and Afghanistan: an expert interview with Colonel Elspeth Cameron Ritchie, MD, MPH. *Medscape Psychiatry & Mental Health, 10*(2).

The New Wellness. (2009). *90% of disease is caused by the well-known problem.* Retrieved January 3, 2012, from www.thenewwellness.com/90-of disease is caused by stress.

Tull, M. (2010). *PTSD in Iraq war veterans.* Retrieved from http://ptsd.about.com/od/prevalence/a/IraqWarPTSD.htm.

WebMD. (2011). *Anxiety & panic disorders health center: posttraumatic stress disorder—symptoms.* Retrieved January 10, 2012, from www.webmd.com./Anxiety panic/tc/post-traumatic-stress-disorder-symptoms.

World Health Organization (1992). *ICD-10 classification of mental and behavioral disorders.* Geneva, Switzerland, Author Retrieved February 2, 2012, from www.mentalhealth.com/ICD/P 22-an.html.

Yoder, E. A. (2010). Compassion fatigue in nurses. *Applied Nursing Research, 23,* 191–197. Retrieved February 15, 2011, from www. Medscape.com/view article/732211.

Zoroya, G. (2010). *Army finds simple blood test to identify mild brain trauma.* Retrieved February 15, 2011, from www.USAtoday.com/your life/health/medical/2011-11-15.

CHAPTER

11

Anxiety, Anxiety Disorders, and Obsessive-Compulsive Disorders

Elizabeth M. Varcarolis

evolve WEBSITE

http://evolve.elsevier.com/Varcarolis/essentials

KEY TERMS AND CONCEPTS

acting-out behaviors, p. 170
acute anxiety, p. 165
agoraphobia, p. 175
altruism, p. 168
anxiety, p. 165
anxiolytic drugs, p. 185
burnout, p. 179
chronic anxiety, p. 173
compassion fatigue/secondary
    traumatic stress, p. 179
compulsions, p. 177
denial, p. 171
devaluation, p. 171
displacement, p. 170
dissociation, p. 170
fear, p. 165
generalized anxiety
    disorder (GAD), p. 176
hoarding, p. 177
idealization, p. 171
mild anxiety, p. 165
moderate anxiety, p. 166

normal anxiety, p. 165
obsessions, p. 177
obsessive-compulsive
    disorder (OCD), p. 177
panic attack, p. 174
panic disorders (PDs), p. 174
panic level of anxiety, p. 167
passive aggression, p. 170
phobia, p. 175
projection, p. 171
rationalization, p. 170
reaction formation, p. 170
repression, p. 170
severe anxiety, p. 167
social phobia, p. 175
somatization, p. 170
specific phobias, p. 175
splitting, p. 171
sublimation, p. 169
suppression, p. 169
undoing, p. 170

SELECTED CONCEPT: **Burnout**

Burnout can occur in any work-related situation. Burnout occurs among health care professionals when feelings of disengagement, blunted emotions, frustration, depression, and negative feelings affect motivation and drive, and results in demoralization. Burnout produces a sense of helplessness and hopelessness.

When working long periods of time in demanding situations, nurses and other healthcare professionals may no longer be able to function effectively and feel constantly overwhelmed, depressed and ineffectual.

(Reese, 2011)

OBJECTIVES

1. Differentiate among normal anxiety, acute anxiety, and chronic anxiety.
2. Contrast and compare the four levels of anxiety in relation to perceptual field, ability to learn, and physical and other defining behavioral characteristics.
3. Summarize five properties of the defense mechanisms.
4. Give a definition for at least six defense mechanisms.
5. Rank the defense mechanisms from harmless to highly detrimental.
6. Describe clinical manifestations of each anxiety disorder.
7. Formulate four NANDA International nursing diagnoses that might be appropriate in the care of an individual with an anxiety disorder.
8. Name three defense mechanisms commonly used in excess by patients with anxiety disorders.
9. Propose realistic outcome criteria for patients with (a) generalized anxiety disorder, (b) panic disorder, and (c) obsessive-compulsive disorder.
10. Discuss three classes of medications that have demonstrated *evidence-based effectiveness* in treating anxiety disorders.
11. Identify the patient's experience and needs when planning *patient-centered care* for a person with obsessive-compulsive disorder.
12. Compare and contrast the differences between hoarding behaviors with obsessive-compulsive disorder (OCD) and hoarding behaviors without OCD.

An understanding of anxiety and anxiety defense mechanisms is basic to the practice of psychiatric nursing. One of the greatest contributions to psychiatric nursing by Hildegard Peplau (1909 to 1999) was the operational definition of the four levels of anxiety and the recommendation of appropriate interventions to treat each level of anxiety. Anxiety is a universal human experience to which no one is a stranger. It is the most basic of emotions. Dysfunctional behavior is often a defense against anxiety. When behavior is recognized as dysfunctional, interventions to reduce anxiety can be initiated by the nurse. As anxiety decreases, dysfunctional behavior will frequently decrease.

ANXIETY

Anxiety and fear are indistinguishable except for the cause. Anxiety can be defined as a feeling of apprehension, uneasiness, uncertainty, or dread resulting from a real or perceived threat whose actual source is unknown or unrecognized. Fear is a reaction to a specific danger. The body reacts in similar ways physiologically and emotionally to both anxiety and fear.

An important distinction between anxiety and fear is that anxiety affects us at a deeper level than does fear. Anxiety invades the central core of the personality. It erodes the individual feelings of self-esteem and personal worth that contribute to a sense of being fully human.

Normal anxiety is a healthy life force that is necessary for survival. It provides the energy needed to carry out the tasks involved in living and striving toward goals. Anxiety motivates people to make and survive change. It prompts constructive behaviors, such as studying for an examination, being on time for a job interview, preparing for a presentation, and working toward a promotion.

Acute anxiety is also referred to as state anxiety. Acute anxiety is precipitated by an imminent loss or change that threatens an individual's sense of security. Acute anxiety is a normal and expected response to stress. For example, many entertainers experience acute anxiety before live concerts or theater performances. Students may experience acute anxiety before an examination. Patients preparing for surgery often experience acute anxiety. The death of a loved one can stimulate acute anxiety when there is great disruption in the life of the bereaved person. In general, crisis involves the experience of acute anxiety.

Pathological anxiety differs from normal anxiety in terms of duration, intensity, and disturbance in a person's ability to function (e.g., the person exhibits dysfunctional behaviors or extreme withdrawal). Pathological anxiety is usually more chronic in nature and is anxiety that a person has experienced for a long time. An understanding of the types, levels, and defensive patterns used in response to anxiety is basic to psychiatric nursing care. This understanding is essential for effectively assessing and planning interventions to help both patients and nurses lower their levels of anxiety. With practice, one becomes more skilled at identifying levels of anxiety, understanding the defenses used to alleviate anxiety, and evaluating the possible stressors contributing to increases in a person's level of anxiety.

LEVELS OF ANXIETY

Levels of anxiety range from mild, to moderate, to severe, to panic. Peplau's classic delineation of these four levels of anxiety (1968) is based on the work by Harry Stack Sullivan in 1953 (American psychiatrist and theorist, 1892 to 1949). Assessment of a patient's level of anxiety is basic to therapeutic intervention in any setting—psychiatric, hospital, general hospital, or community. Identification of a specific level of anxiety can be used as a guideline in selecting interventions. Although four levels of anxiety from mild to panic have been defined, the boundaries between these levels are not distinct, and the behaviors and characteristics shown by individuals experiencing anxiety can and often do overlap these categories. Use Table 11-1 as a guide for making observations.

Mild Anxiety

Mild anxiety occurs in the normal experience of everyday living. A person's ability to perceive reality is brought into sharp focus. A person sees, hears, and grasps more information, and

TABLE 11-1   ANXIETY LEVELS AND THEIR CHARACTERISTICS

MILD	MODERATE	SEVERE	PANIC
Perceptual Field			
May have heightened perceptual field	Has narrow perceptual field; grasps less of what is occurring	Has greatly reduced perceptual field	Unable to focus on the environment
Is alert and can see, hear, and grasp what is happening in the environment	Can attend to more *if pointed out by another* (selective inattention)	Focuses on details or one specific detail	Experiences the utmost state of terror and emotional paralysis; feels he or she "ceases to exist"
Can identify issues that are disturbing and are producing anxiety		Attention scattered	In panic, may have hallucinations or delusions that take the place of reality
		Completely absorbed with self	
		May not be able to attend to events in environment *even when pointed out by others*	
		In severe to panic levels of anxiety, the environment is blocked out. It is as if these events are not occurring.	
Ability to Learn			
Able to work effectively toward a goal and examine alternatives	Able to solve problems but not at optimal ability	Unable to see connections between events or details	May be mute or have extreme psychomotor agitation leading to exhaustion
	Benefits from guidance of others	Has distorted perceptions	Shows disorganized or irrational reasoning
Mild and moderate levels of anxiety can alert the person that something is wrong and can stimulate appropriate action.		*Severe and panic levels prevent problem solving and discovery of effective solutions. Unproductive relief behaviors are implemented, thus perpetuating a vicious cycle.*	
Physical or Other Characteristics			
Slight discomfort	Voice tremors	Feelings of dread	Experience of terror
Attention-seeking behaviors	Change in voice pitch	Ineffective functioning	Immobility or severe hyperactivity or flight
Restlessness	Difficulty concentrating	Confusion	Dilated pupils
Irritability or impatience	Shakiness	Purposeless activity	Unintelligible communication or inability to speak
Mild tension-relieving behavior: foot or finger tapping, lip chewing, fidgeting	Repetitive questioning	Sense of impending doom	Severe shakiness
	Somatic complaints, (e.g., urinary frequency and urgency, headache, backache, insomnia)	More intense somatic complaints (e.g., dizziness, nausea, headache, sleeplessness)	Sleeplessness
	Increased respiration rate	Hyperventilation	Severe withdrawal
	Increased pulse rate	Tachycardia	Hallucinations or delusions; likely out of touch with reality
	Increased muscle tension	Withdrawal	
	More extreme tension-relieving behavior; pacing, banging hands on table	Loud and rapid speech	
		Threats and demands	

problem solving becomes more effective. A person may display physical symptoms such as slight discomfort, restlessness, irritability, or mild tension-relieving behaviors (e.g., nail biting, foot or finger tapping, fidgeting).

Moderate Anxiety

As anxiety escalates, the patient's perceptual field narrows and some details are excluded from observation. An individual experiencing moderate anxiety sees, hears, and grasps less information than someone who is not in that state. Individuals may demonstrate **selective inattention,** in which only certain things in the environment are seen or heard. The ability to think clearly is hampered, but learning and problem solving can still take place, although not at an optimal level. At the moderate level of anxiety, the person's ability to solve problems is enhanced greatly by the supportive presence of another person. Physical symptoms include tension, pounding heart, increased pulse and respiration rates, perspiration, and mild somatic symptoms (e.g., gastric discomfort, headache, urinary urgency). Voice tremors and shaking may be noticed. Mild or moderate anxiety levels can be constructive, because anxiety can be viewed as a signal that something in the person's life needs attention.

Severe Anxiety

The perceptual field of a person experiencing severe anxiety is greatly reduced. A person with severe anxiety may focus on one particular detail or many scattered details. The person will have difficulty noticing events occurring in the environment, even when they are pointed out by another. Learning and problem solving are not possible at this level, and the person may be dazed and confused. Behavior is automatic and aimed at reducing or relieving anxiety. Often the individual complains of increased severity of somatic symptoms (e.g., headache, nausea, dizziness, insomnia), trembling, and pounding heart. The most classic experiences are hyperventilation and a sense of impending doom or dread.

Panic Level of Anxiety

The panic level of anxiety is the most extreme form and results in markedly disturbed behavior. An individual is not able to process events in the environment and may lose touch with reality. The resulting behavior may be confusion, shouting, screaming, or withdrawal. Hallucinations, or false sensory perceptions such as seeing people or objects that are not present, may be experienced by people at panic levels of anxiety. Physical behavior may be erratic, uncoordinated, and impulsive. Automatic behaviors are used to reduce and relieve anxiety, although such efforts may be ineffective. Acute panic may lead to exhaustion. Review Table 11-1 to identify the levels of anxiety and review how the level affects (1) perceptual field, (2) ability to learn, and (3) physical manifestations and other defining characteristics.

INTERVENTIONS

Mild to Moderate Levels of Anxiety

A patient experiencing a mild to moderate level of anxiety is still able to solve problems; however, the ability to concentrate decreases as anxiety increases. The nurse can help the patient focus and solve problems with the use of specific communication techniques, such as employing open-ended questions, giving broad openings, and exploring and seeking clarification. These techniques can be useful to a patient experiencing mild to moderate anxiety. Restricting topics of communication and introducing irrelevant topics can increase a person's anxiety and are tactics that usually make the *nurse*, not the patient, feel better.

Reducing the patient's level of anxiety and preventing escalation of anxiety can be accomplished by being calm, recognizing the anxious patient's distress, and being willing to listen. Evaluation of effective past coping mechanisms is useful. Often the nurse can help the patient consider alternatives to problem situations and offer activities that may temporarily relieve feelings of inner tension. Table 11-2 identifies counseling interventions useful in assisting people experiencing mild to moderate levels of anxiety.

Severe to Panic Levels of Anxiety

A patient experiencing a severe to panic level of anxiety is unable to solve problems and may have a poor grasp of events occurring in the environment. Unproductive relief behaviors may predominate and the person may not be in control of his or her actions. Extreme regression and aimless behaviors are behavioral manifestations of a person's intense psychic pain. The nurse must be concerned with the patient's safety and, at times, with the safety of others. Physical needs (e.g., for fluids and rest) must be met to prevent exhaustion.

Anxiety reduction measures may take the form of moving the person to a quiet environment in which there is minimal stimulation and providing gross motor activities to drain some of the tension. The use of medications may have to be considered, but medications and restraints should be used only after other more personal and less restrictive interventions have failed to decrease anxiety to safer levels. Although communication may be scattered and disjointed, themes can often be heard that the nurse must address. The feeling that one is understood can decrease the sense of isolation and reduce anxiety.

Because individuals experiencing severe to panic levels of anxiety are unable to solve problems, techniques suggested for communicating with people with mild to moderate levels of anxiety are not always effective. Patients experiencing severe to panic anxiety levels are out of control, so they need to know that they are safe from their own impulses. **Firm, short, and simple statements are useful.**

Reinforcing commonalities in the environment and recognition of reality when there are distortions can also be useful interventions for severely anxious persons. Table 11-3 suggests some basic nursing interventions for patients with severe to panic levels of anxiety.

DEFENSE MECHANISMS

Responses to stress and anxiety are affected by factors such as age, gender, culture, life experiences, and lifestyle. Vaillant and Vaillant (2004) identified three classes of coping mechanisms that people use to overcome stressful and anxiety-provoking situations that still remain useful today. It is important to note that social support is one mediating factor that has been heavily researched and has significant implications for nurses and other health care professionals. The fact that strong social supports from significant others can enhance mental and physical health and act as a significant buffer against distress has been well documented in the literature. Numerous studies have found a strong correlation between lower mortality rates and intact support systems.

Defense mechanisms protect people from painful awareness of feelings and memories that can provoke overwhelming anxiety. Adaptive use of defense mechanisms helps people lower anxiety to achieve goals in acceptable ways.

Defense mechanisms operate all the time. However, when an individual is faced with a situation that triggers high levels of anxiety, that person may become more rigid in the use of defense mechanisms and may revert to using less mature defenses. The degree of distortion of reality and disruption in

TABLE 11-2 INTERVENTIONS FOR MILD TO MODERATE LEVELS OF ANXIETY*

NURSING DIAGNOSIS: *Anxiety* (moderate) related to situational event or psychological stress, as evidenced by increase in vital signs, moderate discomfort, narrowing of perceptual field, and selective inattention

INTERVENTION	RATIONALE
1. Help the patient identify anxiety. "Are you comfortable right now?"	1. It is important to validate observations with the patient, name the anxiety, and start to work with the patient to lower anxiety.
2. Anticipate anxiety-provoking situations.	2. Escalation of anxiety to a more disorganizing level is prevented.
3. Use nonverbal language to demonstrate interest (e.g., lean forward, maintain eye contact, nod your head).	3. Verbal and nonverbal messages should be consistent. The presence of an interested person provides a stabilizing focus.
4. Encourage the patient to talk about his or her feelings and concerns.	4. When concerns are stated aloud, problems can be discussed and feelings of isolation decreased.
5. Avoid closing off avenues of communication that are important for the patient. Focus on the patient's concerns.	5. When staff anxiety increases, changing the topic or offering advice is common but leaves the person isolated.
6. Ask questions to clarify what is being said. "I'm not sure what you mean. Give me an example."	6. Increased anxiety results in scattering of thoughts. Clarifying helps the patient identify thoughts and feelings.
7. Help the patient identify thoughts or feelings before the onset of anxiety. "What were you thinking right before you started to feel anxious?"	7. The patient is assisted in identifying thoughts and feelings, and problem solving is facilitated.
8. Encourage problem solving with the patient.*	8. Encouraging patients to explore alternatives increases sense of control and decreases anxiety.
9. Assist in developing alternative solutions to a problem through role play or modeling behaviors.	9. The patient is encouraged to try alternative behaviors and solutions.
10. Explore behaviors that have worked to relieve anxiety in the past.	10. The patient is encouraged to mobilize successful coping mechanisms and strengths.
11. Provide outlets for dissipating excess energy (e.g., walking, playing Ping-Pong, dancing, exercising).	11. Physical activity can provide relief of built-up tension, increase muscle tone, and increase endorphin levels.

*Patients experiencing mild to moderate anxiety levels are still able to problem solve.

interpersonal relationships determines if the use of a defense mechanism is adaptive (healthy) or maladaptive (unhealthy) (Vaillant, 1994).

Sigmund Freud and his daughter Anna outlined most of the defense mechanisms that we recognize today. Five of the most important properties of defense mechanisms are as follows:

1. Defenses are a major means of managing conflict and affect.
2. Defenses are relatively unconscious.
3. Defenses are discrete from one another.
4. Although defenses are often the hallmarks of major psychiatric syndromes, they are reversible.
5. Defenses are adaptive as well as pathological.

All defense mechanisms except sublimation and altruism can be used in both healthy and unhealthy ways. (Sublimation and altruism are commonly very healthy coping mechanisms.) Most people use a variety of defense mechanisms but not always at the same level. Keep in mind that whether the use of defense mechanisms is adaptive or maladaptive is determined for the most part by their *frequency, intensity,* and *duration* of use.

The defense mechanisms are discussed in the following sections starting with the most mature and healthy, followed by those that are less healthy, and then by those that result in a greater degree of reality distortion and disruption in relationships and personal functioning.

Healthy Defenses
Altruism
In altruism, emotional conflicts and stressors are addressed by meeting the needs of others. Unlike in self-sacrificing behavior, in altruism the person receives gratification either vicariously or from the response of others.

VIGNETTE

Six months after losing her husband in a car accident, Jeanette began to spend 1 day a week doing grief counseling with families who had lost a loved one. She found that she was effective in helping others in their grief, and she obtained a great deal of satisfaction and pleasure from helping others work through their pain.

TABLE 11-3 INTERVENTIONS FOR SEVERE TO PANIC LEVELS OF ANXIETY*

NURSING DIAGNOSIS: *Anxiety* (severe, panic) related to severe threat (biochemical, environmental, psychosocial), as evidenced by verbal or physical acting out, extreme immobility, sense of impending doom, inability to differentiate reality (possible hallucinations or delusions), and inability to problem solve

INTERVENTION	RATIONALE
1. Maintain a calm manner.	1. Anxiety is communicated interpersonally. The quiet calm of the nurse can serve to calm the patient. The presence of anxiety can escalate anxiety in the patient.
2. Always remain with the person experiencing an acute severe to panic level of anxiety.	2. Alone with immense anxiety, a person feels abandoned. A caring face may be the patient's only contact with reality when confusion becomes overwhelming.
3. Minimize environmental stimuli. Move to a quieter setting and stay with the patient.	3. Helps minimize further escalation of patient's anxiety.
4. Use clear and simple statements and repetition.	4. A person experiencing a severe to panic level of anxiety has difficulty concentrating and processing information.
5. Use a low-pitched voice; speak slowly.	5. A high-pitched voice can convey anxiety. Low pitch can decrease anxiety.
6. Reinforce reality if distortions occur (e.g., seeing objects that are not there or hearing voices when no one is present).	6. Anxiety can be reduced by focusing on and validating what is happening in the environment.
7. Listen for themes in communication.	7. In severe to panic levels of anxiety, verbal communication themes may be the only indication of the patient's thoughts or feelings.
8. Attend to physical and safety needs when necessary (e.g., need for warmth, fluids, elimination, pain relief, family contact).	8. High levels of anxiety may obscure the patient's awareness of physical needs.
9. Because safety is an overall goal, physical limits may need to be set. Speak in a firm, authoritative voice: "You may not hit anyone here. If you can't control yourself, we will help you."	9. A person who is out of control is often terrorized. Staff must offer the patient and others protection from destructive and self-destructive impulses.
10. Provide opportunities for exercise (e.g., walk with nurse, use a punching bag, play Ping-Pong).	10. Physical activity helps channel and dissipate tension and may temporarily lower anxiety.
11. When a person is constantly moving or pacing, offer high-calorie fluids.	11. Dehydration and exhaustion must be prevented.
12. Assess need for medication or seclusion after other interventions have been tried and been unsuccessful.	12. Exhaustion and physical harm to self and others must be prevented.

*Patients who are experiencing severe to panic levels of anxiety are no longer able to problem solve.

Sublimation

Sublimation is an unconscious process of substituting constructive and socially acceptable activity for strong impulses that are not acceptable in their original form. Often these impulses are sexual or aggressive. A man with strong hostile feelings may choose to become a butcher, or he may participate in rough contact sports. A person who is unable to experience sexual activity may channel this energy into something creative, such as painting or gardening.

Humor

Humor makes life easier. An individual may deal with emotional conflicts or stressors by emphasizing the amusing or ironic aspects of the conflict or stressor through **humor.**

> **VIGNETTE**
> A man goes to an interview that means a great deal to him. He is being interviewed by the top executives of the company. He has recently had foot surgery and, on entering the interview room, he stumbles and loses his balance. There is a stunned silence, and then the man states calmly, "I was hoping I could put my best foot forward." With everyone laughing, the interview continues in a relaxed manner.

Suppression

Suppression is the conscious denial of a disturbing situation or feeling. For example, a student who has been studying for the state board examinations says, "I can't worry about paying my rent until after my exam tomorrow."

Intermediate Defenses
Repression

Repression is the exclusion of unpleasant or unwanted experiences, emotions, or ideas from conscious awareness. Examples include forgetting the name of a former boyfriend or girlfriend or forgetting an appointment to discuss poor grades. Repression is considered the cornerstone of the defense mechanisms, and it is the first line of psychological defense against anxiety.

Displacement

Transfer of emotions associated with a particular person, object, or situation to another person, object, or situation that is nonthreatening is called displacement. The frequently cited example in which the boss yells at the man, the man yells at his wife, the wife yells at the child, and the child kicks the cat demonstrates the successive use of displaced hostility. The use of displacement is common but not always adaptive. Spousal, child, and elder abuse are often cases of displaced hostility.

Reaction Formation

In reaction formation (also termed **overcompensation**), unacceptable feelings or behaviors are kept out of awareness by developing the opposite behavior or emotion. For example, a person who harbors hostility toward children becomes a Boy Scout leader.

Somatization

Transforming anxiety on an unconscious level into a physical symptom that has no organic cause is a form of somatization. Often the symptom functions as an attention seeker or as an excuse.

> **VIGNETTE**
>
> A professor develops laryngitis on the day he is scheduled to defend a research proposal to a group of peers.
> A woman who does not want to go out with the brother of her boss calls to say "her back went out," and she cannot make the date (and, in fact, her back is sore).

Undoing

Undoing compensates for an act or communication (e.g., giving a gift to undo an argument). A common behavioral example of undoing is compulsive hand washing. This can be viewed as cleansing oneself of an act or thought perceived as unacceptable.

Rationalization

Rationalization consists of justifying illogical or unreasonable ideas, actions, or feelings by developing acceptable explanations that satisfy the teller as well as the listener. Common examples are, "If I had Lynn's brains, I'd get good grades, too," or "Everybody cheats, so why shouldn't I?" Rationalization is a form of self-deception.

Immature Defenses
Passive Aggression

A passive-aggressive individual deals with emotional conflict or stressors by indirectly and unassertively expressing aggression toward others. On the surface, there is an appearance of compliance that masks covert resistance, resentment, and hostility. In passive aggression, aggression toward others is expressed through procrastination, failure, inefficiency, passivity, and illnesses that affect others more than oneself. Such passive-aggressive behaviors occur especially in response to assigned tasks or demands for independent action, responsibilities, or obligations.

> **VIGNETTE**
>
> Sam promises his boss that he is working on the presentation for important patients, even though he constantly "forgets" to bring in samples of the presentation. The day of the presentation, Sam calls in sick with the flu.

Acting-Out Behaviors

In acting out, an individual addresses emotional conflicts or stressors by actions rather than by reflections or feelings (APA, 2000). For example, a person may lash out in anger verbally or physically to distract the self from threatening thoughts or feelings. The verbal or physical expression of anger can make a person feel temporarily less helpless or vulnerable. By lashing out at others, an individual can transfer the focus from personal doubts and insecurities to some other person or object. Acting-out behaviors are a destructive coping style.

> **VIGNETTE**
>
> When Harry was turned down a third time for a promotion, he went to his office and tore apart every patient file in his file cabinet. His initial feelings of worthlessness and lowered self-esteem related to the situation were interpreted by Harry to mean "I am no good." This thinking resulted in Harry's quickly transforming these painful feelings into actions of anger and destruction. Temporarily, Harry felt more powerful and less vulnerable.

Dissociation

A disruption in the usually integrated functions of consciousness, memory, identity, or perception of the environment is known as dissociation.

> **VIGNETTE**
>
> A young mother who saw her son struck by a car was taken to a neighbor's house while the police dealt with the accident. Later she told the policeman, "I really don't remember what happened. The last thing I remember is going out the door to check on Johnny." At that moment, to protect herself from an unbearable situation, she separated the threatening event from awareness until she could begin to deal with her feelings of devastation.

Devaluation

Devaluation occurs when emotional conflicts or stressors are handled by attributing negative qualities to self or others (APA, 2000). When devaluing another, the individual then appears good by contrast.

> **VIGNETTE**
>
> A woman who is very jealous of a coworker says, "Oh, yes, she won the award. Those awards don't mean anything anyway, and I wonder what she had to do to be chosen." In this way she minimizes the other woman's accomplishments and keeps her own fragile self-esteem intact.

Idealization

In idealization, emotional conflicts or stressors are addressed by attributing exaggerated positive qualities to others. Idealization is an important aspect of the development of the self. Children who grow up with parents they can respect and idealize develop healthy standards of conduct and morality.

When people idealize and overvalue a person in a new relationship, they are sure to be disappointed when the object of the idealization turns out to be human. This leads to a great deal of disappointment and painful lowering of self-esteem. Such individuals may then devalue and reject the object of their affection to protect their own self-esteem. This pattern can be repeated over and over on a job, in friendships, in intimate relationships, and in marriage.

> **VIGNETTE**
>
> Mary met the most "wonderful and perfect" man. No one could tell Mary that Jim was nice but had some quirks, like everyone else. Mary would not listen. When Jim failed to live up to Mary's expectations of giving her constant attention, adoration, and gifts, Mary was devastated. Shortly thereafter, she started saying that Jim was, like all men, a brute, and that she wanted no more to do with such an insensitive person.

Splitting

Splitting is the inability to integrate the positive and negative qualities of oneself or others into a cohesive image. Aspects of the self and of others tend to alternate between opposite poles; for example, either good, loving, worthy, and nurturing, or bad, hateful, destructive, rejecting, and worthless. Use of this defense mechanism is prevalent in personality disorders, especially in people who have borderline components, and will be discussed at greater length in Chapter 13.

> **VIGNETTE**
>
> Alice viewed her therapist as the most wonderful, loving, and insightful therapist she had ever seen. When her therapist refused to write her a prescription for Valium, Alice shouted at her that she was the "stupidest, most uncaring, and thickheaded person," and she demanded another therapist "right away."

Projection

A person unconsciously rejects emotionally unacceptable personal features and attributes them to other people, objects, or situations through projection. Projection is the hallmark of blaming, scapegoating, prejudicial thinking, and stigmatization. People who always feel that others are out to deceive or cheat them may be projecting onto others those characteristics in themselves that they find distasteful and cannot consciously accept.

Projection of anxiety can often be seen in systems (family, hospital, school, business, politics). In a family in which there are problems, the child is often scapegoated, and the pain and anxiety within the family are projected onto the child: "The problem is Tommy." In a larger system in which anxiety and conflict are present, the weakest members are scapegoated: "The problem is the nurses' aides…the students…the new salesman…the Democrats/Republicans who are to blame for the mess we're in today." When pain and anxiety exist within a system, projection can be an automatic relief behavior. Once the cause of the anxiety is identified, changes in relief behavior can ensue, and the system can become more functional and productive.

Denial

Denial involves escaping unpleasant realities by ignoring their existence. For example, a man believes that physical limitations reflect negatively on one's manhood. Thus he may deny chest pains, even though his family has a history of heart attacks, because of a threat to his self-image as a man. A woman whose health has deteriorated because of alcohol abuse denies she has a problem with alcohol by saying she can stop drinking whenever she wants. Table 11-4 gives examples of adaptive and maladaptive uses of some common defense mechanisms.

ANXIETY DISORDERS

Anxiety is a normal response to threatening situations, and everyone experiences occasional distress. Anxiety becomes a problem when it interferes with adaptive behavior, causes physical symptoms, or exceeds a tolerable level. With people who have anxiety disorders, the experience is often one of considerable functional impairment and distress.

Anxiety is painful. Individuals with anxiety disorders use rigid, repetitive, and ineffective behaviors to try to control anxiety and ward off painful feelings. The common element in anxiety disorders is that individuals experience a degree of anxiety that is so high that it interferes with dysfunction at work, social, and family functions. Anxiety disorders are common and chronic, tend to be persistent, and are usually disabling.

Anxiety can be some of the first symptoms of a medical disorder, which is discussed later in this chapter. However, it is important to note that anxiety disorders can mimic medical illnesses as well. Patients may visit a variety of medical practitioners seeking an explanation for their symptoms when in fact the basis of their complaints is an anxiety disorder. For example, 70% of patients with panic disorder (PD) had seen at least 10 medical practitioners without receiving a diagnosis or adequate treatment (Pollock et al., 2010) and others had developed symptoms of generalized anxiety disorder (GAD) shortly before exhibiting somatic symptoms.

TABLE 11-4   DEFENSE MECHANISMS

DEFENSE MECHANISM	ADAPTIVE	MALADAPTIVE
Repression	Man forgets his wife's birthday after a marital fight.	Woman is unable to enjoy sex after having pushed out of awareness a traumatic sexual incident from childhood.
Sublimation	Woman who is angry with her boss writes a short story about a heroic woman. By definition, use of sublimation is always constructive.	None
Regression	Four-year-old boy with a new baby brother starts sucking his thumb and wanting a bottle.	Man who loses a promotion starts complaining to others, does sloppy work, misses appointments, and arrives late for meetings.
Displacement	Patient criticizes a nurse after his family fails to visit.	Child who is unable to acknowledge fear of his father becomes fearful of animals.
Projection	Man who is unconsciously attracted to other women teases his wife about flirting.	Woman who has repressed an attraction toward other women refuses to socialize. She fears another woman will make homosexual advances toward her.
Compensation	Short man becomes assertively verbal and excels in business.	Individual drinks alcohol when self-esteem is low to diffuse discomfort temporarily.
Reaction formation	Recovering alcoholic constantly preaches about the evils of alcoholic beverages.	Mother who has an unconscious hostility toward her daughter is overprotective to protect daughter from harm, interfering with daughter's normal growth and development.
Denial	Man reacts to news of the death of a loved one by saying, "No, I don't believe you. The doctor said he was fine."	Woman whose husband died 3 years earlier still keeps his clothes in the closet and talks about him in the present tense.
Conversion	Student is unable to take a final examination because of a terrible headache.	Man becomes blind after seeing his wife flirt with other men.
Undoing	After flirting with her male secretary, a woman brings her husband tickets to a show.	Man with rigid and moralistic beliefs and repressed sexuality is driven to wash his hands to gain composure when around attractive women.
Rationalization	Employee says, "I didn't get the raise because the boss doesn't like me."	Father who thinks his son was fathered by another man excuses his malicious treatment of the boy by saying, "He is lazy and disobedient," when that is not the case.
Identification	Five-year-old girl dresses in her mother's shoes and dress and meets her father at the door.	Young boy thinks a neighborhood pimp with money and drugs is someone to emulate.
Introjection	After his wife's death, husband has transient complaints of chest pains and difficulty breathing—the symptoms his wife had before she died.	Young child whose parents were overcritical and belittling grows up thinking that she is inferior. She has taken on her parent's evaluation of her as part of her self-image.
Suppression	Businessman who is preparing to make an important speech later in the day is told by his wife that morning that she wants a divorce. Although visibly upset, he puts the incident aside until after his speech, when he can give the matter his total concentration.	A woman who feels a lump in her breast shortly before leaving for a 3-week vacation puts the information in the back of her mind until after returning from her vacation.

PREVALENCE AND COMORBIDITY

Anxiety disorders are the most prevalent lifetime psychiatric disorders in the United States and are estimated at 28.8% (Kessler et al., 2005), which means that approximately one in four individuals in the United States will experience an anxiety disorder in his or her lifetime. People with anxiety disorders frequently seek health care services for relief of physical symptoms. Women are reported to be more frequently affected than men. Despite the high prevalence of these disorders, they often are unrecognized and untreated.

Anxiety disorders are highly **comorbid/co-occurring** with each other, with major depressive disorders, and with alcohol and/or drug abuse (Martin et al., 2009; Yates, 2011). Major depressive disorder (MDD) co-occurs in approximately up to half of people with anxiety disorders and produces greater impairment and poorer response to treatment. Substance abuse is also frequently present and has a similar negative effect on treatment as well. Anxiety disorders frequently co-occur with many other psychiatric disorders (e.g., eating disorders, bipolar disorders, dysthymia); several studies suggest that up to 90% of people with an anxiety disorder develop another psychiatric disorder during their lifetime.

Other co-occurring conditions that are medical in nature and have been well documented in the literature include cancer, heart disease, high blood pressure, irritable bowel syndrome, kidney and liver dysfunction, reduced immunity, and others. Chronic anxiety is thought to be associated with increased risk for cardiovascular morbidity and mortality (Yates, 2011). Usually anxiety disorders begin in childhood, adolescence, and early adulthood.

THEORY

Anxiety disorders are most likely caused by a complex interaction of biological, psychological, and environmental factors. There is no longer any doubt that biological factors such as genetic vulnerability may interact with stress or trauma to trigger pathological anxiety states in some individuals (e.g., phobias, panic attacks). By the same token, traumatic life events (witnessing spousal abuse, child abuse, muggings, sexual assault), psychosocial factors, and sociocultural factors also are etiologically significant.

Neurobiology

Although the neurobiology of anxiety and anxiety disorders is vastly complex, the following identifies some of the major factors in anxiety that relate directly to evidence-based nursing care. Refer to Chapter 4 for more on the neurotransmitters and how medications work and to Chapter 10 for more information on the stress response.

Certain anatomical pathways (the **limbic system**) provide structure for electrical impulses that either receive or send anxiety-related responses. Neurons release chemicals (neurotransmitters) that convey these messages (Preston et al., 2010). Some patients with anxiety disorders will exhibit an increase in anxiety response, adapt slowly to repeated stimuli, and respond excessively to moderate stimuli (Sadock & Sadock, 2007).

The limbic system, referred to by some as "the emotional brain," consists of the amygdala, septum, cingulate, and hippocampus. The three functions of the limbic system are (Preston et al., 2010, p. 38) as follows:

- The appraisal of emotional stimuli
- The initiation of emotional responses (fight-or-flight response) (Chapter 10)
- The cessation of reactivity after external stressors subside and the restoration of the nervous system to a state of homeostasis

The part of the limbic system most associated with anxiety disorders as well as the obsessive-compulsive disorders is the cingulate, where the neural pathways connect to the limbic system and prefrontal lobes that result in the regulation of emotions. The limbic system is involved in storing memories and creating emotions, and is thought to be a major factor in processing anxiety-related information. Some of the other parts of the brain involved in anxiety and anxiety-related disorders are the following:

- Frontal cortex: cognitive interpretations (e.g., potential threat)
- Hypothalamus: activation of the stress response (fight-or-flight response; refer to Chapter 10)
- Hippocampus: associated with memory related to fear responses
- Amygdala: fear, especially related to phobic and panic disorders

There is a link between anxiety and specific areas of the brain. When anxiety occurs it causes an imbalance in certain neurotransmitters in the brain that regulate anxiety. Based on animal studies and responses to drug treatment, at present there are three main mediators of anxiety in the central nervous system that regulate anxiety responses; these are serotonin (5-HT), norepinephrine (NE), and γ-aminobutyric acid (GABA).

- Serotonin (5-HT): Serotonin level is thought to be decreased in anxiety disorders. Therefore, it is hypothesized that serotonin dysfunction contributes to anxiety disorders. The selective serotonin reuptake inhibitors (SSRIs), which increase serotonin levels in the brain, are often first-line medications for the treatment of many anxiety disorders.
- Norepinephrine (NE): Norepinephrine is known to mediate arousal. When a person feels threatened (real or perceived) the level of norepinephrine (adrenaline) increases and can cause hyperarousal and increased anxiety. In some people with anxiety disorders, it is thought that the noradrenergic system is poorly regulated and can cause bursts of activity. Noradrenergic drugs such as propranolol (which blocks adrenergic receptor activity) and clonidine (which stimulates α-adrenergic receptors) are used to help lower anxiety.
- GABA (γ-aminobutyric acid): GABA is an inhibitory neurotransmitter in the brain. The release of GABA slows neural transmission, which has a calming effect. Binding of the benzodiazepine medications to the benzodiazepine receptors facilitates the action of GABA.

A number of drugs including antianxiety agents, sedative-hypnotics, general anesthetics, and anticonvulsant drugs are the targets of the GABA receptor system (Howland, 2010), thus slowing neural transmission and lowering anxiety. Abnormalities of these benzodiazepine receptors may lead to unregulated anxiety levels.

A **genetic** component is substantiated by numerous studies that find anxiety disorders tend to cluster in families. Twin studies indicate the existence of a genetic component to panic disorders (PDs). For example, there is a high concordance rate in monozygotic twins as compared with dizygotic twins; however, it is still uncertain if the genetic influence is specific to panic disorder or represents general anxiety proneness (Pollock et al., 2010).

People with obsessive-compulsive disorder (OCD) also show genetic components as referred to in the section later in this chapter on OCD (Hemmings & Stein, 2006; Stuart et al., 2008). Twin and family studies report that panic disorder has a heritability of approximately 40% (Taylor et al., 2008).

Cognitive Behavioral Theory

Behavioral Theory

Learning theories provide another view. Behavioral psychologists conceptualize anxiety as a learned response that can be unlearned. Some individuals may learn to be anxious from the modeling provided by parents or peers. For example, a mother who is fearful of thunder and lightning and who hides in closets during storms may transmit her anxiety to her children, who continue to adopt her behavior even into adult life. Such individuals can unlearn this behavior by observing others who react normally to a storm. For example, behavioral therapy in the form of gradually exposing a highly anxious person to a feared object or situation (such as that in agoraphobia) over time with support can help the person overcome his or her fear of the object or situation.

Cognitive Theory

Cognitive theorists believe that anxiety disorders are a result of distortions in an individual's thinking and perceiving. Because individuals with such distortions believe that any mistake they make will have catastrophic results, they experience acute anxiety. Brain scans taken before and after cognitive therapy treatment support the hypothesis that learning to reframe one's thinking can literally change the chemistry and function of the brain. Cognitive behavioral therapy seems to have the best evidence not only for effective psychotherapeutic treatment of anxiety disorders but also for more lasting results in other disorders and problematic situations.

CULTURAL CONSIDERATIONS

Reliable data on the incidence of anxiety disorders among cultures are sparse, but sociocultural variation in symptoms of anxiety disorders has been noted. In some cultures, individuals express anxiety through somatic symptoms, whereas in other cultures cognitive symptoms predominate. Panic attacks in Latin Americans and Northern Europeans often involve sensations of choking, smothering, numbness, or tingling, as well as fear of dying. In other cultural groups, panic attacks involve fear of magic or witchcraft. Social phobias in Japanese and Korean cultures may relate to a belief that the individual's blushing, eye contact, or body odor is offensive to others.

One of the barriers for some cultural groups seeking health care for anxiety disorders is the stigma that various cultures are associated with mental disorders. For example, African Americans are much less likely to seek mental health services than the majority of the population, and Asian Americans even more so (Satcher et al., 2005).

Interestingly, the incidence of anxiety disorders seems to vary among culture and countries. Anxiety disorders also vary among immigrants from generation to generation. One must be aware of the cultural norm before hastily making a diagnosis (e.g., labeling ritualistic behavior as obsessive-compulsive disorder).

CLINICAL PICTURE

The term *anxiety disorders* refers to a number of disorders, including panic disorders, phobias, general anxiety disorders, among others.

Panic Disorders

The panic attack is the key feature of **panic disorders (PDs)**. A **panic attack** is the sudden onset of extreme apprehension or fear, usually associated with feelings of impending doom: "I am going to die." The feelings of terror present during a panic attack are so severe that normal function is suspended, the perceptual field is severely limited, and misinterpretation of reality may occur. Severe personality disorganization is evident. People experiencing panic attacks may believe that they are losing their minds or are having a heart attack; the attacks are often accompanied by highly uncomfortable physical symptoms. Some of the symptoms a person may experience are palpitations, chest pain, diaphoresis, muscle tension, urinary frequency, hyperventilation, breathing difficulties, nausea, feelings of choking, chills, hot flashes, and gastrointestinal symptoms. Typically, panic attacks occur suddenly (not necessarily in response to stress), are extremely intense, last 1 or 2 minutes (occasionally lasting up to 30 minutes), and then subside. During the intervals between panic attacks, the person may experience low-level constant anxiousness and anticipatory anxiety. It is not uncommon for someone rushed to the emergency department (ED) with all the signs and symptoms of a heart attack (chest pain, difficulty breathing, dizziness, excessive fatigue) to have an extensive medical workup that proves negative for cardiac problems. At that point the person needs to be referred to a counselor for potential diagnosis and treatment of an anxiety disorder. Major depression occurs in up to two thirds of the cases of people with PD and complicates the course of the disorder considerably (Pollock et al., 2010).

Panic attacks are usually terrifying and painful for the person who is experiencing them. Increased rates of suicide and suicide attempts are associated in people with panic attacks (Taylor et al., 2008).

Many well-known individuals have been known to suffer from panic attacks, including Sigmund Freud, Princess Diana, Cher, Alfred Lord Tennyson, and Winston Churchill. The incidence of panic attacks over time may lead to complications such as persistent anxiety, phobic avoidance, depression, alcoholism, or other drug overuse (Pollock et al., 2010).

Preston and colleagues (2010, p. 115) cite the following pharmacological treatments as efficacious in the treatment of panic disorders:

- High-potency benzodiazepines, such as alprazolam, clonazepam, and lorazepam
- Antidepressants such as tricyclics and SSRIs
- Monoamine oxidase inhibitors (MAOIs)
- Utilization of cognitive and behavioral therapy in conjunction with medications has been effective in treating some people with panic attacks

Panic Disorder With Agoraphobia

Panic disorder with agoraphobia is a combination of the aforementioned symptoms and agoraphobia. Agoraphobia, a phobic disorder, is intense, excessive anxiety or fear about being in places or situations from which help might not be available, and escape might be either difficult or embarrassing. The feared places are avoided by the individual in an effort to control anxiety. Examples of situations that are commonly avoided by patients with agoraphobia are being alone outside; being alone at home; traveling in a car, bus, or airplane; being on a bridge; and riding in an elevator. Avoidance behaviors can be debilitating and life constricting. Consider the effect on a father whose avoidance renders him unable to leave home and who thus cannot see his child's high school graduation, or the businesswoman whose avoidance of flying prevents her from attending distant business conferences.

Phobias

A phobia is a persistent, irrational fear of a specific object, activity, or situation that leads to a desire for avoidance, or actual avoidance, of the object, activity, or situation.

Specific phobias are characterized by the experience of high levels of anxiety or fear in response to specific objects or situations, such as dogs, spiders, heights, storms, water, blood, closed spaces, tunnels, and bridges. Specific phobias are common and usually do not cause much difficulty because people can contrive ways to avoid the feared object, such as cats or spiders. Clinical names for common phobias are provided in Table 11-5.

There is no evidence that these disorders are related to biological dysfunction and need medication to be treated (Preston et al., 2010). In fact, behavioral therapy seems to be the only therapy effective with specific phobias.

Social anxiety disorders (SADs), or social phobias, are characterized by severe anxiety or fear provoked by exposure to a social situation or a performance situation (e.g., fear of saying something that sounds foolish in public, fear of being unable to answer questions in a classroom, fear of eating in the presence of others, fear of performing on stage). Fear of public speaking is the most common social phobia. Barbra Streisand,

TABLE 11-5	CLINICAL NAMES FOR COMMON PHOBIAS
CLINICAL NAME	**FEARED OBJECT OR SITUATION**
Acrophobia	Heights
Agoraphobia	Open spaces
Astraphobia	Electrical storms
Claustrophobia	Closed spaces
Glossophobia	Talking
Hematophobia	Blood
Hydrophobia	Water
Monophobia	Being alone
Mysophobia	Germs or dirt
Nyctophobia	Darkness
Pyrophobia	Fire
Xenophobia	Strangers
Zoophobia	Animals

the great Laurence Olivier, Richard Burton, and Kim Basinger are but a few well-known performers who suffered from terrific bouts of performance anxiety when appearing in front of an audience.

Social anxiety disorders are believed to be influenced by psychological factors such as the quality of early attachments, the development of appropriate social skills, inadequate experiences interacting with others, and other negative environmental influences (Preston et al., 2010). There is also evidence from twin and high-risk studies that suggests a complex genetic transmission of this disorder. There are currently ongoing biological studies to identify specific neurobiological factors associated with anxiety and fear. The beta-blocker propranolol reduces the physiological symptoms of anxiety, although not the cognitive (e.g., worry). Propranolol is used effectively by many performers or lecturers before appearing on stage to act, conduct, speak, and otherwise make a presentation in front of an audience. More pervasive social anxiety may respond to monoamine oxidase inhibitors (MAOIs) and selective serotonin reuptake inhibitors (SSRIs). Cognitive therapy interventions along with social skills training are helpful for many.

Agoraphobia, described previously, can be the most limiting and debilitating of all of the phobias. In its most extreme form, patients may simply refuse to leave their homes, putting great strain on family and friends and resulting in problems within marriages. Characteristically, phobic individuals experience overwhelming and crippling anxiety when they are faced with the object or situation provoking the phobia. Phobic people go to great lengths to avoid the feared object or situation. A phobic person may not be able to think about or visualize the object or situation without becoming severely anxious. The life of a phobic person becomes more restricted as activities are discontinued so that the phobic object can be avoided. All too frequently, complications ensue when people try to decrease anxiety through self-medication with alcohol or drugs.

This disorder is thought to be primarily due to psychogenic causes leading to a conditioned fear response of fear and anxiety. This conditioned fear response responds well to cognitive behavioral therapy (CBT) and SSRI medications.

Generalized Anxiety Disorder

Generalized anxiety disorder (GAD) is a chronic psychiatric disorder associated with severe distress different from other anxiety disorders in that there is pervasive cognitive dysfunction, impaired functioning, and poor health-related outcomes (Allgulander, 2009; Taylor et al., 2008). Up to two thirds of people with generalized anxiety disorder have comorbid major depression, and up to 25% present with panic disorder. Self-medication may lead to alcohol or substance use disorder (Harvard Mental Health Letter, 2011).

GAD also differs from other anxiety disorders in that patients do not fear a specific external object or situation, and there is no distinct symptomatic reaction pattern. Basically, GAD is characterized by excessive, persistent, and uncontrollable anxiety, and by excessive worrying. It is sometimes referred to as the "worry disease." Accompanying symptoms include restlessness, fatigue, poor concentration, irritability, tension, and sleep disturbance.

The individual's worry is out of proportion to the true effect of the event or situation about which the individual is focused. Examples of worries typical in GAD are inadequacy in interpersonal relationships, job responsibilities, finances, health of family members, household chores, and lateness for appointments. In fact, these excessive worries are conducive to disturbances in relationships and family life, impaired functioning at work, and disturbances in social roles. Sleep disturbance is common because the individual worries about the day's events and real or imagined mistakes, reviews past problems, and anticipates future difficulties during sleep hours. These constant worries leave the limbic system in a perpetual state of alertness. Decision making is difficult because of poor concentration and dread of making a mistake.

GAD is thought by many to be a psychogenic disorder. However, there is also speculation that GAD may be biologically mediated. For example, buspirone and 5-HT serotonin antagonists (SSRIs) are effective in reducing the "what if's" and worrying in GAD patients (Preston et al., 2010). An overview of medications and therapies for specific anxiety disorders is found in Table 11-6.

Anxiety Caused by Medical Conditions

In anxiety attributable to medical conditions, the individual's symptoms of anxiety are a direct physiological result of a medical condition. Examples include the following:

- Respiratory: asthma, hypoxia, pulmonary edema, chronic obstructive pulmonary disease (COPD), pulmonary embolism

TABLE 11-6   DEFENSES USED IN ANXIETY DISORDERS

PHENOMENON	DEFENSE	PURPOSE	EXAMPLE
Phobia	Displacement	In phobias, anxiety is reduced when strong feelings about the original object are directed at a less-threatening object and that object is avoided.	Patient has abnormal fear of cats. In therapy, it is discovered that the patient unconsciously links cats to a feared and cruel mother.
Compulsion	Undoing	Performing a symbolic act cancels an unacceptable act or idea.	Patient performs symbolic rituals (e.g., hand washing, cleaning, and checking). Hand washing removes guilt. Cleaning removes dirty thoughts. Checking protects against hostile thoughts.
Obsession	Reaction formation	Anxiety-producing unacceptable thoughts or feelings are kept out of awareness by the opposite feeling or idea.	Patient with strong aggressive feelings toward husband repeatedly thinks the opposite ("I love him with all my heart") to keep hostile feelings out of awareness.
	Intellectualization	Excessive use of reasoning, logic, or words prevents the person from experiencing associated feelings.	Person talks in detail about parents' funeral but is unable to feel the associated pain of loss.
Posttraumatic stress	Isolation disorder	Facts associated with anxiety-laden events remain conscious, but associated painful feelings are separated from the experience.	Patient describes feeling "numb and empty inside."
Repression			Patient is unable to trust authority figures at work after taking orders from commanding officer to kill civilians while in combat.

- Cardiovascular: cardiac dysrhythmias such as torsades de pointes, angina, congestive heart failure, mitral valve prolapse, hypertension
- Endocrine: hyperthyroidism, hypoglycemia, hypercortisolism, pheochromocytoma
- Neurological: Parkinson's disease, akathisia, postconcussion syndrome, complex partial seizures
- Metabolic: hypercalcemia, hyperkalemia, hyponatremia, porphyria

To determine whether the anxiety symptoms are caused by a medical condition, a careful and comprehensive assessment of multiple factors is necessary. Evidence must be present in the history, physical examination, and/or laboratory findings to diagnose the medical condition.

OBSESSIVE-COMPULSIVE DISORDER (OCD)

At one time the causes of OCD were thought to be psychogenic in origin. Now there is substantial evidence that OCD has biological origins and is thought by many to be a neurologically based disorder. OCD seems to occur more often in patients with other neurological disorders, such as in Huntington's chorea epilepsy, Sydenham's chorea, or brain trauma (Black & Andreasen, 2011). Other factors that support OCD as a neurological disorder include the following (Black & Andreasen, 2011; Preston et al., 2010):

1. Brain imaging studies show an increase in metabolic activity in patients with OCD, specifically hyperactivity in the prefrontal cortex and dysfunction in the basal ganglia. Some researchers speculate that the basal ganglia dysfunction is responsible for the complex motor programs involved in OCD, whereas the tendency to worry and plan excessively is a result of the prefrontal cortex hyperactivity.
2. There is evidence that OCD has a strong genetic component. There is a 7% incident of OCD in first-degree relatives of patients with OCD versus 2.5% in the general population, thus suggesting a strong genetic component.
3. Clinical studies have shown that OCD patients are responsive to selective serotonin reuptake inhibitors (SSRIs) whereas other antidepressants are ineffective. Also, the tricyclic antidepressant clomipramine has proved to be especially effective in people with OCD.

Obsessive-compulsive (OC) symptoms are common, but obsessive-compulsive disorders (OCDs) can be extremely disabling and painful. OCD is no longer considered uncommon.

Obsessions are defined as thoughts, impulses, or images that persist and recur so that they cannot be dismissed from the mind. Obsessions often seem senseless to the individual who experiences them, although they still cause the individual to experience severe anxiety. Common obsessions include fear of hurting a loved one or fear of contamination.

Compulsions are ritualistic behaviors that an individual feels driven to perform in an attempt to reduce anxiety. Common compulsions are repetitive hand washing and checking a door multiple times to make sure it is locked. In doing this we are performing a compulsive act that temporarily reduces high levels of anxiety. The primary gain is achieved by compulsive rituals, but because the relief is only temporary, the compulsive act must be repeated many times.

Although obsessions and compulsions can exist independently of each other, they most often occur together as in obsessive-compulsive disorder (OCD). OCD behavior exists along a continuum. "Normal" individuals may experience mildly obsessive-compulsive behavior. Nearly everyone has experienced having a song playing persistently through the mind, despite attempts to push it away. Many people have had nagging doubts as to whether a door is locked or the stove is turned off. These doubts require the person to go back to check the door or stove. Minor compulsions, such as touching a lucky charm, knocking on wood, and making the sign of the cross upon hearing disturbing news, are not harmful to the individual. Mild compulsions (timeliness, orderliness, and reliability) are valued traits in selective contexts in the U.S. society.

At the more severe end of the continuum are obsessive-compulsive symptoms that typically center on dirtiness, contamination, and germs and occur with corresponding compulsions, such as cleaning and hand washing. A smaller number focus on safety issues and engage in repetitive checking rituals. At the most severe levels are persistent thoughts of sexuality, violence, illness, or death. These obsessions or compulsions cause marked distress to the individual. People often feel humiliation and shame regarding these behaviors. The rituals are time-consuming and interfere with normal routine, social activities, and relationships with others. Severe OCD consumes so much of the individual's mental processes that the performance of cognitive tasks may be impaired.

Hoarding

Is hoarding an obsessive-compulsive disorder? Compulsive hoarding is associated with excessive collecting of items and the failure to discard excessive amounts of these items. Compulsive hoarding is often associated with OCD. About 50% of patients who meet the criteria for compulsive hoarding syndrome have comorbid/co-occurring OCD (Pertusa et al., 2008). Pertusa and colleagues have noted that in people with OCD excessive hoarding is associated with the following:

- Increased Axis I (mental disorders) and Axis II (personality disorder) comorbidities
- Impairment in the performance of activities of daily living
- Reduced insight
- Poor response to standard psychological and pharmacological treatments
- A distinct genetic and neurobiological profile

In most cases compulsive hoarding does not meet the *DSM-IV-TR* criteria for OCD. Although compulsive hoarding can be disabling and result in social isolation, people with compulsive hoarding suffer extreme disruption in daily living and severe distress and often live in unsafe conditions. Therefore the following question is being debated: Is hoarding a distinct variant of OCD or is compulsive hoarding a separate syndrome that may co-occur in some people with OCD?

APPLICATION OF THE NURSING PROCESS

ASSESSMENT

Symptoms of Anxiety

People with anxiety disorders rarely need hospitalization unless they are suicidal or have compulsions causing injury (e.g., cutting self). Therefore most patients prone to anxiety are encountered in a variety of community settings. A common example of an acute anxiety episode occurs when an individual who is taken to an emergency department to rule out a heart attack is found to be experiencing a panic attack. Therefore one of the first things that may need to be determined is whether the anxiety is from a secondary source (medical condition or substances) or a primary source, as in an anxiety disorder.

Defenses Used in Anxiety Disorders

People use a variety of ego defenses and behaviors to lessen the uncomfortable levels of anxiety. Psychodynamic theorists believe that people who suffer from anxiety disorders employ specific defenses (see Table 11-6). A comprehensive and sophisticated assessment is the Hamilton rating scale for anxiety. *A word of caution:* The Hamilton scale highlights important areas in the assessment of anxiety. Because many answers are subjective, experienced clinicians use this tool as a guide when planning care and draw on their knowledge of their patients.

ASSESSMENT GUIDELINES

Anxiety Disorders

1. Ensure that a sound physical and neurological examination is performed to help determine whether the anxiety is primary or secondary to another psychiatric disorder, a medical condition, or substance use.
2. Assess for potential for self-harm and suicide. It is known that people suffering from high levels of intractable anxiety may contemplate, attempt, or complete suicide.
3. Perform a psychosocial assessment. Always ask the person, "What has happened recently that might be increasing your anxiety?" The patient may identify a problem that should be addressed through counseling or therapy (e.g., stressful marriage, recent loss, stressful job or school situation). In some situations, there may be no identifiable recent event.
4. Assess cultural beliefs and background. Differences in culture can affect how anxiety is manifested.

DIAGNOSIS

NANDA International (NANDA-I, 2012-2014) provides many nursing diagnoses that can be considered for patients experiencing anxiety and anxiety disorders. The "related to" component will vary with the individual patient. Table 11-7 identifies potential nursing diagnoses for the anxious patient. Included are the signs and symptoms that might be found on assessment that support the diagnoses.

OUTCOMES IDENTIFICATION

The Nursing Outcomes Classification (NOC) identifies a number of desired outcomes for patients with anxiety or anxiety-related disorders (Moorhead et al., 2008). *Psychiatric–Mental Health Nursing: Scope and Standards of Practice* (ANA, 2007) emphasizes that outcomes should, among other considerations:

- Reflect patient values and ethical and environmental situations.
- Be culturally appropriate.
- Be documented as measurable goals.
- Include a time estimate of expected outcomes.

Table 11-8 identifies short- and long-term outcomes using the criteria from *Psychiatric–Mental Health Nursing: Scope and Standards of Practice* (ANA, 2007).

PLANNING

Anxiety disorders are encountered in numerous settings. Nurses care for people with concurrent anxiety disorders in medical-surgical units and in outpatient settings, such as homes, day programs, and clinics. Usually patients with anxiety disorders do not require admission to inpatient psychiatric units. Therefore, planning for care usually involves selecting interventions that can be implemented in a community setting.

Whenever possible, the patient should be encouraged to participate actively in planning. By sharing decision making with the patient, the nurse increases the likelihood of positive outcomes. Shared planning is especially appropriate for a patient with mild or moderate anxiety. When the patient is experiencing severe levels of anxiety, he or she may be unable to participate in planning, which requires the nurse to take a more directive role.

Self-Care for Nurses

Anxiety is communicated empathetically from person to person. Therefore, it is not surprising that being around an anxiety-disordered patient may cause the nurse to experience very intense and uncomfortable emotions. When working with highly anxious patients, students and new clinicians will do best to work under supervision of a more experienced health care professional. Supervision can help nurses/health care professionals identify and intervene with their emotions when they become negative and problematic. When nurses in any situation feel anger, frustration, or other negative feelings toward the patient, the nurse and patient will most likely experience a situation of mutual withdrawal.

Common responses when working with anxiety-disordered clients include increased anxiety, frustration, anger, and other negative emotions. For example, communication techniques with patients with OCD have to provide clear structure, because these patients tend to correct and clarify repeatedly as though they cannot let go of any topic, often frustrating and/or angering the nurse/clinician. With phobic and agoraphobic patients, angry feelings may arise when the patient does not make rapid progress. Feelings of frustration, anger, and anxiety and negative feelings can cause tension and fatigue from mental strain. These feelings

TABLE 11-7   POTENTIAL NURSING DIAGNOSES FOR THE ANXIOUS PATIENT

SIGNS AND SYMPTOMS	NURSING DIAGNOSES[*]
• Concern that a panic attack will occur • Exposure to phobic object or situation • Presence of obsessive thoughts • Recurrent memories of traumatic event • Fear of panic attacks	Anxiety (moderate, severe, panic) Fear
• High levels of anxiety that interfere with the ability to work, disrupt relationships, and change ability to interact with others • Avoidance behaviors (phobia, agoraphobia) • Hypervigilance after a traumatic event • Inordinate time taken for obsession and compulsions	Ineffective coping Deficient diversional activity Social isolation Ineffective role performance Impaired social interaction Ineffective relationship Post-trauma syndrome
• Difficulty with concentration • Preoccupation with obsessive thoughts • Disorganization associated with exposure to phobic object • Intrusive thoughts and memories of traumatic event • Excessive use of reason and logic associated with overcautiousness and fear of making a mistake	
• Inability to go to sleep related to intrusive thoughts, worrying, replaying of a traumatic event, hypervigilance, fear	Sleep deprivation Disturbed sleep pattern Fatigue
• Feelings of hopelessness, inability to control one's life, low self-esteem related to inability to have some control in one's life	Hopelessness Chronic low self-esteem Spiritual distress
• Inability to perform self-care related to rituals • Skin excoriation related to rituals of excessive washing or excessive picking at the skin • Inability to eat because of constant ritual performance	Self-care deficit Impaired skin integrity Imbalanced nutrition: less than body requirements
• Feeling of anxiety or excessive worrying that overrides appetite and need to eat • Excessive overeating to appease intense worrying or high anxiety levels	Imbalanced nutrition: more than body requirements

[*]Nursing Diagnoses—Definitions and Classification 2012-2014. Copyright © 2012, 1994-2012 by NANDA International. Used by arrangement with Blackwell Publishing Limited, a company of John Wiley & Sons, Inc.

of frustration and mental strain, especially over a period of time, may lead to burnout. **Burnout** is defined as "a state of physical, emotional, and mental exhaustion caused by long-term involvement in emotionally demanding situations" (Pines & Aronson, 1988, p. 9), as opposed to compassion fatigue, described under posttraumatic stress disorder (PTSD) in Chapter 10. Supervision, stress management courses, mindfulness, yoga, exercise, creative activities, and humor are all examples of stress reduction techniques (refer to Box 10-1 for selected stress reduction techniques). As instructors often tell their students, "keep your bucket full," meaning students as well as health care providers need to work at keeping a healthy balance in their personal lives.

IMPLEMENTATION

The nurse follows the *Psychiatric–Mental Health Nursing: Scope and Standards of Practice* (ANA, 2007) when intervening with patients. Whenever possible, interventions should be based on the best evidence available. Overall guidelines for basic nursing interventions are as follows:

1. Identify community resources that can offer specialized treatment that is proven to be highly effective for people with a variety of anxiety disorders.
2. Identify community support groups for people with specific anxiety disorders and their families.
3. Use therapeutic communication, milieu therapy, promotion of self-care activities, psychotherapy, and health teaching and health promotion as appropriate.

Communication Guidelines

Psychiatric mental health nurses use therapeutic communication skills to assist patients with anxiety disorders to reduce anxiety, enhance coping and communication skills, and intervene in crises. When patients request or prefer to use integrative therapies, the nurse performs assessment and teaching as appropriate.

TABLE 11-8	**SHORT- AND LONG-TERM OUTCOMES FOR SPECIFIC ANXIETY DISORDERS**
ANXIETY DISORDER	**SHORT- OR LONG-TERM OUTCOMES**
Phobia	Patients will: • Develop skills at reframing anxiety-provoking situation (date). • Work with nurse/clinician to desensitize self to feared object or situation (date). • Demonstrate one new relaxation skill that works well for them (date).
Generalized anxiety disorder	Patients will: • State increased ability to make decisions and problem solve. • Demonstrate ability to perform usual tasks even though still moderately anxious by (date). • Demonstrate one cognitive or behavioral coping skill that helps reduce anxious feelings by (date).
Obsessive-compulsive disorder	Patients will: • Demonstrate techniques that can distract and distance self from thoughts that are anxiety producing by (date). • Decrease time spent in ritualistic behaviors. • Demonstrate increased amount of time spent with family and friends and on pleasurable activities. • State they have more control over intrusive thoughts and rituals by (date).
Posttraumatic stress disorder	Patients will: • Attend support group at least once a week by (date). • Increase social support by one each month with aid of nurse/counselor. • Report increase in restful sleep periods. • Report decrease in nightmares or flashbacks. • Demonstrate at least one new anxiety reduction technique (cognitive or behavioral) that works well for them.

EXAMINING THE EVIDENCE

Paying Attention To Yourself Can Be Good For You!

I have been hearing more about mindfulness meditation as a new intervention for anxiety and depression that actually changes brain function. What is it and is it really effective?

That is a very good question. Mindfulness meditation (MM) is often used as an integral aspect of cognitive behavioral therapy (CBT), which aims at changing distorted and maladaptive thoughts and feelings toward more realistic/adaptive experiences. Mindfulness meditation (MM) is the practice of paying attention to what you are experiencing from moment to moment without drifting into thoughts about the past or concerns about the future, and without analyzing or making judgments about what is going on around you. It has been reported to produce positive effects on psychological well-being that extend beyond the time the individual is formally meditating (Nalliboff & Frese, 2008).

MM is not a new idea. Religions have preached mindfulness for centuries and it is central to Buddhism and other contemplative traditions. Over the past 30 years, MM has increasingly found a place in mainstream health care because it has been shown not only to reduce symptoms of depression but also to alleviate anxiety, headaches, psoriasis, high

blood pressure, high cholesterol levels, eating disorders, substance abuse, and chronic pain (Holzel & Carmody, 2011). With advances in imaging, scientists have begun to explore the brain mechanisms that may underlie these benefits. MM impacts the synthesis of neurotransmitters, particularly serotonin and norepinephrine, which influences mood, increases activity in telomerase (an enzyme important to the long-term health of cells), and affects the concentration of gray matter in the amygdala (a region of the brain associated with fear, anxiety, and stress). Some studies suggest it can improve immune function (Holzel & Carmody, 2011).

Mindfulness may also rival medication at preventing depression relapse. Clinicians often recommend that the patient continue taking some type of maintenance medication, usually an antidepressant, for extended periods. However, not everyone wants to take medications indefinitely and some—notably pregnant women or people taking other drugs—may have good reason to avoid additional medications. A recent study suggests MM as a possible alternative to medication. Results showed that 38% of those treated with MM relapsed compared with 46% prescribed medication (Segal et al., 2010).

EXAMINING THE EVIDENCE—cont'd

Paying Attention To Yourself Can Be Good For You!

Other studies have also reported mindfulness as promoting the use of personal coping skills, less negative stress responses (Zeidan & Johnson, 2010), self-compassion, and early recognition of potential problems (While, 2009). For many of those who suffer from depression, MM and its focus on positive thoughts and self-compassion can provide an escape from a self-perpetuating pattern of depression where thoughts frequently become unrealistically negative and critical.

Holzel, B., & Carmody, J. (2011). Mindfulness practice leads to increases in regional brain gray matter density. *Psychiatry Research: Neuroimaging, 191,* 36-43.

Nalliboff, B., & Frese, M. (2008). Mind/body psychological treatments for irritable bowel syndrome. *Advance Access, 5*(1), 41-50.

Segal, Z.V., et al. (2010). Antidepressant monotherapy vs sequential pharmacotherapy and mindfulness-based cognitive therapy, or placebo, for relapse prophylaxis in recurrent depression. *Archives of General Psychiatry, 67*(12), 1256-1264.

While, A. (2009). Mindfulness: me time counts. *British Journal of Community Nursing, 15*(11), 570.

Zeidan, F., & Johnson, S. (2010). Effects of brief and sham mindfulness meditation on mood and cardiovascular variables. *Journal of Alternative and Complementary Medicine, 16*(8), 867-873.

Contributed by Lois Angelo.

Refer to the "Applying the Art" feature for an example of a nurse using therapeutic communication with a patient experiencing obsessive-compulsive disorder.

Health Teaching and Health Promotion

Health teaching is a significant nursing intervention for patients with anxiety disorders. Patients may conceal symptoms for years before seeking treatment, with problems frequently being disclosed during examination of a comorbid condition. More than 50% of people who experience panic attacks seek medical treatment at one time or another. Teaching about the specific disorder and available effective treatments is a major step to improving the quality of life of these patients. Giving patients written information about support groups/telephone support groups, Internet sites, nearby clinics, and medication handouts, for example, is all part of health teaching and health promotion.

In the community or hospital setting, the nurse teaches the patient about signs and symptoms of the disorder, theory regarding causes or risk factors, and risk of co-occurrence with other disorders, especially substance abuse and/or depression. Medication to target the individual's specific disorder, use of relaxation exercises, and availability of specialized treatments such as cognitive behavioral therapy are part of health teaching and health promotion.

Patients with anxiety disorders are usually able to meet their own basic physical needs. Sleep, however, can be a real problem. Patients with anxiety disorders often experience sleep disturbance and nightmares. Teaching patients ways to promote sleep (e.g., warm bath, warm milk, relaxing music) and monitoring sleep through a journal are useful interventions.

Milieu Therapy

As mentioned, most patients with anxiety disorders can be treated successfully as outpatients. Hospital admission is necessary only if severe anxiety or symptoms that interfere with the individual's health are present, or if the individual is suicidal. If or when hospitalization is necessary, the following features of the therapeutic milieu can be especially helpful to the patient:

- Structuring the daily routine to offer physical safety and predictability, thus reducing anxiety over the unknown
- Providing daily activities to promote sharing and cooperation
- Providing therapeutic interactions, including one-on-one nursing care and behavior contracts
- Including the patient in decisions about his or her own care

Psychotherapy

Among the most useful therapies are cognitive behavioral therapies (CBTs), which provide education, address cognitive distortions, and present behavioral approaches in an attempt to reduce symptoms and increase involvement with others and the environment. The cognitive element of CBT refers to teaching people to restructure their thinking and examine their assumptions, problems, or concerns so that problems or concerns seem more amenable to change, and hold less negative emotional impact. Essentially, the therapist helps patients correct their faulty conceptions and helps them change their "self signals" or "self talk." Teaching people to successfully redefine their fears and to look at themselves in a new and more positive way can trigger chemical changes in the brain similar to those caused by medications.

CBT essentially challenges core beliefs that are causing a person distress. The following are examples of such beliefs (Sadock & Sadock, 2007):

- Panic attacks: catastrophic misinterpretations of bodily and mental disturbances
- Phobias: danger in specific avoidable situations
- Obsessive-compulsive disorders: repeated warnings or doubting about safety and repetitive acts to ward off threats
- Anxiety disorders: fear of physical or psychological threats

APPLYING THE ART

A Person With Obsessive-Compulsive Disorder

SCENARIO: Eight-year-old Tommy Jansen came to see the school nurse I worked with during my community nursing leadership rotation. His productive cough and a temperature of 101.2° F prompted a call to his mother. While we waited, Tommy looked worried. "Germs make people sick," he said. I nodded. "But how did I get sick when [holding out his red dry hands] I wash my hands lots of times just like Mommy does?" Tommy took a tissue for a cough. "Maybe I got sick because I forgot to use a tissue to hold the doorknob like Mommy does." When Mrs. Jansen arrived, I introduced myself and we talked privately while Tommy's make-up assignments were being gathered.

THERAPEUTIC GOAL: By the end of this interaction, Tommy will acknowledge needing help to manage his anxiety and ritualistic hand washing.

STUDENT-PATIENT INTERACTION	THOUGHTS, COMMUNICATION TECHNIQUES, AND MENTAL HEALTH NURSING CONCEPTS
Mrs. Jansen: "I'm going to get Tommy to his pediatrician this afternoon. He didn't carry a fever this morning, though he did act a little grouchy."	Tommy looked relieved to see his mother. I don't observe any signs of abuse or neglect.
Student's feelings: Poor little guy—I wonder about that.	
Student: "You're concerned about him." *She nods.* "Mrs. Jansen, Tommy worried that he got sick from germs, despite, as he said, 'washing my hands lots of times like Mommy'."	*He's already a worrier at 8 years old. Sounds like he's afraid that getting sick is his fault.*
Student's feelings: I just met this person yet here I am jumping in, which means I might make a mistake. I guess I'd rather make a mistake by trying to help than by saying nothing. Guess I'm anxious.	
Mrs. Jansen: *Looking stricken.* "My poor baby! I didn't want my problem to affect him."	I *give information* about Tommy. From looking at Tommy's hands and from what he is saying, this could be a problem. I am concerned that his mother has some obsessive-compulsive traits.
Student: "Your problem?"	I use *restatement.* Because Mrs. Jansen is able to identify a problem, she may be showing some *insight.*
Mrs. Jansen: "Until now I've been convincing myself that I just wanted my house clean."	She uses *denial* and *rationalization.*
Student's feelings: How could she not see that her behavior represents more than just keeping her house clean?	
Student: "How do you explain all the hand washing and using tissues to not touch doorknobs?"	Although I asked an *open* question, this came out like I was being critical of her, like I'm *challenging* or even accusing her.
Student's feelings: I didn't mean to sound like I'm blaming her. This isn't about a logical decision. It's about a disorder.	
Mrs. Jansen: *Looks down. Silent.*	
Student: "I'm sorry I pushed you for an explanation. This must be so difficult."	I work on restoring trust by attempting to *translate into feelings.*
	I hope I did the right thing by saying I'm sorry.
Mrs. Jansen: *Nods, then makes brief eye contact.* "Since Tommy's dad went to Iraq, I worry all the time. I know I sound crazy, but when I try to stop washing my house, my hands, the doorknobs, I see Tom, Sr. getting blown up by a suicide bomber."	Worrying "all the time" sounds like *generalized anxiety disorder.* The obsessive worry that gets relieved by the washing rituals sounds like *OCD.* Both disorders cause such distress. Her *self-esteem* sounds low, especially about her *mothering role.*
Student's feelings: I would worry too with my loved one in Iraq. She worries about "sounding crazy." The stigma of mental illness interferes with people feeling okay about seeking treatment. I feel concern toward her.	
Student: "You feel kind of scared so often and so alone."	I attempt to *translate* into feelings.
Student's feelings: I want to always show nonjudgmental acceptance. I show empathy when I reflect underlying feelings. I feel sad at all she has to carry. She obviously cares about her son.	

APPLYING THE ART—cont'd

A Person With Obsessive-Compulsive Disorder

STUDENT-PATIENT INTERACTION	THOUGHTS, COMMUNICATION TECHNIQUES, AND MENTAL HEALTH NURSING CONCEPTS
Mrs. Jansen: *Tears in her eyes.* "While I wash things, my mind rests a minute. Then I look at my bloody raw hands! Now, I've worried Tommy. Poor kid deserves better than me." **Student:** "Mrs. Jansen, sounds like you're feeling really down on yourself."	I assess her *self-esteem.* Low self-esteem, *depressed mood,* and *suicide* ideation go hand-in-hand. I *validate* to see if I've understood her meaning.
Mrs. Jansen: "Sometimes I feel panicky...like giving up." **Student:** "Like giving up...as in suicide?" **Student's feelings:** *I feel awkward asking about suicide, but I would rather feel funny asking, than overlook a suicide cue.*	*Asking* about suicide does not plant the idea of suicide.
Mrs. Jansen: "No, never. I wouldn't do that to Tommy, Jr. The only time I can resist cleaning for a while is when Tommy needs me to help him with something at home or when I watch him play soccer." **Student's feelings:** *I'm so relieved that she answered "no" immediately even if the reason is Tommy rather than self.*	She focuses so many of her responses in terms of her son. Mrs. Jansen recognizes that resisting the compulsion is healthy behavior. I *validate* the meaning.
Student: "So sometimes you are able to delay the compulsive washing behavior. How do you feel, then?" **Student's feelings:** *I called the behavior "compulsive." I hope that naming the behavior with the word "compulsive" does not threaten her.*	I *give support* by saying, "you are able to...." I then ask an *open question.*
Mrs. Jansen: "Proud of myself, but also scared for Tom, Sr. You said 'compulsive.' I've heard of that on Dr. Phil."	Mrs. Jansen identified hearing about *OCD* on television. Maybe that helped her readiness to talk about her ritualistic behaviors.
Student: *Nods.* "Obsessive-compulsive disorder responds to medication and therapy. You don't have to do this all by yourself." **Student's feelings:** *I feel hopeful that Mrs. Jansen really will seek treatment.*	I *validate* the meaning and *assess* her feelings. I do a little teaching as I give information that OCD responds to treatment.
Mrs. Jansen: *Looking down at her red raw hands.* "I'm ready for Tommy's sake." *I watch and wait.* "And for myself." *As Tommy rejoins us, Mrs. Jansen asks the school nurse for the community mental health number.*	

There are currently several forms of behavioral therapy, which involves teaching and physical practice of activities to decrease anxious or avoidant behaviors. As noted earlier, one form of behavioral therapy is relaxation training, examples of which include the following:

- *Modeling*—mimicking appropriate behaviors in situations
- *Systematic desensitization*—gradually exposing a person to the feared object or situation until the person is free of incapacitating anxiety
- *Response prevention*—starts with the therapist preventing the compulsion, such as hand washing, and gradually helping the patient limit the time between rituals until the urge dissipates

- *Thought stopping*—examples include snapping a rubber band on one's wrist to stop an obsession or negative thought

Pharmacological, Biological, and Complementary and Alternative Therapies

Anxiety disorders are chronic and incurable conditions, although in most cases treatable, and there are many helpful treatments available. Several classes of medications have been found to be effective in the treatment of anxiety disorders. Psychopharmacology is an important adjunct to use with other therapies, especially cognitive behavioral therapy (CBT). Best evidence research points to the fact that when the serotonergic system is modulated (SSRIs, CBT) by itself, or with the noradrenergic system (serotonin-norepinephrine reuptake inhibitors [SNRIs]), anxiety symptoms are alleviated much more than by using traditional antidepressants (tricyclics) alone. The following medications have been shown to be helpful (Preston et al., 2010; Satcher et al., 2005):

1. Benzodiazepines: Prescribed for *short-term treatment only;* not recommended for use by patients with substance dependence problems
2. Buspirone: Management of anxiety disorders or short-term relief of anxiety symptoms, especially GAD
3. SSRIs: First-line treatment for all anxiety disorders
4. SNRIs: Examples include venlafaxine, milnacipran, and duloxetine; only venlafaxine is currently approved for panic disorder (PD), generalized anxiety disorder (GAD), and social affective disorder (SAD)
5. Tricyclic antidepressants: Second- or third-line use in people with PD, GAD, and SAD; clomipramine is effective in obsessive-compulsive disorder (OCD)

6. MAOIs: Recently being used in people with social anxiety disorder (SAD) and rejection sensitivity

Refer to Table 11-9 for trade and generic names of common medications and Table 11-10 for therapeutic modalities used to treat specific anxiety disorders.

Antidepressants

As stated previously, selective serotonin reuptake inhibitors (SSRIs) are the first-line treatment for anxiety disorders. They are preferable to the tricyclic antidepressants (TCAs) because they have more rapid onset of action, have fewer problematic side effects, and are more effective. Monoamine oxidase inhibitors (MAOIs) are reserved for treatment-resistant conditions because of the risk of life-threatening hypertensive crisis if the patient does not follow dietary restrictions. (Patients cannot eat foods containing tyramine and must be given specific dietary instructions.) Venlafaxine (Effexor) and duloxetine (Cymbalta) are serotonin-norepinephrine reuptake inhibitors (SNRIs) used to treat anxiety disorders.

TABLE 11-9	MEDICATIONS COMMONLY USED IN THE TREATMENT OF ANXIETY DISORDERS	
GENERIC NAME	**TRADE NAME**	**COMMENTS**
Benzodiazepines		
Alprazolam*	Xanax Xanax XR	Anxiolytic effects result from depressing neurotransmission in the limbic system and cortical areas. Useful for short-term treatment of anxiety; dependence and tolerance develop. These drugs are NOT indicated as a primary treatment for OCD or PTSD.
Diazepam	Valium	
Lorazepam*	Ativan	
Oxazepam	Serax	
Chlordiazepoxide	Librium	
Clorazepate	Tranxene	
Buspirone		
Buspirone hydrochloride†	BuSpar	Alleviates anxiety, but works best before benzodiazepines have been tried. Less sedating than benzodiazepines. Does not appear to produce physical or psychological dependence. Requires 3 or more weeks to be effective.
Selective Serotonin Reuptake Inhibitors (SSRIs)		
First Line		
Citalopram	Celexa	
Escitalopram	Lexapro	Escitalopram not useful with SAD or PD
Fluoxetine	Prozac	
Fluvoxamine	Luvox	
Paroxetine	Paxil	
Sertraline	Zoloft	
Dual-Action Reuptake Inhibitors (Serotonin and Norepinephrine) (SNRIs)		
First Line		
Duloxetine	Cymbalta	Acts within 1 to 2 weeks
Venlafaxine	Effexor	

GENERIC NAME	TRADE NAME	COMMENTS
TABLE 11-9	**MEDICATIONS COMMONLY USED IN THE TREATMENT OF ANXIETY DISORDERS—cont'd**	
Tricyclic Antidepressants (TCAs)		
Second or Third Line		
Amitriptyline	Elavil	Clomipramine effective with OCD,
Clomipramine	Anafranil	PD, GAD, SAD; may also respond
Desipramine	Norpramin	to Surmontil
Doxepin	Sinequan	
Imipramine	Tofranil	
Maprotiline	Ludiomil	
Nortriptyline	Pamelor	
Trimipramine	Surmontil	
Amoxapine	Asendin	
Beta-Blockers		
Propranolol	Inderal	Used to relieve physical symptoms of
Atenolol	Tenormin	anxiety, as in performance anxiety (stage fright). Act by attaching to sensors that direct arousal messages.

*Most commonly used benzodiazepines for treating chronic or unpredictable anxiety syndromes.
†Useful as a first-line treatment in GAD.
GAD, Generalized anxiety disorder; *OCD*, obsessive-compulsive disorder; *PD*, panic disorder; *PTSD*, posttraumatic stress disorder; *SAD*, seasonal affective disorder.
Adapted from Varcarolis, E. M. (2006). *Manual of psychiatric mental health nursing care plans* (3rd ed., p. 151). St Louis: Saunders. Benzodiazepine dosages updated from Lehne, R. A. (2007). *Pharmacology for nursing care* (6th ed.). St Louis: Saunders.

Antidepressants have the secondary benefit of treating co-occurring depressive disorders in patients. Because anxiety and depression frequently occur together, these agents may bring welcome benefits to patients. However, there are three notes of caution. First, when treatment is started, low doses of SSRIs must be used because of the activating effect, which temporarily increases anxiety symptoms. Second, in patients with co-occurring bipolar disorder, use of an antidepressant may cause a manic episode, which requires the addition of mood stabilizers or even antipsychotic agents. Third, use of MAOIs is contraindicated in patients with comorbid substance abuse because of the risk of hypertensive crisis with use of stimulant drugs.

Anxiolytics

Anxiolytic drugs (also called *antianxiety drugs*) are often used to treat the somatic and psychological symptoms of anxiety disorders. When moderate or severe anxiety is reduced, patients are better able to participate in treatment directed at their underlying problems. Benzodiazepines are most commonly prescribed because they have a quick onset of action. Because of the potential for dependence, however, these medications should ideally be used for *short periods only* until other medications or treatments reduce symptoms. It is important for the nurse to monitor for side effects of the benzodiazepines, including sedation, ataxia, and decreased cognitive function. Benzodiazepines are not recommended for patients with a known substance use problem and should not be given to women who

are pregnant or breast-feeding. Box 11-1 lists important information on patient and family medication teaching.

Buspirone (BuSpar) is an alternative anxiolytic medication that does not cause dependence; however, 2 to 4 weeks are required for it to become fully effective. Its usefulness in anxiety disorders is probably limited to the treatment of GAD.

Other Classes of Medication

Other classes of medication sometimes used to treat anxiety disorders include beta-blockers, antihistamines, and anticonvulsants. These agents are often added if the first course of treatment is ineffective. Beta-blockers have been used to treat panic disorder and social anxiety disorder (SAD). Anticonvulsants have shown some benefit in the management of GAD, SAD, and co-occurring depression with SAD or panic disorder. See Box 11-1 for information on patient and family medication teaching.

Complementary and Alternative Medicine (CAM)

Among the primary "natural" substances purported to relieve anxiety are kava kava and valerian root. Although randomized controlled studies are underway, available scientific evidence regarding the efficacy of any of these agents in the treatment of anxiety disorders is sparse.

Kava Kava

For hundreds of years, kava kava has been used as part of a ceremonial drink in the Pacific Islands. It has been believed that this

TABLE 11-10   ACCEPTED TREATMENTS FOR SELECTED ANXIETY DISORDERS*

DISORDER	PHARMACOTHERAPY	THERAPEUTIC MODALITY	COMMENTS
Panic disorder (PD)	High-potency benzodiazepines Antidepressants (TCAs and SSRIs)	CBT (cognitive behavioral therapy) • Relaxation techniques • Breathing techniques • Cognitive restructuring • Systematic desensitization • In vivo exposure aimed at eliminating avoidance behaviors	Benzodiazepines (short term) to reduce or eliminate panic attacks in initial phase of treatment Antidepressants may decrease panic episodes and treat underlying depression CBT teaches new coping skills and ways to reframe thinking
Generalized anxiety disorder (GAD)	When medications are indicated: • Buspirone (BuSpar) reduces rumination and worry, not addictive • SSRI and TCA antidepressants effective with chronic anxiety • Gabapentin (antiseizure drug) used to reduce anxiety	Cognitive therapy Behavioral therapy Stress management Relaxation training Aerobic level exercises	Many patients are helped with psychological approaches and may not need medications
Social phobia/ social anxiety disorder (SAD)	SSRIs may help lessen rejection sensitivity Beta-blockers target physical symptoms of anxiety (e.g., propranolol)	Cognitive behavioral therapy	Benzodiazepines can be addictive over the long term and are not really a drug of choice for social anxiety disorder
Obsessive-compulsive disorder (OCD)	SSRIs reduce OCD symptoms directly (e.g., fluvoxamine [Luvox] and fluoxetine [Prozac]) TCAs (e.g., clomipramine [Anafranil])	Exposure and response prevention (emotionally difficult treatment for patients yet up to 75-80% successful) SSRIs reduce OCD symptoms directly	Effective and necessary in addition to serotonergic medications Exposure in vivo plus response prevention are the crucial essential factors Complete remission is not common

MAOI, Monoamine oxidase inhibitor; *SSRI,* selective serotonin reuptake inhibitor; *TCA,* tricyclic antidepressant.
*The sooner the treatment is initiated, the greater the chance of successful recovery.
Updated from Varcarolis, E. (2002). *Foundations of psychiatric mental health nursing* (4th ed., p. 331). Philadelphia: WB Saunders; reprinted with permission; Preston, J.D., O'Neal, J.H., & Talaga, M.C. (2010). *Handbook of clinical psychopharmacology for therapists* (6th ed.). Oakland, CA: New Harbinger Publications; Preston, J., & Johnson, J. (2011). *Clinical psychopharmacology made ridiculously simple* (6th ed.). Miami, FL: MedMaster.

herb can elevate mood, well-being, contentment, and feelings of relaxation. However, now the medical community believes kava kava may increase psychiatric symptoms and can be dangerous. Even though some countries have removed kava kava from the market, it is still available in the United States. However, in March of 2002 the FDA issued a consumer advisory warning of potential risk of liver failure associated with kava kava (UMM, 2009). Kava kava can have multiple drug interactions and potentiate the effects of certain medications, such as anticonvulsants, antianxiety agents, diuretics, and many others.

Valerian

Valerian is used for conditions related to anxiety and psychological stress, but it is most commonly used for insomnia (inability to sleep). Although it has proven effective for insomnia, there is insufficient scientific evidence to rate its safety. Valerian, unlike kava kava, is considered safe for most people when used in medical amounts on a short-term basis. Some side effects of valerian are headaches, excitability, uneasiness, and even insomnia (MEDLINE-plus, 2010).

Herbs and dietary supplements are not subject to the same rigorous testing as prescription medications. Also, herbs and dietary supplements are not required to be uniform, and there is no guarantee of bioequivalence of the active compound across preparations. Problems that can occur with the use of psychotropic herbs include toxic side effects and herb-drug interactions.

BOX 11-1   PATIENT AND FAMILY MEDICATION TEACHING: ANXIOLYTIC DRUGS

1. Caution the patient and family:
   - Not to increase dose or frequency of ingestion without prior approval of therapist
   - That these medications reduce the ability to handle mechanical equipment (e.g., cars, saws, and other machinery)
   - Not to drink alcoholic beverages or take other antianxiety drugs because depressant effects of both would be potentiated
   - To avoid drinking beverages containing caffeine because they decrease the desired effects of the drug
2. Recommend that the patient taking benzodiazepines avoid becoming pregnant because these drugs increase the risk of congenital anomalies.
3. Advise the patient not to breast-feed because these drugs are excreted in the milk and would have adverse effects on the infant.

4. Teach a patient who is taking monoamine oxidase inhibitors about the details of a tyramine-restricted diet.
5. Teach the patient that:
   - Cessation of benzodiazepine use after 3 to 4 months of daily use may cause withdrawal symptoms such as insomnia, irritability, nervousness, dry mouth, tremors, convulsions, and confusion.
   - Medications should be taken with, or shortly after, meals or snacks to reduce gastrointestinal discomfort.
   - Drug interactions can occur: antacids may delay absorption; cimetidine interferes with metabolism of benzodiazepines, causing increased sedation; central nervous system depressants, such as alcohol and barbiturates, cause increased sedation; serum phenytoin concentration may become too high because of decreased metabolism.

EVALUATION

Identified outcomes serve as the basis for evaluation. In general, evaluation of outcomes for patients with anxiety disorders deals with questions such as the following:

- Is the patient experiencing a reduced level of anxiety? Describe the level of anxiety supported by the patient's present symptoms.
- Does the patient recognize symptoms as anxiety related? What symptoms does he or she experience when anxiety levels are rising?
- Does the patient continue to display obsessions, compulsions, phobias, worrying, or other symptoms of anxiety disorders? If so, ask the patient to quantify the number of increased or decreased symptoms during the day/night/situation. How does the patient describe the change in the level of intensity?
- What newly learned behaviors does the patient use to help manage anxiety?
- Can the patient adequately perform self-care activities? Describe changes in ability to manage health care needs.
- Can the patient maintain satisfying interpersonal relations? How does the patient describe close relationships now as compared with before treatment?
- Can the patient assume usual roles? Describe the ways certain role performances have improved, and identify role performances that still require interventions.
- Is the patient compliant with medication?

KEY POINTS TO REMEMBER

- The basic emotion of anxiety is differentiated from fear in that anxiety has an unknown or unrecognized source, whereas fear is a reaction to a specific threat.
- Anxiety can be normal, acute, or chronic, as well as adaptive or maladaptive.
- Peplau operationally defined four levels of anxiety. The patient's perceptual field, ability to learn, and physical or other characteristics are different at each level (see Table 11-1).
- Effective psychosocial interventions are different for people experiencing mild to moderate levels of anxiety and for individuals experiencing severe to panic levels of anxiety. Effective psychosocial nursing approaches are suggested in Tables 11-2 and 11-3.
- Defenses against anxiety can be adaptive or maladaptive. Defenses are presented in a hierarchy from healthy to intermediate to immature. Table 11-4 provides examples of adaptive and maladaptive uses of many of the more common defense mechanisms.

- Anxiety disorders are the most common psychiatric disorders in the United States and frequently co-occur with depression or substance abuse.
- Research has identified genetic and biological factors in the etiology of anxiety disorders.
- Psychological theories, cultural influences, and socioeconomic status also are pertinent to the understanding of anxiety disorders.
- Patients with anxiety disorders suffer from panic attacks, irrational fears, excessive worrying, uncontrollable rituals, or severe reactions to stress.
- People with anxiety disorders are often too embarrassed or ashamed to seek psychiatric help. Instead, they consult their primary care providers about multiple somatic complaints.
- One form of psychotherapy in particular is effective for treating anxiety disorders—cognitive behavioral therapy (CBT).
- Interventions include counseling, milieu therapy, promotion of self-care activities, psychobiological intervention, and health teaching.

APPLYING CRITICAL JUDGMENT

1. Ms. Smith, a patient with OCD, washes her hands until they are cracked and bleeding. Your nursing goal is to promote healing of her hands. What interventions will you plan?

2. This is Mr. Olivetti's third emergency department visit in a week. He is experiencing severe anxiety accompanied by many physical symptoms. He clings to you, desperately crying, "Help me! Help me! Don't let me die!" Diagnostic tests have ruled out a physical disorder. The patient outcome has been identified as "Patient anxiety level will be reduced to moderate/mild within 1 hour." What are some of the effective interventions you should use?

3. Mrs. Zeamans is a patient with GAD. She has a history of substance abuse and is a recovering alcoholic. During a clinic visit, she tells you she plans to ask the psychiatrist to prescribe diazepam (Valium) to use when she feels anxious. She asks whether you think this is a good idea. How would you respond? What other kind of medications might the physician order?

CHAPTER REVIEW QUESTIONS

Choose the most appropriate answer(s).

1. Which nursing action is most effective for severely anxious patients?
   1. Detailing differences among various patients
   2. Encouraging group participation
   3. Providing brief information sessions
   4. Increasing opportunities for making decisions

2. During a panic attack, the client demonstrates rapid breathing and appears pale. What is the initial nursing intervention?
   1. Reorient the patient to person, place, time.
   2. Give an IM injection of Ativan.
   3. Encourage the patient to take deep breaths.
   4. Call the physician.

3. The nurse is aware that a side effect of Xanax is:
   1. adverse reactions with specific foods.
   2. hypertension.
   3. dependency.
   4. photosensitivity.

4. A client continually repeats almost every detail and etiology of his wife's serious illness without any emotion. This behavior indicates the defense mechanism of:
   1. intellectualization.
   2. repression.
   3. displacement.
   4. projection.

5. A young adolescent has a crush on a boy in the neighborhood that keeps avoiding her. However, she tells her mother, "I think that he may love me." This is an example of the defense mechanism of:
   1. suppression.
   2. rationalization.
   3. denial.
   4. projection.

REFERENCES

Allgulander, C. (2009). *Generalized anxiety disorder: between now and DSM-V*. Retrieved February 3, 2011, from www.mdconsult/das/article/body.

American Nurses Association, American Psychiatric Nurses Association, & International Society of Psychiatric-Mental Health Nurses. (2007). *Psychiatric–mental health nursing: scope and standards of practice*. Silver Springs, MD: Nursesbooks.org.

American Psychiatric Association. (2000). *Diagnostic and statistical manual of mental disorders (DSM-IV-TR)* (4th ed., text rev.). Washington, DC: Author.

Beck, C. T. (2011). Secondary traumatic stress in nurses: a systemic review. *Archives of Psychiatric Nursing, 25*(1), 1–10.

Black, D. W., & Andreasen, N. A. (2011). *Introductory textbook of psychology* (5th ed.). Washington, DC: American Psychiatric Publishing.

Harvard Health Publications (2011). *Understanding the stress response.* Retrieved July 27, 2011, from www.health.harvard.edu/newsletters/Harvard_Mental_Health.

Hemmings, S. M. J., & Stein, D. J. (2006). The current status of association studies in obsessive-compulsive disorder. In D. J. Stein (Ed.), Obsessive compulsive spectrum disorders. *Psychiatric Clinics of North America 29*(2), 441–444.

Howland, R. H. (2010). Potential adverse effects of discontinuing psychotropic drugs. *Journal of Psychosocial Nursing, 48*(9), 11–14.

Kessler, R. C., Berglund, P., Demler, O., et al. (2005). Lifetime prevalence and age-of-onset distributions of DSM-IV disorders in the national comorbidity survey replication. *Archives of General Psychiatry, 62*, 593–602.

Martin, E. L., Ressler, K. J., Binder, E., & Nemeroff, C. B. (2009). *The neurobiology of anxiety disorders, brain imaging, genetics, and psychoneurobiology*. Retrieved February 3, 2011, from www.md consult.com/das/article/body 234818638–6/jorg=ccli.

MEDLINEplus, U.S. National Library of Medicine, & NIH. (2010). *Valerian*. Retrieved February 11, 2011, from www.nlm.nih.gov/MEDLINEplus/druginfo/natural/870.html.

Moorhead, S., Johnson, M., Maas, M. L., & Swanson, E. (2008). *Nursing outcomes classification (NOC)* (4th ed.). St Louis: Mosby.

North American Nursing Diagnosis Association International (NANDA-I). (2012). *NANDA nursing diagnoses: definitions and classification 2012-2014*. Philadelphia: Author.

Peplau, H. E. (1968). A working definition of anxiety. In S. F. Burd, & M. A. Marshall (Eds.), *Some clinical approaches to psychiatric nursing*. New York: Macmillan.

Pertusa, A., Fullana, M. A., Singh, S., Alonso, P., Menchon, J. M., et al. (2008). Compulsive hoarding: OCD symptom, distinct clinical syndrome, or both? *American Journal of Psychiatry, 165*, 1289–1298.

Pines, A., & Aronson, E. (2008). Career burnout: causes and cures. New York, New York: Free Press.

Pollock, M. H., Otto, M. W., Whittmann, & Rosenbaum, J. F. (2010). Anxious patients. In T. A. Stern, G. L. Fricchione, N. H. Cassem, M. S. Jellinek, & J. F. Rosenbaum (Eds.), *Massachusetts General Hospital: handbook of general hospital psychiatry* (6th ed.). Philadelphia: Saunders.

Preston, J. D., O'Neal, J. H., & Talaga, M. C. (2010). *Handbook of clinical psychopharmacology for therapists* (6th ed.). Oakland, CA: New Habinger Publications.

Reese, S. M. (2011). *Burned out? How doctors recover their spark.* Retrieved July 28, 2011, from www.medscape.com/viewarticle/746117?src=nl_topic.

Sadock, B. J., & Sadock, V. A. (2007). *Kaplan and Sadock's synopsis of psychiatry* (10th ed.). Philadelphia: Wolters/Lippincott Williams & Wilkins.

Satcher, D., Delgado, P. L., & Masand, P. S. (2005). A surgeon general's perspective on the unmet needs of patients with anxiety disorders. *Medscape Psychiatry & Mental Health, 10*(2).

Stuart, S. E., Dougherty, D. D., Wilhelm, S., Keuthen, N., & Jenike, M. A. (2008). OCD and OCD-related disorders. In T. A. Stern, J. F. Rosenbaum, M. Fava, J. Biedermann, & S. L. Rauch (Eds.), *Massachusetts General Hospital: comprehensive clinical psychology* (pp. 447–464). Philadelphia: Mosby/Elsevier.

Sullivan, H. S. (1953). *The interpersonal theory of psychiatry.* New York: Norton.

Taylor, C. T., Pollack, M. H., LeBeau, R. T., & Simon, N. M. (2008). Anxiety disorders: panic, social anxiety, and generalized anxiety. In T. A. Stern, J. F. Rosenbaum, M. Fava, J. Biederman, & S. L. Rauch (Eds.), *Massachusetts General Hospital: comprehensive clinical psychiatry.* Philadelphia: Saunders.

University of Maryland Medical Center (UMM). (2009). *Kava kava.* Retrieved February 11, 2011, from www.umm.edu/almed/articles/kava-kava-000259.htm.

Vaillant, G. E. (1994). Ego mechanisms of defense and personality psychopathology. *Journal of Abnormal Psychology, 103*(1), 44–50.

Vaillant, G. E., & Vaillant, C. O. (2004). Normality and mental health. In B. J. Sadock, & V. A. Sadock (Eds.), *Kaplan and Sadock's comprehensive textbook of psychiatry* (8th ed., vol. 1, pp. 583–597). Philadelphia: Lippincott Williams & Wilkins.

Yates, W. R. (2011). *Anxiety disorders.* Retrieved January 9, 2012, from http://emedicine.Medscape.com/article/286227-overview.

Yoder, E. A. (2010). Compassion fatigue in nurses. *Applied Nursing Research, 23*, 191–197. Retrieved February 15, 2011, from www.Medscape.com/view article/732211.

12

Somatoform Disorders and Dissociative Disorders

Elizabeth M. Varcarolis

evolve WEBSITE

http://evolve.elsevier.com/Varcarolis/essentials

KEY TERMS AND CONCEPTS

alternate personality (alter) or subpersonality, p. 202
body dysmorphic disorder (BDD), p. 195
depersonalization/derealization disorder, p. 201
dissociative amnesia, p. 201
dissociative disorders, p. 200
dissociative fugue, p. 201
dissociative identity disorder (DID), p. 202

factitious disorder, p. 192
functional neurological disorder (conversion disorder), p. 194
hypochondriasis, p. 194
la belle indifférence, p. 195
malingering, p. 193
pain disorder, p. 194
secondary gains, p. 196
somatoform disorders, p. 191
somatization, p. 191
subpersonality, p. 202

SELECTED CONCEPT: Somatize
To somatize is the tendency to experience and communicate physical symptoms in response to psychological distress. Although medical tests repeatedly demonstrate no medical basis, people continue to seek relief from their somatic symptoms that are causing significant distress and/or dysfunction.

SELECTED CONCEPT: Dissociation
Everyone uses dissociation. Daydreaming, fantasizing, "zoning out" are all examples of healthy dissociation and can be used in creative ways to solve problems.
  However severe traumatic dissociation comes from major trauma, and an individual is unable to integrate the trauma into their psyche. Depending on the severity and impact of the event, a person may be unable to recall a specific event, experience depersonalization and derealization (refer to text), or in severe cases may separate off into fragmented emotional states, partially formed identities, or break off into full formed identities as in dissociative identity disorder (multiple personalities).

1. Compare and contrast the essential characteristics of somatic symptom disorders versus those of dissociative disorders.
2. Differentiate the key characteristic differences among somatic symptom disorders, malingering, and factitious disorders.
3. Applying patient-centered care, identify five appropriate psychosocial interventions for a patient with somatic complaints that have no medical cause.
4. Describe and elaborate on the central components of three dissociative disorders.
5. Giving clinical examples, compare and contrast dissociative amnesia and dissociative fugue.
6. Discuss three specialized elements in the assessment of a patient with a dissociative disorder.
7. List at least three expected outcomes for patients with somatoform disorders (e.g., hypochondriasis).

Somatoform disorders are a group of disorders characterized by the presence of physical symptoms in the absence of known physical findings or medical illnesses that would explain the symptoms. **Somatization** is the tendency to experience and to report physical symptoms that are associated with significant distress and/or dysfunction. Somatization is associated with increased health care use, functional impairment, provider dissatisfaction, psychiatric comorbidity, and failure to respond to standard treatment. In many cases the symptoms occur a few months or later after a stressful event. For some people, somatization progresses to a form of chronic illness behavior. In the most extreme cases of somatization, the sick role becomes the person's predominant mode of relating to the world (e.g., hypochondriasis).

SOMATOFORM DISORDERS

Somatoform disorders are mental disorders that involve physical symptoms (e.g., gastrointestinal, neurological, urological, pain) for which there is no physical explanation. People with these disorders are often extremely and persistently preoccupied with their perceived health issue, demand unnecessary tests, and do not comply with physician recommendations. Presently there are basically five somatoform disorders: somatization disorder, hypochondriasis, pain disorder, conversion disorder, and body dysmorphic disorder. People who are thought to have a somatoform disorder suffer from significant distress and/or dysfunction, and all incur large health care costs, with the person usually failing to respond to standard treatment. These disorders are grouped together because the symptoms suggest a physical disorder, but after thorough physical exams and laboratory tests are completed no clear organic cause or physiological mechanisms can be identified.

When patients do not obtain an answer from a physician concerning their physical distress, they will often visit several medical facilities (referred to as "doctor shopping"). Unfortunately, these individuals often undergo unnecessary surgeries, invasive diagnostic procedures, and drug trials, all of which can be life-threatening (Braun et al., 2010).

It is important to be reminded that these symptoms are not intentional or under the conscious control of the patient (with the exception of the factitious disorders, which are under the control of the patient). Therefore, a diagnosis of the somatoform disorder requires both a thorough medical examination and a mental health evaluation if the physician suspects somatoform disorder. Yates (2012) advises that any primary anxiety disorder or mood disorder should be ruled out before leaning toward a somatoform disorder.

PREVALENCE AND COMORBIDITY

Prevalence rates of somatoform disorders in the general population are unknown. It is estimated that up to 30% of patients seen by their primary care providers present with unexplained symptoms, and of that 30% a large proportion of these patients are diagnosed with no serious medical basis for their symptoms (Black & Andreasen, 2011).

Differentiating somatic symptom disorders from physical disorders and identifying co-occurring/**comorbid conditions** are significant issues for the primary care provider. Research shows that half of all frequent users of medical care have psychological problems. Psychiatric disorders are frequently present in people who have medically unexplained complaints. A **depressive disorder** can be diagnosed between 50% and 60% of the time and an **anxiety disorder** can be diagnosed between 40% and 50% of the time in patients who present with physical complaints that are unexplained medically (Kroenke & Rosmalen, 2006). Excessive co-occurrence of **substance use** is common in an effort to self-medicate when personality disorders are present.

Therefore a comprehensive physical examination with appropriate diagnostic studies is necessary to rule out medical conditions that can be confused with somatic symptom disorders. Along with a comprehensive medical examination, a thorough psychosocial history is required to clarify a somatic symptom disorder diagnosis as well as any co-occurring mental health issues/disorders.

THEORY

Genetic and Familial Factors

There is no direct evidence of a genetic etiology for any one *specific* somatic symptom disorder. However, some physiological data support a genetic theory that somatization disorder tends to occur in families, presenting in 10% to 20% of first-degree female relatives of women with somatization disorder. Twin studies show an increased risk of conversion disorder in monozygotic twin pairs. First-degree biological relatives of people with chronic pain disorder are more likely to have chronic pain, depressive disorder, and alcohol dependence.

Some believe that genetic and familial factors could play a significant role in the predisposition to somatic symptom disorders. These disorders are associated with the following characteristics:

- Low pain threshold
- Poor ability to express emotions (alexithymia)
- Patterns of information processing characterized by distractibility, impulsiveness, and failure to habituate to repetitive stimuli

Genetic and Environmental Origins

A study by Taylor and associates (2006) supports previous twin studies that report somatic symptom disorders are moderately heritable. The study included monozygotic (MZ) as well as dizygotic twin groups. They evaluated for "health anxiety," which ranges from mild to severe, with severe meeting the criteria for hypochondriasis. There are several facets of "health anxiety" that include health-related fears, disease conviction, excessive health-related behaviors (e.g., "doctor shopping"), and impairment in occupational functioning.

Learning and Sociocultural Factors

Research supports the idea that early experiences and learning are the primary factors of somatic sensitivity and bodily preoccupations. One hypothesis is that an adult presenting with somatic symptom disorder may display attentiveness to the same symptoms that were a source of parental attention during the person's childhood. Constant attention to a specific body part enhances the ability of a person to direct sensations to that body part. Therefore symptoms are reinforced by constant parental attention, and the child learns the benefits of the sick role.

Psychological Theory

One theory is that if the parents are unavailable, harsh, or inconsistent and fail to acknowledge the needs of the child during the separation and individuation phases, a process of self-focus ensues. The child, and later adult, learns to focus on the body as a defense against stress and mental pain because emotional and nurturing needs as a child were not met from the outside world.

Interpersonal Model

There is growing evidence that childhood adversity is linked to adult hypochondriasis. Many patients report traumatic events and substance abuse in their families compared with controls. Yates (2010) identified some childhood influences that are thought to contribute to somatization:

- Children raised in homes where there is a high degree of parental somatization may model somatization.
- Early sexual abuse may be associated with increased risk of somatization later in life.

Childhood physical abuse and sexual abuse are also associated with conversion disorder, dissociative disorder, and

many other disorders (Cely-Serrano & Floet, 2006). Table 12-1 provides clinical examples of each of the somatic symptom disorders and their associated defense mechanisms.

CULTURAL CONSIDERATIONS

Cultural factors can influence an individual's tendency to develop somatic symptoms, as well as the types of symptoms that unconsciously might be used. In some cultures, somatic symptoms may be the first symptoms that indicate a patient may have an underlying anxiety or depressive disorder.

Some sources state that the type and frequency of somatic symptoms vary across cultures. The sensation of burning hands and feet or the impression of worms in the head or ants under the skin is more common in Africa and southern Asia than in North America. Alteration of consciousness with falling is a symptom commonly associated with culture-specific religious and healing rituals. Somatization disorder, which is rarely seen in men in the United States, is often reported in Greek and Puerto Rican men, which suggests that cultural mores may permit these men to use somatization as an acceptable approach to dealing with life stress.

In **some** cultures, certain physical symptoms are believed to result from the casting of spells on the individual. Spellbound individuals often seek the help of traditional healers in addition to modern medical staff. The medical provider may diagnose a non–life-threatening somatic symptom disorder, whereas the traditional healer may offer an entirely different explanation and prognosis. The individual may not show improvement until the traditional healer removes the spell.

MAKING A DIAGNOSIS

When a patient presents with severe preoccupation with unexplained physical symptoms that cannot be explained by a medical disorder, substance use, or another mental disorder, then the psychiatric diagnosis of somatoform disorder must be considered. Because anxiety disorders and mood disorders often present with physical symptoms, these disorders must be ruled out, and with successful treatment, the physical symptoms usually dramatically improve (Yates, 2010). Therefore, a diagnosis of somatoform disorder is made with both a medical and a psychological workup.

However, before moving toward a diagnosis of somatoform disorder, two other disorders must be ruled out: **factitious disorder** and **malingering.**

Factitious Disorder

Factitious disorder refers to deliberate fabrication of symptoms or self-injury without obvious gains (e.g., economic incentive). The unconscious motivation is thought to be for the purpose of assuming the sick role and receiving nurturance, comfort, and attention. A person may exaggerate a symptom, fabricate a symptom, or simulate and/or induce a symptom. For example, a person might inject a caustic substance into the skin to form an abscess, exacerbate a wound, use medication inappropriately, or self-induce fever or seizures.

	DEFENSE	
DISORDER	**MECHANISM**	**EXAMPLE**
Functional neurological disorder (conversion disorder)	Conversion	Jan, a 28-year-old former secretary, awakens one morning to find that she has a tingling in both hands and cannot move her fingers. Two days earlier, Jan's husband had told her that he wanted a separation and that she would have to go back to work to support herself. The conversion of anxiety relates to the separation and the increase in dependency needs to "paralysis of her fingers" so that she is unable to work.
Prominent pain	Displacement	Henry, 47, a laborer, "pulled a muscle" in his back 1 year ago. Two weeks before this, his wife, a waitress, told him that she wanted to go back to school to get her bachelor's degree. He suffers severe, constant pain, despite negative results from myelography, computed tomography, magnetic resonance imaging, and examinations. He watches television all day and collects disability. His wife, unable now to return to school, waits on him and has assumed his home responsibilities. Henry displaces his anxiety over the threat to his own self-esteem by his wife's potential change of status onto "pain in his back." The focus of his anxiety is now on his back and not on his threatened self-esteem.
Body dysmorphic disorder	Symbolism and projection	Michele, a young, attractive woman, is preoccupied with her nose, which she considers too long and ugly. She is constantly concerned by and distressed over her perception. Two plastic surgeons she consulted are hesitant to reshape her nose, but this has not altered her thinking that her nose makes her ugly.
Somatization disorder: Prominent somatic complaints	Somatize	Deanna, 27, presents at the physician's office with excessively heavy menstruation. She tells the nurse that recently she experienced pain "first in my back and then going to every part of my body." She states that she is often bothered by constipation and vomiting when she "eats the wrong food." She says that she was "unwell" and had suffered from seizures and still has them occasionally. The nurse becomes confused, not knowing which symptoms Deanna wants the physician to evaluate. Deanna tells the nurse that she lives at home with her parents because her poor health makes it hard for her to hold a job.
Prominent hypochondriasis health anxiety (hypochondriasis)	Denial and somatization	Julio, 52, lost his wife to colon cancer 5 months earlier, which he "took very well." Recently he saw a sixth physician with the same complaint. He believes that he has liver cancer, despite repeated and extensive diagnostic tests, results of which are all negative. He has ceased seeing his friends, has dropped his hobbies, and spends much of his time checking his sclera and "resting his liver." His son finally demands that he see a doctor.
Psychological factors affecting medical conditions	Denial	

Factitious disorder imposed on another (factitious disorder by proxy) has the same criteria as a factitious disorder, except in this case the deliberate fabrication of symptoms or injury is imposed upon another person, often a child.

Munchausen syndrome is the most severe and chronic form of factitious disorder and can result in self-harm severe enough to require hospitalization; "doctor shopping" in attempts to seek surgery and invasive diagnostic tests is also present. ***Munchausen syndrome imposed on another*** is manifested by a caregiver (usually a mother with a health care background) injuring a child to receive attention or sympathy.

Malingering

Malingering, on the other hand, involves a conscious process of intentionally producing symptoms for an obvious benefit; for example, an employee complains of nonexistent back pain to claim disability income. Often, the symptoms the malingerer chooses are highly subjective and difficult to prove or disprove (e.g., back pain, headache). Often malingerers are attempting to obtain pain medication, receive disability benefits, or seek financial reward from filing a lawsuit against their employer. Malingering is not categorized under the heading of somatic symptom disorders.

CLINICAL PICTURE

Somatoform Disorders

Somatoform disorders are relatively more common in those who are unmarried, nonwhite, poorly educated, and from a rural area (Yates, 2010); they are also more prevalent in women than in men. Cognitive behavioral therapy (CBT) seems to be beneficial for lowering anxiety levels, regulating activities, increasing emotional awareness, and providing cognitive restructuring and interpersonal communication skills (Allen et al., 2006; Yates, 2010). However, these disorders are usually chronic and relapsing, characterized by excessive or maladaptive responses to symptoms, and rarely remit completely. Often the following occur in people with somatic disorders:

1. Disproportionate and persistent concerns about the medical seriousness of one's symptoms
2. High levels of health-related anxiety
3. Excessive time and energy devoted to the symptoms or health concerns

Somatization Disorders

A person with somatization disorder usually has a long history of physician visits for complaints of multiple somatic symptoms. The most frequent symptoms are pain (head, chest, **back,** joints, pelvis), dysphagia, nausea, bloating, constipation, palpitations, dizziness, and shortness of breath, although vague symptoms such as fatigue may also be prominent. Sexual symptoms, such as lack of libido or erectile dysfunction, or pseudoneurological symptoms, such as fainting or colorblindness, may also be present. Usually the disorder appears before the age of 30 years. One or more somatic symptoms is distressing or causes significant functional impairment. When describing their symptoms, individuals may describe their symptoms in very exaggerated and colorful ways or have symptoms that do not generally co-occur with a serious disease (e.g., a strange taste in one's mouth). Patients report significant distress and seek multiple providers for medical care—a process that alleviates the patient's concerns. Individuals with somatization disorders often have histories of repeated surgeries, alcohol or drug abuse, marital instability, and suicide attempts. As previously stressed, anxiety and depression are common comorbid conditions with these disorders.

Hypochondriasis

Hypochondriasis is a widespread phenomenon. Patients with this disorder misinterpret innocent physical sensations as evidence of a serious illness. They cannot be reassured by negative diagnostic test findings, and they seek extensive medical care with frustrating results. Most patients refuse referral to a psychiatrist because they believe their symptoms are physical. Hypochondriacal symptoms often occur concomitant with a

mood or anxiety disorder, and when diagnosed they must be treated. Physical symptoms that are caused by an anxiety or depressive disorder often resolve dramatically with treatment (Yates, 2010). People with hypochondriasis experience severe distress, and their ability to function in personal, social, and occupational roles often is impaired.

No specific socioeconomic factors are associated with this disorder. However, as mentioned previously, many patients exhibiting hypochondriacal symptoms have a history of sexual or physical trauma, parental upheaval, or extensive absence from school during childhood for health reasons. The course of the illness is chronic and relapsing, with symptoms exacerbated during times of stress.

Hypochondriasis Without Somatic Symptoms

Most patients with hypochondriasis present with somatic symptoms as well as total preoccupation with the belief of having a devastating sickness or disease. These individuals are thought to have *prominent health anxiety (hypochondriasis), another form of hypochondriasis.* They have minimal or no somatic symptoms but reveal a disproportionate or excessive preoccupation with having a serious illness. The concerns do not involve a specific sign or symptom, but rather reflect a belief of having an underlying and an undetected medical diagnosis.

Pain Disorder

Prominent pain is one of the most frequent reasons people seek medical attention. When testing rules out any identifiable organic cause for the pain and the discomfort leads to significant impairment, pain disorder may be diagnosed. Although most pain can be alleviated, chronic pain results in significant disability and high health care costs. People with these somatoform disorders often have a very low quality of life because they can be severely disabled by their symptoms. They may live like invalids—working infrequently, not attending school, and avoiding social obligations. Pain is often associated with a stressful life event and is potentiated by secondary gains (attention, freedom from responsibilities or from conflict-producing situations, financial rewards). When these secondary gains are reinforced, the symptoms are also reinforced, making it more difficult for the person to relinquish the symptoms. Chronic pain, real or imagined, is extremely disorganizing and distracting and can make life very difficult. Suicide can be a serious risk for these patients.

Pain is difficult to measure objectively, and individuals react differently to the same source of pain. Frequent comorbid conditions include depression, substance dependence, and personality disorders. These patients are at risk for excessive use of narcotic or sedative medications. Some research suggests that a background of sexual abuse, poor social skills, or trauma is common in people with pain disorder.

The course of pain disorder varies according to the acuity of the symptoms. Acute pain disorders have a favorable prognosis, but chronic pain is more difficult to treat. Antidepressants tend to decrease pain intensity for some.

Conversion Disorders

Conversion disorders are essentially functional neurological disorders. Conversion disorders are marked by symptoms or deficits that affect voluntary motor or sensory functions and that suggest a medical condition (Braun et al., 2010). However, the dysfunction does not correspond to current scientific understanding of known neurological and medical illnesses. The symptoms are neither voluntarily controlled nor culturally sanctioned. Many patients show a lack of emotional concern about the symptoms (la belle indifférence), although others are quite distressed. Common symptoms are involuntary movements, seizures, paralysis, abnormal gait, anesthesia, blindness, and deafness.

The long-held view of conversion disorders is based on psychoanalytic theory. Now there seem to be competing etiologies as well as doubt that the etiology is purely psychological in origin. Functional brain imaging studies are pointing to the understanding of conversion disorders as symptoms related to the brain as well as to the mind-body perspective. A number of studies in people with stress-related disorders (e.g., borderline personality disorder with early abuse, depression with early abuse, and posttraumatic stress disorder [PTSD]) have found that in these patients there is often smaller hippocampal volume in the brain. The diagnosis of *"functional neurological disorder"* instead of conversion disorder has been widely supported by clinicians as more accurate terminology. Because there also seem to be brain changes in many patients who have undergone severe stress earlier in life, the notion that the conversion disorders are purely psychological may be scientifically incorrect (Stone et al., 2010).

Conversion disorders are among the most common of the somatic symptom disorders; they are more prevalent in women and seem to be increasing in the elderly population. Black and Andreasen (2011) estimate that from 20% to 25% of patients admitted to neurological units have conversion symptoms. Socioeconomic factors that seem to be related to conversion disorders include lower education and income levels and residence in rural areas (Black & Andreasen, 2011). Some studies have found an association between childhood physical or sexual abuse and conversion disorder. Common comorbid psychiatric conditions include depression, anxiety, other somatic symptoms of unknown origin, and personality disorders. There are also cases in which a comorbid medical or neurological condition exists but the conversion symptoms are an exaggeration of the original problem.

The course of the disorder is related to its acuity: in cases with acute onset during stressful events, the remission rate is very good. If symptoms have been present for more than 6 months the remission rate is about 50%.

Body Dysmorphic Disorder

Body dysmorphic disorder (BDD) is a highly distressing and impairing disorder. Patients with body dysmorphic disorder usually have a normal appearance, although a small number do show minor defects. The average age of onset is younger than 20 years. Preoccupation with an imagined "defective body part" results in obsessional thinking and compulsive behavior, such as mirror checking and camouflaging. Individuals with BDD may feel great shame and hide or withdraw from others. Many will alter their appearance through plastic surgeries, wrongly perceiving themselves as being ugly or having "hideous physical flaws" (and often people with BDD undergo multiple plastic surgeries). Unfortunately, even when cosmetic surgery is sought, there is **no** relief of symptoms.

Normal social activities related to academic or occupational functioning are impaired. Patients are frequently concerned with the face, skin, genitalia, thighs, hips, and hair. Researchers found that about three fourths of surgeries for BDD patients involved facial features (e.g., rhinoplasty) and breast enlargements (HDN, 2010). Common comorbid diagnoses include major depression, substance use disorder, social phobia (Braun et al., 2010), and obsessive-compulsive disorder. Individuals with BDD reported higher rates of suicidal ideation, suicide attempts, and completed suicides than individuals who did not meet criteria for BDD. The disorder is often kept secret for many years, and the patient does not respond to reassurance. The pharmacological agents of choice for people with BDD are selective serotonin reuptake inhibitor (SSRI) antidepressants and clomipramine (a tricyclic antidepressant) (Braun et al., 2010).

In a study conducted at Harvard and Brown University (Bjornsson et al., 2011), psychiatrists determined that the recovery rate for BDD sufferers over 8 years was 76% and the reoccurrence rate was 14%. This is in direct contrast to the belief that BBD was chronic and the response to treatment was limited.

Pseudocyesis

It is worth mentioning that pseudocyesis is the false belief that one is pregnant, while at the same time the woman's body may mimic the signs and symptoms of pregnancy (e.g., abdominal enlargement, sensations of fetal movement, breast engorgement, and even endocrine changes). These changes occur with no explainable medical reason. This process can also be viewed as a form of a somatoform disorder

NURSING PROCESS: SOMATOFORM DISORDERS

Assessment of patients with somatic symptom disorders is a complex process that requires careful and complete medical examination because 13% to 30% of people diagnosed with a somatic symptom disorder eventually developed an organic condition that was related to the original symptom (Braun et al., 2010). The following sections outline several areas that are not normally included in a nursing assessment but are of considerable importance in the assessment of a patient with suspected somatic symptom disorders.

APPLICATION OF THE NURSING PROCESS

ASSESSMENT

Symptoms and Unmet Needs

Assessment should begin with collection of data about the nature, location, onset, character, and duration of the symptom(s).

Often, patients with conversion disorder report having a sudden loss in function of a body part. "I woke up this morning and couldn't move my arm." Patients with somatization disorder, hypochondriasis, or pain disorder usually discuss their symptoms in dramatic terms. They may use colorful metaphors and exaggerations: "The pain was searing, like a hot sword drawn across my forehead" or "My symptoms are so rare that I've stumped hundreds of doctors." Individuals with body dysmorphic disorder are concerned about only one part of the body, display disgust with the offending part, and often seek cosmetic surgery.

Information should be sought about patients' ability to meet their own basic needs. Tachypnea and tachycardia may be instigated by anxiety. Nutrition, fluid balance, and elimination needs should be evaluated because patients with somatization disorders often complain of gastrointestinal distress, diarrhea, constipation, and anorexia. The physiological need for sex may be altered by patient experiences of painful intercourse, pain in another part of the body, or lack of interest in sex.

Rest, comfort, activity, and hygiene needs may be altered as a result of patient problems such as fatigue, weakness, insomnia, muscle tension, pain, and avoidance of diversional activity. Safety and security needs may be threatened by patient experiences of blindness, deafness, loss of balance and falling, and anesthesia of various parts of the body.

Voluntary Control of Symptoms

During assessment it is important to determine if the symptoms are under the patient's voluntary control. People with somatoform disorders do not have voluntary control over their symptoms (with the exception of factitious disorders). The patient does not understand the relationship between symptoms and interpersonal conflicts that may be obvious to others, and often suffers extreme physical discomfort and mental anguish.

Secondary Gains

The nurse tries to identify the benefits a person might be receiving from the symptoms. Secondary gains are those benefits derived from the symptoms alone; for example, in the sick role, the patient is not able to perform the usual family, work, and social functions, and receives extra attention from loved ones. If a patient derives personal benefit from the symptoms, relinquishing the symptoms is more difficult. The clinician works with the patient to achieve the same benefits through healthier avenues (e.g., assertiveness training). One approach to identifying the presence of secondary gains is to ask the patient questions such as the following:

- What abilities have you lost since the development of your symptom(s)?
- How has this problem affected your life?

Cognitive Style

In general, patients with these disorders misinterpret physical stimuli and distort reality regarding their symptoms. For example, sensations a normal individual might interpret as a headache might suggest a brain tumor to a patient with predominant health anxiety (hypochondriasis). Exploring the patient's cognitive style is helpful in distinguishing between predominant health anxiety (hypochondriasis) and predominant somatic complaints (somatization disorder). The patient with predominant health anxiety exhibits more anxiety and an obsessive attention to detail, along with a preoccupation with the fear of serious illness. The patient with predominant somatic complaints is often rambling and vague about the details of his or her many symptoms and gives a disorganized history.

Ability to Communicate Feelings and Emotional Needs

Patients with somatoform disorders have difficulty communicating their emotional needs. As children, many of these patients had difficulty expressing emotions in their families and would use somatization as an unconscious expression of anxiety, depression, or fear. As adults, patients are able to describe their physical symptoms, but are unable to verbalize feelings, especially those related to anger, guilt, and dependence. As a consequence, the somatic symptom may be the patient's chief means of communicating emotional needs. Psychogenic blindness or hearing loss may represent the symbolic statement, "I can't face this knowledge." For example, after a wife overheard friends discussing her husband's sexual infidelity, she developed total deafness.

Dependence on Medication

Individuals experiencing many somatic complaints often become dependent on medication to relieve pain or anxiety or to induce sleep. Physicians prescribe anxiolytic agents for patients who seem highly anxious and concerned about their symptoms. Patients often return to the physician for prescription renewal or seek treatment from numerous physicians. It is important that the nurse assess the type and the amount of medications being used.

ASSESSMENT GUIDELINES

It is always important to ensure that an underlying medical condition has been eliminated from the differential diagnosis. Some important differential diagnostic considerations for hypochondriasis are multiple sclerosis, myasthenia gravis, thyroid or parathyroid disease, and other autoimmune disorders (e.g., systemic lupus erythematosus and others). However, the presence of a general medical condition does not exclude the possibility of a coexisting hypochondriasis.

Somatoform Disorders

1. Ensure that a thorough physical examination with appropriate medical tests has been completed.
2. Assess for nature, location, onset, characteristics, and duration of the symptom(s).
3. Assess the patient's ability to meet basic needs.
4. Assess risks to safety and security needs of the patient as a result of the symptom(s).
5. Determine whether the symptoms are under the patient's voluntary control.
6. Identify any secondary gains that the patient is experiencing from symptom(s).

7. Explore the patient's cognitive style and ability to communicate feelings and needs.
8. Assess type and amount of medication the patient is using.

DIAGNOSIS

Patients with somatic disorders present various nursing problems. *Ineffective Coping* is frequently diagnosed. Causal statements might include the following:
- Distorted perceptions of body functions and symptoms
- Chronic pain of psychological origin
- Dependence on pain relievers or anxiolytics
- Table 12-2 identifies potential nursing diagnoses for patients with somatic symptom disorders.

OUTCOMES IDENTIFICATION

The overall goal in treating somatic symptom disorders is that people with these disorders will eventually be able to live as normal a life as possible. They may never be pain free or free of other symptoms, but it is hoped the quality of their lives can be improved.

The following are examples of potential outcome criteria:
- Patient will articulate feelings such as anger, shame, guilt, and remorse.
- Patient will resume performance of work role behaviors.
- Patient will identify ineffective coping patterns.

- Patient will make realistic appraisal of strengths and weaknesses.
- Patient will allow family to be involved in decision making.

PLANNING

Because patients with somatoform disorders are seldom admitted to psychiatric units specifically because of these disorders, long-term interventions usually take place on an outpatient basis or in the home. Short-term planning may be initiated if the patient is admitted to a medical-surgical unit. Such a stay is usually short, and discharge will occur as soon as diagnostic tests are completed and negative results are received.

Nursing/clinician interventions should focus initially on establishing a helping relationship with the patient. The therapeutic relationship is vital to the success of the care plan, given the patient's resistance to the concept that no physical cause for the symptom exists and the patient's tendency to change caregivers.

To be successful, therapeutic interventions must address ways to help the patient meet needs without resorting to somatization. The secondary gains the patient has derived from illness behaviors become less important to the patient when underlying needs can be met directly. The optimal goal is not only to relieve symptoms (which the patient believes are real) but also, and more importantly, to increase quality of life and independence. Collaboration with family or significant others is essential for success.

TABLE 12-2 POTENTIAL NURSING DIAGNOSES FOR SOMATOFORM DISORDERS

SIGNS AND SYMPTOMS	NURSING DIAGNOSES*
Inability to meet occupational, family, or social responsibilities because of symptoms	*Ineffective Coping* *Ineffective Role Performance*
Inability to participate in usual community activities or friendships because of psychogenic symptoms	*Impaired Social Interaction* *Ineffective Relationship*
Dependence on pain relievers	*Powerlessness*
Distortion of body functions and symptoms	*Disturbed Body Image*
Presence of secondary gains by adoption of sick role	*Pain (Acute or Chronic)*
Inability to meet family role function and need for family to assume role function of the somatic individual	*Interrupted Family Processes* *Ineffective Sexuality Pattern*
Assumption of some of the roles of the somatic parent by the children	*Impaired Parenting*
Shifting of the sexual partner's role to that of caregiver or parent and of the patient's role to that of recipient of care	*Risk for Caregiver Role Strain*
Feeling of inability to control symptoms or understand why he or she cannot find help	*Chronic Low Self-Esteem* *Spiritual Distress*
Development of negative self-evaluation related to losing body function, feeling useless, or not feeling valued by significant others	*Hopelessness*
Inability to take care of basic self-care needs related to conversion symptom (paralysis, seizures, pain, fatigue)	*Those that focus on Self-Care Deficit (e.g., Bathing/Hygiene, Dressing/Grooming, Feeding, Toileting)*
Inability to sleep related to psychogenic pain	*Disturbed Sleep Pattern*

*Nursing Diagnoses—Definitions and Classification 2012-2014. Copyright © 2012, 1994-2012 by NANDA International. Used by arrangement with Blackwell Publishing Limited, a company of John Wiley and Sons, Inc.

IMPLEMENTATION

Communication Guidelines

Generally for patients with somatic symptom disorders, nursing interventions take place in the home or clinic setting. The nurse attempts to help the patient improve overall functioning through the development of effective coping and communication strategies. Remember, when patients complain of physical symptoms, take the symptoms seriously, because even if a medical explanation is not found the symptoms are real and troublesome to the patient. Table 12-3 lists several possible interventions for patients with somatic symptom disorders.

Working with people who have somatoform disorders can be frustrating, and you and other staff may find yourself avoiding interaction with them. However, it is important to note that when people feel they are receiving care and attention, the intensity of their symptoms tends to diminish. As the symptoms are alleviated, it becomes easier to address emotional issues.

Health Teaching and Health Promotion

When somatization is present, the patient's ability to perform self-care activities may be impaired and nursing or caregiving intervention is necessary. In general, interventions involve the use of a straightforward approach to support the highest level of self-care of which the patient is capable. For patients manifesting paralysis, blindness, or severe fatigue, an effective nursing approach is to support patients while expecting them to feed, bathe, or groom themselves. For example, the patient who demonstrates arm paralysis can be expected to eat using the other arm. The patient who is experiencing blindness can be told where foods are located on his or her plate by comparing the plate to a clock face. These strategies are effective in reducing secondary gain.

Assertiveness training is often appropriate to teach patients with somatic symptom disorders. Use of assertiveness techniques gives patients a direct means of meeting needs and thereby decreases the need for somatic symptoms. Teaching

TABLE 12-3 INTERVENTIONS FOR SOMATOFORM DISORDERS	
INTERVENTION	**RATIONALE**
1. Offer explanations and support during diagnostic testing.	1. Reduces anxiety while ruling out organic illness.
2. After physical complaints have been investigated, avoid further reinforcement (e.g., do not take vital signs each time patient complains of palpitations).	2. Directs focus away from physical symptoms.
3. Spend time with patient at times other than when summoned by patient to voice physical complaint.	3. Rewards non–illness-related behaviors and encourages repetition of desired behavior.
4. Observe and record frequency and intensity of somatic symptoms. (Patient or family can give information.)	4. Establishes a baseline and later enables evaluation of effectiveness of interventions.
5. Do not imply that symptoms are not real.	5. Acknowledges that psychogenic symptoms are real to the patient.
6. Shift focus from somatic complaints to feelings or to neutral topics.	6. Conveys interest in patient as a person rather than in patient's symptoms; reduces need to gain attention via symptoms.
7. Assess secondary gains that "physical illness" provides for patient (e.g., attention, increased dependency, and distraction from another problem).	7. Allows these needs to be met in healthier ways and thus minimizes secondary gains.
8. Use straightforward approach to patient exhibiting resistance or covert anger.	8. Avoids power struggles, demonstrates acceptance of anger, and permits discussion of angry feelings.
9. Have patient direct all requests to case manager.	9. Reduces manipulation.
10. Show concern for patient, but avoid fostering dependency needs.	10. Shows respect for patient's feelings while minimizing secondary gains from "illness."
11. Reinforce patient's strengths and problem-solving abilities.	11. Contributes to positive self-esteem; helps patient realize that needs can be met without resorting to somatic symptoms.
12. Teach assertive communication.	12. Provides patient with a positive way of meeting needs; reduces feelings of helplessness and need for manipulation.
13. Teach patient stress reduction techniques, such as meditation, relaxation, and mild physical exercise.	13. Provides alternate coping strategies; reduces need for medication.

an exercise regimen, such as doing range-of-motion exercises for 15 to 20 minutes daily, can help the patient feel in control, increase endorphin levels, and may help decrease anxiety.

Case Management

"Doctor shopping" is common among patients with somatic symptom disorders. The patient constantly changes physicians, clinics, or hospitals, hoping to establish a physical basis for distress. Repeated computed tomography scans, magnetic resonance images, and other diagnostic tests are often documented in the medical record. Case management can help limit health care costs associated with such visits. The case manager can recommend to the physician that the patient be scheduled for brief appointments every 4 to 6 weeks at set times rather than on demand and that laboratory tests be avoided unless they are absolutely necessary. The patient who establishes a relationship with the case manager often feels less anxiety because the patient has someone to contact and knows that someone is "in charge."

Psychotherapy

Cognitive and behavioral approaches can be effective and may prove to be the therapy of choice for patients with somatic symptom disorders (Braun et al., 2010). Behavior modification can provide incentives, motivation, and rewards to help patients control their symptoms. Family and group therapy can increase awareness of communication and interaction patterns and help patients improve interpersonal communication and learn strategies to improve social skills (Cely-Serrano & Floet, 2006). Nurses and other clinicians may be involved with teaching patients alternative coping skills (relaxation techniques, cognitive restructuring, and refocusing) to aid in controlling anxiety and reappraising thinking in an effort to better mediate symptoms. Refer to Table 12-4 for a summary of the characteristics of somatic symptom disorders, their comorbidities, and specific therapeutic approaches that have the potential to improve the quality of life for these patients.

TABLE 12-4 SOMATOFORM DISORDERS

DISORDER	CHARACTERISTICS	COMORBIDITY	THERAPEUTIC APPROACH
Functional neurological disorder (conversion disorder)	One or two neurological symptoms that have no medical basis Symptoms cause significant distress or impairment in functioning	Major depression; dissociative disorder; personality disorder	Behavioral therapy; family therapy; hypnosis; anxiolytics
Predominant somatic complaints (somatization disorder)	Many physical symptoms accompanied by health-related severe anxiety and preoccupation, which takes inordinate periods of time	Major depression; panic disorder; personality disorder; substance dependence	Consultation with primary care provider to arrange regular patient visits, limited tests; group therapy; cognitive behavioral therapy, which focuses on decreasing stress and restructuring in interpersonal communications
Predominant health anxiety (hypochondriasis)	Characterized less by a focus on symptoms than by the patients' beliefs that they have a specific disease	Depressive disorder; anxiety disorder; other somatic symptom disorders	Cognitive behavioral therapy; antidepressants; cognitive group therapy; stress management
Predominant pain (pain disorder)	Symptoms of pain that are either solely related to or significantly exacerbated by psychosocial factors	Anxiety disorder; depressive disorder; substance dependence	Group therapy; family therapy; cognitive behavioral therapy; antidepressants; hypnosis
Body dysmorphic disorder	False belief or exaggerated perception that a body part is defective	Major depression; obsessive-compulsive disorder; social phobia	Cognitive behavioral therapy; SSRI antidepressants
Psychological factors affecting medical conditions	Presence of one or more clinically psychological or behavioral factors that adversely affects a medical condition and negatively influences its course of treatment Examples include denying seriousness of cardiovascular disease, not taking medications because of side effects	Depression; anxiety; substance abuse	Relaxation training; support groups; psychological counseling; psychotherapy; others

Pharmacological Therapies

Currently antidepressants, specifically selective serotonin reuptake inhibitors (SSRIs), show the greatest promise for helping patients suffering from somatic symptom disorders (Black & Andreasen, 2011). Patients may also benefit from short-term use of antianxiety medication, which must be monitored carefully because of the risk of dependence. The nurse may administer these medications in certain settings, but teaching about the medication to patients and families is helpful in all settings.

EVALUATION

Evaluation of patients with somatic symptom disorders is a simple process when measurable behavioral outcomes have been written clearly and realistically. For these patients, nurses often find that goals and outcomes are only partially met. This should be considered a positive finding, because these patients often exhibit remarkable resistance to change. Patients are likely to report the continuing presence of somatic symptoms, but they often state that they are less concerned about the symptoms. Families are likely to report relatively high satisfaction with outcomes, even without total eradication of the patient's symptoms.

DISSOCIATIVE DISORDERS

The hallmark of the dissociative disorders is disturbances in the normally well-integrated continuum of consciousness, memory, identity, and perception. Dissociative disorders include amnesiac states (dissociative amnesia and dissociative fugue) and dissociative identity disorder (DID), formerly known as multiple personality disorder. Dissociation is an unconscious defense mechanism to protect the individual against overwhelming anxiety. Patients with dissociative disorders have intact reality testing; that is, they are not delusional or hallucinating. When the ability to integrate memories is impaired, the individual has *dissociative amnesia*. When the ability to maintain one's identity is affected, the individual may develop a *dissociative fugue* or *dissociative identity disorder*. When there is a persistent or recurrent disruption in perception, the individual has *depersonalization disorder*, with a feeling of detachment from the mind or body.

Dissociative disorders are characterized by altered mind-body connections and possibly brain alterations related to traumatic stress or anxiety (e.g., from early child abuse). For people who use extreme dissociation as a defense against overwhelming anxiety, consciousness itself can be altered in a dramatic way, whereas thinking, feeling, and perceptions are less impaired. These disorders can be quite severe.

We all dissociate. Fantasy, daydreaming, absorption in activities, and night dreaming are considered normative dissociations. For example, we say we are on "automatic pilot" when we drive home from work but cannot recall the last 15 minutes before reaching home. However, these common experiences are distinctly different from the processes of pathological dissociation where the dissociation becomes distorted and interferes with the person's functioning and quality of life (Black & Andreasen, 2011). People with these disorders routinely experience significant emotional pain and struggle with overall functioning and safety.

PREVALENCE AND COMORBIDITY

The actual **prevalence of dissociative disorders** in the general population is difficult to determine. However, a study conducted by Sar and associates (2007) determined the prevalence of dissociative disorders in general psychiatric settings to range from 5% to 20%, and to range between 12% and 29% among outpatients.

Dissociative processes and/or dissociative disorders often exist in patients who present at a psychiatric emergency department with self-harming behaviors (e.g., suicide or self-mutilation), addictions, eating disorders, "rapid cycling" mood changes, pseudoseizures, trauma-related flashbacks, and many other conditions. Often identification of the dissociative process is overlooked by mental health clinicians who are not trained in dissociation or dissociative disorders. **Dissociative disorders can co-occur** with a wide range of other psychiatric disorders. Besides the disorders previously mentioned, potential dissociative processes may occur concomitant with posttraumatic stress disorder, profound body dysmorphic disorder, borderline personality disorders, childhood sexual abuse, attention deficit problems, and others.

THEORY

The actual cause of dissociative disorders is unclear. However, as mentioned earlier, stress seems to play a major role. We have already mentioned that childhood physical, sexual, or emotional abuse and other traumatic life events are associated with adult dissociative symptoms. Several factors related to etiology are reviewed in the following sections.

Biological Factors

Current research suggests that the limbic system is involved in the development of dissociative disorders. Traumatic memories are processed in the limbic system, and the hippocampus stores this information. Animal studies show that early prolonged detachment from the caretaker negatively affects the development of the limbic system. For humans, early trauma or detachment from the caregiver could impair memory processing, leading to dissociation. Significant early trauma and lack of attachment have also been demonstrated to have effects on neurotransmitters, specifically on serotonin.

One study found that people with dissociative identity disorder may have hippocampi that are about 19% smaller and amygdalae that are about 32% smaller as compared with control subjects (Vermetten et al., 2006). The hippocampus is the part of the brain essential for memory and learning, and the amygdala regulates emotion.

Extreme stress can cause alterations in the brain that may manifest as brain scan abnormalities. Therefore it would be prudent to examine dissociative disorders from both a brain and a mind perspective.

Depersonalization disorder and dissociative fugue have a possible neurological link. Altered perceptions of self and fugue states occur with neurological diseases such as brain tumors and epilepsy, especially complex partial seizure disorder. Depersonalization is also experienced by individuals under the influence of certain drugs, such as alcohol, barbiturates, and hallucinogens.

Genetic Factors

Several studies suggest that DID is more common among first-degree biological relatives of individuals with the disorder than in the population at large. There is also evidence that patient histories recount multiple generations of DID and occurrence among siblings (Black & Andreasen, 2011).

Psychosocial Factors

Learning theory suggests that dissociative disorders can be explained as learned methods for avoiding stress and anxiety. The pattern of avoidance occurs when an individual deals with an unpleasant event by consciously deciding not to think about it. The more anxiety-provoking the event, the greater the need not to think about it. The more this technique is used, the more likely it is to become automatically invoked as dissociation. When stress is intolerable—for example, in an abused child—the individual develops dissociation to defend against pain and the memory of the stressful event.

CULTURAL CONSIDERATIONS

Certain culturally bound disorders exist in which there is a high level of activity, a trancelike state, and running or fleeing, followed by exhaustion, sleep, and amnesia regarding the episode. These syndromes include *piblokto* among native people of the Arctic, Navajo *frenzy* witchcraft, and *amok* among western Pacific natives. These syndromes, if observed in individuals native to the corresponding geographical areas, must be differentiated from dissociative disorders.

CLINICAL PICTURE

Depersonalization/Derealization Disorder

Depersonalization is the persistent or recurrent alteration in the perception of self while reality testing remains intact. The person experiencing depersonalization may feel mechanical or dreamy; a sense of unreality, slow movement of time, or detachment from the body may also be experienced. The person feels as if he or she is seeing themselves from a distance or outside the body. Some patients even report the very disturbing perception of their limbs being larger or smaller than normal. In some cases, depersonalization may be preceded by severe stress; in other cases, there may be an association with childhood emotional trauma.

> **VIGNETTE**
>
> Lucinda describes becoming very distressed at perceiving changes in her appearance when she looks in a mirror. She thinks that her image looks wavy and indistinct. Soon after, she describes feeling as though she is floating in a fog with her feet not actually touching the ground. Questioning reveals that Lucinda's son has recently confided to her that he is gay and has just tested positive for human immunodeficiency virus (HIV).

Derealization is a persistent or recurrent experience of unreality of surroundings while reality testing remains intact. There is often an unreal, dreamlike, distance, or distorted experience in familiar surroundings.

> **VIGNETTE**
>
> Miquel had just been forced to resign from a job that he really liked and had mastered. He got this job after being out of work for 9 months. He returned home after he was told that the company was letting the newer employees go for financial reasons. As he walks into his apartment, he looks around, and even though everything is the same, it somehow looks unreal and unfamiliar, distorted and strange.

In both these instances of depersonalization and derealization, the symptoms cause clinically significant distress or impairment in social, occupational, or other important areas of functioning, as specified in the *DSM-5* (APA, 2010a).

Dissociative Amnesia

Psychologically induced memory loss is called dissociative amnesia and is marked by the inability to recall important personal information. The amnesia is reported to occur after a severe physical or psychological stressor. Black and Andreasen (2011) report estimations that between 5% and 20% of combat veterans were amnesic for their combat experience.

> **VIGNETTE**
>
> A young woman is found wandering in a park near where she lives. She is disheveled and poorly nourished. She has no knowledge of what happened to her. Her parents identify her 2 weeks later when she appears on a new TV show searching for missing identities. It is discovered that the woman had recently broken up with her boyfriend of 3 years.

Dissociative Fugue

Dissociative fugue is characterized by sudden, unexpected travel away from the customary locale and inability to recall one's identity and information about some or all of the past. In rare cases, an individual with dissociative fugue assumes a whole new identity. During a fugue state, individuals tend to lead rather simple lives, rarely calling attention to themselves. After a few weeks to a few months, they may remember their former identities and become amnesic of the time spent in the fugue state. Usually a dissociative fugue is precipitated by a traumatic event.

VIGNETTE

A middle-aged woman awakens one morning and notices snow outside the window swirling around unfamiliar buildings and streets. The radio tells her it is December. She is perplexed to find herself in a residential hotel in Chicago with no idea of how she got there. She feels confused and shaken. As she leaves the hotel, she is surprised to find that strangers recognize her and say, "Good morning, Sally." The name Sally does not seem right, but she cannot remember her true identity. She finds her way to a hospital, where she is evaluated and referred to the psychiatric nurse in the emergency department. A day later, "Sally" is able to remember her true identity, Mary Hunt. She tells the nurse tearfully that she can now recall that her husband came home one day and "out of the blue" told her he wanted a divorce to marry a younger woman. Mary calls her sister in New York, who comes to Chicago to take her home.

Dissociative Identity Disorder

The prevalence of dissociative identity disorder is thought to be low. Up to 90% of patients with this disorder are women (Black & Andreasen, 2011). The essential feature of **dissociative identity disorder (DID)**, formerly known as multiple personality disorder, is the presence of two or more distinct personality states that recurrently take control of behavior. Each **alternate personality (alter)**, or **subpersonality**, has its own pattern of perceiving, relating to, thinking about the self and the environment, affect, cognition, behavior, and/or memories. It is believed that severe sexual, physical, or psychological trauma in childhood predisposes an individual to the development of DID. This disruption in personalities may be observed by others or reported by the individual (APA, 2010b).

Typical **cognitive distortions** include the insistence that alternate personalities inhabit separate bodies and are unaffected by the actions of one another. The primary personality or host is usually not aware of the subpersonalities and is perplexed by lost time and unexplained events. Experiences such as finding unfamiliar clothing in the closet, being called a different name by a stranger, or not having childhood memories are characteristic of DID. Subpersonalities are often aware of the existence of each other to some degree. Transition from one personality to another occurs during times of stress and may range from a dramatic to a barely noticeable event. Some patients experience the transition when awakening. Shifts may last from minutes to months, although shorter periods are more common. People diagnosed with DID may meet the criteria for one or several other psychiatric disorders,

such as borderline personality disorder, past diagnosis of schizophrenia, or psychotic mood disorder.

The constant disruption of the main personality causes significant distress or impairment in social, occupational, or other important areas of functioning.

VIGNETTE

Andrea, a conservative 28-year-old electrical engineer, is the primary personality. Three alternate personalities coexist and vie for supremacy:

- Michele is a 5-year-old girl who is sometimes playful and sometimes angry. She speaks with a slight lisp and with the facial expressions, voice inflections, and vocabulary of a precocious child. She likes to play on swings, draw with a crayon, and eat ice cream. She likes to cuddle a teddy bear and occasionally sucks her thumb. Her favorite outfit is jeans and a Mickey Mouse sweatshirt.
- Ann is an accomplished ballet dancer. She is shy but firm about needing time to practice. When she is dominant, she likes to wear white and fixes her hair in a severe, pulled-back style. She does little but dance when she is in control.
- Bridget is near Andrea's age, although she says a lady never tells her age. She dresses seductively in bright colors, wears her hair tousled, and likes to frequent bars and stay out late. She often drinks to excess and has several male admirers. Bridget has many moods. She states that she would like to get rid of Ann and Andrea because they're such "goody-goodies."

Andrea does not drink or dance, hates ice cream, and sees herself as somewhat awkward. She is a paid soloist in a church choir. Andrea takes public transportation, but Ann and Bridget have driver's licenses. Andrea goes to bed and arises early, but Bridget and Michele like to stay up late.

Andrea seeks treatment when she finds herself behind the wheel of a moving car and realizes that she does not know how to drive. She has been concerned for some time because she has found strange clothes in her closet. She has also received phone calls from men who insist that she has flirted with them in bars. She sometimes misses appointments and cannot account for periods of time. Although she goes to bed early, she is often unaccountably tired in the morning.

APPLICATION OF THE NURSING PROCESS

ASSESSMENT

Medical Workup

In order for one of the dissociative disorders to be diagnosed, medical and neurological illnesses, substance use, and other coexisting psychiatric disorders must be ruled out or identified as coexisting with a dissociative disorder. Medical personnel

EXAMINING THE EVIDENCE

Proving Multiple Personality Disorder

How do we know that dissociative identity disorder (DID)/multiple personality disorder actually exists?

There continues to be no clear consensus on the concept of dissociation and scientific interest is waning. While dissociation, trauma, and psychosis were theorized as being intricately connected in the early 1900s, the relationship slowly eroded in the ensuing 100 years. Literature on trauma and psychosis has become prevalent in recent years; this is not the case with the concept of dissociation (Moscowitz et al., 2008). There are currently many disagreements among current specialists regarding the etiology and treatment of dissociative disorders. The *DSM* currently lists dissociation as a "disorder" yet the *Psychodynamic Diagnostic Manual* lists it as "dissociative personality" (Dell & O'Neil, 2010). Less than 40% of psychiatrists in the United States support the inclusion of DID in the *DSM* and nearly 70% question it as a valid diagnosis (Escobar, 2004).

Sybil was a hugely popular book and film in the 1970s; it recounted the case of a woman named Sybil who was abused by her mother and "dissociated" into 16 different personalities. This paved the way for an explosion of multiple personality disorder diagnoses in the 1980s. Since that time there have been allegations that Sybil's symptoms were a result of suggestions made by her therapist.

This confusion has raised concerns in the treatment of dissociation. One new theory stresses impaired parent-child attachment patterns, another theory emphasizes trauma-based disruptions, and another links maladaptive attachment patterns directly to dysfunctional brain development (Weber, 2009). Although dissociative states have traditionally been considered anxiety spectrum disorders, antianxiety agents have rarely been successful. A recent patient study discusses the precipitation of a "possessed state" by the use of the antidepressant nortriptyline (Prakash et al., 2008).

Nurses are often on the frontlines of the health care team and may be in ideal practice environments, such as school settings, for first-line identification of key features of dissociation in children and adolescents. Early identification and care of children and adolescents are main determinants of improved prognosis; however, the continued controversy among practitioners can often hinder much needed treatment (Weber, 2009). As our diagnostic procedures and understanding of the concept of dissociation are studied further, perhaps we will learn if Sybil was either a very talented actress or the unwilling host of 16 personalities.

Escobar, J. I. (2004). Transcultural aspect of dissociative and somatoform disorders. *Psychiatric Times, 21*, 5.
Dell, P., & O'Neil, J. (2010). *Dissociation and the dissociative disorders: DSM-V and beyond.* New York: Routledge.
Moscowitz, A., et al. (2008). *Psychosis, trauma, and dissociation.* Philadelphia: Wiley-Blackwell.
Prakash, R., et al. (2008). *Possession states precipitated by nortriptyline.* The Royal Australian and New Zealand College of Psychiatrists.
Weber, S. (2009). Treatment of trauma and abuse related dissociative symptoms in children and adolescents. *Journal of Child and Adolescent Psychiatric Nursing, 22*(1), 2–6.
Contributed by Lois Angelo.

collect objective data from physical examination, electroencephalography, imaging studies, projective tests, structured personality tests, and specific questionnaires designed to identify dissociative symptoms.

Identity and Memory

Assessing patients' ability to identify themselves requires more than asking patients to state their names. Changes in patient behavior, voice, and dress might signal the presence of an alternate personality. Referring to self by another name or in the third person and using the word *we* instead of *I* are indications that the patient may have assumed a new identity. The nurse should consider the following when assessing memory:

- Can the patient remember recent and past events?
- Is the patient's memory clear and complete or is it partial and fuzzy?
- Is the patient aware of gaps in memory, such as lack of memory for events such as a graduation or a wedding?
- Do the patient's memories place the self with a family, in school, in an occupation?

Patients with amnesia and fugue may be disoriented with regard to time and place as well as person. Relevant assessment questions include the following:

- Do you ever lose time or have blackouts?
- Do you find yourself in places with no idea how you got there?

Patient History

The nurse must gather information about events in the person's life. Has the patient sustained a recent injury, such as a concussion? Does the patient have a history of epilepsy, especially temporal lobe epilepsy? Does the patient have a history of early trauma, such as physical, mental, or sexual abuse? If DID is suspected, pertinent questions include the following:

- Have you ever found yourself wearing clothes that you cannot remember buying?
- Have you ever had strange people greet and talk to you as though they were old friends?
- Does your ability to engage in things such as athletics, artistic activities, or mechanical tasks seem to change?
- Do you have differing sets of memories about childhood?

Mood

Is the individual depressed, anxious, or unconcerned? Many patients with DID seek help when the primary personality is depressed. The nurse also observes for mood shifts. When subpersonalities of DID assume control, their predominant moods may be different from that of the principal personality. If the subpersonalities shift frequently, marked mood swings may be noted.

Use of Alcohol and Other Drugs

Specific questions should be asked to identify drug or alcohol use. Dissociative episodes may be associated with recent use of alcohol or other substances—such as cocaine, opioids, sedatives, or stimulants.

Effect on Patient and Family

Has the patient's ability to function been impaired? Have disruptions in family functioning occurred? Is secondary gain evident? In fugue states, individuals often function adequately in their new identities by choosing simple, undemanding occupations and having few intimate social interactions. The families of patients in fugue states report being highly distressed over the patient's disappearance. Patients with amnesia may be more dysfunctional. Their perplexity often renders them unable to work, and their memory loss impairs normal family relationships.

Families often direct considerable attention toward the patient but may exhibit concern over having to assume roles that were once assigned to the patient. Patients with DID often have both family and work problems. Families find it difficult to accept the seemingly erratic behaviors of the patient. Employers dislike the lost time that may occur when subpersonalities are in control. Patients with depersonalization disorder are often fearful that others may perceive their appearance as distorted and may avoid being seen in public. If they exhibit high anxiety, the family is likely to find it difficult to keep relationships stable.

Suicide Risk

Whenever a patient's life has been substantially disrupted, he or she may have thoughts of suicide. The nurse gathering data should be alert for expressions of hopelessness, helplessness, or worthlessness and for verbalization or other behavior of a subpersonality that indicates the intent to engage in self-destructive or self-mutilating behaviors.

ASSESSMENT GUIDELINES

Dissociative Disorders

1. Assess for a history of a similar episode in the past with benign outcomes.
2. Establish whether the person suffered abuse, trauma, or loss as a child.
3. Identify relevant psychosocial distress issues by performing a basic psychosocial assessment. (See Chapter 7 for information on the basic psychosocial assessment.)

DIAGNOSIS

Nursing diagnoses for patients with dissociative disorders are suggested in Table 12-5.

OUTCOMES IDENTIFICATION

Outcomes must be established for each nursing diagnosis. General goals are to develop trust, correct faulty perceptions, and encourage the patient to live in the present instead of dissociating. NOC outcomes potentially appropriate for patients with

TABLE 12-5 **POTENTIAL NURSING DIAGNOSES FOR DISSOCIATIVE DISORDERS**	
SIGNS AND SYMPTOMS	**NURSING DIAGNOSES***
Amnesia or fugue related to a traumatic event	*Disturbed Personal Identity*
Symptoms of depersonalization; feelings of unreality or body image distortions	*Disturbed Body Image*
Alterations in consciousness, memory, or identity	*Ineffective Coping*
Abuse of substances related to dissociation	*Ineffective Role Performance*
Disorganization or dysfunction in usual patterns of behavior (absence from work, withdrawal from relationships, changes in role function)	*Ineffective Coping* *Ineffective Family Coping*
Disturbances in memory and identity	*Interrupted Family Processes*
Interrupted family processes related to amnesia or erratic and changing behavior	*Impaired Parenting* *Ineffective Impulse Control*
Feeling of being out of control of memory, behaviors, and awareness	*Anxiety*
Inability to explain actions or behaviors when in altered state	*Spiritual Distress* *Risk for Other-Directed Violence* *Risk for Self-Directed Violence*
Obsessive fear of contracting or having a serious or terminal illness	*Death Anxiety*

*Nursing Diagnoses—Definitions and Classification 2012-2014. © Copyright 2012, 1994-2012 by NANDA International. Used by arrangement with Blackwell Publishing Limited, a company of John Wiley and Sons, Inc.

dissociative disorders include *Identity, Role Performance, Coping, Anxiety Self-Control, Self-Mutilation Restraint,* and *Aggression Self-Control* (Moorhead et al., 2008). Specific examples of indicators that the outcomes are being achieved include the following:

- Patient will verbalize clear sense of personal identity.
- Patient will report decrease in stress (using a scale of 1 to 10).
- Patient will report comfort with role expectations.
- Patient will plan coping strategies for stressful situations.
- Patient will refrain from injuring self.

PLANNING

The planning of nursing care for the patient with a dissociative disorder is influenced by the setting and presenting problem. Nurses may encounter such a patient in times of crisis either in the emergency department or when the patient is admitted to the hospital for suicidal or homicidal behavior. The care plan will focus on safety and crisis intervention. The patient also may seek treatment of a comorbid depressive or anxiety disorder in the community setting. Planning will address the major complaint with appropriate referrals for treatment of the dissociative disorder.

IMPLEMENTATION

Most of the time the DID patient is treated in the community. However, a patient with DID is admitted to a psychiatric unit when suicidal or in need of crisis stabilization. At that time, the nurse gathers specific information about identity, memory, consciousness, life events, mood, suicide risk, and the effect of the disorder on the patient and the family.

Communication Guidelines

Nurses can offer emotional presence during the recall of painful experiences, provide a sense of safety, and encourage an optimal level of functioning. Table 12-6 offers examples of interventions for patients with dissociative disorders.

Health Teaching and Health Promotion

Patients with dissociative disorders need teaching about the illness and instruction in coping skills and stress management. They may need to develop a plan to interrupt a dissociative episode, such as singing or doing a specific activity. Staff and significant others are made aware of the plan in order to foster their cooperation. Patients need to keep a daily journal to increase their awareness of feelings and to identify triggers to dissociation. If a patient has never written a journal, the nurse should suggest beginning with a 5- to 10-minute daily writing exercise.

Milieu Therapy

When the patient is in a crisis that requires hospitalization, providing a safe environment is fundamental. Other desirable characteristics include that the environment be quiet, simple, structured, and supportive. Confusion and noise increase

TABLE 12-6 INTERVENTIONS FOR DISSOCIATIVE DISORDERS

INTERVENTION	RATIONALE
1. Ensure patient safety by providing safe, protected environment and frequent observation.	1. Sense of bewilderment may lead to inattention to safety needs; some subpersonalities may be thrill seeking, violent, or careless.
2. Provide nondemanding, simple routine.	2. Reduces anxiety.
3. Confirm identity of patient and orientation to time and place.	3. Supports reality and promotes ego integrity.
4. Encourage patient to do things for self and make decisions about routine tasks.	4. Enhances self-esteem by reducing sense of powerlessness and reduces secondary gain associated with dependence.
5. Assist with other decision making until memory returns.	5. Lowers stress and prevents patient from having to live with the consequences of unwise decisions.
6. Support patient during exploration of feelings surrounding the stressful event.	6. Helps lower the defense of dissociation used by patient to block awareness of the stressful event.
7. Do not overwhelm patient with data regarding past events.	7. Memory loss serves the purpose of preventing severe to panic levels of anxiety from overtaking and disorganizing the individual.
8. Allow patient to progress at own pace as memory is recovered.	8. Prevents undue anxiety and resistance.
9. Provide support during disclosure of painful experiences.	9. Can be healing while minimizing feelings of isolation.
10. Accept patient's expression of negative feelings.	10. Conveys permission to have negative or unacceptable feelings.
11. Teach stress reduction methods.	11. Provides alternatives for anxiety relief.

anxiety and the potential for depersonalization, delayed memory return, or shifts among subpersonalities. Task-oriented therapy or occupational and art therapy can be useful for these patients if used in isolation from one another.

Psychotherapy

Psychotherapy has been proven to be the primary and most effective treatment modality in dissociative identity disorder patients (Lowenstein & Putnam, 2005). Therapists who treat this population need special training in dissociation. Turkus and Kahler (2006) state that therapy needs to be very flexible. From their years of experience they found applying specific techniques within an overall psychodynamic framework effective. Such techniques include psychoeducation, "talking through," traumatic re-enactment, safety planning, journaling, and artwork.

APPLYING THE ART

A Person With Dissociative Disorder

SCENARIO: Last week I noticed 25-year-old Sammy restlessly reading a magazine while she waited for her teenage brother to finish his outpatient psychotherapy with the advanced practice nurse. Today she again made eye contact with me, and she looked like she had been crying. I offered her a tissue as I sat near her in the waiting area, empty except for the receptionist at the far end.

THERAPEUTIC GOAL: By the end of this interaction, Sammy will express at least one indication that she is ready to access help for feelings related to trauma.

STUDENT-PATIENT INTERACTION	THOUGHTS, COMMUNICATION TECHNIQUES, AND MENTAL HEALTH NURSING CONCEPTS
Student: "Hi. We've smiled at each other before. I'm _____, a nursing student from _____. May I sit with you while you wait?" ***Student's feelings:*** *I remember her. Who would think that smiling and making eye contact could open a nurse-patient interaction a week later?*	Even though this relationship has not been planned, the *contract* sets boundaries. I will need to let her know about confidentiality as soon as possible.
Sammy: *Nods and takes the tissue.* "I'm Samantha, 'Sammy,' here with my 14-year-old brother. Sometimes I wonder if I'm not the one who should be seeing someone. But I need to be the strong one."	
Student: "I've found that sometimes a person still qualifies as 'the strong one' yet lets it be okay to get a little help along the way." ***Student's feelings:*** *It's frustrating that mental illness still carries so many stigmas.* *Sammy glances at me, holding eye contact 1 or 2 seconds.*	I chose *restatement* because her words "the strong one" are significant to her self-esteem.
Student's feelings: *I hope I didn't push that too much. I keep thinking about my friend who almost waited too long to get help. Good timing that my clinical teacher made rounds just now.*	I need to think about HIPAA (patient confidentiality, the Health Insurance Portability and Accountability Act) at all times.
Sammy: "I've sort of been a mother to my brother his whole life. When he was born I was just starting middle school."	
Student: "You really care about your brother. I want to listen, but let's move to that side of the room so the receptionist can still see you to tell us when your brother's done." *We move and the receptionist lets my instructor know where I am.*	I use *reflection* and *offer self*. The patient cannot feel safe if I do not feel safe, so I stay in visual range and let my instructor know where I am.
Sammy: *Doodles on scrap paper as she talks.* "I don't know what I'd do if anything ever happened to my brother. He's only 14, you know."	
Student's feelings: *I feel that way about my family, too.*	
Student: "That's the second time you've told me he's only 14. His age seems important to you."	I use *validation*. Is her brother's age a *theme*?

APPLYING THE ART—cont'd

A Person With Dissociative Disorder

STUDENT-PATIENT INTERACTION	THOUGHTS, COMMUNICATION TECHNIQUES, AND MENTAL HEALTH NURSING CONCEPTS
Sammy: *Eyes widen.* "Fourteen is how old I was when my dad left for good."	
Student: "You still remember how rough that time was."	Using *reflection* shows *empathy.*
Student's feelings: *Sad. So young to lose her dad.*	
Sammy: "Yeah. My 'nice' mom turned into a mean and bitter mom. I tried to help her all I could, especially after we lost the house and had to move."	
Student: "That must've been scary to lose your dad, your home, and your 'nice' mom all at once."	I use *reflection* and *restatement.* "Loss" is definitely a *theme.* I wonder to what extent she has been able to work through the *grief process.*
Student's feelings: *I feel overwhelmed just thinking about all she lost when just a young teen.*	
Sammy: "First, I lost my 'nice' mom, then last year she really dies and Billy moved into my apartment." *Eyes tearing.* "He just couldn't handle everything and started messing up and getting in fights at school."	I remember that *depression* may manifest as irritability in teens.
Student's feelings: *No wonder Billy had trouble.*	
Student: "You say your mother really died. Sounds like you believe part of her died long before last year."	I use *restatement.*
Student's feelings: *My mother loves me, and I know this even when we argue. I need to keep tuning into Sammy.*	
Sammy avoids eye contact. Suddenly her doodles become purposeful as she now draws with dark lines.	
Student: "What are you drawing?"	I use an *open question* as Sammy's attention turns to the drawing.
Sammy: *Silently draws a simple house. She gives only one of the windows a shade, which she darkens with forceful scribbles.*	
Student: "Sammy, you seem upset. I am concerned about what you are going through. Talk a little about what is going on with you."	Her *anxiety level* starts to escalate. I *reflect* and then assess with an *open question.*
Student's feelings: *Whatever is going on, I feel Sammy's intensity. I hope I can handle this.*	
Sammy: "It was in that room." *She points to the picture of the closed window shade.* "I'm just...." *Sobs, wrings her hands, and breathes rapidly.*	Is she having an *abreaction?*
Student's feelings: *Should I stop and go get my teacher? I don't want to interrupt the process. I'm scared of what's happening but others are nearby. I can get help. I'm not alone.*	
Student: "I'm _____. I'm right here with you, Sammy."	I *offer self.*
Sammy: *Suddenly rapidly looks around over each shoulder.* "Don't make me do that! Please, Mommy! Make him stop touching there." *She holds her cheek like she's just been slapped, then whimpers.*	She is hyperventilating, *hypervigilant,* and appears unaware of her present environment. She seems to be escalating into *severe levels of anxiety.* I think she is reliving something awful that she had *dissociated.* Is this a *flashback?*
Student: "Sammy, you are a grownup now. You are safe here at the clinic. No one can hurt you like that now." *I wait quietly while leaning toward her.*	I use *attending behavior.*
Student's feelings: *I don't know if I'm saying the right things but I have to try.*	

Continued

APPLYING THE ART—cont'd

A Person With Dissociative Disorder

STUDENT-PATIENT INTERACTION	THOUGHTS, COMMUNICATION TECHNIQUES, AND MENTAL HEALTH NURSING CONCEPTS
Sammy: *Sobs loudly, then cries, then looks up and breathes more slowly.* "I feel like I want to vomit. I'm scared. I don't want to think about that ever again! What's happening to me?" *Wringing hands.*	Could she have *posttraumatic stress disorder*?
Student's feelings: *Something sexual happened. I feel like I could vomit, too. Was she forced to have oral sex?*	
Student: "I don't know for sure, but it seems like you recovered a memory from a time when you were younger. Something terribly hurtful happened."	I *give information* and use *reflection*.
Student's feelings: *I really feel for Sammy.*	
Sammy: *Nods, cries softly.* "I've always felt so dirty. My mom had lots of boyfriends. One of them...maybe more than one of them...it's just too awful." *Shudders.*	How would a nurse be able to intervene therapeutically if Sammy's mother were the patient? What about if the perpetrator were the patient? Would I be able to care about either of them? Could I be therapeutic?
Student's feelings: *I feel furious at Sammy's mother!*	
Student: "You are safe now. You're in charge of you. You decide how much, if, and when you feel ready to visit those memories."	I remember that working through *repressed dissociated trauma* takes a long, painful time.
Sammy: "I've always felt different from other women, like I'm not good enough. I should've been strong enough to stop it."	I remember that sometimes women who are raped blame themselves so they at least feel some sense of control. In other words, the trauma will not reoccur if only I do this or do not do that.
Student's feelings: *I grieve for her. She was raped. Probably repeatedly. Imagine how terrified and powerless a young girl would feel.*	
Student: "Whatever happened when you were a child was not your fault. You did the best you could. These feelings are left over from your childhood when you felt powerless."	*Support* is therapeutic whereas *reassurance* is nontherapeutic, like I am trying to talk her into something. She will feel like it is not okay to say and feel whatever she needs to feel. I think interspersing rather than saying all that at once would be better.
Student's feelings: *I so want to make this all better and I can't! I believe all I've said but I must not overdo or I'm reassuring rather than supporting her. This is not about me; I cannot protect her. I can support her to empower herself.*	
Sammy: "I can't handle all this."	
Student: "You don't have to handle it alone. Let me get my instructor. She works here part-time."	I think it is okay for me to briefly leave Sammy. My teacher knows all the resources here at the clinic.
Student's feelings: *We got through the deeply emotional part. I'm relieved, but ready for my instructor's help.*	
Sammy nods. I ask the receptionist to page my instructor.	
Student: "That took courage to let some of your feelings out."	
Sammy: *Shudders.* "I have a lot more stuff where that came from." *She manages a small smile at me.* "I guess I was assaulted or something." *Looks to me as though checking my reaction.*	Her anxiety level is returning to *mild*.
Student: "I'm so sorry for all this pain in your life." *I wait.*	I show *empathy*.
Student's feelings: *She needs my nonjudgmental acceptance.*	
Sammy nods, stifles a sob.	

APPLYING THE ART—cont'd

A Person With Dissociative Disorder

STUDENT-PATIENT INTERACTION	THOUGHTS, COMMUNICATION TECHNIQUES, AND MENTAL HEALTH NURSING CONCEPTS
Student: "I see strength in you. You are here helping your brother and somehow coping with all this in your life despite such trauma."	*Offering support* and *making an observation.*
Student's feelings: *I really feel she's pretty amazing. I don't know if I'd do so well, though I know this is only the beginning of all she has to go through as she heals.*	
Sammy: *Surprised.* "I guess I am. Thanks. It really helps to talk." *She breathes deeply and stops crying.*	
My instructor comes, and after a while Sammy agrees to see an advanced practice nurse–psychotherapist and maybe later a group for adult survivors of child sexual abuse.	A *group for survivors* could really help Sammy find meaning and support from others with similar trauma.
Sammy: "I feel worn out."	
Student: "No wonder! Sammy, you took some giant steps today. It's exhausting to feel so much, so intensely."	I give *support* and use *reflection* again. I think these are becoming my favorites.
Student's feelings: *I probably shouldn't have said "no wonder." But really—no wonder!*	
Sammy: "Yes. Thanks."	
Student: "Thank you."	
Student's feelings: *I'd like to work with her again, but the work she has to do requires an advanced practice nurse. Still, I helped her connect with help, and that feels good!*	

Pharmacological, Biological, and Integrative Therapies

There are no specific medications for dissociative disorders, but appropriate antidepressants or anxiolytic medications are given for comorbid conditions. Substance use disorders and suicidal risk, which are common, must be assessed carefully if medication is prescribed. In the acute setting, the nurse may witness dramatic memory retrieval in patients with dissociative amnesia or fugue after treatment with intravenous benzodiazepines (Ballew et al., 2003).

EVALUATION

Treatment is considered successful when outcomes are met. In the final analysis, the evaluation is positive when the following are achieved:
- Patient safety has been maintained.
- Anxiety has been reduced and the patient has returned to a functional state.
- Conflicts have been explored.
- New coping strategies have permitted the patient to function at a better level.
- Stress is handled adaptively, without the use of dissociation.

KEY POINTS TO REMEMBER

- Somatic symptom disorders are characterized by the presence of multiple, real physical symptoms for which there is no evidence of medical illness.
- Dissociative disorders involve a disruption in consciousness with a significant impairment in memory, identity, or perceptions of self.
- The emergence of somatic symptom disorders and dissociative symptoms is believed to be a response to psychological stress, along with possible brain changes.
- Patients with somatic symptom disorders and dissociative disorders often have a number of comorbid psychiatric illnesses, primarily depression, anxiety and substance abuse, and borderline personality disorder as well as many others.

- The course of these disorders may be brief, with acute onset and spontaneous remission, or chronic, with a gradual onset and prolonged impairment.
- Because these patients may not seek psychiatric treatment, the nurse does not usually see them in the acute psychiatric setting, except during a period of crisis such as suicidal risk.
- The nursing assessment is especially important to clarify the history and course of past symptoms, as well as to obtain a complete picture of the current physical and mental status.
- Although these patients do respond to crisis intervention, they usually require referral for psychotherapy, including CBT to attain sustained improvement in level of functioning.

APPLYING CRITICAL JUDGMENT

1. A patient with suspected somatization disorder has been admitted to the medical-surgical unit after an episode of chest pain with possible electrocardiographic changes. While on the unit, she frequently complains of palpitations, asks the nurse to check her vital signs, and begs staff to stay with her. Some nurses measure her pulse and blood pressure when she asks. Others evade her requests. Most staff try to avoid spending time with her. Consider why staff wish to avoid her. Discuss what you could do when you felt like you wanted to avoid her. Design interventions to cope with the patient's behaviors. Give rationales for your interventions.

2. A patient with body dysmorphic disorder talks incessantly about how big her nose is, how those around her are offended by her appearance, and how her appearance has negatively affected her employment and her social life. What are some of the interventions you could take to reduce her anxiety?

3. A patient with DID has been admitted to the crisis unit for a short-term stay after a suicide threat. On the unit, the patient has repeated the statement that she will kill herself to get rid of "all the others," meaning her subpersonalities. The patient refuses to sign a "no harm" contract. Design a care plan to meet her safety and security needs.

CHAPTER REVIEW QUESTIONS

Choose the most appropriate answer(s).

1. Nurses working with patients with somatization and dissociative disorders can expect that these patients will fit on the continuum of psychobiological disorders at the:
   1. mild level.
   2. moderate to severe level.
   3. severe to psychotic level.
   4. They do not belong on the continuum, because anxiety has been reduced by ego defense mechanisms.

2. Mr. R. presents with a history of having assumed a new identity in a distant locale. He has no recollection of his former identity. Which *DSM-IV-TR* diagnosis can the nurse expect the psychiatrist to make?
   1. Hypochondriasis
   2. Conversion disorder
   3. Dissociative fugue
   4. Depersonalization disorder

3. When considering a diagnosis of somatic symptom disorder, which information, among the four types listed below, is *least* likely to require detailed assessment by the nurse?
   1. Patient's level of ability to voluntarily control symptoms
   2. Results of patient's diagnostic laboratory tests
   3. Patient's limitations in carrying out activities of daily living
   4. Patient's potential for violent behavior

4. Nurse S is developing outcome criteria with her patient, who has a nursing diagnosis of *Ineffective coping*. The diagnosis is related to the patient's dependence on pain relievers to treat chronic pain of psychological origin. Which of the following are appropriate outcome criteria?
   1. Patient will resume performance of work role behaviors.
   2. Patient will identify ineffective coping patterns.
   3. Patient will make realistic appraisal of strengths and weaknesses.
   4. Patient will make realistic appraisal of family's capacity to be involved in decision making.

5. Which sign or symptom would be *least* likely to occur for a patient with hypochondriasis?
   1. Impairment in occupational functioning
   2. Repetitive, time-consuming rituals
   3. Misinterpretation of physical sensations
   4. Loss of interest in formerly pleasurable activities

REFERENCES

Allen, L. A., Woolfolk, R. I., Escobar, J. I., et al. (2006). Cognitive behavioral therapy for somatization disorder: a randomized controlled trial. *Archives of Internal Medicine, 166*, 1512–1518.

American Psychiatric Association (APA). (2010a). *Depersonalization/derealization disorder.* Retrieved August 1, 2011, from www.DSM5.org/ProposeRevision/Pages/proposed.

American Psychiatric Association (APA). (2010b). *Dissociative identity disorder.* Retrieved August 2, 2011, from www.dsm5.org/Propose Revision/Pages/proposed revision.aspx?rid=57.

Ballew, L., Morgan, Y., & Lippmann, S. (2003). Intravenous diazepam for dissociative disorder: memory lost and found. *Psychosomatics, 44*, 346–347.

Bjornsson, A. S., Dyek, I., Moitra, E., et al. (2011). The clinical course of body dysmorphic disorder in the Harvard/Brown Anxiety Research Project (HARP). *Journal of Nursing and Mental Disease, 199*(1), 55–57.

Black, D. W., & Andreasen, N. C. (2011). *Introductory textbook of psychiatry* (5th ed.). Washington, DC: American Psychiatric Publishing.

Braun, I. M., Greenberg, D. B., Smith, F. A., & Cassem, N. H. (2010). Functional somatic symptoms, deception syndromes, and somatic symptom disorders. In T. A. Stern, G. L. Friccione, N. H. Cassem, M. S. Jellinek, & J. F. Rosenbaum (Eds.), *Massachusetts General Hospital handbook of general hospital psychiatry* (6th ed.). Philadelphia: Saunders/Elsevier.

Cely-Serrano, M. S., & Floet, A. M.W. (2006). *Somatic symptom disorder: hypochondriasis.* Retrieved July 5, 2007, from www.emedicine.com/ped/topic2911.htm.

HDN-Health Day News. (2010). *Cosmetic surgery not a help for body dysmorphic disorder.* Retrieved March 7, 2011, from http://Medi cineNet.com/script/main/art.asp?articlekey=118.

Kroenke, K., & Rosmalen, J. G. M. (2006). Symptoms, syndromes, and the value of psychiatric diagnostics, in patients who have functional somatic disorders. *Medical Clinics of North America, 90*, 603–626.

Lowenstein, R. J., & Putnam, R. W. (2005). Dissociative disorders, dissociative identity disorder. In B. J. Sadock, & V. A. Sadock (Eds.), *Comprehensive textbook of psychiatry* (8th ed., Vol. 1, pp. 1844–1901). Philadelphia: Lippincott Williams & Wilkins.

Moorhead, S., Johnson, M., Maas, M. L., & Swanson, E. (2008). *Nursing outcomes classification (NOC)* (4th ed.). St Louis: Mosby.

Sar, V., Lpuimca, A., Ozturk, E., et al. (2007). Dissociative disorders in the psychiatric emergency ward. *General Hospital Psychiatry, 29*, 45–50.

Stone, J., LaFrance, C., Levenson, J. L., & Sharp, M. (2010). Issues for DSM-5: conversion disorder. *American Journal of Psychiatry, 167*, 626–627. Retrieved February 23, 2011, from http://ajp.psychiatry online.org/cgi/content/full/167/6/626.

Taylor, S., Thordarson, D., Jang, K. L., & Asmundson, G. J. G. (2006). Genetic and environmental origins of health anxiety: a twin study. *World Psychiatry, 5*(1), 47–50.

Turkus, J. A., & Kahler, J. A. (2006). Therapeutic interventions in the treatment of dissociative disorders. *Psychiatric Clinics of North America, 29*, 245–262.

Vermetten, E., Schmahl, C., Lindner, S., et al. (2006). Hippocampal and amygdalar volumes in dissociative identity disorder. *American Journal of Psychiatry, 163*, 630–636.

Yates, W. R. (2010). *Somatic symptom disorders: treatment and medication.* Updated 2010. Retrieved February 18, 2011, from http://emedicine.Medscape.com/article/294908-treatment.

Personality Disorders

Elizabeth M. Varcarolis

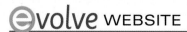evolve WEBSITE

http://evolve.elsevier.com/Varcarolis/essentials

KEY TERMS AND CONCEPTS

antisocial personality disorder
  (dyssocial), p. 215
avoidant personality disorder,
  p. 217
borderline personality disorder,
  p. 215
dialectical behavior therapy
  (DBT), p. 226
entitlement, p. 215
manipulation, p. 215

narcissistic personality disorder,
  p. 217
obsessive-compulsive personality
  disorder, p. 218
passive-aggressive traits, p. 219
personality, p. 213
personality disorder (PD), p. 213
schizotypal personality disorder,
  p. 215
splitting, p. 216

SELECTED CONCEPT: Personality

Attitude and behavior are just part of a person's character. Our mental, emotional, spiritual, and cultural influences and physical well-being are all aspects of what we call our personality (Exforsys, 2010).

"Personality, as defined, is an enduring pattern of relating, and thinking about the environment and oneself that is seen in a wide range of social and personal situations" (Blaise et al, 2008, p. 525).

Personality is essentially an enduring pattern of perceiving; interacting with others, modes of thought, responses to stress and opportunity, and ways we perceive and interact with the world. Mayer (2005) identified three psychological qualities needed to guide a person toward effective social and interpersonal functioning:

- A stable and realistic sense of self.
- A system for the interpretation of social situations and the understanding of the relational motives and actions of others.
- The capacity to serve the self as it relates with others.

OBJECTIVES

1. Summarize four characteristics shared by people with personality disorders.
2. Describe at least four co-occurring conditions that are often present in people with a personality disorder.
3. Define and differentiate among at least three examples of primitive or immature defenses.
4. Compare and contrast the behaviors seen in borderline personality disorder and narcissistic personality disorder.
5. Applying self-care, identify some of the feelings that are experienced by health care professionals when working with a person with a personality disorder.
6. Discuss how you would use teamwork and collaboration when working with a patient who is extremely manipulative.
7. In planning patient-centered care with a patient who has impulsive behaviors, identify four communication guidelines you would use.

Personality is essentially an enduring pattern of perceiving, relating, and thinking about the environment. In other words, personality is the "style" a person adopts to deal with the world. Personality traits are stylistic peculiarities that all people bring to social relationships, including shyness, seductiveness, rigidity, suspiciousness, or passive-aggressive traits. In ordinary/nonpathological states, personality traits are flexible and adaptive.

In people with a personality disorder (PD), these traits are exaggerated and rigid to the point that they cause dysfunction in their relationships (Black & Andreasen, 2011).

People with PDs present the most complex, difficult behavioral challenges for themselves and people around them. In the health care community a "difficult patient" is almost always an individual with a PD. Personality disorders are among the most frequently treated disorders by psychiatrists and mental health practitioners, although the initial focus of treatment is usually a co-occurring symptom or disorder (e.g., anxiety disorder, depressive disorder, substance abuse disorder, eating disorder, or a medical condition). Personality disorders range from mild to severe based on functionality.

All people with PDs share common characteristics:
- *Inflexible and maladaptive responses to stress.* Individuals have difficulty responding flexibly and adaptively to the environment and to the changing demands of life. They often are unable to cope with stress and react by using maladaptive behaviors, which exposes the disorder.
- *Disability in work and personal relationships, which is generally more serious and pervasive than the similar disability found in other disorders.*

Individuals with PDs assume that everyone thinks and functions as they do; therefore, within relationships they do not view their behavior as a problem; they do not see a need to make changes or accommodate others. They believe that they are normal and that others have a problem. This thinking leads to problems with self-concept, relationships, and ability to function in society. Although some individuals with PDs may desire closer relationships with others, the following are some of the reasons personal and work relationships often fail for individuals with PDs:
- Avoidance and fear of rejection
- Blurring of boundaries between the self and others so that closeness seems to lead to fusion, which may terrify both parties
- Insensitivity to the needs of others
- Demanding and fault finding
- Inability to trust
- Lack of individual accountability
- Passive-aggressive traits
- Tendency to evoke intense interpersonal conflict: People with PDs fail to see themselves objectively, and they lack the desire to alter aspects of their behavior to enrich or maintain important relationships. Relationships are often marked by intense emotional upheavals and hostility that lead to serious interpersonal conflict, and in some cases violence (self-violence or violence toward others).
- Capacity to "get under the skin" of others: People with PDs often have an uncanny ability to merge personal boundaries with others, which has an intense and undesirable effect on others.

Most people with PDs do suffer. Their relationships with others are problematic, and they rarely reach their potential. They are often socially isolated because of their rigidity, maladaptive coping skills, and control issues that complicate their interactions with society. These patients can act bizarre, anxious, withdrawn, manipulative, or violent, and their behaviors tend to alienate them from the population. Because they are unaware that their personalities cause problems, they often blame others for their difficulties or even deny they have a problem.

PREVALENCE AND COMORBIDITY

Black and Andreasen (2011) state that epidemiological studies in the general population estimate that between 9% and 16% meet the criteria for a personality disorder. However, in the clinical population of people already diagnosed with a psychiatric disorder, studies find that between 30% and 50% have a co-occurring personality disorder. For example, some studies indicate that up to 50% of people with a major depressive disorder and more than 60% of people with generalized anxiety disorder may have a comorbid personality disorder (Black & Andreasen, 2011).

A number of PDs are associated with significant emotional disability as well as problems with social functioning and occupational impairment, in particular avoidant and antisocial

PDs. Interestingly, many people with obsessive-compulsive personality disorder seem to be high functioning, with no correlation to high disability.

Comorbid/Co-occurring Disorders

Personality disorders often co-occur with other PDs, with other Axis I disorders (e.g., substance abuse, somatic symptom disorders, eating disorders, posttraumatic stress disorder [PTSD], depression, anxiety disorders), or with general medical conditions. In fact, comorbidity seems to be the rule and not the exception. The co-occurrence of personality disorder with an Axis I disorder often portends a poor response to treatment.

Because most people with PDs do not believe there is anything wrong with them and that problems with their lives are caused by outside people or events, they rarely enter treatment for their disorder alone. Most often the disorder is not the initial focus of treatment. Many clinicians advocate that PDs should be evaluated in all psychiatric patients because their presence can influence the course and treatment of an Axis I disorder or a medical disorder for which the patient sought help initially.

THEORY

It is unlikely that there is any single cause for a discrete PD. Personality traits and their exaggerations are probably largely caused by a combination of hereditary temperamental traits and environmental and neurodevelopmental events. The contribution of genetic, biological, and environmental factors will vary with each specific disorder. The personality traits are thought to be present from infancy, but in most cases it is not until adolescence that the disorder emerges.

Genetic Factors

PDs have historically been considered to be environmentally mediated. However, research results support a more dominant role of genetics. In a definitive study of 128 pairs of twins who were raised apart, identical twins were found to have more similar personality traits than fraternal twins (Markon et al., 2002).

Genetics seem to play a significant role in the development of schizotypal personality disorder, which is more common in families with a history of schizophrenia. Obsessive-compulsive personality disorder seems to have a genetic link as well. A strong genetic factor is found through family and adoption studies of the etiology of borderline and antisocial personality disorders (Black & Andreasen, 2011).

Neurobiological Factors
Impulsive and Aggressive Behaviors

Disturbances in levels of the neurotransmitter serotonin (5-hydroxytryptamine, 5-HT) have been linked with irritability, impulsivity, and hypersensitivity. Brain imaging studies suggest abnormalities in prefrontal, corticostriatal, and limbic networks that may be related to lower serotonin neurotransmission (5-HT) and behavioral disinhibition in people with borderline and antisocial personality disorders (Oldham,

2005). Excessive aggressive behaviors are triggered by a failure of cortical "top-down" control of the limbic emotional system, which then triggers frustration, anger, or fear (Siever & Weinstein, 2009).

Affective Instability

Affective instability, seen in borderline personality disorder, is characterized by brief shifts of mood from depression, to irritability, to anxiety lasting up to a couple of hours in length (Siever & Weinstein, 2009). Affective instability is thought to be a result of excessive limbic reactivity in GABAergic/glutamatergic/cholinergic circuits. "These shifts are dramatic and trigger impulsive aggression and self destructive behavior, including drug and alcohol abuse, reckless driving, promiscuity, direct self injurious actions, as well as suicidal gestures or attempts" (Siever & Weinstein, 2009, p. 370).

Psychological Influences

Children suffering from abuse or trauma or children living in homes in which there is domestic abuse, divorce, separation, or parental absence are at risk for development of personality disorders; neglect seems to be particularly damaging (Black & Andreasen, 2011). Childhood trauma may be a risk factor for any personality disorder in general and for borderline and antisocial personality disorders in particular (Black & Andreasen, 2011). Patients diagnosed with antisocial personality disorder often have a history including excessively harsh or erratic discipline, alcoholic parent(s), or an abusive or chaotic home life.

This is particularly true for people with borderline personality disorder (BPD). There is consistent evidence that sexual abuse is a common risk factor for BPD, which also may entail significant parental conflict or loss. Linehan (1993), an early pioneer in the successful treatment of people with borderline personality disorder, made the observation that those with borderline personality disorder frequently were raised in families in which they were subjected to constant belittling, devaluation, and validation. If the history of sexual abuse was before the age of 13, posttraumatic stress disorder (PTSD) may also be present with borderline traits or diagnoses.

Cultural Considerations

It is important when making a psychiatric diagnosis to be aware of the cultural implications and what is considered normal so that culturally unsanctioned behaviors can be differentiated. This is especially true when a clinician is making a diagnosis of personality disorder. However, it appears that certain groups of the population are at a greater risk than others for certain PDs. In general, other risk factors include being Native American or African American, being a young adult, having low socioeconomic status, and being divorced, separated, widowed, or never married.

Cross-cultural studies indicate low rates of antisocial personality disorder in Taiwan, China, and Japan, as well as in Jewish families, which might be attributed to their strong family ties (Black & Andreasen, 2011).

CLINICAL PICTURE

In the following clinical picture, the major pathological personality traits are identified.

Schizotypal Personality Disorder
Pathological Personality Traits

Individuals with schizotypal personality disorders avoid interpersonal relationships, have unusual beliefs, and may be indifferent to the reactions of others in their lives.

These individuals exhibit markedly strange behavior. They most closely resemble people with schizophrenia. They are perceived by others as strikingly odd, strange, or eccentric (Sadock & Sadock, 2010). Individuals with schizotypal personality disorders may have magical thinking and rituals, or hold beliefs that they can control the actions of others. Their speech is peculiar in phrasing and syntax and may have meaning only to them. Reactions of confusion by others to their apparent illogical speech may cause these individuals to become suspicious of others and eventually to develop paranoid thinking. Their eccentric and unkempt appearances, strange behaviors, and nonadherence to social conventions make it impossible for them to have give-and-take conversations. Because of these odd styles of behavior and inattention to social conventions, they lack friends. People with this disorder are genuinely unhappy about their lack of relationships and their social anxiety and unhappiness increase over time. Under increased stress, these individuals may exhibit psychotic symptoms (Sadock & Sadock, 2010).

Up to 10% of people with schizotypal personality disorder commit suicide and some may develop schizophrenia (Black & Andreasen, 2011). These individuals enter the health care system either because of a co-occurring disorder or because of a psychotic episode.

> **VIGNETTE**
> Ms. Sands is 36 years old, lives alone, and is a "writer" on social security benefits. She goes out every night, only at night, to a nearby grocery store (because "their magic does not work at night"). She dresses in several layers of multicolored and mismatched clothes even in warmer weather. She wears a turban on her head to "keep them from seeing my thoughts." Each night she tells the grocer in a flat and formal manner that she is going to be a famous director and star. She knows this because "it hasn't snowed yet, and that means the coast is clear."

Antisocial Personality Disorder (Dyssocial Personality)
Pathological personality traits

Dyssocial personality (antisocial personality disorder) is characterized by deceit, manipulation, revenge, and harm to others with an *absence of remorse for hurting others*.

People with antisocial PD have a sense of entitlement, which means they believe they have the right to hurt others, take what they want, treat others unfairly, destroy the property of others, and so on (**callousness**). They do not adhere to traditional values or standards of morality as boundaries for their actions. Therefore, there is no restraint on their behavior, nor do they feel any sense of responsibility for their actions. People who have dyssocial personality disorders lack regard for the law and the rights of others and have a history of persistent lying, use of aliases, conning others for personal profit or pleasure, and stealing (**deceitfulness**). However, they do count on others to conform to the social norms.

Verbally these patients may be charming, engaging, and uncanny in their ability to find just the right angle to lure a person into their intrigue with the intent to exploit them for money, favors, or more sadistic purposes (**manipulation**). Promiscuity, reckless disregard for the safety of others, failure to honor work or financial commitments, and drunk driving are common events in their lives. Their lives are marked by chronic irresponsibility and unreliability. They may have a history of violence, partner abuse, child abuse, anger in response to minor slights, and vindictive behavior toward others that can result in physical or emotional pain. General reckless disregard for the safety of others is a common trait of these individuals. However, this same recklessness applies to themselves as well in their pursuit of thrill-seeking activities. People with antisocial personality disorder often become bored and engage in risky and dangerous sports or other activities, some claiming they participate in such behaviors just to "feel alive."

> **VIGNETTE**
> Mr. Jones has been extorting money from lonely widows by charming them, "helping them with their finances," promising to marry them, and then taking off with their money. When in court, he laughed when he was asked if he felt guilty for taking the life savings of these elderly lonely widows, "Hey, I gave them what they wanted." Fingerprints revealed that his name was really Oliver Torres, with a long list of aliases, as well as a history of assault and burglary. He had abandoned his wife and three children 4 years previously.

Borderline Personality Disorder (BPD)

People with borderline personality disorder have up to a 90% chance of having another psychiatric disorder and up to 40% may have two or more psychiatric disorders (Black & Andreasen, 2011). People with BPD are frequently raised in families in which they were subjected to constant belittling, devaluation, and invalidation (Linehan, 1993). Central to the character of people with borderline personality disorder is their instability of affect marked by unstable and frequent mood changes. Feelings of anxiety, dysphonia, and irritability can be intense though short lived (**emotional lability**). Chronic depression is common. Linehan (1993) refers to the patterns of high emotional sensitivity, acute responsiveness, and slow return to normal as "emotional dysregulation." This cycle may lead to feelings of deadness, panic, and fury as well as *self-mutilation* and *suicide-prone behaviors*. These are common responses to threats of separation or rejection. People with BPD desperately seek relationships to avoid feelings of abandonment and chronic feelings of emptiness. However, their excessive demands, impulsive behavior, or uncontrolled anger drives others away. Their relationships are stormy, marked by intense neediness and lack of trust. Their perception of the person in the relationship alternates between idealization/devaluation and overinvolvement/withdrawal. When relationships end, the person with borderline personality disorder is often left with feelings of deadness, panic, and fury. A person with BPD can experience dissociative states under stress. Recurrent suicide attempts or self-mutilation make suicide a significant risk in these patients. Their frequent use of the defense of splitting not only strains personal relationships but also creates turmoil in health care settings.

> **VIGNETTE**
>
> Mrs. Kit is twice divorced and has been hospitalized several times for suicidal ideation. She is also prone to injuring herself by cutting her inner thighs and arms with a razor when anxious or experiencing feelings of abandonment. She has arrived for today's therapy session. Mrs. Kit's nurse therapist is leaving for a 2-week vacation and has been preparing Mrs. Kit for the separation for more than 2 months. The therapist has given Mrs. Kit the name and phone number of another therapist to call and see while she is away. Mrs. Kit arrives at the office with fresh razor marks on her arms and tells the nurse that she is quitting therapy because the nurse really does not like her anyway and she might as well kill herself: "Go, have a good time; I might not be here when you get back." Mrs. Kit then storms out of the office and refuses to answer her phone all day.

EXAMINING THE EVIDENCE

Are Personality Disorders Treatable?

Borderline Personality Disorder—A Climate of Hope
I spent time with a patient diagnosed with borderline personality disorder (BPD) during my clinical rotation on a psych unit. This was her fourth hospitalization for attempted suicide and self-injury, and the cost of hospitalization for these patients must be soaring, as well as their suffering. Is there anything that can be done to help?

Hospitalization is always expensive, and yes, there are some new developments. It is estimated that approximately 1% of the population may have BPD. Because BPD patients have difficulty managing their emotions and frequently take extremes measures to deal with them—by harming themselves, using drugs, or considering and attempting suicide—there is much hope for a variety of treatment approaches. However, it is true that there is often continued psychological suffering as well as a financial burden placed on mental health services/insurance companies and often patients and families. The development of effective treatment services is a top health care priority (Barnicot & Katsakou, 2011).

BPD patients requiring hospital admission for attempted suicide have an increased risk of adverse outcomes and require careful clinical monitoring. Classic psychiatric hospitalization is of unproven value for suicide prevention among BPD patients. A recent study claims that short-term hospitalization at a general hospital may be the best alternative to psychiatric inpatient care. This intensive treatment includes interventions with the family/friends to clarify communication processes, decrease acute conflicts, and teach the patient and family adapted coping behaviors. A combination of this brief, intensive emergency-type treatment that readily connects to a comprehensive outpatient program may be a cost-effective alternative to inpatient hospitalization (Berrino & Ohlendorf, 2011).

For outpatient treatment, dialectical behavior therapy (DBT) (developed by Marsha Linehan), which involves replacing extremes of emotion and behavior with more moderate responses, has been widely successful. A new, effective strategy is the DBT Coach, which utilizes a smartphone application as an adjunct to standard DBT. The DBT Coach is designed to provide increased support in "opposite action" (OA). OA focuses on changing unwanted negative emotions in the moment by behaving in ways that are counter to the emotion's action urge. When users are experiencing a difficult emotion they are led to emotion-specific branching of possible responses by the DBT Coach. Next, users are asked if they are willing to work on changing the emotion. If they respond "yes," they are directed to specific coaching tools. If they respond "no," several screens help the user evaluate the pros and cons of changing the emotion. In cases where users were not willing to work on reducing the emotion, the program instructs them to call their therapist (Rizvi & Linehan, 2011).

Another outgrowth of standard DBT is DBT for Adolescents (DBT-A), a 16-week behavioral program that includes individual therapy, family therapy, and multifamily skills training in an outpatient setting. A recent study showed a significant reduction in suicidal ideation and BPD symptoms at the end of the session. Inpatient studies have shown that DBT-A could be successfully modified for use on inpatient units as well (Fleischhaker & Bohme, 2011).

New, effective treatments for persons with BPD assist mental health professionals in dealing with what used to be a very frustrating diagnosis. In addition, BPD is the only major psychiatric disorder for which psychosocial

EXAMINING THE EVIDENCE—cont'd

Are Personality Disorders Treatable?

interventions remain the primary treatment. Mental health professionals who make a serious investment treating patients with BPD can expect to become proud of their professional skills (of their personal growth in tolerance and empathy) and to experience a deeply appreciated, life-changing role for their patients (Gunderson, 2009).

Barnicot, K., & Katsakou, C. (2011). Treatment completion in psychotherapy for borderline personality disorder—a systematic review and meta-analysis. *Acta Psychiatrica Scandinavica, 123,* 327-338.

Berrino, A., & Ohlendorf, P. (2011). Crisis intervention at the general hospital: an appropriate treatment of choice for acutely suicidal borderline patients. *Psychiatry Research, 186,* 287-292.

Fleischhaker, C., & Bohme, R. (2011). Dialectical Behavioral Therapy for Adolescents (DBT-A): a clinical trial for patients with suicidal and self-injurious behavior and borderline symptoms with a one-year follow-up. *Child and Adolescent Psychiatry and Mental Health, 5*(3), 1-10.

Gunderson, J. (2009). Borderline personality disorder: ontogeny of a diagnosis. *American Journal of Psychiatry, 166,* 530-538.

Rizvi, S., & Linehan, M. (2011). A pilot study of the DBT Coach: an interactive mobile phone application for individuals with borderline personality disorder and substance use disorder, *Behavior Therapy, 10,* 1016.

Contributed by Lois Angelo.

Narcissistic Personality Disorder
Pathological Personality Traits

Narcissistic personality disorder is a maladaptive social response characterized by a person's grandiose sense of personal achievements. People with this disorder consider themselves special and expect special treatment. Their demeanor is arrogant and haughty and their sense of entitlement is striking (**grandiosity**). They lack empathy for the needs or feelings of others and in fact exploit others to meet their own needs. If they are at fault in some way, they always blame others for the problems they themselves have caused. At times, people who have narcissistic PD are admired and envied by others for what appears to be a rich and talented life. However, they require this admiration in greater and greater quantities (**attention seeking**). On the other hand, narcissistic PD patients often envy others their successes or possessions, believing that they deserve the admiration and privileges more. Because of their fragile self-esteem, they are prone to depression, interpersonal difficulties, occupational problems, and rejection (Sadock & Sadock, 2010). Their relationships are shallow and superficial and based on what the other person can do for them. Common characteristics of narcissistic people are manipulation, the use of the defense mechanism splitting, tantrums, and arrogance with sadistic and often paranoid tendencies.

Avoidant Personality Disorder
Pathological Personality Traits

People with avoidant personality disorder have high levels of anxiety and outward signs of fear and feelings of low self-worth. People with avoidant PDs are hypersensitive to criticism or rejection; therefore they tend to avoid situations that require socialization. Even though they have a strong desire for affection, they are fearful of rejection, disappointment, criticism, or ridicule. Therefore they can spend most of the time in self-imposed social isolation. They are inhibited and are fearful or reluctant to express irritation and anger with others even when it is justified. However, unlike a person with a borderline PD, they do not respond with anger to rejection, but rather withdraw. They view themselves as personally unappealing or inferior to others and consequently they have very low self-esteem. They are openly distressed by their isolation and their difficulty relating to others, as well as their low self-esteem, which adds to their inability to feel any joy or obtain any pleasure out of life. Because of their constant anxiety and feelings of low self-worth, they are unable to feel empathy with others since they are consumed with their own self-deprecation. Virtually all people with avoidant PDs have social phobias.

VIGNETTE

Mr. Chad is the vice president of a successful business. He is very arrogant and always reminds people of what he has done for the company and where it would be without him. As an aside, he will say that it is he who really runs the company, and it is he who should be the president. When employees disagree with him or have a different or novel way to implement change or progress, he takes their ideas and plans and then "lets the employee go," later taking credit for the good idea. He is known to lose his temper on the slightest provocation such as having to wait for someone to start a meeting, but by the same token, he is usually late for meetings and appointments.

VIGNETTE

Keith is a 32-year-old computer programmer. He is excessively shy, and rarely speaks with his coworkers other than perfunctory "hellos." He has never had a relationship with a woman, and tries to avoid situations in which he will be alone with any of the female employees. Sometimes the group goes out after work for a drink, and when Keith is asked he becomes very anxious and makes excuses for why he must decline. His sense of loneliness has become intolerable, and he finally seeks psychotherapy, not knowing where else to turn.

Obsessive-Compulsive Personality Disorder
Pathological Personality Traits

People with obsessive-compulsive personality disorder are preoccupied with orderliness, perfectionism, control, neatness, and the achievement of perfection. They are cautious and consider all choices in a methodical and inflexible manner. They are obsessed with rules and details and follow them rigidly, believing there is only one way to do things correctly. They have great difficulty incorporating new ideas or viewpoints (**rigid perfectionism**). They are often unable to make decisions and may have trouble completing tasks, since they persistently pursue tasks long after their actions have any consequence, and even in the face of repeated failures (**perseveration**). They are high achievers and do well in the sciences and intellectually demanding fields that require attention to detail, and they obtain their sense of self-worth from work and productivity, so much so that their devotion to work may exclude pleasurable activities and friendships.

They often have a very formal demeanor, lack a sense of humor, and have limited interpersonal skills. Although they are excessive in verbosity, these patients are miserly with material goods and emotions. They are uncomfortable with their feelings, relationships, and situations they cannot control or in which events are unpredictable. Even though they may have deep and genuine affection for others, their intimacy in *relationships is superficial* and rigidly controlled. People with obsessive-compulsive personality disorder are financially extremely stingy, and it is difficult for them to part with personal objects even if they are broken or worthless. Unlike people with the Axis I obsessive-compulsive disorder (OCD) (refer to Chapter 11), people with this disorder do not display unwanted obsessions and ritualistic behavior.

> **VIGNETTE**
>
> Mike is a 45-year-old middle manager for a microchip company. He works late and sometimes on the weekends, avoiding social and recreational activities. He has a need to get everything done to perfection, which has pushed back the deadline on many projects. He has experienced some heartburn now for a month, and his wife has been insisting he see a physician. He tells her when this project is finished he will go but hates to "waste" his money on physicians. In the physician's office he says he does not have time to take a treadmill test. When the physician tells Mike that he cannot make a diagnosis until he gets all the test results, Mike becomes very anxious.

PERSONALITY DISORDER TRAITS

Paranoid Personality Disorder Traits
Pathological Personality Traits

People with paranoid personality disorder traits are not strangers to the health care system. Nurses encounter people who are hostile, irritable, angry, injustice collectors, pathologically jealous of their partner, and litigious cranks; they are constantly suspicious and believe that others are lying, cheating, exploiting, or trying to harm them in some way. Often people with these characteristics are referred to as having paranoid personality traits (Sadock & Sadock, 2010). They lack warmth, pay close attention to power and rank, and express disdain to those who are weak, sickly, and impaired. Although they may appear businesslike and efficient, they often generate fear and conflict in others (Sadock & Sadock, 2010). People with paranoid traits are constantly suspicious of the intentions of others, and find hidden malicious meaning in benign comments and behaviors (ideas of reference). They usually make others uncomfortable; they are keenly aware of the weaknesses of others and exploit these weaknesses to keep interpersonal distance. It has been said that individuals with personality traits "lack the milk of human kindness."

> **VIGNETTE**
>
> Mr. Cole, a 58-year-old man, comes into the emergency department (ED) with chest pains. He refuses to give background information "because the information could be used against me" and is haughty and demeaning to the nurse, saying "Get someone in here who knows something." When the nurse turned her back to Mr. Cole to speak to the physician, Mr. Cole shouted, "What lies is she telling you about me? Do either one of you know what you are doing?" "Are you both in this together?"

Schizoid Personality Traits
Pathological Personality Traits

People with schizoid personality traits are seen by others as eccentric, isolated, or lonely. They may exist on the periphery of society content to avoid relationships of even the most superficial nature. Their affect is usually flat, which projects emotional coldness. They appear indifferent to praise or criticism by others. Although they invest no interest or energy into human relationships of any kind, they may invest enormous energy into nonhuman interests such as mathematics and astronomy. Typically loners, they spend much time daydreaming and are often very attached to animals. There is some evidence that people with schizoid personality traits may later develop schizophrenia or a delusional disorder. Although aloof, some individuals with schizoid traits have conceived, developed, and given our world genuinely original and creative ideas.

> **VIGNETTE**
>
> Mr. Ortiz, a 38-year-old unmarried bookkeeper, was assaulted on his way home from work. A bystander called 911 and Mr. Ortiz was taken to the ED in an unconscious state. Once awake, he answers questions in a monotone and avoids making eye contact. He often looks away and does not respond at all. He is compliant and remains a passive recipient of his treatment. Mr. Ortiz rejects all nursing interventions aimed at increasing socialization.

Histrionic Personality Disorder Traits

People with histrionic personality disorders manipulate others through their dramatic, charming, flamboyant, and sexually seductive behaviors. Their excessively emotional behavior is an attempt to seek the kind of constant attention, love, and admiration that they require. They may act out with displays of temper, tears, and accusations when they are not getting the attention or praise they believe they deserve. Interactions are often characterized by a seductiveness or provocation to draw others into a relationship or work project, but the person's attention is usually short-lived since they are subject to constant, sudden emotional shifts and emotional lability. Their relationships tend to be superficial and shallow and usually do not last long because of their constant need for attention and their insensitivity to the needs of others. Histrionic people lack insight about their role in the failure of relationships. They may seek treatment for depression or another comorbid condition.

> **VIGNETTE**
> Ms. Miller, a 45-year-old woman, meets her therapist, Dr. Jim, for the first time dressed in a tight top and short skirt and wearing a lot of makeup. She becomes flirtatious with him and tells Dr. Jim that she wants extra time today because her story is so long and she is most likely more interesting than his other patients. When he reiterates the terms of the contract and reminds her that they have 20 minutes remaining in today's session to discuss her issues, she becomes angry and insulting and tells Dr. Jim he better admit her to the hospital immediately or she will commit suicide.

Dependent Personality Disorder Traits

People with dependent personality disorder traits believe they are incapable of surviving if left alone. They solicit caretaking by clinging and being perversely and excessively submissive. By early adulthood, these people perceive themselves as being unable to separate from others, work independently, or function at all on their own. If others do not initiate or take responsibility for them, their needs remain neglected. Their intense fear of being alone is so great that they tolerate poor, even abusive treatment in order to stay in a relationship, and once a relationship ends there is an urgent need to get into another. They obsessively ruminate and fantasize about abandonment even when it is not threatened. Their high levels of anxiety intensify their inability to complete anything on their own; they are unable to make decisions without excessive advice and reassurance.

The patient with dependent personality disorder traits is at greater risk for anxiety and mood disorders, and this disorder can occur with borderline, avoidant, and histrionic personality disorders. This condition commonly occurs in individuals who have a general medical condition or disability that requires them to be dependent on others.

> **VIGNETTE**
> Mr. Martin, 49 years old, has lived with his mother since high school. His mother cooks, cleans, and shops for him. He works as a shipping dock clerk and has had the job for 30 years. He even has to ask his mother's advice on what to wear each day for work. He has become extremely anxious and fearful because his mother has been scheduled for surgery and will be away from the home for 5 days. He is terrified that he cannot cope without her there to care for him.

Passive-Aggressive Personality Traits

The *Diagnostic and Statistical Manual of Mental Disorders*, edition 5, is proposing passive-aggressive personality traits as a diagnosis under personality disorders.

People with passive-aggressive personality traits are chronically irritable and unjustifiably blame others. They are verbally aggressive, hostile, and manipulative, and their interpersonal relationships are usually marked by ambivalence and conflict. They resent being asked to do anything for anyone else either in work or in social situations, and their key traits are negativism and obstructiveness. Their demeanor is usually sullen and their work is often characterized by procrastination and inefficiency. People with passive-aggressive behavioral traits are more likely to express their negative/hostile feelings indirectly. Although they may openly agree to another's demands or requests, they rarely complete that demand or request. In fact, the actions of people with passive-aggressive personality traits are usually the opposite of their promises. Therefore, a person with passive-aggressive traits often disrupts or sabotages other people's projects or plans. Dealing with people with passive-aggressive personality traits is usually very difficult.

> **VIGNETTE**
> A nursing instructor who is perceived by others to constantly complain, be irritable, and avoid responsibility in any way has volunteered to be in charge of one of the committees involved with an upcoming accreditation visit. As the months before the accreditation visit passed, it became more noticeable that this instructor had canceled many of the meetings for her committee, missed deadlines, and failed to complete her committee work. In fact, the day the draft was to be compiled, she called in sick. When one of the committee members suggested that the accreditation material was in her office, it was discovered that absolutely nothing had been done on the report. When the nursing instructor realized that others had been in her office, she became furious that anyone should invade her privacy. She then took the next 2 weeks off from work, essentially jeopardizing the project.

APPLICATION OF THE NURSING PROCESS

ASSESSMENT

Primitive Defenses

People with personality disorders often exhibit outrageous and troublesome behaviors because they are unable to use higher level defense mechanisms to modulate painful feelings and to channel needs or aggression into creative outlets; ambivalence is poorly tolerated and impulse control is dismal (Groves, 2004). "Normal people," or at least those who live full and satisfying lives amid the inevitable personal crises and challenging circumstances that naturally constitute life, have at their disposal a variety of higher level defense mechanisms that they use to help them through such events and eventually continue with their lives. The "ego weakness" of people with PDs relies on more immature or primitive defenses (e.g., splitting, dissociation, psychotic thinking). (See Chapter 11 for definitions of immature or primitive defenses.)

These extreme and outrageous behaviors are thought to arise from intense affect, distorted cognitions, and inadequate or primitive defenses (Groves, 2004). Figure 13-1 identifies the unmodulated affects (rage, envy, shame), some of the challenging behaviors, and the cognitive processes that contribute to some of these behaviors. To add to the difficulties, personal boundaries are often blurred in many people with PDs. Closeness can seem like fusion, and the boundaries where one person begins and where another person ends are blurred. Needs are experienced as rage, and sexuality and dependency are confused with aggression (Groves, 2004).

The intense and inappropriate behaviors that characterize the lives of people with PDs tend to uproot their relationships in all settings, and are no less disruptive in the health care setting. These primitive defenses are an attempt to control their inner chaos.

For nurses, clinicians, and other health care workers, much of the challenge is dealing with many of the PD defenses and **behaviors.** This is especially true with patients who have borderline and antisocial (dyssocial) PD because nurses encounter these patients frequently in all medical settings.

Personality disorders are difficult to diagnose; people with these disorders usually present because of their comorbidity with other PDs and other complicated problems, and their response to psychotherapy and medication is unpredictable.

It is observed that often many of the problematic symptoms and behaviors may decline over time. However, even when these individuals stop meeting the *DSM* criteria for a PD, their functional scores do not change. They continue to have serious problems.

Assessment Tools

Several structured interview tools are used to diagnose PDs. These tools are not used in all clinical settings because of the need for lengthy interviews (2 hours or longer) and evaluation.

Assessment of History

Taking a full medical history can help determine if the problem is psychiatric, medical, or both. Medical illness should never be ruled out as the cause for problem behavior until the data support this conclusion. Important issues in assessment for PDs include the following: a history of suicidal or aggressive ideation or actions, current use of medicines and illegal substances, ability to handle money, and legal history.

Important areas that should be investigated include current or past physical, sexual, or emotional abuse and level of

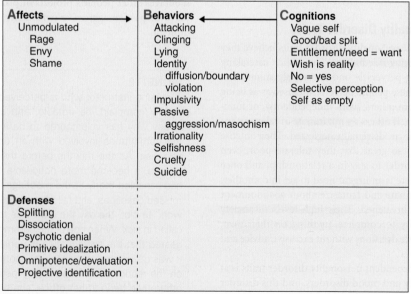

Affects	Behaviors	Cognitions
Unmodulated	Attacking	Vague self
Rage	Clinging	Good/bad split
Envy	Lying	Entitlement/need = want
Shame	Identity	Wish is reality
	diffusion/boundary	No = yes
	violation	Selective perception
	Impulsivity	Self as empty
	Passive	
	aggression/masochism	
	Irrationality	
	Selfishness	
	Cruelty	
	Suicide	
Defenses		
Splitting		
Dissociation		
Psychotic denial		
Primitive idealization		
Omnipotence/devaluation		
Projective identification		

FIGURE 13-1 ABCs of difficult patients' problem behaviors: how troublesome behaviors arise. (From Groves, J.E. [2004]. Personality disorders I: approaches to difficult patients. In T.A. Stern, J.B. Herman, & P.E. Slavin [Eds.], *Massachusetts General Hospital guide to primary care psychiatry* [2nd ed.]. New York: McGraw-Hill.)

current risk of harm from self or others. At times, immediate interventions may be needed to ensure the safety of the patient or others. Information regarding prior use of any medication, including psychopharmacological agents, is important. This information gives evidence of other contacts the patient has made for help and indicates how the health care provider found the patient at that time.

ASSESSMENT GUIDELINES
Personality Disorders

1. Assess for suicidal or homicidal thoughts. If these are present, the patient will need immediate attention.
2. Determine whether the patient has a medical disorder or another psychiatric disorder that may be responsible for the symptoms (especially a substance use disorder).
3. View the assessment of personality functioning from within the person's ethnic, cultural, and social background.
4. Ascertain whether the patient experienced a recent important loss. PDs are often exacerbated after the loss of a significant supporting person or as the result of a disruptive social situation.
5. Evaluate for a change in personality in middle adulthood or later, which signals the need for a thorough medical workup or assessment for unrecognized substance use disorder.
6. Be aware of the strong negative emotions these patients may evoke in you.

Self-Care for Nurses

Finding an approach for helping patients with PDs who have overwhelming needs can be daunting for health care workers. The intense feelings evoked in the nurse/clinician often mirror the feelings being experienced by the patient. Health care workers may feel confused, helpless, angry, and frustrated. These patients are often hostile, calling the nurse inadequate or incompetent; they are abusive of authority and are often successful in using splitting behaviors with the staff—praising or disparaging the nurse to peers in such a way that the peers begin to react negatively toward each other. Usually this is the patient's attempt to defend against his or her own feelings of frustration and powerlessness, but when staff are split, the result is often substantial conflict within the treatment team.

Untrained and unsupported staff may easily regress or become vengeful in response to a difficult patient's sense of entitlement, manipulativeness, dependency, ingratitude, impulsivity, and rage (Zimmerman & Groves, 2010). Frequent communication among staff and continuous availability of supervision and support are vital in times when the behaviors of these patients start to affect the confidence, feelings, behaviors, and effectiveness of staff members.

Nurses and other health care workers should practice self-health management. This includes acknowledging and accepting their own emotional responses, and attempting to ensure personal well-being.

DIAGNOSIS

As previously mentioned, people with PDs are usually admitted to psychiatric institutions because of presenting symptoms, Axis I comorbid disorders, dangerous behavior, or a court order for treatment. Borderline personality disorder (BPD) as well as antisocial personality disorders present a challenge for health care providers. Patients with these conditions are most often seen in the treatment setting and the behaviors central to these disorders often cause the most disruption in psychiatric and medical-surgical settings. The nursing care of BPD and antisocial behaviors is emphasized. It is safe to say that most or all people with personality disorders or severe negative personality traits have ineffective relationships and ineffective coping styles. Emotions such as anxiety, rage, and depression and behaviors such as withdrawal, paranoia, and manipulation are among the most frequent manifestations that health care workers need to address. See Table 13-1 for common potential nursing diagnoses.

OUTCOMES IDENTIFICATION

Realistic goal setting is based on the perspective that personality change involves one behavioral solution and one learned skill at a time. This can be expected to take much time and repetition. No matter how intelligent these patients may appear or how insightful they can be about themselves and others, PD patients find that change is slow and occurs via trial and error with the support of affect management and much interpersonal reinforcement—there are no shortcuts. In permanent change the learning can be integrated at the cellular level. Often these patients may have already seen several caregivers, taking what they need from one nurse or counselor before moving on to the next caregiver. Their road to recovery is long and circuitous, and the nurse is their most recent attempt to find healing.

Because larger steps are not realistic, outcomes need to be very modest and obtainable. For some individuals, overall outcome criteria might include the following:

- Minimizing self-destructive or aggressive behaviors
- Reducing the effect of manipulating behaviors
- Linking consequences to functional as well as dysfunctional behaviors
- Practicing the substitution of functional alternatives during a crisis
- Initiating functional alternatives to prevent a crisis
- Practicing ongoing management of anger, anxiety, shame, and happiness
- Creating a lifestyle that prevents regression

PLANNING

Basically, patients with PDs do not voluntarily seek treatment. Because people with antisocial and borderline PDs usually present to health care settings for other reasons, staff will benefit from in-service instruction and supervision regarding both acknowledging and coping with the behaviors of these disorders and learning techniques to prevent disruptions in the health care setting.

TABLE 13-1	POTENTIAL NURSING DIAGNOSES FOR PERSONALITY DISORDERS
SIGNS AND SYMPTOMS	**NURSING DIAGNOSES***
Crisis, high levels of anxiety	*Ineffective Coping* *Risk for Disturbed Personal Identity*
Anger and aggression; child, elder, or spouse abuse	*Risk for Other-Directed Violence* *Ineffective Coping* *Impaired Parenting* *Disabled Family Coping* *Risk for Impaired Attachment* *Ineffective Impulse control* *Post-Trauma Syndrome*
Withdrawal	*Impaired Social Isolation*
Paranoia	*Fear* *Disturbed Sensory Perception* *Disturbed Thought Processes* *Defensive Coping*
Depression	*Hopelessness* *Risk for Suicide* *Risk for Self-Mutilation* *Chronic Low Self-Esteem* *Risk for Spiritual Distress*
Difficulty in relationships, manipulation	*Ineffective Coping* *Impaired Social Interaction* *Defensive Coping*
Dysfunctional family processes	*Interrupted Family Processes* *Disturbed Personal Identity* *Risk for Loneliness* *Ineffective Relationship*
Failure to keep medical appointments, late arrival for appointments, failure to follow prescribed medical procedure or medication regimen	*Ineffective Self-Health Management* *Noncompliance*

*Nursing Diagnoses—Definitions and Classifications 2012-2014. Copyright © 2012, 1994-2012 by NANDA International. Used by arrangement with Blackwell Publishing Limited, a company of John Wiley and Sons, Inc.

IMPLEMENTATION

It is often difficult to create a therapeutic relationship with patients with PDs. Because most have experienced a series of interrupted therapeutic alliances, their suspiciousness, aloofness, and hostility can be a setup for failure. The guarded and secretive style of many of these patients tends to produce an atmosphere of combativeness. When patients blame and attack others, the nurse needs to understand the context of their complaints; these attacks develop from feeling threatened, and the more intense the complaints, the greater the fear of potential harm or loss.

Lacking the ability to trust, patients require a sense of control over what is happening to them. Giving them choices—whether to come to a clinic appointment in the morning or afternoon, for example—may enhance compliance with treatment. Because these individuals are hypersensitive to criticism yet have no strong sense of autonomy, the most effective teaching of new behaviors builds on their own existing skills.

When people with PDs exhibit fantasies that attribute malevolent intentions to the nurse or others, it is important to orient them to reality. They need to know that even though they have insulted or threatened their caregiver, they will still be helped and protected from being hurt. When they are hurt by others, as naturally happens in everyday life, the nurse takes time to dissect the situation with them, asking when, where, and how it happened, and honestly describes for them how people, systems, families, and relationships work. It is important to be honest about their limitations and assets. The patient may already be aware of them, but acknowledging them demonstrates trustworthiness.

Communication Guidelines

People with PDs may be excessively dependent, demanding, manipulative, or stubborn, or they may self-destructively refuse treatment. Nurses greatly enhance their ability to be therapeutic when they combine limit-setting, trustworthiness, manipulation management, and authenticity with their own natural style. People with borderline PD are impulsive (e.g., suicidal, self-mutilating), aggressive, manipulative, and even psychotic under periods of stress. People with antisocial PD most often are seen in the health care systems through court order. They are also manipulative, aggressive, and impulsive.

Refer to Table 13-2 for interventions for manipulation and Table 13-3 for interventions for impulsive behaviors.

Milieu Therapy

Individuals with PDs may at times be treated within a therapeutic milieu: inpatient, partial hospital, or day treatment settings. The primary therapeutic goal of milieu therapy is affect management in a group context. Community meetings, problem-solving groups, coping skills groups, and socializing groups are all areas in which patients can interact with peers, consider relationship problems, delegate and take responsibility for certain tasks, discuss goals, collectively deal with problems that arise in the milieu, and learn problem-solving skills.

Through desensitization via social group experience, overwhelming and painful internal states can be felt and endured, even while the task of the group is accomplished. When a patient acts out unconscious thoughts and needs inappropriately, the therapeutic goal is to make those needs/thoughts conscious. Then the person can learn to verbally communicate more clearly their thoughts or needs to others, instead of acting them out in a socially unacceptable (e.g., antagonistic) manner.

TABLE 13-2 INTERVENTIONS FOR MANIPULATION

INTERVENTION	RATIONALE
1. Assess your own reactions toward patient. If you feel angry, discuss with peers ways to reframe your thinking to defray feelings of anger.	1. Anger is a natural response to being manipulated. It is also a block to effective nurse-patient interaction.
2. Assess patient's interactions for a short period before labeling as manipulative.	2. A patient might respond to one particular, high-stress situation with maladaptive behaviors, but use appropriate behaviors in other situations.
3. Set limits on any manipulative behaviors, e.g., • Arguing or begging • Flattery or seductiveness • Instilling guilt, clinging • Constantly seeking attention • Pitting one person, staff, group against another • Frequently disregarding the rules • Constant engagement in power struggles • Angry, demanding behaviors	3. From the beginning, limits need to be clear. It will be necessary to refer to these limits frequently because it is to be expected that the patient will test these limits repeatedly.
4. Intervene in manipulative behavior. • All limits should be adhered to by all staff involved. • Objective physical signs in managing clinical problems should be carefully documented. • Behaviors should be documented objectively (give time, dates, circumstances). • Provide clear boundaries and consequences. • Enforce the consequences.	4. Patients will test limits, and, once they understand the limits are solid, this understanding can motivate them to work on other ways to meet their needs. It is hoped that this will be done with the nurse clinician by following problem-solving alternative behaviors and learning new effective communication skills.
5. Be vigilant; **avoid:** • Discussing yourself or other staff members with the patient • Promising to keep a secret for the patient • Accepting gifts from the patient • Doing special favors for the patient	5. Patients can use this kind of information to manipulate you and/or split staff. Decline all invitations in a firm, but straightforward manner; for example: "I am here to focus on you." "I cannot keep secrets from other staff. If you tell me something I may have to share it." "I cannot accept gifts, but I am wondering what this means to you." "You are to return to the unit by 4 PM on Sunday, period."

TABLE 13-3 INTERVENTIONS FOR IMPULSIVE BEHAVIORS

INTERVENTION	RATIONALE
1. Identify the needs and feelings preceding the impulsive acts.	1. Identify triggers to impulsive actions.
2. Discuss current and previous impulsive acts.	2. Helps link pattern of thoughts or events that trigger impulsive action.
3. Explore effects of such acts on self and others.	3. Helps patients evaluate the results of their behaviors on self and others—may motivate change.
4. Recognize cues of impulsive behaviors that may injure others.	4. Once cues are recognized, planning alternatives to impulsive actions is possible.
5. Identify situations that trigger impulsivity, and discuss alternative behaviors.	5. Once aware of cause and effect, patient can make choices.
6. Teach or refer patient to appropriate place to learn needed coping skills (e.g., anger management, assertive skills).	6. Special skills training can potentiate positive change in behaviors.

APPLYING THE ART

A Person With Borderline Personality Disorder

SCENARIO: Maria is an 18-year-old female who has already met with me three times on the young adult unit. She always wore long sleeves even though the unit was warm. The last time we met, Maria shared her poetry, which expressed themes of loneliness amid the beauty of nature. Each time she seemed glad to see me while simultaneously disparaging the evening shift staff.

THERAPEUTIC GOAL: By the end of this interaction, Maria will choose to express her feelings using a nondestructive form of communication rather than through self-mutilating behavior.

STUDENT-PATIENT INTERACTION	THOUGHTS, COMMUNICATION TECHNIQUES, AND MENTAL HEALTH NURSING CONCEPTS
Maria: "I wondered if you'd actually come back."	According to her chart, she has many reasons to mistrust, starting with her dad, who sexually abused her. She started self-mutilating in middle school when her parents divorced.
Student: "Hi, Maria. I came back as I said I would, but next Tuesday is my last day here." ***Student's feelings:*** *Sometimes I feel guilty to enter my patients' lives only to leave again. I don't want to be one more person to let her down.*	I *give information* reminding Maria of our *original nurse-patient contract.* Maria reacts with surprise, but avoids any discussion about *termination* of the *nurse-patient relationship.*
Maria: Avoids eye contact. "Read this." Hands me her poem. ***Student's feelings:*** *I feel okay about her bossiness. I recognize that I'm in charge of my own boundaries. Actually I'm relieved that Maria and I get along. She gets in so much trouble with the staff. I've seen the staff get frustrated with Maria.*	Maria says, "Read this" almost as a command. The abuse in her childhood left her feeling powerless. She needs to feel in charge of something.
Student: "Your poem describes the mother as 'daisy.' 'Daisy deigning to decorate my life.'" Maria nods. "The 'my life' person might feel lonely with such a powerful mother who drops by to decorate only." We make eye contact. "Is this about you, Maria?"	I reflect the feeling "lonely" and seek to clarify that the poem actually refers to Maria and her mother.
Maria: "She loves me, she loves me not." ***Student's feelings:*** *I'm beginning to feel a little lost in the poetry. I need to pay better attention in my English classes!*	Through the poem, Maria uses *symbolism* to safely express her thoughts and sad feelings.
Student: "At first I didn't catch the meaning of 'daisy' in your poems. 'She loves me, she loves me not.' You're sharing about your mother." ***Student's feelings:*** *I feel so sad that she's so young yet still must battle this mental torment that so disrupts her life and her happiness. She shows so much talent in her writings.*	
Maria: "She says I can't come back to live with her! She's such a ____!"	Maria shows anger in her swearing. Fear and loss fuel her anger. Her mood changes so fast! *Labile,* that's the term.
Student: "You feel abandoned. Maybe thrown away like the daisy petals." ***Student's feelings:*** *I know from her history the chaos evident in her family. I also recognize that Maria pulls people close and then pushes them away. Still, I can't image not being able to turn to my family. I feel lonely at the thought.*	I use *reflection,* remembering that patients with *borderline personality disorder* vacillate between feeling *engulfed* by the person they move close to and needing to push that person away to *individuate* self again. Unfortunately, they often *devalue* the other person, get rejected, and then experience *abandonment depression* until once again they move too close.

APPLYING THE ART—cont'd

A Person With Borderline Personality Disorder

STUDENT-PATIENT INTERACTION	THOUGHTS, COMMUNICATION TECHNIQUES, AND MENTAL HEALTH NURSING CONCEPTS
Maria: "I don't feel anything. Just numb. I have to go to the bathroom." **Student:** "Okay." *When Maria leaves, I tell my instructor and the nurse what just happened. The nurse immediately goes to find Maria.* **Student's feelings:** *I feel upset with myself for not immediately understanding that after this exchange Maria might cut herself!*	Maria says she is numb, not *depressed*. The numbness *isolates* her feelings from awareness. I probably should have gone with her or asked if she felt like cutting when she said she felt numb. Self-mutilation breaks through the numbness that has its roots in Maria's past. As a child Maria had to *dissociate* to survive the sexual abuse.
Maria: *Standing in front of me.* "You told on me!" *Raises voice but sits down two chairs away.* **Student's feelings:** *I feel uncomfortable being yelled at, and my anxiety level begins to elevate some.* **Student:** "Maria, I told the nurse that you felt upset about your mom and maybe about my leaving. I was concerned that you would be okay." **Student's feelings:** *I feel anxious, but I know that in reporting, I did the right thing. I want Maria to know I am concerned for her safety.*	I understand her behavior; it will just take me a while to not take a patient's behavior so personally and look beyond the behavior to the patient's reason for the behavior. When Maria confronts me, I *give truthful information.* When we *contracted* I said I would need to share important information with the *treatment team.*
Maria: "I don't want to talk to you anymore." **Student's feelings:** *I feel sad as Maria rejects me. I know this isn't really about me, but still I feel sad.* **Student:** *Quietly.* "You're really upset at me and at your mother, yet you were still able to stop from cutting yourself." **Student's feelings:** *I feel good that so far I'm able to contain my feelings in light of her angry and rejecting behavior toward me. I do know she needs me to stay calm and not be pushed away no matter how hard she tries.*	I *reflect* feelings and make an observation and give *support* by identifying her nondestructive choice and that she has some control over not cutting herself.
Maria: "I'm so ____ at you. A fine nurse you'll be!" *Storms away.*	With the sarcasm, Maria *devalues* me. I remember devaluing as the other pole to *idealizing* others, also part of the disorder. Nevertheless, using words to express her anger shows some progress. She uses *withdrawal* in leaving me. The closeness threatens her safety by encroaching on her *ego boundaries.* Maria's deeper loss, which pertains to her mother, gets *displaced* into the anger at me.
I stay seated about 5 minutes. I notice Maria glancing over at me a few times before she leaves for lunch. **Student's feelings:** *Maria acts so very angry at me. I feel my heart rate pick up (guess it makes me anxious). Okay, I'll take some mindful breaths. It's hard to wait here but I want Maria to know she's worth waiting for.* *I leave to debrief with my clinical group.*	Because I promised Maria that the 45 minutes we contracted was for her, I will make myself available to her for the contracted period of time.
Student's feelings: *I hope Maria will let me talk to her later today or at least on the last day I come.*	Maria's self-esteem and even her sense of identify are fragile. She restores some kind of control or power by leaving me before I terminate with her.

Psychotherapy

Several psychotherapies have been shown to be effective in treating personality disorders, although they are lengthy and expensive.

Psychodynamic Psychotherapy

This approach may help patients recognize their responsibility in the existence of turmoil in their lives and learn healthier ways of reacting to other people and problems. Individual, family, and group therapy all can be helpful.

Cognitive Behavioral Therapy

This form of therapy helps people become aware of their thought processes so that they can recognize how they draw faulty conclusions. The focus is then on reframing one's faulty thinking into a rational and realistic way of thinking about the world. Behavioral techniques include social skills training and assertiveness training, and helping patients learn more effective ways to deal with their feelings, frustrations, and interpersonal issues.

Dialectical Behavior Therapy

Dialectical behavior therapy (DBT) is another approach to cognitive behavioral therapy, which was developed by Marsha Linehan (1993) for the parasuicidal individual with borderline PD. Its theory and philosophy borrow from biological, social, cognitive behavioral and spiritual orientations. It is a four-stage treatment. In stage 1 the primary focus is on stabilizing the patient and achieving behavioral control, emotional regulation, distress tolerance skills, and constant crisis interventions. According to Blennerhassett and O'Raghallaigh (2005), the following are target behaviors:

- Decreasing life-threatening suicidal behaviors
- Decreasing therapy-interfering behaviors
- Decreasing quality-of-life–interfering behaviors
- Increasing behavioral skills

Dialectical behavior therapy has been extremely effective in helping borderline individuals gain hope and quality of life. Advanced practice nurses are now learning these skills and techniques for use in their practice.

Systems Training for Emotional Predictability and Problem Solving (STEPPS)

This is a relatively new supplement approach in the treatment of borderline personality disorder. One approach to STEPPS is a 20-week manual-driven program in which the results of two studies demonstrated that this program was useful in reducing the intensity of core aspects of borderline personality disorder (Ness, 2009). Although it does not appear to reduce hospital utilization or suicidal ideation, it did seem to reduce the number of suicide attempts and emergency department (ED) visits (Ness, 2009).

Pharmacological, Biological, and Integrative Therapies

There are no medications for the treatment of these disorders, but at times treating the symptoms is helpful. Generally, benzodiazepines for anxiety are not appropriate because the potential is great for abuse, as well as overdose. Many of these patients present with comorbid substance abuse problems. Most people do not seek treatment, but those with borderline (suicidal or self-harm behaviors) and antisocial PDs (remanded by the courts) are most frequently seen in health care settings.

Because of their propensity for suicidal gestures and self-harm, medications with low toxicity are appropriate for patients with borderline PD. Because borderline patients may become psychotic under stress, a second-generation atypical antipsychotic can be helpful. Depression is highly comorbid in these patients; therefore the selective serotonin reuptake inhibitors (SSRIs) trazodone and venlafaxine are good choices because they are the least toxic in overdose (Preston et al, 2010). The SSRIs can also help borderline patients who have comorbid panic attacks. Carbamazepine (anticonvulsant) to help target impulsivity, uncontrolled behaviors, and self-harm has been useful. Some people with antisocial PD have problems with anger and acting out. Lithium, anticonvulsants, or SSRIs may be helpful to minimize aggression. Anticonvulsants may be used with other PDs as well to help curb impulsive and aggressive behaviors.

People with schizotypal PD, although they rarely voluntarily seek treatment, may be helped with low-dose antipsychotic medications, which help ameliorate anxiety and psychosis-like features associated with this disorder. Obsessive-compulsive PD is often helped with clomipramine (a tricyclic antidepressant) and SSRIs to ameliorate obsessional thinking and comorbid depression.

EVALUATION

Evaluating treatment effectiveness in this patient population is difficult. Health care providers may never know the real results of their interventions, particularly in acute care settings. Even in long-term outpatient treatment, many patients find the relationship too intimate an experience to remain long enough for successful treatment. However, some motivated patients may be able to learn to change their behavior, especially if positive experiences are repeated. Each therapeutic episode offers an opportunity for patients to observe themselves interacting with caregivers who consistently try to teach positive coping skills. Perhaps effectiveness can be measured by how successfully the nurse is able to be genuine with the patient, maintain a helpful posture, offer substantial instruction, and still care for the patient. Specific short-term outcomes may be accomplished and, overall, the patient can be given the message of hope that quality of life can always be improved.

KEY POINTS TO REMEMBER

- People with personality disorders (PDs) present with the most complex, difficult behavioral challenges for themselves and the people around them.
- People with PDs have inflexible and maladaptive ways of handling stress; demonstrate disabilities in both work and intimate relationships; evoke strong, intense personal conflict with those around them; and have difficulty managing impulses.
- PDs often co-occur with other Axis I disorders (e.g., depression, substance abuse, somatization, eating disorders, PTSD, anxiety disorders), other personality disorders, and general medical conditions.
- It is unlikely there is any single cause for discrete PDs—most seem to have genetic and environmental risk factors.
- People with these disorders respond to stress (e.g., frustration, anger, loneliness) with more primitive defenses, resulting in outrageous behaviors unmodified by "normal" defenses.
- Needs are experienced as rage, and sexuality and dependency are confused with aggression.
- Self-assessment is an important part of assessment when working with a person with a PD. When personal feelings are not recognized or confronted, substantial interpersonal conflict will ensue.

- Determining if there is a history of suicide/homicide/self-mutilation, and if there are co-occurring disorders as well, is a vital part of the initial assessment interview.
- Nursing diagnoses are given and reflect the problematic behaviors of the PD at the time.
- Communication guidelines for manipulative and impulsive behaviors are outlined.
- Careful evaluation for antidepressants, anticonvulsants (for aggressive and impulsive behaviors), and antipsychotics (for stress-induced psychotic thinking) may offer the patient relief.
- Therapy has been used for patients with PDs; however, there is little evidence-based research comparing the efficacy of different therapies with different disorders, except for dialectical behavior therapy (DBT), which has been extremely effective in people with borderline PD.
- Much needs to be done to better understand PDs:
  - Conducting more and better biological research
  - Completing prospective community studies of psychosocial risk factors such as trauma
  - Developing medications specifically for borderline PD
  - Creating a common approach to psychotherapy

APPLYING CRITICAL JUDGMENT

1. Ms. Pemrose is brought to the ED after slashing her wrist with a razor. She has previously been in the ED for drug overdose and has a history of addictions. Ms. Pemrose can be sarcastic, belittling, and aggressive to those who try to care for her. She has a history of difficulty with interpersonal relationships at her job. When the psychiatric triage nurse comes in to see her, Ms. Pemrose is at first adoring and compliant, telling him, "You are the best nurse I've ever seen, and I truly want to change." But when he refuses to support her request for diazepam (Valium) and meperidine (Demerol) for "pain," she yells at him, "You are a stupid excuse for a nurse. I want a physician immediately." Ms. Pemrose has borderline PD.

   A. What defense mechanism is Ms. Pemrose using?

   B. How could the nurse best handle this situation in keeping with setting limits and offering concern and useful interventions?

   C. When you research Ms. Pemrose's records, what might you expect to find in her history, including behavioral issues, family history, and potential comorbidities?

   D. In terms of safety, explain what you feel is the primary initial concern when planning care.

   E. If Ms. Pemrose agreed to accept treatment, describe the treatment regimen that has been determined to be helpful in people with borderline personality disorders.

   F. When Ms. Pemrose becomes manipulative, identified specific steps that can help minimize negative effects for manipulation.

   G. A nurse working with someone like Ms. Pemrose, who exhibited impulse behavior, identify the kinds of nursing interventions might help.

CHAPTER REVIEW QUESTIONS

Choose the most appropriate answer(s).

1. Which of the following best describes people with PDs?
   1. They readily assume the roles of compromiser and harmonizer.
   2. They often seek help to change maladaptive behaviors.
   3. They have the ability to tolerate high levels of anxiety.
   4. They have difficulty working and loving.

2. After completing an assessment of a client diagnosed with borderline personality disorder, the nurse finds which of the following to be true?
   1. Flexible coping skills
   2. Socially appropriate behavior
   3. Eagerness to learn new coping skills
   4. Self defeating cycle of behavior

3. For the nurse working with patients with PDs, which nursing intervention must be an ongoing priority?
   1. Offering professional advice
   2. Probing for etiological factors
   3. Encouraging diversional activity
   4. Setting appropriate limits

4. Which interventions are appropriate to demands from a client with borderline personality disorder?
   1. Assign two staff members per shift to this client.
   2. Design a strict activity schedule.
   3. Hold frequent staff meetings.
   4. Be consistent in response to client demands.

5. Impulsive behavior is characterized by:
   1. postponing gratification to appropriate time.
   2. manipulation and control.
   3. short periods between thoughts and actions.
   4. loud, frequent outbursts.

REFERENCES

Black, D. W., & Andreasen, N. C. (2011). Personality disorders. In *Introductory textbook of psychiatry.* (5th ed.). Washington, DC: American Psychiatric Publishing, pp. 295–318.

Blaise, M. A., Smallwood, P., Groves, J. E., & Rivas-Vazquez, R. A. (2008). Personality and personality disorders. In Stern et al: *Massachusetts General Hospital Comprehensive Clinical Psychiatry.* Philadelphia: Saunders/Elsevier.

Blennerhassett, R. C., & O'Raghallaigh, J. W. (2005). Dialectical behavior therapy in the treatment of borderline personality disorder. *British Journal of Psychiatry, 186,* 278–280.

Exforsys, Inc. (2010). What is personality? Retrieved March 31, 2012, from http://www.exforsys.com/careercenter/personality development/whatispersonality.html.

Groves, J. E. (2004). Personality disorders I: approaches to difficult patients. In T. A. Stern, J. B. Herman, & P. E. Slavin (Eds.), *Massachusetts General Hospital guide to primary care psychiatry* (2nd ed.). New York: McGraw-Hill.

Linehan, M. M. (1993). *Understanding borderline personality disorder: a dialectical approach.* New York: Guilford.

Markon, K. E., Krueger, R. F., Bouchard, T. J., & Gottesman, I. I. (2002). Normal and abnormal personality traits: evidence for genetic and environmental relationships in the Minnesota study of twins reared apart. *Journal of Personality and Social Psychology, 70,* 661–694.

Mayer, J. D. (2005). A tale of two visions: can a new view of personality help integrate psychology? *Am J Psychol 60,* 294–307.

Ness, T. M. (2009). *STEPPS: a viable supplement to treatment of borderline personality.* Retrieved August 5, 2011, from: www.psychiatrictimes.com/print/articles/10168/142-5290?printable= true.

Oldham, J. M. (2005). *Guidelines watch: practice guideline for the treatment of patients with borderline personality disorder.* Arlington: American Psychiatric Association.

Preston, J. D., O'Neal, J. H., & Talaga, M. C. (2010). *Handbook of clinical psychopharmacology for therapists* (6th ed.). Oakland, CA: New Harbinger Publications.

Sadock, B. J., & Sadock, V. A. (2010). Personality disorders. In J. Sadock, & V. A. Sadock (Eds.), *Kaplan & Sadock's pocket handbook of clinical psychiatry* (5th ed.). Philadelphia: Lippincott Williams & Wilkins.

Siever, L. J., & Weinstein, L. N. (2009). The neurobiology of personality disorders: implications for psychoanalysis. *Journal of the American Psychoanalytic Association, 57,* 361. Retrieved February 25, 2011, from www.sagepub/content/57/2/361.refs.html.

Zimmerman, D. J., & Groves, J. E. (2010). Difficult patients. In T. A. Stern, et al. (Eds.), *Massachusetts General Hospital handbook of general hospital psychiatry* (6th ed.). Philadelphia: Saunders/Elsevier.

Eating Disorders

Kathleen Ibrahim

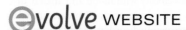 WEBSITE

http://evolve.elsevier.com/Varcarolis/essentials

KEY TERMS AND CONCEPTS

anorexia nervosa, p. 230
binge eating disorder (BED), p. 230
bulimia nervosa, p. 230
cachectic, p. 233
cognitive distortions, p. 235

ideal body weight, p. 234
lanugo, p. 233
purging, p. 233
refeeding syndrome, p. 234

SELECTED CONCEPT: Cognitive Distortion—Eating Disorder
People with eating disorders have cognitive distortions that are the result of processing errors in the brain. It is important to determine which cognitive distortions were present before the eating disorder, and which ones are the result of semi starvation.

Although the eating behavior is targeted, the underlying emotions of anxiety, dysphoria, low self-esteem, and feelings of lack of control are also addressed through cognitive behavioral therapy.
(http://www.anorexia-reflections.com/cognitive-distortions.html)

OBJECTIVES

1. Compare and contrast the signs and symptoms of anorexia nervosa and bulimia nervosa.
2. Apply knowledge of patient safety needs when assessing for at least two life-threatening conditions that may develop for a patient with anorexia, and at least two for a patient with bulimia.
3. Identify examples of therapeutic interventions that are appropriate for the acute phase and those that are appropriate for the long-term phase of treatment when planning patient-centered care for a patient with anorexia nervosa.
4. Describe what you know about evidence-based practice in the optimal treatment of eating disorders.
5. Distinguish between effective treatments when planning patient-centered care for patients with acute bulimia and for individuals in long-term therapy for bulimia.
6. Discuss the teamwork and collaboration needed to effectively treat eating disorders.
7. Differentiate between the long-term prognosis of anorexia nervosa, bulimia nervosa, and binge eating disorder.

For the majority of people, eating provides nourishment for the body as well as the soul. Families and friends gather around the table to break bread as they celebrate, mourn, laugh, cry, share, and demonstrate love. However, for some individuals, eating loses its communal value and becomes hidden and shrouded in secrecy and shame. People with eating disorders experience severe disruptions in normal eating patterns and a significant disturbance in the perception of body shape and weight.

Diagnostic categories included in this chapter are anorexia nervosa, bulimia nervosa, and binge eating disorders. Individuals with anorexia nervosa engage in self-starvation, express intense fear of gaining weight, and have a disturbance in self-evaluation of weight and its importance; females with anorexia often experience amenorrhea. There are two subtypes of anorexia—those with one subtype restrict their intake of food, whereas those with the other subtype engage in binge eating and/or purging.

Individuals with bulimia nervosa engage in repeated episodes of binge eating followed by inappropriate *compensatory* behaviors such as self-induced vomiting; misuse of laxatives, diuretics, or other medications; fasting; or excessive exercise.

Individuals with eating disorders may display a mixture of anorectic and bulimic behaviors.

In the fifth edition of the *Diagnostic and Statistical Manual of Mental Disorders (DSM-5)* binge eating disorder will become a bona fide eating disorder. Binge eating disorder is diagnosed when individuals engage in repeated episodes of binge eating after which they experience significant distress. These individuals do not regularly use the compensatory behaviors seen in patients with bulimia nervosa.

According to the Academy for Eating Disorders (AED, 2011) the most effective care involves a *multidisciplinary* team approach that enlists the expertise of various health care sectors, including medical physicians, psychologists, psychiatrists, nutritionists, and psychopharmacologists. In addition, families and spouses are always encouraged to participate.

PREVALENCE AND COMORBIDITY

Eating disorders are culturally influenced disorders with varying prevalence depending on the culture and its social norms. The actual number of individuals with eating disorders is not known because these disorders may exist for a long time before the person either willingly or unwillingly seeks help.

The estimated lifetime prevalence rate among women for developing anorexia nervosa is about 1% and the rate among men is 0.3%. For bulimia nervosa, the lifetime prevalence rate for women is 1.5% and for men it is 0.5% (Hudson et al., 2007). Female as well as male athletes demonstrate an increased incidence of eating disorders.

Anorexia nervosa has an average age of onset in early to middle adolescence whereas bulimia nervosa more typically appears in late adolescence. The course for both disorders may be a single episode but more frequently the pattern is intermittent and often chronic in nature, particularly for anorexia nervosa. There is a prevalent crossover pattern from anorexia nervosa

restricting subtype, to anorexia nervosa binge/purge subtype, and then crossing over to bulimia nervosa (Peat et al., 2009).

The issue of an increasing incidence and diagnosis of eating disorders in midlife has been researched. McLean and colleagues (2010) studied women ages 35 to 65 and found that developmental factors (age-related changes in appearance and role changes) potentially increased risk for body dissatisfaction and disordered eating. Scholtz and colleagues (2010) found no evidence of late-onset anorexia nervosa but instead an exacerbation in midlife of a previously established dormant form of anorexia.

Eating disorders are almost always comorbid with other psychiatric illnesses. More than 50% of people with anorexia have one other concurrent psychiatric disorder, and almost 95% of people with bulimia have another psychiatric disorder. For example, anorexia nervosa is associated with social phobia (34% of cases), depression (65% of cases), and obsessive-compulsive disorder (26% of cases) (Sadock & Sadock, 2007). There is a significant comorbidity with mood and anxiety disorders, substance abuse, body dysmorphic disorders, impulse control disorders, and personality disorders, especially borderline and obsessive-compulsive personality disorders. The AED (2011) advises to always assess for psychiatric risk, including suicidal and self-harm thoughts, plans, and/or intent. Up to one third of deaths related to eating disorders are attributable to suicide.

A history of sexual abuse is more common in those with eating disorders than in the general population. Women with a history of eating disorders and sexual abuse have a higher rate of other comorbid psychiatric illnesses than women diagnosed solely with eating disorders.

THEORY

The etiology of eating disorders is varied and complex. It appears that these disorders include a biological vulnerability or predisposition that is activated by psychological, environmental, and cultural factors.

Neurobiological and Neuroendocrine Models

Neuroendocrine abnormalities are noted in both anorexia nervosa and bulimia nervosa (Bailer & Kaye, 2011). These abnormalities are of "the chicken or the egg" quality because we are not certain if they cause the eating disorder or if the eating disorder causes them. There is some support for a primary pathology because people with active illness and people who have recovered have exactly the same abnormalities. Brain imaging studies demonstrate unusual activity in various regions of the brain including the frontal, cingulate, temporal, and parietal areas. In both anorexia nervosa and bulimia nervosa, serotonin pathways are abnormal. Researchers believe that this altered serotonin pathway may be key to anxiety responses, inhibition, and even distortions in body image. Brain scans also reveal altered serotonin receptors and transporters. This may be the basis for mood problems, reduced impulse control, and the motivation for eating and enjoying food.

Genetic Models

Results of family, twin, and adoption studies of individuals with anorexia nervosa, bulimia nervosa, and binge eating disorder have shown that genetic factors contribute to the risk of developing an eating disorder (Thornton et al., 2011). For example, there is an approximately 70% concordance rate for identical twins, and only about 20% for nonidentical twins (Black & Andreasen, 2011). Female relatives of people with eating disorders are up to 12 times more likely to develop an eating disorder. Kaye and colleagues (2008) are conducting linkage analyses—studying pedigrees of individuals with multiply affected family members. These results (genetic markers) can be used to explore chromosomal regions that are known to contain genetic variation affecting risk. What is inherited is not clear. Both individuals with anorexia nervosa and individuals with bulimia nervosa have a characteristic phenotype—a constellation of personality traits that have been shown to be moderately heritable. Genetic vulnerability might stem from an underlying neurotransmitter dysfunction, or perhaps the vulnerability is one of inherited temperament, cognitive style, mood-regulating tendencies, and unique weight set point.

Psychological Models

Although biology may create a predisposition for eating disorders, psychological determinants may play a role in activating them. Anorexia nervosa results in amenorrhea in females and physiological changes that interfere with the development of an age-appropriate sexual role. Psychoanalytic theorists long believed that fear of sexual maturity and the need to maintain a childlike body were primary beliefs for people with anorexia. The "core psychopathology" in both anorexia and bulimia is thought to be low self-esteem and self-doubts about personal worth. These feelings produce harsh self-judgment focused solely on the issue of weight. The overvalued ideas about weight, shape, and control are critical to maintaining the eating-disordered behaviors (Fairburn, 2008).

Family theorists have long believed that specific dynamics converge to create individuals with eating disorders. For anorexia, these families are seen as controlling, emphasizing perfection, achievement, and compliance. Bulimic families are seen as chaotic and emotionally expressive, particularly in terms of conflict and negativity. Critics of these theories emphasize that these characteristics may not be the cause of the problem, but rather part of the genetic makeup related to the disorder. For example, the perfectionist and controlling qualities of anorectic families may be a result of obsessive genetic tendencies. However, The Academy for Eating Disorders has published a position paper based on current knowledge strongly opposing any theoretical model that states family dynamics are the primary cause of anorexia nervosa or bulimia nervosa (Le Grange et al., 2010).

CULTURAL CONSIDERATIONS

The assumption that eating disorders are rare in non-Western countries and among ethnic minorities in the United States is no longer valid. Globalization has exposed minorities and non-Western societies to the value of the thin beauty ideal. Food refusal in non-Western societies may not be motivated by fat phobia but rather dieting may reflect personal meaning based on religious or ascetic values. However, the non–fat phobic profile of eating disorders in some Asian countries appears to be changing and increasingly conforming more to the Western profile that includes drive for thinness and fear of weight gain (Becker et al., 2009).

SELF-CARE FOR NURSES

The nurse caring for the anorectic patient may find it difficult to appreciate the compelling force of this illness, regarding it as trivial (compared to a mental illness such as schizophrenia), incorrectly believing that weight restriction, bingeing, and purging are self-imposed. The nurse may believe that the patient "chooses" to engage in behaviors that are risky and blame the patient for his or her health problems. In addition, the common personality traits of these clients—including perfectionism, obsessive thoughts and actions relating to food, and the need to control their therapy in such a way that they are in almost constant conflict with their caregivers—pose challenges to the nurse.

In the effort to motivate the patient and take advantage of the decision to seek help and be healthier, the nurse must take care not to cross the line toward authoritarianism and assumption of a parental role in the relationship. As the nurse struggles to build a therapeutic alliance and be empathetic, the patient's terror at gaining weight and resistance to nursing interventions may engender significant frustration. Nurses must guard against any tendency to be coercive in their approach and must be aware that one of the primary goals of treatment—weight gain—is the very outcome the client fears. Frequent acknowledgment of the situation for the client and of the constant struggle that so characterizes the treatment will help during times of extreme resistance. If countertransference/personal feelings are not recognized and examined, withdrawal may result to avoid feelings of frustration. Being supervised by a competent, supportive, more experienced clinician and sharing with peers help minimize feelings of frustration and can contribute to therapeutic growth in the nurse.

CLINICAL PICTURE

Anorexia nervosa and bulimia nervosa are two separate syndromes and as such they present two clinical pictures. Box 14-1 identifies the signs and symptoms of these disorders.

Eating disorders are serious and in extreme cases can lead to death. Box 14-2 identifies a number of complications that can occur and the laboratory findings that may result in individuals with eating disorders. Because the eating behaviors in these conditions are so extreme, hospitalization may become necessary. Box 14-3 identifies when an individual should be hospitalized; often hospitalization is via the emergency department (ED).

In treating patients who have been sexually abused or who have otherwise been the victim of boundary violations, it is

BOX 14-1   POSSIBLE SIGNS AND SYMPTOMS OF ANOREXIA NERVOSA AND BULIMIA NERVOSA

Anorexia Nervosa
- Terror of gaining weight
- Preoccupation with thoughts of food
- View of self as fat even when emaciated
- Peculiar handling of food:
  - Cutting food into small bits
  - Pushing pieces of food around plate
- Possible development of rigorous exercise regimen
- Possible self-induced vomiting; use of laxatives and diuretics
- Cognition is so disturbed that the individual judges self-worth by his or her weight
- Controls what he or she eats to feel powerful to overcome feelings of helplessness

Bulimia Nervosa
- Binge eating behaviors
- Often self-induced vomiting (or laxative or diuretic use) after bingeing
- History of anorexia nervosa in one fourth to one third of individuals
- Depressive signs and symptoms
- Problems with:
  - Interpersonal relationships
  - Self-concept
  - Impulsive behaviors
- Increased levels of anxiety and compulsivity
- Possible chemical dependency
- Possible impulsive stealing
- Controls/undoes weight after bingeing, which is motivated by feelings of emptiness

BOX 14-2   SOME MEDICAL COMPLICATIONS OF ANOREXIA NERVOSA AND BULIMIA NERVOSA

Anorexia Nervosa
- Bradycardia
- Orthostatic changes in pulse rate or blood pressure
- Cardiac murmur—one third with mitral valve prolapse
- Sudden cardiac arrest caused by profound electrolyte disturbances
- Prolonged QT interval on electrocardiogram
- Acrocyanosis
- Symptomatic hypotension
- Leukopenia
- Lymphocytosis
- Carotenemia (elevated carotene levels in blood), which produces skin with yellow pallor
- Hypokalemic alkalosis (with self-induced vomiting or use of laxatives and diuretics)
- Elevated serum bicarbonate levels, hypochloremia, and hypokalemia
- Electrolyte imbalances, which lead to fatigue, weakness, and lethargy
- Osteoporosis, indicated by decrease in bone density
- Fatty degeneration of liver, indicated by elevation of serum enzyme levels
- Elevated cholesterol levels
- Amenorrhea
- Abnormal thyroid functioning
- Hematuria
- Proteinuria

Bulimia Nervosa
- Cardiomyopathy from ipecac intoxication (medical emergency that usually results in death)
- Cardiac dysrhythmias
- Sinus bradycardia
- Sudden cardiac arrest as a result of profound electrolyte disturbances
- Orthostatic changes in pulse rate or blood pressure
- Cardiac murmur; mitral valve prolapse
- Electrolyte imbalances
- Elevated serum bicarbonate levels (although can be low, which indicates metabolic acidosis)
- Hypochloremia
- Hypokalemia
- Dehydration, which results in volume depletion, leading to stimulation of aldosterone production, which in turn stimulates further potassium excretion from kidneys; thus there can be an indirect renal loss of potassium as well as a direct loss through self-induced vomiting
- Severe attrition and erosion of teeth producing irritating sensitivity and exposing the pulp of the teeth
- Loss of dental arch
- Diminished chewing ability
- Parotid gland enlargement associated with elevated serum amylase levels
- Esophageal tears caused by self-induced vomiting
- Severe abdominal pain indicative of gastric dilation
- Russell's sign (callus on knuckles from self-induced vomiting)

CRITERIA FOR HOSPITAL ADMISSION OF INDIVIDUALS WITH EATING DISORDERS

Physical Criteria

- Weight loss more than 30% over 6 months
- Rapid decline in weight
- Inability to gain weight with outpatient treatment
- Severe hypothermia caused by loss of subcutaneous tissue or dehydration (body temperature lower than 36° C or 96.8° F)
- Heart rate less than 40 beats per minute
- Systolic blood pressure less than 70 mm Hg
- Hypokalemia (less than 3 mEq/L) or other electrolyte disturbances not corrected by oral supplementation
- Electrocardiographic changes (especially dysrhythmias)

Psychiatric Criteria

- Suicidal or severely irrepressible, self-mutilating behaviors
- Uncontrollable use of laxatives, emetics, diuretics, or street drugs
- Failure to comply with treatment contract
- Severe depression
- Psychosis
- Family crisis or dysfunction

critical that the nurse and other health care workers maintain and respect clear boundaries. Fundamental to the care of individuals with eating disorders is the establishment and maintenance of a therapeutic alliance. This will take time as well as diplomacy on the part of the nurse.

APPLICATION OF THE NURSING PROCESS: ANOREXIA NERVOSA

ASSESSMENT

The nurse assessing a patient with anorexia observes a cachectic (severely underweight with muscle wasting) male or female who may have lanugo (a growth of fine, downy hair on the face and back); mottled, cool skin on the extremities; and low blood pressure, pulse, and temperature readings. All of these findings are consistent with a malnourished and dehydrated state.

Cardinal symptoms for anorexia nervosa include dangerously low body weight measurements relative to the age and gender of the patient. Various standards help define significantly low body weight, including pediatric growth tables and Metropolitan Life Insurance tables. However, calculations based on body mass index (BMI) (weight in kilograms divided by height in meters squared) are more precise. Ideal BMIs are thought to be between 19 and 25. Automatic calculators of BMI are widely available on the Internet.

Individuals with the binge/purge type of anorexia nervosa may have prominent parotid glands—the largest of the salivary glands, located in each cheek in front of the ears—because of hyperstimulation from repeated vomiting. Furthermore, they may present with severe electrolyte imbalance as a result of purging, which may be in the form of vomiting, abusing laxatives or diuretics, or using enemas. These individuals may be dangerously ill and often begin treatment in an intensive care unit.

As with any comprehensive psychiatric nursing assessment, a complete evaluation of biopsychosocial function is mandatory. The areas to be covered include the following patient characteristics:

- Perception of the problem
- Eating habits
- History of dieting
- Methods used to achieve weight control (restricting, purging, exercising)
- Value attached to a specific shape and weight
- Interpersonal and social functioning
- Mental status and physiological parameters

ASSESSMENT GUIDELINES

Anorexia Nervosa

1. Determine if medical or psychiatric condition warrants hospitalization (see Box 14-3).
2. Assess level of family understanding about the disease and where to receive support.
3. Assess acceptance of therapeutic modalities.
4. Perform a thorough physical examination with appropriate bloodwork.
5. Check for other medical conditions.
6. Determine the family and patient's need for teaching or information regarding the treatment plan (e.g., psychopharmacological interventions, behavioral therapy, cognitive therapy, family therapy, individual psychotherapy).
7. Assess the patient's and family's desire to participate in a support group.

VIGNETTE

Tina, a 16-year-old girl who is 60% of ideal body weight, is cachectic on admission to an inpatient psychiatric unit. She has lanugo over most of her body and prominent parotid glands. She is further assessed to be hypotensive (86/50 mm Hg) and dehydrated. In addition, she has a low serum potassium level and dysrhythmias that appear on an electrocardiogram (ECG). A decision is made to transfer her to the intensive care unit until she is medically stabilized. As an intravenous catheter is inserted, her severe weight phobia and fear of being overweight are underscored when she cries, "There's not going to be sugar in the IV, is there?" The nurse responds, "I hear how frightened you are. We need to do what's necessary to get you past this crisis."

DIAGNOSIS

Imbalanced nutrition: less than body requirements is usually the most compelling nursing diagnosis initially for individuals with anorexia. It generates further nursing diagnoses; for example, *Decreased cardiac output, Risk for injury* (electrolyte imbalance), and *Risk for imbalanced fluid volume,* which would have first priority when problems are addressed. Other nursing diagnoses include *Disturbed body image, Anxiety, Chronic low self-esteem, Deficient knowledge, Ineffective coping, Powerlessness,* and *Hopelessness.*

OUTCOMES IDENTIFICATION

Outcomes need to be measurable and include a time estimate for attainment (ANA, 2007). Some common outcome criteria for patients with anorexia nervosa include the following (fill in the appropriate time [e.g., within 3 weeks, by discharge]); the patient will:

- Refrain from self-harm.
- Normalize eating patterns, as evidenced by eating 75% of three meals per day plus two snacks.
- Achieve 85% to 90% of ideal body weight.
- Be free of physical complications.
- Demonstrate two new, healthy eating habits.
- Demonstrate improved self-acceptance, as evidenced by verbal and behavioral data.
- Address maladaptive beliefs, thoughts, and activities related to the eating disorder.
- Participate in treatment of associated psychiatric symptoms (defects in mood, self-esteem).
- Demonstrate at least one behavior and one interest that are appropriate to age.
- Participate in long-term treatment to prevent relapse.

PLANNING

Planning is affected by the acuity of the patient's situation. In the case of a patient with anorexia who is experiencing extreme electrolyte imbalance or whose weight is less than 75% of ideal body weight, the plan is to provide immediate stabilization, most likely in an inpatient unit (APA, 2000a). Inpatient hospitalization is usually brief, attempts limited weight restoration, and addresses only acute complications (such as electrolyte imbalance and dysrhythmias) and acute psychiatric symptoms (such as significant depression). Some hospitalized patients experience refeeding syndrome, a potentially catastrophic treatment complication in which the demands of a replenished circulatory system overwhelm the capacity of a nutritionally depleted cardiac muscle, which results in cardiovascular collapse (APA, 2000a).

Once a patient is medically stable, the plan begins to address the issues underlying the eating disorder. These issues are usually treated on an outpatient basis and will include individual, group, and family therapy as well as psychopharmacological therapy during different phases of the illness. The nature of the treatment is determined both by the intensity of the symptoms—which

may vary over time—and by the experienced disruption in the patient's life.

The following are the three main goals for all eating disorders:

1. Restore the patient's nutritional state (Black & Andreasen, 2011).
   a. For anorexia nervosa this means restoring weight within normal range.
   b. For bulimia this means ensuring a balanced metabolic state.
2. Modify the patient's distorted eating behaviors.
3. Help change distorted and erroneous beliefs about weight loss and body image.

IMPLEMENTATION

See Table 14-1 for specific interventions regarding anorexia nervosa.

Acute Care

Patients with eating disorders may be admitted to intensive care, coronary care, and medical and special eating disorders units. Typically when an individual with an eating disorder is admitted to any of these units, the person is in a crisis state. The nurse is challenged to establish trust and monitor the eating pattern. Weight restoration and weight monitoring create opportunities to counter the distorted ideas that maintain the illness. Nurses and other health care providers provide milieu therapy, counseling, health teaching, and medication management. Within special eating disorder units and general psychiatric units, patient privileges may be linked to weight gain and treatment plan compliance.

Communication Guidelines

The nurse on a behavioral health inpatient unit may have to operate as both primary nurse and group leader. The initial focus depends on the results of a comprehensive assessment. Interventions include milieu therapy, teaching, and psychotherapy. Any acute psychiatric symptoms, such as suicidal ideation, are addressed immediately. At the same time, a patient with anorexia begins a weight restoration program that allows for incremental weight gain. Based on the patient's height, a treatment goal is set at 90% of ideal body weight, the weight at which most women are able to menstruate.

In the effort to motivate the patient and take advantage of the decision to seek help and be healthier, the nurse must avoid authoritarianism and assumption of a parental role. As the nurse struggles to build a therapeutic alliance and be empathic, the patient's terror at gaining weight and resistance to nursing interventions may engender significant frustration. As previously stated, nurses must appreciate the compelling force of this illness and be aware that one of the primary goals of treatment—weight gain—is the very outcome the patient fears. Frequent acknowledgment of the difficulty of the situation for the patient and of the constant struggle that characterizes the treatment will help during times of extreme resistance.

Establishing a therapeutic alliance with a person with anorexia is challenging because the compelling force of the

TABLE 14-1 INTERVENTIONS FOR ANOREXIA NERVOSA

INTERVENTION	RATIONALE
1. Acknowledge the emotional and physical difficulty the patient is experiencing.	1. A first priority is to establish a therapeutic alliance.
2. Assess for suicidal thoughts/self-injurious behaviors.	2. The potential for a psychiatric crisis is always present.
3. Monitor physiological parameters (vital signs, electrolyte levels) as needed.	3. The life-threatening effect of weight restriction and/or purging needs to be monitored.
4. Weigh patient wearing only bra and panties/underwear only on a routine basis (same time of day after voiding and before drinking/eating). Some protocol includes weighing with the patient's back to the scale.	4. Weights are a high-anxiety time. The underweight patient might try to manipulate the weight by drinking fluids or placing heavy objects in clothing before being weighed. Discussion of weight gain (or loss) may be postponed for the primary therapist.
5. Monitor patient during and after meals to prevent throwing away food and/or purging.	5. The compelling force of the illness makes it difficult to stop certain behaviors.
6. Recognize the patient's distorted image/overvalued ideas of body shape and size without minimizing or challenging patient's perceptions.	6. A straightforward statement that the nurse's perceptions are different will help to avoid a power struggle. Arguments and power struggles intensify the patient's need to control.
7. Educate the patient about the ill effects of low weight and resultant impaired health.	7. The treatment goal of gaining weight is what the patient most resists. Focus on the benefits of improved health and increased energy at a more normalized weight.
8. Work with patients to identify strengths.	8. When patients are feeling overwhelmed, they no longer view their lives objectively.

illness runs counter to therapeutic interventions. As patients begin to refeed, ideally they begin to participate in milieu therapy, in which the cognitive distortions that perpetuate the illness are consistently confronted by all members of the interdisciplinary team. Box 14-4 identifies some common types of cognitive distortion characteristic of people with eating disorders. Although the eating behavior is targeted, the underlying emotions of anxiety, dysphoria, low self-esteem, and feelings of lack of control are also addressed through counseling.

Health Teaching and Health Promotion

Self-care activities are an important part of the treatment plan. These activities include learning more constructive coping skills, improving social skills, and developing problem-solving and decision-making skills. The skills become the focus of therapy sessions and supervised food shopping trips. As patients approach their goal weight, they are encouraged to expand the repertoire to include eating out in a restaurant, preparing a meal, and eating forbidden foods.

Discharge planning is a critical component in treatment. Often family members benefit from counseling. The discharge planning process must address living arrangements and school and work plans, as well as the feasibility of independent financial status, applications for state and/or federal program assistance (if needed), and follow-up outpatient treatment.

Milieu Therapy

Individuals admitted to an inpatient unit designed to treat eating disorders participate in a program provided by an interdisciplinary team and consisting of a combination of therapeutic

BOX 14-4 COGNITIVE DISTORTIONS RELATED TO EATING DISORDERS

Overgeneralization: A single event affects unrelated situations.
- "He didn't ask me out. It must be because I'm fat."
- "I was happy when I wore a size 6. I must get back to that weight."

All-or-nothing thinking: Reasoning is absolute and extreme, in mutually exclusive terms of black or white, good or bad.
- "If I have one Popsicle, I must eat five."
- "If I allow myself to gain weight, I'll blow up like a balloon."

Catastrophizing: The consequences of an event are magnified.
- "If I gain weight, my weekend will be ruined."
- "When people say I look better, I know they think I'm fat."

Personalization: Events are overinterpreted as having personal significance.
- "I know everybody is watching me eat."
- "People won't like me unless I'm thin."

Emotional reasoning: Subjective emotions determine reality.
- "I know I'm fat because I feel fat."
- "When I'm thin, I feel powerful."

Adapted from Bowers, W. A. (2001). Principles for applying cognitive-behavioral therapy to anorexia nervosa. *Psychiatric Clinics of North America, 24*(2), 293-303.

APPLYING THE ART

A Person With an Eating Disorder: Anorexia

SCENARIO: I met 15-year-old Stacie on the eating disorders unit. A "straight A" student, Stacie was 5 feet 7 inches tall and weighed 90 pounds. Her mother was a physician and her father a college professor. Her older brother quarterbacked his college team. We had set up the contract that morning and she had just finished the post-lunch focus group.

THERAPEUTIC GOAL: By the end of this interaction, Stacie will express at least one painful feeling directly instead of acting out with self-destructive behavior.

STUDENT-PATIENT INTERACTION	THOUGHTS, COMMUNICATION TECHNIQUES, AND MENTAL HEALTH NURSING CONCEPTS
Stacie: "They think we're going to all go and vomit after lunch so they keep us talking. Like that's going to help."	I should *clarify indefinite pronouns*. She used "they" a lot but I am guessing she means the staff. Her feelings take precedence right now.
Student's feelings: *I am feeling a bit overwhelmed. Where to start! She looks like a skeleton, and here I am always struggling with my own weight.*	
Student: "You sound pretty frustrated."	*Reflection* rarely fails to continue the interaction. I am aware of my own potential for *countertransference* in this situation.
Student's feelings: *Her thinness scares me.*	
Stacie: "I am! Sometimes I feel like a piece of taffy being pushed and pulled and stretched by everyone else."	Control sounds like a key issue. She is revisiting *autonomy versus shame and doubt*. I remember that adolescents re-encounter all of Erikson's earlier stages as part of *identity versus role confusion*.
Student's feelings: *I'm feeling some anxiety about being able to figure this out. She shares how controlled she feels by making an analogy to candy. Is her whole life about food?*	
Student: "Pushed and pulled?"	*Restatement* and *encouraging her to elaborate*. I hope this shows Stacie I am really listening by using her exact words.
Stacie: "Try being in that family of mine! You can't stay unless you're at the top of your game."	I wonder which carries the most emotional impact for her: achievement or staying in the family.
Student's feelings: *I am feeling drawn into her story. How overwhelming for her.*	
Student: "You feel a lot of pressure to excel…at everything?"	I *restate* again. *Love and belonging* to precedes *self-esteem needs*. Still, do I need to assess further with my *direct question* about how high she sets the bar for herself? If she sees herself as a constant failure and food becomes the only area she can control, then despair, even suicide, becomes a possibility.
Student's feelings: *I feel uncertain here. I probably should have focused first on the family part. Hope we can get back to her family stuff, too.*	
Stacie: "My mom would say, 'Honey, just be yourself,' but she'd really mean, 'as long as you get straight A's and make the family proud, like your brother does!'"	
Student's feelings: *I kind of feel intimidated by her straight A's. She accomplishes more than I do in my own studies. Why can't that be enough? I feel sad that she never feels good enough.*	
Student: "Somehow you never quite feel good enough." *Concerned look, leaning toward her.*	I reflect back her feelings. I hope to convey *empathy* with my nonverbal behavior.
Stacie: "That's it, exactly." *Eyes fill with tears. I pause to let her cry.*	When a person is crying, feelings are very close to the surface. Saying comforting things might help her push her feelings down. Expressing emotions directly is much healthier for her than using food to *displace* feelings.
Student's feelings: *I want to comfort her but I stop myself because the tears are healthy. She actually lets herself feel frustration and now sadness.*	

APPLYING THE ART—cont'd

A Person With an Eating Disorder: Anorexia

STUDENT-PATIENT INTERACTION	THOUGHTS, COMMUNICATION TECHNIQUES, AND MENTAL HEALTH NURSING CONCEPTS
Stacie: *Crying.* "I can't tell you how long it's been since I actually cried." **Student's feelings:** *I'm glad she could unbottle some of her feelings and that she felt safe to do so with me.* **Student:** "Maybe crying is not such a bad thing."	I ask an *indirect question.* Maybe she will see that she can let out some of her painful feelings and that it is okay.
Stacie: "It's not done in my family." **Student's feelings:** *Seems like she never lets go of the pressures she feels from her family. In some ways I understand that, with all my family does to keep me plugging through nursing, I feel like I'd really let them down if I failed.* **Student:** "I wonder if a person can stay in the family yet still feel and do things a little differently than everyone else." **Student's feelings:** *I feel like Stacie really made some progress and we can build a foundation for the next time we talk. I feel more hopeful for her.*	The family theme pervades her thoughts. Again, an *indirect question* asks Stacie to ponder without feeling interrogated. The work of *identity versus role confusion* means separating and *individuating* oneself as distinct from one's family.
Stacie: "Maybe. I never thought of it that way." *Takes the tissue I offer, looking thoughtful.*	I'll report this to my instructor and chart about her being able to cry.

---

modalities. These modalities are designed to normalize eating patterns and to begin to address the issues raised by the illness. The milieu of an eating disorder unit is purposefully organized to assist the patient in establishing more adaptive behavioral patterns, including normalization of eating.

The highly structured milieu includes precise mealtimes, adherence to the selected menu, observation during and after meals, and regularly scheduled weighings. Close supervision of patients includes monitoring of all trips to the bathroom after eating to ensure that there is no self-induced vomiting. Patients may also need monitoring on bathroom trips after seeing visitors and after any hospital pass. The latter is to ensure that the patient has not had access to and ingested any laxatives or diuretics.

Therapy groups are led by nurses and other interdisciplinary team members (especially dietitians) and are tailored to the issues of patients with eating disorders.

Psychotherapy

The patient may be involved in a variety of therapies as a multimodal approach to address different issues (Olmsted et al., 2010). The following therapies are used in all of the eating disorders and are geared to the recovery point of the patient:

- **Cognitive behavioral therapy** is used to diminish errors in the patient's thinking and perceptions that result in distorted attitudes and eating-disordered behaviors. The patient practices new ways of examining cognitions and self-monitors behaviors.

- **Dialectical behavioral therapy** is a form of cognitive behavioral therapy adapted to address problems associated with emotional dysregulation.
- **Psychodynamic therapy** explores the underpinnings of the disorder.
- **Group therapy** offers support to patients who feel isolated while offering an arena in which to explore the eating disorder.
- **Family therapy** is especially efficacious in early-onset and short-duration anorexia. It supports parent refeeding of children and identifies family dynamics that may be contributing to the problem.

These therapies may take place in a variety of settings, including a partial hospitalization program, community mental health center, psychiatric home care program, or more traditional outpatient treatment. Regardless of the setting, the goals of treatment remain the same: weight restoration with normalization of eating habits and initiation of the treatment of the psychological, interpersonal, and social issues that are integral to the experience of the patient.

Often the nurse and other health care workers might contract with the patient regarding the terms of treatment. For example, outpatient treatment can continue only if the patient maintains a weight that has been negotiated by both the patient and the health care team. If the patient's weight falls below the goal, other treatment arrangements must be made until the patient returns to the goal weight. This highly structured approach to treatment of patients whose weight is less than 75% of ideal body weight is essential. Techniques such as assisting the patient with a daily meal plan, reviewing a journal of meals and dietary intake, and providing for weekly weighing (ideally two or three times a week) are essential in order to reach a medically stable weight.

Families often report feeling powerless in the face of such mystifying behavior. For instance, patients are often unable to experience compliments as supportive and therefore are unable to internalize the support. They often seek attention from others but feel scrutinized when they receive it. Patients express that they want their families to care about them but are unable to recognize expressions of care. When others do respond with love and support, patients do not perceive this as positive. Consequently, families experience the tension of saying or doing the wrong thing and then feeling responsible if a setback occurs. Psychiatric nurse clinicians have an important role in assisting families and significant others to develop strategies for improved communication and to search for ways to be comfortably supportive to the patient.

Pharmacological, Biological, and Integrative Therapies

Numerous studies of pharmacological intervention have failed to demonstrate efficacy for any one agent (Black & Andreasen, 2011; Kaplan & Howlett, 2010). The improvement in weight gain and appetite is facilitated through the treatment of the underlying anxiety. Olanzapine, the second-generation antipsychotic increasingly being reported in the literature, has been shown to affect weight gain and improve cognition and body image. Numerous studies of fluoxetine have shown mixed results in maintaining weight and preventing relapse.

Long-Term Treatment

Anorexia nervosa is a chronic illness that waxes and wanes. Recovery is evaluated as a stage in the process rather than a fixed event. Factors that influence the stage of recovery include percentage of ideal body weight that has been achieved, the extent to which self-worth is defined by shape and weight, and the amount of disruption existing in the patient's personal life. The patient will require long-term treatment that might include periodic brief hospital stays, outpatient psychotherapy, and pharmacological interventions. The combination of individual, group, couples, and family therapy (especially for the younger patient) provides the anorectic patient with the greatest chance for a successful outcome.

EVALUATION

The process of evaluation is incorporated into the outcomes specified by the goals. Evaluation is ongoing, and short-term and intermediate goals are revised as necessary to achieve the treatment outcomes established. The goals provide a daily guide for evaluating success and must be continually re-evaluated for their appropriateness. Generally, the long-term outcome for anorexia nervosa in terms of symptom recovery is less favorable than that for bulimia nervosa.

APPLICATION OF THE NURSING PROCESS: BULIMIA NERVOSA

ASSESSMENT

People with bulimia nervosa may not initially appear to be physically or emotionally ill. They are often at or slightly above or below ideal body weight. However, as the assessment continues and the nurse makes further observations, physical and emotional problems become apparent. On inspection, the patient may demonstrate enlargement of the parotid glands and dental erosion and caries if the patient has been inducing vomiting. The history may reveal difficulties with impulsivity as well as compulsivity. Family relationships may be chaotic and reflect a lack of nurturing. These individuals' lives reflect instability and troublesome interpersonal relationships as well. It is not uncommon for patients to have a history of impulsive stealing of items such as food, clothing, or jewelry. Refer to Box 14-1 for a listing of the characteristics of bulimia nervosa and anorexia nervosa.

ASSESSMENT GUIDELINES

Bulimia Nervosa

1. Medical stabilization is the first priority. Problems resulting from purging are disruptions in electrolyte and fluid balance and cardiac function. Therefore a thorough medical examination is vital.
2. Medical evaluation usually includes a thorough physical examination as well as pertinent laboratory testing of the following:
   - Electrolyte levels
   - Glucose level
   - Thyroid function tests
   - Complete blood count
   - Electrocardiogram (ECG)
3. Psychiatric evaluation is advised because treatment of psychiatric comorbidity is important to outcomes (depression and suicide are concerns).

VIGNETTE

I was a three-sport athlete throughout high school and then played volleyball in college. How did the bingeing and purging start, and how did it happen to me? I began to down thousands of calories at my parents' house and secretly go to the bathroom and purge, and then start all over again. By the time I went to college, I would go to several fast-food restaurants and order cheeseburgers, french fries, tacos, and milkshakes; consume them all by the time I got home; and then induce vomiting the minute I walked through the door. As time went by, the cycles became worse. I despised what I was doing and what it was doing to me, breaking blood vessels in my face, causing my eyes to swell, and causing me to deceive everyone. I hated it so much that each time I binged and purged, I swore to myself that it would never happen again.—Carly

DIAGNOSIS

Assessment of the patient with bulimia nervosa may reveal the need for multiple potential nursing diagnoses as a result of many disordered eating and weight control behaviors. Problems resulting from purging are a first priority because electrolyte and fluid balance and cardiac function are affected. Common nursing diagnoses include *Decreased cardiac output, Disturbed body image, Powerlessness, Chronic low self-esteem, Anxiety,* and *Ineffective coping* (substance abuse, impulsive responses to problems).

OUTCOMES IDENTIFICATION

Some useful measurable outcome criteria for patients with bulimia nervosa follow (fill in the timeframe [e.g., in 1 week, by discharge]); the patient will:

- Refrain from binge/purge behaviors.
- Demonstrate at least two new skills for managing stress/anxiety/shame (triggers to binge/purge behaviors).
- Obtain and maintain normal electrolyte balance.
- Be free of self-directed harm.
- Express feelings in a non–food-related way.
- Verbalize desire to participate in ongoing treatment.
- State feels good about self and about who he or she is as a person.
- Name two personal strengths.

PLANNING

The criteria for inpatient admission of a patient with bulimia nervosa are included in the criteria for inpatient admission of a patient with an eating disorder, which is presented in Box 14-3. As with anorexia nervosa, the patient with bulimia may be treated for life-threatening complications, such as gastric rupture (rare), electrolyte imbalance, and cardiac dysrhythmias, in an acute care unit of a hospital. If the patient is admitted to a general inpatient psychiatric unit because of acute suicidal risk, only the acute psychiatric manifestations are addressed short term. Planning will also include appropriate referrals for continuing outpatient treatment.

IMPLEMENTATION

See Table 14-2 for intervention guidelines for a patient with bulimia nervosa.

Acute Care

A patient who is medically compromised as a result of bulimia nervosa is referred to an inpatient unit for comprehensive treatment of the illness. The cognitive behavioral model of treatment is highly effective and frequently serves as the cornerstone of the therapeutic approach. Inpatient units designed to treat eating disorders are especially structured to interrupt the cycle of binge eating and purging and to normalize eating habits. Therapy is begun to examine the underlying conflicts and distorted perceptions of shape and weight that sustain the

TABLE 14-2 INTERVENTIONS FOR BULIMIA NERVOSA	
INTERVENTION	**RATIONALE**
1. Assess mood and presence of suicidal thoughts/behaviors.	1. Emotional dysregulation is at the core of bulimic behaviors and there is always the risk for self-destructive behaviors.
2. Monitor physiological parameters (vital signs, electrolyte levels) as needed.	2. The life-threatening effect of weight restriction and/or purging needs to be monitored.
3. Explore dysfunctional thoughts that maintain the binge/purge cycle.	3. Nonjudgmental reframing can balance and combat distorted thinking and challenge automatic behaviors.
4. Educate the patient that fasting can lead to continuation of bingeing and the binge/purge cycle, emphasizing its self-perpetuating nature.	4. The binge/purge cycle is maintained by the pattern of restricting, hunger, bingeing and purging accompanied by feelings of shame, then repetition of the cycle.
5. Monitor patient during and after meals to prevent throwing away food and/or purging.	5. A straightforward statement that the nurse's perceptions are different will help avoid a power struggle. Arguments and power struggles intensify the patient's need to control.
6. Acknowledge the patient's overvalued ideas of body shape and size without minimizing or challenging patient's perceptions.	6. Cognitive behavioral approaches can be very effective in helping the patient identify irrational beliefs about self and body image.
7. Encourage patient to keep a journal of thoughts and feelings.	7. A journal can provide information to identify irrational thinking and identify triggers that induce disordered eating behaviors. Reframing distorted beliefs and thinking can lead to healthier behaviors.

illness. Evaluation for treatment of comorbid disorders, such as major depression and substance abuse, is also undertaken. In most cases of substance dependence, the treatment of the eating disorder must occur after the substance dependence is treated.

Communication Guidelines

Compared with the food-restricting patient with anorexia, the patient with bulimia nervosa often more readily establishes a therapeutic alliance with the nurse because the eating behaviors are so ego-dystonic, or against what they want. The therapeutic alliance allows the nurse, along with other members of the interdisciplinary team, to provide counseling that gives useful feedback regarding the distorted beliefs held by the patient. See Box 14-4 for a list of common cognitive distortions.

In working with a patient who has bulimia, the nurse needs to be aware that the patient is sensitive to the perceptions of others. The patient may feel significant shame and totally out of control. In building a therapeutic alliance, the nurse needs to empathize with feelings of low self-esteem, unworthiness, and dysphoria (sadness or unease). The nurse may suspect dishonesty when the patient does not report bingeing or purging. An accepting, non-judgmental approach, along with a comprehensive understanding of the subjective experience of the patient, will help to build trust.

Milieu Therapy

The highly structured milieu of an inpatient unit has as its primary goals the interruption of the binge/purge cycle and the prevention of the disordered eating behaviors. Interventions such as observation during and after meals to prevent purging, normalization of eating patterns, and maintenance of appropriate amounts of exercise are integral elements of treatment. The interdisciplinary team uses a comprehensive approach to address the emotional and behavioral problems that arise when the patient is no longer binge eating or purging. The interruption of the binge/purge pattern allows underlying feelings to surface and be examined.

Health Teaching and Health Promotion

Health teaching focuses not only on the eating disorder but also on the importance of meal planning, use of relaxation techniques, maintenance of a healthy diet and exercise, implementation of coping skills, and knowledge of the physical and emotional effects of bingeing and purging as well as the effects of cognitive distortions. This preparation lays the foundation for the second phase of treatment, in which there are carefully planned challenges to the patient's newly developed skills. For instance, the patient is expected to have a meal while on pass outside the hospital. On return to the unit, the patient can share the experience.

On discharge from the hospital, the individual is referred for long-term care to solidify the goals that have been achieved, address the attitudes and the perceptions that maintain the eating disorder, and deal with the psychodynamic issues that attend the illness. The patient and family could benefit from connecting with a national network that addresses eating disorders—Anorexia Nervosa and Related Eating Disorders (ANRED; www.anred.com).

Psychotherapy

A cognitive behavioral approach is the most effective treatment for bulimia nervosa. Patients with bulimia nervosa, because of possible coexisting depression, substance abuse, and personality disorders, often undergo various therapies. Although the specific eating-disordered behaviors may not be targeted in some therapies, it is those very behaviors that are responsible for much of the patient's emotional distress. It is imperative that irrational attitudes and perceptions of weight and shape be addressed. Therefore restructuring faulty perceptions and helping individuals develop accepting attitudes toward themselves and their bodies is a primary focus of therapy. When patients do not indulge in these bulimic behaviors, issues of self-worth and interpersonal functioning become more prominent (Fairburn, 2008).

Pharmacological, Biological, and Integrative Therapies

Fluoxetine (Prozac) has been approved by the Food and Drug Administration (FDA) for the treatment of bulimia nervosa and has been regarded as the "gold standard" in the treatment of this disorder. Either alone or in combination with other behavioral treatments, binge eating and purging behaviors are noted to be significantly decreased. Fluoxetine has a very favorable side effect profile compared to other pharmacological agents; however, as a selective serotonin reuptake inhibitor (SSRI), it contains the Black Box warning indicating increased risk of suicidal ideation (Broft et al., 2010).

EVALUATION

The process of evaluation is built into the outcomes specified by the goals. Evaluation is ongoing, and short-term and intermediate goals are revised as necessary to achieve the treatment outcomes established. The goals provide a daily guide for evaluating success and must be continually reevaluated for their appropriateness.

BINGE EATING DISORDER

Binge eating disorder (BED) is a variant of compulsive overeating. Although considerable controversy exists over whether this proposed diagnosis constitutes a separate eating disorder, 20% to 30% of obese individuals seeking treatment report binge eating as a pattern of overeating. These individuals report recurrent episodes of eating a large amount of food in a short period of time, and usually feeling guilty or shameful after bingeing. The pattern is not unlike bulimia nervosa; however, in binge eating disorder there are no compensatory mechanisms used (e.g., self-induced vomiting, inappropriate use of diuretics/laxatives, etc.) Although considerable controversy existed in *DSM-IV-TR* over whether this proposed diagnosis constituted a separate eating disorder, binge eating disorder is thought to be formally recognized as a specific disorder in *DSM-5*.

EXAMINING THE EVIDENCE

Obesity—More Attention to the Psychological Distress

I find it so alarming that obesity seems to be a huge issue worldwide; however, all I can find to answer patients' queries are referrals to nutritionists and lectures on exercise. Is there any chance that obesity will be considered an eating disorder so I can suggest behavioral services equal to those with anorexia/bulimia nervosa? You are right on target with your concern regarding the growing rates of obesity. If the current trends continue, an estimated 9 out of 10 adults will be overweight or obese by 2050. The consequences of obesity both to the people concerned and to the public service systems/insurance companies have been widely publicized. Obesity is associated with a range of serious health problems, including type 2 diabetes, cardiovascular disease, and some forms of cancer (Yilmaz, 2011). At present in the United States, only 8 states cover obesity treatment for adults, and 10 states reimburse for obesity treatment for children (Lee & Sheer, 2010). Currently, obesity is excluded as a diagnosis from the *DSM-5*, but according to the American Psychiatric Association, there may be a possibility of including some kind of overeating syndrome distinct from binge eating in the future since a number of studies show that people who eat excessively also have biological similarities, in terms of neural firing patterns, to those with substance disorders (Gever, 2010). Although obesity is not classified as an eating disorder, it is on the continuum of food misuse, at the other end of the spectrum from dietary-restricting eating disorders (Yilmaz, 2011).

This is not to say that everyone who is obese has an eating disorder, but many people who are obese show disordered eating patterns. About one third of obese people engage in binge eating and use food as a means of regulating painful emotions. Overeating behavior becomes a way of coping with problems similar to more readily recognized eating disorders such as anorexia and bulimia (Yilmaz, 2011).

Theories designed to understand binge eating may serve to understand loss of control/overeating. Future research should investigate more thoroughly the role of psychopathology in overweight children (Goosens et al., 2010).

There does seem to be some movement in the right direction. The Institute of Medicine (IOM) recommends multiple interventions, such as adopting healthy eating practices, increasing exercise, decreasing sedentary activities, and monitoring weight. However, psychological measures such as individual/group therapies, understanding of eating triggers and social/occupational support are not included (Birch, 2011). Recently, studies have shown the effectiveness of cognitive behavioral therapy (CBT) in the treatment of obesity; CBT concentrates on the reasons why people find weight loss difficult together with the psychological processes central to weight regain, such as unrealistic goals and expectations. CBT can lead to longer term weight loss after 1-year follow-up, especially if dietary and exercise reinforcement sessions are included (Goosens et al., 2010).

Although eating disorders characterized by very low body weight or the use of purging behaviors continue to receive attention in the popular media, a focus on these comparatively uncommon disorders may detract from the recognition of the more common, often disabling condition of obesity. The epidemic of obesity calls for greater awareness of the significance of eating-disordered behavior in the context of obesity prevention initiatives. Obesity prevention programs that focus on body weight to the exclusion of body image/self-esteem may be counterproductive and potentially harmful. Given the conspicuous links between eating-disordered behavior and overweight, a more logical approach would be to develop programs that integrate obesity with eating disorders. Psychological distress associated with negative body image warrants greater attention when considering the public health burden of obesity (Mond et al., 2009).

Birch, L., Chair, Committee on obesity prevention policies for young children, Port Brief: early childhood obesity prevention policies (2011). Institute of Medicine of the National Academies.

Gever, J. (2010). APA: obesity rejected as a psychiatric diagnosis. *MedPage*, May 29, 2010.

Goosens, L., et al. (2010). Relations of dietary restraint and depressive symptomatology to loss of control over eating in overweight youngsters. *European Child and Adolescent Psychiatry*, *19*, 587-596.

Lee, J., & Sheer, J. (2010). Coverage of obesity: a state by state analysis of Medicaid and state insurance laws. *Public Health Reports*, *125*(4), 598-604.

Mond, J., et al. (2009). Comparing the health burden of eating-disordered behavior and overweight in women. *Journal of Women's Health*, *18*(7), 1081-1088.

Yilmaz, J. (2011). Adopting a psychological approach to obesity. *Nursing Standard*, *25*(21), 43-45.

Contributed by Lois Angelo.

Overeating is frequently noted as a symptom of a depression (i.e., atypical depression). High rates of mood disorders and personality disorders are found among binge eaters. Binge eaters also report a history of major depression significantly more often than non–binge eaters. They further report that binge eating is soothing and helps to regulate their moods. Although dieting is almost always an antecedent of binge eating in bulimia nervosa, in approximately 50% of a sample of obese binge eaters, no attempt to restrict dietary intake occurred before bingeing (APA, 2000). An effective program for those with binge eating disorder must integrate modification of the disordered eating with reported events and associated mood changes, working towards the ultimate goal of a more appropriate weight for the individual (Fairburn, 2008).

There is limited evidence to suggest that antidepressant, antiobesity, and other medications affect long-term improvement in the frequency of binge eating or in mood symptoms. Although cognitive behavioral therapy alone has resulted in significant improvement, the addition of medication has been shown to improve outcomes in some individuals (Bodell & Devlin, 2010).

KEY POINTS TO REMEMBER

- A number of theoretical models help explain risk factors for the development of eating disorders.
- Neurobiological theories identify an association between eating disorders, depression, and neuroendocrine abnormalities.
- Psychological theories explore issues of control in anorexia and affective instability and poor impulse control in bulimia, but these are not considered causes of eating disorders.
- Genetic theories postulate the existence of vulnerabilities that may predispose people toward eating disorders, and increasingly twin studies confirm genetic liability, which perhaps interacts with environmental mechanisms.
- Sociocultural models look both at our present societal ideal of being thin and at the ideal feminine role model in general.
- Eating disorders are now appearing in populations in which they had been rare. The dynamics—the stress of acculturation versus identification with the new culture—are being examined.
- Anorexia nervosa is a possibly life-threatening eating disorder that includes being severely underweight; having low blood pressure, pulse, and temperature measurements; being dehydrated; and having low serum potassium level and dysrhythmias. Anorexia may be treated in an inpatient treatment setting—in which milieu therapy, psychotherapy (cognitive), development of self-care skills, and psychobiological interventions can be implemented.
- Eating disorders thought to occur only in preteen or teenage groups are now being diagnosed in people ages 35 to 65.
- Long-term treatment is provided on an outpatient basis and aims to help patients maintain healthy weight; it includes treatment modalities such as individual therapy, family therapy, group therapy, psychopharmacology, and nutrition counseling.
- Individuals with bulimia nervosa are typically within the normal weight range, but some may be slightly below or above ideal body weight.
- Assessment of a patient with bulimia may show enlargement of the parotid glands, dental erosion, and dental caries if the patient has induced vomiting.
- Acute care may be necessary when life-threatening complications are present, such as gastric rupture (rare), electrolyte imbalance, and cardiac dysrhythmias.
- The primary goal of interventions for a patient with bulimia is to interrupt the binge/purge cycle.
- Psychotherapy as well as self-care skill training is included.
- Long-term treatment focuses on therapy aimed at addressing any coexisting depression, substance abuse, and/or personality disorders that are causing the patient distress and interfering with quality of life. Self-worth and interpersonal functioning eventually become issues that are useful to target.
- Eating disorders not otherwise specified (EDNOS) include a variety of patterns (binge eating disorder was introduced in this chapter).
- Binge eaters report a history of major depression significantly more often than non–binge eaters.
- Effective treatment for obese binge eaters integrates modification of the disordered eating, improvement of depressive symptoms, and achievement of an appropriate weight for the individual.

APPLYING CRITICAL JUDGMENT

1. Tom Shift, a 19-year-old model, has experienced a rapid decrease in weight over the past 4 months, after his agent told him he would have to lose weight or lose a coveted account. Tom is 6 feet 2 inches tall and weighs 132 pounds, down from his usual 176 pounds. He is brought to the emergency department with a pulse rate of 40 beats per minute and severe dysrhythmias. His laboratory workup reveals severe hypokalemia. He has become extremely depressed, saying, "I'm too fat...I won't take anything to eat. If I gain weight my life will be ruined. There is nothing to live for if I can't model." Tom's parents are startled and confused, and his best friend is worried and feels powerless to help Tom. "I tell Tom he needs to eat or he will die. I tell him he is a skeleton, but he refuses to listen to me. I don't know what to do."

A. Which physical and psychiatric criteria suggest that Tom should be immediately hospitalized? What other physical signs and symptoms may be found on assessment?
B. What are some of the questions you would eventually ask Tom when evaluating his biopsychosocial functioning?
C. What are your feelings toward someone with anorexia? Can you make a distinction between your thoughts and feelings toward women with anorexia and toward men with anorexia?
D. What are some things you could do for Tom's parents and Tom's friend in terms of offering them information, support, and referrals? Identify specific referrals.

APPLYING CRITICAL JUDGMENT—cont'd

E. Explain the kinds of interventions or restrictions that may be used while Tom is hospitalized (e.g., weighing, observation after eating or visits, exercise, therapy, self-care).

F. How would you describe partial hospitalization programs or psychiatric home care programs when asked if Tom will have to be hospitalized for a long time?

G. What are some of Tom's cognitive distortions that would be a target for therapy?

H. Identify at least five criteria that, if met, would indicate that Tom was improving.

2. You and your close friend Mary Alice have been together since nursing school and you are now working on the same surgical unit. Mary Alice told you that in the past she has made several suicide attempts. Today you accidentally come upon her bingeing off unit, and she looks embarrassed and uncomfortable when she sees you. Several times you notice that she spends time in the bathroom and you hear sounds of retching. In response to your concern, she admits that she has been bingeing/purging for several years but that now she is getting out of control and feels profoundly depressed.

A. Although Mary Alice does not show any physical signs of bulimia nervosa, what would you look for when assessing an individual with bulimia?

B. What kinds of emergencies could result from bingeing and purging?

C. What would be the most useful type of psychotherapy for Mary Alice initially and what issues would need to be addressed?

D. What kinds of new skills does a person with bulimia need to learn to lessen the compulsion to binge and purge?

E. What would be some signs that Mary Alice is recovering?

CHAPTER REVIEW QUESTIONS

Choose the most appropriate answer(s).

1. Which of the following is an example of all-or-nothing thinking, which is a frequent cognitive distortion of patients with an eating disorder?
   1. "If I allow myself to gain weight, I'll become immense."
   2. "I'm unpopular because I'm fat."
   3. "When I'm thin, I'm powerful."
   4. "When people say I look better, they're really thinking I look fat."

2. Typical goals of inpatient hospitalization for an anorectic patient do not include:
   1. stabilization of the patient's immediate condition.
   2. limited weight restoration.
   3. determination of the causes for the eating disorder.
   4. restoration of normal electrolyte balance.

3. Which patient with an eating disorder would be at greatest risk for hypokalemia? A patient with:
   1. anorexia who loses weight by restricting food intake.
   2. anorexia or bulimia who purges to promote weight loss.
   3. bulimia whose predominant pathological behavior is excessive nocturnal eating.

4. an eating disorder who exercises intensely more than 4 hours per day but maintains a normal electrolyte balance.

4. Which medication is likely to be used in the treatment of patients with eating disorders? An:
   1. SSRI such as fluoxetine.
   2. antipsychotic such as risperidone.
   3. anxiolytic such as alprazolam.
   4. anticonvulsant such as carbamazepine.

5. Which of the following is least likely to contribute to building an effective therapeutic alliance between the nurse and an anorectic patient?
   1. Establishing disciplined eating through the nurse's authoritarian approach with the patient
   2. Avoiding the stance of a parental role in order to foster a sense of empowerment
   3. Offering a highly structured approach in treating severely underweight patients
   4. Contracting with the outpatient person about treatment terms

REFERENCES

Academy for Eating Disorders (AED). (2011). *Eating disorders: critical points for early recognition and medical risk management in the care of individuals with eating disorders* (2nd ed.). Retrieved August 8, 2011, from Academy for Eating Disorders: www.aedweb.org.

American Nurses Association, American Psychiatric Nurses Association, & International Society of Psychiatric-Mental Health Nurses. (2007). *Psychiatric-mental health nursing: scope and standards of practice.* Silver Springs, MD: Nursesbooks.org. Retrieved August 9, 2011, from www.dsm5.org/proserevision/Pages/FeedingandEating Disorders.aspx.

American Psychiatric Association (APA). (2000). *Practice guidelines for the treatment of psychiatric disorders: compendium 2000.* Washington, DC: Author.

Bailer, U. F., & Kaye, W. H. (2011). Serotonin: imaging findings in eating disorders. *Current Topics in Behavioral Neurosciences,* 6, 59–79.

Becker, A. E., Thomas, J. J., & Pike, K. M. (2009). Should nonfat-phobic anorexia nervosa be included in DSM-V? *International Journal of Eating Disorders, 42*(7), 620–635.

Black, D. W., & Andreasen, N. C. (2011). *Introductory textbook of psychiatry* (5th ed.). Washington, DC: American Psychiatric Publishing.

Bodell, L. P., & Devlin, M. J. (2010). Pharmacotherapy for binge-eating disorder. In C. M. Grilo, & J. E. Mitchell (Eds.), *The treatment of eating disorders: a clinical handbook* (pp. 402–413). New York: Guilford Press.

Broft, A., Berner, L. A., & Walsh, B. T. (2010). Pharmacotherapy for bulimia nervosa. In C. M. Grilo, & J. E. Mitchell (Eds.), *The treatment of eating disorders: a clinical handbook* (pp. 388–401). New York: Guilford Press.

Engel, S. G., & Wonderlich, S. A. (2010). New technologies in treatments for eating disorders. In C. M. Grilo, & J. E. Mitchell (Eds.), *The treatment of eating disorders: a clinical handbook* (pp. 500–509). New York: Guilford Press.

Fairburn, C. G. (2008). *Cognitive behavior therapy and eating disorders.* New York: Guilford Press.

Hudson, J. I., Hiripi, E., Harrison, G. P., & Kessler, R. C. (2007). The prevalence and correlates of eating disorders in the national comorbidity survey replication. *Biological Psychiatry, 61,* 348–358.

Kaplan, A. S., & Howlett, A. (2010). Pharmacotherapy for anorexia nervosa. In C. M. Grilo, & J. E. Mitchell (Eds.), *The treatment of eating disorders: a clinical handbook* (pp. 175–186). New York: Guilford Press.

Kaye, W. H., Bulik, C. M., Plotnicov, K., Thornton, L., Devlin, B., et al. (2008). The genetics of anorexia nervosa collaborative study: methods and sample description. *International Journal of Eating Disorders, 41*(4), 289–300.

Le Grange, D., Lock, J., Loeb, K., & Nicholls, D. (2010). Academy for eating disorders position paper: the role of the family in eating disorders. *International Journal of Eating Disorders, 43*(1), 1–5.

McLean, S. A., Paxton, S. J., & Wertheim, E. H. (2010). Factors associated with body dissatisfaction and disordered eating in women in midlife. *International Journal of Eating Disorders, 43*(6), 527–536.

Olmsted, M. P., McFarlane, T. L., Carter, J. C., Trottier, K., Woodside, B. D., et al. (2010). Inpatient and day hospital treatment for anorexia nervosa. In C. M. Grilo, & J. E. Mitchell (Eds.), *The treatment of eating disorders: a clinical handbook* (pp. 388–401). New York: Guilford Press.

Peat, C., Mitchell, J. E., Hoek, H. W., & Wonderlich, S. A. (2009). Validity and utility of subtyping anorexia nervosa. *International Journal of Eating Disorders, 42*(7), 590–594.

Sadock, J. B., & Sadock, V. A. (2007). *Kaplan and Sadock's synopsis of psychiatry* (10th ed.). Philadelphia: Wolters/Lippincott Williams & Wilkins.

Scholtz, S., Hill, L. S., & Lacey, H. (2010). Eating disorders in older women: does late onset anorexia nervosa exist? *International Journal of Eating Disorders, 43*(5), 393–397.

Thornton, L. M., Mazzeo, S. E., & Bulik, C. M. (2011). The heritability of eating disorders: methods and current findings. *Current Topics in Behavioral Neuroscience, 6,* 141–156.

Mood Disorders: Depression

Elizabeth M. Varcarolis

evolve WEBSITE

http://evolve.elsevier.com/Varcarolis/essentials

KEY TERMS AND CONCEPTS

anergia, p. 249

anhedonia, p. 249

atypical antidepressants, p. 265

deep brain simulation, p. 271

dual action reuptake inhibitor
   (SNRI) antidepressants, p. 268

dysthymia, p. 252

electroconvulsive therapy (ECT),
   p. 259

hypersomnia, p. 256

light therapy, p. 271

major depressive disorder (MDD),
   p. 251

mood, p. 251

psychomotor agitation, p. 255

psychomotor retardation, p. 255

rapid transcranial magnetic stimulation (rTMS), p. 271

S-adenosylmethionine (SAMe),
   p. 272

selective serotonin reuptake
   inhibitor (SSRI), p. 264

St. John's wort, 272

tricyclic antidepressants (TCAs),
   p. 264

vagus nerve stimulation (VNS),
   p. 270

vegetative signs of depression,
   p. 255

SELECTED CONCEPT: Self Esteem

NANDA's definition of self esteem is "a pattern of perceptions or ideas about the self that is sufficient for well-being and can be strengthened."

Situational low self esteem refers to a negative perception of self which may occur when our behavior is inconsistent with our values, when we fail at something, when we experience a significant loss/rejection etc.

Chronic low self esteem, however, "is long-standing negative self evaluating/ feelings about self or self capabilities." These painful feelings often present in people with depression. Depression can be demoralizing, and painful levels of low self-esteem can erode a person's quality of life, and belief in self, which can dampen the spirit and contribute to hopelessness and helplessness for the future.

Therapies that help biologically to lower depressive feelings, and talking therapies that help change a person's perceptions of their self-concept have helped to decrease depression, increase quality of life, and an increase functioning and productivity for many people.

(NANDA, 2012-2014)

OBJECTIVES

1. Differentiate between major depressive disorder (MDD) and dysthymia disorder (DD).
2. Summarize the links between the stress model of depression and the biological model of depression.
3. Apply patient-centered care during an assessment of a depressed individual's behaviors in each of the following areas: (a) affect, (b) thought processes, (c) feelings, (d) physical characteristics, and (e) communication.
4. Apply communication strategies that are useful for depressed patients in a nursing care plan for a depressed individual.
5. Describe the evidence-based practice relating to the advantages versus the disadvantages of both the selective serotonin reuptake inhibitors (SSRIs) and the tricyclic antidepressants (TCAs).
6. Explain the unique attributes of two atypical antidepressants for use in specific circumstances.
7. Discuss at length, using a step-by-step approach, the role of monoamine oxidase (MAO) in our brain and explain why special dietary/medication restrictions have to be maintained when a monoamine oxidase inhibitor (MAOI) is prescribed.
8. Relate why the selegiline transdermal system (STS) is such a breakthrough MAOI.
9. Identify potential safety issues regarding the adverse reactions of the SSRIs, especially in older adults.
10. Applying the knowledge of evidence-based practice, explain identification of the types of depression for which electroconvulsive therapy (ECT) is most helpful.
11. Explain all the ways that teamwork and collaboration are useful in the treatment of depression.

It is impossible to convey adequately the personal pain and suffering experienced by an individual going through a severe depressive episode. All races, all ages, and both genders are susceptible to depressive episodes, although some individuals are more vulnerable than others. The following chapter will help you in understanding this complex group of disorders so that you will be able to provide optimal care for a depressed person.

PREVALENCE AND COMORBIDITY

In terms of chronic conditions seen in medical practice, depression is secondary only to hypertension (Cassano et al., 2010). Approximately 16.5% of people older than age 18 in this country will have a major depressive episode in their lifetime. The 12-month prevalence of a major depressive disorder (MDD) is 6.7%. Women are 70% more likely to experience a depressive episode during their lifetime than are men (National Institute of Mental Health [NIMH], 2010a).

Chronic depressive disorder (dysthymia) occurs in about 2.5% of the population over a lifetime (Kessler et al., 2005). Major depression disorder (MDD) (a depression without manic symptoms) may or may not eventually meet the criteria for a bipolar disorder (BD) in any given year, or even a co-occurring chronic depressive disorder in any 1 year (*Depression Facts and Statistics,* 2009; Rihmer & Angst, 2009).

A depressive syndrome frequently accompanies other psychiatric disorders such as anxiety disorders, schizophrenia, substance abuse, eating disorders, and schizoaffective disorder. People with anxiety disorders (e.g., panic disorder, generalized anxiety disorder, obsessive-compulsive disorder) commonly present with depression, as do people with personality disorders (particularly borderline personality disorder), adjustment disorders, and brief depressive reactions.

People with co-occurring chronic medical problems (e.g., hypertension, backache, diabetes, heart problems, arthritis) are at a higher risk for depression than those in the general population (Cassano et al., 2010). Depression is often secondary to a medical condition. Depression also may be secondary to use of substances such as alcohol, cocaine, marijuana, heroin, and even anxiolytics and other prescription medications. Depression also can be a sequela of bereavement and grief (refer to Chapter 25).

Mixed anxiety–depression is perhaps one of the most common psychiatric presentations. Symptoms of anxiety frequently co-occur with cases of major depression, chronic depression, or any other depressive syndrome (Rihmer & Angst, 2009). The presence of comorbid anxiety disorder and depression has a negative effect on the disease course and these patients are significantly less likely to benefit from antidepressant medication than those without anxiety (NIMH, 2008). Comorbidity has been shown to result in a higher rate of suicide, greater severity of depression, and greater impairment in social and occupational functioning as well as including more coexisting illnesses, both medical and psychiatric (Fava et al., 2008).

Children and Adolescents

Children as young as 3 years of age have been diagnosed with depression. MDD is said to occur in as many as 18% of preadolescents, which is perhaps a low estimate because depression in this age-group is often underdiagnosed. At age 10 years, children have a 14% chance of suffering from a MDD in their lifetime; from ages 13 to 18, individuals have an 11.2% chance of being afflicted with a depressive disorder and a 3.3% lifetime prevalence of a severe depressive disorder (Kessler et al., 2005; NIMH, 2010b). Major depression among adolescents is often associated with substance abuse and antisocial behavior, both of which can obscure accurate diagnosis. Unfortunately, approximately 50 years ago the average age of onset of depression was approximately 29 years, and presently the average age of onset is just 14.5 years (*Depression Facts and Statistics,* 2009).

MDDs in children and adolescents have a high recurrence rate, and those with very severe depression, a sense of hopelessness, anxiety, and family conflict are less likely to achieve remission, but early treatment with medication and cognitive behavioral therapy (CBT) in the first 12 weeks can help in achieving remission (NIMH, 2010c; Yellowlees, 2011a). Children in families with other depressed members seem to become depressed earlier (ages 12 to 13 years) than children in families with no other depressed members (16 to 17 years). Even before adolescence, girls are more vulnerable to depression than boys.

Older Adults

Depression among older adults (65 or older) is approximately 6% to 9% for major depression and 17% to 18% for chronic depression (dysthymia). In fact, a disproportionate number of depressed older Americans are likely to die by suicide, accounting for a disparate amount of all suicides, and the incidence appears to increase with age (Rosenbaum & Covino, 2006). The symptoms in older adults with depression often are unrecognized because many masquerade as medical symptoms. Depression in older adults is often associated with chronic illnesses, and depression can remain undiagnosed approximately 50% of the time. Between 13% and 27% of older adults have some form of clinical depression that does not meet the *Diagnostic and Statistical*

Manual of Mental Disorders (DSM) criteria, and these older adults are more prone to an increased risk for major depression, physical disability, medical illness, and high use of health services (*Depression Facts and Statistics,* 2009). The good news is that efforts to improve recognition of depression and education have led to positive treatment response among older adults. However, research suggests that use of antidepressant medication in those 65 and older can be risky (Lowry, 2011). Some studies show that falls, stroke, seizure, and other adverse outcomes are associated with the use of antidepressants in older adults. Those taking the selective serotonin reuptake inhibitors (SSRIs) fared worse than older adults administered tricyclic antidepressants (TCAs), which were introduced to the market before SSRIs (see Chapter 28 for more on depression in the older adult) (Lowry, 2011).

THEORY

Many theories attempt to explain the cause of depression; however, basically depression is thought to involve changes in receptor-neurotransmitter relationships in the following areas of the brain:

1. Limbic system (emotional alterations)
2. Prefrontal cortex (decreased mood, problems concentrating)
3. Hippocampus (memory impairments; feelings of worthlessness, hopelessness, and guilt)
4. Amygdala (anxiety and reduced motivation)

EXAMINING THE EVIDENCE

Antidepressants and Suicide Risk

I have been hearing about children, adolescents, and even young adults having problems with suicidal thoughts and even attempts after taking antidepressants. Should they continue to take these drugs?
That is a good question. This has been a controversial topic for nearly 10 years. In 2004 the U.S. Food and Drug Administration (FDA) ordered all pharmaceutical companies to add a serious warning, or a "Black Box," to all antidepressant advertising, stating: "Antidepressants increase the risk of suicidal thinking and behavior in children and adolescents with major depressive disorder and other psychiatric disorders." This warning was provoked by testimony from grieving parents whose children had committed suicide while taking antidepressants. It resulted in an extensive review by the FDA of the literature and of studies describing clinical trials of antidepressants in children. Findings from the review revealed that among the more than 2000 children taking SSRIs there were no completed suicides, yet about 4% of these children experienced suicidal thinking for behavior, a rate twice that of children taking placebos.

Despite the widespread use of antidepressant medications since 2004, particularly SSRIs, there is inconsistent

evidence that increased antidepressant use has reduced the prevalence of suicidal ideation or suicide attempts during the past decade. Although the FDA raised concerns, it has not provided patients, clinicians, or policymakers with adequate guidance on the treatment decisions they face and several studies face criticism for channeling bias (Schneeweiss et al., 2010).

A U.S. district court awarded more than $3 million to the family of a patient who hanged herself at age 15 after being treated with an SSRI antidepressant (Prozac). The ruling stated that "Prozac is capable of causing chemical imbalances in the brains of certain adolescents that can lead them to take their own lives when they would not otherwise do so. Other events in the patient's life, an argument followed by a breakup with her boyfriend and her alleged participation in the Goth subculture, were not sufficiently traumatic to account for her suicide. The FDA has warned that pediatric patients being treated with antidepressants need to be watched closely for worsening during the first few months after starting the medication or after changing the dosage up or down which was not done in this case. Face to face meetings should occur regularly with the health care provider, pediatric patient and the

Continued

EXAMINING THE EVIDENCE—cont'd
Antidepressants and Suicide Risk

patient's family. Attention must be paid to specific signs of suicidality as well as unusual changes in general behavior" (Snyder, 2011).

Antidepressants have proven to be highly successful and effective in dealing with depression in many patients. However, treatment decisions should be based on efficacy, and clinicians should be highly vigilant in monitoring each patient after initiating therapy with any antidepressant agent. Compared with the SSRI class, none of the other antidepressant classes differed significantly in the risk of suicidality, including serotonin-norepinephrine reuptake inhibitors, tricyclic agents, and newer and atypical antidepressants (Schneeweiss et al., 2010). Thus all commonly used antidepressants carry a similar risk of suicide among children, adolescents, and young adults, supporting the FDA advisory of 2004 (Dolder, 2010).

Dolder, C. (2010). Pharmacological and clinical profile of newer antidepressants, *Drugs and Aging, 27*(8), 625-640.
Schneeweiss, S., et al. (2010). Variation in the risk of suicide attempts and completed suicides by antidepressant agent in adults. *Archives of General Psychiatry, 67*(5), 497-506.
Snyder, K. (2011). Court faults nurse practitioner's prescription of Prozac for adolescent patient, *Floyd v US, Legal Newsletter,* January 2011.
Contributed by Lois Angelo.

BOX 15-1   PRIMARY RISK FACTORS FOR DEPRESSION

- History of prior episodes of depression
- Family history of depressive disorder, especially in first-degree relatives
- History of suicide attempts or family history of suicide
- Female gender
- Age 40 years or younger
- Postpartum period
- Chronic medical illness
- Absence of social support
- Negative, stressful life events
- Active alcohol or substance abuse
- History of sexual abuse

The primary neurotransmitters involved with depression are serotonin and norepinephrine, although dopamine is also related to depression.

It is becoming evident that depression is a heterogeneous, systemic illness involving an array of different neurotransmitters, neuronal pathways, hereditary processes, and/or traumatic life events.

It is commonly accepted that genetic predisposition to the illness combined with childhood stress may lead to significant changes in the central nervous system (CNS) that result in depression. However, there are common risk factors for depression that may signal the presence of this common and serious psychiatric illness (Box 15-1).

Biological Theories
Genetic Factors
Twin studies consistently show that genetic factors play a role in the development of depressive disorders. Various studies reveal that the average concordance rate for unipolar depression mood disorders among monozygotic twins (twins sharing the same genetic constitution) is 50%. That is, if one twin is affected, the second has a 50% chance of being affected. The percentage for dizygotic twins (different genetic constitution) is 20%. Thus identical twins (monozygotic) have a greater concordance rate than dizygotic twins (Gelder et al., 2006). However, because concordance rates in monozygotic twins are not 100% it appears that other factors also must be involved.

Adoptive studies also have pointed to genetic contribution for the development of depression. For example, the risk for the development of depression in children born to parent(s) with a depressive illness is the same when these children are adopted by a nondepressive family. Although some studies are inconclusive, most studies are supportive of a genetic link concluding that mood disorders are heritable for some people (Kelsoe, 2009). Increased heritability is associated with an earlier age of onset, greater rate of comorbidity (especially alcoholism and psychosis), and increased risk of recurrent illness (Kelsoe, 2009). However, any genetic factors that are present must interact with environmental and neurobiological preconditions for depression to develop.

Biochemical Factors
The brain is a highly complex organ that contains billions of neurons. There is much evidence to support the concept that depression is a biologically heterogeneous disorder; that is, many CNS neurotransmitter abnormalities can probably cause clinical depression. These neurotransmitter abnormalities may be the result of inherited or environmental factors, or even of other medical conditions, such as cerebral infarction, hypothyroidism, acquired immunodeficiency syndrome, or drug use. Whatever the etiological contribution, depression is ultimately mediated through changes in the brain's neurochemistry and the circuitry involved in emotional regulations.

Neurobiological investigations in depression have focused on the monoamine neurotransmitters (serotonin, noradrenaline, and dopamine). Specific neurotransmitters in the brain are believed to be related to altered mood states. **Serotonin** (5-hydroxytryptamine or 5-HT) **and norepinephrine (NE) are**

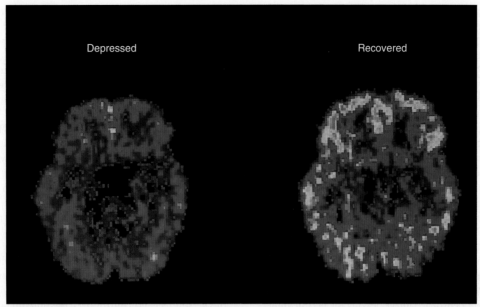

FIGURE 15-1 Positron emission tomography (PET) scans of a 45-year-old woman with recurrent depression. The scan on the left was taken when the patient was not taking medication and was very depressed. The scan on the right was taken several months later when the patient was well, after she had been treated with medication for her depression. Note that her entire brain, particularly the left prefrontal cortex, is more active when she is well. (Courtesy Mark George, MD, Biological Psychiatry Branch, National Institute of Mental Health.)

two major neurotransmitters involved in depression. Serotonin is an important regulator of sleep, appetite, and libido. A serotonin circuit dysfunction can result in poor impulse control, low sex drive, decreased appetite, disturbed regulation of body temperature, and irritability. Decreased levels of NE in the medial forebrain bundle (MFB) may account for anergia (reduction in or lack of energy), anhedonia (an inability to find meaning or pleasure in existence), decreased concentration, and diminished libido in depression.

The dopamine (DA), acetylcholine, and γ-aminobutyric acid (GABA) systems are believed to be involved in the pathophysiology of a major depressive episode. Dopamine neurons in the mesolimbic system are thought to play a role in the reward and incentive behavior processes, emotional expression, and learning processes that are disrupted in depression. This is particularly true in melancholic states (severe MDD).

Serotonin and norepinephrine are also involved in the perception of **pain** by modifying the effects of substance P, glutamate, GABA, and other pain mediators (Narasimhan & Campbell, 2010). There is considerable overlap in the biological underpinnings of both major depression and chronic pain. For example, genetics and neurotransmitter functionality are similar in both (Narasimhan & Campbell, 2010). In some cases chronic painful physical conditions (**CPPCs**) such as backaches or headaches may be due to MDD rather than chronic pain, and in some cases these conditions may present as the only sign of depression (Hall-Flavin, 2010; Narasimhan & Campbell, 2010).

Another theory to explain the dysfunction of the neurotransmitters NE, DA, and 5-HT is abnormalities in the number of receptor sites, which could increase or decrease the activity of neurotransmitters. It is important to keep in mind that the neurotransmitters specific to depression (norepinephrine, serotonin, and dopamine) have many subtypes, accounting for the complexity in treatment and varied patient responses to attempts to increase levels of these neurotransmitters through medications. The relationships among the serotonin, norepinephrine, dopamine, acetylcholine, and GABA systems are complex and need further assessment and study. However, medication that helps regulate these neurotransmitters has proved empirically successful in the treatment of many patients. Figure 15-1 shows a positron emission tomography (PET) scan of the brain of a woman with depression before and after taking medication.

Image Findings

Magnetic resonance imaging (MRI) scans show some patients who are depressed have smaller frontal lobes and smaller caudate nuclei compared to control subjects (Sadock & Sadock, 2010). Computed tomography (CT) scans show large cerebral ventricles in some patients with psychotic depression, and diminished basal ganglia blood flow in some depressed patients (Sadock & Sadock, 2010).

In cases of inherited depression, research funded by NIMH found that tissue thickness–specific areas of the right half of the brain may increase the risk for developing depression. The same changes found on the left side of the brain are more apt to signal the severity of a person's depression or anxiety symptoms (Proceedings of the National Academy of Sciences, 2009).

PSYCHOSOCIAL THEORIES

The Stress-Diathesis Model of Depression

The stress-diathesis model of depression is a psychological theory that explains depression from an environmental, interpersonal, and life-events perspective combined with biological vulnerability or predisposition (diathesis). It is well-known that psychosocial stressors and interpersonal events trigger certain neurophysical and neurochemical changes in the brain. Early life trauma may result in long-term hyperactivity of the corticotropin-releasing factor (CRF) and norepinephrine systems of the CNS with a consequent neurotoxic effect on the hippocampus that leads to neuronal loss. Because norepinephrine, serotonin, and acetylcholine play a role in stress regulation, when these neurotransmitters become overtaxed through stressful events, neurotransmitter depletion may occur and cause permanent neuronal damage, leaving the person vulnerable to depression later in life (Sadock & Sadock, 2010). An analysis by Karg and colleagues (2011) of 54 studies published from 2001 to 2009 found there is evidence for a "depression gene." People who possess a "short" version of the serotonin transporter gene (*5-HTTLPR*) are at a higher risk of depression when they become stressed, especially if they have been maltreated as children and/or have unusually severe medical illness in childhood (WebMD, 2011). However, people with the "long" or protected version of the gene who underwent multiple life stressors experienced no more depression than people in the general population.

Therefore life events (psychosocial stressors and interpersonal events) may influence the development and recurrence of depression through the psychological and biological experience of stress in some people, which results in changes in the connections among nerve cells in the brain.

Cognitive Theory

Aaron T. Beck, one of the early proponents of cognitive therapy, applied cognitive behavioral theory to depression. Beck proposed that people acquire a psychological predisposition to depression through early life experiences. These experiences contribute to negative, illogical, and irrational thought processes that may remain dormant until they are activated during times of stress (Beck & Rush, 1995).

Beck found that depressed people process information in negative ways, even in the midst of positive factors that affect the person's life. Beck believed that three automatic negative thoughts—called **Beck's cognitive triad**—are responsible for the development of depression:

1. *A negative, self-deprecating view of self:* "I really never do anything well; everyone else seems smarter."
2. *A pessimistic view of the world:* "Once you're down, you can't get up. Look around, poverty, homelessness, sickness, war, and despair are every place you look."
3. *The belief that negative reinforcement (or no validation for the self) will continue:* "It doesn't matter what you do; nothing ever gets better. I'll be in this stupid job the rest of my life."

The phrase *automatic negative thoughts* refers to thoughts that are repetitive, unintended, and not readily controllable. This cognitive triad seems to be consistent in all types of depression, regardless of clinical subtype.

The goal of cognitive behavioral therapy (CBT) is to change the way a patient thinks, which will in turn help relieve the depressive syndrome. This is accomplished by assisting the patient in the following:

1. Identifying and testing negative cognition
2. Developing alternative thinking patterns
3. Rehearsing new cognitive and behavioral responses

Learned Helplessness

Martin Seligman's theory is that of learned helplessness. Seligman (1973) stated that although anxiety is the initial response to a stressful situation, anxiety is replaced by depression if the person feels no control over the outcome of a situation. People who believe that an undesired event is their fault and that nothing can be done to change it are prone to depression. The theory of learned helplessness has been used to explain the development of depression in certain social groups, such as older adults, people living in impoverished areas, and women.

CULTURAL CONSIDERATIONS

According to the Cross-National Collaborative Group, the prevalence rate of depressive disorders in Asian Americans was the lowest in comparison to whites, African Americans, and Hispanics (Rihmer & Angst, 2009). Prevalence rates for MDD in whites are significantly higher than those in African Americans and Mexican Americans, although the opposite is true for chronic/dysthymic disorder (DD) (Riolo et al., 2005). We know that, compared to men, women are twice as likely to be diagnosed with depression and also that divorced or single people are more vulnerable to depression than married individuals. However, according to Sadock and Sadock (2010), there is no correlation with socioeconomic status or between races or religious groups.

CLINICAL PICTURE

Mood disorders can range from mild to severe. There are distinct differences between the *DSM* diagnostic criteria for a major depressive disorder and those for a chronic depressive disorder (dysthymia), which are two of the most common depressive disorders seen in medical practice. Depression can be manifested in a variety of other symptoms that are called specifiers. Other subgroups are being researched as well (Table 15-1).

All forms of depression share common symptoms, which can make it difficult to make a correct diagnosis. Preston and

TABLE 15-1   SOME FEATURES OF DEPRESSIVE DISORDERS BY CLINICAL SYMPTOMS

DISORDER	SYMPTOMS
Major depressive disorder (MDD)	Symptoms represent a change from usual functioning
	Associated with high mortality rate
	Significant in physical, social, and role functioning, as well as increased potential for pain and physical illness
With melancholic features	Depression with complete loss of pleasure in life and inability to feel better
	Marked by early morning awakening, feels worse in the morning, movements are agitated or very slow, substantial weight loss, or extreme feelings of guilt
	Occurs in severe depressions and one with psychotic features
With postpartum onset	Indicates onset within 4 weeks after childbirth
	Can present with or without psychotic features
	Severe ruminations or delusional thoughts about infant signify increased risk of harm to infant
With seasonal pattern	Indicates that episodes mostly begin in fall or winter and remit in spring
	Characterized by anergia, hypersomnia, overeating, weight gain, and craving for carbohydrates Responds to light therapy
With anxiety, mild-severe	Significant amounts of anxiety along with depression
With suicide risk severity	
With catatonic features	Includes some of the following: echopraxia, echolalia, grimacing, stereotyped movements, posturing, negativism, stupor, waxy flexibility, agitation, mutism, mannerisms
With atypical features	Long-standing sensitivity to rejection, substantial weight gain or increased appetite, sleeping too much, body feels heavier, feels weighted down
	Personality and anxiety disorders are also co-occurring
Dysthymia	A depressed mood for most of the day, more days than not, lasting for at least 2 years
	Mood is not a change from usual behavior
With atypical features	Indicates mood reactivity (can be cheered with positive events) and rejection sensitivity (pathological sensitivity to perceived interpersonal rejection) that are present throughout life and result in functional impairment
	Other symptoms include hypersomnia, hyperphagia (overeating), leaden paralysis (feeling weighed down in extremities)

colleagues (2010) identify the following core symptoms common to all types of depression:

- Mood of sadness, despair, emptiness
- Loss of ability to experience pleasure in life (anhedonia)
- Low self-esteem
- Apathy, low motivation, and social withdrawal
- Excessive emotional sensitivity
- Irritability
- Suicidal ideation

Major Depressive Disorder (Single Episode or Recurrent)

Patients with a major depressive disorder (MDD) experience substantial pain and suffering, as well as psychological, social, and occupational disability. Basically, the individual is unable to function normally. A patient with MDD presents with a history of one or more major depressive episodes and no history of manic or hypomanic episodes. In some cases, the patient's history of depression may include psychotic features. MDD with psychotic symptoms is a severe form of mood disorder that is characterized by delusions or hallucinations. For example, patients might have delusional thoughts that interfere with their nutritional status (e.g., "God put snakes in my stomach and told me not to eat.").

The emotional, cognitive, physical, and behavioral symptoms an individual exhibits during a major depressive episode represent a change in the person's usual functioning.

The course of MDD is variable. An average episode may last about 9 months, although it has been shown that 20% of individuals will not have recovered by that time. Long-term studies indicate that after 5 years there is a 70% recurrence rate and an 80% recurrence rate after 8 years (Psychdirect.com, 2006).

According to the Mayo Clinic (2012) and NIMH (2009), the characteristics of an individual with a major depressive disorder may include the following:

- Substantial pain, suffering, and intolerable sadness
- Inability to carry out normal social or occupational functions (e.g., getting out of bed in the morning)
- Excessive feelings of guilt
- In severe cases psychotic delusions may be present
- Extreme fatigue, tiredness, and loss of energy (anergia)
- Slowed thinking, speaking, or body movements
- Insomnia common, often marked by early-morning wakefulness in MDD
- Inability to find any pleasure in previous pleasurable activities (anhedonia)
- Symptoms (emotional, cognitive, physical, and behavioral) represent a change in usual patterns of functioning
- May have recurrent thoughts of death or taking one's own life
- Physical changes (vegetative signs) in eating patterns (has no appetite), bowel patterns, loss of sexual drive, difficulty sleeping (insomnia or hypersomnia)
- Crying spells for no apparent reason
- Irritability
- Trouble thinking, concentrating, and making decisions, as well as memory difficulties
- May complain of pain, such as backache or headache, that does not seem to have a physical cause

---

VIGNETTE

Sally, a bright, successful, 34-year-old businessperson, finds her world is changing. Over the past few weeks she has become more and more withdrawn. Her life has become empty of meaning. She has great difficulty getting out of bed in the mornings, but finds it hard to sleep more than 3 to 4 hours a night, waking at 2 or 3 AM. She is constantly exhausted.

Sally finds it impossible to concentrate at work and has called in sick the past 2 days, unable to find the energy to dress, bathe, groom, or even eat. She has not eaten for 3 days except for some water and a few glasses of milk and a few crackers she found in a neglected box tucked away in the pantry. She has lost considerable weight.

When her best friend calls to find out why she has not shown up for work, Sally tells her, "I don't know. I just can't concentrate; I can't focus on anything. Nothing seems to be worth doing. I feel so heavy and empty inside. I don't see things getting any better." When her friend tries to coax her out of her mood, Sally snaps at her and tells her to mind her own business and leave her alone. Later, Sally is filled with remorse, telling herself she is a horrible person and does not deserve her friend's concern and loyalty. She wonders what it would be like if she no longer had to deal with all this pain; could she take this much longer?

Refer to Assessment for a more thorough discussion of the signs and symptoms in depression.

Subtypes Seen in MDD

The diagnosis for MDD may include a specifier in patients with specific symptoms. Specifiers are listed in Table 15-1, including additions from the *DSM-5* proposed revisions (APA, 2011a,b).

Dysthymia

Dysthymic disorder (DD) is characterized by depressive symptoms that have been present for at least 2 years. Because dysthymic disorder is more chronic in nature, it cannot be distinguished from the person's usual pattern of functioning: "I've always been this way." It's just the way I *am*." Although people with dysthymia suffer from social and occupational distress, it is not usually severe enough to warrant hospitalization unless the person becomes suicidal. The age of onset is usually from early childhood and teenage years to early adulthood. Patients with chronic depression are at risk for developing MDD as well as other psychiatric disorders, often referred to as double depression.

Even though there are specific indicators in making a diagnosis between major depression (MDD) and the more chronic dysthymic disorder (DD), it can be difficult because all forms of depression share the similar core symptoms previously listed. The major differences between major depressive disorders and chronic/dysthymic disorders are the level of severity, duration, and persistence. In the severity of the symptoms, chronic depression is much less severe than an episode of MDD. In terms of duration, dysthymic depression can endure for years. In addition to the core symptoms of depression just listed, there are other notable symptoms of dysthymia.

According to WebMed (2012) and Preston and colleagues (2010), the characteristics seen in an individual with a dysthymic/chronic depression may include the following:

- Able to function at work and in social situations but not at optimal level
- Chronic low; great sadness
- Eating too much or too little
- Difficulty with sleeping; in dysthymia there is often difficulty getting to sleep; excessive sleeping seems to be more common in chronic depression
- Loss of energy, fatigue, and chronic tiredness even for simple tasks
- Decreased capacity to experience pleasure, enthusiasm, or motivation
- Irritability
- Negative thinking
- Low self-esteem
- Shared symptoms include thoughts of death or self-harm; unexplained pain at times of the presenting symptom; feelings of worthlessness, helplessness, hopelessness, and low self-esteem

Refer to Assessment for a more thorough discussion of the signs and symptoms in depression.

VIGNETTE

Sam had another bad week at work. He just cannot seem to perform the way he thinks he should—he never gets things right. Although his work seems acceptable to others, he constantly puts himself down. He wanted to take a class to improve his computer skills, but cannot seem to find the energy or the time. His weekends are filled with 'hanging around' his apartment. "Nothing much going on...there is never much going on. Life is dull; has it ever been otherwise?" His brother is always telling him that he has a face as long as a football field. "What's the matter with you, bro? You're good looking, smart. Go find a girl and have some fun in life. Why can't you just enjoy anything?" Sam just sighs. Who could be interested in him? He gets a cold beer from the fridge and continues watching reruns on TV.

APPLICATION OF THE NURSING PROCESS

ASSESSMENT

Undiagnosed and untreated depression is often associated with more severe presentation of depression, greater suicidality, somatic problems, and severe anxiety or co-occurring anxiety disorders. Depression in older adults is often missed, especially if there are coexisting medical problems. Depression in children and adolescents may remain undiagnosed when attention is focused on behavioral problems ("just a stage"). Racial and economic disparities in health care, among other factors, lead to underdiagnosis and undertreatment of African Americans, Hispanics, and other minorities.

A study by Bijl and associates (2004), still relevant today, concluded that depressed individuals who sought treatment manifesting psychological symptoms were recognized as depressed 90% of the time; in contrast, those who presented with only somatic symptoms (e.g., chronic pain, insomnia) were recognized as depressed 50% of the time. In those who had a medical disorder, depression was identified 20% of the time.

Assessment Tools

Numerous standardized screening tools can help the clinician assess the type of depression a person may be experiencing, for example, the Beck Depression Inventory, the Hamilton Depression Scale, the Geriatric Depression Scale, and Zung's Self-Rating Depression Scale. Refer to Figure 15-2 for an example of the signs and symptoms clinicians assess for before making a diagnosis of depression.

The National Mental Health Association (NMHA) has a website (www.depression-screening.org) that enables people to take a confidential screening test for depression online and find reliable information on the illness.

Assessment of Suicide Potential

A patient with depression should always be evaluated for suicidal or homicidal ideation. White males complete more than 78% of all suicides (Andrews and Benner, 2012). It is also the third leading cause of death among people ages 15 to 24 and the second leading cause of death in college students (Andrews and Benner, 2012). However, all patients diagnosed with depression should have an initial suicide evaluation. An evaluation might include the following statements or questions:

- "You have said you are depressed. Tell me what that is like for you."
- "When you feel depressed, what thoughts go through your mind?"
- "Have you ever thought about taking your own life in the past? Now? Do you have a plan? Do you have the means to carry out your plan? Is there anything that would prevent you from carrying out your plan?"

Refer to Chapter 23 for more on suicide prevention and intervention.

Areas to Assess

Mood

A depressed mood and **anhedonia** (lack of enjoyment in life) are the key symptoms in depression. Nearly 97% of people with depression have **anergia** (lack of energy). **Anxiety,** a common symptom in depression, is seen in about 60% to 90% of depressed patients. Some feelings that may be inherent in a depressed mood are as follows:

- Feelings of **worthlessness** range from feeling inadequate to having an unrealistic evaluation of self-worth. These feelings reflect the low self-esteem that is a painful partner to depression. Statements such as "I am no good, I'll never amount to anything" are common. Themes of one's inadequacy and incompetence are repeated relentlessly.
- **Guilt** is a common accompaniment to depression. A person may ruminate over present or past failings. Extreme guilt can assume psychotic proportions: "I have committed terrible sins." "I have caused terrible pain and destruction to everyone I have ever known and now I'm paying for it."
- **Helplessness** is evidenced by believing that everything is too difficult to accomplish (e.g., grooming, housework, working, caring for children). With feelings of helplessness come feelings of **hopelessness.** Even though most depressive states are usually time limited, during a depressed period people believe that things will never change, which leads some to consider suicide as a way to escape the constant mental pain. Hopelessness is one of the core characteristics of depression and suicide, as well as a characteristic of schizophrenia, alcoholism, and physical illness. Hopelessness results in negative expectations for the future and loss of control over future outcomes.
- **Anger** and **irritability** are natural outcomes of profound feelings of helplessness. Anger in depression is often expressed inappropriately. For example, anger may be expressed in destruction of property, hurtful verbal attacks, or physical aggression toward others. Anger may also be directed toward the self in the form of suicidal or self-destructive behaviors (e.g., alcohol abuse, substance abuse, overeating, smoking). These behaviors often result in feelings of low self-esteem and worthlessness.

Patient's Name

Date of Assessment

To rate the severity of depression in patients who are already diagnosed as depressed, administer this questionnaire. The higher the score, the more severe the depression.

For each item, write the correct number on the line next to the item. (Only one response per item)

1. **DEPRESSED MOOD** (Sadness, hopeless, helpless, worthless)

____ 0= Absent
1= These feeling states indicated only on questioning
2= These feeling states spontaneously reported verbally
3= Communicates feeling states non-verbally—i.e., through facial expression, posture, voice, and tendency to weep
4= Patient reports VIRTUALLY ONLY these feeling states in his spontaneous verbal and non-verbal communication

2. **FEELINGS OF GUILT**

____ 0= Absent
1= Self reproach, feels he has let people down
2= Ideas of guilt or rumination over past errors or sinful deeds
3= Present illness is a punishment. Delusions of guilt
4= Hears accusatory or denunciatory voices and/or experiences threatening visual hallucinations

3. **SUICIDE**

____ 0= Absent
1= Feels life is not worth living
2= Wishes he were dead or any thoughts of possible death to self
3= Suicidal ideal or gesture
4= Attempts at suicide (any serious attempt rates 4)

4. **INSOMNIA EARLY**

____ 0= No difficulty falling asleep
1= Complains of occasional difficulty falling asleep—i.e., more than 1/2 hour
2= Complains of nightly difficulty falling asleep

5. **INSOMNIA MIDDLE**

____ 0= No difficulty
1= Patient complains of being restless and disturbed during the night
2= Waking during the night—any getting out of bed rates 2 (except for purposes of voiding)

6. **INSOMNIA LATE**

____ 0= No difficulty
1= Waking in early hours of the morning but goes back to sleep
2= Unable to fall asleep again if he gets out of bed

7. **WORK AND ACTIVITIES**

____ 0= No difficulty
1= Thoughts and feelings of incapacity, fatigue or weakness related to activities; work or hobbies
2= Loss of interest in activity; hobbies or work—either directly reported by patient, or indirect in listlessness, indecision and vacillation (feels he has to push self to work or activities)
3= Decrease in actual time spent in activities or decrease in productivity
4= Stopped working because of present illness

8. **RETARDATION: PSYCHOMOTOR** (Slowness of thought and speech; impaired ability to concentrate; decreased motor activity)

____ 0= Normal speech and thought
1= Slight retardation at interview
2= Obvious retaradation at interview
3= Interview difficult
4= Complete stupor

9. **AGITATION**

____ 0= None
1= Fidgetiness
2= Playing with hands, hair, etc.
3= Moving about, can't sit still
4= Hand wringing, nail biting, hair-pulling, biting of lips

10. **ANXIETY (PSYCHOLOGICAL)**

____ 0= No difficulty
1= Subjective tension and irritability
2= Worrying about minor matters
3= Apprehensive attitude apparent in face or speech
4= Fears expressed without questioning

11. **ANXIETY SOMATIC:** Physiological concomitants of anxiety, (i.e., effects of autonomic overactivity, "butterflies," indigestion, stomach cramps, belching, diarrhea, palpitations, hyperventilation, paresthesia, sweating, flushing, tremor, headache, urinary frequency. Avoid asking about possible medication side effects (i.e., dry mouth, constipation).

____ 0= Absent
1= Mild
2= Moderate
3= Severe
4= Incapacitating

FIGURE 15-2 The Hamilton Rating Scale for Depression. (Hamilton, M. (1960). A rating scale for depression. *Journal of Neurology, Neurosurgery and Psychiatry, 23*, 56-62.)

12. SOMATIC SYMPTOMS (GASTROINTESTINAL)

____ 0= None
1= Loss of appetite but eating without encouragement from others. Food intake about normal
2= Difficulty eating without urging from others. Marked reduction of appetite and food intake

13. SOMATIC SYMPTOMS GENERAL

____ 0= None
1= Heaviness in limbs, back or head. Backaches, headache, muscle aches. Loss of energy and fatigability
2= Any clear-cut symptom rates 2

14. GENITAL SYMPTOMS (Symptoms such as: loss of libido; impaired sexual performance; menstrual disturbances)

____ 0= Absent
1= Mild
2= Severe

15. HYPOCHONDRIASIS

____ 0= Not present
1= Self-absorption (bodily)
2= Preoccupation with health
3= Frequent complaints, requests for help, etc.
4= Hypochondriacal delusions

16. LOSS OF WEIGHT

____ A. When rating by history:
0= No weight loss
1= Probably weight loss associated with present illness
2= Definite (according to patient) weight loss
3= Not assessed

17. INSIGHT

____ 0= Acknowledges being depressed and ill
1= Acknowledges illness but attributes cause to bad food, climate, overwork, virus, need for rest, etc.
2= Denies being ill at all

18. DIURNAL VARIATION

____ A. Note whether symptoms are worse in morning or evening. If NO diurnal variation, mark none
0= No variation
1= Worse in A.M
2= Worse in P.M
____ B. When present, mark the severity of the variation. Mark "None" if NO variation
0= None
1= Mild
2= Severe

19. DEPERSONALIZATION AND DEREALIZATION (Such as: Feelings of unreality; Nihilistic ideas)

____ 0= Absent
1= Mild
2= Moderate
3= Severe
4= Incapacitating

20. PARANOID SYMPTOMS

____ 0= None
1= Suspicious
2= Ideas of reference
3= Delusions of reference and persecution

21. OBSESSIONAL AND COMPULSIVE SYMPTOMS

____ 0= Absent
1= Mild
2= Severe

Total Score _____

FIGURE 15-2, cont'd The Hamilton Rating Scale for Depression.

Physical Changes

A person who is depressed sees the world through gray-colored glasses. Posture is poor, and the patient may look older than the stated age. Facial expressions convey sadness and dejection, and the patient may have frequent bouts of weeping. Conversely, the patient may say that he or she is unable to cry. Feelings of **hopelessness** and **despair** are readily reflected in the person's affect. For example, the patient may not make eye contact, may speak in a monotone, may show little or no facial expression (flat affect), and may answer with only yes or no responses. Frequent sighing is common.

People who are depressed often complain of lack of energy (**anergia**). Lethargy and fatigue can result in psychomotor retardation. Movements are slow, facial expressions are decreased, and gaze is fixed. The continuum in psychomotor retardation may range from slowed and difficult movements

to complete inactivity and incontinence. At other times the nurse may note psychomotor agitation. For example, patients may constantly pace, bite their nails, smoke, tap their fingers, or engage in some other tension-relieving activity. At these times, patients feel fidgety and unable to relax.

Grooming, dress, and personal hygiene are markedly neglected. People who usually take pride in their appearance and dress may be poorly groomed and allow themselves to look shabby and unkempt.

Vegetative signs of depression are universal. Vegetative signs of depression are the somatic changes and alterations in those activities necessary to support physical life and growth (e.g., eating, sleeping, elimination, sex). For example, **changes in eating patterns** are common. About 60% to 70% of people who are depressed report having anorexia; overeating occurs more often in chronic depression (dysthymia).

Changes in sleep patterns are a cardinal sign of depression. Often, people have **insomnia,** waking at 3 or 4 AM and staying awake, or sleeping only for short periods. The light sleep of a depressed person tends to prolong the agony of depression over a 24-hour period. For some, sleep is increased (hypersomnia) and provides an escape from painful feelings. This is more common in young depressed individuals or those with bipolar tendencies. In any event, sleep is rarely restful or refreshing.

Changes in bowel habits are common. Constipation is seen most frequently in patients with psychomotor retardation. Diarrhea occurs less frequently, often in conjunction with psychomotor agitation. **Interest in sex declines** (loss of libido) during depression. Some men experience impotence, and a declining interest in sex often occurs among both men and women, which can further complicate marital and social relationships.

Approximately 50% to 75% of people suffering from depression complain of **pain** with or without reporting psychological symptoms. People who suffer from **chronic pain** need careful assessment for possible depression.

Cognition

When people are depressed, their thinking is slow and their memory and concentration are usually affected. Depressed people dwell on and exaggerate their perceived faults and failures and are unable to focus on their strengths and successes. As mentioned, identifying the presence of suicidal thoughts and suicide potential has the highest priority in the initial assessment. Approximately two thirds of depressed people contemplate suicide, and up to 15% of untreated or inadequately treated patients actually follow through with the suicide ideation (see Chapter 23).

When depressed, a person's ability to solve problems and think clearly is negatively affected. Judgment is poor, and indecisiveness is common. The individual may claim that the mind is slowing down. Evidence of delusional thinking may be seen in a person with major depression. Common statements of delusional thinking are "I have committed unpardonable sins," and "I am wicked and should die."

Self-Care for Nurses

People who are depressed often reject the presence, friendship, or interactions with others. Over time, family, friends, and health care workers can experience feelings of frustration, hopelessness, ineffectiveness, and annoyance. When working with depressed patients, nurses often experience the following:

- **Unrealistic expectations of self.** Often we have unrealistic expectations of ourselves or the depressed individual. Unmet expectations usually result in the nurse feeling anxious, hurt, angry and helpless, or incompetent. Identifying realistic expectations for oneself and for the patient is one way to decrease feelings of helplessness and can increase the nurse's self-esteem and therapeutic potential.
- **Becoming depressed while caring for a depressed patient.** We have all experienced a feeling of hopelessness or depression when around a person who is depressed, but once away from that person your mood is elevated and those feelings disappear. Some clinicians assume this is a diagnostic sign of patient depression—that is, feeling depressed around somebody who is depressed regardless of whether the person shows any symptoms. Often, however, we do not recognize that those feelings of hopelessness/helplessness/depression do not originate in us but rather we are experiencing what the other person/patient is experiencing via empathy. If the nurse is not able to identify that these feelings originate in the patient, and are not the nurse's own feelings, the usual result is the nurse withdraws from the patient, and consequently experiences feelings of inadequacy, ineffectiveness, and increased anxiety. Once again, sharing your feelings with a more experienced clinician can help the nurse separate his or her feelings from the patient's feelings, allowing the nurse to provide optimal therapeutic care for the depressed individual.

In all cases it is extremely important for the nurse to share his or her negative feelings toward a patient, ideally with a mentor or supervisor. Sharing with a more experienced nurse or mentor can help you understand the source of your negative feelings, which will increase your ability to work with the patient and therapeutically grow as a nurse.

ASSESSMENT GUIDELINES

Depression

1. Always evaluate the patient's risk of harm to self or others. Overt hostility is highly correlated with suicide (see Chapter 23).
2. A thorough medical and neurological examination helps determine if the depression is primary or secondary to another disorder. Depression can be secondary to a host of medical or other psychiatric disorders, as well as medications. Essentially, evaluate the following:
   - If the patient is psychotic
   - If the patient has used drugs or alcohol
   - If comorbid medical conditions are present
   - If the patient has a history of a comorbid psychiatric disorder (e.g., eating disorder, borderline personality disorder, anxiety disorder)
3. Assess history of depression. If the patient has a history, determine therapies used previously that were effective. Some of the following questions can be asked:
   - "Have you ever gone through or felt anything like this before?"
   - "What seemed to help you at that time?"
4. Assess support systems, family, and significant others and the need for information and referrals.
   - "With whom do you live?"
   - "Whom do you trust?"
   - "To whom do you talk when you are upset?"
5. Assess for any events that might have "triggered" a depressive episode.
   - "Has anything happened recently to upset you?"
   - "Have you had any major changes in your life?"
   - "Have you had any recent losses: job, divorce, loss of partner, child moving away, deaths?"

6. Include a psychosocial assessment that includes cultural beliefs and spiritual practices related to mental health and treatment. Determine if the depression is affecting the patient's beliefs and practice.
   - "How do you view depression?"
   - "Have you tried taking any over-the-counter remedies (e.g., herbs) to help with your depression?"
   - "Do you find solace in spiritual activities or a place of worship (e.g., church, temple, mosque)?"

DIAGNOSIS

Depression is complex; depressed individuals have a variety of needs and there are many nursing diagnoses. However, during the initial assessment, a high priority for the nurse is identification of the presence of suicide potential. Therefore the nursing diagnosis of *Risk for Suicide* is always considered. Other key targets for nursing interventions are represented by the diagnoses of *Hopelessness, Ineffective Coping, Social Isolation, Spiritual Distress*, and one or more of the *Self-Care Deficits (e.g., bathing/hygiene, dressing/grooming, feeding, toileting)*. Table 15-2 identifies signs and symptoms commonly experienced in depression and offers possible nursing diagnoses.

OUTCOMES IDENTIFICATION

Outcomes should include goals for safety. Even if the patient is not having self-destructive thoughts, one goal should be to name a person who the patient will contact if such thoughts arise. Goals for the outcomes of vegetative or physical signs of

TABLE 15-2 POTENTIAL NURSING DIAGNOSES FOR DEPRESSION

SIGNS AND SYMPTOMS	NURSING DIAGNOSES*
Previous suicidal attempts, putting affairs in order, giving away prized possessions, suicidal ideation (has plan, ability to carry it out), overt or covert statements regarding killing self, feelings of worthlessness, hopelessness, helplessness	*Risk for Suicide* *Risk for Self-Mutilation*
Lack of judgment, memory difficulty, poor concentration, inaccurate interpretation of environment, negative ruminations, cognitive distortions	*Decisional Conflict* *Impaired Memory* *Acute Confusion*
Difficulty with simple tasks, inability to function at previous level, poor problem solving, poor cognitive functioning, verbalizations of inability to cope	*Ineffective Coping* *Interrupted Family Processes* *Risk for Impaired Parent/Infant/Child Attachment* *Ineffective Role Performance*
Difficulty making decisions, poor concentration, inability to take action	*Decisional Conflict*
Feelings of helplessness, hopelessness, powerlessness	*Hopelessness*
Feelings of inability to make positive change in one's life or have a sense of control over one's destiny	*Powerlessness* *Ineffective Coping*
Questioning meaning of life and own existence, inability to participate in usual religious practices, conflict over spiritual beliefs, anger toward spiritual deity or religious representatives	*Spiritual Distress* *Impaired Religiosity* *Risk for Impaired Religiosity*
Feelings of worthlessness, poor self-image, negative sense of self, self-negating verbalizations, feeling of being a failure, expressions of shame or guilt, hypersensitivity to slights or criticism	*Chronic Low Self-Esteem* *Situational Low Self-Esteem*
Withdrawal, noncommunicativeness, speech that is only in monosyllables, avoidance of contact with others	*Impaired Social Interaction* *Social Isolation* *Risk for Loneliness*
Vegetative signs of depression: changes in sleeping, eating, grooming and hygiene, elimination, sexual patterns	*Self Neglect (bathing/hygiene, dressing/grooming)* *Imbalanced Nutrition: Less Than Body Requirements* *Disturbed Sleep Pattern* *Constipation* *Sexual Dysfunction*

*Nursing Diagnoses—Definitions and Classification 2012-2014. Copyright © 2012, 1994-2012 by NANDA International. Used by arrangement with Blackwell Publishing Limited, a company of John Wiley and Sons, Inc.

TABLE 15-3	INTERVENTIONS FOR SEVERELY WITHDRAWN INDIVIDUALS: COMMUNICATION
INTERVENTION	**RATIONALE**
1. When a patient is mute, use the technique of *making observations:* "There are many new pictures on the wall" or "You are wearing your new shoes."	1. When a patient is not ready to talk, direct questions can raise the patient's anxiety level and frustrate the nurse. Pointing to commonalities in the environment draws the patient into, and reinforces, reality.
2. Use simple, concrete words.	2. Slowed thinking and difficulty concentrating impair comprehension.
3. Allow time for the patient to respond.	3. Slowed thinking necessitates time to formulate a response.
4. Listen for covert messages and ask about suicide plans: "Have you had thoughts of harming yourself in any way?"	4. People often experience relief and decrease in feelings of isolation when they share thoughts of suicide.
5. Avoid platitudes such as, "Things will look up" or "Everyone gets down once in a while."	5. Platitudes tend to minimize the patient's feelings and can increase feelings of guilt and worthlessness because the patient cannot "look up" or "snap out of it."

depression (e.g., *reports adequate sleep*) are formulated to show, for example, evidence of weight gain, return to normal bowel activity, sleep of 6 to 8 hours per night, or return of sexual desire.

PLANNING

The planning of care for patients with depression is geared toward the phase of depression the person is in and the particular symptoms the person is exhibiting. At all times the nurse and members of the health care team are cognizant of the potential for suicide, and assessment of risk for self-harm (or harm to others) is ongoing during the care of the depressed person. There is evidence that a combination of therapeutic (cognitive, behavioral, interpersonal [IP]) and psychopharmacological interventions can be an effective approach in treating depression.

Nurses and clinicians need to assess and plan for any vegetative signs of depression, as well as changes in concentration, activity level, social interaction, or personal appearance, for example. Therefore the planning of care for a patient who is depressed is based on the individual's symptoms and attempts to encompass a variety of areas in the person's life. Safety is always the highest priority.

IMPLEMENTATION

Communication Guidelines

A person who is depressed may speak and comprehend very slowly. The lack of an immediate response by the patient to a remark does not mean that the patient has not heard or chooses not to reply; rather, the patient just needs a little more time to compose a reply. In extreme depression, however, a person may be mute.

Some depressed patients are so withdrawn that they are unwilling or unable to speak. Nurses may feel uncomfortable with silence and not being able to "do anything" to effect immediate change. However, just sitting with a patient in silence may be a valuable intervention. It is important to be aware that this time spent together can be meaningful to the depressed person, especially if the nurse has a genuine interest in learning about the depressed individual.

> **VIGNETTE**
> Doris, a senior nursing student, is working with a depressed, suicidal, withdrawn woman. The instructor notices in the second week that Doris spends a lot of time talking with other students and their patients and little time with her own patient. In post conference, Doris acknowledges feeling threatened and useless and says that she wants a patient who will interact with her. After reviewing the symptoms of depression and its behavioral manifestations as well as the needs of depressed individuals, Doris turns her attention back to her patient and spends time rethinking her plan of care. After 4 weeks of sharing her feelings in post conferences, working with her instructor, and trying a variety of approaches with her patient, Doris is rewarded. On the day of discharge, the patient tells Doris how important their time together was for her: "I actually felt someone cared."

It is difficult to say when a withdrawn or depressed person will be able to respond. However, certain techniques are known to be useful in guiding effective nursing interventions. Some communication interventions to use with a severely withdrawn patient are listed in Table 15-3. Communication interventions to use when caring for depressed patients are offered in Table 15-4.

Health Teaching and Health Promotion

It is important for patients and their families to understand that depression is a legitimate medical illness over which the patient has no voluntary control. Depressed patients and their families need to learn about the biological symptoms of depression as well as the psychosocial and cognitive changes. Families

TABLE 15-4   INTERVENTIONS FOR DEPRESSION: COMMUNICATION

INTERVENTION	RATIONALE
1. Help the patient question underlying assumptions and beliefs and consider alternate explanations to problems.	1. Reconstructing a healthier and more hopeful attitude about the future can alter depressed mood.
2. Work with the patient to identify cognitive distortions that encourage negative self-appraisal. For example:	2. Cognitive distortions reinforce a negative, inaccurate perception of self and world.
a. Overgeneralizations	a. The patient takes one fact or event and makes a general rule out of it ("He always..."; "I never...").
b. Self-blame	b. The patient consistently blames self for everything perceived as negative.
c. Mind reading	c. The patient assumes others do not like him or her, and so forth, without any real evidence that assumptions are correct.
d. Discounting of positive attributes	d. The patient focuses on the negative.
3. Encourage activities that can raise self-esteem. Identify need for (a) problem-solving skills, (b) coping skills, and (c) assertiveness skills.	3. Many depressed people, especially women, are not taught a range of problem-solving and coping skills. Increasing social, family, and job skills can change negative self-assessment.
4. Encourage exercise, such as running and/or weight-lifting. Initially walking 10 to 15 minutes a day 3 or 4 times a week has short-term benefits.	4. Exercise can help alleviate depression and anxiety, improve self-concept, and shift neurochemical balance.
5. Encourage formation of supportive relationships, such as through support groups, therapy, and peer support.	5. Such relationships reduce social isolation and enable the patient to work on personal goals and relationship needs.
6. Provide information referrals, when needed, for spiritual/religious information (e.g., readings, programs, tapes, community resources).	6. Spiritual and existential issues may be heightened during depressive episodes—many people find strength and comfort in spirituality or religion.

must recognize the overt and covert signs of suicidal ideation and know precautionary measures to take if the warning signs of suicidal thinking or planning occur (see Chapter 23). Review of the patient's medications and their adverse reactions helps families evaluate clinical changes and maintain alertness for reactions that might affect patient compliance. Adverse effects of antidepressants and specific areas to be emphasized in patient and family teaching are presented later in this chapter.

If the patient is hospitalized, predischarge counseling should begin early and be carried out with the patient and the patient's significant others. One purpose of this counseling is to clarify the interpersonal stresses and to discuss steps that can alleviate tension in the family system. Including significant others in discharge planning facilitates progress in the following ways:

- Increases the understanding and acceptance of the depressed family member during the aftercare period
- Increases the patient's use of aftercare facilities in the community
- Contributes to higher overall adjustment in the patient after discharge
- Increases understanding of symptoms that signal the need for relapse prevention

Health teaching also may include teaching and interventions for self-care deficits. In addition to experiencing intense feelings of hopelessness, despair, low self-worth, and fatigue, the depressed person also may have physical deficits related to the depression. Some effective interventions targeting the physical needs of the depressed patient are listed in Table 15-5.

Milieu Therapy

When a person is acutely and severely depressed, the structure of the hospital setting may be necessary. The depressed person needs protection from suicidal acts in a supervised environment where antidepressant medications can be closely regulated. If a patient is thought to be suicidal, finding a safe environment may be the first action taken. Hospitals have protocols for suicidal observation and protection. If a patient is highly suicidal, refusing food, becoming debilitated, or exhibiting psychotic depression, then electroconvulsive therapy (ECT) may be administered.

Psychotherapy

CBT, interpersonal therapy (IPT), and behavioral therapy have been proven effective in the treatment of depression. However, only CBT and IPT demonstrate superiority in the maintenance phase. CBT helps people change their negative styles of thinking and behaving, whereas IPT focuses on working through personal relationships that may contribute to depression. Outcome research has consistently found that CBT and medication are largely comparable. CBT helps guard against relapse, because people learn skills of how to reshape their thinking and behaviors.

TABLE 15-5	INTERVENTIONS TARGETING THE PHYSICAL NEEDS OF THE DEPRESSED PATIENT
INTERVENTION	**RATIONALE**
Nutrition—Anorexia	
1. Offer small, high-calorie and high-protein snacks frequently throughout the day and evening.	1. Low weight and poor nutrition render the patient susceptible to illness. Small, frequent snacks are more easily tolerated than large plates of food when the patient is anorectic.
2. Offer high-protein and high-calorie fluids frequently throughout the day and evening.	2. These fluids prevent dehydration and can minimize constipation.
3. When possible, encourage family or friends to remain with the patient during meals.	3. This strategy reinforces the idea that someone cares, can raise the patient's self-esteem, and can serve as an incentive to eat.
4. Ask the patient which foods or drinks he or she likes. Offer choices. Involve the dietitian.	4. The patient is more likely to eat the foods provided.
5. Weigh the patient weekly and observe the patient's eating patterns.	5. Monitoring the patient's status gives the information needed for revision of the intervention.
Sleep—Insomnia	
1. Provide periods of rest after activities.	1. Fatigue can intensify feelings of depression.
2. Encourage the patient to get up and dress and to stay out of bed during the day.	2. Minimizing sleep during the day increases the likelihood of sleep at night.
3. Encourage the use of relaxation measures in the evening (e.g., tepid bath, warm milk).	3. These measures induce relaxation and sleep.
4. Reduce environmental and physical stimulants in the evening—provide decaffeinated coffee, soft lights, soft music, quiet activities.	4. Decreasing caffeine and epinephrine levels increases the possibility of sleep. Playing relaxing music can help the patient sleep.
Self-Care Deficits	
1. Encourage the use of toothbrush, washcloth, soap, makeup, shaving equipment, and so forth.	1. Being clean and well groomed can temporarily increase self-esteem.
2. When appropriate, give step-by-step reminders such as, "Wash the right side of your face, now the left."	2. Slowed thinking and difficulty concentrating make organizing simple tasks difficult.
Elimination—Constipation	
1. Monitor intake and output, especially bowel movements.	1. Many depressed patients are constipated. If the condition is not checked, fecal impaction can occur.
2. Offer foods high in fiber and provide periods of exercise.	2. Roughage and exercise stimulate peristalsis and help evacuation of fecal material.
3. Encourage the intake of fluids.	3. Fluids help prevent constipation.
4. Evaluate the need for laxatives and enemas.	4. These measures prevent fecal impaction.

Some studies indicate that psychotherapy alone (CBT or IPT), especially in individuals with early life traumas (child abuse), is more effective than pharmacology alone. CBT combined with medications is proven effective in people with chronic depressions (Feldman, 2007).

Mindfulness-Based Cognitive Therapy (MBCT)

There are increasing studies reported in the literature about the use of mindfulness-based cognitive therapy (MBCT) and its effectiveness in treating people who are experiencing relapse/reoccurrence of major depressive disorder (MDD). MBCT is a combination of cognitive behavioral therapy (CBT) and mindfulness-based stress reduction (MBSR). Mindfulness is

a form of meditation, and mindfulness-based stress reduction (MBSR) was developed by Kabat-Zinn at the University of Massachusetts in the early 1970s. Mindfulness is a meditation technique that has been used successfully in patients coping with medical or mental health disorders; it shows promise as an effective tool to prevent relapse in patients with major depression disorders (MDDs) (Kuyken et al., 2008).

Group Therapy

Group therapy is a widespread modality for the treatment of depression; it increases the number of people who can receive treatment at a decreased cost per individual. Another advantage is that groups offer patients an opportunity to socialize and to

APPLYING THE ART

A Person With Depression

SCENARIO: After a medical workup revealed no physical problems, Nadia, a 39-year-old mother of three, admitted herself voluntarily to the inpatient psychiatric unit, stating she no longer had the energy to care for her children or her marriage, saying, "I am not fit to be a mother or wife." I saw Nadia 3 days later and set up a contract to meet with her after breakfast, expecting that later we would attend group therapy and then meet for one-to-one discussion. Instead Nadia, after missing group, reluctantly met with me in the day room.

THERAPEUTIC GOAL: By the conclusion of this interaction, Nadia will state she understands that depression is a treatable disorder and that her symptoms were the cause of her despondent behavior.

STUDENT-PATIENT INTERACTION	THOUGHTS, COMMUNICATION TECHNIQUES, AND MENTAL HEALTH NURSING CONCEPTS
Nadia: *Speaking slowly, eyes downcast.* "I couldn't face all those people."	
Student: "You're looking down like you are sad." *No response from Nadia.* "I wonder what facing the group means to you."	Depression slows everything: thoughts, feelings, and responses to others. I *make an observation* and *attempt to translate into feelings,* then shift to an *indirect question.* Because depression hinders Nadia's processing of information, I need to slow my pace. Allow more silence.
Student's feelings: I should have stayed with "sad." I aimed for her feelings, then did not wait for her to share any feelings.	
Nadia: *Slowly shakes her head back and forth. Silent for 3 minutes. No eye contact.*	
Student: *With a concerned look.* "You shake your head as if you are saying no."	I use *silence* along with attending behavior. I *make an observation* and then use *restatement.*
Student's feelings: I know it's the right thing to do, but waiting during the silence makes me so anxious. I need to stay mindfully alert and attentive. I can endure the silence for Nadia's sake.	
Nadia: "Everybody in group makes progress. I just keep sinking deeper."	
Student: "Sinking deeper?"	Nadia has just started taking antidepressant medication. Most affect *serotonin or norepinephrine neurotransmitter levels,* but therapeutic effectiveness takes 2 to 3 weeks. I use *restatement* to encourage Nadia to say more.
Nadia: "Into depression. I can't pull it together even though I know my kids need me." *Makes eye contact.*	Depression erodes self-esteem, and low self-esteem in turn exacerbates depression.
Student's feelings: I know from experience that it's hard to pull anything together when you feel depressed.	
Student: "You care about your children." *She nods.* "Sounds like you find it difficult at this time to care about yourself very much."	I *attempt to translate into feelings* adding "at this time" to imply a temporary state (e.g., she will again find self-caring as she heals).
Student's feelings: I've noticed that sometimes, like Nadia, nurses find it easier to care for others than take care of self, even basic self-care or prevention measures.	
Nadia: *Sustaining eye contact.* "I can't do anything right. I have nothing to show for my life."	

Continued

APPLYING THE ART—cont'd

A Person With Depression

STUDENT-PATIENT INTERACTION	THOUGHTS, COMMUNICATION TECHNIQUES, AND MENTAL HEALTH NURSING CONCEPTS
Student: "Think about what you've accomplished! You have your children, your marriage, your teaching career." *Nadia shrugs, eyes downcast.*	I inadvertently minimized her feelings by giving *approval* and *advice,* which is *nontherapeutic.* Even though all the things I pointed out may be valid, none of it rings true for Nadia right now.
Student's feelings: She has so much going for her. Why can't she see that?	One step that helps with depression would be for Nadia to problem solve and work through any cognitive distor-
My response causes Nadia to pull away by withdrawing eye contact. When I deliver positives about Nadia before she feels more positive about herself, I discount her experience, which interferes with trust.	tions (e.g., "I can't do anything right"). *Cognitive behavioral therapy,* like antidepressant medication, takes time, but depression is a treatable disorder.
I need to remember that support and nonjudgmental acceptance provide the foundation for the nurse-patient relationship.	
Student: *After waiting for 2 minutes.* "Nadia, I am here to be with you right where you are at this moment. No pressure."	I offer self and acceptance.
Nadia: *Looking up.* "Thank you. You don't know how much that means. I do want to get better and not feel like depression consumes who I am."	
Student: *Nods.* "You want to get better. You were able to take the first courageous step. In deciding to get admitted, you acknowledge that your symptoms are a problem, and they are the symptoms of depression, a disorder."	I *give support.* Separating oneself as distinct from the disorder of depression restores some sense of control to Nadia.
Student's feelings: Nadia feels swallowed up (consumed) by the depression. I want her to know that depression need not be her life.	
Nadia: "Oh, I never thought of it that way...as a first step, not a sign of failure. My symptoms are from the depression."	
Student's feelings: As a nurse, my belief in Nadia's ability to battle the depression offers hope.	
Student: *Nods.* "A treatable disorder." I continue to sit with Nadia in silence for a short while.	At some level, Nadia acknowledges a self not fully consumed by depression.
Nadia: "Yes, depression is a disorder, not all that I am."	Hope will grow as Nadia begins to take charge of her disorder through active investment in treatment.

share common feelings and concerns as well as provide patients with the opportunity to reach out and support others. Belonging to a group can help decrease feelings of isolation, hopelessness, helplessness, and alienation. Medication groups for patients and families can increase understanding of medications, including ways to handle various side effects and compliance.

Pharmacological, Biological, and Integrative Therapies

Antidepressant Medication Therapy

Antidepressant therapy benefits about 65% to 80% of people with nondelusional unipolar depression. ECT has shown a 75% to 85% efficacy rate for those patients who are delusional

or melancholic. It is believed by many that depressed individuals without psychotic features benefit most from a combination of specific psychotherapies (e.g., CBT, IPT, behavioral) and antidepressant medications, compared to either psychotherapy or psychopharmacological treatment alone. In fact, it is believed that the combination and continuation of at least two of these therapies may reduce the risk of recurrence or relapse of MDD and DD. Essentially, the core symptoms of depression improve with antidepressant therapy, and quality-of-life measures improve with certain psychotherapies. Antidepressant drugs can positively alter poor self-concept, degree of withdrawal, vegetative signs of depression, and activity level. Target symptoms include the following:

- Sleep disturbance
- Appetite disturbance (decreased or increased)
- Fatigue
- Decreased sex drive
- Psychomotor retardation or agitation
- Diurnal variations in mood (often worse in the morning)
- Impaired concentration or forgetfulness
- Anhedonia (loss of ability to experience joy or pleasure in living)

One drawback to the use of antidepressant medication is that improvement in mood may take 1 to 3 weeks or longer. If a patient is acutely suicidal, this may be too long to wait. At these times, ECT may be a consideration.

A note about safety. The possibility that antidepressant medication might contribute to suicidal behavior has been well covered in the media and caused grave concerns among the professional community and general public (refer to the Examining the Evidence feature in this chapter). However, there has not been any conclusive evidence to support this concern. To the contrary, review of the use of selective serotonin reuptake inhibitors (SSRIs) in 27 countries over time saw a strong association between increased antidepressant prescribing and reduction in suicide (Ludwig & Marcotte, 2005). A study conducted at five U.S. academic medical centers examining the association between use of antidepressants and suicide concluded that suicide attempts or completions were reduced by 20% among those taking an antidepressant (Yellowlees, 2011b). On the other hand, a recent study in Nottingham, England, found that adults older than age 65 taking the newer generation antidepressants (e.g., SSRIs) are more at risk for strokes, fractures, epilepsy, and even death (ScienceDaily, 2011).

Therefore it should be concluded that all treatments have potential risks. At present, there is no conclusive evidence that either the newer or the older antidepressants *precipitate* suicide; however, there are no data disproving that antidepressants may *contribute* to suicide. The safest path is for physicians/clinicians to consider each patient individually when prescribing antidepressants. Presently, The U.S. Food and Drug Administration (FDA) has Black Box warnings on the SSRIs and is still evaluating data from numerous studies; the FDA recommends that all consumers of antidepressants be observed carefully for worsening of depression and suicidal thoughts. This is especially true for children, adolescents, and older adults.

Choosing an antidepressant. All antidepressants work equally well, although they certainly do not all work well for all individuals. Because the complex interplay of neurotransmitters responsible for depression is unique for different individuals, a variety of antidepressants or a combination of antidepressants may need to be tried before the most effective regimen is found. Each antidepressant has adverse effects as well as cost, safety, and maintenance considerations. The following are some of the primary and secondary considerations when choosing a specific antidepressant:

Primary considerations
- Side effect profile (e.g., sexual dysfunction, weight gain)
- Ease of administration

- Past response
- Safety and medical considerations
- Specific depressive symptoms (e.g., anxiety, irritability, hypersomnia, insomnia)
- Medical considerations (diabetes, high cholesterol, cardiac disease)

Secondary considerations
- Neurotransmitter specificity
- Family history of response
- Cost

The neurotransmitters and receptor sites in the brain are the targets of pharmacological intervention (Table 15-6). While reading the following section, see if you can identify potential side effects caused by the blockage of the given neurotransmitter.

TABLE 15-6	POTENTIAL EFFECTS OF RECEPTOR BLOCKADE	
	RECEPTOR BLOCKED	**POTENTIAL EFFECTS**
NE	Norepinephrine	Decreased depression
		Tremors
		Tachycardia
		Erectile and/or ejaculatory dysfunction
α_1	Specific receptor for epinephrine	Antipsychotic effect
		Postural hypotension
		Dizziness
		Reflux tachycardia
		Ejaculatory dysfunction and/or impotence
		Memory dysfunction
α_2	Specific receptor for norepinephrine	Priapism
5-HT	Serotonin	Decreased depression
		Antianxiety effects
		Gastrointestinal disturbance
		Sexual dysfunction
5-HT_2	Serotonin	Decreased depression
		Decreased suicidal behavior
		Antipsychotic effects
		Hypotension
		Ejaculatory dysfunction
		Weight gain and carbohydrate craving
DA	Dopamine reuptake blocked	Decreased psychosis
		Psychomotor agitation
		Parkinsonian effect
Ach	Acetylcholine	Anticholinergic effects
H_1	Histamine	Sedation
		Weight gain
		Cognitive impairment

Studies that compare the SSRIs to the older tricyclic anti-depressants (TCAs) fail to find support for one group over the other. The difference lies in the quality and quantity of adverse effects, complications, and patient compliance. Basic antide-pressant classes include the following:

First-line agents
- Cyclic antidepressants (e.g., TCAs)
- SSRIs and SNRIs
- Atypical antidepressants

Second-line agents
- Monoamine oxidase inhibitors (MAOIs)

Tricyclic antidepressants. The tricyclic antidepressants (TCAs) inhibit the reuptake of norepinephrine and serotonin by the presynaptic neurons in the CNS. Therefore the amount of time that norepinephrine and serotonin are available to the post-synaptic receptors is increased. This increase in norepinephrine and serotonin levels in the brain is believed to be responsible for mood elevations when TCAs are given to depressed people.

The sedative effects of TCAs are attributed to antihistamine (H_1 receptor) actions and somewhat to anticholinergic actions. Patients must take therapeutic doses of TCAs for 10 to 14 days or longer before they become effective. The full effects may not be evident for 4 to 8 weeks. An effect on some symptoms of depres-sion, such as insomnia and anorexia, may be noted sooner. A person who has shown a positive response to TCA therapy would probably be maintained on that medication for 6 to 12 months to prevent an early relapse. Choice of TCA is based on the following:
- The drug that has proven effective for the patient or a family member in the past
- The drug's adverse effects

For example, a patient who is lethargic and fatigued may have the best results with a more stimulating TCA, such as desipramine (Norpramin) or protriptyline (Vivactil). If a more sedating effect is needed for agitation or restlessness, drugs such as amitriptyline (Elavil) and doxepin (Sinequan) may be more appropriate choices. **Regardless of which TCA is given, the dosage should always be low initially and should be increased gradually.** Caution should be used, especially in older adults because slow drug metabolism may be a problem. The accepted practice for older adults is always, **"Start low, go slow."**

Common adverse reactions. The chemical structure of TCAs is similar to that of antipsychotic medications. Therefore the **anti-cholinergic** effects (e.g., dry mouth, blurred vision, tachycardia, constipation, urinary retention, and esophageal reflux) are simi-lar. These side effects are more common and more pronounced in patients taking antidepressants. These adverse effects are usually not serious and are often transitory, but **urinary retention and severe constipation warrant immediate medical attention.**

The α-adrenergic blockade of TCAs can produce postural orthostatic hypotension and tachycardia. Postural hypotension can lead to dizziness and increase the risk of falls.

Administering the total daily dose of the TCA at night is beneficial for two reasons. First, most TCAs have sedative effects and thereby aid sleep. Second, the minor side effects occur dur-ing sleep, which increases compliance with drug therapy. Table 15-7 reviews side effects of TCAs that are commonly prescribed.

Potential toxic effects. The most serious side effects of the TCAs are cardiovascular: dysrhythmias, tachycardia, myocar-dial infarction, and heart block. Because the cardiac side effects are so serious, TCA use is considered a risk in patients with cardiac disease and in older adults. Patients should have a thor-ough cardiac workup before beginning TCA therapy. The risk of a lethal overdose with a TCA should always be taken into consideration when choosing an antidepressant.

Drug interactions. Individuals taking TCAs can have adverse reactions to numerous other medications. A few of the more common medications usually *not* given while TCAs are being used are listed in Box 15-2. A patient who is taking any of these medications along with a TCA should have a medi-cal clearance beforehand because some of the reactions can be fatal.

Use of antidepressants may precipitate a psychotic episode in a person with schizophrenia. An antidepressant can precipi-tate a manic episode in a patient with bipolar disorder (BD). Depressed patients with BD often receive lithium along with the antidepressant.

Contraindications. Individuals who have recently had a myocardial infarction (or other cardiovascular problems), those with narrow-angle glaucoma or a history of seizures, and pregnant women should not be treated with TCAs, except with extreme caution and careful monitoring.

Patient teaching. Teaching patients and their significant others about medications is an expected nursing responsibil-ity. Medication teaching is begun in the hospital. The nurse or another qualified health care provider must review the medica-tions, possible side effects, and necessary patient precautions. Areas for the nurse to discuss when teaching patients and their families about TCA therapy are presented in Box 15-3. Patients and significant others need to have written information for all medications that will be taken at home.

Selective serotonin reuptake inhibitors. The introduction of Prozac, the first selective serotonin reuptake inhibitor (SSRI), in 1988 heralded an important advance in pharmacotherapy. Essen-tially, the SSRIs selectively block the neuronal uptake of serotonin (e.g., 5-HT, 5-HT_1 receptors), thereby leaving more serotonin available at the synaptic site. (See Chapter 4 for detailed informa-tion on the mechanism of action of SSRIs.)

SSRI antidepressant drugs have a lower incidence of anti-cholinergic side effects (e.g., dry mouth, blurred vision, urinary retention), less cardiotoxicity, and faster onset of action than the TCAs. Patients are more likely to comply with a regimen of SSRIs than of TCAs because of the more favorable side effect profile, and compliance is a crucial step toward recovery or remission. The SSRIs seem to be effective in depression with anxiety fea-tures as well as in depression with psychomotor agitation.

Because the SSRIs cause fewer adverse effects and have low cardiotoxicity, they are less dangerous when they are taken in overdose. The SSRIs, serotonin-norepinephrine reuptake inhibitors (SNRIs), and newer atypical antidepressants have a low lethality risk in suicide attempts compared with the TCAs, which have a very high potential for lethality with overdose. As mentioned previously, the SSRIs do have Black Box warnings

<table>
<tr><td colspan="2">

BOX 15-2 DRUGS TO BE USED WITH CAUTION IN PATIENTS TAKING A TRICYCLIC ANTIDEPRESSANT

- Phenothiazines
- Barbiturates
- Monoamine oxidase inhibitors
- Disulfiram (Antabuse)
- Oral contraceptives (or other estrogen preparations)
- Anticoagulants
- Some antihypertensives (clonidine, guanethidine, reserpine)
- Benzodiazepines
- Alcohol
- Nicotine

</td><td>

BOX 15-3 PATIENT AND FAMILY TEACHING ABOUT TRICYCLIC ANTIDEPRESSANTS

- The patient and family should be informed that improvement in mood may take from 7 to 28 days after initiation of treatment. Up to 6 to 8 weeks may be required for the full effect to be reached and for major depressive symptoms to subside. The family should reinforce this frequently to the depressed family member because depressed people have trouble remembering and respond to ongoing reassurance.
- The patient should be reassured that drowsiness, dizziness, and hypotension usually subside after the first few weeks.
- When the patient starts taking tricyclic antidepressants (TCAs), the patient should be cautioned to be careful working around machines, driving cars, and crossing streets because of possible altered reflexes, drowsiness, or dizziness.
- Alcohol can block the effects of antidepressants. The patient should be told to refrain from drinking alcohol.
- If possible, the patient should take the full dose at bedtime to reduce the experience of side effects during the day.
- If the patient forgets the bedtime dose (or the once-a-day dose), the next dose should be taken within 3 hours; otherwise, the patient should wait until the usual medication time the next day. The patient should *not* double the dose.
- Suddenly stopping TCAs can cause nausea, altered heartbeat, nightmares, and cold sweats in 2 to 4 days. The patient should call the physician or take one dose of TCA until the physician can be contacted.

</td></tr>
</table>

that there may be an increase in suicidal thinking and/or behavior when taking the medication.

Indications. The SSRIs have a broad base of clinical use. In addition to their use in treating depressive disorders, the SSRIs have been prescribed with success to treat some of the anxiety disorders, in particular, obsessive-compulsive disorder and panic disorder (see Chapter 11). Fluoxetine (Prozac) has been found to be effective in treating some women who suffer from late luteal phase dysphoric disorder and bulimia nervosa.

Common adverse reactions. Agents that selectively enhance synaptic serotonin within the CNS may induce agitation, anxiety, sleep disturbance, tremor, sexual dysfunction (primarily anorgasmia), or tension headache. The effect of SSRIs on sexual performance may be the most significant undesirable outcome reported by patients.

Autonomic reactions (e.g., dry mouth, sweating, weight change, mild nausea, and loose bowel movements) also may be experienced with the SSRIs. See Table 15-7 for a general side effect profile of the SSRIs.

Potential toxic effects. One rare and life-threatening event associated with the SSRIs is **serotonin syndrome.** This is thought to be related to overactivation of the central serotonin receptors, caused either by too high a dose or by interaction with other drugs. Symptoms include abdominal pain, diarrhea, sweating, fever, tachycardia, elevated blood pressure, altered mental state (delirium), myoclonus (muscle spasms), increased motor activity, irritability, hostility, and mood change. Severe manifestation can induce hyperpyrexia (excessively high fever), cardiovascular shock, or death.

The risk of this syndrome seems to be the greatest when an SSRI is administered in combination with a second serotonin-enhancing agent, such as an MAOI. For example, a person taking fluoxetine would have to discontinue this medication for a full 5 weeks before starting an MAOI (5 weeks is the half-life for fluoxetine). If a person is already taking an MAOI, the person should wait at least 2 weeks before starting fluoxetine therapy. Other SSRIs have shorter periods of activity; for example, sertraline and paroxetine have half-lives of 2 weeks, so there

would need to be a 2-week gap between the administration of different medications.

A recent Swedish study found that there was a link between use of SSRIs during pregnancy and lung hypertension in newborns (Lowry, 2012). More research is needed; however, it should be noted that the women who participated in this study were considerably older and also smoked cigarettes. Caution in the use of SSRIs for the elderly population has already been mentioned; it will be discussed further in Chapter 28. Despite more recent studies of the suicidal potential for adolescents using SSRIs, caution should always be observed when prescribing psychotropics for any individual.

Box 15-4 lists the symptoms of serotonin syndrome and gives emergency treatment guidelines. Box 15-5 is a useful tool for patient and family teaching about SSRIs.

Atypical and dual action reuptake inhibitor (SNRI) antidepressants. Many of the more recently released antidepressants affect a variety of neurotransmitters. These antidepressants are all effective agents. Table 15-7 introduces both atypical

TABLE 15-7 CHARACTERISTICS OF SPECIFIC ANTIDEPRESSANTS*

GENERIC NAME	TRADE NAME	POTENTIAL SIDE EFFECTS	ADVANTAGES OF SELECTIVE DRUGS	DISADVANTAGES OF SELECTIVE DRUGS
Selective Serotonin Reuptake Inhibitors (SSRIs): Most Popular Type of Antidepressants*				
Citalopram[†]	Celexa	**Common side effects include:** • Headache, which usually dissipates in a few days • Nausea, which usually dissipates in a few days • Sleeplessness and/or drowsiness during day, which usually dissipates in a few weeks • Tremors and/or dizziness • Sexual problems: reduces sexual drive, problems having and enjoying sex • Agitation, feeling jittery and nervous; rare serotonin syndrome; rare activation of suicidal ideation	Minimal interaction with other drugs, minimal weight gain, sedation	Possible initial anxiety
Escitalopram[†]	Lexapro		Minimal interaction, sedation, and weight gain	Possible initial anxiety 18 yr or older; 12-17 yr for MDD
Fluoxetine[†]	Prozac		Activating (energizing)	Possible interaction with other drugs, initial anxiety 8 yr or older
Fluvoxamine	Luvox			8 yr or older for OCD only
Paroxetine[†]	Paxil		Good antianxiety benefit	Weight gain, interacts with other meds, contraindicated in pregnancy Prone to gastrointestinal (GI) upset
Sertraline[†]	Zoloft		Not too sedating, nor prone to increased anxiety	6 yr and older only for OCD
Atypical Antidepressants				
Bupropion	Wellbutrin	Anxiety, insomnia, nausea, headache, dizziness, anorexia	Energizing, few sexual side effects, less weight gain	Rare seizures, doses over 400 mg; possible increased anxiety/insomnia
Nefazodone	Serzone	Nausea, headache, anxiety, sedation, dizziness	Good at reducing anxiety, fewer sexual side effects	*Has been associated with liver toxicity, and is associated with drug interactions; there is a warning against its use with Xanax*
Buspirone	BuSpar	Anxiety, nausea, headache, dizziness	Mainly used in treatment of anxiety; can be antidepressant in higher doses Can act like an antidepressant in higher doses	Plus side: very useful augmenting drug for antidepressants
Dual Action Reuptake Inhibitors (Serotonin and Norepinephrine) (SNRIs)				
Mirtazapine	Remeron	Dry mouth, abnormal dreams, confusion, sedation, influenza-like symptoms, hypotension	Good for severe depression, insomnia, less sexual dysfunction	High weight gain and sedation Rare: induction of mania, suicidal thoughts or behaviors
Duloxetine	Cymbalta	Nausea, diarrhea, decreased appetite, sexual dysfunction, increased blood pressure, inappropriate secretion of antidiuretic hormone, hyponatremia	Good for severe depression	Possible nausea, sedation Rare: induction of hypomania
Venlafaxine	Effexor	Headache, nervousness, insomnia, decreased appetite, sexual dysfunction, inappropriate secretion of antidiuretic hormone, hyponatremia	Good for severe depression, social anxiety disorder, generalized anxiety disorder	Possible high blood pressure, GI upset Rare: induction of hypomania Rare: activation of suicidal ideation

Drug/Class	Generic/Brand	Comments	Age FDA approved
	Desvenlafaxine Pristiq	Nausea, insomnia, dry mouth, nervousness, anorexia, constipation, and increased blood pressure	Rare: induction of hypomania Rare: activation of suicidal ideation or behavior
Selective Norepinephrine Reuptake Inhibitors (Selective NRIs)			
Atomoxetine	Strattera	Not yet FDA approved for depression	Good for cognitive symptoms, low side effect profile
Reboxetine	Vestra	Not yet available in United States	Effective in improving energy and cognition

Tricyclic Antidepressants (TCAs)

Amitriptyline	Elavil
Clomipramine	Anafranil
Desipramine	Norpramin
Doxepin	Sinequan
Imipramine	Tofranil
Maprotiline	Ludiomil
Nortriptyline	Pamelor
Protriptyline	Vivactil
Trimipramine	Surmontil
Amoxapine	Asendin

Common side effects include:
- Dry mouth
- Constipation
- Bladder problems (hard to empty bladder, weak urine stream, men with enlarged prostate may be more affected)
- Sexual problems include reduced sex drive, problems having and enjoying sex
- Blurred vision, which usually dissipates quickly
- Drowsiness

10 yr or older only for OCD

12 yr and older

6 yr and older (for bedwetting)

Monoamine Oxidase Inhibitors (MAOIs)

Isocarboxazid	Marplan
Phenelzine[‡]	Nardil
Tranylcypromine[‡]	Parnate
Selegiline	Eldepryl, EMSAM Transdermal Patch

- MAOIs are always used as second-line treatment and only used in depressions that are resistant to other medications and treatments
- MAOIs have high risk of hypertensive crisis
- If taken with any foods high in tyramine or any sympathomimetic drugs can lead to cerebral hemorrhage or death (refer to Table 15-9)

Most used[‡]
Most used[‡]

Inhibits type B MAO

Used in Parkinson's patients and FDA approved for depression

*Age FDA approved: all are 18 or older unless otherwise specified and stated in last column.
[†]Anticholinergic side effects include dry mouth, blurred vision, constipation, urinary retention, tachycardia, and possible confusion.
[‡]Most use MAO inhibitors.
From Preston, J.D., O'Neal, J.H., & Talaga, M.C. (2010). *Handbook of clinical psychopharmacology for therapists* (6th ed.). Oakland, CA: New Harbinger Publications; *Journal of Psychosocial Nursing and Mental Health Services.* (2011). Clip & save: drugs to treat depression. *Journal of Psychosocial Nursing and Mental Health Services, 49*(7), 15-16; National Institute of Mental Health (NIMH). (2011). *What medications are used to treat depression?* Retrieved August 11, 2011, from www.nimh.nih.gov/health/publications/mental-health-medications/what-medications; National Institute of Mental Health (NIMH). *Major depressive disorder among adults.* Downloaded February 26, 2011, at www.nimh.nih.gov/statistics/1MDD_ADULT.shtm1.

BOX 15-4 SYMPTOMS AND INTERVENTIONS FOR SEROTONIN SYNDROME

Symptoms

- Hyperactivity or restlessness
- Tachycardia → cardiovascular shock
- Fever → hyperpyrexia
- Elevated blood pressure
- Altered mental status (e.g., delirium)
- Irrationality, mood swings, hostility
- Seizures → status epilepticus
- Myoclonus, incoordination, tonic rigidity
- Abdominal pain, diarrhea, bloating
- Apnea → death

Emergency Measures

1. Discontinue offending agent(s)
2. Initiate symptomatic treatment:
   - Serotonin receptor blockade: cyproheptadine, methysergide, propranolol
   - Cooling blankets, chlorpromazine for hyperthermia
   - Dantrolene, diazepam for muscle rigidity or rigors
   - Anticonvulsants
   - Artificial ventilation
   - Paralysis

antidepressants and dual action reuptake inhibitor (SNRI) antidepressants and identifies their strengths and side effect profiles. Each of these agents blocks different neurotransmitters and transmitter subtypes, which accounts for their strengths in targeting unique populations of depressed individuals as well as for their efficacy in treating other conditions.

Monoamine oxidase inhibitors. MAOIs are second-line medications but have proven benefits for patients who have not responded to other medications or to ECT treatment. They also have been found useful in re-refractory anxiety states. In particular, MAOIs have established efficacy in treatment of those with **atypical depression** (see Table 15-7).

In addition to being effective with atypical depression and MDD, MAOIs can be useful in treating other disorders such as panic disorder, social phobia, generalized anxiety disorder, obsessive-compulsive disorder, posttraumatic stress disorder, and bulimia. Essentially, MAOIs prevent the breakdown of norepinephrine, serotonin, and dopamine in the brain, thereby increasing the levels of these brain amines and resulting in elevated mood. (See Chapter 4 for detailed information on the mechanism of action of MAOIs.) Common adverse reactions and potential toxic effects of MAOIs are outlined in Table 15-8.

Unfortunately, the MAOIs also inhibit the breakdown of tyramine in the liver. Increased levels of tyramine can lead to high blood pressure, hypertensive crisis, and eventually cerebrovascular accident and death. Therefore people taking MAOIs must restrict their intake of tyramine so that their

BOX 15-5 PATIENT AND FAMILY TEACHING ABOUT SELECTIVE SEROTONIN REUPTAKE INHIBITORS

- Selective serotonin reuptake inhibitors (SSRIs) may cause sexual dysfunction or lack of sex drive. Inform nurse or physician.
- SSRIs may cause insomnia, anxiety, and nervousness. Inform nurse or physician.
- SSRIs may interact with other medications. Be sure physician knows other medications patient is taking (e.g., digoxin, warfarin). SSRIs should not be taken within 14 days of the last dose of a monoamine oxidase inhibitor (MAOI).
- No over-the-counter drug should be taken without first notifying physician.
- Common side effects include fatigue, nausea, diarrhea, dry mouth, dizziness, tremor, and sexual dysfunction or lack of sex drive.
- Because of the potential for drowsiness and dizziness, patient should not drive or operate machinery until these side effects are ruled out.
- Alcohol should be avoided. SSRIs may act synergistically, and people report increased effects of alcohol (e.g., one drink can seem like two). Alcohol is also a central nervous system (CNS) depressant that may work against the desired effect of the SSRI.
- Liver and renal function tests should be performed and blood counts checked periodically.

- Medication should not be discontinued abruptly. People report such effects as dizziness, nausea, diarrhea, muscle jerkiness, and tremors. If side effects from the SSRIs become bothersome, patient should ask physician about changing to a different drug. Abrupt cessation can lead to serotonin withdrawal.
- SSRIs should be used with caution in the elderly and in pregnant women. The physician should take into account the benefits versus the risk in these populations, as well as all patients taking SSRIs or any kind of antidepressant.
- Any of the following symptoms should be reported to a physician immediately:
  - Increase in depression or suicidal thoughts
  - Rash or hives
  - Rapid heartbeat
  - Sore throat
  - Difficulty urinating
  - Fever, malaise
  - Anorexia and weight loss
  - Unusual bleeding
  - Initiation of hyperactive behavior
  - Severe headache

TABLE 15-8   COMMON ADVERSE REACTIONS TO AND TOXIC EFFECTS OF MONOAMINE OXIDASE INHIBITORS

ADVERSE REACTIONS	COMMENTS
• Hypotension • Sedation, weakness, fatigue • Insomnia • Changes in cardiac rhythm • Muscle cramps • Anorgasmia or sexual impotence • Urinary hesitancy or constipation • Weight gain	Hypotension is the most critical side effect (10%); older adults, especially, may sustain injuries from falls.

TOXIC EFFECTS	COMMENTS

Hypertensive crisis*
• Severe headache
• Stiff, sore neck
• Flushing; cold, clammy skin
• Tachycardia
• Severe nosebleeds, dilated pupils
• Chest pain, stroke, coma, death
• Nausea and vomiting
	1. Patient should go to local emergency department immediately—blood pressure should be checked.
	2. One of the following may be given to lower blood pressure:
	  • 5 mg intravenous phentolamine (Regitine) *or*
	  • Oral chlorpromazine *or*
	  • Nifedipine (Procardia) (calcium channel blocker), 10 mg sublingually

*Related to interaction with foodstuffs and cold medication.

blood pressure does not rise to dangerous levels. See Table 15-9 for a list of foods that are high in tyramine.

Until 2006 the MAOIs commonly used in the United States were phenelzine (Nardil) and tranylcypromine sulfate (Parnate). In 2006 the FDA approved an MAOI that is delivered transcutaneously by way of a patch called the *selegiline transdermal system (STS)*. STS is able to inhibit monoamine oxidase in the central nervous system, increasing the availability of norepinephrine, serotonin, and dopamine, while at the same time avoiding the breakdown of tyramine in the liver and digestive tract. When STS is applied in doses of 6 mg over 24 hours by way of a skin patch, it does **not** require a tyramine-restricted diet (Nemeroff et al., 2007). At higher doses (9 or 12 mg), dietary restrictions must be observed.

See Table 15-7 for an overview of MAOIs in current use and a description of their adverse effects. Patients who do not improve with initial therapy often show improvement when switched to another class of antidepressants or when a drug from another class is added to the therapy. Box 15-6 can be used as a teaching guide for patients and their families regarding MAOIs.

Contraindications. Use of MAOIs may be contraindicated when one of the following is present:
- Cerebrovascular disease
- Hypertension and congestive heart failure
- Liver disease
- Consumption of foods containing tyramine, tryptophan, and dopamine (see Table 15-8)
- Use of certain medications (Box 15-7)
- Recurrent or severe headaches
- Surgery in the previous 10 to 14 days
- Age younger than 16 years

Brain Stimulation Therapies
Somatic Treatments

Electroconvulsive therapy. Electroconvulsive therapy (ECT) remains one of the most effective treatments for major depression with psychotic symptoms, and for treatment of patients with life-threatening psychiatric conditions (e.g., self-harm). Today ECT is mostly reserved for people with treatment-resistant (TR) depression, accounting for between 20% and 30% of depressed individuals. Treatment-resistant depression exists when pharmacological interventions fail or when the side effects are too uncomfortable.

Although stigmatized for many years, ECT is safe and effective, and can achieve a 70% to 90% remission rate in depressed patients within 1 to 2 weeks. The following list describes when ECT may be indicated:
- There is a need for a rapid, definitive response when a patient is suicidal or homicidal.
- The patient is in extreme agitation or stupor.
- The patient develops a life-threatening illness because of refusal of foods and fluids.
- The patient has a history of poor drug response, a history of good ECT response, or both.
- Standard medical treatment has no effect.

ECT is useful in treating patients with major depressive and bipolar depressive disorders, especially when psychotic symptoms are present (e.g., delusions of guilt, somatic delusions, or delusions of infidelity). Patients who have depression with marked psychomotor retardation and stupor also respond well. However, ECT is not necessarily effective in patients with chronic depression, atypical depression, personality disorders, drug dependence, or depression secondary to situational or social

TABLE 15-9	**FOODS THAT CAN INTERACT WITH MONOAMINE OXIDASE INHIBITORS**	
CATEGORY	**UNSAFE FOODS (HIGH TYRAMINE CONTENT)**	**SAFE FOODS (LITTLE OR NO TYRAMINE)**
Foods That Contain Tyramine		
Vegetables	Avocados, especially if overripe; fermented bean curd; fermented soybean; soybean paste; broad beans (fava bean pods); sauerkraut	Most vegetables
Fruits	Figs, especially if overripe; bananas in large amounts (banana peel is extremely high in tyramine)	Most fruits
Meats	Meats that are fermented, smoked, cured, or otherwise aged; spoiled meats; liver, unless very fresh	Meats that are known to be fresh (exercise caution in restaurants; meats may not be fresh)
Sausages	Fermented varieties: bologna, pepperoni, salami, air-dried sausages, others	Nonfermented varieties
Fish	Pickled herring and smoked salmon negligible; lungfish row, sliced schmaltz herring in oil, salmon mousse; dried, pickled, or cured fish; fish that is fermented, smoked, or otherwise aged; spoiled fish	Fish that is known to be fresh; vacuum-packed fish, if eaten promptly or refrigerated only briefly after opening
Milk, milk products	Practically all cheeses, especially hard cheeses	Milk, yogurt, cottage cheese, cream cheese
Foods with yeast	Yeast extract (e.g., Marmite, Bovril)	Baked goods that contain yeast
Beer, wine	Some imported beers, tap (draft) beers, some wines, Chianti	Major domestic brands of beer; most white wines
Other foods	Protein dietary supplements; soups (may contain protein extract); shrimp paste; soy sauce	

Foods That Contain Other Vasopressors

FOOD	COMMENTS
Chocolate	Contains phenylethylamine, a pressor agent; large amounts can cause a reaction.
Fava beans	Contain dopamine, a pressor agent; reactions are most likely with overripe beans.
Ginseng	Headache, tremulousness, and mania-like reactions have occurred.
Caffeinated beverages	Caffeine is a weak pressor agent; large amounts may cause a reaction.

From Lehne, R.A. (2007). *Pharmacology for nursing care* (6th ed.). St Louis: Saunders; Preston, J.D., O'Neal, J.H., & Talaga, M.C. (2010). *Handbook of clinical psychopharmacology for therapists* (6th ed.). Oakland, CA: New Harbinger Publications.

difficulties. The usual course of ECT for a depressed patient is 2 or 3 treatments per week to a total of 6 to 12 treatments.

Procedure. The procedure is explained to the patient, and informed consent is obtained if the patient is being treated voluntarily. When informed consent cannot be obtained from a patient treated involuntarily, permission may be obtained from the next of kin, although in some states treatment must be court ordered. Use of a general anesthetic and muscle-paralyzing agents has revolutionized the comfort and safety of ECT.

Potential adverse reactions. On awakening from ECT, the patient may be confused and disoriented. The nurse and significant others may need to orient the patient frequently during the course of treatment. Many patients state that they have memory deficits for the first few weeks after treatment. Memory usually, although not always, recovers. ECT is not a permanent cure for depression, and maintenance treatment with TCAs or lithium decreases the relapse rate. Maintenance

ECT (once a week to once a month) may also help to decrease relapse rates for patients with recurrent depression.

It should be noted, however, that only 60% of patients will respond to treatment, which includes available pharmacotherapies, cognitive behavioral therapies, and ECT (Scicurious, 2012). Therefore other methods are desperately needed to treat the 40% of depressed individuals who do not respond to available therapies.

Vagus nerve stimulation. Vagus nerve stimulation (VNS) was FDA approved in 2009 as an adjunctive, long-term treatment for patients with **treatment-resistant depression (TRD)** (those with chronic or recurrent MDD who have failed a minimum of four antidepressant medication trials or ECT, or both) (Mayo Staff, 2010; Sadock & Sadock, 2007). ECT is considered by many the most effective acute intervention for TRD, but TRD patients often relapse during the first year following ECT.

The exact mechanism of action of VNS is not totally understood. VNS does affect blood flow to specific parts of the brain

BOX 15-6 PATIENT AND FAMILY TEACHING ABOUT MONOAMINE OXIDASE INHIBITORS

- Tell the patient and the patient's family to avoid certain foods and all medications (especially cold remedies) unless prescribed by and discussed with the patient's physician (see Table 15-9 and Box 15-7 for specific food and drug restrictions).
- Give the patient a wallet card describing the monoamine oxidase inhibitor (MAOI) regimen.
- Instruct the patient to avoid Chinese restaurants (where soy sauce, sherry, brewer's yeast, and other contraindicated products may be used).
- Tell the patient to go to the emergency department immediately if he or she has a severe headache.
- Ideally, monitor the patient's blood pressure during the first 6 weeks of treatment (for both hypotensive and hypertensive effects).
- Instruct the patient that after the MAOI is stopped, dietary and drug restrictions should be maintained for 14 days.

BOX 15-7 DRUGS THAT CAN INTERACT WITH MONOAMINE OXIDASE INHIBITORS

Use of the following drugs should be restricted in patients taking monoamine oxidase inhibitors (MAOIs):
- Over-the-counter medications for colds, allergies, or congestion (any product containing ephedrine, phenylephrine hydrochloride, or phenylpropanolamine)
- Tricyclic antidepressants (e.g., imipramine, amitriptyline)
- Narcotics
- Antihypertensives (e.g., methyldopa, guanethidine, reserpine)
- Amine precursors (e.g., levodopa, L-tryptophan)
- Sedatives (e.g., alcohol, barbiturates, benzodiazepines)
- General anesthetics
- Stimulants (e.g., amphetamines, cocaine)

and affects neurotransmitters including serotonin and norepinephrine, which are implicated in depression. Vagus nerve stimulation does not seem to significantly relieve depression for most people; however, it does make a noteworthy difference for some individuals (Mayo Staff, 2010). The treatments are rather expensive and not covered by most insurance companies. VNS involves surgically implanting a device called a pulse generator into the upper left chest. The pulse generator is connected by a wire to the left vagus nerve; when the generator is stimulated electrical impulses are transmitted to areas of the brain that affect mood centers. When successful, there is an improvement

of depressive symptoms. "Wearable" devices are being developed and tested. Because the vagus nerve affects many functions of the brain, VNS is being studied for other conditions as well (e.g., anxiety disorder, Alzheimer's disease, migraines, and chronic pain/fibromyalgia). Even though it is an FDA-approved therapy for bouts of depression, results have been mixed and there is still controversy concerning its effectiveness.

Rapid transcranial magnetic stimulation (rTMS). Rapid transcranial magnetic stimulation (rTMS), FDA approved in 2008, applies the principles of electromagnetism to deliver an electrical field to the cerebral cortices, but unlike ECT, the waves do not result in generalized seizure activity. An electrical magnetic coil is placed on the scalp, not implanted. Pulsed high-intensity current passes through the coil, creating powerful magnetic fields that change the way brain cells function. Daily treatments last for approximately 40 minutes, resulting in very low incidence of side effects (Mrazek, 2010). rTMS demonstrated significant antidepressant effect in individuals with medication-resistant depression; however, those with moderate depression did not show notable improvement and some individuals had no response at all (Mrazek, 2010). Other factors limiting the use of rTMS include that it can take several weeks to become effective and it is very expensive.

Deep brain stimulation. Deep brain stimulation (DBS) has been used in the treatment of Parkinson's patients for some time, followed by its utilization to treat patients with chronic pain. More recently, DBS has been used experimentally in patients with severe, treatment-resistant depression or obsessive-compulsive disorder (OCD) (NIMH, 2009; Scicurious, 2012). Therefore, the procedure has been employed and refined for many years. Implementation of DBS is considered major surgery because individual electrodes must be implanted into the chosen brain areas. In the treatment of depression the area of implantation is called the subcallosal cingulate (SCC). An insulated wire is connected to an impulse generator, which is connected to a battery-powered device that generates stimulation. The battery-powered device is usually placed under the skin, most often near the clavicle. Once implanted and activated the impulse generator can transmit signals that depolarize the local group of neurons near the implanted electrodes (Scicurious, 2012). A recent, though small, study provides positive data regarding DBS use in patients with treatment-resistant depression, including those with bipolar disorder (Anderson, 2012).

Complementary and Integrative Therapies

Light therapy. Light therapy is the first-line treatment for seasonal affective disorder with or without medication (see Table 15-1). Full-spectrum wavelength light is the specific type of light used. People with seasonal affective disorder often live in climates in which there are marked seasonal differences in the amount of daylight. Seasonal variations in mood disorders in the Southern Hemisphere are the reverse of those in the Northern Hemisphere. Light therapy also may be useful as an adjunct to medications in treating chronic MDD or dysthymia with seasonal exacerbations.

Light therapy is thought to be effective because of the influence of light on melatonin. Melatonin is secreted by the pineal gland

and is necessary for maintaining and shifting biological rhythms. Exposure to light suppresses the nocturnal secretion of melatonin, which seems to have a therapeutic effect on people with seasonal affective disorder. Treatments consist of exposure to light balanced to replicate the effects of sunlight for 30 to 60 minutes a day.

St. John's wort. St. John's wort (*Hypericum perforatum*) is a whole plant product with antidepressant properties that is not regulated by the FDA. In numerous studies, St. John's wort demonstrated efficacy comparable with placebo and was generally comparable in effect to low-dose TCAs, and less so to SSRIs (Mischoulon, 2007). The herb is not to be taken by certain patient populations, such as those who have MDD or are pregnant. To date, any efficacy is found for people who have mild depression. St. John's wort poses potentially harmful drug interactions that can result in significant toxic effects on the liver. Some drugs that need to be avoided when taking St. John's wort are amphetamines or other stimulants, other antidepressants (MAOIs, SSRIs), warfarin, theophylline, digoxin, and other prescription and over-the-counter drugs. Although there is some information regarding drug interactions, there is a lack of accurate information available (Preston et al., 2010).

S-Adenosylmethionine (SAMe). In a new study, S-adenosylmethionine (SAMe), an over-the-counter dietary supplement that is well tolerated and safe, was found to be effective as an adjunct treatment in people with major depressive disorder (MDD) who are resistant to other treatment. There have been 40 previous studies, but the most recent study was a double-blind, placebo study conducted by Harvard Medical School and Massachusetts General Hospital. The administrators found that response rates and remission rates were higher for patients treated with medication and adjunctive SAMe (36.1% and 25.8%, respectively) than adjunctive placebo (17.6% and 11.7%, respectively). Although the study warrants replication, SAMe may play a big role as adjunctive treatment for people with major depressive disorder who are nonresponsive to medications (Papakostas et al., 2010).

Peer support. We all experience positive results when talking to good friends regarding a problem or situation that is causing us difficulty; therefore it is no surprise that peer support/support groups can make a difference in people's lives. Researchers led by Dr. Paul Pfeiffer and associates at the University of Michigan Medical School in Ann Arbor examined 14 studies involving depression and peer support. Their findings found that support groups were "superior" to regular care, but not to cognitive behavioral therapy. Pfeiffer's team suggested the reason could be support groups decrease feelings of isolation, provide a buffer against stressful events, increase health information, and offer role models (Dotinga, 2011).

Exercise. There is substantial evidence that exercise can enhance mood and reduce symptoms of depression and anxiety (Mayo Foundation for Medical Education and Research, 2005). It may take at least 30 minutes a day for at least 3 to 5 days a week in order to reduce the symptoms of depression and anxiety; however, shorter periods of time (10 to 15 minutes) have shown to reduce depression and anxiety in the short term (Mayo Foundation for Medical Education and Research, 2005).

The Future of Treatment

There is a great need for earlier detection and intervention, achievement of remission, prevention of progression, and integration of neuroscience and behavioral science in the treatment of depression High-risk ages and groups, including the following, are in need of screening:

- Individuals in late adolescence and early adulthood
- Women in their reproductive years
- Adults and older adults with medical problems
- People with a family history of depression

There is also a need for education, particularly about the linkage between physical symptoms and depression. Psychopharmacological treatment should be augmented with cognitive behavioral therapies, and there is a need for more supplementary strategies, such as the following:

- Promotion of sleep hygiene
- Increase in exercise
- Better total health care

Continual research will result in more genetic screening tools and understanding of the pharmacogenetics of depression; the use of neuroimaging will become a common diagnostic tool and will not be restricted to research.

Brain imaging. A study from the University of Wisconsin–Madison (Johnstone et al., 2007), perhaps the first study to use brain imaging, revealed a breakdown in normal patterns of emotional processing in people who are depressed. Using a functional magnetic resonance imaging scanner, the researchers found that healthy people are able to regulate their negative emotions through conscious efforts, such as envisioning a more positive outcome or reframing a negative situation. The scan revealed that high levels of regulatory activity correlated with low levels of activity in the emotional response centers. They found that some depressed individuals lacked the ability to regulate emotions. In these individuals, high levels of regulatory activity did not change the levels of activity in the emotional centers, demonstrating the neural circuits regulating emotion in some depressed individuals are dysfunctional.

EVALUATION

Short-term indicators and outcome criteria are frequently evaluated. For example, if the patient presents to the unit with suicidal thoughts, the nurse evaluates whether the patient still has suicidal thoughts, is able to state alternatives to suicidal impulses in the future, and is able to explore thoughts and feelings that precede suicidal impulses. Outcomes relating to thought processes, self-esteem, and social interactions are frequently formulated because these areas are often problematic in people who are depressed.

Physical needs also warrant nursing or medical attention. If a person has lost weight because of anorexia, is the appetite returning? If a person was constipated, are the bowels now functioning normally? If the person was suffering from insomnia, is he or she now getting 6 to 8 hours of sleep per night? If the indicators have not been met, an analysis of the data, nursing diagnoses, goals, and planned nursing interventions is made. The patient should be reassessed and the care plan reformulated when necessary.

KEY POINTS TO REMEMBER

- Depression is the most commonly seen psychiatric disorder in the health care system.
- There are a number of subtypes of depression and depressive clinical phenomena. Two primary depressive disorders are major depressive disorder (MDD) and chronic depressive disorder (dysthymic disorder).
- The symptoms in major depression are usually severe enough to interfere with a person's social or occupational functioning (inability to experience pleasure [anhedonia], significant weight loss, insomnia or hypersomnia, extreme fatigue [anergia], psychomotor agitation or retardation, diminished ability to think or concentrate, feelings of worthlessness, recurrent thoughts of death).
- A person with MDD may or may not have psychotic symptoms, and the symptoms a person usually exhibits during a major depression are different from the characteristics of the normal premorbid personality.
- In chronic depression the symptoms last for at least 2 years and are usually considered mild to moderate. Usually, a person's social or occupational functioning is not as greatly impaired as they are in major depressive disorder (MDD), although they may cause significant distress or some impairment in these areas. The symptoms in a chronic/dysthymic depression are often congruent with the person's usual pattern of functioning.
- Many theories exist about the cause of depression. The most accepted is the psychophysiological theory; however, cognitive theory, learned helplessness theory, and psychodynamic and life events issues help explain triggers to depression and maintenance of depressive thoughts and feelings.
- Nursing assessment includes the evaluation of affect, thought processes (especially suicidal thoughts), feelings, physical behavior, and communication. The nurse also needs to be aware of the symptoms that mask depression.
- Nursing diagnoses can be numerous. Depressed individuals are always evaluated for *Risk for Suicide*. Some other common nursing diagnoses are *Disturbed Thought Processes, Chronic Low Self-Esteem, Imbalanced Nutrition, Constipation, Disturbed Sleep Pattern, Ineffective Coping, Spiritual Distress,* and *Disabled Family Coping.*
- Interventions with patients who are depressed involve several approaches, including using specific principles of communication, planning activities of daily living, administering or participating in psychopharmacological therapy, maintaining a therapeutic environment, and teaching patients about the biochemical aspects of depression and medication teaching.
- Several short-term psychotherapies are effective in the treatment of depression, including IPT, CBT, and some forms of group therapy.
- Electroconvulsive therapy (ECT) is an effective treatment for people with major depression with psychotic features and for patient's refractory to other treatments. Vagus nerve stimulation (VNS) can be a valuable adjunctive treatment in treatment-resistant depression. Light therapy is the first line of treatment for seasonal affective disorder (SAD).
- Evaluation is ongoing throughout the nursing process, and patients' outcomes are compared with the stated outcome criteria and short-term and intermediate goals. The care plan is revised by use of the evaluation process when desired outcomes are not being met.

APPLYING CRITICAL JUDGMENT

1. You are spending time with Mr. Plotsky, who is being given a workup for depression. He avoids eye contact, he slouches in his seat, and his expression appears blank, but sad. Mr. Plotsky has suffered from numerous bouts of major depression in the past and says to you, "This will be my last depression. I will never go through this again."
   A. If safety is the first concern, what are the appropriate questions to ask Mr. Plotsky at this time?
   B. Give an example of the kinds of signs and symptoms you might find when you assess a patient with depression in terms of behaviors, thought processes, activities of daily living, and ability to function at work and at home?
   C. Mr. Plotsky tells you that he has tried every medication there is but that none have worked. He asks you about the herb St. John's wort. What is some information he should have about its effectiveness for severe depression, its interactions with other antidepressants, and its regulatory status?
   D. What might be some somatic options for a person who is resistant to antidepressant medications?
   E. Mr. Plotsky asks what causes depression. In simple terms, how might you respond to his query?
   F. Mr. Plotsky tells you that he has never tried therapy because he thinks it is for babies. What information could you give him about various therapeutic modalities that have proven effective for some other depressed patients?
2. When you are teaching Ms. Mac about her SSRI sertraline (Zoloft), she asks you, "What makes this such a good drug?"
   A. What are some of the positive attributes of SSRIs? What is one of the most serious, although rare, side effects of the SSRIs?
   B. Devise a teaching plan for Ms. Mac.

CHAPTER REVIEW QUESTIONS

Choose the most appropriate answer(s).

1. Which statement from a depressed patient might precede a suicide attempt?
   1. I want to be the best I can be.
   2. I have decided to solve all my problems.
   3. I have the most horrendous family.
   4. I will try and work with staff.

2. Which response to a patient experiencing depression would be helpful from the nurse?
   1. "Don't worry, we all get down once in a while."
   2. "Don't consider suicide. It's an unacceptable option."
   3. "Try to cheer up. Things always look darkest before the dawn."
   4. "I can see you're feeling down. I'll sit here with you for a while."

3. A patient diagnosed with major depression appears tired and lethargic, but states he will try a group activity. What nursing intervention best assists this patient to integrate into the milieu?
   1. Have the patient sit outside of groups until he is ready to fully participate.
   2. Encourage the patient to choose which of several groups he might like to attend.
   3. Arrange for the patient to participate in a structured group activity.
   4. Do nothing and allow the patient to take the initiative in joining a group.

4. Electroconvulsive therapy (ECT): (select all that apply)
   1. is useful in treatment of patients with depressive disorders.
   2. can cause memory deficits.
   3. has a usual course of therapy that includes 2-3 treatments.
   4. can achieve 90% remission rate in 1-2 months.

5. When the nurse is caring for a depressed patient, the problem that should receive the highest nursing priority is:
   1. powerlessness.
   2. suicidal ideation.
   3. inability to cope effectively.
   4. anorexia and weight loss.

REFERENCES

American Psychiatric Association (APA). (2011a). *Major depressive disorder, recurrent.* Retrieved August 8, 2011, from www.dsm5.org/ProposeRevision/Pages/proposerevision.aspx?rid=45.

American Psychiatric Association (APA). (2011b). *Catatonic specifier.* Retrieved August 11, 2011, from www.dsm5.org/ProposedRevision/Pages/proposerevision.aspx?=445.

Anderson, P. (2012). *More good news and deep brain stimulation and depression.* Retrieved January 25, 2012, from www.Medscape.com/view article/756474_print.

Andrew, L. B., & Brenner B. E. (2012). Depression and suicide. Retrieved March 31, 2012, from emedicine.medscape.com/article/805495-overview.

Beck, A. T., & Rush, A. J. (1995). Cognitive therapy. In H. I. Kaplan, & B. J. Sadock (Eds.), *Comprehensive textbook of psychiatry/VI* (6th ed., vol. 2, pp. 1847–1856). Baltimore: Williams & Wilkins.

Bijl, D., van Marwijk, H. W., de Haan, M., et al. (2004). Effectiveness of disease management programs for recognition, diagnosis and treatment of depression in primary care. *European Journal of General Practice, 10*(1), 6–12. abstract.

Cassano, P., Cassem, N. H., Papkosteas, G. I., Fava, M., & Stern, T. A. (2010). In T. A. Stern, G. L. Fricchione, N. H. Cassem, M. S. Jellinek, & J. F. Rosenbaum (Eds.), *Massachusetts General Hospital handbook of general hospital psychiatry* (6th ed.). Philadelphia: Saunders/Elsevier.

Depression facts and statistics. (2009). Retrieved February 27, 2011, from www.depressionperception.com/depression/depression_facts.

Dotinga, R. (2011). *Peer support beats usual care for depression, analysis finds.* Retrieved from MedlinePlus atwww.nln.nih.gov.Medlineplus/news/full story_109010.html.

Fava, M., et al. (2008). Difference in treatment outcome in outpatients with anxious versus non-anxious depression: A STAR*D Report. *American Journal of Psychiatry.* Retrieved February 27, 2011, from www.nimh.nih.gov/science–news/2008/co-/occurring/anxiety.

Feldman, G. (2007). Cognitive and behavioral therapies for depression: overview, new directions and practical recommendations for dissemination. *Psychiatric Clinics of North America, 30*(1), 39–50.

Gelder, M., Harrison, P., & Cowen, P. (2006). *The shorter Oxford textbook of psychiatry* (5th ed.). London: Oxford University Press.

Hall-Flavin, D. K. (2010). *Pain and depression. Is there a link?* Retrieved March 1, 2011, from Mayo Clinic at www.MayoClinic.com/health/pain-and depression/AN01449.

Johnstone, T., van Reekum, C. M., & Urry, H. L. (2007). Failure to regulate: counterproductive recruitment of top-down prefrontal-subcortical circuitry in major depression. *Journal of Neuroscience, 27*(33), 8877–8884.

Journal of Psychosocial Nursing and Mental Health Services. (2011). Clip & save: drugs to treat depression. *Journal of Psychosocial Nursing and Mental Health Services, 49*(7), 15–16.

Karg, K., Burnmeister, M., Shudden, K., & Sen, S. (2011). *The serotonin transporter promoter variant (5-httlpr), stress, and depression meta-analysis revisited: Evidence of genetic moderation.* Retrieved March 31, 2011, from www.archgen.com at University of Pittsburgh.

Kelsoe, J. R. (2009). Mood disorder: genetics. In B. J. Sadock, V. A. Sadock, & P. Ruiz (Eds.), *Kaplan & Sadock's comprehensive textbook of psychiatry* (9th ed., vol. 1, pp. 1653–1664). Baltimore: Williams & Wilkins.

Kessler, R. C., Berglund, P., Demler, O., et al. (2005). Lifetime prevalence and age of onset distributions of *DSM-IV* disorders in the national comorbidity survey replication. *Archives of General Psychiatry, 62*(6), 592–602.

Kuyken, W., Byrod, S., Taylor, R. S., Watkins, E., et al. (2008). Mindfulness-based cognitive therapy to prevent relapse in recurrent depression. *Journal of Consulting and Clinical Psychology, 76*(6), 966–978.

Lowry, F. (2011). *Newer antidepressants in older patients may be risky.* Retrieved August 11, 2011, from www.medscape.com/viewarticle/747592?src=nl_topic.

Lowry, F. (2012). *SSRIs in pregnancy linked to lung hypertension in newborns.* Retrieved January 25, 2012, from www.medscape.com/view article/756875_print.

Ludwig, J., & Marcotte, D. E. (2005). Antidepressants, suicide and drug regulation. *Journal of Policy, Analysis and Management, 24,* 249–272.

Mayo Clinic Staff. (2005). *Depression and anxiety: exercise eases symptoms.* Retrieved August 21, 2007, from http://mayoclinic.com/health/depression-and-exercise/MH00043.

Mayo Clinic Staff. (2010). *Electroconvulsive therapy (ECT): Why is it done?* Retrieved March 31, 2012, from http://www.mayoclinic.com/health/electroconvulsive-therapy/MyOO129//DSECTION=why.

Mayo Clinic Staff. (2012). *Depression (Major depression).* Retrieved February 16, 2012, from http://www.mayoclinic.com/health/depression/DS00175/DSECTON=symptoms.

Mischoulon, D. (2007). Update and critique of natural remedies as antidepressant treatments. *Psychiatric Clinics of North America, 30*(1), 51–68.

Mrazek, D. (2010). *Transcranial magnetic stimulation can treat depression.* Retrieved August 11, 2011, from www.mayoclinic.com/health/transcranial-magnetic-stimulation/MY01466.

Narasimhan, M., & Campbell, N. (2010). A tale of two comorbidities: understanding the neurobiology of depression and pain. *Indian Journal of Psychiatry, 52,* 127–130.

National Institute of Mental Health (NIMH). (2008). *Co-occurring anxiety contemplates treatment response for those with major depression.* Retrieved February 27, 2011, from www.nimh.nih.gov/science–news/2008/co-occurring anxiety.

National Institute of Mental Health (NIMH). (2011). *What medications are used to treat depression?* Retrieved August 11, 2011, from www.nimh.nih.gov/health/publications/mental-health-medications/what-medications.

National Institute of Mental Health (NIMH). (2010a). *Major depressive disorder among adults.* Retrieved February 26, 2011, from www.nimh.nih.gov/statistics/1MDD_ADULT.shtml.

National Institute of Mental Health (NIMH). (2010b). *Dysthymic disorder among children.* Retrieved February 26, 2011, from www.nimh.gov/statistics/1DD_CHILD.shtml.

National Institute of Mental Health (NIMH). (2010c). *Early treatment decisions crucial for teens with treatment-resistant depression.* Retrieved February 27, 2011, from www.nimh.nih.gov/science–news/2010/earliest–treatment–dec.

National Institute of Mental Health (NIMH). (2009). *Women and depression: discovering hope/what are the different forms of depression?* Retrieved March 2, 2011, from http://www.nih.gov/health/publication/woman-and-depression-discovering-hope/.

Nemeroff, C., DeVane, L., & Lydiard, B. (2007). *Emerging trends for monoamine oxidase inhibition in the management of depression: a patient-focused, interactive program.* Charleston, SC: CME, Office of Continuing Education, Medical University of South Carolina (MUSC).

Papakostas, G. I., Mischoulon, D., Shyu, I., Albert, J. E., & Fava, M. (2010). S-Adenosyl methionine (SAMe) augmentation of serotonin reuptake inhibitors were antidepressant nonresponders with major depressive disorder: a double-blind, randomized clinical trial. *American Journal of Psychiatry.* Retrieved March 1, 2011, from www.psychiatryonline.org/CGI/content/abstract/167/8/942.

Preston, J. D., O'Neal, J. H., & Talaga, M. C. (2010). *Handbook of clinical psychopharmacology for therapists* (6th ed.). Oakland, CA: New Harbinger Publications.

Proceedings of the National Academy of Sciences. (2009). *Thinning tissue in right half of brain signals increase risk of inherited depression.* Retrieved February 27, 2011, from www.nimh.nih.gov/science-news/2009/thinning-tissue-in-r.

Psych Direct Evidenced Based Mental Health Education and Information. (2006). *Mood disorders: professional audiences.* Retrieved August 8, 2006, from www.psychdirect.com/depression/depression_pro, htm#Anchor-DOES-49425.

Rihmer, Z., & Angst, J. (2009). Mood disorders: epidemiology. In B. J. Sadock, V. A. Sadock, & P. Ruiz (Eds.), *Kaplan and Sadock's comprehensive textbook of psychiatry.* (9th ed., vol. 1). Philadelphia: Wolters Kluwer/Lippincott Williams & Wilkins.

Riolo, S., Nguyen, T. A., & Greden, J. F. (2005). Prevalence of depression by race/ethnicity: findings from the National Health and Nutrition Examination survey. *American Journal of Public Health, 95*(6), 998–1000.

Rosenbaum, J. F., & Covino, J. M. (2006). Depression in geriatric patients. *Medscape Psychiatry and Mental Health.* Retrieved August 6, 2006, from www.medscape.com/viewarticle/520524.

Sackheim, H. A., Brannan, S. K., Rush, A. J., et al. (2007). Durability of antidepressant response to vagus nerve stimulation (VNS). *International Journal of Neuropsychopharmacology, 9,* 1–10.

Sadock, B. J., & Sadock, V. A. (2010). *Kaplan & Sadock's pocket handbook of clinical psychiatry* (5th ed.). Philadelphia: Wolters Kluwer/Lippincott Williams & Wilkins.

Sadock, B. J., & Sadock, V. A. (2007). *Kaplan & Sadock's synopsis of psychiatry* (10th ed.). Philadelphia: Lippincott Williams & Wilkins.

Sicurious. (2012). *Deep brain stimulation for major depression: miracle therapy or just another treatment?* Retrieved January 29, 2012, from http://blogs. Scientific American.com/scicurious-brain/2012/01/09/deep-brain-stimulation–for.

ScienceDaily. (2011). *New antidepressants can increase risk for elderly, study suggests.* Retrieved January 26, 2012, from www.sciencedaily.com/releases/2011/08/110802184544.htm.

Seligman, M. E. (1973). Fall into hopelessness. *Psychology Today, 7,* 43.

U.S. Department of Veterans Affairs. (2006). *Evidence-based depression treatment.* Retrieved August 8, 2006, from www.va.gov/tides_waves/page.cfm?pg20.

WebMD. (2012). *Depression Health Center: dysthymia (mild chronic depression).* Retrieved February 16, 2012, from http://www.webmd.com/depression/guide/chronic-depression-dysthymia?print=true.

WebMD. (2011). *Depressive gene link to response to stress.* Retrieved March 2, 2011, from www.webmd/depression/news/20110104/depression–link–to–response–to–stress.

Yellowlees, P. (2011a). *Recurrence of major depression in adolescents.* Retrieved August 11, 2011, from www.medscape.com/view article/747180?src=nl_topic.

Yellowlees, P. (2011b). *A closer look at suicide and antidepressants.* Retrieved January 25, 2012, from www.Medscape.com/view article/755801_print.

Bipolar Spectrum Disorders

Elizabeth M. Varcarolis

evolve WEBSITE

http://evolve.elsevier.com/Varcarolis/essentials

KEY TERMS AND CONCEPTS

SELECTED CONCEPT: Genetic Findings Potential for New Medications? Reappraisal of *DSM* Diagnosis?

A trio of genome-wide studies have definitively identified genetic links between bipolar illness and schizophrenia (NIMH, 2009). These shared genetic roots are hoped to provide new insight into the cause of both of these chronic disabling disorders. Existing therapies for these groups of people are ineffective as long-term options. This information is hoped to lead to improved treatment and quality of life for these patients. These findings raise two questions for further research:

1. Do these shared genetic causes call into question the correctness of using two distinct diagnostic entities?
2. Can an understanding of these common genetic variants lead to future medications that will target these specific genes?

(NIMH, 2009; Dallas, 2011; McKeever, 2009)

OBJECTIVES

1. Discuss the progression of behaviors, speech patterns, and thought processes of a person escalating from hypomania to mania to delirious mania. Act these out in your study group.
2. Apply best-known evidence-based practice to identify interventions for each of the progressions from hypomania to mania to delirious mania.
3. Describe in detail the physical, safety, personal, and legal considerations a nurse must be aware of during a patient's manic phase.
4. Discuss the rationale for at least five communication strategies that are effective with patients in acute mania.
5. Identify specific incidences when teamwork and collaboration are key for a patient in an acute phase of mania and those for a patient in delirious mania.
6. Apply knowledge of safety in establishing a milieu for a hospitalized patient in acute mania.
7. Using informatics identify expected side effects of lithium therapy.
8. Compare and contrast the differences between the signs and interventions for early and severe lithium toxicity.
9. Using evidence-based knowledge, identify the bipolar clinical subtypes that may respond better to anticonvulsant therapy as well as those that may respond better to lithium therapy. List the medications most appropriate for pregnant women with bipolar disorder.
10. Develop a patient-centered teaching plan for a patient with bipolar disorder who is in the continuation phase of treatment.
11. Compare and contrast the focus of treatment for a person in the acute manic phase and that for a person in the continuation or maintenance phase of a bipolar I disorder.
12. Teach a classmate how to evaluate the differences between a unipolar depression and a bipolar depression.

Bipolar spectrum disorders (BSDs), formerly called manic-depressive illness, are among the most serious of the mental health disorders and rank sixth among the world's most disabling illnesses (Black & Andreasen, 2011). Bipolar disorders are chronic, recurrent, and life-threatening illnesses that require lifetime monitoring. However, they all too frequently are undiagnosed, with some individuals living 8 to 10 years before obtaining proper treatment, if at all. Bipolar spectrum disorders are characterized by two opposite poles. One pole is mania, an exaggerated euphoria or irritability, and the other pole is depression. Bipolar disorders are a group of disorders with different courses and treatments. Alternating mood episodes are characterized by mania, hypomania, depression, and concurrent mania and depression (i.e., mixed episodes in which depressive symptoms occur during a manic attack). Periods of normal functioning may alternate with periods of illness (highs, lows, or mixed highs and lows).

Unfortunately slightly less than half of individuals with bipolar disorder regain full occupational, interpersonal, and/or social functioning, even during remission. Individuals with BSD have significant morbidity and mortality rates. It is estimated that between 25% and 50% of people with BSD attempt suicide and 11% succeed in ending their life (Soreff & McInnes, 2011). BSDs are close to the top of disorders with the highest lifetime rate of suicide.

Although it is now recognized that bipolar illness spans a wide spectrum of behaviors, we will focus on the most commonly identified disorders. The following are based on severity and patterns, listed from most to least severe:

- Bipolar I disorder: At least one episode of mania alternating with major depression. Psychosis may accompany the manic episode.
- Bipolar II disorder: Hypomanic episode(s) alternating with major depression. Psychosis is not present in bipolar II. The hypomania of bipolar II tends to be euphoric and the depression tends to place the patient at particular risk for suicide.
- Cyclothymia: Hypomanic episodes alternating with minor depressive episodes (at least 2 years in duration). Individuals with cyclothymia tend to have irritable hypomanic episodes.
- Bipolar disorder NOS (not otherwise specified) is a designation that includes disorders with bipolar features that do not meet criteria for any of the previously specified disorders.

The specifier rapid cycling bipolar disorder (four or more mood episodes in a 12-month period) is used to indicate more severe symptoms such as poorer global functioning, higher recurrence risk, and greater resistance to conventional somatic treatments. Mania or hypomania with mixed features (a mixed features specifier) is used when a patient in a full bipolar or hypomanic mood displays at the same time depressive symptoms—for example, increased activity or agitation and feelings of worthlessness or suicidal ideation at the same time (Preston et al., 2010). The distinction between bipolar I and bipolar II diagnoses in conjunction with the rapid cycling or mixed mania specifiers is crucial. Each dictates specific treatment implications and appropriate medical interventions (Preston & Johnson, 2009).

Studies indicate that there are striking differences between unipolar and bipolar depression.

- Unipolar depression affects women more than men and appears later in life. Sleep disturbances manifest as general insomnia, difficulty falling asleep, or waking repeatedly at night. A loss of appetite and diminished interest in eating are common. Depression may be agitated (e.g., pacing and restlessness) and episodes often last longer.
- Bipolar depression affects men and women more equally than unipolar depression. Onset is usually much younger,

in the vicinity of 18 years old. Disturbances in sleep manifest as hypersomnia, excessive tiredness, and difficult morning waking. Changes in appetite often take the form of binge eating and cravings for carbohydrates, which may alternate with loss of appetite. Bipolar depression is more often marked by psychomotor retardation. Patients with bipolar depression are also at higher risk of drug abuse and suicide than those with unipolar depression (BPhoenix, 2010).

PREVALENCE AND COMORBIDITY

The lifetime prevalence of bipolar spectrum disorder (BSD) varies around the world but in the U.S. population it is estimated to be 4.4% with a 12-month prevalence of 2.8% (Brauser, 2011). Whereas major depression usually appears between 25 and 30 years of age, bipolar disorders emerge between childhood and 50 years, with most cases manifesting between 15 and 19 years (Soreff & McInnes, 2011). People with BSD are occasionally diagnosed with major depression disorder; these individuals may indeed have a bipolar disorder in which the first manic episode does not appear until they are older than 50 (Soreff & McInnes, 2011). The male to female ratio for bipolar I is 1:1 whereas for bipolar II it is 1:2.

Cyclothymia usually begins in adolescence or early adulthood and has a lifetime prevalence of 2.5% (Kessler et al., 2005). There is a 15% to 50% risk that an individual with cyclothymia will subsequently develop bipolar I or bipolar II disorder.

A study assessing World Health Organization (WHO) surveys found that at least 76.5% of respondents with BSD have a comorbid disorder. According to the study the most common co-occurring disorders are anxiety disorders (62%), in particular panic attacks (49.8%), behavioral disorders (44.8%), and substance use disorders (36.6%). The only difference in the U.S. population versus other countries was that the incidence of behavioral disorders was substantially higher in the United States (Brauser, 2011). Substance-abusing individuals with bipolar disorder seem to experience more rapid cycling and more mixed or dysphoric mania (anger and irritability) and report more hospitalizations. Comorbid substance and anxiety disorders worsen the prognosis and greatly increase the risk of suicide.

The bipolar spectrum disorders also have a high rate of *medical* comorbidity, especially cardiovascular, cerebrovascular, and metabolic diseases. There are also medical conditions that are associated with manic symptoms such as central nervous system (CNS) tumors or trauma, hypothyroidism, seizure disorders, and some infectious diseases (e.g., human immunodeficiency virus [HIV]).

THEORY

The results of an international study confirmed that bipolar illness manifests itself in many ways and exists on a spectrum. Merikangas and colleagues (2011) stress it is more important to attend to each individual's suffering than it is to determine if the individual conforms to the current definitions of bipolar disorders.

Because of increasingly sophisticated neuroimaging and genetic research, our knowledge of the neurobiology of bipolar disorder is one of complexity. It is a disorder involving complex disturbances in relationships and marked disruption in sleep patterns, linking environmental and genetic influences, neural systems and behaviors, and high rates of certain psychological and medical comorbidities. BSDs are now defined as a multisystem of disorders involving disturbances in all of these aforementioned domains. The etiology or pathophysiology of BSDs has not yet been determined, nor are there any specific biological or genetic markers that correspond with this disease state (Soreff & McInnes, 2011).

Biological Theories
Genetic Factors

Twin, family, and adoption studies provide significant evidence to support the view that bipolar disorders have a strong genetic component. However, the inheritance of the bipolar disorders is not a matter of "one gene, one illness" but an expression of multiple genes and chromosomes. An early age of onset is associated with hereditability, which increases with the amount of shared genetic material. Therefore identical twins have greater heritable risk (33% to 90%) (Soreff & McInnes, 2011) than fraternal twins (18% to 35%) (Kelsoe, 2009). First-degree relatives are seven times more likely to develop bipolar disorder than people in the general population (Soreff & McInnes, 2011). Because the concordance rates for most disorders in twins are not 100%, it is strongly accepted that any genetic basis for bipolar disorder does have a strong underpinning. However, it is likely that multiple genes on a variety of chromosomes are interacting in, as yet, unknown ways (Preston et al., 2010).

Increasingly, researchers are finding evidence that there is a genetic link on specific chromosomes that point to a susceptibility to both bipolar disorder I and schizophrenia. A study by Lichtenstein and colleagues (2009) demonstrated that both bipolar disorder and schizophrenia definitely share a common genetic cause.

Neurobiological Factors

The interrelationships in the neurotransmitter system are complex. Mood disorders are most likely a result of complex interactions among numerous chemicals, including neurotransmitters and hormones. Neurotransmitters (norepinephrine, serotonin, and dopamine) have been implicated as causal factors in mania and depression. During a manic episode, patients with bipolar disorder demonstrate significantly higher plasma levels of norepinephrine and epinephrine, and people with depression have decreased levels of epinephrine and norepinephrine.

One study reported that people with bipolar disorder have about one third more neurotransmitters in two major areas of the brain, which may cause an overstimulation in the brain. Neuroreceptor oversensitivity also has been identified as a cause of bipolar disorder symptoms.

Neuroendocrine Factors

The hypothalamic-pituitary-adrenal (HPA) axis, which modulates the stress response and is involved in maintaining homeostasis, has been closely scrutinized in people with mood disorders for decades. The severity of manic episodes seems to be highly correlated to the degree of neuroendocrine alteration. A study suggested that disruption in the hypothalamic-pituitary-adrenal axis (HPA axis) and hormonal imbalances can contribute to the clinical outcome of bipolar disorder. This study offered evidence that hormonal exacerbations of mood symptoms in bipolar women may be a clinical marker of the severity of this disorder during their reproductive period (Dias, 2011).

Neuroanatomical Factors

Some studies with patients with severe recurrent bipolar disorders have identified ventricular enlargement, cortical atrophy, and sulcal widening. The higher resolution magnetic resonance imaging (MRI) scans identify reduced volumes in the hippocampus, medial orbital cortex, and anterior cingulum (Thase, 2009). Increased illness severity, bipolarity, and increased cortical levels are associated with diffuse and focal areas of atrophy (Thase, 2009).

Brain pathways implicated in the pathophysiology of bipolar disorder are in subregions of the prefrontal cortex (PFC) and medial temporal lobe (MTL). Dysregulation in the neurocircuits surrounding these areas has been viewed through functional imaging (e.g., positron emission tomography, magnetic resonance imaging) (Pollock & Kuo, 2004).

Psychological Influences

Although there is increasing evidence for genetic and biological vulnerabilities in the etiology of the mood disorders, stressful life events can trigger symptoms of bipolar disorder. Family atmosphere suggests an association between high expressed emotion and relapse. Bipolar individuals who suffered abuse as children revealed earlier onset of bipolar disorder, faster cycling frequencies, and an increase in comorbid disorders such as substance abuse (Garno et al., 2005).

CULTURAL CONSIDERATIONS

At the best of times, BSDs are often missed, especially in lower socioeconomic groups, and may remain untreated for years or for the patient's lifetime. Unipolar depression is a common misdiagnosis, as well as anxiety disorders or substance abuse disorders, which may or may not be co-occurring with a bipolar disorder. Cultural differences and beliefs can vastly complicate the issue. Spiritual/religious beliefs in many cultures or religions may include ghosts, spirits, or even the hearing of voices as a sign of divinity or being special. Clinicians not familiar with the culture often miss important cues and misinterpret the actuality of what is being reported. All too many times minority groups are misdiagnosed as having schizophrenia.

CLINICAL PICTURE

Mania may begin gradually over the course of a few weeks, but more typically it has an abrupt onset. Excessive activity over time can result in cardiac disorders and exhaustion. With effective treatment, the prognosis of any one manic episode is good. Unfortunately, reoccurrence is likely. A manic episode may last for a few days to months, and may be followed by a depressed episode that may occur suddenly. During this time there may be remorse for inappropriate behavior (marital infidelity, catastrophic business decisions, and financial ruin) during the manic episode; therefore the risk for suicide may be high. Suicide can occur in both manic and depressed phases of the bipolar disorder.

APPLICATION OF THE NURSING PROCESS

ASSESSMENT

Figure 16-1 presents the Mood Disorder Questionnaire (MDQ). This is *not* a diagnostic test; rather, it is a helpful screening device for assessment purposes.

Level of Mood

The euphoric mood associated with a bipolar illness is unstable. During euphoria patients may state they are experiencing "an intense feeling of well-being," are "cheerful in a beautiful world," or are becoming "one with God." This mood may change to irritation and quick anger when the elated person is thwarted. The irritability and belligerence may be short-lived, or it may become the prominent feature of a person's manic illness. When the person is elated, the overjoyous mood may seem out of proportion to what is occurring in the person's environment, and a cheerful mood may be inappropriate to the circumstances.

People in a manic state may laugh, joke, and talk in a continuous stream, with uninhibited familiarity. During mania people demonstrate boundless enthusiasm, treat everyone with confidential friendliness, and incorporate everyone into their plans and activities. They know no strangers. Energy and self-confidence seem boundless.

Elaborate schemes to get rich and famous and acquire unlimited power may be frantically pursued, despite objections and realistic constraints. Excessive phone calls and e-mails are made, often to famous and influential people all over the world. People in the manic phase are busy all hours of the day and night furthering their grandiose plans and wild schemes. To the manic person, no aspirations are too high and no distances are too far. No boundaries exist in reality to curtail the elaborate schemes.

In the manic state, a person often gives away money, prized possessions, and expensive gifts. The manic person throws lavish parties, frequents expensive nightclubs and restaurants, and spends money freely on friends and strangers alike. This spending, excessive use of credit cards and high standards of living continue even in the face of bankruptcy. Intervention is often needed to prevent financial ruin.

As the clinical course progresses, sociability and euphoria are replaced by a stage of hostility, irritability, and paranoia. The vignette on p. 281 is a patient's description of this experience (Jamison, 1995a, p. 67).

MOOD DISORDER QUESTIONNAIRE

Instructions: Please answer each question as best you can.

	Yes	No
1. **Has there ever been a period of time when you were not your usual self and....**		
you felt so good or so hyper that other people thought you were not your normal self or you were so hyper that you got into trouble?	○	○
you were so irritable that you shouted at people or started fights or arguments?	○	○
you felt much more self-confident than usual?	○	○
you got much less sleep than usual and found you didn't really miss it?	○	○
you were much more talkative or spoke much faster than usual?	○	○
thoughts raced through your head or you couldn't slow down your mind?	○	○
you were so easily distracted by things around you that you had trouble concentrating or staying on track?	○	○
you had much more energy than usual?	○	○
you were much more active or did many more things than usual?	○	○
you were much more social or outgoing than usual; for example, you telephoned friends in the middle of the night?	○	○
you were much more interested in sex than usual?	○	○
you did things that were unusual for you or that other people might have thought were excessive, foolish, or risky?	○	○
spending money got you or your family into trouble?	○	○
2. **If you answered "Yes" to more than one of the above, have several of these ever happened during the same period of time?**	○	○

3. **How much of a problem did any of these cause you — like being unable to work; having family, money, or legal troubles; or getting into arguments or fights? Please select one response only.**

    ○ No problem   ○ Minor problem   ○ Moderate problem   ○ Serious problem

	Yes	No
4. **Have any of your blood relatives (children, siblings, parents, grandparents, aunts, uncles) had manic-depressive illness or bipolar disorder?**	○	○
5. **Has a health care professional ever told you that you have manic-depressive illness or bipolar disorder?**	○	○

Criteria for Results: Answering "Yes" to 7 or more of the events in question 1, answering "Yes" to question 2, and answering "Moderate problem" or "Serious problem" to question 3 is considered a positive screen result for bipolar disorder.

FIGURE 16-1 The Mood Disorder Questionnaire. (From Hirschfeld, R.M.A., et al. [2000]. Development and validation of a screening instrument for bipolar spectrum disorder: the Mood Disorder Questionnaire. *American Journal of Psychiatry, 157*[11], 1873-1875. Copyright © 2004 Eli Lilly and Company.)

VIGNETTE

At first when I'm high, it's tremendous...ideas are fast, like shooting stars you follow until brighter ones appear. All shyness disappears; the right words and gestures are suddenly there. Uninteresting people and things become intensely interesting. Sensuality is pervasive; the desire to seduce and be seduced is irresistible. Your marrow is infused with unbelievable feelings of ease, power, well-being, omnipotence, euphoria...you can do anything. But somewhere this changes.

The fast ideas become too fast and there are far too many. Overwhelming confusion replaces clarity. You stop keeping up with it—memory goes. Infectious humor ceases to amuse—your friends become frightened...everything now is against the grain. You are irritable, angry, frightened, uncontrollable, and trapped in the blackest caves of the mind—caves you never knew were there. It will never end. Madness carves its own reality.

Refer to Table 16-1 for the characteristics of a person experiencing different phases of mania.

Behavior
During Mania

When in full-blown mania, a person constantly switches from one activity to another, one place to another, and one project to another. Many projects may be started, but few, if any, are completed. Inactivity is impossible, even for the shortest period of time. Hyperactivity may range from mild, constant motion to frenetic, wild activity. The writing of flowery and lengthy letters and the making of excessive long-distance telephone calls are accentuated. Individuals become involved in pleasurable activities that can have painful consequences. For example, spending large sums of money on frivolous items, giving money away indiscriminately, or making foolish business investments can leave a family penniless. Sexual indiscretion can dissolve relationships and marriages.

Bipolar individuals can be manipulative, profane, fault finding, and adept at exploiting others' vulnerabilities. They constantly push limits. These behaviors often alienate family, friends, employers, health care providers, and others.

When people are hypomanic they have voracious appetites for food as well as for indiscriminate sex. Although the constant activity of the hypomanic prevents proper sleep, short periods of sleep are possible. However, all patients experiencing mania sleep less, and some patients may not sleep for several days in a row. The person is too busy to eat, sleep, or engage in sexual activity. **This nonstop physical activity and the lack of sleep and food can lead to physical exhaustion and even death if not treated and therefore constitutes an emergency.**

Modes of dress often reflect the person's grandiose yet tenuous grasp of reality. Dress may be described as outlandish, bizarre, colorful, and noticeably inappropriate. Makeup may be garish or overdone. Manic people are highly distractible. Concentration is poor, and individuals move from one activity to another without completing anything. Judgment is poor, and impulsive marriages and divorces often take place.

TABLE 16-1   MANIA ON A CONTINUUM

HYPOMANIA	ACUTE MANIA	DELIRIOUS MANIA
Communication		
1. Talks and jokes incessantly, is "life of the party," and gets irritated when not center of attention	1. May change suddenly from laughing to anger or depression; *mood is labile*	1. Totally out of touch with reality
2. Treats everyone with familiarity and confidentiality; often borders on crude	2. Becomes inappropriately demanding of people's attention, and intrusive nature repels others	—
3. Talk is often sexual—can reach obscene, inappropriate propositions to total strangers	3. Speech may be marked by profanities and crude sexual remarks to everyone (nursing staff in particular)	—
4. Talk is fresh; flits from one topic to the next; marked by *pressure of speech*	4. Speech marked by *flight of ideas*, in which thoughts race and fly from topic to topic; may have *clang associations*	4. Most likely has clang associations
Affect and Thinking		
1. Full of pep and good humor, feelings of euphoria and sociability; may show inappropriate intimacy with strangers	1. Good humor gives way to increased irritability and hostility, short-lived period of rage, especially when not getting his or her way or when controls are set on behavior. May have quick shifts of mood from hostility to docility	1. May become destructive or aggressive—totally out of control

Continued

TABLE 16-1   MANIA ON A CONTINUUM—cont'd

HYPOMANIA	ACUTE MANIA	DELIRIOUS MANIA
2. Feels boundless self-confidence and enthusiasm. Has elaborate schemes for becoming rich and famous. Initially, schemes may seem plausible.	2. Grandiose plans are totally out of contact with reality. Thinks he or she is a musician, prominent businessman, great politician, or religious figure, without any basis in fact.	2. May experience undefined hallucinations and delirium
3. Judgment often poor. Gets involved with schemes in which job, marriage, or financial status may be destroyed.	3. Judgment is extremely poor	—
4. May write large quantities of letters to rich and famous people regarding schemes or may make numerous worldwide telephone calls	—	—
5. Decreased attention span to internal and external cues	5. Decreased attention span and distractibility are intensified	—
Physical Behavior		
1. Overactive, distractible, buoyant, and busily occupied with grandiose plans (not delusions); goes from one action to the next	1. Extremely restless, disorganized, and chaotic. Physical behavior may be difficult to control. May have outbursts, such as throwing things or becoming briefly assaultive when crossed.	1. *Dangerous state.* Incoherent, extremely restless, disoriented, and agitated. Hyperactive. Motor activity is totally aimless (must have physical or chemical restraints to prevent exhaustion and death).
2. Increased sexual appetite; sexually irresponsible and indiscreet. Illegitimate pregnancies in hypomanic women and venereal disease in both men and women are common. Sex used for escape, not for relating to another human being	2. No time for sex—too busy. Poor concentration, distractibility, and restlessness are severe.	2. Same as in acute mania but in the extreme
3. May have voracious appetite, eat on the run, or gobble food during brief periods	3. No time to eat—too distracted and disorganized	3. Same as in acute mania but in the extreme
4. May go without sleeping; unaware of fatigue. However, may be able to take short naps	4. No time for sleep—psychomotor activity too high; if unchecked, can lead to exhaustion and death	—
5. Financially extravagant, goes on buying sprees, gives money and gifts away freely, can easily go into debt	5. Same as in hypomania but in the extreme	5. Too disorganized to do anything

After Mania

People often emerge from a manic state startled and confused by the shambles of their lives. The following description conveys one patient's experience (Jamison, 1995a, p. 68):

Thought Processes

Approximately 50% of patients during the manic phase have psychotic symptoms (Black & Andreasen, 2011). Grandiose delusions are common. For example, a manic individual may think he or she has special powers and special abilities. At other times or concurrently, the delusions may be of a paranoid nature.

> **VIGNETTE**
> Now there are only others' recollections of your behavior—your bizarre, frenetic, aimless behavior. At least mania has the grace to dim memories of itself...now it's over, but is it? Incredible feelings to sort through. Who is being too polite? Who knows what? What did I do? Why? And most hauntingly, will it, when will it, happen again? Medication to take, resist, resent, forget...but always to take. Credit cards revoked...explanations at work...bad checks and apologies overdue...memory flashes of vague men (what did I do?)...friendships gone, a marriage ruined.

Sensory perceptions may become altered as the mania escalates, and hallucinations may occur. However, in hypomania, no evidence of delusions or hallucinations is present.

Flight of ideas is a nearly continuous flow of accelerated speech with abrupt changes among topics that are usually based on understandable associations or a play on words. At times the attentive listener can keep up with the changes, even though direction changes constantly. Speech is rapid, verbose, and circumstantial (including minute and unnecessary details). When the condition is severe, speech may be disorganized and incoherent. The incessant talking often includes joking, puns, and teasing:

> "How are you doing, kid, no kidding around, I'm going home… home sweet home…home is where the heart is…the heart of the matter is I want out, and that ain't hay…hey, Doc…get me out of this place."

The content of speech is often sexually explicit and ranges from grossly inappropriate to vulgar. Themes in the communication of the manic individual may revolve around extraordinary sexual prowess, brilliant business ability, or unparalleled artistic talents (e.g., writing, painting, and dancing). The person may actually have only average ability in these areas.

Speech is not only profuse but also loud, bellowing, or even screaming. One can hear the force and energy behind the rapid words. As mania escalates, flight of ideas may give way to clang associations. Clang associations are the stringing together of words because of their rhyming sounds, without regard to their meaning:

> "Cinema I and II, last row. Row, row, row your boat. Don't be a cutthroat. Cut your throat. Get your goat. Go out and vote. And so I wrote."

Grandiosity (inflated self-regard) is apparent in both the ideas expressed and the person's behavior. People with mania may exaggerate their achievements or importance, state that they know famous people, or believe that they have great powers. The boast of exceptional powers and status can take delusional proportions in mania.

Cognitive Function

The onset of bipolar disorder is often preceded by comparatively high cognitive function. In fact, bipolar illness is often associated with creativity and high achievement (Black & Andreasen, 2011). However, there is growing evidence that about one third of patients who are bipolar display significant and persistent cognitive difficulties that include problems with verbal memory, sustained attention, and occasionally executive functioning as the disease progresses. These deficits often persist, even in remission. Cognitive impairment appears to be a core feature of bipolar disorder and a contributing factor to poor psychosocial outcomes (Robinson & Ferrier, 2006).

The potential cognitive dysfunction among a large subgroup of patients with bipolar disorder has specific clinical implications:

- Cognitive function greatly affects overall function.
- Cognitive deficits correlate with greater number of manic episodes, history of psychosis, chronicity of illness, and poor functional outcome.

- Early diagnosis and treatment are crucial to prevent illness progression, cognitive deficits, and poor outcome.
- Medication selection should consider not only the efficacy of the drug in reducing mood symptoms but also the cognitive effect of the drug on the patient.

ASSESSMENT GUIDELINES

Bipolar Disorder

1. Assess whether the patient is a danger to self and others:
   - Manic behaviors can be exhaustive to the patient to the point of death.
   - Patients may not eat or sleep, often for days at a time.
   - Poor impulse control may result in harm to others or self.
   - Uncontrolled spending may occur.
2. Assess for need for controls. Controls may be needed to protect patient in mania from bankruptcy because during this time patients may give away all of their money or possessions.
3. Assess for need for hospitalization to safeguard and stabilize the patient.
4. Assess medical status:
   - A person in acute untreated mania may become dehydrated or exhausted, which has led to severe dehydration and cardiac collapse. Therefore cardiac status, signs of dehydration (poor skin turgor, dark and scant urinary output), and poor skin integrity—which may develop into infections—should be assessed.
   - A thorough medical examination helps to determine whether mania is primary (bipolar disorder or cyclothymia) or secondary to another condition.
     - Mania can be secondary to a general medical condition (e.g., brain disease, certain infections including HIV, and endocrine disorders).
     - Mania can be substance induced (caused by use or abuse of a drug or substance, or by toxin exposure).
5. Assess for any coexisting medical or other condition that warrants special intervention (e.g., substance abuse, anxiety disorder, metabolic disease, cardiac problems, legal or financial crises).
6. Assess the patient's and family's understanding of bipolar disorder, knowledge of medications, and knowledge of support groups and organizations that provide information on bipolar disorder and patient and family support.

DIAGNOSIS

Nursing diagnoses vary for a patient with a bipolar disorder. A primary consideration for a patient in acute mania is the prevention of exhaustion and death from cardiac collapse. Because of the patient's poor judgment, excessive and constant motor activity, probable dehydration, and difficulty evaluating reality, *Risk for Injury* is a likely and appropriate diagnosis if the patient's activity level is dangerous to his or her health. During the continuation phase, assessment of areas such as compliance to medication, risk for suicide, optimizing family support, and availability of social support can be invaluable in achieving

EXAMINING THE EVIDENCE

Bipolar Disorder—No Longer a Stigma, Now a Style?

Bipolar disorder (BD) seems to be making the news quite a bit lately. Recently, I have noticed a lot of people in the creative arts, such as film and television celebrities, who are diagnosed with BD. Is there a connection between BD and creativity?

That has been the supposition for many years. More recently, there has been renewed interest in the diagnosis of bipolar disorder. After 30 years of research, there is persuasive evidence linking creativity with bipolar disorders—about 75% of studies link creative and artistic occupations with BD (Tremblay & Grosskopf, 2010). Affective disorders tend to be overrepresented in the creative artist population. The rate of mood disorders, suicide, and institutionalization was 20 times that of the normal population in a study of major British and Irish poets between 1705 and 1805 (Glazer, 2009).

There is a new and unusual phenomenon where patients present to the psychiatrist with self-diagnosed BD. The increasing popularity of BD as a self-diagnosis may be attributed to widespread media coverage of celebrities with BD and their willingness to share their personal experiences with the media. Most of them state that the increased energy, new ideas, and powerful high mood would be difficult to relinquish. Over the years, stigma attached to mood disorders may have lessened following the change in name from manic-depressive illness (mania conjured up negativity) to BD about 20 years ago. Often unknown to the public are the difficulties associated with BD—medical risks of mood stabilizers/antidepressants, acute emotional distress at times, predisposition to other mental illnesses, and increased risk for suicide (Chan & Sireling, 2010).

Three core features of the creative process—fluency of association, use of cognitive imagery, and positive affect—are commonly reported in bipolar disorder. Abnormalities of dopamine function may be shared with bipolar disorder and the creativity process, and associated positive traits help explain creative cognitive styles (Murray & Johnson, 2010). Creativity seems to start by a person plunging into a state of deep concentration, of dissociation. Once into dissociation there is heightened activity in certain frontal and inferior temporal regions of the brain (Arehart, 2011). However, some features of the creative careers—intermittent unemployment, substance misuse, irregular sleep and activity schedules—can be counterproductive for people with BD. Creating a career in the arts is highly competitive and can lead to long-term stress. Negative life events and chronic stressors can predict greater severity of depressive symptoms (Murray & Johnson, 2010).

There is also substantive evidence of a link between creativity and BD in a variety of occupations, not just the entertainment business. Productivity gains from enhanced creativity outweigh losses from BD such as absenteeism and lack of energy during depressive states. The extent to which persons with BD contribute to the workforce has implications for society's response to the inevitable identification and understanding of genetic markers for BD. The creative benefits of the disease weigh against its elimination via genetic engineering or selective abortion. The development of medication that reduces social and private costs of the illness without inhibiting creativity might be a fruitful social investment (Tremblay & Grosskopf, 2010).

Arehart, J. (2011). What's going on in brains of creative people? *Psychiatric News, 46*(13), 15-25.
Chan, D., & Sireling, L. (2010). I want to be bipolar… a new phenomenon. *Psychiatrist, 34,* 103-105.
Glazer, E. (2009). Rephrasing the madness and creativity debate: what is the nature of the creativity construct? *Personality and Individual Differences, 46,* 755-764.
Murray, G., & Johnson, S. (2010). The clinical significance of creativity in bipolar disorder. *Clinical Psychology Review, 30,* 721-732.
Tremblay, C., & Grosskopf, S. (2010). Brainstorm: occupational choice, bipolar illness and creativity. *Economics and Human Biology, 8,* 233-241.
Contributed by Lois Angelo.

relapse prevention. Refer to Table 16-2 for a list of potential nursing diagnoses for bipolar disorders.

OUTCOMES IDENTIFICATION

Phase I (Acute Mania)

The overall goal during the acute manic phase is to prevent injury. Outcomes in phase I reflect physiological as well as behavioral issues (stated in measurable terms within safe timeframes). For example, the patient will:

- Be well hydrated within 24 hours—as evidenced by good skin turgor—and within normal limits of urinary output, concentration, and dilution.
- Maintain stable cardiac status, as evidenced by stable vital signs within normal limits (by *date*).
- Maintain or obtain tissue integrity, as evidenced by absence of infection or absence of untreated cuts or abrasions (by *date*).
- Get sufficient sleep and rest while in the hospital, as evidenced by 4 to 6 hours sleep at night and 10-minute rest periods every hour.
- Demonstrate self-control with aid of staff or medication, as evidenced by absence of harm to others (*state the behaviors*) (by *date*).
- Make no attempt at self-harm with aid of staff or medication, as evidenced by physical safety checked with regularity throughout period of acute mania.

TABLE 16-2	POTENTIAL NURSING DIAGNOSES FOR BIPOLAR DISORDERS
SIGNS AND SYMPTOMS	**NURSING DIAGNOSES***
Excessive and constant motor activity Poor judgment Lack of rest and sleep Poor nutritional intake (excessive or relentless mix of above behaviors can lead to cardiac collapse)	*Risk for Injury*
Loud, profane, hostile, combative, aggressive, demanding behaviors Intrusive and taunting behaviors Inability to control behavior Rage reaction	*Risk for Other-Directed Violence* Risk *for Self-Directed Violence* *Risk for Suicide* *Interrupted Family Processes* *Ineffective Coping* *Ineffective Impulse Control*
Manipulative, angry, or hostile verbal and physical behaviors Impulsive speech and actions Property destruction or lashing out at others in a rage reaction	*Defensive Coping* *Ineffective Coping* *Disabled Family Coping* *Ineffective Relationship*
Racing thoughts, grandiosity, poor judgment	*Disturbed Thought Processes* *Ineffective Coping*
Giving away valuables, neglecting family, making impulsive major life changes (divorce, career changes) Continuous pressured speech jumping from topic to topic *(flights of ideas)*	*Interrupted Family Processes* *Caregiver Role Strain* *Impaired Verbal Communication*
Constant motor activity, going from one person or event to another Annoyance or taunting of others; loud and crass speech Provocative behaviors	*Impaired Social Interaction* *Risk for Injury*
Failure to eat, groom, bathe, dress self because too distracted, agitated, and disorganized	*Imbalanced Nutrition: Less Than Body Requirements* *Deficient Fluid Volume* *Self-Care Deficit (bathing/hygiene, dressing/grooming)*
Inability to sleep because too frantic and hyperactive (sleep deprivation can lead to exhaustion and death)	*Disturbed Sleep Pattern* *Risk for Activity Intolerance* *Risk-Prone Health Behavior*

**Nursing Diagnoses—Definitions and Classification 2012-2014.* Copyright © 2012, 1994-2012 by NANDA International. Used by arrangement with Blackwell Publishing Limited, a company of John Wiley and Sons, Inc.

Phase II (Continuation of Treatment)

The continuation phase lasts for approximately 2 to 6 months. Although the overall outcome of this phase is relapse prevention, many other outcomes must be accomplished to achieve relapse prevention. These outcomes include the following:

- Patient and family will attend psychoeducational classes that discuss a variety of topics and give directions to patients and families to help prevent relapse
  - Knowledge of disease process
  - Knowledge of early signs of relapse
  - Knowledge of medication
  - Consequences of substance addictions for predicting future relapse
  - Knowledge of early signs and symptoms of relapse

- Support groups or therapy (psychoeducational groups and cognitive behavioral therapy [CBT], interpersonal social rhythm therapy [IPSRT], and family-focused therapy [FFT] are all evidence-based treatment modalities)
- Communication and problem-solving skills training

Phase III (Maintenance Treatment)

The overall outcomes for the maintenance phase continue to focus on prevention of relapse and to limit the severity and duration of future episodes.

- Participation in learning interpersonal strategies related to work, interpersonal, and family problems
- Participation in psychotherapy group or other ongoing supportive therapy modality that has evidence-based support

- Relapse prevention
- Medication compliance
- Family psychoeducation or therapy
- Increased social support
- Attendance at bipolar or substance use support groups

PLANNING

The planning of care for an individual with bipolar disorder usually is targeted toward the particular phase of mania (e.g., acute mania, continuation of treatment, or maintenance treatment) as well as any other co-occurring issues identified in the assessment (e.g., risk of suicide, risk of violence to person or property, family crisis, legal crises, substance abuse, risk-taking behaviors, issues of medical compliance).

Acute Phase

During the acute phase (up to first 2 months), planning focuses on medically stabilizing the patient while maintaining safety. When mania is acute, hospitalization is usually the safest place for a patient. Nursing care is often geared toward decreasing physical activity, increasing food and fluid intake, ensuring at least 4 to 6 hours of sleep per night, alleviating any bowel or bladder problems, and intervening to see that self-care needs are met. Some patients may require seclusion or even electroconvulsive therapy, and they certainly need careful medication management.

Continuation Phase

During the continuation phase (2 to 6 months), planning focuses on maintaining compliance with the medication regimen and preventing relapse. Interventions are planned in accordance with the assessment data regarding the patient's interpersonal and stress reduction skills, cognitive functioning, employment status, substance-related problems, and social support systems, for example. During this time, psychoeducational teaching is a priority for patient and family. The need for referrals to community programs, groups, and support for any co-occurring disorders or problems (e.g., substance abuse, family problems, legal issues, and financial crises) is evaluated.

Evaluation of the need for communication skills training and problem-solving skills training is important. People with bipolar disorders often have interpersonal problems that affect their work, family, and social lives, as well as other emotional problems. Residual problems resulting from reckless, violent, withdrawn, or bizarre behavior that may have occurred during a manic episode often leave lives shattered and family and friends hurt and distant. For some patients, specific psychotherapy (in addition to medication management) is needed to address these issues, although the focus of psychotherapeutic treatment will vary over time for each person.

Maintenance Phase

The maintenance phase begins at about 6 months, and planning focuses on preventing relapse and limiting the severity and duration of episodes. Patients with bipolar disorders require medications over long periods of time, if not a lifetime. Specific psychosocial

therapies, support or psychoeducational groups, and periodic evaluations all help patients maintain their family and social lives in order to continue employment, and minimize relapse rates.

IMPLEMENTATION

Self-Care for Nurses

During the manic phase, a patient can elicit numerous intense, unpleasant, and negative emotions in health care professionals. During mania, the patient is out of control and resists being controlled. The patient may use humor, manipulation, power struggles, or demanding behavior to prevent or minimize the staff's ability to set limits or control dangerous behaviors. The **consistent setting of limits,** followed by the whole staff, is the main theme in treating a person in mania. The patient may use a variety of ways to distract the staff, loosen the limits, and continue to escalate.

For example, the patient might get involved in power plays with the staff, by pointing out faults or oversights and drawing negative attention to one or more staff members. Alternatively, the patient may become aggressively demanding, shouting to staff. This is done in a loud, shrill, and disruptive manner, provoking staff to become defensive, frustrated, and exasperated. When staff start losing control, it allows the manic behavior to go unchecked, and escalate further.

The patient can also use **splitting** as a way to distract staff and loosen staff limits. For example, the patient turns staff members against other staff members, or against groups of staff (e.g., day staff versus night staff). The patient might tell one staff member, "Ms. Diaz, you are the best. You are the only nurse who listens to me, and seems to care, unlike Mr. Peters, who hardly looks at me and says such unfair things about you." Meanwhile the patient tells Mr. Peters, "Thank God you are here. Ms. Diaz is so cold and uncaring, and I hate to say this but she says terrible things about you." Now dissension among staff members loosens the staff's enforcement of limits, and the patient remains in control. This tactic of splitting is used by other patient groups as well (e.g., borderline personality disorder, antisocial personality disorder, substance abusers).

Because consistent setting of limits by all staff is imperative for treatment to be effective, nurses, physicians, and all health care workers need to communicate with each other and reestablish limit setting.

Patients with bipolar disorders are often ambivalent about treatment. They may minimize the destructive consequences of their behaviors or deny the seriousness of the disease. Some are reluctant to relinquish the increased energy, euphoria, and heightened sense of self-esteem of hypomania, before the devastating features of full-blown mania commence. Unfortunately, nonadherence to the regimen of mood-stabilizing medication is a major cause of relapse. Therefore establishing a therapeutic alliance with the bipolar individual is crucial.

Acute Phase

Hospitalization provides safety for a patient in acute mania (bipolar I disorder), imposes external controls on destructive behaviors, and provides medical stabilization.

Communication Guidelines

Communicating with a patient who is acutely manic can be challenging, but there are some specific and effective approaches for communicating with a person in the manic phase of bipolar disorder (Table 16-3).

Milieu Therapy

Seclusion. Control during the acute phase of hyperactive behavior almost always includes immediate treatment with an antipsychotic. However, when a patient is dangerously out of control, seclusion or restraints also may be indicated. Seclusion provides comfort and relief to many patients who can no longer control their own behavior, and seclusion serves the following purposes:

- Reduces overwhelming environmental stimuli
- Protects a patient from injuring self, others, or staff
- Prevents destruction of personal property or property of others

Seclusion is warranted when documented data collected by the nursing and medical staff reflect the following points:

- Substantial risk of harm to others or self is clear.
- The patient is unable to control his or her actions.
- Problematic behavior has been sustained (continues or escalates despite other measures).
- Other measures (e.g., setting limits beginning with verbal de-escalation or using chemical restraints) have failed.

The use of seclusion or restraints is associated with complex therapeutic, ethical, and legal issues. Most state laws prohibit the use of unnecessary physical restraint or isolation. Barring an emergency, the use of seclusion and restraints warrants the patient's consent; therefore most hospitals have well-defined protocols for treatment with seclusion. Seclusion protocol includes a proper reporting procedure through the chain of command when a patient is to be secluded. Refer to Chapter 24 for more on seclusion and restraint and accepted protocols and to Chapter 6 for more on the legal parameters.

Safety and physical needs. Specific strategies can help maintain the safety of the patient during the hospitalized period. Staff members continually set limits in a firm, non-threatening, and neutral manner to prevent further escalation of mania and to provide safe boundaries for the patient and others (Table 16-4).

Pharmacological, Biological, and Integrative Therapies

During the acute phase, medications are vital to bring the patient to a safe physical and psychological level of functioning. However, medications are pivotal and vital through all phases of treatment, and for many patients they are a lifelong protection against the pain and destruction of relapse.

Antimanic Bipolar Medications (Mood Stabilizers)

Individuals with bipolar disorder often require multiple medications. There may be times when an antianxiety agent can help reduce agitation or anxiety or an antipsychotic agent (e.g., olanzapine) can help alleviate psychomotor activity and delusions or hallucinations. Antianxiolytics or antipsychotics may be used for a limited time, but mood stabilizers are considered lifetime maintenance therapy for bipolar patients (Preston et al., 2010). Most

TABLE 16-3 INTERVENTIONS FOR ACUTE MANIA: COMMUNICATION	
INTERVENTION	**RATIONALE**
1. Use firm and calm approach: "John, come with me. Eat this sandwich."	1. Structure and control are provided for patient who is out of control. Feelings of security can result: "Someone is in control."
2. Use short and concise explanations or statements.	2. Short attention span limits comprehension to small bits of information.
3. Remain neutral; avoid power struggles and value judgments.	3. Patient can use inconsistencies and value judgments as justification for arguing and escalating mania.
4. Be consistent in approach and expectations.	4. Consistent limits and expectations minimize potential for patient's manipulation of staff.
5. Have frequent staff meetings to plan consistent approaches and to set agreed-on limits.	5. Consistency of all staff is needed to maintain controls and minimize manipulation by patient.
6. With other staff, decide on limits, tell patient in simple, concrete terms with consequences; for example, "John, do not yell at or hit Peter. If you cannot control yourself, we will help you" or "The seclusion room will help you feel less out of control and prevent harm to yourself and others."	6. Clear expectations help patient experience outside controls as well as understand reasons for medication, seclusion, or restraints (if unable to control behaviors).
7. Hear and act on legitimate complaints.	7. Underlying feelings of helplessness are reduced, and acting-out behaviors are minimized.
8. Firmly redirect energy into more appropriate and constructive channels.	8. Distractibility is the nurse's most effective tool during the patient's manic phase.

APPLYING THE ART

A Person With Bipolar Disorder

SCENARIO: I approached Gloria, a 33-year-old woman who had seemed edgy and distracted when we talked earlier. She had been admitted to the hospital for the third time after becoming angry and threatening suicide over losing a job she loved—exercising and caring for the animals at a pet store. She is on suicide precautions.

THERAPEUTIC GOAL: By the end of this session, Gloria will show increased ability to problem solve as evidenced by insight that stopping medication exacerbates the disorder.

STUDENT-PATIENT INTERACTION	THOUGHTS, COMMUNICATION TECHNIQUES, AND MENTAL HEALTH NURSING CONCEPTS
Student: *Smiling.* "Hi, Gloria. Would you talk some more about your feelings when you heard you were going to be fired from your job?"	I know that "could" or "would" acts like an *indirect question* rather than a *direct question,* meaning I will get more than a yes or no answer.
Gloria: "Get the _____ away from me! I'm sick of you people asking about that _____ job." *Clenching fists, practically yelling.*	
Student's feelings: *I forgot to tune in to Gloria as a person before I jumped in with questions. She's loud, but I'm okay. Her fear and loss fuel all that anger. Okay, self, mindfully breathe.*	I forgot to *assess* first! I must remember, she is afraid and *displacing* her frustration onto me. Each time she gets admitted means starting over. If only she had kept taking her Depakote and Abilify.
Student: *Quiet and concerned.* "Gloria, I'm _____, your nursing student. You've been through such a rough time. You feel upset at the job and anyone that asks you about it."	Using *reflection* makes sense because I hope that reflecting the feelings lets my *empathy* get through to her.
Student's feelings: *I can do this. I'll step back a little, slow things down, and keep telling myself that her anger is not really about me. I care about Gloria so I'm not going to be pushed away that easily.*	
Student's feelings: *I'm struggling with anxiety, too.*	I remember now. *Anxiety* is communicated interpersonally.
Gloria: "I need to walk." *Starts pacing quickly down the hall.*	Gloria is using walking as a healthy relief behavior for her anxiety.
Student's feelings: *I hope she'll let me walk with her. Walking will help my anxiety, too!*	
Student: "Good idea. Let's walk together. Tell me what's happening inside." *We quickly walk down the hall.*	I am offering myself by walking with her. Using an indirect question often helps the patient talk without feeling interrogated.
Student's feelings: *As she responds while we walk, I'm feeling calmer, too.*	
Gloria: "I feel like, why even try anymore? While I worked at the pet store, I felt like my life meant something. Then I go and stop taking my medicine. It's just so expensive. I'm such a loser." *Eyes fill with tears.*	
Student's feelings: *I feel so sad for her. She struggles so hard, and then seems to give in by quitting her medication. Sometimes I feel like a loser. Sometimes I feel like nursing school pressures me too much, especially when I bomb a test. I need to put my own "failure worries" on hold to handle later and refocus to fully tune in to Gloria.*	
Student: "Sounds like right now you're blaming yourself for what you've lost." *I pause, handing her a tissue.* "Gloria, I care about what happens to you. When you say, 'why even try' you mean...?"	By saying "right now" I plant the idea that she may not always choose to see herself as a failure. I must stay alert for countertransference. Using Gloria's name and reminding her who I am factor in that she is probably experiencing moderate anxiety, so her *perceptual field* of what she is able to take in decreases. I need to assess even a *covert reference* to *suicide,* especially with Gloria's history.

APPLYING THE ART—cont'd

A Person With Bipolar Disorder

STUDENT-PATIENT INTERACTION	THOUGHTS, COMMUNICATION TECHNIQUES, AND MENTAL HEALTH NURSING CONCEPTS
Gloria: "Don't worry. I don't want to kill myself anymore. But I just keep screwing up! I even let my animals down." *Glancing at me.* **Student's feelings:** *I wish she could see the survivor I see when I'm with her. I'm relieved Gloria recognizes she wants to live now. I have so much hope inside for her.* **Student:** "Talk some more about your animals."	When Gloria tells me not to worry she may be using *projection* in that she may still have some latent concern about her suicide potential. She is still on *16-minute checks*, which continues to be necessary, and I will report and chart about all this. By using a *focusing* approach, I remind her of what she values. She may also remember what she was able to do well, which may help her *self-esteem*. She said, "my animals," so I deliberately *restated*, "your animals" because they are so important to her.
Gloria: "I loved caring for all of the animals, but especially the puppies. One little beagle had such sad eyes, I took him home. That's when I got in trouble. I know I wouldn't have done that if I'd kept taking my meds." **Student:** "So you recognize a link between stopping your meds and doing some things you wouldn't usually do when you take charge of your bipolar disorder by staying on your meds?" **Student's feelings:** *I feel kind of proud of myself for knowing to praise her about the meds.* **Gloria:** "I still get mad too easily, but I'm starting to think more clearly since my Abilify's been upped. I've been wondering if my boss would give me a second chance. I did well with the animals. My boss said so before I got sick again. My case manager made sure the beagle pup got back okay." **Student:** "I hear you reminding yourself that your skills in pet care endure even through this bout in the hospital."	Was Gloria using *identification*? The beagle's "sad" eyes may have resonated with Gloria's own sadness. I am using the *behavior modification technique of positive reinforcement* by *attending* to Gloria's insight when she connects her impulsive behavior with stopping her psychotropics. I am also empowering her by deliberately associating taking her medications with taking charge of her disorder. Gloria's actually able to problem solve now, so that means her anxiety has *decreased to mild*. I think the animals provide some of Gloria's *love and belonging needs*, which precede *self-esteem* needs. I *validate* with Gloria about her pet care skills. The treatment team will be doing discharge planning.
Gloria: "I really love those animals. I'm going to run this idea past the nurse and work out when and how to phrase things to call my boss." **Student's feelings:** *She's taking charge of this. Wow! I feel honored that Gloria trusted me. I'm beginning to trust myself some, too.* **Student:** "You are able to find a goal to work toward, maybe even begin to believe in yourself a little." **Gloria:** *Nods.*	I give Gloria support by naming her mentally healthy verbalizations as a goal. I am careful to add qualifiers—"maybe," "begin to," and "a little"—to insert the idea about believing in herself without overwhelming her.

treatment guidelines advocate lithium and divalproex (Depakote) as first-line mood-stabilizing agents (Preston et al., 2010).

For individuals whose recent episode was manic or hypomanic, lithium and olanzapine seem to have the largest body of evidence supporting their effectiveness as mood stabilizers. For those with recent episodes of depression, lamotrigine (Lamictal), olanzapine-fluoxetine combination (Symbyax), and quetiapine are useful in combination with an antidepressant (Preston & Johnson, 2009). Most successful treatment (up to 90%) is with a combination of antipolar medications (e.g., lithium and quetiapine) (Preston & Johnson, 2009).

Lithium carbonate. Lithium carbonate ($LiCO_3$) is effective in the acute treatment of mania and depressive episodes and in the prevention of recurrent mania and depressive episodes. Once primary acute mania has been diagnosed, lithium is most often the first choice of treatment.

Lithium aborts 60% to 80% of acute manic and hypomanic episodes within 10 to 21 days. Lithium is less effective in people

TABLE 16-4 INTERVENTIONS FOR ACUTE MANIA: SAFETY AND PHYSICAL NEEDS

INTERVENTION	RATIONALE
Structure in a Safe Milieu	
1. Maintain low level of stimuli in patient's environment (e.g., away from bright lights, loud noises, and people).	1. Decreases escalating anxiety.
2. Provide structured solitary activities with nurse or aide.	2. Structure provides security and focus.
3. Provide frequent high-calorie fluids.	3. Prevents dangerous levels of dehydration.
4. Provide frequent rest periods.	4. Prevents exhaustion.
5. Redirect violent behavior through physical exercise (e.g., walking)	5. Physical exercise can decrease tension and provide focus.
6. When warranted in acute mania, use antipsychotics and seclusion to minimize physical harm via physician's order.	6. Exhaustion and death can result from dehydration, lack of sleep, and constant physical activity.
7. Observe for signs of lithium toxicity.	7. There is a small margin of safety between therapeutic and toxic doses.
8. Protect patient from giving away money and possessions. Hold valuables in hospital safe until rational judgment returns.	8. Patient's "generosity" is in fact a symptom of the disease and can lead to catastrophic financial ruin for patient and family.
Nutrition	
1. Monitor intake, output, and vital signs.	1. Adequate fluid and caloric intakes are ensured; development of dehydration and cardiac collapse is minimized.
2. Offer frequent high-calorie protein drinks and finger foods (e.g., sandwiches, fruit, milkshakes).	2. Constant fluid and calorie replacement are needed. Patient may be too active to sit at meals. **Finger foods** allow "eating on the run."
3. Frequently remind patient to eat. "Tom, finish your milkshake." "Sally, eat this banana."	3. During mania the patient is unaware of bodily needs and is easily distracted. Needs supervision to eat.
Sleep	
1. Encourage frequent rest periods during the day.	1. Lack of sleep can lead to exhaustion and death.
2. Keep patient in areas of low stimulation.	2. Relaxation is promoted and manic behavior is minimized.
3. At night, provide warm baths, soothing music, and medication when indicated. Avoid giving patient caffeine.	3. Promotes relaxation, rest, and sleep.
Hygiene	
1. Supervise choice of clothes; minimize flamboyant and bizarre dress (e.g., garish stripes or plaids and loud, unmatching colors).	1. The potential is decreased for ridicule, which lowers self-esteem and increases the need for manic defense. The patient is helped to maintain dignity.
2. Give simple step-by-step reminders for hygiene and dress. "Here is your razor. Shave the left side...now the right side. Here is your toothbrush. Put the toothpaste on the brush."	2. Distractibility and poor concentration are countered through simple, concrete instructions.
Elimination	
1. Monitor bowel habits; offer fluids and foods that are high in fiber. Evaluate need for laxative. Encourage patient to go to the bathroom.	1. Fecal impaction resulting from dehydration and decreased peristalsis is prevented.

with mixed mania (elation and depression), those with rapid cycling, and those with atypical features. Lithium is particularly effective in reducing the following:

- Elation, grandiosity, and expansiveness
- Flight of ideas
- Irritability and manipulativeness
- Anxiety

To a lesser extent, lithium controls the following:

- Insomnia
- Psychomotor agitation
- Threatening or assaultive behavior
- Distractibility
- Hypersexuality
- Paranoia

TABLE 16-5	LITHIUM SIDE EFFECTS AND SIGNS OF LITHIUM TOXICITY	
LEVEL	**SIGNS**	**INTERVENTIONS**
Expected Side Effects		
<0.4 to 1 mEq/L (therapeutic level)	Fine hand tremor, polyuria, and mild thirst Mild nausea and general discomfort Weight gain	Symptoms may persist throughout therapy. Symptoms often subside during treatment. Weight gain may be helped with diet, exercise, and nutritional management.
Early Signs of Toxicity		
<1.5 mEq/L	Nausea, vomiting, diarrhea, thirst, polyuria, slurred speech, muscle weakness	Medication should be withheld, blood lithium levels measured, and dosage re-evaluated.
Advanced Signs of Toxicity		
1.5 to 2 mEq/L	Coarse hand tremor, persistent gastrointestinal upset, mental confusion, muscle hyperirritability, electroencephalographic (EEG) changes, incoordination	Interventions outlined above or below should be used, depending on severity of circumstances.
Severe Toxicity		
2 to 2.5 mEq/L	Ataxia, serious EEG changes, blurred vision, clonic movements, large output of dilute urine, tinnitus, blurred vision, seizures, stupor, severe hypotension, coma; death is usually secondary to pulmonary complications	There is no known antidote for lithium poisoning. The drug is stopped, and excretion is hastened. If patient is alert, an emetic is administered. Otherwise, gastric lavage and treatment with urea, mannitol, and aminophylline hasten lithium excretion.
>2.5 mEq/L	Symptoms may progress rapidly; coma, cardiac dysrhythmia, peripheral circulatory collapse, proteinuria, oliguria, and death	In addition to the interventions above, hemodialysis may be used in severe cases.

Data from Lehne, R.A. (2007). *Pharmacology for nursing care* (6th ed.). St Louis: Saunders; Skidmore-Roth, L. (2008). *Mosby's nursing drug reference* (21st ed.). St Louis: Mosby; Preston, J.D., O'Neal, J.H., & Talaga, M.C. (2010). *Handbook of clinical psychopharmacology for therapists* (6th ed.). Oakland, CA: New Harbinger Publications.

Initially in the treatment of acute mania, an antipsychotic or benzodiazepine can help calm symptoms. Antipsychotics act promptly to slow speech, inhibit aggression, and decrease psychomotor activity. The immediate action of the antipsychotic or benzodiazepine medication serves to prevent exhaustion, coronary collapse, and death until lithium reaches therapeutic levels.

Lithium must reach therapeutic levels in the patient's blood to be effective. This usually takes from 7 to 14 days, or longer for some patients. As lithium becomes effective in reducing manic behavior, the antipsychotic agents are usually discontinued. Although lithium is an effective intervention for treating the manic phase of a bipolar disorder, it is not a cure. Many patients receive lithium with or without another mood stabilizer for maintenance indefinitely and experience manic and depressive episodes if the drug is discontinued.

Trade names for lithium carbonate include Lithane, Eskalith, and Lithonate. During the *active phase,* 600 to 900 mg by mouth is given two or three times a day to reach a clear therapeutic result, or a lithium level of 0.8 to 1.2 mEq/L. **The actual maintenance blood levels should range between 0.4 and 1.3 mEq/L.** However, levels of 0.6 mEq/L for bipolar I to 0.8 mEq/L for bipolar II may be effective for many. To avoid serious toxicity, lithium levels should *not* exceed 1.5 mEq/L. At serum levels greater than 1.5 mEq/L, early signs of toxicity can occur; at 1.5 to 2 mEq/L, advanced signs of toxicity may be seen; and at 2 to 2.5 mEq/L or more, severe toxicity can occur, and emergency measures should be taken immediately.

Cases of severe lithium toxicity with levels of 2 mEq/L or greater constitute a life-threatening emergency. In such cases, gastric lavage and treatment with urea, mannitol, and aminophylline can hasten lithium excretion. Hemodialysis also may be used in extreme cases.

Adverse reactions. An extremely narrow window exists between the therapeutic and the toxic dosage of lithium. Initially, blood levels are measured weekly or biweekly until the therapeutic level has been reached. After therapeutic levels have been reached, blood levels are determined every month. After 6 months to 1 year of stability, measurement of blood levels every 3 or more months may suffice. Blood should be drawn 8 to 12 hours after the last dose of lithium is taken. Refer to Table 16-5 for side effects, signs of lithium toxicity, and interventions.

For older adult patients, the principle of **"start low and go slow"** still applies. Levels are often monitored every 3 or 4 days. Some older adults may respond to a dose low enough to maintain a blood level of 0.3 to 0.4 mEq/L. As mentioned, toxic effects are usually associated with lithium levels of 2 mEq/L or higher, but they can occur at much lower levels (even within a therapeutic range).

Maintenance therapy. Some clinicians suggest that patients with bipolar disorder need to be given lithium for 9 to 12 months, but most advocate lifelong lithium maintenance to prevent further relapses.

Lithium is unquestionably effective in preventing both manic and depressive episodes in patients with bipolar disorder. However, complete suppression occurs in only 50% or fewer patients, even with compliance with the maintenance therapy regimen. Therefore both the person with a bipolar disorder and his or her significant other should be given careful instructions about (1) the purpose and requirements of lithium therapy, (2) its adverse effects, (3) its toxic effects and complications, and (4) situations in which the physician should be contacted. The patient and family also should be advised that suddenly stopping lithium can lead to relapse and recurrence of mania. Box 16-1 outlines patient and family teaching regarding lithium therapy.

Patients need to know that **two major long-term risks of lithium therapy are hypothyroidism and impairment of the kidneys' ability to concentrate urine.** Therefore a person receiving lithium therapy must have periodic follow-ups to assess thyroid and renal function. Health care providers need to stress to patients with bipolar disorder and their families the importance of discontinuing maintenance therapy gradually.

Contraindications. Before lithium is administered, a medical evaluation is performed to assess the patient's ability to tolerate the drug. In particular, baseline physical and laboratory examinations should include assessment of renal function; determination of thyroid status, including levels of thyroxine and thyroid-stimulating hormone; and evaluation for dementia or neurological disorders, which presage a poor response to lithium. Other clinical and laboratory assessments, including an electrocardiogram, are performed as needed depending on the individual's physical condition.

Lithium therapy is generally contraindicated in people with cardiovascular disease and in those who have brain damage, renal disease, thyroid disease, or myasthenia gravis. Lithium also may harm a fetus and, whenever possible, is not given to women who are pregnant. Both the fear of pregnancy and the wish to become pregnant are major concerns for many bipolar women taking lithium. Lithium use is also contraindicated in mothers who are breast-feeding and in children younger than 12 years of age.

Anticonvulsants Drugs

Approximately 20% to 40% of bipolar patients may not respond or respond insufficiently to lithium, or they may not tolerate it.

BOX 16-1   PATIENT AND FAMILY TEACHING ABOUT LITHIUM THERAPY

The patient and the patient's family should receive the following teaching. (They should be encouraged to ask questions and given the material in written form as well.)

- Lithium can treat your current emotional problem and helps prevent relapse. Therefore it is important to continue taking the drug after the current episode is over.
- Because therapeutic and toxic dosage ranges are so close, it is important to monitor lithium blood levels very closely—more frequently at first, then once every several months after that.
- Lithium is not addictive.
- It is important to eat a normal diet with normal salt and fluid intake (1500-3000 mL/day or six 12-ounce glasses of fluid). Lithium decreases sodium reabsorption in the kidneys, which could lead to a sodium deficiency.
- Watch sodium levels. A low sodium intake leads to a relative increase in lithium retention, which could produce toxicity.
- You should stop taking lithium if you have excessive diarrhea, vomiting, or sweating. All of these symptoms can lead to dehydration. Dehydration can raise lithium levels in the blood to toxic levels. **Inform your physician if you have any of these problems.**
- Do not take diuretics (water pills) while you are taking lithium.

- Lithium is irritating to the lining in your stomach. It helps to take lithium with meals.
- Lithium can cause renal damage. Kidney function should be assessed before treatment and once a year thereafter.
- Lithium can promote goiter (thyroid enlargement) and frank hypothyroidism. Plasma levels of T_3, T_4, and thyroid-stimulating hormone (TSH) should be measured before treatment and yearly thereafter.
- Do not take any over-the-counter medicines without checking first with your physician.
- If you find that you are gaining a lot of weight, you may need to consult your physician or nutritionist.
- Many self-help groups are available to provide support for people with bipolar disorder and their families. The local self-help group is (give name and telephone number).
- You can find out more information by calling (give name and telephone number).
- Keep a list of side effects and toxic effects handy (see Table 16-5) along with the name and number of a contact person.
- If lithium is to be discontinued, your dosage will be tapered gradually to minimize risk of early relapse.

Some subgroups of bipolar patients may not respond well to lithium but may do well when treated with anticonvulsant drugs.

Three anticonvulsants have demonstrated efficacy for the treatment of mood disorders—carbamazepine (Tegretol), divalproex (Depakote), and lamotrigine (Lamictal) (Preston et al., 2010)—and have been found to have other uses as well. A sustained-release form of carbamazepine (Equetro), Depakote, and Lamictal are all FDA approved (Preston et al., 2010). Anticonvulsants used in bipolar and other disorders are especially effective in the following:

- Beneficial in controlling mania (within 2 weeks) and depression (within 3 weeks or longer)
- Superior in **dysphoric mania** (depressive thoughts and feelings during manic episodes)
- Superior in **rapid cycling** (four or more episodes a year)
- Drugs of choice for bipolar depression
- More effective when there is no family history of bipolar disease
- Effective at dampening affective swings in schizoaffective patients
- Effective at diminishing impulsive and aggressive behavior in some nonpsychotic patients
- Helpful in cases of alcohol and benzodiazepine withdrawal

Divalproex (Depakote). Valproic acid/valproate is useful in treating lithium nonresponders who are in acute mania, who experience rapid cycles, who are in dysphoric mania, or who have not responded to carbamazepine. It is also helpful in preventing manic episodes. As with carbamazepine, it is important to monitor liver function and platelet count periodically, although serious complications are rare. A new study demonstrates that women taking valproate run the risk of developing polycystic ovarian syndrome and that valproate use may lead to birth defects and developmental delays in children exposed in utero (Wisner et al., 2011). Therefore, careful consideration by both the physician and the patient is mandatory for bipolar treatment in women during childbearing years.

Carbamazepine (Tegretol). Some patients with treatment-resistant bipolar disorder improve after taking carbamazepine and lithium or carbamazepine and an antipsychotic. Carbamazepine seems to work better in patients with rapid cycling and in severely paranoid and angry patients with mania than in euphoric, overactive, and overfriendly manic behaviors. It is also thought to be more effective in patients who present with mixed bipolar disorders.

Blood levels of carbamazepine should be monitored at least weekly for the first 8 weeks of treatment because the drug can increase the levels of liver enzymes that accelerate its own metabolism. In some instances this can cause bone marrow suppression and liver inflammation.

Lamotrigine (Lamictal). Lamotrigine is a first-line treatment for bipolar depression and is approved for acute and maintenance therapy. It is generally well tolerated, but there are two concerns with this agent. One is a rare but serious dermatological reaction: a potentially life-threatening rash. Patients should be instructed to seek immediate medical attention if a rash appears, although in most cases rashes are benign (Preston et al., 2010). Another problem with lamotrigine is that in August of 2010, the U.S. Food and Drug administration (FDA) announced that aseptic meningitis is another rare but serious side effect of lamotrigine (FDA, 2010).

Newer anticonvulsant drugs. Other popular anticonvulsants may be used in the treatment of refractory bipolar disorder. However, except for topiramate (Topamax) and oxcarbazepine (Trileptal), other anticonvulsants fail to demonstrate efficacy in practice and/or lack evidence-based studies to support their use (Preston et al., 2010). Topiramate is helpful in mania and does not appear to cause weight gain. Oxcarbazepine, a structural variant of carbamazepine, has the advantage of being better tolerated and has a more favorable drug interaction profile than other anticonvulsants (Preston et al., 2010). See Table 16-6 for commonly prescribed antiepileptic drugs (AEDs) and their adverse reactions.

Anxiolytics

Clonazepam (Klonopin) and lorazepam (Ativan). Clonazepam and lorazepam are useful in the treatment of acute mania in some patients with treatment-resistant mania. These drugs are also effective in managing the psychomotor agitation seen in mania. They should be avoided, however, in patients with a history of substance abuse.

Second-Generation Antipsychotics

In addition to showing sedative properties during the early phase of treatment, which may help with insomnia, anxiety, and agitation, the newer atypical antipsychotics seem to have mood-stabilizing properties. The four FDA-approved second-generation antipsychotics recommended as primary agents in the treatment of both acute mania and mixed mania are olanzapine (Zyprexa), risperidone (Risperdal), aripiprazole (Abilify), and ziprasidone (Geodon). Quetiapine (Seroquel) is FDA approved for acute mania but not for mixed mania. Of the aforementioned medications only aripiprazole and olanzapine are presently approved for maintenance therapy in bipolar disorders (Preston & Johnson, 2009).

Electroconvulsive Therapy

Electroconvulsive therapy (ECT) is used to subdue severe manic behavior. It is especially helpful in patients with treatment-resistant mania and patients with rapid cycling (i.e., those who experience four or more episodes of illness in 1 year). ECT is effective in patients with bipolar disorder who experience paranoid-destructive features (who often respond poorly to lithium therapy) and in those patients who are acutely suicidal (Chapter 23).

Continuation Phase

The treatment continuation phase is a crucial one for patients and their families. The outcome for this phase is to prevent relapse. Community resources are chosen based on the needs of the patient, the appropriateness of the referral, and the availability of resources. Frequently, it is a case manager who evaluates appropriate follow-up care for patients and their families.

TABLE 16-6   ANTIEPILEPTIC DRUGS

DRUG	MAJOR ADVERSE EFFECTS
Carbamazepine (Tegretol)	• **Agranulocytosis** and **aplastic anemia** are most serious adverse reactions • Blood levels should be monitored throughout first 8 weeks because drug induces liver enzymes that speed its own metabolism. Dosage may need to be adjusted to maintain serum level of 6-8 mg/L. • Immediate action when severe adverse reactions appear (e.g., confusion, difficulty breathing, irregular heartbeat, skin rash or hives, jaundice)
Equetro	• A sustained-release form of carbamazepine
Divalproex/valproate (Depakote)	• **Baseline liver function tests should be performed and results monitored** at regular intervals. Hepatitis, although rare, has been reported, with fatalities in children • Severe adverse reactions include fever, chills, right upper quadrant pain, dark urine, malaise, jaundice/confusion, significant drowsiness • Best use for men and older women. Can cause birth defects in pregnant women
Lamotrigine (Lamictal)	• **Life-threatening** rash reported in 3 out of every 1000 individuals (Stevens-Johnson syndrome) • **Rare but potential** septic meningitis risk with lamotrigine • Use caution when renal, hepatic, or cardiac function is impaired
Topiramate (Topamax)	• Used in acute mania or in combination with other drugs • Adverse effects include weight loss, cognitive side effects, fatigue, dizziness, and paresthesia • **Used off-label; not presently FDA approved** for bipolar disorder
Oxcarbazepine (Trileptal)	• Structural variant of carbamazepine • Thought to have better side effect profile and more favorable drug interaction profiles • Not yet FDA approved for bipolar disorders • Used off-label

Medication compliance during this phase is perhaps the most important treatment outcome. This follow-up is frequently handled in a mental health center. However, adherence to the medication regimen is also addressed in day hospitals and in psychiatric home care visits. Some patients may attend day hospitals if they are not too excitable and are able to tolerate a certain level of stimuli. In addition to medication oversight, day hospitals offer structure, decrease social isolation, and help patients channel their time and energy. If a patient is homebound and unable to get to a mental health center or day hospital, then psychiatric home care is the appropriate modality for follow-up care.

Health Teaching and Health Promotion

Patients and families need information about bipolar illness with particular emphasis on the chronic and highly recurrent nature of the illness. They also need to be taught the symptoms of impending episodes. For example, changes in sleep patterns are especially important because they usually precede, accompany, or precipitate mania. Even a single night of unexplainable sleep loss can be taken as an early warning of impending mania. Health teaching stresses the importance of establishing regularity in sleep patterns, meals, exercise, and other activities.

Psychoeducation includes a rich combination of tools to improve functional outcomes for patients and their families (Box 16-2). At the very least, psychoeducation increases compliance by improving the regularity of daily life and sleep habits and by providing clear guidelines for both patients and families to follow.

Maintenance Phase

Maintenance therapy is aimed at preventing recurrence. Not only are some of the community resources cited earlier helpful, but patients and their families often greatly benefit from mutual support and self-help groups.

Psychotherapy

Pharmacotherapy and psychiatric management are essential in the treatment of acute manic attacks. Individuals with bipolar disorder suffer from the psychosocial consequences of their past episodes and their vulnerability to experiencing future episodes. People who have bipolar disease also have to face the burden of long-term treatments that may involve some unpleasant side effects.

During the course of their illness, many patients have sustained strained interpersonal relationships, marriage and family problems, academic and occupational problems, and legal or other social difficulties. Psychotherapy can help people work through these difficulties, which not only decreases some of the psychic distress but also increases self-esteem. Psychotherapeutic treatments in conjunction with psychopharmacology also can help patients improve their functioning between episodes and attempt to decrease the frequency of future episodes.

A study by Miklowitz and colleagues (2007) demonstrated that intensive psychotherapy given weekly and biweekly for up to 30 sessions in 9 months using cognitive behavioral therapy (CBT), interpersonal and social rhythm therapy (IPSRT), and family-focused therapy (FFT) was far superior in higher

---

BOX 16-2 PSYCHOEDUCATION FOR PATIENTS WITH BIPOLAR DISORDER AND THEIR FAMILIES

Patients with bipolar disorder and their families need to know the following:

1. The chronic and episodic nature of bipolar disorder.
2. The fact that bipolar disorder is a long-term illness and that maintenance treatment therefore will require that one or more mood-stabilizing agents be taken for a long time.
3. The expected side effects and toxic effects of the prescribed medication, as well as whom to call and where to go in case of a toxic reaction.
4. The signs and symptoms of relapse that may "come out of the blue."
5. The role of family members and others in preventing a full relapse.
6. The phone numbers of emergency contact people, which should be kept in an easily accessed place.
7. The use of alcohol, drugs of abuse, even small amounts of caffeine, and over-the-counter medications can produce a relapse.
8. Good sleep hygiene is critical to stability. Frequently, the prodrome of a manic episode is lack of sleep. In some cases, mania may be averted by the use of sleep medications (e.g., temazepam [Restoril]).
9. Psychosocial strategies are important for dealing with work, interpersonal, and family problems; lowering stress; enhancing a sense of personal control; and increasing community functioning.
10. Group and individual psychotherapy is invaluable for gaining insight as well as skills in relapse prevention, providing social support, increasing coping skills in interpersonal relations, improving compliance with the medication regimen, reducing functional morbidity, and decreasing rehospitalizations.

Health care workers need to remember the following:

1. Minimization and denial are common defenses that require gradual introduction of facts.
2. Anger and abusive remarks, although aimed at the health care provider, are symptoms of the disease and are not personal.

Adapted from Zerbe, K.J. (1999). *Women's mental health in primary care.* Philadelphia: Saunders; Milkowitz, D.J. (2003). Bipolar disorder. In D.H. Barlow (Ed.), *Clinical handbook of psychological disorders* (pp. 523-560). New York: Guilford Press.

---

year-end recovery rates and resulted in shorter recovery times than those in a control group. The control, called "collaborative therapy," consisted of brief psychoeducational intervention consisting of three sessions in 6 weeks. CBT, IPSRT, and FFT are three very effective psychosocial therapies used in conjunction with medication that can greatly benefit individuals suffering from bipolar conditions.

Psychotherapy is an important treatment in bipolar illness and results in greater compliance with the lithium regimen (Jamison, 1995b). Often patients receiving medication and psychotherapy place more value on psychotherapy than do clinicians. Moreover, patients treated with cognitive therapy are more likely to take their medications as prescribed than patients who do not participate in therapy (Jamison, 1995a; Lam et al., 2003).

One patient describes her feelings about drug therapy and psychotherapy as follows (Jamison, 1995b):

VIGNETTE

I cannot imagine leading a normal life without lithium. From starting and stopping of it, I now know it is an essential part of my sanity. Lithium prevents my seductive but disastrous highs, diminishes my depressions, clears out the weaving of my disordered thinking, slows me, gentles me out, keeps me in my relationships, in my career, out of a hospital, and in psychotherapy. It keeps me alive, too.

But psychotherapy heals, it makes some sense of the confusion, it reins in the terrifying thoughts and feelings, it brings back hope and the possibility of learning from it

all. Pills cannot, do not, ease one back into reality. They bring you back headlong, careening, and faster than can be endured at times. Psychotherapy is a sanctuary, it is a battleground, and it is where I have come to believe that someday I may be able to contend with all of this. No pill can help me deal with the problem of not wanting to take pills, but no amount of therapy alone can prevent my manias and depressions. I need both.

Cognitive behavioral therapy. Cognitive behavioral therapy, an adaptation of Beck's cognitive therapy treatment for depression, is a skills oriented form of therapy. **Cognitive behavioral therapy (CBT)** has been found valuable in helping patients with bipolar disorder accept their illness and the need for medical treatment. Some studies have pointed out that cognitive techniques have also been shown to be effective in decreasing affective symptoms, increasing social functioning, reducing the rate of relapse, and reducing the number of hospital admissions.

CBT focuses mainly on medication adherence, early detection and intervention, and stress and lifestyle management using a variety of CBT techniques. These interventions have been found most effective with patients who have bipolar I disorder (PsychEducation, 2007). CBT is typically used as an adjunct to pharmacotherapy and involves identifying maladaptive cognitions and behaviors that may be barriers to a person's recovery and ongoing mood stability. It is also being used for bipolar disorder in children.

Interpersonal and social rhythm therapy. **Interpersonal and social rhythm therapy (IPSRT)**, a formalized psychotherapy, is based on the idea that problems in interpersonal relationships and disruptions in daily routines can contribute to the recurrence of manic and depressive episodes in an individual with a bipolar disorder. IPSRT has been found effective in shortening a depressive episode in bipolar I patients (Scott & Colom, 2005). The interpersonal aspects of IPSRT derive from interpersonal psychotherapy and focus on resolutions of interpersonal problems (e.g., unresolved grief, disputes, and role transitions) and prevention of further disputes. IPSRT is effective in the acute as well as the maintenance phases of treatment.

Family-focused therapy. Behavioral family management, family therapy, and psychoeducation help families stay together, lead to lower rates of rehospitalization, and improve family functioning. Family-focused therapy (FFT) combines many of the key target areas of CBT and IPSRT (PsychEducation, 2007), including:

- Psychoeducation
- Relapse drill (prevention)
- Ways to make the diagnosis of bipolar disorder more acceptable to the patient

FFT is different from CBT and IPSRT in that it includes the family in therapy. FFT focuses on communication within the family, teaches communication skills, and prepares the entire family for relapse episodes (PsychEducation, 2007).

Support Groups

Patients with bipolar disorder, as well as their friends and families, benefit from forming mutual support groups, such as those sponsored by the Depression and Bipolar Support Alliance (DBSA), the National Alliance for the Mentally Ill (NAMI), the National Mental Health Association, and the Manic-Depressive Association.

EVALUATION

Outcome criteria often dictate the frequency of evaluation of short-term and intermediate indicators. For example, does the patient have stable vital signs? Is the patient well hydrated within safe time limits? Is the patient able to control his or her own behavior or respond to external controls? Is the patient able to sleep for 4 or 5 hours per night or take frequent short rest periods during the day? Does the family have a clear understanding of the patient's disease and need for medication? Do the patient and family know which community agencies may help them?

If outcomes or related indicators are not achieved satisfactorily, the preventing factors are analyzed. Were the data incorrect or insufficient? Were nursing diagnoses inappropriate or outcomes unrealistic? Was intervention poorly planned? After the outcomes and care plan are reassessed, the plan is revised if indicated. Longer-term outcomes include compliance with the medication regimen; resumption of functioning in the community; achievement of stability in family, work, and social relationships and in mood; and improved coping skills for reducing stress.

■ KEY POINTS TO REMEMBER

- Biological factors appear to play a role in the etiology of the bipolar disorders. Strong genetic correlates have been revealed, especially through twin studies.
- Little doubt exists that an excess and/or imbalance in neurotransmitters is also related to bipolar mood swings, which supports the existence of neurobiological influences.
- Neuroendocrine and neuroanatomical findings support evidence for biological influences.
- Bipolar disorder often remains unrecognized, and early detection can help diminish comorbid substance abuse, suicide, and decline in social and personal relationships, and may help promote more positive outcomes.
- The nurse assesses the patient's level of mood (hypomania, acute mania, delirious mania), behavior, and thought processes and is alert to cognitive dysfunction.
- Some nursing diagnoses appropriate for a patient who is manic are *Risk for Violence, Defensive Coping, Ineffective Coping, Disturbed Thought Processes,* and *Situational Low Self-Esteem.*
- During the acute phase of mania, physical needs often take priority and demand nursing interventions. Therefore deficient fluid volume and imbalanced nutrition or elimination, as well as disturbed sleep pattern, are usually addressed in the nursing plan.

- The diagnosis *Interrupted family processes* is vital. Support groups, psychoeducation, and guidance for the family can greatly affect the patient's compliance with the medication regimen.
- Planning nursing care involves identifying the specific needs of the patient and family during the three phases of mania.
- Antimanic medications are available. Lithium has a narrow therapeutic index, which necessitates thorough patient and family teaching and regular follow-up. AEDs such as carbamazepine and valproic acid are useful, especially in treating people with disease refractory to lithium therapy; newer AEDs are also useful in treating patients who need rapid de-escalation and do not respond to other treatment approaches.
- Antipsychotic agents may be needed because of their sedating and mood-stabilizing properties, especially during initial treatment.
- For some patients, ECT may be the most appropriate medical treatment.
- Patient and family teaching takes many forms and is most important in encouraging compliance with the medication regimen and reducing the risk of relapse.
- Evaluation includes examining the effectiveness of the nursing interventions, changing the outcomes as needed, and reassessing the nursing diagnoses. Evaluation is an ongoing process and is part of each of the other steps in the nursing process.

APPLYING CRITICAL JUDGMENT

1. Kioshi Sung is taken into the emergency department after threatening in a loud voice to, "Blow up the world to save the poor, and many more, where's the door? No more, no more. Let me loose." He had attacked a bartender who would not give him any more to drink. He has not eaten or slept for more than 1 week and only takes sips of fluids when offered. He talks nonstop, moving constantly, flailing his arms, and bumping into objects as he walks rapidly.

   A. Identify Mr. Sung's immediate needs (in terms of a nursing diagnosis). Describe the interventions you would plan for his physiological safety and his milieu (safe environment).

   B. Discuss the most appropriate communication techniques and approaches for Mr. Sung at this time. Give examples of what you would say and how you would say it.

   C. What possible medications would Mr. Sung most likely be given immediately? Long term?

   D. Write a medication treatment plan for Mr. Sung and his family.

   E. Describe at least four evidence-based therapeutic modalities for a bipolar patient.

   F. What symptoms would help you evaluate if a bipolar client was in hypomania, mania, or stream media?

   G. Name the most important interventions you would institute for each of the three phases of mania.

CHAPTER REVIEW QUESTIONS

Choose the most appropriate answer(s).

1. In communicating with a patient who is experiencing an elated mood, which of the following interventions by the nurse is most appropriate?
   1. Use a calm, firm approach.
   2. Give expanded explanations.
   3. Make use of abstract concepts.
   4. Encourage lighthearted optimism.

2. Which food selection best meets the needs of the manic patient?
   1. Pineapple, bananas, popcorn
   2. Chicken and mashed potatoes
   3. Corn chowder and spinach
   4. Peanut butter sandwich and carrots

3. A positive characteristic that assists the nurse in the care of the manic patient is:
   1. flight of ideas.
   2. racing thoughts.
   3. taunting behavior.
   4. distractibility.

4. Which activity has a calming effect on the manic patient?
   1. Writing on a notepad
   2. Reading a book
   3. Discussion of current events
   4. Watching a movie

5. A patient has a lithium level of 1.1 mEq/L. This level is:
   1. below the therapeutic level.
   2. above the therapeutic level.
   3. within the therapeutic range.
   4. not needed as lithium does not require blood levels.

REFERENCES

Black, D. W., & Andreasen, N. C. (2011). *Introductory textbook of psychiatry* (5th ed.). Washington, DC: American Psychiatric Publishing.

BPhoenix. (2010). *Unipolar versus bipolar depression.* Retrieved March 15, 2011, from www.angelfire.com/home/bphoenix1/courses.html.

Brauser, D. (2011). *Severity of bipolar disorder rates similar worldwide.* Retrieved March 10, 2011, from www.medscape.com/view article/738747_print.

Dias, R. (2011). Fluctuating hormones linked to more severe bipolar symptoms. *American Journal of Psychiatry, news release.* Retrieved March 12, 2011, from www.nih.gov/mrdlneplus/news/full story08850.html.

Garno, J. L., Goldberg, J. F., Ramirez, P. M., & Ritzler, B. A. (2005). Impact of childhood abuse and the clinical course of bipolar disorder. Retrieved April 4, 2012, from http://bjp.rcpsych.org. Published by the Royal College of Physicians.

Jamison, K. R. (1995a). *An unquiet mind.* New York: Knopf.

Jamison, K. R. (1995b). *Psychotherapy of bipolar patients.* Paper presented at the U.S. Psychiatric and Mental Health Congress, November 18, 1995, New York.

Kelsoe, J. R. (2009). Mood disorders: genetics. In B. J. Sadock, V. A. Sadock, & P. Ruiz (Eds.), *Kaplan and Sadock's comprehensive textbook of psychiatry* (19th ed., vol. pp. 1653–1674). Philadelphia: Wolters Kluwer/Lippincott Williams & Wilkins.

Kessler, R. C., Berglund, P., Dember, O., et al. (2005). Lifetime prevalence and age-of-onset distributions of *DSM-IV* disorders in the National Comorbidity Survey Replication. *Archives of General Psychiatry, 62*(6), 593–602.

Lam, D. H., Watkins, E. R., Hayward, P., et al. (2003). A randomized controlled study of cognitive therapy for relapse prevention for bipolar affective disorder: outcome of the first year. *Archives of General Psychiatry, 60,* 145–152.

Lehne, R. A. (2007). *Pharmacology for nursing care* (6th ed.). St Louis: Saunders.

Lichtenstein, P., Yip, B. H., Bjork, C., et al. (2009). Common genetic determinants of schizophrenia and bipolar disorder in Swedish families: a population-based study. *Lancet, 373*(9659), 234–239. Abstract.

Merikangas, K. R., Jin, R., He, J. -P., et al. (2011). Prevalence and correlates of bipolar spectrum disorder in the world mental health survey initiative. *Archives of General Psychiatry, 68*(3), 241–251.

Miklowitz, M. J., Otto, M. W., Frank, E., et al. (2007). Psychosocial treatments for bipolar depression: a 1-year randomized trial from the systemic treatment enhancement program. *Archives of General Psychiatry, 64*(4), 419–426.

Pollock, R., & Kuo, I. (2004). *Neuroimaging in bipolar disorder.* Paper presented at the 5th Invitational Congress of Biological Psychiatry, February 9-13, 2004, Sydney, Australia.

Preston, J., & Johnson, J. (2009). *Clinical psychopharmacology made ridiculously simple* (5th ed.). Miami: MedMasters.

Preston, J. D., O'Neal, J. H., & Talaga, M. C. (2010). *Handbook of clinical psychopharmacology for therapists* (6th ed.). Oakland, CA: New Harbinger Publications.

PsychEducation. (2007). *Psychotherapy for bipolar disorder.* Retrieved August 28, 2007, from www.psycheducation.org/depression/Psychotherapy.htm.

Robinson, L. J., & Ferrier, I. N. (2006). Evolution of cognitive impairment in bipolar disease: a systematic review of cross-sectional evidence. *Bipolar Disorder, 8*(2), 103–116.

Scott, J., & Colom, F. (2005). Psychosocial treatments for bipolar disorders. In E. Sherwood Brown (Ed.), *Psychiatric Clinics of North America, 28*(2), pp. 371–384.

Skidmore-Roth, L. (2008). *Mosby's nursing drug reference* (21st ed.). St Louis: Mosby.

Soreff, S., & McInnes, L. A. (2011). *Bipolar affective disorder.* Retrieved January 21, 2011, from http://emedicine.com.medscape.com/article/286342–overview.

Thase, M. E. (2009). Mood disorders: neurobiology. In B. J. Sadock, V. A. Sadock, & P. Ruiz (Eds.), *Kaplan and Sadock's comprehensive textbook of psychiatry* (19th ed., pp. 1664–1674). Philadelphia: Wolters Kluwer/Lippincott Williams & Wilkins.

U.S. Food and Drug Administration (FDA). (2010). *Lamictal (lamotrigine): label change—risk of aseptic meningitis.* Retrieved March 14, 2011, from www.fda.gov/Safety/MedWatch/SafetyInformation/Safety.

Wisner, K. L., Lockmen-Westin, E., Finnerty, M., & Essock, S. M. (2011). Valproate prescription prevalence among women of childbearing age. *Psychiatric Services, 62,* 218–220. Retrieved June 16, 2011, from psychservices.psychiatryonline.org/cgi/content/abstract/62/.

Zerbe, K. J. (1999). *Women's mental health in primary care.* Philadelphia: Saunders.

Schizophrenia Spectrum Disorders

Elizabeth M. Varcarolis

evolve WEBSITE

http://evolve.elsevier.com/Varcarolis/essentials

KEY TERMS AND CONCEPTS

acute dystonia, p. 325
affect, p. 309
akathisia, p. 325
associative looseness (LOA), p. 306
atypical (second-generation)
   antipsychotics, p. 320
clang association, p. 307
cognitive symptoms, p. 304
concrete thinking, p. 306
conventional (first-generation)
   antipsychotics, p. 320
delusions, p. 305
echolalia, p. 310
echopraxia, p. 310
extrapyramidal symptoms (EPS),
   p. 324
hallucinations, p. 307
ideas of reference, p. 309

illusions, p. 307
negative symptoms, p. 308
neologisms, p. 307
neurocognitive symptoms, p. 309
neuroleptic malignant syndrome
   (NMS), p. 325
paranoia, p. 309
positive symptoms, p. 305
projection, p. 309
pseudoparkinsonism, p. 325
psychotic, p. 300
stereotyped behavior, p. 309
tardive dyskinesia (TD), p. 325
thought broadcasting, p. 306
thought insertion, p. 306
thought withdrawal, p. 306
waxy flexibility, p. 310
word salad, p. 307

CONCEPTS: Psychoeducation
An effective approach with patients and
families with a schizophrenic member is
a **psychoeducational approach.** Psychoeducation brings educational and behavioral approaches into family treatment.
The psychoeducational approach recognizes that families are secondary victims
of a biological illness. In family therapy
sessions, fears, faulty communication
patterns, and distortions are identified.
Improved problem-solving skills can be
taught, and healthier alternatives to situations of conflict can be explored.

   On an individual level psychoeducation
seems to reduce relapse, encourage medication adherence, reduce readmission,
and cut down on length of hospital stay
(Xia et al, (2011).
(Text), (Xia et al, 2011)

OBJECTIVES

1. Describe the prodromal (early) symptoms that a person
   with schizophrenia may exhibit during the prepsychotic
   phase.
2. Identify evidence-based data that support the
   neurobiological-anatomical-nongenetic findings that
   support the premise that schizophrenia is a neurological
   disease.
3. Compare and contrast the positive and negative symptoms
   of schizophrenia with regard to (a) their effect on quality
   of life, (b) their significance for the prognosis of the disease, and (c) their side effect profile.
4. Delineate ways that neurocognitive impairments impact
   a person who is struggling with schizophrenia; include
   prognosis and quality-of-life indicators.

OBJECTIVES—cont'd

5. Identify the numerous areas in which health care workers need to apply safety interventions for a person with schizophrenia during the different phases of treatment.
6. Demonstrate with classmates the best evidence-based practice we currently have for communicating with a person who is (a) hallucinating, (b) paranoid, and (c) experiencing delusions.
7. Teach a classmate, group, or friend the differences between the properties of typical versus atypical antipsychotic drugs regarding the following: (a) target symptoms, (b) indications for use, (c) adverse effects and toxic effects, (d) need for patient and family teaching and follow-up, and (e) potential for medical compliance.
8. Discuss evidence-based psychosocial therapies for patients with schizophrenia and their families.

9. Differentiate among the three phases of schizophrenia in terms of symptoms, focus of care, and intervention needs using Table 17-5 as a guide.
10. Identify specific times when teamwork and collaboration with other health care professionals are paramount for the implementation of safe and effective care for a patient with schizophrenia.
11. Using informatics, search for available resources for patients and families coping with schizophrenia in your area (e.g., Mental Health America [www.nmha.org] or National Alliance on Mental Illness [NAMI] [www.nami.org/]).
12. Identify some other primary psychotic disorders.

Schizophrenia is a devastating brain disease that targets young people in their teens or early twenties at the beginning of their productive lives. It profoundly disrupts an individual's ability to perceive reality accurately, to think clearly, to use language appropriately, to experience normal emotions, or to engage in normal social/occupational experiences. Schizophrenia spectrum disorders are a group of psychotic disorders.

Psychosis is not a diagnosis but a symptom. **Psychosis** refers to a total inability to recognize reality—for example, experiencing delusions (profoundly believing in ideas with no basis in fact, such as "I have the power to save the world") and hallucinations (experiencing sensory perceptions that are not based in reality, such as hearing voices that tell you to jump in front of a train or that you are a bad person).

Schizophrenia is not just one rigid disorder. People with schizophrenia may vary in terms of their disabilities, presentations, and quality of life. Therefore schizophrenia is often thought of as a spectrum of disorders. Often, individuals have varying degrees of neurocognitive impairments evidenced by disorganized thinking and disorganized speech. The neurocognitive aspects are perhaps one of the most destructive features of schizophrenia. People with these disorders are usually socially isolated or alienated and have deep feelings of inadequacy. Other primary psychotic disorders are identified in Box 17-1.

Some people with schizophrenia function well with the aid of medications and social supports. Others are more disabled, and need a higher level of support in terms of housing, health maintenance, monetary aid, and more. Although schizophrenia is treatable, it is not curable and is a severe mental illness (SMI). Refer to Chapter 27 for a broader understanding of all people with a severe mental illness.

PREVALENCE AND COMORBIDITY

The lifetime prevalence of schizophrenia is 1% worldwide with no differences related to race, social status, culture, gender, or environment (Sadock & Sadock, 2010). A premorbid condition can be an indication of the potential complexity and eventual outcome for an individual who is later diagnosed with schizophrenia. For example, individuals with an early age of onset (18 to 25 years) are more often male and have poorer premorbid adjustment, more evidence of structural brain abnormalities, and more prominent negative symptoms. Individuals with a later onset (25 to 35 years) are more likely to be female, have less evidence of structural brain abnormalities, and have better outcomes. The younger the patient is at the onset of schizophrenia, the more discouraging the prognosis.

An abrupt onset of symptoms with good premorbid functioning is usually a favorable prognostic sign. A slow, insidious onset over a period of 2 or 3 years is more ominous. Those whose prepsychotic personalities show good social, sexual, and occupational functioning have a greater chance for remission or complete recovery. A childhood history of withdrawn, reclusive, eccentric, and tense behavior is an unfavorable diagnostic sign.

Substance abuse disorders occur in more than 40% of individuals with schizophrenia (Sadock & Sadock, 2010). Substance abuse is associated with a variety of negative outcomes, including incarceration, homelessness, violence, suicide, and infection with human immunodeficiency virus (HIV), and is linked with a poorer prognosis. **Nicotine** dependence is very common in people with schizophrenia, and 75% to 85% of people with schizophrenia smoke (Evins et al., 2005). Smoking results in significant morbidity and mortality and is linked with a high rate of emphysema and other pulmonary and cardiac problems. These risks are even greater in people with schizophrenia because they tend to smoke two to three times more than the average smoker.

Depressive symptoms occur frequently in schizophrenia. **Suicide** is the leading cause of premature death in this population, accounting for about 10% of deaths in those who have schizophrenia (Sadock & Sadock, 2010). The rate of comorbid **anxiety disorders** in individuals with schizophrenia also has been found to be higher than the rate of anxiety disorders in the general population.

Psychosis-induced polydipsia is the compulsive drinking of water (between 4 and 10 L/day). Polydipsia is associated with

---

BOX 17-1 OTHER PSYCHOTIC DISORDERS

Schizophreniform Disorder

The essential features of schizophreniform disorder are exactly the same as those of schizophrenia except the symptoms may only last a short time, and impaired social or occupational functioning is usually not apparent.

Brief Psychotic Disorder

Brief psychotic disorder is characterized by a sudden onset of psychotic symptoms (delusions, hallucinations, disorganized speech) or grossly disorganized or catatonic behavior. The episode is usually short-lived and the person returns to his or her premorbid level of functioning. These disorders are usually precipitated by extremely stressful life events.

Schizoaffective Disorder

Schizoaffective disorder is characterized by an uninterrupted period of illness during which time there is a major depressive, manic, or mixed episode, concurrent with symptoms that meet the criteria for schizophrenia. The symptoms must not be a result of any substance use or abuse or be attributable to a general medical condition.

Delusional Disorder

Delusional disorder involves nonbizarre delusions (situations that occur in real life, such as being followed, infected, loved at a distance, deceived by a spouse, or having a disease) of at least 1 month's duration. The person's ability to function is not markedly impaired, nor is the person's behavior obviously odd or bizarre. Common types of delusions seen in this disorder are of grandeur, persecution, or jealousy; somatic delusions; and mixed delusions.

Shared Psychotic Disorder *(Folie à Deux)*

A shared psychotic disorder is a condition in which an individual who is in a close relationship with another individual who has a psychotic disorder with a delusion eventually comes to share the delusional beliefs either in total or in part. Apart from the shared delusion, the behavior of the person who assumes the other's delusional behavior is not odd or unusual. Impairment of the person who shares the delusion is usually much less than that of the person who has the psychotic disorder with the delusion. The cult phenomenon is an example, as was demonstrated at Waco and Jonestown.

Substance-Induced Psychotic Disorder

Psychosis may be induced by substances (drugs of abuse, alcohol, medications, or toxins) or caused by the physiological consequences of a general medical condition (delirium, neurological conditions, metabolic conditions, hepatic or renal diseases, and many others). Medical conditions and substances of abuse must always be ruled out before a primary diagnosis of schizophrenia or other psychotic disorder can be made.

Psychotic Disorder Associated With a Known General Medical Condition

A psychotic condition caused by medical causes.

Catatonic Disorder Associated With a Known General Medical Condition

A psychotic condition with catatonic features (see text) that has been determined to be caused by a general medical condition.

---

psychological disturbances and occurs in some people with a chronic severe mental illness (SMI). There are clearly increased rates of polydipsia in people with schizophrenia, which may result in severe hyponatremia, cerebral edema, and even death.

THEORY

Determining the causes of schizophrenia is clearly a complicated matter. What is known is that brain chemistry and brain activity are different in a person with schizophrenia than in a person without schizophrenia. Schizophrenia most likely occurs as a result of a combination of **inherited genetic factors** and extreme **nongenetic factors** (e.g., virus infection, birth injuries, nutritional factors), which can affect the genes governing the brain or injure the brain directly. Both of the above-mentioned factors may alter the structures of the brain, affect the brain's neurotransmitter system, and disrupt the neural circuits, resulting in impairment in cognition.

Neurobiological Factors

For many years the **dopamine hypothesis** was the most widely accepted explanation for the biochemical pathophysiology in schizophrenia. The dopamine hypothesis concluded there was a hyperactivity of the neurotransmitter dopamine in the limbic regions of the brain. This theory was derived from the study of the action of the antipsychotic drugs that block the activity of dopamine (D_2) and, in doing so, reduce some of the symptoms of schizophrenia. This theory is enhanced by the fact that amphetamines, cocaine, methylphenidate (Ritalin), and levodopa are drugs that increase the activity of dopamine in the brain. These drugs can exacerbate the symptoms of schizophrenia in psychotic patients and simulate symptoms of paranoid schizophrenia in a person without schizophrenia.

With the development of the atypical antipsychotic drugs that block serotonin (5-hydroxytryptamine, $5\text{-}HT_2$) it became apparent that **serotonin** might also play a role in causing some of the symptoms of schizophrenia. Another hypothesis postulates a role for other neurotransmitter systems in the pathophysiology of schizophrenia. One is glutamate or γ-aminobutyric acid (GABA). The glutamate hypothesis theory suggests that there is hypofunction in N-methyl-ᴅ-aspartate (NMDA) receptors in the glutamate system that leads to a combination of excitotoxin toxicity and impaired neural plasticity (Black & Andreasen,

EXAMINING THE EVIDENCE

Blood Testing for Schizophrenia

I have noticed in my psych clinical that it seems to take quite some time for clinicians to agree on a diagnosis of schizophrenia, because there may be overlap between bipolar disorder or other psychotic disorders. There are so many blood tests for most diseases; is there any hope for one for schizophrenia?

Yes, definitely! A blood-based marker for schizophrenia has been recently developed, validated, and marketed in the United States. This test, VeriPsych, uses multiple immunoassay technologies that profile the disease. This test has been found to be 83% sensitive and specific in distinguishing persons with schizophrenia from those without the disease. The study in which the test's validity was established included more than 500 patients in the developmental stage of the illness and 800 patients in the validation stage (Kelly, 2011).

Scientists study biomarkers in the skin, immune cells, and serum to find samples that give a real-time picture of schizophrenia. This is a scientific breakthrough since previous studies of schizophrenia have focused on examining potential biomarkers in brain tissue harvested at autopsy. Now scientists can trace central nervous system abnormalities in the peripheral nervous system (Cassels, 2010).

Despite years of investigation, the pathophysiology of schizophrenia, which affects approximately 2 million Americans, is still not completely understood. There have been advances, however, in diagnosing schizophrenia using standardized systems such as the DSM-IV/DSM-5 and structured interviews, which entail a subjective assessment of clinical symptoms. In addition, diagnosis can be hindered by factors such as substance abuse or other medical conditions. Such complications can lead to delays and inaccuracies in diagnosis, resulting in delayed treatment and a poorer outcome for the individual. The most effective use of blood tests would be to use them as a confirmatory diagnostic aid in conjunction with a clinical assessment by a psychiatric specialist (Schwarz et al., 2011).

Interest in the blood test is not primarily just to confirm a clinical diagnosis of schizophrenia, but also to help a patient accept the illness. It is hoped that serum tests could be used as an aid in helping these individuals who may lack insight or acceptance of their disease (typical in people with thought disorders) better understand the need for treatment (Kelly, 2011). It is accepted that the longer a person with psychosis remains untreated, the poorer their prognosis will be. An accurate blood test may enable earlier treatment intervention, improve patient quality of life, and provide reduction in morbidity, suffering, and health care costs (Schwarz et al., 2011).

Cassels, C. (2010). Blood test for schizophrenia may be on the horizon. Chemical and Engineering News, 88(26).
Kelly, D. (2011). A new blood based diagnostic aid for schizophrenia. Psychiatric Services, 62(9), 1107.
Schwarz, E., et al. (2011). Identification of a biological signature for schizophrenia in serum. Molecular Psychiatry, 12 April 2011. doi:10.1038/mp.2011.42.
Submitted by Lois Angelo.

2011). Phencyclidine hydrochloride (PCP) induces a state that closely resembles schizophrenia. This observation led to sustained interest in the N-methyl-D-aspartate (NMDA) receptor complex and the possible role of **glutamate** in the pathophysiology of schizophrenia.

Genetic Factors

Numerous studies have substantiated over time that schizophrenia has a strong genetic component. Although most people with schizophrenia do not have a family history of the disease, schizophrenia and schizophrenia-like symptoms occur in about 10% of siblings of schizophrenic patients. A child who has one parent with schizophrenia has a 5% to 6% chance of developing the disease whereas a child of two schizophrenic parents has a 46% likelihood of schizophrenia (Black & Andreasen, 2011). Numerous studies of twins (fraternal and identical) emphasize a significantly higher probability of a gene involvement, with close to 46% of identical twins versus 14% of fraternal twins being at risk of schizophrenia (Black & Andreasen, 2011). For identical twins reared apart the concordance rate for schizophrenia is similar, between 40% and 50%, a rate that substantiates a strong genetic component. However, because identical twins do not share a 100% concordance rate, there is obviously more involved than just genes.

Similar to gene involvement with bipolar spectrum disorders, schizophrenia is not a "one gene, one illness" disease, but rather caused by the involvement of multiple genes and other factors. Researchers have begun to identify many regions on chromosomes that are probably related to the development of schizophrenia spectrum disorder.

Neuroanatomical Factors

Disruptions in the connections and communication within neural circuitry (communication pathways) are thought to be severe in schizophrenia. Therefore it is conceivable that structural cerebral abnormalities cause disruption to the entire circuitry of the brain. Numerous brain imaging techniques—such as computed tomography (CT), magnetic resonance imaging (MRI), functional MRI (fMRI), and positron emission tomography (PET)—provide substantial evidence that some people with schizophrenia have structural brain abnormalities. For example, MRI and CT scans demonstrate lower brain volume, larger lateral and third ventricles, atrophy in the frontal lobe, and more cerebrospinal fluid, among other findings, in some people with schizophrenia. PET scans show a low rate of blood flow and glucose metabolism in the frontal lobes of the cerebral cortex, which govern planning, abstract thinking, social adjustment, and decision making. These are just a few of the many findings on brain imaging. Black and Andreasen (2011) state the current thinking on the neuroanatomical findings of schizophrenia suggests a disease of multiple disturbed circuits in the brain.

These findings and many others raise many questions. For example, is schizophrenia neurodevelopmental in origin? If not, what causes these changes to occur? Why do brain changes progress as the disease progresses in some people and not in others? Why do some people show neuroanatomical changes and others do not?

Nongenetic Risk Factors

Infants for whom there is a history of perinatal complications (e.g., birth complications/injury) are at increased risk for developing schizophrenia as adults. Prenatal risk factors include viral infection (influenza, toxoplasmosis, and genital/reproductive infection), poor nutrition or starvation, or exposure to toxins. Lack of oxygen during birth is also considered a risk factor for the development of schizophrenia. Essentially any early insult to the brain of a developing fetus or child (e.g., viral infections, environmental toxins, presence of certain genes) can lead to brain abnormalities. These brain abnormalities can be biochemical, structural, or functional, which may lead to biological vulnerability.

Stress (social, psychological, and physical), although not a cause of schizophrenia, may precipitate the illness in vulnerable individuals and play a role in the severity and course of the disease. The use of street drugs such as cannabis, methamphetamine, and lysergic acid diethylamide (LSD) increases the risk of developing schizophrenia, especially for those younger than age 21 whose brains are still developing.

CULTURAL CONSIDERATIONS

Although the developmental pattern of schizophrenia is consistent across cultures, studies find that some symptoms of schizophrenia as well as prognoses were more severe in industrialized nations than in developing countries (PBS, 2002).

Different cultural groups may view and interpret symptoms seen in schizophrenia in entirely different ways. What is considered normal or acceptable in one culture may be seen as pathological in another. In some subculture groups, "visions" or "voices" are an integral and expected part of various religious experiences (USDHHS, 1999). In some cultural settings, people who experience hallucinations may be perceived as gifted or special. In another culture a person experiencing the same phenomena may be perceived as being possessed or evil and is therefore taunted, isolated, or punished. In either of these two scenarios, effective treatment may be prolonged or never obtained.

A person's cultural background can influence the content and form of the positive and negative symptoms of schizophrenia.

For example, in Ireland where religious piety is highly valued, delusions may include sainthood and religious content. In industrial advanced countries (e.g., America) that focus on surveillance and sinister uses of technology, delusions may assume a more paranoid flavor (e.g., being spied on by their televisions or being under surveillance by the FBI). In Japan, one's honor and social conformity is prized; therefore delusions centering around slander or fear of being humiliated publicly are much more common (PBS, 2002). Therefore it would not be surprising in a culture that believes in ghosts, witches, or evil spirits for delusions to contain ancestral ghosts or witches.

It is important, therefore, to understand how family groups from different subcultures view a family member's "beliefs," "voices," or "visions." Knowing how the family views these symptoms and how they treat such phenomena in their cultural group can provide important information as to how mental health professionals can best approach and reframe treatment to the family and patient to make it more acceptable.

CLINICAL PICTURE

The signs and symptoms of schizophrenia are more numerous than presented here and not all symptoms apply to all individuals with schizophrenia. These symptoms are discussed in more detail under an assessment portion of Application of the Nursing Process. The basic symptoms of schizophrenia, according to the National Alliance on Mental Illness (2009) and Preston and colleagues (2010), are listed in Box 17-2.

BOX 17-2 SYMPTOMS OF SCHIZOPHRENIA

- **Positive symptoms:** Psychotic symptoms are the most obvious (e.g., delusions, hallucinations, and perceptions that are not based on reality).
- **Thought disorder:** Schizophrenia has a profound effect on an individual's ability to think clearly or to use language appropriately (looseness of association).
- **Negative symptoms:** Include poverty of thought, loss of motivation, inability to experience pleasure or joy, feelings of emptiness, and blunted affect.
- **Cognitive symptoms:** Include the inability to understand and process information, trouble focusing attention, and problems with working memory. These are the symptoms that most profoundly affect the individual's ability to engage in normal social/occupational experiences.
- **Characterological symptoms:** Most often people with schizophrenia are *isolated or alienated* from others. These patients have *deep feelings of inadequacy* and *poorly developed social skills*.
- Schizophrenia is a **severe mental illness (SMI)** and people with schizophrenia comprise a large percentage of our homeless population (refer to Chapter 27).

APPLICATION OF THE NURSING PROCESS

ASSESSMENT

Course of the Disease

The course of schizophrenia usually includes recurrent acute exacerbations of psychosis. However, the previous belief of schizophrenia as a disease with an unalterable advancement to progressive deterioration might be inaccurate. A decade's worth of longitudinal studies demonstrated that early and aggressive treatment with antipsychotics may alter the course of the schizophrenias when given at the time of the first psychotic break (Perkins et al., 2006). Prevention of relapse can be more important than the risk of side effects from medications because most side effects are reversible, whereas the consequences of relapse may be irreversible. *With each relapse of psychosis, there is an increase in residual dysfunction and deterioration* (Lewis et al., 2005).

The following are the phases in the course of the disease:

- **Prodromal phase:** Signs and symptoms that precede the acute, fully manifested signs and symptoms of disease. Prodromal symptoms occur in up to 80% to 90% of people with schizophrenia before the emergence of frank psychosis (acute phase). Early prodromal symptoms include social withdrawal and deterioration in function and depressive mood, followed by perceptual disturbances, magical thinking, and peculiar behavior, among others. Prodromal symptoms may appear a month to

a year before the first psychotic break and represent a clear deterioration in previous functioning. Essentially, the symptoms include perceptual difficulties; increased stress, depression, anxiety, and sleep disturbances; and declined functional ability (Addington, 2006). Speech may be characterized by obscure symbolism. Late in the phase, words and phrases may become indecipherable. Frequently, the history of a person with schizophrenia reveals that during adolescence the person was withdrawn from others, lonely or perhaps depressed, and expressed vague or unrealistic plans regarding the future.

- **Acute phase:** Periods of florid positive symptoms (more fully developed and flagrant) (e.g., hallucinations, delusions) as well as negative symptoms (e.g., apathy, withdrawal, lack of motivation) and cognitive symptoms
- **Maintenance phase:** Period in which acute symptoms decrease in severity, particularly the positive symptoms
- **Stabilization phase:** Period in which symptoms are in remission, although there might be milder persistent symptoms

Treatment-Relevant Dimensions of Schizophrenia

The major symptoms of schizophrenia can be grouped into positive, negative, and cognitive. Depression is a frequent comorbidity and can negatively affect the patient's long-term prognosis and the severity of emotional pain and confusion. Figure 17-1 presents an overview of these major

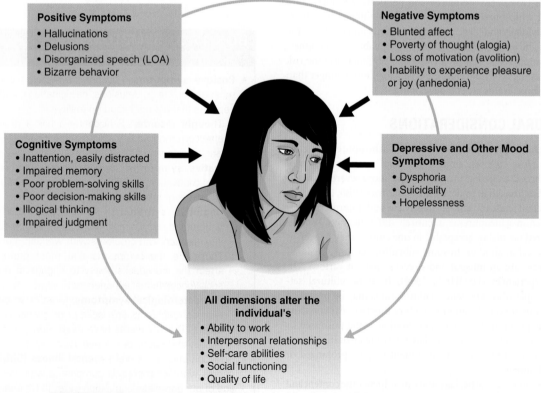

FIGURE 17-1 Treatment-relevant dimensions of schizophrenia. *LOA,* Looseness of association.

symptom groups and the ways in which they can affect an individual's life.

Positive symptoms (e.g., hallucinations, delusions, bizarre behavior, and paranoia) are referred to as *florid psychotic symptoms;* they are the ones that capture our attention. Three decades of analysis of treatment and study findings indicate that perhaps these florid psychotic symptoms may not be the core deficiency after all. Actually, the crippling negative symptoms (e.g., apathy, lack of motivation, anhedonia, and poor thought processes) persist and seem to be the most destructive because they render a person inert and unmotivated. The greater the degree of negative and cognitive symptoms the more likely it is for the person to be unable to function on a job, engage in social activities, and care for self adequately and safely. Refer to Box 17-3 for a list of positive and negative symptoms.

Positive Symptoms

Positive symptoms—such as hallucinations, delusions, bizarre behavior, and paranoia—are associated with an acute onset,

normal premorbid functioning, normal CT findings, normal neuropsychological test results, and favorable response to antipsychotic medications.

The positive symptoms appear early in the first phase of the illness and often precipitate hospitalization. They are, however, the least important prognostically and usually respond to antipsychotic medication. The positive symptoms are presented here in terms of alterations in thinking, speech, perception, and behavior.

Alterations in Thinking

Delusions. Alterations in thinking can take many forms. Delusions are most often defined as false fixed beliefs that cannot be corrected by reasoning. They may be simple beliefs or part of a complex delusional system. In schizophrenia, delusions are often loosely organized and may be bizarre. Most commonly, delusional thinking involves the following themes: ideas of reference, persecution, grandiosity, somatic sensations, jealousy, and control. Table 17-1 provides definitions and examples of delusions.

BOX 17-3 POSITIVE AND NEGATIVE SYMPTOMS OF SCHIZOPHRENIA

Positive Symptoms

Hallucinations
- Auditory
  - Voices commenting
  - Voices conversing
  - Voices commanding
- Somatic-tactile
- Olfactory
- Visual
- taste

Delusions
- Persecutory delusions
- Jealous delusions
- Grandiose delusions
- Religious delusions
- Somatic delusions
- Delusions of reference
- Delusions of being controlled
- Delusions of mind reading
- Thought broadcasting, insertion, withdrawal

Bizarre Behavior
- Clothing, appearance
- Social and sexual behavior
- Aggressive, agitated behavior
- Repetitive, stereotyped behavior

Positive Formal Thought Disorder and Speech Patterns
- Derailment
- Tangentiality
- Incoherence
- Illogicality
- Circumstantiality
- Pressure of speech
- Distractible speech
- Clang associations

Negative Symptoms

Affective Flattening
- Unchanging facial expression
- Decreased spontaneous movements
- Paucity of expressive gestures
- Poor eye contact
- Inappropriate affect
- Lack of vocal inflections

Alogia
- Poverty of speech
- Poverty of content of speech
- Blocking

Avolition, Apathy
- Impaired grooming and hygiene
- Lack of persistence at work or school
- Physical anergia

Anhedonia, Asociality
- Few recreational interests or activities
- Little sexual interest or activity
- Impaired intimacy and closeness
- Few relationships with friends or peers

Attention Deficits
- Social inattentiveness

TABLE 17-1 SUMMARY OF DELUSIONS*

TYPE OF DELUSION	DEFINITION	EXAMPLE
Ideas of reference	Misconstruing trivial events and remarks and giving them personal significance	When Maria saw the doctor and nurse talking together, she believed they were plotting against her. When she heard on the radio that a hurricane was coming, she believed this was really a message that harm was going to befall her.
Persecution	The false belief that one is being singled out for harm by others; this belief often takes the form of people in power conspiring against the person or following the person, or being persecuted by friends or colleagues	Sam believed that the Secret Service was planning to kill him. He believed that the Secret Service was poisoning his food. Therefore he would only eat food that he was certain was safe.
Grandeur	The false belief that one is a very powerful and important person, having special abilities, possessing great wealth or beauty	Sally believed that she was Mary Magdalene and that Jesus controlled her thoughts and was telling her how to save the world.
Somatic delusions	The false belief that the body is changing in an unusual way (e.g., rotting inside, heart is no longer beating)	David told the doctor that his brain was rotting away.
Jealousy	The false belief that one's mate is unfaithful; may have so-called proof	Harry accused his girlfriend of going out with other men, even though this was not the case. His "proof" was that she came home from work late twice that week. He persisted in his belief, even when the girl-friend's boss explained that everyone had worked late.

*A false belief held and maintained as true, even with evidence to the contrary. This does not include unusual beliefs maintained by one's culture or subculture.

Approximately 75% of people with schizophrenia experience delusions at some time during their illness. The most common delusions are persecutory and grandiose, as well as those involving religious or hypochondriacal ideas. A person experiencing delusions is convinced that what he or she believes to be real *is* real. The person's thinking often reflects feelings of great fear and isolation: "I know the doctor talks to the FBI about getting rid of me" or "Everyone wants me dead." Delusions may reflect the person's feelings of low self-worth through the use of reaction formation (observed as grandiosity). "I'm the only one who can save the world, but they won't let me."

At times, delusions hold a kernel of truth. One patient came into the hospital acutely psychotic. He repeatedly told the staff that the mafia was out to kill him. Later, the staff learned that the patient had been selling drugs, had not paid his contacts, and gang members were trying to find him to hurt or even kill him.

Other common delusions observed in schizophrenia include the following:

- Thought broadcasting—belief that one's thoughts can be heard by others (e.g., "My brain is connected to the world mind. I can control all heads of state through my thoughts.")
- Thought insertion—belief that thoughts of others are being inserted into one's mind (e.g., "They make me think bad thoughts.")
- Thought withdrawal—belief that thoughts have been removed from one's mind by an outside agency (e.g., "The devil takes my thoughts away and leaves me empty.")
- **Delusion of being controlled**—belief that one's body or mind is controlled by an outside agency (e.g., "There is a man from darkness who controls my thoughts with electrical waves") and made to feel emotions or sensations (e.g., sexual) that are not one's own.

Concrete thinking. Concrete thinking refers to an overemphasis on specific details and impairment in the ability to use abstract concepts. For example, during an assessment, the nurse might ask what brought the patient to the hospital. The patient might answer "a cab" rather than explaining the reason for seeking medical or psychiatric aid. When asked to give the meaning of the proverb "People in glass houses shouldn't throw stones," the person with schizophrenia might answer, "Don't throw stones or the windows will break." The answer is literal; the ability to use abstract reasoning is absent.

Alterations in speech

Associative looseness. Associations are the threads that tie one thought to another and one concept to another. In schizophrenia, these threads are missing, and connections are interrupted. In associative looseness (or looseness of association [LOA]), thinking becomes haphazard, illogical, and confused.

TABLE 17-2	SUMMARY OF HALLUCINATIONS*	
TYPE OF HALLUCINATION	**DEFINITION**	**EXAMPLE**
Auditory	Hearing voices or sounds that do not exist in the environment but are projections of inner thoughts or feelings	Anna "hears" the voice of her dead mother call her a whore and a tramp.
Visual	Seeing a person, object, or animal that does not exist in the environment	Charles, who is experiencing alcohol withdrawal delirium, "sees" hungry rats coming toward him.
Olfactory	Smelling odors that are not present in the environment	Theresa "smells" her insides rotting.
Gustatory	Tasting sensations that have no stimulus in reality	Sam will not eat his food because he "tastes" the poison the FBI is putting in his food.
Tactile	Feeling strange sensations where no external objects stimulate such feelings; common in delirium tremens	Jack suffers from paranoid schizophrenia. He "feels" electrical impulses controlling his mind.

*A hallucination is a false sensory perception for which no external stimulus exists. Hallucinations are different from illusions in that illusions are misperceptions or misinterpretations of a real experience. For example, a man sees his coat hanging on a coat rack and believes it to be a bear about to attack him. He does see something real but misinterprets it.

Zelda Fitzgerald wrote her husband, the writer F. Scott Fitzgerald, an account of going mad:

Then the world became embryonic in Africa—and there was no need for communication…. I have been living in vaporous places peopled with one-dimensional figures and tremulous buildings until I can no longer tell an optical illusion from a reality…head and ears incessantly throb and roads disappear (Vidal, 1982).

Neologisms. Neologisms are made-up words that have special meaning for the person, for example: "I was going to tell him the *mannerologies* of his hospitality just won't do." "I want all the *vetchkisses* to leave the room and let me be." Children and creative writers often make up their own words, but their creation of neologisms is imaginative, constructive, and adaptive. Neologisms in people with schizophrenia represent a disruption in thought processes.

Echolalia. Echolalia is the pathological repeating of another's words by imitation and is often seen in people with catatonia. Echolalia is the counterpart of **echopraxia,** mimicking of the *movements* of another, which is also seen in catatonia.

Clang association. Clang association is the meaningless rhyming of words, often in a forceful manner ("On the track…have a Big Mac…or get the sack"), in which the rhyming is often more important than the context of the word. This form of speech pattern may be seen in individuals with schizophrenia; however, it may also be seen in people in the manic phase of a bipolar disorder or in individuals with a cognitive disorder, such as Alzheimer's disease or HIV-related dementia.

Word salad. Word salad is a term used to identify a jumble of words that is meaningless to the listener and perhaps to the speaker as well. It may include a string of neologisms. For example, "I sang out for my mother…for this to hell I went. How long is road? These little said three hills hop aboard, share

the appetite of the Christmas mice spread…within three round moons the devil will be washed away."

Alterations in perception

Hallucinations. Hallucinations, especially auditory hallucinations, are the major example of schizophrenic alteration in perception. Hallucinations can be defined as sensory perceptions for which no external stimulus exists. The most common types of hallucination are the following:
- Auditory—hearing voices or sounds
- Visual—seeing persons or things
- Olfactory—smelling odors
- Gustatory—experiencing tastes
- Tactile—feeling bodily sensations

Table 17-2 provides examples of these common types of hallucinations and describes the difference between hallucinations and illusions.

It is estimated that up to 90% of people with schizophrenia experience hallucinations at some time during their illness. Although manifestations of hallucination are varied, auditory hallucinations are most common in schizophrenia. Voices may seem to come from outside or inside the person's head. The voices may be familiar or strange, single or multiple. Voices speaking directly to the person or commenting on the person's behavior are most common. A person may believe that the voices are from God, the devil, deceased relatives, or strangers. The auditory hallucinations may occasionally take the form of sounds other than voices.

Command hallucinations must be assessed carefully because the voices may command the person to hurt self or others. For example, a patient might state that "the voices" are saying "jump out the window" or "take a knife and kill your child." Command hallucinations are often terrifying for the individual. Command hallucinations may signal a psychiatric emergency. Patients who can give an identity to the hallucinated voice are at somewhat greater risk of compliance with the hallucinated command than are those who cannot (Junginger, 1995).

Evidence of possible auditory hallucinatory behavior is turning or tilting of the head—as if the patient is listening to someone—or frequent blinking of the eyes and grimacing. Sometimes, patients verbally respond to "unseen others." Visual hallucinations occur less frequently in people with schizophrenia and are more likely to occur in people with organic disorders.

Personal boundary difficulties. People with schizophrenia often lack a sense of where their bodies end in relationship to where others begin. Patients might say that they are merging with others or are part of inanimate objects. For example, **depersonalization** is a nonspecific feeling that a person has lost his or her identity; the self is different or unreal. People may be concerned that body parts do not belong to them, or they may have an acute sensation that the body has drastically changed. For example, a woman may see her fingers as snakes or her arms as rotting wood. A man may look in a mirror and state that his face is that of an animal. **Derealization** is the false perception by a person that the environment has changed. For example, everything seems bigger or smaller, or familiar surroundings have become strange and unfamiliar.

Alterations in behavior. Bizarre and agitated behaviors are associated with schizophrenia and may have a variety of manifestations. **Bizarre behavior** may take the form of a stilted, rigid demeanor and eccentric dress, grooming, and rituals. Many of these behaviors are associated with catatonic schizophrenia but may be seen in other conditions as well (e.g., brain damage, extreme manic phase of bipolar disorder).

- **Extreme motor agitation** is excited physical behavior, such as running about, in response to inner and outer stimuli, which can be harmful to self as well as to others.
- **Stereotyped behaviors** are motor patterns that originally had meaning to the person (e.g., sweeping the floor, washing windows) but are now mechanical and lack purpose.
- **Automatic obedience** is the performance by a catatonic patient of all simple commands in a robot-like fashion.

- **Waxy flexibility,** seen in catatonia, is evidenced by excessive maintenance of posture. Patients can hold unusual postures for long periods.
- **Stupor** refers to a state in which the catatonic patient is motionless for long periods and may even appear to be in a coma.
- **Negativism** is equivalent to resistance. In *active negativism*, the patient does the opposite of what he or she is told to do. When a person does not perform activities that are normal expectations, such as getting out of bed, dressing, and eating, the behavior is termed *passive negativism (catatonia).*

When patients with schizophrenia are acutely ill, impulse control is lacking. Frequently the lack of impulse control is expressed in socially inappropriate **agitated behaviors** such as grabbing another's cigarette, throwing food on the floor, and obtaining the television remote control and changing channels abruptly.

Negative Symptoms

Negative symptoms—such as apathy, anhedonia, poor social functioning, and poverty of thought—are most likely a result of the neurocognitive defects and are associated with an insidious onset, premorbid history of emotional problems, chronic deterioration, demonstration of atrophy on CT scans, abnormal results on neuropsychological tests, and poor response to antipsychotic therapy.

The negative symptoms of schizophrenia develop over a long period of time. These are the symptoms that most interfere with the individual's adjustment and ability to survive. The presence of negative symptoms impedes the person's ability to initiate and maintain relationships and conversations, hold a job, make decisions, and maintain adequate hygiene and grooming.

The presence of negative symptoms contributes to the person's poor social functioning and social withdrawal. During an acute psychotic episode, negative symptoms are difficult to assess because the positive and more florid symptoms, such as delusions and hallucinations, dominate. Some of the negative phenomena are outlined in Table 17-3.

TABLE 17-3	NEGATIVE SYMPTOMS OBSERVED IN SCHIZOPHRENIA
PHENOMENON	**EXPLANATION**
Affective blunting	In *affective blunting*, severe reduction in the expression, range, and intensity of affect occurs; in *flat affect* no facial expression of emotion is present
Anergia	Lack of energy: passivity, lack of persistence at work or school
Anhedonia	Inability to experience any pleasure in activities that usually produce pleasurable feelings; result of profound emotional barrenness
Avolition	Lack of motivation: inability to initiate tasks, such as social contacts, grooming, and other aspects of activities of daily living
Poverty of content of speech	Speech that is adequate in amount but conveys little information because of vagueness, empty repetitions, or use of stereotypes or obscure phrases
Poverty of speech	Restriction in the amount of speech—answers range from brief to monosyllabic one-word answers
Thought blocking	May be signaled when a patient stops talking in the middle of a sentence and remains silent. After a patient stops abruptly: *Nurse:* "What just happened now?" *Patient:* "I forgot what I was saying. Something took my thoughts away."

Affect is the observable behavior that expresses a person's emotions. In people with schizophrenia, affect may not coincide with inner emotions. Affect can usually be categorized in one of three ways: flat or blunted, inappropriate, or bizarre. A **flat affect** (immobile facial expression or a blank look) or **blunted affect** (minimal emotional response) is commonly seen in schizophrenia. **Inappropriate affect** refers to an emotional response to a situation that is not congruent with the tone of the situation. For example, a young man breaks into laughter when told that his father has died. **Bizarre affect** is especially prominent in the disorganized form of schizophrenia and includes grimacing, giggling, and mumbling to oneself. Bizarre affect is marked when the patient is unable to relate logically to the environment.

Neurocognitive Symptoms

Neurocognitive symptoms represent the third dimension and affect at least 40% to 60% or more of people with schizophrenia. Neurocognitive symptoms disrupt all aspects of the patient's life. Cognitive impairment destroys a patient's ability to hold a job, initiate or maintain a social support system, or live on his or her own. Cognitive impairment also causes difficulty with attention, memory, and executive functions (e.g., decision making and problem solving); impedes the person's ability to manage his or her own health care and/or participate fully in relapse prevention programs; and generally devastates the person's quality of life.

The degree of cognitive deficit is associated with the severity of negative symptoms; **disorganized thinking** reflects the degree to which disorganized speech, disorganized behavior, or inappropriate affect is present. Good verbal memory is one cognitive indicator that the individual eventually can function within the community because it helps with acquisition of psychosocial skills or learning and with retention of skills. These are all necessary for eventual rehabilitation (Beng-Choon et al., 2004).

Depressive and Other Mood Symptoms

Depressive symptoms increase the suffering of patients with schizophrenia and are all too common. Recognition of depression during assessment is crucial because it can increase the likelihood of suicide and substance abuse as well as impaired functioning.

Presentations of Schizophrenia Spectrum Disorders

People with schizophrenia have different neuroanatomical findings, distinct courses of disease development, and various prognoses for their future. For example, patients with different prominent symptoms (e.g., paranoid, catatonic, disorganized, undifferentiated, or residual) will have different presentations. Although not all patients will meet all *DSM* criteria for schizophrenia disorders, it is helpful to be aware of the possible symptoms and to understand how each symptom can present. This knowledge will help determine the optimal approaches to guidance and treatment of each patient.

Paranoid

Any intense and strongly defended irrational suspicion can be regarded as paranoia. Paranoid ideas cannot be corrected by experiences and cannot be modified by facts or reality. Projection is the most common defense mechanism used by people who are paranoid. For example, when paranoid individuals feel self-critical, they experience others as being harshly critical toward them. When they feel *angry*, they experience others as being unjustly angry at them, as if to say, "I'm not angry, you are!"

Because people who are paranoid are unable to trust the actions of those around them, they are usually guarded, tense, and reserved. Although patients may keep themselves aloof from interpersonal contacts, impairment in actual functioning may be minimal. To ensure interpersonal distance, they may adopt a superior, hostile, and sarcastic attitude. A common defense used by paranoid individuals to maintain self-esteem is to disparage others and dwell on the shortcomings of others. The patient frequently misinterprets the messages of others or gives private meaning to the communications of others (ideas of reference). For example, a patient might see his or her nurse talking to the physician and believe that they are planning to harm him or her in some manner. Minor oversights are often interpreted as personal rejection.

People with prominent paranoia usually have a later age of onset of the disease (late twenties to thirties). In some cases, the presence of paranoid schizophrenia is associated with a good outcome or with recovery. People with strong paranoid features usually have their cognitive abilities intact, since psychotic paranoia usually appears later in life. When such a person is amenable to psychopharmacology, their paranoid delusions are usually lessened to a great degree. Thus, they are often able to work, often in jobs that require a high degree of cognitive skills; however, they usually perform better in solitary pursuits and projects where their paranoia is less likely to be stimulated.

> **VIGNETTE**
>
> Sam stares at the nurse as she explains how to replace a bandage after minor surgery on his face. He frequently looks at the door and places himself near it. His general demeanor is condescending, and he becomes sarcastic when the nurse drops a bandage asking, "Are you the best they could give me?" When the nurse answers the phone, he says, "So they got to you, too. You are all plotting against me" *(ideas of reference)*. He starts to mutter to himself and looks to his side as if he is talking to someone *(auditory hallucinations)*.

Paranoid states may occur in numerous mental or organic disorders. For example, people experiencing psychotic depression, a manic episode, or certain physical conditions (e.g., organic brain disease, drug intoxications) also may exhibit paranoid symptoms.

Catatonic

Although we tend to think of catatonia in terms of immobility, the essential feature of catatonia is extreme abnormal motor behavior. In fact, patients exhibit either extreme motor agitation or extreme psychomotor retardation (with mutism, or even stupor) in this *rare* form of schizophrenia.

During the very withdrawn phase, the person does not move or eat, thus becoming vulnerable to pressure ulcers, contractures, and malnutrition. Patients may exhibit bizarre **posturing**—such as holding arms or legs rigidly or bent at severe angles for a long period of time. Also, waxy flexibility may occur—for example, when a leg or arm is placed in an awkward position by someone else, the patient will hold that position for an uncomfortable length of time.

Another trait of catatonia is stereotyped behavior or following a routine obsessively, such as continually arranging and rearranging objects; extreme negativism and resistance as well as automatic obedience are other characteristics of catatonia. Speech patterns may include echolalia (persistently repeating the words of others), and echopraxia (mimicking the movements or gestures of others) may also be present.

During the extreme motor activity phase, the patient may run about ceaselessly and without purpose, leading to exhaustion, cardiac difficulties, or physical collapse. The onset of catatonia is usually abrupt, and the prognosis is favorable. Fortunately, with the advances in pharmacotherapy and improved individual management, severe catatonic symptoms are rarely seen today.

VIGNETTE

Mary has been motionless and has not spoken for days. When her husband raises her arm to dress her and take her to the hospital, it stays raised in the air until he lowers it *(waxy flexibility)*. When she starts to move, she does everything she is told to do (get up, sit down) and only moves on command *(automatic obedience)*. When he speaks to her, she repeats everything he says (e.g., "Mary drink this water," "Mary drink this water" *(echolalia)*.

Refer to the Evolve site for a case study of a patient who has catatonia.

Disorganized

Disorganized components of schizophrenia represent the most regressed and socially impaired of all the schizophrenias. People who are diagnosed with this severe mental illness (SMI) are often homeless, making them easy targets for maltreatment. A person diagnosed with disorganized schizophrenia may have marked looseness of associations, grossly inappropriate affect, bizarre mannerisms, and incoherence of speech, and may display extreme social withdrawal. Although delusions and hallucinations are present, they are fragmentary and poorly organized. Behavior may be considered odd, and giggling or grimacing in response to internal stimuli is common.

Disorganized schizophrenia has an earlier age of onset (early to middle teens) and often develops insidiously. It is associated with poor premorbid functioning, a significant family history of psychopathological disorders, and a poor prognosis. Often, these patients are in state hospitals and can live in the community safely only in a structured and well-supervised setting. Unfortunately a large portion of the homeless population consists of people with this disorder. Families living with a person with disorganized schizophrenia need significant community support, respite care, and day hospital affiliations.

VIGNETTE

Pete pushes his grocery cart down the street loaded with rags, bottles, bags, and such. He appears disheveled, dressed in a dirty plaid shirt, a dirty baseball hat, and ragged jeans. He is giggling and laughing to himself. Once in a while he shouts out something, "Alms for the poor me...howdy to you all.... Where is it? Where is it?" *(looseness of association)*. He goes from garbage can to garbage can rummaging for food.

Undifferentiated

In the undifferentiated type of schizophrenia, active signs of the disorder (positive or negative symptoms) are present, but the individual does not meet the criteria for paranoid, catatonic, or disorganized type. As with disorganized schizophrenia, undifferentiated schizophrenia begins early and has an insidious onset (early to middle teens). However, the premorbid state is less predictable, and the disability remains fairly stable, although persistent, over time.

Residual

In the residual type of schizophrenia, active-phase symptoms are no longer present, but evidence of two or more residual symptoms persists. Residual symptoms include lack of initiative, social withdrawal, inability to work or study, vague or lack of content of speech, and magical thinking or odd beliefs.

ASSESSMENT GUIDELINES

Schizophrenia and Other Psychotic Disorders

1. Determine if the patient had a medical workup; if so, was medical or substance-induced psychosis ruled out?
2. Verify whether the patient is dependent on alcohol or drugs.
3. Assess for command hallucinations (e.g., voices telling the person to harm self or another). If present, ask the patient:
   - Do you plan to follow the command?
   - Do you believe the voices are real?
   - Do you recognize the voices?

4. Review the patient's belief system. Is it fragmented? Is it poorly or well organized? Is it systematized? Is the system of beliefs unsupported by reality (delusion)? If yes, then find out if:
   - Delusions focus on someone trying to harm the patient.
   - The patient is planning to retaliate against a person or organization.
   - Precautions need to be taken.
5. Assess for co-occurring disorders including:
   - Depression
   - Suicidality
   - Anxiety
   - Substance dependency
   - History of violence
6. Inventory the patient's medications and assess whether the patient is adhering to the medication regimen.
7. Determine the family's response to increased symptoms. Are they overprotective? Hostile? Suspicious?
8. Assess the manner in which family members and the patient relate.
9. Review the support system. Is the family well-informed about the disease? Does the family understand the need for medication adherence? Is the family familiar with support groups available in the community or locations where respite and family support may be offered? Have family members received or been referred for psychoeducation?
10. Assess the patient's global functioning (using the Global Assessment of Functioning [GAF] Scale) (see Chapter 2).

DIAGNOSIS

People with schizophrenia have multiple disturbing and disabling symptoms that necessitate a multifaceted approach to care and treatment of the patient as well as the family. Table 17-4 lists potential nursing diagnoses for a person with schizophrenia.

TABLE 17-4 POTENTIAL NURSING DIAGNOSES FOR SCHIZOPHRENIA

SYMPTOM	NURSING DIAGNOSES*
Positive Symptoms	
Hallucinations	
Hears voices that others do not	Disturbed Sensory Perception: auditory or visual[†]
	Impaired Environmental Interpretation Syndrome
	Fear
Hears voices telling him or her to hurt self or others (command hallucinations)	Risk for Self-Directed/Other-Directed Violence
	Ineffective Impulse Control
Distorted Thinking Not Based on Reality	
Persecution: Thinks that others are trying to harm self	Disturbed Thought Processes[†]
Jealousy: Thinks that spouse or lover is being unfaithful, or thinks others are jealous of self when they are not	Defensive Coping
	Disturbed Personal Identity
Grandeur: Incorrectly thinks he or she has powers and talents or is someone powerful or famous	Impaired Environmental Interpretation Syndrome
Reference: Believes that all events within the environment are directed at or hold special meaning for self	
Looseness of association: Shows loose association of ideas	Impaired Verbal Communication
Clang association: Uses words that rhyme in a nonsensical fashion	Disturbed Thought Processes[†]
Echolalia: Repeats words that are heard	
Mutism: Does not speak	
Circumstantiality: Delays getting to the point of communication because of unnecessary and tedious details	
Concrete thinking: Unable to abstract; uses literal translations concerning aspects of the environment	
Negative Symptoms	
Uncommunicative, withdrawn, makes no eye contact	Social Isolation
Preoccupied with own thoughts	Impaired Social Interaction
Expresses feelings of rejection or aloneness (lies in bed all day, positions back to door)	Risk for Loneliness
	Ineffective Relationship
Is stigmatized for diagnosis of schizophrenia	Risk for Compromised Human Dignity
Talks about self as "bad" or "no good"	Chronic Low Self-Esteem
Feels guilty because of "bad thoughts"; extremely sensitive to real or perceived slights	Risk for Self-Directed Violence
	Risk for Suicide

Continued

TABLE 17-4 POTENTIAL NURSING DIAGNOSES FOR SCHIZOPHRENIA—cont'd	
SYMPTOM	**NURSING DIAGNOSES***
Shows lack of energy **(anergia)**	*Ineffective Coping*
Shows lack of motivation **(avolition),** unable to initiate tasks (social contact, grooming, and other aspects of daily living)	*Bathing Self-Care Deficit*
	Dressing Self-Care Deficit
	Self-Neglect
	Constipation
	Deficient Diversional Activity
Other	
Families and significant others become confused or overwhelmed, have lack of knowledge about disease or treatment, feel powerless in coping with patient at home	*Compromised Family Coping*
	Impaired Parenting
	Caregiver Role Strain
	Deficient Knowledge
	Deficient Community Health
Nonadherence to medication and treatment	*Nonadherence*
Patient stops taking medication (often from side effects), stops going to therapy groups, family and significant others not aware of need for medications and treatments	

*Nursing Diagnoses—Definitions and Classification 2012-2014. Copyright © 2012, 1994-2012 by NANDA International. Used by arrangement with Blackwell Publishing Limited, a company of John Wiley and Sons, Inc.

†Disturbed Sensory Perception: auditory or visual and Disturbed Thought Processes are not included the 2012-2014 edition of Nursing Diagnoses—Definitions and Classification. However, because schizophrenia and so many other mental disorders are caused by disturbances in neurological functioning, Disturbed Sensory Perception: auditory or visual appeared to be the most accurate diagnosis to use for hallucinations and delusions, and because schizophrenia is known as a thought disorder, the diagnosis Disturbed Thought Processes seems to be ideal. Therefore, they are included here but probably should not appear on your nursing care plan.

OUTCOMES IDENTIFICATION

Phase I (Acute)

During the acute phase of the illness, the overall goal is **patient safety and medical stabilization.** Therefore if the patient is at risk for violence to self or others, initial outcome criteria should address safety issues (e.g., *patient consistently refrains from inflicting serious injury to self or others*). Another outcome might be *patient consistently refrains from acting on delusions or hallucinations.* Medication adherence is a vital outcome for all phases of recovery. Ideally, outcomes should focus on enhancing the patient's strengths and minimizing the patient's deficits.

Phase II (Maintenance) and Phase III (Stabilization)

Outcome criteria during the maintenance and stabilization phases focus on helping the patient to adhere to medication regimens, understand schizophrenia, and participate in available psychoeducational activities for both the patient and the family.

During the stabilization phase, goals are directed toward continual recovery, improvement in functioning, and enhancement of the individual's quality of life. Improvement in functioning includes the ability to participate in social, vocational, or self-care skills' training and involvement in social groups at various levels.

It is also important to include outcomes that address anxiety control and relapse prevention. Desired outcomes to reduce the patient's vulnerability to psychosis include the following: maintain a regular sleep pattern; reduce alcohol, drug, and caffeine intake; keep in touch with supportive friends and family; stay active (engage in exercise, hobbies, employment); have a routine daily and weekly schedule including enjoyable activities; and take medication regularly.

PLANNING

Phase I (Acute)

During the acute phase of schizophrenia, brief hospitalization is frequently indicated if the patient is considered a danger to self or others, refuses to eat or drink, or is too disorganized to provide self-care. Another indication for hospitalization is the need for specific observation, neurological workup, or other medically related tests or treatments. The planning process focuses on the best strategies to ensure patient safety and provide symptom stabilization.

At this time the treatment team identifies aftercare needs for follow-up and support, as well as the appropriate referrals that will benefit the patient and family. Discharge planning considers not only external factors, such as the patient's living arrangement, economic resources, social supports, and family relationships, but also the internal factor of the patient's vulnerability to stress. Because relapse can be devastating to long-term functioning, vigorous efforts are made to connect the patient with community agencies that provide social supports and programs designed to help the patient remain well.

Phase II (Maintenance) and Phase III (Stabilization)

Planning during the maintenance and stabilization phases of treatment focuses on strategies to provide patient and family education and skills training (psychosocial education). **Relapse prevention skills are vital.** Planning identifies the social, interpersonal, coping, and vocational skills needed, as well as how and where these needs can best be met within the community. **Interventions are always geared toward the patient's strengths and healthy functioning as well as areas of deficiency.**

IMPLEMENTATION

Self-Care for Nurses

A person who is psychotic is intensely anxious, lonely, dependent, and distrustful. The intensity of these emotions often evokes similar emotions in others. Another challenge is trying to understand what the person is saying or means to say when his or her language is incomprehensible to you (LOA). Knowing how to deal with people who are actively hallucinating, or have strong delusional systems (e.g., paranoid), can be very frightening for people who have not been exposed to this before. Usually the hallucinations and delusions are most pronounced when the individual is experiencing extreme levels of anxiety. Anxiety can be transferred to the nurse, clinician, and physician. Initially, students and nurses new to working with people with severe mental health problems need guidance and support. Without the support of more experienced nurses to explore these reactions, the novice nurse may adopt defensive behaviors such as denial or withdrawal and avoidance. For nurses new to the psychiatric setting, especially for student nurses, supportive supervision must be available if learning is to occur. The student's part in the supervisory process is a willingness to discuss and identify personal feelings and problem behaviors. This can be, and often is, accomplished in group supervision; experienced psychiatric nurses call this peer group supervision.

Phase I (Acute)

As with outcomes identification and planning, interventions are geared toward the phase of schizophrenia (Table 17-5). During phase I the clinical focus is on crisis intervention, acute symptom stabilization (medication), and safety. As a result of the recent trend toward decreasing the length of hospital stays, alternatives such as partial hospitalization, halfway houses, and day treatment centers are frequently used as cost-effective alternatives to hospitalization. **Acute-phase interventions** include acute psychopharmacological treatment (psychobiological intervention), supportive and directive communications, limit setting (milieu management

and counseling), and psychiatric, medical, and neurological evaluation.

Phase II (Maintenance) and Phase III (Stabilization)

Once the acute symptoms are somewhat stabilized, the hospitalized patient is discharged to the community, where appropriate treatment can be carried out during the maintenance and stabilization phases. Effective long-term care of an individual with schizophrenia relies on a three-pronged approach: medications, nursing interventions, and community support. **Family psychoeducation, as well as community support, is a key component of effective treatment.**

Phase II and phase III interventions include the following:
Health teaching:
- For the patient and family about the disease
- For the patient and family about medication management
- In cognitive and social skills enhancement
- Of strategies to minimize stress and to control anxiety levels

Health promotion and maintenance:
- To identify signs of relapse and take preventive steps
- To improve deficits in self-care, social, and work functioning
- To encourage participation in nonthreatening activities
- To encourage social relationships
- To encourage family interaction

Communication Guidelines

Therapeutic strategies for communicating with patients with schizophrenia focus on lowering the patient's anxiety, decreasing defensive patterns, encouraging participation in therapeutic and social events, raising feelings of self-worth, and increasing medication compliance. Familiarity with the principles used for dealing with phenomena such as hallucinations, delusions, paranoia, and looseness of association is helpful for establishing rapport and being effective.

Hallucinations

Because hearing voices is the most common hallucinatory experience reported by patients, the nurse initially should try to understand what the voices are saying or telling the person to do. Suicidal or homicidal messages necessitate initiation of safety measures for all members of the health care team.

Hallucinations are real to the person who is experiencing them. Nurses should approach patients who are hallucinating in a nonthreatening and nonjudgmental manner. It is thought that when a person is hallucinating, the individual is experiencing anxiety, fear, loneliness, and low self-esteem, and the brain is not processing stimuli accurately.

During the acute phase of the illness, the nurse should maintain eye contact, call the patient by name, and speak simply but in a louder voice than usual.

Patient: "I hear my mother's voice saying terrible things about me. She says I am no good and should be punished."

Nurse: "That must be very upsetting, Tom. Are you feeling upset?" (*Nurse waits for a response.*)

TABLE 17-5	TREATMENT FOCUS AT DIFFERENT PHASES OF SCHIZOPHRENIA		
PHASE I		**PHASE II**	**PHASE III**
ACUTE: ONSET, EXACERBATION, OR RELAPSE	SUBACUTE OR CONVALESCENT	MAINTENANCE ADAPTIVE PLATEAU	STABLE PLATEAU
Clinical Focus			

Crisis intervention
Safety
Acute symptom
  stabilization
	Social supports
	Stress and vulnerability
	  assessment
	Living arrangements
	Daily activities
	Economic resources
		Understanding and
		  acceptance of illness
			Social, vocational, and
			  self-care skills
			Learning or relearning
			Identification of realistic
			  expectations
			Adaptation to deficits

Intervention			

Acute psychopharmacological
  treatment
Limit setting
Supportive and directive
  care
Psychiatric, medical, neurological
  evaluation
Meeting with family
	Psychosocial evaluation
	Linkage with:
	• Social services
	• Human services
	• Community treatment
	  agencies
	Psychoeducational
	  interventions with
	  families
		Support and teaching
		Medication teaching and
		  side effect management
		Direct assistance with
		  situational problems
		Identification of prodromal
		  and acute symptoms and
		  signs of relapse
		Continued psychoeduca-
		  tional work with families
		  as needed
			Attention to details of
			  self-care, social, and
			  work functioning
			Direct intervention with
			  family and/or employers
			Cognitive and social skills
			  enhancement
			Medication maintenance
			Continued psychoeduca-
			  tional intervention with
			  families as needed

Professional Collaboration			

Inpatient treatment team
Residential alternative to
  hospitalization
Community crisis intervention
Internist
Neurologist
	Social work department
	Health and human
	  services
	Day treatment or a variety
	  of community support
	  services
		Community support staff
		Family support groups
		Group therapists and
		  self-help groups
		Practitioners of behavioral
		  therapies using educational
		  models and cognitive
		  restructuring
			Group therapists
			Social, vocational, and
			  self-care providers
			Family, employer,
			  community support
			staff

Adapted from Gabbard, G. O. (2001). *Treatments of psychiatric disorders* (3rd ed.). Washington, DC: American Psychiatric Publishing.

Patient: "Yes, I feel bad."

Nurse: "Let's go over here and play gin. I hear you are a very good gin player."

Here the nurse tries to identify the feelings the patient is experiencing and then distract his attention to something he can do well. Table 17-6 lists interventions for hallucinations.

Delusions

Delusions reflect the misperception of cognitive stimuli. When the nurse attempts to see the world as it appears through the eyes of the patient, it is easier to understand the patient's delusional experience.

Patient: "I see now…you are in on the CIA plot to drain my brain…you all want me destroyed."

Nurse: "I don't want to hurt you, Tom. Thinking that everyone wants to destroy you must be very frightening."

In this example, the nurse clarifies the reality of the patient's experience and empathizes with the patient's apparent experience and feelings of fear. The nurse avoids being drawn into the conversation regarding the content of the delusion (CIA and plot to destroy) but attempts to identify the feelings that the patient is experiencing. Talking about the person's feelings is helpful; talking about delusional material is not.

It is *never* useful to argue with or try to "reason" with the patient regarding the content of the delusion. Doing so can intensify the patient's retention of irrational beliefs. However, it is helpful for the nurse to clarify misinterpretations of the environment.

Patient: "I see the doctor is here, and he is part of this plan to destroy me."

Nurse: "It is true the doctor wants to see you, but he wants to talk to you about your treatment. Would you feel more comfortable talking to him in the day room?"

Interacting with the patient about concrete realities in the environment helps minimize the time available for the patient to focus on delusional thoughts. Performance of specific manual tasks within the scope of the patient's abilities is also useful

TABLE 17-6 INTERVENTIONS FOR HALLUCINATIONS

INTERVENTION	RATIONALE
1. Watch patients for cues that they may be hallucinating (e.g., eyes darting to one side, muttering, or staring sideways; changes in facial expressions).	1. Patients are usually in high levels of anxiety at this time. Early intervention may help interrupt hallucinatory process and lessen patient's anxiety and potential for harm.
2. Ask patients directly if they are hallucinating. "Are you hearing voices?" "What are they saying to you?"	2. The content of the "voices" can help both you and the patient discover patient's feelings (e.g., fear, anger, worthlessness). The nurse can then address the feelings.
3. If voices are telling patient to harm self or others *(command hallucinations):* a. Notify appropriate authority (e.g., police, physician, administrator) according to unit protocols. b. If in the community, evaluate need for hospitalization.	3. People often obey hallucinatory commands to kill self or others. Early assessment and intervention could save lives.
4. **Document:** what patients say, if they are a threat to self or others, who was contacted and notified and when.	4. If patient threatens self or others, documentation shows that correct legal protocols were followed. Otherwise, nurses, physicians, and institutions can be held legally responsible.
5. Accept the fact that the voices are real to the patient, but explain that you do not hear the voices. Refer to the voices as "your voices" or "the voices that you hear."	5. Validating that your reality does not include voices may help patients cast doubt on their voices.
6. Present a calm demeanor and stay with patient while he or she is hallucinating. At times you can tell the patient to tell the "voices they hear" to go away.	6. When patients feel comfortable with a nurse, they can sometimes learn to push the voices aside when given repeated instruction.
7. Keep patients focused on simple, basic, reality-based topics. Help patient focus on one idea at a time.	7. Hallucinating patients are confused and disorientated; helps patient focus on people and happenings in reality.
8. Help patient identify times and situations when hallucinations are the most prevalent and intense.	8. Helps nurse and patient identify situations and times that are the most threatening and find ways to mitigate perceived threats.
9. Assess for signs of increase in anxiety, fear, or agitation and intervene as soon as possible.	9. The earlier intervention takes place, the easier it is to calm patient and prevent harm.

in distracting the patient from delusional thinking. The more time the patient spends engaged in reality-based activities or with people, the more opportunity the patient has to become comfortable with reality. Table 17-7 lists interventions for a patient experiencing delusions.

Paranoia

A paranoid individual may make offensive yet accurate criticisms of the nurse or the unit policies. It is important that the staff not react to these criticisms with anxiety or rejection of the patient. Staff conferences, peer groups, and clinical supervision are effective ways of looking beyond the behaviors to the motivations of the patient. This provides the opportunity to reduce the patient's anxiety and increase staff effectiveness.

It is important to approach a patient who is paranoid in a nonjudgmental, respectful manner and use clear and simple language, which helps minimize the opportunity for the patient to misconstrue the meaning of a message. Be honest and consistent with the patient regarding expectations and in enforcing rules. Suspicious people are quick to discern dishonesty.

Honesty and consistency increase stability and decrease tension. Explaining to the patient what you are going to do prepares the patient and minimizes the opportunity for misinterpreting your intent as hostile or aggressive. Avoid laughing, whispering, or talking quietly when the patient cannot hear what is being said. Suspicious patients will automatically think that they are the target of the interaction and interpret it in a negative manner *(ideas of reference).*

Associative Looseness

The symptom of associative looseness often mirrors the patient's autistic thoughts and reflects the person's poorly organized thinking. An increase in this type of communication often indicates that the patient is feeling increased anxiety and an inability to respond to internal and external stimuli. The patient's ramblings also may confuse and frustrate the nurse. The following communication guidelines are useful with a patient whose speech is confused and disorganized:

- Do not pretend that you understand the patient's communications when you are confused by words or meanings.

TABLE 17-7 INTERVENTIONS FOR DELUSIONS

INTERVENTION	RATIONALE
1. Assess if external controls are needed: if patient is agitated and believes someone is going to harm him/her or if patient must harm someone else to survive; use safety measures.	1. Beliefs are real for the patient and delusional thinking might dictate a need for self-defense. Evaluate least restrictive alternatives (confer with others if helpful).
2. Be aware that patients' delusions represent the way that they are experiencing reality.	2. Identifying patients' experience helps the nurse to understand patients' feelings.

3. Identify feelings:
  a. If belief is an attempt to "get" patient, then patient is experiencing *fear*.
  b. If belief is someone is controlling patient's thoughts, then the patient is experiencing *helplessness*.
	3. The nurse can focus on feelings, not delusional content.
	  a. "If you believe the CIA is out to kill you, you must feel frightened; are you feeling frightened?"
	  b. "If you believe your thoughts are being controlled, are you feeling helpless?"

4. Do not argue with patient's beliefs or try to correct false beliefs with logic or facts.	4. Arguing will only increase patient's defensive position, thereby reinforcing false beliefs.
5. Do not touch patient; use gestures very carefully, particularly if patient is paranoid.	5. Give delusional patient lots of space. Touching may be perceived as an aggressive or sexual attempt; gestures may be misconstrued to support their delusional thinking.
6. A paranoid patient might not eat or drink, thinking the food is poisoned. Offer food and fluids in closed containers such as a can of soda, a carton of yogurt, unpeeled fruit, or a hardboiled egg.	6. Food that has not "been tampered with" is "safe" to eat, and some nutritional intake is possible.
7. After understanding the patient's underlying feelings (e.g., fear, helplessness), engage patient in reality-based activities such as cards or crafts.	7. When patients are focused on reality-based activities, then their minds are not focused on their delusional thinking; thus the feelings that result with that thinking are momentarily lessened.
If a patient is paranoid, often intellectual functions are higher and may respond better to more intellectually taxing noncompetitive activities.	The more a person is focused in reality, the greater the delusions can be minimized during that time.
8. Observe for events that trigger delusions.	8. Essentially, observe for events that make the patient anxious and fearful. Problem solve ways to mitigate the effect of these situations or events.
9. If anxiety begins to escalate out of control use least restrictive interventions (e.g., one-to-one therapy, prn medications, or seclusion). Always follow unit protocol and provide careful documentation.	9. The whole idea is to lower patients' anxiety. Usually a calm nonthreatening presence during high levels of anxiety helps lower anxiety levels.

- Tell the patient that you are having difficulty understanding.
- Place the difficulty in understanding on yourself, *not* on the patient. For example, say, "I am having trouble following what you are saying," *not* "You are not making any sense."
- Look for recurring topics and themes in the patient's communications. For example, "You've mentioned trouble with your brother several times. Tell me about your brother and your relationship with him."
- Emphasize what is going on in the patient's immediate environment (here and now) and involve the patient in simple reality-based activities. These measures can help the patient better focus thoughts.
- Tell the patient what you do understand, and reinforce clear communication and accurate expression of needs, feelings, and thoughts.

Health Teaching and Health Promotion

The family needs to be included in any psychological strategies aimed at reducing exacerbation of psychotic symptoms. Education is an essential strategy and includes teaching the patient and family about the illness (causes, medications, medication side effects, prevention of relapse); helping the patient and family recognize the effect of stress; ensuring an understanding of the importance of medication to a good outcome; encouraging involvement in psychosocial activities; and identifying sources for ongoing support in dealing with the illness. Some hospitals and clinics offer medication groups for patients (and sometimes family members as well). Medication groups can help patients deal more effectively with troubling side effects, alert the nurse to possible adverse or toxic reactions, and increase adherence to the medication regimen.

APPLYING THE ART

A Person With Schizophrenia

SCENARIO: I noticed Aaron standing barefooted in the hallway with both shoes in his outstretched hand. He almost looked like a statue with his blank, unaware demeanor. He deliberately picked up each foot and then slowly rubbed the ball of each foot against the carpet.

THERAPEUTIC GOAL: By the end of the present encounter, Aaron will demonstrate increased comfort with the student nurse as evidenced by voluntarily walking together in the hallways of the psychiatric unit.

STUDENT-PATIENT INTERACTION	THOUGHTS, COMMUNICATION TECHNIQUES, AND MENTAL HEALTH NURSING CONCEPTS
Student: "Aaron, I am _____, one of the nursing students. Aaron, I'm standing next to you, on your right side."	With *schizophrenia* it is important to say his name and say my own name to make clear our separateness.
Student's feelings: *I'm kind of nervous. How scary and lonely his world must be.*	
Aaron: *Quietly murmuring.* "Don't know left, right, right, correct. I can't quite gather first one, last one. Can't last long…long…long lost soul. Soul train."	He may have an *ego boundary* disturbance. He also holds his shoes far away from his body. What are the clues inside his *loose associations?* He looks stuck just standing there yet he holds his shoes like he is *ambivalent* about going somewhere.
Student's feelings: *I wonder why he rubs each foot against the floor like he really needs to feel where the floor is.*	
Student's feelings: *That part, "long lost soul" makes me feel sad. I felt lost when I first arrived here at school without a single friend. When I let myself know what I'm feeling, memories of the losses in my childhood begin to stir.*	I need to focus on Aaron and deal with potential *countertransference* later. His most intense words are "lost soul." That phrase is near the end of his rambling associations. He may remember the last words he spoke at some level. I will *restate* and then use *reflection* of feelings.
Student: "Long lost soul. You're feeling kind of lost right now. It's hard to decide what to do next."	Maybe he wants to get away on his own "soul train." Is he an *elopement* risk? Probably not. He is too confused right now to plan anything, though he may follow easily. I'll give some structure to meet *safety needs.*
Student: "Aaron, it's _____. Come with me and we'll figure out how to help you. *I touch his arm to direct him toward the day area.*	
Aaron: *Abruptly tilts his head toward opposite wall. He begins mumbling like he's responding back to an unseen other.*	The touch violated his precarious *ego boundary.* He's *hallucinating*—my touch tipped him from *moderate to severe anxiety.* I need to speak in short sentences with lots of pauses to slow this down.
Student's feelings: *I'm so upset with myself. I acted without thinking about how threatening my touch would be without asking first. I so want to help him and now I've scared him. I want to say, "I'm sorry" but that's my need. I'll tell him later when he's able to process information. Okay, keep focused. He needs to feel safe more than anything.*	
Student: "Aaron, I'm here. I'll stay with you."	I *offer self.*
Aaron: *Mumbles.* "The mistop…don't…can't…." *Looks panicked.*	He is approaching *panic level* anxiety. "Mistop." What is that? Is it a *neologism?*
Student: "Aaron, talk to me. What are the voices saying?"	
Student's feelings: *My first job is to stay calm myself. He looks terrified. I need to let him know he's safe. I am okay. Even if I don't say everything right, I do care.*	
Aaron: *Shakes his head.* "Soul train, blame, shame, going to the end of the line…supine…surprise…demise."	He is making *clang associations.* I hear covert references that may be to suicide. I will *restate* and then ask a *direct question* to assess suicide potential.

Continued

APPLYING THE ART—cont'd

A Person With Schizophrenia

STUDENT-PATIENT INTERACTION	THOUGHTS, COMMUNICATION TECHNIQUES, AND MENTAL HEALTH NURSING CONCEPTS
Student: "The end of the line; demise. Aaron, are the voices telling you to hurt yourself or someone else?" ***Student's feelings:*** *Overwhelmed, I can't do this alone. Maybe medication will help. I hope at some level he will feel safer.* **Aaron:** *Mumbles.* **Student:** *Without crowding him, I position myself so he can see my face. Quiet and concerned.* "Let's go together to talk to the nurse." **Aaron:** *Slowly walks with me.*	He probably cannot *reality test* enough to tell me whether the voices tell him to kill himself. I must report this now, but I also do not want to leave him alone if there is the slightest potential for suicide. He needs *close constant observation.* Before he did not come with me. Now he is walking beside me. He feels more comfortable with me now.

When people lack understanding of the disease and its symptoms, they may misinterpret the patient's apathy and lack of drive as laziness. This erroneous assumption can foster hostility by family members, caregivers, or others in the community. Thus further teaching about the negative and positive symptoms of schizophrenia can reduce these tensions.

It is vital that nurses, physicians, and social workers be aware of the community support resources and makes this information available to discharged patients as well as to their families. Examples of such resources include community mental health services, home health services, work support programs, day hospitals, social skills and support groups, family educational skills groups, and respite care.

Milieu Therapy

Effective hospital care involves more than protection from family, social, or work environments that are stressful or disruptive. Many patients need the structure provided by hospitalization. In fact, patients in the acute phase of schizophrenia improve more on a unit with a structured milieu than on an open unit that allows greater freedom. Partial hospitalization programs, halfway houses, and day treatment centers also provide a structured milieu. A therapeutic milieu provides safety, useful activities, resources for resolving conflicts, and opportunities for learning social and vocational skills.

Safety

A schizophrenic patient, especially in the acute phase, is prone to physical violence, often in response to hallucinations (voices telling them others are out to harm/kill them) or delusions (believing that another is out to harm/kill them). During this time, measures need to be taken to protect the patient and others. If verbal de-escalation efforts and chemical restraints (antipsychotic medication) fail to lessen the patient's aggression, physical restraints and seclusion may be indicated (see Chapters 6, 15, and 23).

With the shifting of care for the seriously mentally ill from inpatient to community-based treatment centers, the need for transitional care is heightened, and the role of the nurse in providing a therapeutic milieu is broadened. Alternatives to hospitalization include partial hospitalization, halfway houses, and day treatment programs:

- **Partial hospitalization:** Patients sleep at home and attend treatment sessions during the day or evening.
- **Halfway houses:** Patients live in the community with a group of other patients, sharing expenses and responsibilities. Staff are present in the house 24 hours a day, 7 days a week.
- **Day treatment programs:** Patients live in a halfway house or on their own, sometimes with home visits, or in residential programs. Patients attend a structured program during the day.

Some of these programs may include group therapy, supervised activities, individual counseling, or specialized training and rehabilitation.

Psychotherapy

Program for Assertive Community Treatment

Program for Assertive Community Treatment (PACT) or Assertive Community Treatment (ACT) is designed for the most marginally adjusted and poorly functioning patients. Its aim is to prevent relapse, maximize social and vocational functioning, and keep the individual in the community. It emphasizes the patient's strengths in adapting to the community, provides support and assertive outreach, and involves almost all aspects of the patient's life (e.g., food, shelter, schooling, grooming, budgeting, and transportation). PACT/ACT programs provide mobile crisis intervention, supportive cognitive and behavioral therapy, and substance abuse treatment, to name a few. These programs have been shown to reduce hospital admissions and improve quality of life for many of these patients (Black & Andreasen, 2011). PACT is a team approach available around the clock. Medication adherence is emphasized.

BOX 17-4   PSYCHOEDUCATIONAL STRATEGIES FOR PATIENT AND FAMILY

1. Learn all you can about the illness.
   - Attend psychoeducational groups.
   - Attend support groups.
   - Join the National Alliance on Mental Illness (NAMI).
   - Contact the National Institute of Mental Health (NIMH).
2. Develop a relapse prevention plan.
   - Know the early warning signs of relapse (e.g., social withdrawal, trouble sleeping, increased bizarre or magical thinking).
   - Know whom to call and where to go when early signs of relapse appear.
   - Relapse is part of the illness, not a sign of failure.
3. Take advantage of all psychoeducational tools.
   - Participate in family, group, individual therapy.
   - Learn new behaviors and cognitive coping skills to help handle intrafamily stress and interpersonal, social, and vocational difficulties. Get information from health care workers (nurse, case manager, physician), NAMI, community mental health groups, or a hospital.
   - Everyone needs a place to address their fears and losses, and to learn new ways of coping.
4. Comply with treatment.
   - Research has determined that people who do the best in coping with the disease comply with treatment that works for them.
   - Tell your health care worker (nurse, caseworker, physician, social worker) about troubling side effects (e.g., sexual problems, weight gain, "feeling funny"). Most side effects can be treated.
   - Keeping side effects a secret or stopping medication can prevent you from having the best quality of life. Share your concerns.
5. Avoid alcohol and drugs; they can act on the brain and precipitate a relapse.
6. Keep in touch with supportive people.
7. Keep healthy—stay in balance.
   - Self-care deficit is reflected in high rates of medical comorbidity.
   - Maintain a regular sleep pattern.
   - Maintain self-care (e.g., diet and hygiene).
   - Keep active (hobbies, friends, groups, sports, job, special interests).
   - Learn ways to reduce stress.

Patients and family members should be given telephone numbers and addresses of local support groups that are affiliated with NAMI (www.nami.org).

Data from Zerbe, K. J. (1999). *Women's mental health in primary care.* Philadelphia: Saunders/Baillière Tindall; Tandon, R., et al. (2003). *Beyond symptoms control: moving towards positive patient outcomes.* Paper presented at the American Psychiatric Association 55th Institute on Psychiatric Services, October 31, 2003, Boston. Retrieved January 21, 2005, from www.medscape.com/viewprogram/2835_pnt.

Family Therapy

All evidence-based approaches emphasize the value of family participation in treatment. Families with members who are struggling with schizophrenia often endure considerable hardships while coping with the psychotic and residual symptoms of the illness. Often these families become isolated from their relatives and communities. Families are perhaps the most consistent factor in patients' lives. More than half of patients discharged from a psychiatric facility return to their family of origin. The following example shows how a family came to distinguish between "Martha's problem" and "the problem caused by schizophrenia."

VIGNETTE

It was a good idea, us all meeting in the comfort of our own home to discuss my sister's illness. We were all able to say how it felt, and for the first time I realized that I knew very little about what she was suffering from or how much—the word *schizophrenia* meant nothing to me before but it's much clearer now. I used to think she was just being lazy until she told me in the meeting what it was really like (Gamble & Brennan, 2000).

Programs that provide support, education, coping skills training, and social network development are extremely effective. Medication and psychosocial treatments with family interventions have been shown to reduce relapse rates in the treatment of early schizophrenia (Brauser, 2010); a popular approach with patients and families is a **psychoeducational approach.** It brings educational and behavioral approaches into family treatment. The psychoeducational approach recognizes that families are secondary victims of a biological illness. In family therapy sessions, fears, faulty communication patterns, and distortions are identified. Improved problem-solving skills can be taught, and healthier alternatives to situations of conflict can be explored. Family guilt and anxiety can be lessened, which facilitates change.

Families that receive psychoeducational treatment in multiple-family groups do even better than those treated in single-family groups. Although single- and multiple-family treatments are cost-effective, multiple-family groups are even more so and are the most beneficial both to families and to family members with schizophrenia. Improvement seems to stem from an expansion of the social network available to the family and patient as well as an expansion in problem-solving capacity afforded by a group. Multiple-family groups also decrease emotional overinvolvement while increasing the overall positive tone, which is characteristic of such groups. Box 17-4 lists psychoeducational strategies for the patient and family.

Cognitive Behavioral Therapy

Data support the efficacy of cognitive behavioral therapy (CBT) in conjunction with medication for reducing the frequency and intensity of delusions and hallucinations (positive symptoms), promoting treatment resistance, improving insight and compliance, and alleviating aggression in patients with schizophrenia (Brauser, 2010; Rathod et al., 2010). People with schizophrenia or delusional disorders that seem to benefit most are usually chronic outpatients with treatment-resistant forms of the disease who often have distressing delusions or hallucinations. Usually several months are required, although treatment can last years.

Social Skills Training

Social skills training (SST) can improve the level of social activity, foster new social contacts, improve quality of life, and help lower anxiety. Complex behaviors used in daily living are divided into discrete behavioral techniques (e.g., how to properly answer the phone and take a message, how to initiate a social dialogue, how to order a meal). SST has shown to improve social competence in patients with schizophrenia (Brauser, 2010), especially in those newly diagnosed with the disease.

Pharmacological, Biological, and Integrative Therapies

Drugs used to treat psychotic disorders are called *antipsychotic medications*. Although they may alleviate many of the symptoms of schizophrenia, they cannot cure the underlying psychotic processes. Therefore when patients stop taking their medications, psychotic symptoms usually return. An additional concern is that with each relapse following medication discontinuation it takes longer to achieve remission after restarting medications. This leads to the possibility that the patient will eventually become unresponsive to treatment.

There are two groups of antipsychotic drugs: conventional (traditional), or the dopamine antagonists (D_2 receptor antagonists); and atypical (second-generation), or the serotonin-dopamine antagonists (5-HT_{2A} and 5-HT_{2C} receptor antagonists). In addition, some drugs are used to augment the antipsychotic agents for treatment-resistant patients.

All antipsychotic drugs are effective for most acute exacerbations of schizophrenia and for preventing or mitigating relapse. The conventional (first-generation) antipsychotics target the positive symptoms of schizophrenia, and the atypical (second-generation) antipsychotics are thought to diminish some of the negative symptoms as well. The atypical agents have fewer side effects and thus are better tolerated. The newer atypical agents also help with symptoms of anxiety and depression, decrease suicidal behavior, and are thought to increase neurocognitive functioning.

Although most individuals prefer oral medications, those who are nonadherent to medication therapy and are prone to frequent relapse are candidates for long-lasting injectable formulations.

Antipsychotic agents usually take effect 3 to 6 weeks after the regimen is started. Most patients with schizophrenia respond at least partially to antipsychotic drug therapy. However, without drug treatment, up to 70% to 80% of individuals will relapse within a year.

Because the atypical agents (except for clozapine, which can cause toxic side effects) are generally the treatment of choice for patients experiencing their first episode of schizophrenia, these drugs are discussed first.

Atypical (Second-Generation) Antipsychotics

The atypical antipsychotics (AAPs) first emerged in the early 1990s with clozapine (Clozaril). Unfortunately, clozapine produces agranulocytosis in 0.8% to 1% of people who take it; the drug also increases the risk for seizures. However, clozapine may be used for treatment-refractory patients. The AAPs developed after clozapine do not share these same disadvantages.

The atypical antipsychotics permit more than just control of the most alarming symptoms of schizophrenia (e.g., hallucinations, delusions); they also allow for improvement in the quality of life. Although there does seem to be more use of the conventional (first-generation) antipsychotics, **the atypical antipsychotics are still often chosen as first-line antipsychotics** because they have the following characteristics:

- Have better tolerability with patients than the conventional (first-generation) antipsychotics
- Provide reduction of negative symptoms
- Improve the neurocognitive defects associated with schizophrenia
- May decrease affective symptoms (e.g., anxiety and depression)
- Thought to decrease suicidal behavior
- Reduce neuroanatomical changes/enlargement of the lateral ventricles
- Improve cognition
- Are associated with lower relapse rates

One significant disadvantage of the AAPs is that they all (with the exception of ziprasidone and aripiprazole) have a tendency to cause significant weight gain. Weight gain is a serious metabolic side effect and is associated with a cascade of additional side effects, including:

- Glucose dysregulation, which increases the propensity for diabetes
- Hypercholesterolemia, which increases the propensity for cardiovascular disease
- Hypertension
- Diminished self-esteem related to weight, which leads to problems in adherence to the medication regimen

There have been some cases when the first indication of metabolic syndrome was discovered when the patient developed diabetic coma (Table 17-8).

Conventional (First-Generation) Antipsychotics

The typical antipsychotic agents are becoming much less widely used because of their troubling side effects; however, the conventional antipsychotics are being revisited because of the concern over the metabolic side effects of the AAPs. The National

TABLE 17-8　ATYPICAL (SECOND-GENERATION) ANTIPSYCHOTIC AGENTS (AAPS)

DRUG NAME, GENERIC (TRADE)	ROUTE(S)	INDICATION FOR USE	EPS	ACH	OH	SED	COMMENTS/NOTABLE ADVERSE REACTIONS
Clozapine (Clozaril, Leponex)	PO ODT*: FazaClo	Treatment-resistant schizophrenia and schizophrenia-related suicide behavior	No	High	High	High	• **Not first line;** refractory cases only • Agranulocytosis in 0.8-1%; scheduled WBC required • High seizure rate • Increased risk for diabetes • Significant weight gain (67%) • High lipid abnormalities • Excessive salivation • Tachycardia
Risperidone (Risperdal, Risperdal Consta)	PO ODT*: Risperdal M-TAB Consta Injection (long-acting)	Schizophrenia	Mild (dose-related)	Very low	Moderate	Low	• Hypotension/dizziness • Insomnia • Sedation • Rarely NMS, TD • Sexual dysfunction • Weight gain (18%) • Moderate lipid abnormalities • Increased risk for diabetes
Paliperidone (Invega) Invega Sustena)	Extended release Long-acting intramuscular injection	Schizophrenia and schizoaffective disorder	Mild (dose-related)	Very low	Moderate	Low	• Has same side effects as risperidone • Better tolerated than risperidone • Not approved for elderly, especially those with dementia
Olanzapine† (Zyprexa, Relprevv)	PO ODT*: Zyprexa Long-acting IM injection	Schizophrenia and agitation	Low	Moderate	Moderate	Low	• Significant weight gain (34%) • High lipid abnormalities • Increased risk for diabetes • Drowsiness • Hyperprolactinemia • Agitation and restlessness • Insomnia • Hypotension • Seizures at initiation of therapy • Possibly akathisia or parkinsonism

Continued

TABLE 17-8   ATYPICAL (SECOND-GENERATION) ANTIPSYCHOTIC AGENTS (AAPS)—cont'd

DRUG NAME, GENERIC (TRADE)	ROUTE(S)	INDICATION FOR USE	EPS	Ach	OH	SED	COMMENTS/NOTABLE ADVERSE REACTIONS

Quetiapine (Seroquel, Seroquel XL)	PO	Schizophrenia	Low	Mild	Moderate	Moderate	• Weight gain (23%)
							• Moderate lipid abnormalities
							• May increase risk for diabetes
							• **Serious side effects:**
							  • Cardiac dysrhythmias
							  • Syncope
							  • NMS
							  • Seizures

Ziprasidone (Geodon) Injectable (short acting)	PO
	Short-acting IM injection
		Schizophrenia and acute agitation	Low	Mild	Mild	Low	• **Serious side effects:**
							  • ECG changes‡
							  • QT prolongation, not to be used with other drugs known to prolong QT interval
							• Low propensity for weight gain
							• May cause extrapyramidal side effects (EPS)
							• Targets depressive symptoms

Aripiprazole (Abilify)	PO
	ODT
	Short-acting IM injection
		Schizophrenia and acute agitation	Low	Low to mild	Low to mild	Low	• Little or no weight gain; no increase in glucose, HDL, LDL, or triglyceride levels
							• Can cause anxiety, especially initially
							• May cause dizziness, insomnia, akathisia, sedation
							• **Serious side effects:**
							  • Prolonged QT interval
							  • Diabetic ketoacidosis
							  • Dyskinesia
							  • NMS may occur

Iloperidone (Fanapt)	PO		Low to moderate (dose-dependent)	Low to mild	Low to moderate	Low to moderate	• Weight gain • May affect cardiac QTc interval • Not for use in patients with cardiac conditions as first line • May increase risk for diabetes and dyslipidemia • Severe APS can cause NMS and TD

| Asenapine (Saphris) | Sublingual tablets (ODT*) | Schizophrenia | Low to moderate (dose-dependent) | No | No | Moderate | • May increase risk for diabetes
• Newer drug, at this writing-clinical use will tell; drug trials show favorable side effect profile
• Severe EPS can cause NSM and TD
• Metabolic changes (high blood glucose and diabetes)
• High cholesterol and triglycerides
• Weight gain
• Low white blood cell count
• More sensitive to heat; may take time to cool down
• Most common reactions: sleepiness, inner restlessness (akathisia), movement abnormalities, muscle stiffness (Parkinson-like symptoms) |
| Lurasidone HCl (Latuda) | PO | | High | | | | |

*An orally disintegrating tablet (ODT) is a fast-disintegrating tablet or wafer that dissolves on the tongue.
†The safety of olanzapine at dosages >20 mg/day and quetiapine at dosages >800 mg/day has not been evaluated in clinical trials.
‡Ziprasidone use may carry a risk for QT prolongation in patients with preexisting cardiac disease, low electrolyte levels, or family history of QTc syndrome or in patients taking other drugs that cause long QTc profiles.

Ach, Anticholinergic side effects (dry mouth, blurred vision, urinary retention, constipation, agitation); ECG, electrocardiogram; EPS, extrapyramidal symptoms; HDL, high-density lipoprotein; IM, intramuscular; LDL, low-density lipoprotein; NMS, neuroleptic malignant syndrome; ODT, orally disintegrating tablet; OH, orthostatic hypotension; PO, by mouth; Sed, sedation; TD, tardive dyskinesia; WBC, white blood cell count.

Institute of Mental Health has conducted groundbreaking clinical antipsychotic trials of intervention effectiveness (CATIE) studies to compare continuation rates of typical and atypical antipsychotics. Important findings so far are that people quit taking older medications because of side effects, and that they quit taking the newer ones because of weight gain. There has been some newer interesting evidence. Review of data from 1996 to 2007 revealed that those receiving conventional depo (long-lasting intramuscular injections) as compared to risperidone (atypical antipsychotic) long-acting injections seem to fare better in terms of number of hospital admissions (Lowry, 2011).

Dopamine (D_2) neurotransmission plays a role in psychosis. The conventional antipsychotics are antagonists at the D_2 receptor site in both the limbic and the motor centers. This blockage of D_2 receptor sites in the motor areas is responsible for some of the most troubling side effects of the conventional antipsychotics, namely, the extrapyramidal symptoms (EPS) of akathisia, dystonia, parkinsonism, and tardive dyskinesia. Other adverse reactions include anticholinergic effects, orthostasis, and lowered seizure threshold. It should be noted, however, that the difference between the first generation and the second generation of antipsychotic drugs as far as the extrapyramidal side effects might not be as significant as one thought (Peluso et al, 2012).

When these agents are used, the specific drug is often chosen for its side effect profile. For example, chlorpromazine (Thorazine) is the most sedating agent and has fewer EPS than do other antipsychotic agents, but it causes hypotension at large dosages. Haloperidol (Haldol) is the least sedating and is often used in large dosages to reduce assaultive behavior but has a high incidence of EPS. The value of haloperidol for treating violent behaviors is its effectiveness in controlling hallucinatory phenomena with a low incidence of hypotension. People who are functioning at work or at home may prefer less-sedating drugs; patients who are agitated or excitable may do better with a more sedating medication.

All of the traditional antipsychotic drugs can cause tardive dyskinesia, and should be used with caution in people who have seizure disorders because they can lower the seizure threshold. Table 17-9 identifies drugs according to low, medium, and high

TABLE 17-9　CONVENTIONAL (FIRST-GENERATION) ANTIPSYCHOTICS

DRUG NAME, GENERIC (TRADE)	ROUTE(S) OF ADMINISTRATION	INDICATION FOR USE	SPECIAL CONSIDERATIONS
High Potency: More Sedating, Lower Ach,* and Less Extrapyramidal Side Effects (EPS)			
Haloperidol (Haldol)	Tablet, oral concentrate, short-acting intramuscular injection, long-acting intramuscular injection (lasts 3-4 weeks)	Schizophrenia, acute agitation	Has **low** sedative properties; is used in large doses for assaultive patients to avoid the severe side effect of hypotension Lessens the chance of falls from dizziness or hypotension **High** EPS NMS Ach Tardive dyskinesia
Trifluoperazine (Stelazine)	Capsule, oral concentrate, short-acting intramuscular injection	Schizophrenia	**Low** sedative effect—good for symptoms of withdrawal or paranoia **High** incidence of EPS: akathisia, dystonia, Parkinson-like symptoms, tardive dyskinesia, etc. NMS may occur Anticholinergic side effects (Ach)
Fluphenazine (Prolixin)	Tablet, oral concentrate, short-acting intramuscular injection, long-acting intramuscular injection (every 2-4 weeks)	Schizophrenia	Akathisia, tardive dyskinesia, dystonia, etc. Ach
Medium Potency			
Loxapine (Loxitane)	Capsule, oral concentrate, short-acting intramuscular injection	Schizophrenia	EPS: akathisia, dystonia, Parkinson-like symptoms, tardive dyskinesia, etc. NMS may occur Anticholinergic side effects (Ach) Possibly associated with weight reduction

TABLE 17-9	CONVENTIONAL (FIRST-GENERATION) ANTIPSYCHOTICS—cont'd		
DRUG NAME, GENERIC (TRADE)	**ROUTE(S) OF ADMINISTRATION**	**INDICATION FOR USE**	**SPECIAL CONSIDERATIONS**
Molindone (Moban)	Tablet	Schizophrenia	EPS: akathisia, dystonia, Parkinson-like symptoms, tardive dyskinesia, etc. NMS may occur Ach Same as loxapine Possibly associated with weight reduction
Perphenazine (Trilafon)	Tablet, oral concentrate, short-acting intramuscular injection	Schizophrenia	Can help control severe vomiting Associated with weight gain EPS: akathisia, dystonia, Parkinson-like symptoms, tardive dyskinesia, etc. Ach
Low Potency: More Extrapyramidal Side Effects and Less Sedating			
Chlorpromazine (Thorazine)	Tablet, oral solution, suppository capsule, short-acting intramuscular injection	Schizophrenia	Increases sensitivity to sun (as do other phenothiazines) Highest sedative and hypotensive effects; least potent Ach symptoms May cause irreversible retinitis pigmentosa at ≥800 mg/day EPS: akathisia, dystonia, Parkinson-like symptoms, tardive dyskinesia, etc.
Thioridazine (Mellaril)	Tablet, oral concentrate		Not recommended as first-line antipsychotic Dose-related severe ECG changes (prolonged QTc intervals); may cause sudden death

Ach, Anticholinergic side effects, including dry mouth, dry eyes, blurred vision (especially near vision), urinary retention, intestinal slowing (causing constipation), agitation, sedation, and sexual dysfunction; *ECG,* electrocardiogram; *EPS,* extrapyramidal side effects (parkinson-like side effects, dystonia, akathisia). Refer to Table 17-10.

potency; gives dosages for treatment of acute symptoms and usual maintenance dosages; and lists other considerations.

Tardive dyskinesia (TD) is an EPS that usually appears after prolonged treatment, is more serious, and is not always reversible. Tardive dyskinesia consists of involuntary tonic muscular spasms that typically involve the tongue, fingers, toes, neck, trunk, or pelvis. This potentially serious EPS is most frequently seen in women and older patients, and affects up to 50% of individuals receiving long-term high-dose therapy. Tardive dyskinesia varies from mild to moderate and can be disfiguring or incapacitating.

Early symptoms of tardive dyskinesia are fasciculations of the tongue or constant lip smacking. These early oral movements can develop into uncontrollable biting, chewing, or sucking motions; an open mouth; and lateral movements of the jaw. In many cases, the early symptoms of tardive dyskinesia disappear when the antipsychotic medication is discontinued. In other cases, however, early symptoms are not reversible and may progress. No proven cure for advanced tardive dyskinesia exists. The National Institute of Mental Health developed a brief test for the detection of tardive dyskinesia referred to as the Abnormal Involuntary Movement Scale (AIMS).

Three of the more common EPS are acute dystonia (muscle cramps of the head and neck), akathisia (internal restlessness and external restless pacing or fidgeting), and pseudoparkinsonism (stiffening of muscular activity in the face, body, arms, and legs). The AIMS mentioned in Chapter 7 is one of the tools nurses and physicians can use to detect these EPS.

Neuroleptic malignant syndrome (NMS) occurs in about 0.2% to 1% of patients who have taken antipsychotic agents. It is believed that the acute reduction in brain dopamine activity plays a role in the development of NMS, which is fatal in about 10% of cases. It usually occurs early in the course of therapy but has been reported in people after 20 years of treatment.

Neuroleptic malignant syndrome is characterized by decreased level of consciousness, greatly increased muscle tone, and autonomic dysfunction, including hyperpyrexia, labile hypertension, tachycardia, tachypnea, diaphoresis, and drooling. Treatment consists of early detection, discontinuation of the antipsychotic agent, management of fluid balance, reduction of temperature, and monitoring for complications. Mild cases of neuroleptic malignant syndrome are treated with bromocriptine (Parlodel), whereas more severe cases are treated with intravenous dantrolene (Dantrium) and even with electroconvulsive therapy in some cases. See Table 17-10 for the side effects, onset, and nursing measures for EPS and NMS.

Agranulocytosis is also a serious side effect and can be fatal. Liver involvement also may occur. Nurses need to be aware of the prodromal signs and symptoms of these side effects and teach them to their patients and patients' families.

Side effects often appear early in therapy and can be minimized with treatment. Treatment usually consists of lowering the dosage or prescribing antiparkinsonian drugs, especially centrally acting anticholinergic drugs. Commonly used drugs include trihexyphenidyl (Artane),

TABLE 17-10	NURSING MEASURES FOR EXTRAPYRAMIDAL SYMPTOMS AND NEUROLEPTIC MALIGNANT SYNDROME: CONVENTIONAL (FIRST-GENERATION) ANTIPSYCHOTICS		
SIDE EFFECT		**ONSET**	**NURSING MEASURES**
All conventional antipsychotics share similar side effects, but differ in terms of potency as well as personal reaction to drug. • Anticholinergic side effects (Ach) • Antiadrenergic side effect = orthostatic hypotension (drop in blood pressure upon standing, may lead to falls and injury) • Lower seizure threshold • May raise prolactin levels, causing lactation • **Rarer: agranulocytosis, hyperthermia, neuroleptic malignant syndrome (NMS)**			
Extrapyramidal Symptoms (EPS)			
1. **Pseudoparkinsonism:** masklike facies, stiff and stooped posture, shuffling gait, drooling, tremor, "pill-rolling" phenomenon		5 hours to 30 days	1. Alert medical staff. An anticholinergic agent (e.g., trihexyphenidyl [Artane] or benztropine [Cogentin]) may be used.
2. **Acute dystonic reactions:** acute contractions of tongue, face, neck, and back (tongue and jaw first) • **Opisthotonos:** tetanic heightening of entire body, head and belly up • **Oculogyric crisis:** eyes locked upward		1-5 days	2. First choice: diphenhydramine hydrochloride (Benadryl) 25-50 mg IM/IV. Relief occurs in minutes. Second choice: benztropine 1-2 mg IM/IV. Prevent further dystonias with any anticholinergic agent (see Table 17-11). Experience is very frightening. Take patient to quiet area and stay with him or her until medicated.
3. **Akathisia:** motor inner-driven restlessness (e.g., tapping foot incessantly, rocking forward and backward in chair, shifting weight from side to side)		2 hours to 60 days	3. Physician may change antipsychotic agent or give antiparkinsonian agent. Tolerance does not develop to akathisia, but akathisia disappears when neuroleptic is discontinued. Propranolol (Inderal), lorazepam (Ativan), or diazepam (Valium) may be used.
4. **Tardive dyskinesia** • **Facial:** protruding and rolling tongue, blowing, smacking, licking, spastic facial distortion, smacking movements 　• **Limbs** 　• **Choreic:** rapid, purposeless, and irregular movements 　• **Athetoid:** slow, complex, and serpentine movements • **Trunk:** neck and shoulder movements, dramatic hip jerks and rocking, twisting pelvic thrusts		Months to years	4. No known treatment. Discontinuing the drug does not always relieve symptoms. Possibly 20% of patients taking these drugs for more than 2 years may develop tardive dyskinesia. Nurses and physicians should encourage patients to be screened for tardive dyskinesia at least every 3 months.

TABLE 17-10	NURSING MEASURES FOR EXTRAPYRAMIDAL SYMPTOMS AND NEUROLEPTIC MALIGNANT SYNDROME: CONVENTIONAL (FIRST-GENERATION) ANTIPSYCHOTICS—cont'd	
SIDE EFFECT	**ONSET**	**NURSING MEASURES**
Neuroleptic Malignant Syndrome (NMS) Somewhat rare, potentially fatal. • **Severe extrapyramidal:** severe muscle rigidity, oculogyric crisis, dysphasia, flexor-extensor posturing, cogwheeling • **Hyperpyrexia:** elevated temperature (>103° F [39° C]) • **Autonomic dysfunction:** hypertension, tachycardia, diaphoresis, incontinence	Can occur in the first week of drug therapy but often occurs later. Rapidly progresses over 2 to 3 days after initial manifestation. **Risk factors:** • Concomitant use of psychotropics • Older age • Female gender (3:2) • Presence of a mood disorder (40%) • Rapid dose titration	Stop neuroleptic. Transfer stat to medical unit. Bromocriptine (Parlodel) can relieve muscle rigidity and reduce fever. Dantrolene (Dantrium) may reduce muscle spasms. Cool body to reduce fever. Maintain hydration with oral and IV fluids. Correct electrolyte imbalance. Dysrhythmias should be treated. Small doses of heparin may decrease possibility of pulmonary emboli. Early detection increases patient's chance of survival.

Ach, Anticholinergic side effects, including dry mouth, dry eyes, blurred vision (especially near vision), urinary retention, intestinal slowing (causing constipation), agitation, sedation, and sexual dysfunction; *IM,* intramuscular; *IV,* intravenous; *stat,* immediately.

benztropine mesylate (Cogentin), diphenhydramine hydrochloride (Benadryl), biperiden (Akineton), and amantadine hydrochloride (Symmetrel). However, treatment with antiparkinsonian drugs is not completely benign because the anticholinergic side effects of the antipsychotics may be intensified (e.g., urinary retention, constipation, failure of visual accommodation [blurred vision], cognitive impairment, and delirium).

Most patients develop tolerance to EPS after a few months. Effective nursing and medical management are important encourage compliance with the medication regimen until the major side effects have been properly managed. Table 17-11 identifies some of the drugs most commonly used for the treatment of EPS.

Adjuncts to Antipsychotic Drug Therapy

Antidepressants. Antidepressants are added to antipsychotics when the symptoms meeting the criteria for major depression cause severe distress, including suicidal thoughts, or when depression is disabling (APA, 2004). In fact, a study by Tiihonen and associates (2012) found that the use of antidepressants was associated with markedly decreased suicidal deaths.

Other drugs

Lithium. Lithium and other mood stabilizers help reduce aggressive behavior, but their effectiveness has not been determined adequately (Beng-Choon et al., 2004). The same is true of propranolol and other beta-blockers. Randomized controlled studies did not find evidence to support their use as adjunctive treatment in schizophrenia (Beng-Choon et al., 2004).

Benzodiazepines. Although benzodiazepines have been used in the past as an adjunct to antipsychotics, a new study

TABLE 17-11	TREATMENT OF ACUTE EXTRAPYRAMIDAL SIDE EFFECTS
DRUG	**CHEMICAL TYPE**
Trihexyphenidyl* (Artane)	ACA
Benztropine mesylate* (Cogentin)	ACA
Biperiden* (Akineton)	ACA
Diphenhydramine hydrochloride (Benadryl)	Antihistamine
Bromocriptine mesylate (Parlodel)	D₂ dopamine agonist

*Antiparkinsonian drug.
ACA, Anticholinergic agent (after 1 to 6 months of long-term maintenance antipsychotic therapy, most ACAs can be withdrawn).

demonstrated that benzodiazepine use was associated with marked increase in morbidity (Tiihonen et al, 2012).

EVALUATION

Evaluation is always an important step in the planning of care and is especially important for people who have chronic psychotic disorders. Frequently, outcomes are too ambitious and serve only to discourage patient and staff alike. It is critical for staff to remember that change is a process that occurs over time; for a person diagnosed with schizophrenia, the period may be prolonged.

It is important to schedule regular evaluations for chronically ill patients so that new data can be considered and the patient's problems can be reassessed. Questions to be asked include the following:

- Is the patient not progressing because a more important need is not being met?
- Is the staff using the patient's strengths and interests to achieve the outcomes?
- Are more appropriate interventions available for this patient to facilitate progress?
- If a newer antipsychotic agent is being tried, is there evidence of improvement or a regression in functioning?

- Is the family involved? Are family members supportive? Do they understand the patient's disease and treatment issues?
- Are the patient and family aware of relapse issues (prodromal symptoms of relapse, medication compliance)?
- Are the patient and family working with effective community supports and treatments?

Active staff involvement and interest in the patient's progress communicate concern, help the patient to form and sustain interest, and prevent feelings of helplessness and burnout. Input from the patient can offer valuable information about why a certain desired behavior or situation has not occurred.

KEY POINTS TO REMEMBER

- Schizophrenia is a devastating brain disease. It is not one disorder but a group of disorders. Psychotic symptoms in schizophrenia are more pronounced and disruptive than are symptoms found in other disorders. The basic differences are in the degree of severity of withdrawal, alteration in affect, impairment of intellect, and ability to function in the world.
- Neurochemical (catecholamines and serotonin), genetic, and neuroanatomical findings help explain the symptoms of schizophrenia. However, at present no one theory accounts for all phenomena found in schizophrenic disorders.
- When the nurse works with patients with schizophrenia, four specific groups of symptoms may be evident. No one symptom is found in all cases. The positive, negative, and cognitive symptoms of schizophrenia are three major categories of symptoms. Depression is almost always present.
- The positive symptoms are more florid (hallucinations, delusions, looseness of associations) and respond to antipsychotic drug therapy.
- The negative symptoms (poor social adjustment, lack of motivation, withdrawal) are more debilitating and do not respond as well to antipsychotic therapy.
- The cognitive degree of impairment warrants careful assessment and interventions to increase the person's quality of life and ability to function in the community.

- Comorbid depression needs to be identified and treated to lower the potential for suicide, substance abuse, and relapse.
- Some nursing diagnoses are offered for positive symptoms (delusions and hallucinations), some are for negative symptoms (withdrawal, lack of energy), and some are family focused (see Table 17-4).
- Planning of outcomes proceeds by identifying the phase of schizophrenia and assessing the patient's individual needs based on functional ability, and involves identifying short-term and intermediate indicators.
- Interventions for people with schizophrenia include communication guidelines, health teaching and health promotion, milieu management and strategies, psychotherapy, and pharmacological, biological, and integrative therapies.
- Specific communication strategies are necessary when dealing with a patient who is hallucinating, delusional, or paranoid.
- Because antipsychotic medication is essential, the nurse must understand the properties, adverse effects, toxic effects, and dosages of the traditional, atypical, and other medications used to treat schizophrenia. This information must be shared with the patient and family.

APPLYING CRITICAL JUDGMENT

1. Differentiate between the short-term and long-term needs of people with schizophrenia. Identify the basic focus and interventions for the different phases.
2. Jamie, a 29-year-old woman, is being discharged in 2 days from the hospital after her first psychotic break (paranoid schizophrenia). Jamie is recently divorced and has been working as a legal secretary; recently, her work had become erratic and her suspicious behavior was calling attention to herself at work. Jamie will be discharged in her mother's care until she is able to resume working. Jamie's mother is overwhelmed and asks the nurse how

she is going to cope. "Jamie has become so distant, and she always takes things the wrong way. I can hardly say anything to her without her misconstruing everything. She is very mad at me because I called 911 and had her admitted after she told me she was going to get justice back in the world by blowing up evil forces that have been haunting her life and then proceeded to try to run over her ex-husband, thinking he was the devil. She told me there is nothing wrong with her, and I am concerned she won't take her medication once she is discharged. What am I going to do?"

APPLYING CRITICAL JUDGMENT—cont'd

3. Answer the following questions related to the case study just given. It is best if you can discuss and analyze responses to such situations with your classmates or instructor.

   A. What are some of the priority concerns that the nurse could address in the hospital setting before Jamie's discharge?

   B. How would you explain to Jamie's mother some of the symptoms that Jamie is experiencing? What suggestions could you give her to handle some of her immediate concerns?

   C. What issues could you raise to the staff about Jamie's medication compliance? What would be some ways to deal with this issue?

   D. What are some of the community resources that the case manager could contact to help support this family and increase the chances of continuity of care? Identify some useful community referrals that would be supportive for Jamie and her mother. Choose at least three and describe how they could be supportive to this family.

   E. What do you think of the prognosis for Jamie? Support your hypothesis with data regarding influences on the course of schizophrenia.

   F. Use the computer to access the NAMI (National Alliance on Mental Illness) website (www.NAMI.org). List places in your community that are available to help people with severe mental illnesses (e.g., day care centers, respite centers, group homes).

CHAPTER REVIEW QUESTIONS

Choose the most appropriate answer(s).

1. Which of the following rationales is most important to understand when working with schizophrenic patients?
   1. Environmental stimulation can improve thought process.
   2. Providing external control assists their self control.
   3. Increasing daily social contacts increases their self esteem.
   4. Non-structured group therapy enhances their energy level.

2. Previous to being hospitalized, a patient diagnosed with schizophrenia was reported to be unresponsive, mute and refusing food for several days. What is the highest priority for this patient upon admission to the hospital?
   1. Contacting family members
   2. List of current medications
   3. Assessment of intake and output
   4. Assign patient to a room near the nurses' station

3. Which symptoms of schizophrenia are most amenable to treatment with both low- and high-potency antipsychotic medications?
   1. Hallucinations and delusions
   2. Lack of motivation and initiative
   3. Inadequate hygiene and grooming
   4. Social withdrawal and isolation

4. A patient with paranoid schizophrenia is delusional, unkempt and annoying to other patients. The priority intervention for this patient is to:
   1. encourage the patient to maintain ADLs.
   2. provide a safe environment.
   3. determine the frequency of the delusions.
   4. assess need for a private room.

5. Which nursing diagnosis is universally applicable to patients with schizophrenia?
   1. Noncompliance
   2. Disturbed body image
   3. Disturbed thought processes
   4. Risk for other-directed violence

REFERENCES

Addington, J. (2006). *An ounce of prevention: identifying patients with prodromal symptoms.* Retrieved August 8, 2006, from www.medscap.com/viewprogram/5298_pnt.

American Psychiatric Association (APA). (2004). *Practice guidelines for the treatment of patients with schizophrenia* (2nd ed.). Washington, DC: Author.

American Psychiatric Association (APA). (2000). *Diagnostic and statistical manual of mental disorders (DSM-IV-TR)* (4th ed., text rev.). Washington, DC: Author.

Beng-Choon, H., Black, D. W., & Andreasen, N. C. (2004). Schizophrenia and other psychotic disorders. In R. E. Hales, & S. C. Yudofsky (Eds.), *Essentials of clinical psychiatry* (2nd ed., p. 200). Washington, DC: American Psychiatric Publishing.

Black, D. W., & Andreasen, N. C. (2011). *Introductory textbook of psychiatry* (5th ed.). Washington, DC: American Psychiatric Publishing.

Brauser, D. (2010). *Better outcomes with antipsychotics plus psychosocial treatment for early schizophrenia.* Retrieved August 15, 2011, from www.medscape.com/viewarticle/728337.

Evins, A. E., Cather, C., & Deckersbach, T. (2005). A double-bind placebo-controlled trial of bupropion sustained-release for smoking cessation in schizophrenia. *Journal of Clinical Psychopharmacology, 25*(3), 218–225. Abstract.

Gamble, C., & Brennan, G. (2000). Working with families and informed careers. In C. Gamble, & G. Brennan (Eds.), *Working with serious mental illness: a manual for clinical practice.* London: Baillière Tindall.

Junginger, J. (1995). Common hallucinations and predictions of dangerousness. *Psychiatric Services, 46*(9), 911.

Lewis, M. M., Lockwood, A., et al. (2005). Prognosis: review: longer duration of untreated psychosis is associated with worse outcome in people with first episode psychosis. *Archives of General Psychiatry, 62,* 975–983.

Lowry, F. (2011). *Older antipsychotics tromp newer agents for schizophrenia: newer not necessarily better, researchers say.* Retrieved August 15, 2011, from www.medscape.com/viewarticle/744755_print.

Maxmen, J. S., & Ward, N. G. (2002). *Psychotropic drugs: fast facts* (2nd ed.). New York: Norton.

National Alliance on Mental Illness (NAMI). (2009). *Schizophrenia: PACT: Program of Assertive Community Treatment.* Retrieved March 18, 2011, from www.nami.org/template.CFM?Section= schizophrenia.

PBS. (2002). *The secret life of the brain.* Retrieved March 22, 2011, from www.pbs.org/wnet/brains/episode3/cultures/index.html.

Peluso, M. J., Lewis, S. W., Barnes, T. R., & Jones, P. B. (2012). Retrieved June 6, 2012, from http://reference.Medscape.com/ MEDLINE/abstract/22442101?src=nlbest.

Perkins, D. O., Johnson, J. L., Hamer, R. M., et al. (2006). Predictors of antipsychotic medication adherence in patients recovering from a first psychotic episode. *Schizophrenia Research, 83*(1), 53–63. Abstract.

Preston, J. D., O'Neal, J. H., & Talaga, M. C. (2010). *Handbook of clinical psychopharmacology for therapists* (6th ed.). Oakland, CA: New Harbinger Publications.

Rathod, S., Phiri, P., & Kingdon, D. (2010). Cognitive behavioral therapy for schizophrenia. *Psychiatric Clinics of North America, 33*(3). Retrieved March 20, 2011, from www.mdconsult.com/das/ article/body/237614148–;2/jorg=c.

Sadock, B. J., & Sadock, V. A. (2010). *Kaplan & Sadock's pocket handbook of clinical psychiatry* (5th ed.). Philadelphia: Wolters Kluwer/ Lippincott Williams & Wilkins.

Tandon, R., Stuck, Z. G., Kujawa, M. J., et al. (2003). *Beyond symptoms control: moving towards positive patient outcomes.* Paper presented at the American Psychiatric Association 55th Institute on Psychiatric Services, October 31, 2003, Boston. Retrieved January 21, 2005, from www.medscape.com/viewprogram/2835.

Tiihonen, J., Suokas, J. T., Suvisaari, J. M., Haukka, J., & Korhonen, P. (2012). *Polypharmacy with antipsychotics, antidepressants, benzodiazepines, and mortality in schizophrenia.* Retrieved June 13, 2012, from http://reference.Medscape.com/MEDLINE/abstract/ 22566579?src=nlbest.

U.S. Department of Health and Human Services (USDHHS). (1999). *Mental health: a report of the Surgeon General.* Rockville, MD: Author, Center for Mental Health Services, National Institutes of Health.

Vidal, G. (1982). *The second American revolution and other essays (1976-1982).* New York: Random House.

Xia, J., Mirender, L. B., Belgamwar, M. R. (2011). *Psychoeducation for schizophrenia.* Retrieved/August 15, 2011, from medscape.com/ viewarticle/735323.

Neurocognitive Disorders

Elizabeth M. Varcarolis

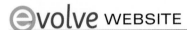

WEBSITE

http://evolve.elsevier.com/Varcarolis/essentials

KEY TERMS AND CONCEPTS

agnosia, p. 341

agraphia, p. 343

Alzheimer's disease (AD), p. 340

aphasia, p. 341

apraxia, p. 341

cognition, p. 332

confabulation, p. 340

delirium, p. 332

dementia, p. 332

hallucinations, p. 335

hypermetamorphosis, p. 343

hyperorality, p. 343

hypervigilance, p. 335

illusions, p. 335

mild cognitive syndrome, p. 332

perseveration, p. 340

primary dementia, p. 332

pseudodementia, p. 343

sundown syndrome, p. 333

tau protein, p. 340

SELECTED CONCEPT: Cognition

Cognition is the operation of the mind that includes "the mental faculty of knowing, perceiving, recognizing, conceiving, judging, reasoning, and imagining" *(American Heritage Medical Dictionary, 2007).*

Cognitive processing has a direct relationship to activities of daily living. Although primarily an intellectual and perceptual process, cognition is closely integrated with an individual's emotional and spiritual values. When human beings can no longer understand facts or connect the appropriate feelings to events, they have trouble responding to the complexity of life's challenges.

OBJECTIVES

1. Using descriptive words, describe the behavior, cognitive abilities, clinical picture, and types of feelings a person with delirium might experience.
2. Discuss the critical safety needs of a patient with delirium.
3. Demonstrate in a nursing care plan interventions and rationales for the care of a person experiencing delirium.
4. Describe the four A's, the defense mechanisms, and the signs and symptoms occurring in each of the four stages of Alzheimer's disease (AD).
5. Identify best evidence with rationales for the various interventions for each of the following categories when caring for a patient with Alzheimer's disease or teaching family members: (a) communication, (b) health maintenance, (c) safe environment.

6. Discuss the kinds of teamwork and collaboration needed in the community to support both patients with AD and their families (list at least four kinds of community service and different kinds of in-home service).
7. Applying informatics, find different types of family supports and individual supports for a patient with AD in your own community.

Cognitive processing has a direct relationship to activities of daily living. Although primarily an intellectual and perceptual process, cognition is closely integrated with an individual's emotional and spiritual values. When human beings can no longer understand facts or connect the appropriate feelings to events, they have trouble responding to the complexity of life's challenges.

Cognition is the operation of the mind that includes "the mental faculty of knowing, perceiving, recognizing, conceiving, judging, reasoning, and imagining" (*American Heritage Medical Dictionary*, 2007). Cognitive disorders are those disorders that impair the brain's ability to carry out normal cognitive functioning. The term cognitive disorders can be used interchangeably with the term *neurocognitive disorders,* because these disorders affect the brain's ability to function intellectually, emotionally, socially, and certainly occupationally. In extreme cases of a neurocognitive disorder, such as Alzheimer's disease, almost all aspects of brain function are destroyed, in time leaving a shell of a once vital, functioning human being whose personality, life memories, and abilities are gone forever.

For our purposes here we will discuss three main categories of the cognitive/neurocognitive disorders: (1) delirium; (2) dementia (a major neurocognitive disorder); and (3) mild cognitive impairments (MCI). MCI is actually a syndrome and will be addressed in the next section.

PREVALENCE AND COMORBIDITY

Delirium is defined by The Free Dictionary as "a state of mental confusion that develops quickly and usually fluctuates in intensity." There is a reduced awareness and responsiveness to the environment. The person is often disoriented and incoherent and has severe memory disturbance. Hallucinations and delusions are not uncommon, and ideas of reference are frequent (The Free Dictionary.com). Delirium is a syndrome and is always secondary to another condition, such as a general medical condition or substance use (drugs of abuse, a medication, or toxin exposure),

or it may have multiple causes. It is a transient disorder, and if the underlying medical cause is corrected, complete recovery should occur. However, health care workers need to be very cognizant of the fact that delirium may easily occur in a patient with dementia.

Delirium, one of the most commonly encountered medical disorders in medical practice, is often overlooked or misdiagnosed. It is a significant risk for all hospitalized older patients. Delirium is present in up to 60% of nursing home residents who are 75 years or older, and as many as 75% to 85% of people with a terminal illness develop delirium near death.

Dementia is much more serious in nature and is a major neurocognitive disorder. Dementia usually develops more slowly than delirium and is characterized by multiple cognitive deficits that include impairment in memory without impairment in consciousness. More than 80% of dementias are irreversible; those dementias that have a reversible component are **secondary** to other pathological processes (e.g., neoplasms, trauma, infections, and toxin exposure). When the underlying causes are treated, the dementia often improves. However, most dementias, such as dementias of the Alzheimer's type, are related to a **primary** encephalopathy. Alzheimer's disease (AD) accounts for 60% to 80% of all dementias in the United States and is the seventh leading cause of death in adults and the fifth leading cause of death in those older than 65. The average lifetime prevalence of Alzheimer's disease is about 12.5% in people 65 years or older, and jumps to 14% in people older than 71 (Alzheimer's Association, 2010). Primary dementia has no known cause or cure; thus it is progressive and irreversible. Examples of other dementias include vascular dementia, Pick's disease, Huntington's disease, Creutzfeldt-Jakob disease, Lewy body disease, and Parkinson's disease.

Mild cognitive impairment (MCI) is a syndrome in which people have mild cognitive impairments (MCI), but this category excludes people with dementia and age-associated memory impairment. For example, a person older than 65 may have a cognitive decline greater than that typically experienced by others

Notes on the Use of the Brief Neurocognitive Mental Status Exam

1. *Behavior observations*
   a. Look for signs of drowsiness or fluctuating degrees of alertness.
   b. This may be formally tested by administering a digit span test or by careful observation during the interview.
   c. Make note of slurred speech or word-finding problems.
   d. Watch for unsteady gait and poor gross motor coordination.

2. *Orientation* – Ask: "What is the date (month, day, year), and what time of day is it now?" "Can you tell me where you are right now? Please be specific." Ask the patient to identify relatives who have accompanied him or her.

3. *Recent memory* – Present three items and ask for immediate recall. Then after a period of five minutes, ask the patient to again recall the three items. Most normal adults should be able to recall three items. Inability to do so may suggest recent memory problems. A second trial may be conducted later in the interview.

4. *Calculations* – Ask the patient to begin with the number 100 and subtract 7 from this number, then subtract 7 again, and so forth. This test provides a rough measure of concentration.

5. *Reproduction of cross and cube* – Present stimulus illustrations shown below. You can copy them onto a 3-by-5-inch, unlined, white index card. Allow the patient to copy the designs one at a time onto a blank sheet of paper. Drawing performance can be compared to samples (see below) to derive rough estimates of the patient's constructional ability.

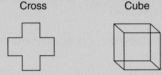

Cross   Cube

6. *Thinking/Speech* – Note the presence of incoherent or irrelevant speech.

FIGURE 18-1 Neurocognitive mental status exam. (From Preston, J., O'Neal, J., & Talaga, M.A. [2010]. *Handbook of clinical psychopharmacology for therapists* [6th ed., pp. 301-302]. Oakland, CA: New Harbinger Publications.)

similar in age and education level. The impairment primarily involves memory difficulties. A person might forget things more often, such as important events or appointments, or have difficulty following a conversation or a plot in a book or movie. At times, the person may have trouble finding his or her way around familiar places and often becomes overwhelmed by previously easy tasks (Gauthier et al., 2006; Mayo Clinic, 2011). Therefore, memory impairment is the predominant symptom. However, it does not interfere with the individual's general cognitive functioning nor does it interfere with the individual's activities of daily living and socialization. Although mild cognitive impairment does not affect the individual's daily living, it might result in greater effort being required to perform tasks and the use of compensatory strategies. Noteworthy, however, is that it has been estimated that approximately 12% of people with such mild cognitive impairments progress to dementia in 1 year (Black & Andreasen, 2011).

In all disorders in which a patient experiences a change in cognitive functioning, a mental status exam (Figure 18-1) and a thorough medical workup are vital (e.g., history, physical, neurological exam, lab tests, scans, x-rays).

DELIRIUM (A POTENTIALLY REVERSIBLE NEUROCOGNITIVE DISORDER)

Nurses frequently encounter delirium on medical and surgical units in the general hospital setting. During certain phases of a hospital stay, confusion may be noted (e.g., after surgery or after the introduction of a new drug). The second or third hospital day may herald the onset of confusion and difficulty adjusting to an unfamiliar environment.

Delirium occurs more frequently in older patients. Surgery, drugs, urinary tract infections, pneumonia, cerebrovascular disease, and congestive heart failure are some of the most common causes. Delirium is also commonly seen in children with fever and in terminally ill patients.

A delayed or missed diagnosis can have serious implications because the longer a condition remains untreated, the greater the risk that the condition can cause permanent damage. Depression often masquerades as dementia, and can even co-occur with dementia; therefore a clear definition of the three can be useful during assessment. Table 18-1 offers some guidelines for distinguishing among delirium, depression, and dementia.

The essential feature of delirium is a disturbance in consciousness coupled with cognitive difficulties. Thinking, memory, attention, and perception are typically disturbed. The clinical manifestations of delirium develop over a short period (hours to days) and tend to fluctuate during the course of the day. Sundown syndrome, in which symptoms and problem behaviors become more pronounced in the evening, may occur in both delirium and dementia.

Because delirium increases psychological stress, supportive interventions that lower anxiety and promote calm and security

TABLE 18-1 COMPARISON OF DELIRIUM, DEMENTIA, AND DEPRESSION

	DELIRIUM	DEMENTIA	DEPRESSION
Onset	Sudden, over hours to days	Slowly, over months	May have been gradual with exacerbation during crisis or stress
Cause or contributing factors	Hypoglycemia, fever, dehydration, hypotension; infection, other conditions that disrupt body's homeostasis; adverse drug reaction; head injury; change in environment (e.g., hospitalization); pain; emotional stress	Alzheimer's disease, vascular disease, human immunodeficiency virus infection, neurological disease, chronic alcoholism, head trauma	Lifelong history, losses, loneliness, crises, declining health, medical conditions
Cognition	Impaired memory, judgment, calculations, attention span; can fluctuate through the day	Impaired memory, judgment, calculations, attention span, abstract thinking; agnosia	Difficulty concentrating, forgetfulness, inattention
Level of consciousness	Altered	Not altered	Not altered
Activity level	Can be increased or reduced, restlessness; behaviors may worsen in evening (sundown syndrome); sleep-wake cycle may be reversed	Not altered; behaviors may worsen in evening (sundown syndrome)	Usually decreased; lethargy, fatigue, lack of motivation; may sleep poorly and awaken in early morning
Emotional state	Rapid swings; can be fearful, anxious, suspicious, aggressive, have hallucinations and/or delusions	Flat; delusions	Extreme sadness, apathy, irritability, anxiety, paranoid ideation
Speech and language	Rapid, inappropriate, incoherent, rambling	Incoherent, slow (sometimes due to effort to find the right word), inappropriate, rambling, repetitious	Slow, flat, low
Prognosis	Reversible with proper and timely treatment	Not reversible; progressive	Reversible with proper and timely treatment

can foster a sense of control. Patients with delirium may appear withdrawn, agitated, or psychotic. Also, underlying personality traits often become exaggerated. For example, a person can become more paranoid or display more disinhibition.

Box 18-1 lists common causes of delirium. Nursing interventions center on the following:

- Performing a comprehensive nursing assessment to aid in identifying the cause
- Preventing physical harm as a result of confusion, aggression, or electrolyte and fluid imbalance
- Using supportive measures to relieve distress

APPLICATION OF THE NURSING PROCESS: DELIRIUM

ASSESSMENT

Generally the nurse suspects the presence of delirium when a patient abruptly develops a disturbance in consciousness that is manifested in reduced clarity of awareness of the environment. The person may have difficulty with orientation—first to time, then to place, and last to person. For example, a man

with delirium may think that the year is 1972, that the hospital is home, and that the nurse is his wife. Orientation to person is usually intact to the extent that the person is aware of self-identity. *Level of awareness is disturbed and the ability to focus, sustain, or shift attention is impaired.* Questions need to be repeated because the individual's attention wanders, and the person might easily need to be refocused. Conversation is made more difficult because the person may be easily distracted by irrelevant stimuli.

Fluctuating levels of consciousness are unpredictable. Disorientation and confusion are usually markedly worse at night and during the early morning (sundowning). In fact, some patients may be confused or delirious only at night and may remain lucid during the day. Some clinicians use the Mini-Mental State Examination to screen or follow the progress of an individual with delirium. Nursing assessment includes (1) cognitive and perceptual disturbances, (2) physical needs, and (3) moods and physical behaviors.

Cognitive and Perceptual Disturbances

It may be difficult to engage patients in conversation while they are delirious because they are easily distracted and

BOX 18-1   COMMON CAUSES OF DELIRIUM

Postoperative states

Drug intoxications and withdrawals

- Alcohol, anxiolytics, opioids, and central nervous system stimulants (e.g., cocaine, crack cocaine, and others)

Infections

- Systemic: pneumonia, typhoid fever, malaria, urinary tract infection, and septicemia
- Intracranial: meningitis and encephalitis

Metabolic disorders

- Dehydration
- Hypoxia (pulmonary disease, heart disease, and anemia)
- Hypoglycemia
- Sodium, potassium, calcium, magnesium, and acid-base imbalances
- Hepatic encephalopathy or uremic encephalopathy
- Thiamine (vitamin B_1) deficiency (Wernicke's encephalopathy)
- Endocrine disorders (e.g., thyroidism or parathyroidism)
- Hypothermia or hyperthermia
- Diabetic acidosis

Drugs

- Digitalis, steroids, lithium, levodopa, anticholinergics, benzodiazepines, central nervous system depressants, tricyclic antidepressants
- Central anticholinergic syndrome as a result of using multiple drugs with anticholinergic side effects

Neurological diseases

- Seizures
- Head trauma
- Hypertensive encephalopathy

Tumor

- Primary cerebral

Psychosocial stressors

- Relocation or other sudden changes
- Sensory deprivation or overload
- Sleep deprivation
- Immobilization
- Pain

---

display marked attention deficits, and because their memory is impaired. In mild delirium, memory deficits are noted on careful questioning. In more severe delirium, memory problems usually take the form of obvious difficulty in processing and remembering recent events. For example, the person might ask when a son is coming to visit, even though the son left only an hour earlier. Perceptual disturbances are also common. Perception is the processing of information about one's internal and external environment. Various misinterpretations of reality may take the form of illusions or hallucinations.

Illusions are errors in perception of sensory stimuli. For example, a person may mistake folds in the bedclothes for white rats or the cord of a window blind for a snake. The stimulus is a real object in the environment; however, it is misinterpreted and often becomes the object of the patient's projected fear. Illusions, unlike delusions or hallucinations, can be explained and clarified for the individual.

Hallucinations are false sensory stimuli (see Chapter 17 for guidelines in dealing with hallucinations). *Visual* hallucinations are common in delirium. *Tactile* hallucinations may also be present. For example, delirious individuals may become terrified when they "see" giant spiders crawling over the bedclothes or "feel" bugs crawling on their bodies. Auditory hallucinations occur more often in other psychiatric disorders, such as schizophrenia and psychotic depression.

The delirious individual generally has awareness that something is very wrong. For example, the delirious person may state, "My thoughts are all jumbled." When perceptual disturbances are present, the emotional response is one of fear and anxiety. Verbal and psychomotor signs of agitation should be noted.

Physical Needs

Physical Safety

A person with delirium becomes disoriented and may try to "go home." Alternatively, a person may think that he or she *is* home and may jump out of a window in an attempt to get away from "invaders." Wandering, pulling out intravenous lines and Foley catheters, and falling out of bed are common dangers that require nursing intervention.

An individual experiencing delirium has difficulty processing stimuli in the environment. Confusion magnifies the inability to recognize reality. The physical environment should be made as simple and as clear as possible. Objects such as clocks and calendars can maximize orientation to time. Eyeglasses, hearing aids, and adequate lighting without glare can maximize the person's ability to more accurately interpret the environment. The nurse should interact with the patient whenever the patient is awake. Short periods of social interaction help reduce anxiety and misperceptions.

Biophysical Safety

Autonomic signs, such as tachycardia, sweating, flushed face, dilated pupils, and elevated blood pressure, are often present. These changes must be monitored and documented carefully and may require immediate medical attention.

Changes in the sleep-wake cycle usually are noted, and in some cases, a complete reversal of the night-day sleep-wake cycle can occur. The patient's level of consciousness may range from lethargy to stupor or from semicoma to hypervigilance. In hypervigilance, patients are extraordinarily alert and their eyes constantly scan the room; they may have difficulty falling asleep or may be actively disoriented and agitated throughout the night.

It is also important that the nurse assess all medications because the nurse is in a position to recognize drug reactions or potential interactions before delirium actually occurs.

Moods and Physical Behaviors

The delirious individual's behavior and mood may change dramatically within a short period. Moods may fluctuate from fear, anger, and anxiety to euphoria, depression, and apathy. These labile moods are often accompanied by physical behaviors associated with feeling states. A person may strike out from fear or anger or may cry, call for help, curse, moan, and tear off clothing and then within a minute become apathetic or laugh uncontrollably. In short, behavior and emotions are erratic and fluctuating. Lack of concentration and disorientation complicate interventions. The following vignette illustrates the fear and confusion a patient may experience when admitted to an intensive care unit (ICU). Read the following and analyze the nurse's approach.

VIGNETTE

A 55-year-old married man, Mr. Arnold, is admitted to the ICU after having cardiac surgery, a three-vessel coronary artery bypass graft. Mr. Arnold's surgery took longer than usual and has necessitated his remaining on a cardiac pump for 3 hours. He arrives in the ICU without further complications. On awakening from the anesthesia, he hears the nurse exclaim, "I need to get a gas." Another nurse answers in a loud voice, "Can you take a large needle for the injection?" During this period, Mr. Arnold experiences the need to urinate and asks the nurse very calmly if he can go to the bathroom. Her reply is, "You don't need to go; you have a tube in." He again complains about his discomfort and assures the nurse that if she will let him go to the bathroom, he will be fine. The nurse informs Mr. Arnold that he cannot urinate and that he has to keep the "mask" on so that she can get the "gas" and check his "blood levels." On hearing this, Mr. Arnold begins to implore more loudly and states that he sees the bathroom sign. He assures the nurse that he will only take a minute. In reality, the sign is an exit sign.

To prove to him that a bathroom does not exist in the ICU and that the sign does not indicate a bathroom, the nurse takes off the restraints so that Mr. Arnold's head can be raised to see the sign. He abruptly breaks away from the nurse's grasp and runs toward the entrance of the ICU. He discovers a door, which is the entrance to the nurses' lounge; Mr. Arnold barricades himself in the room and pulls out his chest tube, Foley catheter, and intravenous lines. He finds the bathroom that is connected to the lounge. Ten minutes later, the nurses and security personnel break through the barricade and escort Mr. Arnold back to bed.

When he becomes fully alert and oriented a day later, Mr. Arnold tells the nurses his perception of the previous day's events. Initially, he had thought he had been kidnapped and was being held against his will (the restraints had been tight). When the nurse yelled out about blood gas, he had thought she was going to kill him with noxious gas through his facemask (the reason he did not want to wear the facemask). All he could think about was escaping his tormentor and executioner. In this case, the nurse had not assessed the alteration in Mr. Arnold's mental status and allowed him to get out of bed. The medical jargon and loud voices had perpetuated his confusion and distortion of reality.

The nurses could have told Mr. Arnold where he was and that the nursing staff was caring for him; they could have better explained the function of his Foley catheter. What else could the nurses have done to help orient and comfort Mr. Arnold?

ASSESSMENT GUIDELINES
Delirium

1. Assess for fluctuating levels of consciousness, which is key in delirium.
2. Interview family or other caregivers to establish the patient's normal level of consciousness and cognition.
3. Assess for past confusional states (e.g., prior dementia diagnosis).
4. Identify other disturbances in medical status (e.g., infection, dyspnea, edema, presence of jaundice).
5. Identify any electroencephalographic, neuroimaging, or laboratory abnormalities documented in the patient's record.
6. Assess vital signs, level of consciousness, and neurological signs.
7. Assess potential for injury (e.g., falls, wandering).
8. Assess the need for comfort measures (e.g., to address pain or cold, to improve positioning).
9. Monitor factors that worsen or improve symptoms.
10. Assess for availability of immediate medical interventions to help prevent irreversible brain damage.
11. Remain nonjudgmental. Confer with other staff readily when questions arise.

DIAGNOSIS

Safety needs play a substantial role in nursing care. If fever and dehydration are present, fluid and electrolyte balance will need to be managed. If the underlying cause of the patient's delirium results in fever, decreased skin turgor, decreased urinary output or fluid intake, and dry skin or mucous membranes, then the nursing diagnosis of *Deficient Fluid Volume* is appropriate.

Any condition that alters brain activity, including metabolic imbalances, infections, altered sleep, substance abuse, and medication use, can be viewed as a *Risk for Acute Confusion*. Perceptions are disturbed during delirium and may be acted

TABLE 18-2 **POTENTIAL NURSING DIAGNOSES FOR THE CONFUSED PATIENT**	
SYMPTOMS	**NURSING DIAGNOSES***
Wanders, has unsteady gait, acts out fear from hallucinations or illusions, forgets things (leaves stove on, doors open) Awake and disoriented during the night *(sundown syndrome),* frightened at night	*Risk for Injury* *Wandering* *Disturbed Sleep Pattern* *Fear* *Acute Confusion*
Too confused to take care of basic needs	*Bathing Self-Care Deficit (specify)* *Bowel Incontinence* *Dressing Self-Care Deficit* *Feeding Self-Care Deficit* *Functional Urinary Incontinence* *Imbalanced Nutrition: Less Than Body Requirements* *Deficient Fluid Volume* *Ineffective Self-Health Management*
Sees frightening things that are not there *(hallucinations),* mistakes everyday objects for something sinister and frightening *(illusions),* may become paranoid and think that others are doing things to confuse him or her *(delusions)*	*Fear* *Defensive Coping* *Impaired Environmental Interpretation Syndrome* *Ineffective Impulse Control* *Powerlessness*
Does not recognize familiar people or places, has difficulty with short- and/or long-term memory, forgetful and confused Has difficulty with communication, cannot find words, has difficulty in recognizing objects and/or people, incoherent Devastated over losing place in life as known (during lucid moments), fearful and overwhelmed by what is happening to him or her	*Impaired Memory* *Impaired Environmental Interpretation Syndrome* *Acute* or *Chronic Confusion* *Impaired Verbal Communication* *Ineffective Relationship* *Spiritual Distress* *Hopelessness* *Situational Low Self-Esteem* *Grieving*
Family and loved ones overburdened and overwhelmed, unable to care for patient's needs	*Disabled Family Coping* *Interrupted Family Processes* *Impaired Home Maintenance* *Caregiver Role Strain* *Chronic Sorrow* *Deficient Community Health*

**Nursing Diagnoses—Definitions and Classification 2012-2014.* Copyright © 2012, 1994-2012 by NANDA International. Used by arrangement with Blackwell Publishing Limited, a company of John Wiley and Sons, Inc.

on by the patient. For example, if feeling threatened or thinking that common medical equipment is harmful, the patient may pull off an oxygen mask, pull out an intravenous or nasogastric tube, or try to leave the health care facility. Hallucinations, distractibility, illusions, disorientation, agitation, restlessness, and/or misperception are major aspects of the clinical picture. When some of these symptoms are present, *Risk for Injury, Fear,* and *Acute Confusion* are appropriate nursing diagnoses.

Because the sleep-wake cycle may be disrupted, the patient may be less responsive during the day and may become disruptively wakeful during the night. Therefore, *Disturbed Sleep Pattern* related to impaired cerebral oxygenation or disruption in consciousness is a likely diagnosis.

Sustaining communication with a delirious patient is difficult. *Impaired Verbal Communication* related to cerebral hypoxia or decreased cerebral blood flow, as evidenced by confusion or clouding of consciousness may be diagnosed.

Other nursing diagnoses include *Self-Care Deficit, Impaired Environmental Interpretation Syndrome,* and *Impaired Social Interaction.* Table 18-2 identifies nursing diagnoses for any confused patient (delirium or dementia).

OUTCOMES IDENTIFICATION

The overall outcome is that the delirious patient will return to the premorbid level of functioning. Although the patient can demonstrate a wide variety of needs, *Risk for Injury* is always present and foremost. Appropriate outcomes are as follows:

- Patient will remain safe and free from injury while in the hospital.

- During periods of lucidity, patient will be oriented to time, place, and person with the aid of nursing interventions, such as the provision of clocks, calendars, maps, and other types of orienting information.
- Patient will remain free from falls and injury while confused with the aid of nursing safety measures throughout hospital stay.
- Patient's tubes (e.g., nasogastric [NG], intravenous [IV], O_2) will remain in place with aid of nurse, family, and/or medication as needed.

Because levels of consciousness can change throughout the day, the patient needs to be checked for orientation (time, place, and person) frequently during different times of the day.

IMPLEMENTATION

Medical management of delirium involves treating the underlying organic causes. If the underlying cause of delirium is not treated, permanent brain damage may result. Judicious use of antipsychotic or antianxiety agents may also be helpful in controlling behavioral symptoms.

A patient in acute delirium should never be left alone. Because most hospitals and health facilities are unable to provide one-to-one supervision of the patient, family members can be encouraged to stay with the patient. Refer to Table 18-3 for guidelines in caring for a patient with delirium.

EVALUATION

Evaluation includes identifying if the long-term outcome criteria have been met. Long-term outcome criteria for a person with delirium include the following:
- Patient will remain safe.
- Patient will be oriented to time, place, and person by discharge.
- Underlying cause will be treated and ameliorated.
- Patient will return to premorbid level of functioning

However, the short-term goals need constant assessment. Are the vital signs stable? Is the patient's skin turgor and urine specific gravity within normal limits?

▌DEMENTIA

Because Alzheimer's disease (AD) is the primary diagnosis for dementia and the assessments and nursing interventions are primarily the same for all patients with dementia, this section will focus on Alzheimer's disease.

Cultural Considerations

Although AD is not affected by ethnicity in terms of behaviors (e.g., wandering, insomnia, incontinence, and possibly aggression), there do seem to be differences regarding incidents of AD in different ethnic groups. For example, older African Americans are almost twice as likely to develop Alzheimer's disease as white Americans. Hispanic Americans are about 1.5 times as likely to develop Alzheimer's disease as white Americans. Although at this point there does not seem to be any genetic correlation, there are other correlations. African Americans and Hispanics are more prone to high blood pressure and diabetes, which are significant risk factors for Alzheimer's disease. Many African Americans and Hispanics live at lower economic levels and have less access to education and health care, which are also risk factors for AD (Alzheimer's Association, 2010).

Although the behaviors resulting from Alzheimer's disease are similar, attitudes and perceptions of such behaviors can vary greatly among cultural groups. The emotions of frustration, anger, guilt, anxiety, and conflict are closely tied to the cultural value placed on the ability to maintain control.

Native American cultures are more likely to accept their lack of control over the situation. Therefore they may be far more likely to respond to their family members' situation with a sense of *loss* that life with their loved one, and life as their loved one knew it, is gone forever. Among many in the white population, there is more a belief that people should be able to alter or influence a situation, which results in stronger feelings of anger, guilt, anxiety, and conflict over having no impact on the course of AD.

Health care workers who are able to assess and understand the cultural aspects of caregiving behaviors may be able to offer services and training that are more congruent with the caregiver's culture. Health care workers have a long way to go to become more proficient in understanding the nuances of culture and how it relates to the quality of care that patients and families may ultimately accept. The issue is complicated by the fact that patients and families from a minority group may be composed of many different subcultural groups. A good example is the Hispanic population, which shares Spanish as a language; however, Hispanics comprise Mexicans, Cubans, Puerto Ricans, Salvadorans, and Nicaraguans, who all come from very distinct cultural backgrounds.

Risk Factors for Alzheimer's Disease
Age and Gender
Age seems to be the most important risk factor for AD. Women are much more susceptible to developing AD than men. For example, 17.2% of women versus 9.1% of men develop AD at age 65. At age 75, 18.5% of women versus 10.2% of men will be diagnosed with Alzheimer's disease.

Other common risk factors. People with Alzheimer's disease have much higher rates of diabetes and high blood pressure than do people who do not develop Alzheimer's disease. Also, it is noted that people at lower educational levels seem to have increased risk for Alzheimer's disease than those with higher educational levels. Socioeconomic levels seem to affect the aforementioned statistics. Generally, people at lower socioeconomic levels appear to be more prone to AD than people with a higher standard of living. This may be explained in part by lack of adequate medical care (e.g., past head trauma) and poor dietary intake.

TABLE 18-3   INTERVENTIONS FOR A PATIENT WITH DELIRIUM

INTERVENTION	RATIONALE
1. Work with treatment team to reduce or eliminate factors causing delirium.	1. Underlying factors can lead to dementia if not reversed.
2. Monitor neurological signs on an ongoing basis.	2. Track progression or reversal of neurological disequilibrium.
3. Introduce self and call patient by name at the beginning of each contact.	3. With short-term memory impairment, person is often confused and needs frequent orienting to time, place, and person.
4. Maintain face-to-face contact.	4. If patient is easily distracted, he or she needs help to focus on one stimulus at a time.
5. Use short, simple, concrete phrases.	5. Patient may not be able to process complex information.
6. Briefly explain everything you are going to do before doing it.	6. Explanation prevents misinterpretation of action.
7. Encourage family and friends (one at a time) to take a quiet, supportive role.	7. Familiar presence lowers anxiety and increases orientation.
8. Keep room well lit.	8. Lighting provides accurate environmental stimuli to maintain and increase orientation.
9. Keep head of bed elevated.	9. Helps provide important environmental cues.
10. Provide clocks and calendars.	10. These cues help orient patient to time.
11. Encourage family members to bring in meaningful articles from home (e.g., pictures or figurines).	11. Familiar objects provide comfort and support and can aid orientation.
12. Encourage patient to wear prescribed eyeglasses or hearing aid.	12. Helps increase accurate perceptions of visual auditory stimuli.
13. Make an effort to assign the same personnel on each shift to care for patient.	13. Familiar faces minimize confusion and enhance nurse-patient relationships.
14. When hallucinations are present, clarify reality; for example, "I know you are frightened; I do not see spiders on your sheets. I'll sit with you for a while."	14. Person feels understood and reassured while reality is validated.
15. When illusions are present, clarify reality; for example, "This is a coat rack, not a man with a knife...see? You seem frightened. I'll stay with you for a while."	15. Misinterpreted objects or sounds can be clarified, once pointed out.
16. Inform patient of progress during lucid intervals.	16. Consciousness fluctuates: patient feels less anxious knowing where he or she is and who you are during lucid periods.
17. Ignore insults and name calling, and acknowledge how upset the person may be feeling. For example: *Patient:* "You incompetent jerk, get me a real nurse, someone who knows what they are doing." *Nurse:* "You are very upset. What you are going through is very difficult. I'll stay with you."	17. Terror and fear are often projected onto environment. Arguing or becoming defensive only increases patient's aggressive behaviors and defenses.
18. If patient behavior becomes physically abusive, first, set limits on behavior. For example: *Nurse:* "Mr. Jones, you are not to hit me or anyone else. Tell me how you feel." *Nurse:* "Mr. Jones, if you have difficulty controlling your actions, we will help you gain control." Second, check orders for use of chemical or physical restraints.	18. Clear limits need to be set to protect patient, staff, and others. Often, patient can respond to verbal commands. Chemical and physical restraints are used as a last resort, if at all.

More risk factors include a history of head injury, a first-degree relative with AD, a family history of AD (a genetic polymorphism on chromosome 19 apolipoprotein E gene [*APOE*]; discussed under Genetic Theories), obesity, insulin resistance, vascular factors, inflammatory markers, hypertension, and Down syndrome (Anderson & Hoffman, 2012).

THEORY

As yet, a single cause of AD has not been identified. Most likely, several genetic and nongenetic factors—that affect each person differently—may interact to cause AD.

Genetic Theories

One genetic risk factor consistently related to Alzheimer's disease is the cholesterol-carrying apolipoprotein E gene *(APOE E4)* on chromosome 19. The *APOE* gene provides instructions to manufacture proteins needed to help transport cholesterol in the bloodstream. *APOE* has several forms or alleles: *APOE E2* is rare and may provide protection against AD, *APOE E3* is believed to play a neutral role in AD, and *APOE E4* occurs in about 40% of all people who develop late-onset AD and is considered a risk factor for AD (ADEAR, 2010; Anderson & Hoffman, 2012).

Genetic factors associated with early-onset Alzheimer's disease consist of mutations in three genes. Early-onset AD is relatively rare, develops in people ages 30 to 60, and accounts for only 5% of people with the disease (ADEAR, 2010). Early-onset genetic defects that relate to **Alzheimer's** include the gene *APP* on chromosome 21, the gene *PS-1* on chromosome 14, and the gene *PS-2* on chromosome 1 (ADEAR, 2010).

Anatomical Pathology of Alzheimer's Disease

Alzheimer's disease (AD) is a complex disease that begins to damage the brain long before the symptoms appear. AD affects processes that keep the neurons healthy, such as (1) communication, (2) metabolism, and (3) repair. In a healthy brain neurons are supported by microtubules, which guide nutrients and molecules between the cell body and the axon terminals. A special protein called tau protein is responsible for the stability of the microtubules. In AD tau protein is subjected to chemical changes, which result in neurofibrillary tangles and cause disintegration of the microtubules, thus collapsing the neuron's transport system. This disintegration of the neuron transport system results in malfunction of communication between neurons, and eventually leads to neural cell death. It is the destruction and death of the cells that causes memory failure, personality changes, problems in carrying out daily activities, and other features of the disease (Anderson & Hoffman, 2011).

The anatomical pathology of Alzheimer's disease includes senile plaques (SNs) and neurofibrillary tangles (NFTs). It is believed that the disease begins with the buildup of beta-amyloid protein, resulting in **senile plaques,** which are also called **beta-amyloid plaques.** These plaques are cores of degenerated neuron material that lie free of the cell bodies on the ground substances of the brain. The quantity of plaques has been correlated with the degree of mental deterioration.

The **neurofibrillary tangles** are the damaged remains of microtubules that allow the flow of nutrients through the neurons. These neurofibrillary tangles form in the hippocampus, which is the part of the brain responsible for recent (short-term) memory.

Granulovascular degeneration is another active process in the disease and it results in the filling of brain cells with fluid and granular material. Increased degeneration accounts for increased loss of mental function. **Brain atrophy** is observable with wider cortical sulci and enlarged cerebral ventricles, as demonstrated by computed tomography (CT) and magnetic resonance imaging (MRI) scans. Imaging techniques reveal significant loss of cells and volume in the regions of the brain devoted to memory and higher mental functioning.

APPLICATION OF THE NURSING PROCESS: DEMENTIA

ASSESSMENT

Overall Assessment

AD is commonly characterized by progressive deterioration of cognitive functioning. Initially, deterioration may be so subtle and insidious that others may not notice. In the early stages of the disease, the affected person may be able to compensate for loss of memory. Some people may have superior social graces and charm that give them the ability to hide severe deficits in memory, even from experienced health care professionals. This hiding is actually a form of **denial,** which is an unconscious protective defense against the terrifying reality of losing one's place in the world. Family members may also unconsciously deny that anything is wrong as a defense against the painful awareness that a loved one is deteriorating. As time goes on, symptoms become more obvious, and other defensive maneuvers become evident.

Another defense mechanism is confabulation—the making up of stories or answers to maintain self-esteem when the person does not remember. For example, the nurse addresses a patient who has remained in a hospital bed all weekend:

> *Nurse:* "Good morning, Ms. Jones. How was your weekend?"
> *Patient:* "Wonderful. I discussed politics with the President, and he took me out to dinner."
> *or*
> *Patient:* "I spent the weekend with my daughter and her family." *(less grandiose)*

Confabulation is not the same as lying. When people are lying, they are aware of making up an answer; confabulation is an **unconscious** attempt to maintain self-esteem.

Perseveration (the repetition of phrases or behavior) is eventually seen and is often intensified under stress. The avoidance of answering questions is another mechanism by which the patient is able to maintain self-esteem unconsciously in the face of severe memory deficits. Therefore, (1) denial, (2) confabulation, (3) perseveration, and (4) avoidance of questions are four defensive behaviors the nurse might notice during assessment.

Dementia is a syndrome of impaired cognitive function marked by slowly deteriorating social and occupational functioning although levels of alertness are generally not disturbed (Black & Andreasen, 2011). Cognitive impairment involves the four A's:

- **Amnesia or memory impairment.** Initially, the person has difficulty remembering recent events. Gradually, deterioration progresses to include both recent and remote memory.
- Aphasia (loss of language ability), which progresses with the disease. Initially, the person has difficulty finding the correct word, then is reduced to a few words, and finally is reduced to babbling or mutism.
- Apraxia (loss of purposeful movement in the absence of motor or sensory impairment). The person is unable to perform once-familiar and purposeful tasks. For example, in apraxia of gait, the person loses the ability to walk. In apraxia of dressing, the person is unable to put clothes on properly (may put arms in trousers or put a jacket on upside down).
- Agnosia (loss of sensory ability to recognize objects). For example, the person may lose the ability to recognize familiar sounds (auditory agnosia), such as the ring of the telephone, a car horn, or the doorbell. Loss of this ability extends to the inability to recognize familiar objects (visual or tactile agnosia), such as a glass, magazine, pencil, or toothbrush. Eventually, people are unable to recognize loved ones or even parts of their own bodies.

There are also disturbances in executive functioning (planning, organizing, abstract thinking). The clumping of neurons in the brain results in the deterioration of working components in the brain. These cells contain memories, receive sights and sounds, activate hormone secretion, produce emotions, and command muscles into motion.

Assessing Stages of AD

AD is classified according to the stage of the degenerative process. The number of stages defined ranges from three to seven, depending on the source. This text will present four stages of Alzheimer's disease to help illustrate the progression of symptoms while they develop over the course of this tragic deteriorating mind disease. Table 18-4 can be used as a guide to review the four stages of AD and highlight the deficits associated with each stage.

The rate of progression varies individually. Some persons in stage 1 decline quickly and may die within 3 years. Others, although their condition worsens, may still function in the community with support. Still others may remain at this level for 3 years or more. The duration of the disease from onset of symptoms to death averages 8 to 10 years but can range from 3 to 20 years (APA, 2000).

Stage 1: Mild Alzheimer's disease

The loss of intellectual ability is insidious. The person with mild Alzheimer's disease loses energy, drive, and initiative and has difficulty learning new things. Because personality and social behavior remain intact, others tend to minimize and underestimate the loss of the individual's abilities. The individual may still continue to work, but the extent of the dementia becomes evident in new or demanding situations. Depression may occur early in the disease but usually lessens as the disease progresses. Activities such as grocery shopping or managing finances are noticeably impaired during this phase.

> **VIGNETTE**
>
> Mr. Collins, a 56-year-old lineman for a telephone company, feels that he is getting old. He keeps forgetting things and writes notes to himself on scraps of paper. One day on the job, he forgets momentarily which wires to connect and connects all the wrong ones, causing mass confusion for a few hours. At home, Mr. Collins becomes very upset when his wife suggests that they invite the new neighbors for dinner. It is hard for him to admit that anything new confuses him, and he often forgets names *(aphasia)* and sometimes loses the thread of conversations. Once he even forgot his address when his car stopped working on the highway. He is moody and depressed and becomes indignant when his wife finds 3 months' worth of unpaid bills stashed in his sock drawer. Mrs. Collins is bewildered, upset, and fearful that something is terribly wrong.

Stage 2: Moderate Alzheimer's disease

Deterioration becomes evident during the moderate phase. Often the person with moderate AD cannot remember his or her address or the date. There are memory gaps in the person's history that may fluctuate from one moment to the next. Hygiene suffers, and the ability to dress appropriately is markedly affected. The person may put on clothes backward, button the buttons incorrectly, or not fasten zippers *(apraxia)*. Often, the person has to be coaxed to bathe.

Mood becomes labile, and the individual may have bursts of paranoia, anger, jealousy, and apathy. Activities such as driving are hazardous, and families are faced with the difficulty of taking away the car keys from their loved one. Care and supervision become full-time jobs for family members. Denial mercifully takes over and protects people from the realization that they are losing control, not only of their minds but also of their lives. Along with denial, people with AD begin to withdraw from activities and from others because they often feel overwhelmed and frustrated when they try to do things that once were easy. They may also have moments of becoming tearful and sad.

As important as it is to recognize all of the deficits of stage 2, it is helpful for caretakers to realize that the patient still retains abilities that influence care.

TABLE 18-4   STAGES OF ALZHEIMER'S DISEASE

STAGE	HALLMARKS
Stage 1 (Mild) Forgetfulness	Shows short-term memory loss; loses things, forgets Memory aids compensate: lists, routine, organization Aware of the problem; concerned about lost abilities Depression common—worsens symptoms Disease is not diagnosable from the symptoms
Stage 2 (Moderate) Confusion	Shows progressive memory loss; short-term memory impaired; memory difficulties interfere with all abilities Withdrawn from social activities Shows declines in instrumental activities of daily living (ADLs), such as money management, legal affairs, transportation, cooking, housekeeping Denial common; fears "losing his or her mind" Depression increasingly common; frightened because aware of deficits; covers up for memory loss through confabulation Problems intensified when stressed, fatigued, out of own environment, ill Commonly needs day care or in-home assistance
Stage 3 (Moderate to severe) Ambulatory dementia	Shows ADL losses (in order): willingness and ability to bathe, grooming, choosing clothing, dressing, gait and mobility, toileting, communication, reading, and writing skills Shows loss of reasoning ability, safety planning, and verbal communication Frustration common; becomes more withdrawn and self-absorbed Depression resolves as awareness of losses diminishes Has difficulty communicating; shows increasing loss of language skills Shows evidence of reduced stress threshold; institutional care usually needed
Stage 4 (Late) End stage	Family recognition disappears; does not recognize self in mirror Nonambulatory; shows little purposeful activity; often mute; may scream spontaneously Forgets how to eat, swallow, chew; commonly loses weight; emaciation common Has problems associated with immobility (e.g., pneumonia, pressure ulcers, contractures) Incontinence common; seizures may develop Most certainly institutionalized at this point Return of primitive (infantile) reflexes

From Hall, G.R. (1994). Caring for people with Alzheimer's disease using the conceptual model of progressively lowered stress threshold in the clinical setting. *Nursing Clinics of North America, 29*(1), 129-141.

VIGNETTE

Mr. Collins is transferred to a less complicated work position after his inability to function is recognized. His wife drives him to work and picks him up. Mr. Collins often forgets what he is doing and stares blankly. He accuses the supervisor of spying on him. Sometimes he disappears at lunch and is unable to find his way back to work. The transfer lasts only a few months, and Mr. Collins is forced to take an early retirement. At home Mr. Collins sleeps in his clothes. He loses interest in reading and watching sports on television and often breaks into angry outbursts, seemingly over nothing. Often he becomes extremely restless and irritable and wanders around the house aimlessly.

Stage 3: Moderate to Severe Alzheimer's disease

At the moderate to severe stage, the person is often unable to identify familiar objects or people, even a spouse (*severe agnosia*). The person needs repeated instructions and directions to perform the simplest tasks (*advanced apraxia*): "Here is the face cloth, pick up the soap. Now, put water on the face cloth and rub the face cloth with soap." Often the individual cannot remember where the toilet is and becomes incontinent. Total care is necessary at this point, and the burden on the family can be emotionally, financially, and physically devastating. The world is very frightening to the person with AD because nothing makes sense any longer. Agitation, violence, paranoia, and delusions are commonly seen. Another problem that is frightening to family members and caregivers is wandering behavior. It is estimated that about 60% of people with AD wander and are at risk for becoming lost (Mayo Clinic, 2010).

Institutionalization may be the most appropriate recourse at this time because the level of care is so demanding, and violent outbursts and incontinence may be burdens that the family can no longer handle. The following are some criteria that indicate the need for placement in a skilled nursing facility:

- Wandering
- Danger to self and others
- Incontinence
- Behavior affects the sleep and general health of others
- Total dependence on others for physical care

> **VIGNETTE**
> Mr. Collins is terrified. Memories come and then slip away. People come and go, but they are strangers. Someone is masquerading as his wife, and it is hard to tell what is real. Things never stay in the same place. Sometimes people hide the bathroom where he cannot find it. He in turn hides things to keep them safe, but he forgets where he hides them. Buttons and belts are confusing, and he does not know what they are doing there anyway. Sometimes he tries to walk away from the terrifying feelings and the strangers. He tries to find something he has lost long ago...if he could only remember what it is.

Stage 4: Late Alzheimer's disease

Late in AD the following symptoms may occur: agraphia (inability to read or write), hyperorality (the need to taste, chew, and put everything in one's mouth), blunting of emotions, visual agnosia (loss of ability to recognize familiar objects), and hypermetamorphosis (manifested by touching of everything in sight). At this stage, the ability to talk, and eventually the ability to walk, is lost. The end stage of AD is characterized by stupor and coma. Death frequently is secondary to infection or choking.

> **VIGNETTE**
> Mrs. Collins and the children keep Mr. Collins at home until his outbursts become frightening. Once, he is lost for 2 days after he somehow unlocks the front door. Finally, Mrs. Collins has her husband placed in a Veterans Administration (VA) hospital. When his wife comes to visit, Mr. Collins sometimes cries. He never talks and is always tied into his chair when she comes to see him. The staff explains to her that although Mr. Collins can still walk, he keeps getting into other people's beds and scaring them. They explain that perhaps he wants comfort and misses human touch. They encourage her visits, even though Mr. Collins does not seem to recognize her. He does respond to music. His wife brings him a small CD player, and plays the country and western music he has always loved; at those times Mr. Collins nods and claps his hands.

> Mrs. Collins is torn between guilt and love, anger and despair. She is confused and depressed. She is going through the painful process of mourning the loss of the man she has loved and shared a life with for 34 years. Three months after his admission to the VA hospital, and 8 years after the incident of the crossed wires at the telephone company, Mr. Collins chokes on some food, develops pneumonia, and dies.

Diagnostic Tests for Dementia

A wide range of problems may masquerade as dementia and may be mistaken for AD. For example, depression and dementia in the older adult present with similar symptoms. It is important that nurses and other health care professionals be able to assess some of the important differences among depression, dementia, and delirium. See Table 18-1 for important differences among these three phenomena. It is important to emphasize that depression and dementia or depression and delirium can coexist in the same person. Therefore it is important that a complete and thorough medical exam (neurological, medical, psychiatric history, review of medications, and nutritional evaluation) be performed.

Other disorders that often mimic dementia include drug toxicity, metabolic disorders, infections, and nutritional deficiencies. A disorder that mimics dementia is sometimes referred to as a pseudodementia. That is, although the symptoms may suggest dementia, a careful examination may reveal another diagnosis altogether, usually depression. This reinforces the importance of performing a comprehensive assessment (including laboratory tests) when symptoms of dementia are present to identify nondementia causes.

No definitive test presently exists to diagnose AD and we must rely on symptoms; in fact, a confirmation of the disease can only be made on autopsy. However, preliminary evidence suggests that positron emission tomography (PET) and single photon emission computed tomography (SPECT) scans can aid in the diagnosis. Studies using magnetic resonance imaging (MRI) to measure the size of brain structures are illuminating; a recent study showed that about 12% of people with smaller brain structures and only mild minor cognitive symptoms will eventually progress to dementia (Black & Andreasen, 2011). Researchers have recently discovered 23 proteins in cerebrospinal fluid that may be biomarkers for AD and are optimistic that diagnosing the disease may be possible (Finehout et al., 2007).

CT, PET, and other developing scanning technologies have diagnostic capabilities because they reveal brain atrophy and rule out other conditions, such as neoplasms. The use of mental status questionnaires such as the Mini-Mental State Examination in people older than 75 is sometimes recommended to increase earlier detection.

ASSESSMENT GUIDELINES

Dementia

1. Identify and treat any general medical conditions that might contribute to the dementia.

2. Evaluate potential of suicide or aggression toward others.

3. Explore how well the family is prepared for and informed about the progress of the patient's dementia (e.g., the phases and course of AD, vascular dementia, acquired immunodeficiency syndrome [AIDS]-related dementia, or dementia associated with multiple sclerosis, lupus erythematosus, or brain injury).

4. Review the medications the patient is currently taking, including over-the-counter (OTC) remedies, herbs, complementary agents, and recreational drugs.

5. Evaluate the patient's current level of cognitive functioning.

6. Discuss with family members how they are coping with the patient and their main issues at this time.

7. Assess evidence of neglect or abuse.

8. Review the resources available to the family. Ask the family members to describe the help they receive from other family members, friends, and community resources. Determine if caregivers are aware of community support groups and resources.

9. Determine the appropriate safety measures needed by the patient and arrange for them to be implemented.

10. Evaluate the safety of the patient's home environment (e.g., with regard to wandering, eating inedible objects, falling, engaging in provocative behaviors toward others).

11. Identify the needs of the family for teaching and guidance (e.g., how to manage catastrophic reactions, lability of mood, aggressive behaviors, and nocturnal delirium and increased confusion and agitation at night, or sundown syndrome).

DIAGNOSIS

One of the most important areas of concern is the patient's *safety*. Many people with AD wander and may be lost for hours or days. Wandering, along with behaviors such as rummaging, may be perceived as purposeful to the patient. Wandering may result from changes in the physical environment, fear caused by hallucinations or delusions, or lack of exercise.

Seizures may occur in the later stages of this disease. Injuries from falls and accidents can occur during any stage as confusion and disorientation progress. The potential for burns exists if the patient is a smoker or is unattended when using the stove. Prescription drugs can be taken incorrectly, or bottles of noxious fluids can be mistakenly ingested, which results in a medical crisis. Therefore, *Risk for Injury* is always present.

As the person's ability to recognize or name objects is decreased, *Impaired Verbal Communication* becomes a problem. As memory diminishes and disorientation increases, *Impaired Environmental Interpretation Syndrome, Impaired Memory,* and *Chronic Confusion* occur.

During the course of the disease, people show personality changes, increased vulnerability, and often inappropriate behaviors. Common behaviors include hoarding, regression, and being overly demanding. Therefore nurses and family members often intervene in behaviors that signal *Ineffective Coping*. Family caregivers may experience *Compromised* or even *Disabled Family Coping*.

Additional family issues may emerge. Perhaps some of the most crucial aspects of the patient's care are support, education, and referrals for the family. The family loses an integral part of its unit. Family members lose the love, function, support, companionship, and warmth that this person once provided. *Caregiver Role Strain* is always present and planning with the family and offering community support are integral parts of appropriate care. *Anticipatory Grieving* is also an important phenomenon to assess and may be an important target for intervention. Helping the family grieve can make the task ahead somewhat clearer and, at times, less painful. See Table 18-2 for potential nursing diagnoses for confused patients with dementia.

OUTCOMES IDENTIFICATION

Families who have a member with dementia are faced with an exhaustive list of issues that need addressing. Self-care needs, impaired environmental interpretation, constant confusion, ineffective individual coping, and role strain of the caregiver are just a few of the areas nurses and other health care members will need to target (Box 18-2).

PLANNING

The planning of care for a patient with dementia is geared toward the patient's immediate needs. Figure 18-2 presents the Functional Dementia Scale, which can be used by nurses and families to plan strategies for addressing immediate needs and to track progression of the dementia.

Identifying level of functioning and assessing caregivers' needs help the nurse identify appropriate community resources. Does the patient or family need the following?

- Transportation services
- Supervision and care when primary caregiver is out of the home
- Referrals to day care centers
- Information on support groups within the community
- Meals on Wheels
- Information on respite and residential services
- Telephone numbers for help lines
- Home health aides
- Home health services
- The Alzheimer's Association's Safe Return program (www.alz.org)
- Additional teaching or psychopharmaceutical aids to manage distressing or harmful behaviors when appropriate

Because stress is a common occurrence when working with persons with cognitive impairments, the health care staff needs to be proactive in minimizing its effects as well as in teaching and providing guidelines to caregivers and loved ones. Reducing stress can be facilitated by the following measures:

- **Have a realistic understanding of the disease** so that expectations for the patient are realistic.

BOX 18-2   SUGGESTED OUTCOME CRITERIA FOR DEMENTIA*

Injury
- Patient will remain safe in the hospital or at home.
- With the aid of an identification bracelet and neighborhood or hospital alert, patient will be returned within 1 hour of wandering.
- Patient will remain free of danger during seizures.
- With the aid of interventions, patient will remain burn-free.
- With the aid of guidance and environmental manipulation, patient will not be hurt if a fall occurs.
- Patient will ingest only correct doses of prescribed medications and appropriate food and fluids.

Communication
- Patient will communicate needs.
- Patient will answer yes or no appropriately to questions.
- Patient will state needs in alternative modes when aphasic (e.g., will signal correct word on hearing it or will refer to picture or label).
- Patient will wear prescribed glasses or hearing aid each day.

Caregiver Role Strain
- Family members will have the opportunity to express "unacceptable" feelings in a supportive environment.
- Family members will have access to professional counseling.
- Family members will name two organizations within their geographical area that can offer support.

Caregiver Role Strain (continued)
- Family members will participate in patient's plan of care, with encouragement from staff.
- Family members will state that they have outside help that allows them to take personal time for themselves each week or month.
- Family members will have the names of three resources that can help with financial burdens and legal considerations.

Impaired Environmental Interpretation: Chronic Confusion
- Patient will acknowledge the reality of an object or a sound that was misinterpreted (illusion), after it is pointed out.
- Patient will state that he or she feels safe after experiencing delusions or illusions.
- Patient will remain nonaggressive when experiencing paranoid ideation.

Self-Care Needs
- Patient will participate in self-care at optimal level.
- Patient will be able to follow step-by-step instructions for dressing, bathing, and grooming.
- Patient will put on own clothes appropriately, with aid of fastening tape (Velcro) and nursing supervision.
- Patient's skin will remain intact and free from signs of pressure.

*Not an exhaustive list.

- **Establish realistic outcomes** for the patient and recognize when they are achieved. These outcomes may be as minor as *patient feeds self with spoon*, yet it must be remembered that even the smallest achievement can be a significant accomplishment for the impaired individual.
- **Maintain good self-care.** Nurses and caregivers need to protect themselves from the negative effects of stress by obtaining adequate sleep and rest, eating a nutritious diet, exercising, engaging in relaxing activities, and addressing their own spiritual needs.

IMPLEMENTATION

The needs of a patient with dementia are complex, change over time, and can take place in a variety of settings during various stages of the disease. Care settings include the emergency department, general hospital, home settings, long-term care settings, and the community.

The nurse's attitude of unconditional positive regard is the single most effective tool in caring for patients with dementia. It induces patients to cooperate with care, reduces catastrophic outbreaks, and increases family members' satisfaction with care. A warm, empathic, and nonjudgmental approach using calm, unhurried, clear communications can help allay confusion and agitation. The nurse and others should always introduce themselves with each encounter. Expectations should be clear and explained in simple, step-by-step instructions. To help patients maintain a sense of self-control, they should be given simple and appropriate choices in their care (e.g., "Do you want to wash your face before or after you brush your teeth?").

Because a considerable number of individuals with dementia have secondary behavioral disturbances (e.g., depression, hallucinations, delusions, agitation, insomnia, and wandering), there is an increase in the need for supervision. Many of these situations respond well to the interventions listed in Tables 18-5 and 18-6. For example, a woman who is 78 years old believes that she is 23 and has babies at home would not be calmed by being told that she is 78 and has no babies. It is most helpful to reflect back to patients their feelings and to show understanding and concern for their plight (Alverez, 2002). For example, "Mrs. Green, you miss your children, and this can be a lonely place."

Intervention with family members is critical. The effects of losing a family member to dementia—that is, watching the deterioration of a person who has had an important role

FUNCTIONAL DEMENTIA SCALE

Circle one rating for each item:
1. None or little of the time
2. Some of the time
3. Good part of the time
4. Most or all of the time

Client: _____
Observer: _____
Position or relation to patient: _____
Facility: _____
Date: _____

1	2	3	4	1. Has difficulty in completing simple tasks on own (e.g., dressing, bathing, doing arithmetic).
1	2	3	4	2. Spends time either sitting or in apparently purposeless activity.
1	2	3	4	3. Wanders at night or needs to be restrained to prevent wandering.
1	2	3	4	4. Hears things that are not there.
1	2	3	4	5. Requires supervision or assistance in eating.
1	2	3	4	6. Loses things.
1	2	3	4	7. Appearance is disorderly if left to own devices.
1	2	3	4	8. Moans.
1	2	3	4	9. Cannot control bowel function.
1	2	3	4	10. Threatens to harm others.
1	2	3	4	11. Cannot control bladder function.
1	2	3	4	12. Needs to be watched so doesn't injure self (e.g., by careless smoking, leaving the stove on, falling).
1	2	3	4	13. Destructive of materials around him/her (e.g., breaks furniture, throws food trays, tears up magazines).
1	2	3	4	14. Shouts or yells.
1	2	3	4	15. Accuses others of doing bodily harm or stealing his or her possessions — when you are sure the accusations are not true.
1	2	3	4	16. Is unaware of limitations imposed by illness.
1	2	3	4	17. Becomes confused and does not know where he or she is.
1	2	3	4	18. Has trouble remembering.
1	2	3	4	19. Has sudden changes of mood (e.g., gets upset, angered, or cries easily).
1	2	3	4	20. If left alone, wanders aimlessly during the day or needs to be restrained to prevent wandering.

FIGURE 18-2 Functional Dementia Scale. (From Moore, J.T., et al. [1983]. A functional dementia scale. *Journal of Family Practice, 16,* 498.)

TABLE 18-5 INTERVENTION GUIDELINES FOR DEMENTIA: COMMUNICATION

INTERVENTION	RATIONALE
1. Always identify yourself and call the person by name at each meeting.	1. Patient's short-term memory is impaired—requires frequent orientation to time and environment.
2. Speak slowly.	2. Patient needs time to process information.
3. Use short, simple words and phrases.	3. Patient may not be able to understand complex statements or abstract ideas.
4. Maintain face-to-face contact.	4. Verbal and nonverbal clues are maximized.
5. Be near patient when talking, one or two arm-lengths away.	5. This distance can help patient focus on speaker as well as maintain personal space.
6. Focus on one piece of information at a time.	6. Attention span of patient is poor and patient is easily distracted—helps patient focus. Too much data can be overwhelming and can increase anxiety.
7. Talk with patient about familiar and meaningful things.	7. Self-expression is promoted and reality is reinforced.
8. Encourage reminiscing about happy times in life.	8. Remembering accomplishments and shared joys helps distract patient from deficit and gives meaning to existence.
9. When patient is delusional, acknowledge patient's feelings and reinforce reality. Do not argue or refute delusions.	9. Acknowledging feelings helps patient feel understood. Pointing out realities may help patient focus on realities. Arguing can enhance adherence to false beliefs.

TABLE 18-5 INTERVENTION GUIDELINES FOR DEMENTIA: COMMUNICATION—cont'd

INTERVENTION	RATIONALE
10. If a patient gets into an argument with another patient, stop the argument and separate individuals. After a short while (5 minutes), explain straightforwardly to each patient why you had to intervene.	10. Escalation to physical acting out is prevented. Patient's right to know is respected. Explaining in an adult manner helps maintain self-esteem.
11. When patient becomes verbally aggressive, acknowledge patient's feelings and shift topic to more familiar ground (e.g., "I know this is upsetting for you, because you always cared for others. Tell me about your children.").	11. Confusion and disorientation easily increase anxiety. Acknowledging feelings makes patient feel more understood and less alone. Topics patient has mastery over can remind him or her of areas of competent functioning and can increase self-esteem.
12. Have patient wear prescription eyeglasses or hearing aid.	12. Environmental awareness, orientation, and comprehension are increased, which in turn increases awareness of personal needs and the presence of others.
13. Keep patient's room well lit.	13. Environmental clues are maximized.
14. Have clocks, calendars, and personal items (e.g., family pictures or Bible) in clear view of patient while he or she is in bed.	14. These objects assist in maintaining personal identity.
15. Reinforce patient's pictures, nonverbal gestures, X's on calendars, and other methods used to anchor patient in reality.	15. When aphasia starts to hinder communication, alternate methods of communication need to be instituted.

TABLE 18-6 INTERVENTION GUIDELINES FOR DEMENTIA: HEALTH TEACHING AND HEALTH PROMOTION

INTERVENTION	RATIONALE
Dressing and Bathing	
1. Always have patient perform all tasks within his or her present capacity.	1. Maintains patient's self-esteem and uses muscle groups; impedes staff burnout; minimizes further regression.
2. Always have patient wear own clothes, even if in the hospital.	2. Helps maintain patient's identity and dignity.
3. Use clothing with elastic, and substitute fastening tape (Velcro) for buttons and zippers.	3. Minimizes patient's confusion and eases independence of functioning.
4. Label clothing items with patient's name and name of item.	4. Helps identify patient if he or she wanders and gives patient additional clues when aphasia or agnosia occurs.
5. Give step-by-step instructions whenever necessary (e.g., "Take this blouse…put in one arm…now the next arm…pull it together in the front…now ….").	5. Patient can focus on small pieces of information more easily; allows patient to perform at optimal level.
6. Make sure that water in faucets is not too hot.	6. Judgment is lacking in patient; patient is unaware of many safety hazards.
7. If patient is resistant to performing self-care, come back later and ask again.	7. Moods may be labile, and patient may forget but often complies after short interval.
Nutrition	
1. Monitor food and fluid intake.	1. Patient may have anorexia or be too confused to eat.
2. Offer finger foods that patient can take away from the dinner table.	2. Increases input throughout the day; patient may eat only small amounts at meals.
3. Weigh patient regularly (once a week).	3. Monitors fluid and nutritional status.
4. During periods of hyperorality, watch that patient does not eat nonfood items (e.g., ceramic fruit or food-shaped soaps).	4. Patient puts everything into mouth; may be unable to differentiate inedible objects made in the shape and color of food.

Continued

TABLE 18-6   INTERVENTION GUIDELINES FOR DEMENTIA: HEALTH TEACHING AND HEALTH PROMOTION—cont'd

INTERVENTION	RATIONALE
Bowel and Bladder Function	
1. Begin bowel and bladder program early; start with bladder control.	1. Establishing same time of day for bowel movements and toileting—in early morning, after meals and snacks, and before bedtime—can help prevent incontinence.
2. Evaluate use of disposable diapers.	2. Prevents embarrassment.
3. Label bathroom door as well as doors to other rooms.	3. Additional environmental clues can maximize independent toileting.
Sleep	
1. Because patient may awaken, be frightened, or cry out at night, keep area well lit.	1. Reinforces orientation, minimizes possible illusions.
2. Maintain a calm atmosphere during the day.	2. Encourages a calming night's sleep.
3. Medications are not recommended for sleep. The use of nonmedical interventions has proven most helpful in many cases. When medications have been prescribed, low-dose tricyclic antidepressants, neuroleptics with sedative properties (e.g., haloperidol [Haldol]), benzodiazepines, and others may be ordered.	3. Helps clear thinking and sedates. However, psychotic medications should be used with extreme care, and other methods should be applied first
4. Avoid the use of restraints.	4. Can cause patient to become more terrified and fight against restraints until exhausted to a dangerous degree.

within the family unit and who is loved and a vital part of his or her family's history—are devastating, exhausting, and painful. Nurses can teach families about the progression of the illness, give them guidelines for safely caring for their family member who lives at home (Tables 18-7 and 18-8), and find appropriate support for families who are grieving.

Communication Guidelines

How nurses choose to communicate with patients with dementia affects the patient's maintenance of self-esteem and ability to participate in care. People with dementia often find it difficult to express themselves. They:

- Have difficulty finding the right words.
- Use familiar words repeatedly.
- Invent new words to describe things (neologisms).
- Frequently lose their train of thought.
- Rely on nonverbal gestures.

See Table 18-5 for a variety of nursing interventions and guidelines integral for communicating with a cognitively impaired person. These interventions and guidelines also can be taught to family members.

Health Teaching and Health Promotion

Educating families who have a cognitively impaired member is one of the most important areas for nurses. Families who are caring for a member in the home need to know about strategies for communicating and structuring self-care activities (see Table 18-6).

Most important, families need to know where to get help. Help includes professional counseling and education regarding the process and the progression of the disease. Families need to know about and be referred to community-based groups that can help bear this tremendous burden (e.g., day care centers, senior citizen groups, organizations providing home visits and respite care, and family support groups). A list with definitions of some of the types of services available in the patient's community, as well as the names and telephone numbers of the providers of these services, should be given to the family.

The Alzheimer's Association (www.alz.org) is a national umbrella agency that provides various forms of assistance to people with the disease and their families. The Alzheimer's Association has launched Safe Return to help locate and return missing people with AD and other memory impairments. Wandering is a common behavior during the second and third stages of AD, and the Safe Return program offers peace of mind to families. Some communities are instituting small GPS systems that can be attached by a wristband or armband to help locate a person with AD.

Information regarding housekeeping, home health aides, and companions is also available through this organization. Such outside resources can help prevent the total emotional and physical fatigue of family members. Types of resources that might be available in some communities are found in Table 18-7. When the nurse is unable to provide the relevant information, proper referrals by the social worker are needed. Information regarding advance directives, durable power of attorney, guardianship, and conservatorship should be included in the communication with the family.

TABLE 18-7	SERVICES FOR PEOPLE WITH DEMENTIA AND THEIR FAMILIES OR CAREGIVERS
TYPE OF SERVICE	**SERVICES PROVIDED**
Family or caregiver Some patients may live by themselves in the community; active case management is vital when this is the case.	Caregivers have a right to: • Easy access to services • Respite care • Full involvement in decision making • Assessment of the needs of the caregiver as well as those of the patient • Information and referral • Case management: coordination of community resources and follow-up
Community **services**	• Adult day care: provides activities, socialization, supervision • Physician services • Protective services: prevent, eliminate, and/or remedy effects of abuse or neglect • Recreational services • Transportation • Mental health services • Legal services
Home care	• Meals on Wheels • Home health aide services • Homemaker services • Hospice services • Occupational therapy • Paid companion or sitter services • Physical therapy • Skilled nursing • Personal care services: assistance in basic self-care activities • Social work services • Telephone reassurance: regular telephone calls to individuals who are isolated and homebound* • Personal emergency response systems: telephone-based systems to alert others that a person who is alone is in need of emergency assistance*

*Vital for those living alone.

Milieu Therapy

Interventions and guidelines for families in structuring a safe environment and planning appropriate activities are found in Table 18-8.

Pharmacological, Biological, and Integrative Therapies

Neurocognitive Impairment

Although there is no cure for Alzheimer's disease, there are a number of prescription drugs currently approved by the Food and Drug Administration (FDA) for Alzheimer's disease patients. For example, medications called cholinesterase inhibitors can help delay or prevent symptoms from becoming worse for a limited time, and are useful in people with mild to moderate Alzheimer's disease. They work by preventing the breakdown of acetylcholine, and they stimulate nicotinic receptors to release more acetylcholine into the brain. Examples of cholinesterase inhibitors are galantamine hydrobromide (Razadyne), rivastigmine tartrate (Exelon), and donepezil hydrochloride (Aricept). Another drug, tacrine (Cognex), has been FDA approved but is rarely used today because of its deleterious side effects (ADEAR, 2010). These first FDA-approved agents demonstrated positive effects not only on cognition but also on behavior and function in activities of daily living for patients with mild to moderate AD. All of these medications are effective for a limited period—until the stores of acetylcholine have been depleted. At that point, the functioning of the person with AD may deteriorate drastically.

Memantine hydrochloride (Namenda), an N-methyl-D-aspartate (NMDA), is an antagonist at the NMDA-glutamatergic ion channels. This drug works by blocking the toxic effects associated with excess glutamate and regulates glutamate activation. It is the first drug to target symptoms of AD during the moderate

TABLE 18-8   INTERVENTIONS FOR A SAFE MILIEU IN THE HOME

INTERVENTION	RATIONALE
Safe Environment	
1. Gradually restrict use of the car.	1. Even mild dementia increases risk of vehicular accident (APA, 2008).
2. Remove throw rugs and other objects in person's path.	2. Minimizes tripping and falling.
3. Minimize sensory stimulation.	3. Decreases sensory overload, which can increase anxiety and confusion.
4. If patient becomes verbally upset, listen briefly, give support, then change the topic.	4. Goal is to prevent escalation of anger. When attention span is short, patient can be distracted to more productive topics and activities.
5. Label all rooms and drawers. Label often-used objects (e.g., hairbrushes and toothbrushes).	5. May keep patient from wandering into other patients' rooms. Increases environmental clues to familiar objects.
6. Install safety bars in bathroom.	6. Prevents falls.
7. Supervise patient when he or she smokes.	7. Danger of burns is always present.
8. If patient has history of seizures, educate family on how to deal with seizures.	8. Seizure activity is common in advanced Alzheimer's disease.
Wandering	
1. If patient wanders during the night, put mattress on the floor.	1. Prevents falls when patient is confused.
2. Have patient wear MedicAlert bracelet that cannot be removed (with name, address, and telephone number). Provide police department with recent pictures.	2. Patient can easily be identified by police, neighbors, or hospital personnel.
3. Alert local police and neighbors about patient wandering.	3. May reduce time necessary to return patient to home or hospital.
4. If patient is in the hospital, have him or her wear brightly colored vest with name, unit, and phone number printed on back.	4. Makes patient easily identifiable.
5. Put complex locks on door.	5. Reduces opportunity to wander.
6. Place locks at top of door.	6. In moderate and late Alzheimer's-type dementia, ability to look up and reach upward is lost.
7. Encourage physical activity during the day.	7. Physical activity may decrease wandering at night.
8. Explore the feasibility of installing sensor devices or GPS system.	8. Sensor provides warning if patient wanders. GPS can help locate patient.
9. Use a bed monitor.	9. Alerts staff if patient has left his or her bed during the night.
Useful Activities	
1. Provide picture magazines and children's books when patient's reading ability diminishes.	1. Allows continuation of usual activities that patient can still enjoy; provides focus.
2. Provide simple activities that allow exercise of large muscles.	2. Exercise groups, dance groups, and walking provide socialization as well as increased circulation and maintenance of muscle tone.
3. Encourage group activities that are familiar and simple to perform.	3. Activities such as group singing, dancing, reminiscing, and working with clay and paint all help to increase socialization and minimize feelings of alienation.

to severe stages of the disorder. Like the cholinesterase inhibitors, the benefits of memantine (Namenda) are time limited. Ergoloid mesylates such as Hydergine, an ergot alkaloid, have been approved for use in people with AD and stroke. There are many new drugs in the pipeline for treating Alzheimer's disease—for example, results of a pilot study using a nasal spray form of insulin over a 4-month period resulted in stabilized or improved cognitive function for mild to moderate AD (Brooks, 2011).

Targeting Behavioral Symptoms of Alzheimer's Disease

Cognitive behavioral approaches and nursing interventions mentioned in this text are often helpful in lowering anxiety, dealing with physical agitation, and intervening with hallucinations and delusions. At times, other medications may be useful in managing behavioral symptoms of dementia, but these need to be used with extreme caution. Age alters the metabolism, absorption, and elimination of many medications, and older

EXAMINING THE EVIDENCE

Activating the Environment—For Each Patient

I just completed a clinical rotation in a long term care facility and noticed that many of the patients with dementia participated in "sit down" groups that exercised only their arms and upper torso. That seemed kind of boring. Is there anything else that might liven it up?

There is good news for long term care nurses who are eager to advocate for the individual needs of their patients—the organizational structure, rules, and regulations in long term care have all dramatically changed during the past decade and continue to do so. Emphasis is now placed on "person appropriate" activity relevant to needs, interests, culture, and background. Large-group programming that dominated the activities' calendar Monday through Friday is no longer sufficient (Smith et al., 2009).

Commonly called "culture change," this movement to improve the quality of life among older adults has gained considerable momentum (Smith et al., 2009). Additional treatments have been implemented that include intensified physical routines and outdoor and work-related activities; also, alternative therapies, such as acupressure (noninvasive variation of acupuncture) and massage, have been used to manage agitation and increase relaxation in patients with dementia (Lin et al., 2009).

Activation and rehabilitation in outdoor environments for individual treatment of persons with cognitive impairment are highly recommended. For persons with Alzheimer's disease outdoor physical activities can play an important part of everyday life by creating meaningful routines and improving well-being and health (Cedervall et al., 2010). Gardening activities, such as watering, weeding, raking, and planting, and outdoor walks are enjoyable experiences for all patients, but the degree of independence varied (Thelandes et al., 2008). In the Netherlands, Green Care Farms have been successfully developed to provide some vigorous physical outdoor activities to meet the needs of home-bound cognitively impaired adults (deBruen, 2009).

Also, small work-related indoor groups assisted cognitively impaired persons more than activities that were not related to "meaningful work." Sorting activities, stamping, and folding towels tapped into past role identity and feelings familiar to residents in a nursing home (Mansfield et al., 2009). In addition, utilization of specific past learned skills of a patient, such as playing instruments, knitting, and singing songs, resulted in decreased anxiety levels and reduction in nonconforming behaviors (Zec et al., 2008). Another successful activity combined exercise and music for patients with AD just before mealtimes. This activity was linked to slower decline in eating ability and decreased apathy overall (Moore, 2010).

Thus with some outside pressure and interest from governmental and consumer groups, along with advocacy from the nurse, the living environment—both indoors and out—for the cognitively impaired patient can be activated to individualize the needs of each patient with the goal of an improved quality of life.

Cedervall, Y., et al. (2010). Physical activity and implications on well-being in mild Alzheimer's disease: a qualitative case study in 2 men with dementia and their spouses. *Physiotherapy Theory and Practice, 26*(4), 226-239.

deBruen, S.R. (2009). Green care farms promote activity in elderly people with dementia. *Journal of Housing for the Elderly, 23*(4), 368-389.

Lin, L., et al. (2009). Using acupressure and Montessori based activities to decrease agitation for residents with dementia: a cross over trial. *Journal of American Geriatrics Society, 57*(6).

Mansfield, J., et al. (2009). The impact of stimulus on engagement of nursing home residents with dementia. *Archives of Gerontology and Geriatrics, 49*(1).

Moore, J. (2010). *Familiar physical activity to familiar music: the effects on apathy, agitation, eating and dietary intake of institutionalized older adults with dementia.* University of Massachusetts/Amherst doctoral dissertation.

Smith, M., et al. (2009). Beyond bingo: meaningful activities for persons with dementia in nursing homes. *Annals of Long Term Care, 17.*

Thelandes, V., et al. (2008). Gardening activities for nursing home residents with dementia. *Advances in Physiotherapy, 10,* 53-56.

Zec, R., et al. (2008). Non-pharmacological and pharmacological treatment of the cognitive and behavioral symptoms of Alzheimers. *Neurorehabilitation, 23,* 425-438.

Courtesy of Lois Angelo.

APPLYING THE ART

A Person With Dementia

SCENARIO: I met 75-year-old Mr. Samson on our geriatric rotation. He had recently been moved to the Memory Disorder Unit of the nursing facility. His wife of 50 years, whom he called Darlin' (her name was Darlene), had resided on the assisted living side of the facility until her sudden death from a myocardial infarction 3 weeks earlier. Mr. Samson and I regularly used the pictures in the memory wallet that his wife and the staff had assembled to remind him about his life.

THERAPEUTIC GOAL: By the end of this encounter, Mr. Samson will begin to process the reality of his wife's death as evidenced by referring to her and their life together in the past tense at least part of the time.

STUDENT-PATIENT INTERACTION	THOUGHTS, COMMUNICATION TECHNIQUES, AND MENTAL HEALTH NURSING CONCEPTS
Student: "Mr. Samson, what's wrong?" **Mr. Samson:** *Crying.* "My Darlin', what's wrong with my Darlin'?" *He gestures toward the sign of the memorial service to be held for "Mrs. Darlene Samson" and one other resident who had died the previous month.*	I knew from the chart that Mr. Samson had attended his wife's funeral. I should have said my name and reminded him that we had talked a few times before, but I was worried because he was sitting in the lobby sobbing. He is crying like he just discovered "his Darlin'" died. How awful to not be able to hold on to your own life and what matters most in your memories.
Student: "Mr. Samson, I'm _____, your nursing student. You feel worried seeing your wife's name on the sign. *He nods.* Let's use your memory wallet to remember together about your Darlin'." *I wait until he makes eye contact and takes the wallet out of his hip pocket.* **Student's feelings:** *I am feeling a little anxious now. I hope I did okay in calling Mrs. Samson Darlin' as he does. I hope he'll remember if I show him the picture the staff put in the wallet showing Mr. Samson standing and looking at his wife in the casket. Seems unkind in some ways.*	I *introduce* myself again and use *reflection.* Diverting to the task of looking through the memory wallet provides structure to help meet *safety needs.*
Student: *Smiling encouragingly.* "Tell me about the pictures."	I know that the mental health focus needs to include helping with *reality orientation* for as long as his progressive *dementia* will allow.
Mr. Samson: *No longer crying.* "This was our house. Darlin' keeps such a great garden. I used to love her tomatoes the best. *He points to the tall plants beside the house.* **Student's feelings:** *He's trying so hard. I admire him. I never knew either of my grandfathers.*	He uses the present tense "keeps...garden," but the past tense for "was our house" and "used to love her tomatoes." He is having trouble sorting out the present from the past.
Student: "You still love tomatoes! I helped you make the tomato salad for lunch. None tastes as good as Darlin's did, I bet." **Student's feelings:** *I did well here by reminding him of still liking tomatoes.*	I make an *observation.* I refer to Mrs. Samson's tomatoes in the past tense to *reinforce reality.*
Mr. Samson: "Right. I wonder if Darlin' picked the tomato salad. We meet in the solarium every day." **Student's feelings:** *I feel frustrated that he's talking about Darlin' like she's alive. Two days ago he talked like he remembered that Mrs. Samson died 3 weeks ago.*	
Student: "Look at this next picture." *I wait as he absorbs the funeral home picture.* **Student's feelings:** *Was that too direct? I didn't know what to say when he talked about meeting her in the solarium.*	How nontherapeutic. I sound like I am giving a command. I should have started with, "I have some sad news."

APPLYING THE ART—cont'd

A Person With Dementia

STUDENT-PATIENT INTERACTION	THOUGHTS, COMMUNICATION TECHNIQUES, AND MENTAL HEALTH NURSING CONCEPTS
Mr. Samson: "Oh God, oh God. She died. She's gone. When did she die? How can I go on without her?" *He buries his head in his hands, sobbing.*	
Student's feelings: *He's experiencing this as though for the first time. I feel ready to cry.*	
Student: "I am with you. May I hold your hand? *He nods.* It's so painful to say goodbye."	Touch communicates caring. I *reflect feelings* about saying goodbye.
	I ask permission before touching.
Mr. Samson: "We were married 50 years. She's the love of my life. Darlin' was my soul mate."	Again he mixes past and present tenses. How can he progress through the grief process when he keeps moving back to the denial stage?
	I cannot imagine 50 years with one person. What an accomplishment.
Student: "You're really struggling with letting yourself know she died. You say, Darlin' was your soul mate. You miss her so much."	I use *reflection.* I also carefully *restate* to emphasize his use of the past tense. I wonder what effect the memorial service will have on him. When he comes to the point of grieving anew every time, we will have to take out the funeral picture and emphasize feelings using *validation therapy.*
Student's feelings: *I'll talk with the treatment team. He may need some extra support as his memory impairment grows and as he faces the memorial service.*	
Mr. Samson: "I do, every minute of every day." *He makes eye contact as we continue talking until he's calmer and no longer crying.*	
Student's feelings: *I like him and I feel so sad about his situation.*	
Student: "Are you ready to walk together back to your room so you can get ready for reminiscence group?" *He nods.*	Giving him a choice empowers him.

adults are more sensitive to these effects. The basic rule for older patients is: **"start low and go slow."**

In patients with coexisting depression, the choice of agents is usually based on the side effect profile. Selective serotonin reuptake inhibitors (SSRIs) have a low side effect profile and appear better tolerated. Bupropion (Wellbutrin), venlafaxine (Effexor), and mirtazapine (Remeron) are also good choices. Agents with anticholinergic side effects should be avoided (APA, 2008).

The use of restraints and medications to control disruptive behavior in patients with dementia is often associated with falls, worsening cognitive impairment, oversedation, and other adverse drug reactions. Physical restraints are rarely indicated. In 2008 the APA suggested using structural education programs for staff to help manage disruptive behaviors through behavioral interventions and/or cognitive techniques in order to reduce use of both medications and restraints (APA, 2008).

Atypical antipsychotic medications (particularly risperidone [Risperdal], olanzapine [Zyprexa], and quetiapine fumarate [Seroquel]) have been used extensively for treating

behavioral symptoms of AD. Some of these troubling symptoms are (1) psychoses (hallucinations and delusions), (2) severe mood swings, (3) anxiety (agitation), and (4) verbal or physical aggression (combativeness). However, current research questions the advisability of using the expensive atypical antipsychotics, none of which are FDA approved for treating AD, for these behaviors. In fact, in 2005 the FDA issued a Black Box warning that stated, "Treatment of behavioral disorders in elderly patients with dementia with atypical antipsychotic medication is associated with increased mortality" (Science News, 2011). It is generally accepted that whatever modest benefit this classification of medication may provide is negated by the side effects. It is recommended that atypical antipsychotics be used sparingly for the few patients who benefit from them. Anxiety, agitation, and delusional behaviors can often be tempered by timely, appropriate use of nursing interventions. The updated APA guidelines (APA, 2008) for treating patients with dementia strongly suggest that nonpharmacological treatment should be tried first. The use of antipsychotics in all settings (home, long-term care) should be limited.

EVALUATION

Outcomes need to be stated in measurable terms, be within the capability of the patient, and be evaluated frequently. As the person's condition continues to deteriorate, outcomes need to be altered to reflect the person's diminished functioning. Frequent evaluation and reformulation of outcome criteria and short-term indicators also help diminish staff and family frustration, as well as minimize the patient's anxiety by ensuring that tasks are not more complicated than the person can accomplish. The overall outcomes for treatment are to promote the patient's optimal level of functioning and to retard further regression, whenever possible. Working closely with family members and providing them with the names of available resources and support sources may help increase the quality of life for both the family and the patient.

KEY POINTS TO REMEMBER

- *Neurocognitive disorder* is a term that refers to disorders marked by disturbances in orientation, memory, intellect, judgment, and affect resulting from changes in the brain.
- Delirium, major neurocognitive disorders, and minor neurocognitive disorders encompass the cognitive disorders in patients that are under our care as health care workers.
- Delirium is marked by acute onset, disturbance in consciousness, and symptoms of disorientation and confusion that fluctuate by the minute, hour, or time of day.
- Delirium is always secondary to an underlying condition; therefore, it is temporary, transient, and may last from hours to days once the underlying cause is treated. If the cause is not treated, permanent damage to neurons can result.
- Dementia (a major neurocognitive disorder) usually has a more insidious onset than delirium. There is global deterioration of cognitive functioning (e.g., memory, judgment, ability to think abstractly, and orientation) that is often progressive and irreversible, depending on the underlying cause.
- Dementia may be primary (e.g., Alzheimer's disease, vascular dementia, Pick's disease, Lewy body disease). In this case, the disease is irreversible. Or it may be secondary to other causes and when treated may be reversed.
- Alzheimer's disease accounts for up to 70% to 80% of all cases of dementia, and vascular dementia accounts for up to 20%.

- There is little known about the actual causes of AD. There are a number of risk factors including advancing age, head trauma, obesity, diabetes, low socioeconomic status and educational levels, and the presence of apolipoprotein E4 (*APOE E4* allele) among others.
- Signs and symptoms change according to the four stages of Alzheimer's disease: stage 1 (mild), stage 2 (moderate), stage 3 (moderate to severe), and stage 4 (late).
- The behavioral manifestations of AD include confabulation, perseveration, aphasia, apraxia, agnosia, and hyperorality.
- No known cause or cure exists for AD, although a number of drugs that increase the brain's supply of acetylcholine (a nerve communication chemical) are helpful in slowing the progress of the disease for a limited period of time.
- People with AD have many unmet needs and present many management challenges to their families as well as to health care workers.
- Mild cognitive impairment (MCI) is a syndrome in which there is a decline in the previous level of cognitive functioning, however, it does not interfere with the person's ability to function and maintain independence in their life.
- Specific nursing interventions for cognitively impaired individuals can increase communication, safety, and self-care, as well as minimize confusion. The need for family teaching and support is crucial.

APPLYING CRITICAL JUDGMENT

1. Mrs. Kendel is an 82-year-old woman who has progressive Alzheimer's disease. She lives with her husband, who has been trying to care for her in their home. Mrs. Kendel often wears evening gowns in the morning, places her blouse on backward, and sometimes wears her bra on backward outside her blouse. She often forgets the location of objects. She makes an effort to cook but often confuses frying pans and pots and sometimes has trouble turning on the stove. Once in a while, she cannot find the bathroom in time, often mistaking it for a broom closet. She becomes frightened of noises and is terrified when the telephone or doorbell rings. At times she cries because she is aware that she is losing her sense of her place in the world. She and her husband have always been close, loving companions, and he wants to keep her at home as long as possible.

A. Help Mr. Kendel by making a list of suggestions that he can try at home that might help facilitate (a) communication, (b) activities of daily living, and (c) maintenance of a safe home environment.

B. Identify at least seven interventions that are appropriate to this situation for each of the areas cited in the previous question.

C. Identify possible types of resources available for maintaining Mrs. Kendel in her home for as long as possible. Provide the name of one self-help group that you would urge Mr. Kendel to join.

D. Share with your clinical group the name and function of at least three community agencies in your area that could be an appropriate referral for a family in your neighborhood.

CHAPTER REVIEW QUESTIONS

Choose the most appropriate answer(s).

1. A nurse assessing a patient with suspected delirium will expect to find that the patient's symptoms developed:
   1. over a period of hours to days.
   2. over a period of weeks to months.
   3. with no relationship to another condition.
   4. during middle age.

2. Of the following outcomes, which one is most appropriate for a patient with cognitive impairment related to delirium?
   1. Patient will participate fully in self-care from admission on.
   2. Patient will have stable vital signs 6 hours after admission.
   3. Patient will participate in simple activities that bring enjoyment.
   4. Patient will return to the premorbid level of functioning.

3. A patient diagnosed with dementia has been eating very little during mealtimes since admission to the nursing home 2 days ago. Select the priority nursing intervention.
   1. Obtain a detailed nutritional history.
   2. Sit with the patient and prompt her to eat.
   3. Report the need for diet changes to the MD.
   4. Encourage the family to bring in home cooked meals.

4. Nursing staff that care for cognitively impaired patients can develop burnout. Strategies to avoid the development of burnout include:
   1. setting realistic patient goals.
   2. insulating self from emotional involvement with patients.
   3. sedating patients to promote rest and minimize catastrophic episodes.
   4. encouraging the family to permit the use of restraints to promote patient safety.

5. A daughter of a patient diagnosed with Alzheimer's disease states she feels guilty and wants to take her father home from the nursing home as soon as possible. The best response by the nurse would be:
   1. "This would definitely help your family with the huge expense of long-term care."
   2. "Your father might really enjoy the familiar surroundings of your home."
   3. "What a kind gesture for you to make!"
   4. "It is most likely that patients with Alzheimer's disease will continue to deteriorate."

REFERENCES

Alverez, C. (2002). Anger and aggression. In E. M. Varcarolis (Ed.), *Foundations of psychiatric mental health nursing: a clinical approach* (4th ed.). Philadelphia: Saunders.

Alzheimer's Association. (2010). *2010 Alzheimer's disease facts and figures.* Chicago, IL: Author.

Alzheimer's Disease Education and Referral Center (ADEAR). (2010). Retrieved January 7, 2012.

American Heritage Medical Dictionary. (2007). Boston, MA: Houghton Mifflin.

American Psychiatric Association (APA). (2008). *Practice guideline for the treatment of patients with Alzheimer's disease and other dementias* (2nd ed.). Retrieved from www.psychiatryonline.com/popup.aspx?aID=152238.

American Psychiatric Association (APA). (2011). *Diagnostic and statistical manual of mental disorders (DSM-IV-TR)* (4th ed., text rev.) Washington, DC: Author.

Anderson, H. S., & Hoffman, M. (2011). *Alzheimer's disease.* Retrieved April 9, 2012, from http://emedicine.medscape.com/article/1134817-overview.

Black, D. W., & Andreasen, N. C. (2011). *Introductory textbook of psychiatry* (5th ed.). Washington, DC: American Psychiatric Publishing.

Brooks, M. (2011). *Intranasal insulin promising for MCI, Alzheimer disease.* Retrieved April 9, 2012, from www.medscape.com/viewarticle/749616.

Finehout, E. J., Franck, Z., Choe, L. H., et al. (2007). Cerebrospinal fluid proteomic biomarkers for Alzheimer's disease. *Annals of Neurology, 61*(2), 120–129.

Gauthier, S., et al. (2006). Mild cognitive impairment. *Lancet, 367,* 2006. Retrieved February 6, 2012, from www.thelancet.com.

Mayo Clinic. (2011). *Mild cognitive impairment (MCI).* Retrieved February 2, 2012, from www.MayoClinic.com/health/mild cognitive impairment/DS00553/DSECTION=symps.

Mayo Clinic. (2010). *Caregivers.* Retrieved April 17, 2011, from www.mayoclinic.com/health/Alzheimers/HQ 00218.

Science News. (2011). *Use of atypical antipsychotics in treatment of dementia declined after FDA warning.* Retrieved July 4, 2011, from http://esciencenews.com/articles/2011/02/07/use.atypical.antipsychotics.treatment.dementia.

The Free Medical Dictionary. Retrieved February 6, 2012, from http://medical-dictionary.thefree dictionary.com/p/delirium.

Addictions and Compulsions

Elizabeth M. Varcarolis

⊖volve WEBSITE

http://evolve.elsevier.com/Varcarolis/essentials

KEY TERMS AND CONCEPTS

abuse, p. 357
addiction, p. 357
Al-Anon, p. 378
Alateen, p. 378
Alcoholics Anonymous (AA),
    p. 379
antagonistic effect, p. 365
blood alcohol level (BAL), p. 366
club drugs, p. 372
codependence, p. 364
cognitive impairment, p. 358
dependence, p. 357

enabling, p. 364
flashbacks, p. 364
motivational incentives, p. 378
motivational interviewing, p. 378
Recovery Paradigm, p. 378
relapse prevention, p. 373
SMART, p. 379
substance-abuse intervention, p. 373
synergistic effects, p. 365
tolerance, p. 364
toxicology screen, p. 366
withdrawal, p. 364

SELECTED CONCEPT: Substance-Induced Cognitive Impairment

All patients with substance use disorders share common cognitive deficits in core executive functions. For example all substance users have difficulty with planning, working memory, inhibition, and decision-making. There are also alterations in selective attention, episodic memory, and difficulties with emotional processing. After three months of abstinence executive functions increase about 30% in people with moderate to severe impairment, and increases up to 70% in those with mild impairment.

(Verdejo-Garcia, A., 2011)

OBJECTIVES

1. Compare and contrast the differences between substance abuse and substance dependence.
2. Relate how substances of abuse affect dopamine release in the brain and how this effect can lead to the progression of an addiction (dependence on the drug).
3. Discuss the cognitive deficits that occur in all individuals with substance use disorders.
4. While planning patient-centered care, identify four components of the assessment process you would apply with a chemically dependent individual.
5. Discuss the rationale for inclusion of motivation and spirituality into planning care and how that may impact your patient's progress toward sobriety.
6. Compare and contrast the clinical picture of an individual in alcohol withdrawal with that of an individual experiencing alcohol delirium.
7. Describe how reporting an impaired colleague to the proper authorities would protect the safety of patients; then discuss the resultant impact on the health professional's future ability to practice as well as his or her physical health and personal relationships.
8. Explain how teamwork and collaboration contribute to helping an impaired colleague as well as providing safety for the patients under his or her care.
9. Describe aspects of enabling behaviors and give examples.
10. While planning patient-centered care, list clinical manifestations you would find on assessment regarding the signs and symptoms of intoxication, overdose, and withdrawal for at least two substances of abuse.
11. List signs and symptoms you would observe in a hospital unit (e.g., medical-surgical unit, labor and delivery, intensive care unit) for a person who is withdrawing from alcohol and describe the appropriate nursing care and pharmacological therapy.
12. Describe assessment strategies for people with alcohol and drug problems.
13. Identify differences between the conventional treatment of people with addictions versus the recovery models (e.g., 12-step programs, SMART).
14. For each phase of recovery, plan patient-centered care for relapse prevention in a recovering patient.

Mind-altering substances have been used since ancient times. People throughout the centuries have known that the leaves of certain plants, fermented fruit juice or certain kinds of mushrooms, for example, could produce feelings of well-being and/or altered states of consciousness. The degree to which use of mind-altering substances is either accepted or condemned varies among cultures. For example, adult use of alcohol, nicotine, and caffeine is acceptable in most segments of American society.

Most of you may choose not to practice in the field of psychiatric mental health nursing. As a new graduate you may seek a career in the emergency department, medical-surgical unit, obstetrics and gynecology, or a clinic setting, for example. In all settings patients come from a cross section of society, and presently there is an epidemic proportion of alcohol and other drugs being inappropriately used and abused in our society. As a nurse you need to be aware of the signs and symptoms of impending withdrawal from alcohol or other substances in whatever health care setting you choose. As you read this chapter, become familiar with the behaviors of impending withdrawal of various substances, since your observations may at the very least help your patient obtain safety during withdrawal and at most save your patient's life.

Although the use and abuse of substances extends across social and economic boundaries, adolescents and young adults are among the most vulnerable population of substance abusers. Marijuana, prescription drugs, and over-the-counter medications account for most of the top drugs abused by twelfth graders in the past year. Caffeine-laced alcoholic-flavored drinks have been removed from the market and even just drinks that contain higher levels of caffeine are of concern, because teenagers and young adults often add alcohol to these drinks. The use of ecstasy (club drug) increased among eighth to tenth graders from 2009 to 2010 (National Institute on Drug Abuse [NIDA], 2010a). A multitude of uncontrolled designer chemicals is easily available to teens and young adults through the Internet, health food stores, and drugstores. Among them, "bath salts" is a stimulant and contains a combination of the worst effects of several different drugs (e.g., hallucinogenic-delusional properties, extreme agitation, and feelings of superhuman strength and combativeness, as well as the hyperaddictive qualities of cocaine and methamphetamines) (Volkow, 2010). Although "bath salts" were first introduced to young adults, all age-groups are at risk of dependence from this drug. However, even though bath salts have been removed from the market by the FDA, they seem to still be available, in addition to even more dangerous designer chemicals.

Abuse is the habitual use of a substance that falls outside of medical necessity or social acceptance for the single purpose of altering one's mood, emotion, or state of consciousness (*American Heritage Medical Dictionary*, 2007) and resulting in adverse effects to the abuser or to others. **Addiction/ dependence** is a "habitual psychological and physiological dependence on the substance or practice beyond one's voluntary control" (*American Heritage Medical Dictionary*, 2002). In physical addiction, in which there is a "physical or psychological need for a habit-forming substance," a tolerance develops when the body adapts to the substance and gradually requires increasing amounts of the substance to reproduce the effects originally produced by smaller doses. Addiction also applies to a "habitual compulsive involvement in activity, such as gambling" (*The American Heritage Science Dictionary*, 2002). Therefore, a person has to take increasing quantities of the drug to "stay normal" or prevent withdrawal. At this point, the person no longer has control over their substance use or compulsive involvement in an activity, even when it is interfering with functioning and well-being. This dependence on addiction to a drug is progressive and can even be fatal.

We are all aware that there are many behaviors that have compulsive and addictive-like qualities—compulsive cell phone texting or sexting, compulsive overeating, compulsive shopping, sex addictions, compulsive gambling, and compulsive Internet use (e.g., porn, online gambling) are just a few examples (refer to Table 19-1 for a short list of compulsive behaviors).

For our purposes here, we will use an operational definition of addiction called **the three C's:**

1. Behavior that is motivated by emotions ranging along the spectrum of **"craving to compulsive use"**
2. **Continued use** despite adverse consequences to health, mental state, relationships, occupation, or finances
3. **Loss of control**

There is another **"C"** that could be added to this list: cognitive impairment. All patients with substance use disorders share common cognitive deficits in core executive functions. For example, all substance users have difficulty with planning, working memory, inhibition, and decision making. There are also alterations in selective attention, episodic memory, and emotional processing (Verdejo-Garcia, 2011).

See Table 19-1 for an overview of common nonchemical compulsions with addiction-like behaviors.

TABLE 19-1 SOME COMPULSIVE-ADDICTIVE LIKE BEHAVIORS

DEFINITION	COMMENTS
Gambling Compulsive gambling is when a person has uncontrollable urges to gamble despite negative consequences, such as spending all his/her money on gambling, failing to repay loans, telling lies, and even resorting to theft or fraud Compulsive gambling can destroy lives and families	• 4-6% of gamblers become pathological gamblers (PGs) or problem gamblers • PG and major depression often co-occur • Presence of gambling opportunities can double the prevalence of PG and problem gamblers • Youth (11-19 years old) show a 4-7% prevalence rate of problem gambling • Internet gambling has increased access to all age-groups, and for some it has led to financial ruin
Shopping and Spending Pattern of chronic, repetitive purchasing that becomes difficult to stop and results in harmful consequences	• 6% prevalence rate • Compulsive shoppers get a "high" caused by increase in levels of endorphins and dopamine, reinforcing the desire to spend • May coexist in people with mood disorders, substance abuse, or eating disorders
Internet Abuse Compulsive Internet use provides a high, and the person needs that high to feel normal Internet becomes the predominant priority in a person's life and negatively affects relationships, work or school, marriages, finances Large subgroup participates in sexual encounters, resulting in divorces, separations, and problems at home	• About 5-10% of Internet users are compulsive users • More than 50% of people "addicted" to the Internet suffer from other addictions (drugs, sex, alcohol, and smoking) • Types of Internet addictions include cyber porn, sexual encounters, Internet gambling, online gaming, auctions, excessive e-mailing
Sexual Addiction Pursuit of persistent and escalating patterns of sexual behavior despite negative consequences to self and others	• 19-24 million Americans are addicted to sex • Sexual addictions include compulsive masturbation, anonymous sex with multiple partners, multiple affairs outside a committed relationship, computer sex, cell phone sexting, and more • Sexual compulsivity often co-occurs with other addictive behaviors

PREVALENCE AND COMORBIDITY

Prevalence of Substance Abuse

In 2007 (the latest year for which data are available), 38,371 people died of direct drug-induced causes, and there is a drug-induced death in the United States every 15 minutes (Office of National Drug Control Policy [ONDCP], 2010).

Alcohol

Alcohol use disorder is the most common substance-abuse problem in the United States. About 66% of American adults occasionally drink alcoholic beverages; 12% are heavy drinkers. For our purposes, a heavy drinker is described as a person who drinks every day, and becomes intoxicated several times a month (Black & Andreasen, 2011). There are about two to three men for every woman who becomes an alcoholic, and 16 and 30 years is the usual age range of onset. Black and Andreasen (2011) state that from 25% to 50% of medical-surgical patients in general hospitals are alcohol dependent. With psychiatric inpatients, that percentage increases to 50% to 60% alcohol dependence/addiction.

Illicit Drugs

Marijuana is still the most commonly abused illicit drug in the United States (SAMHSA, 2010b). However, there has been a dramatic increase in substances often referred to as **club drugs.** These substances include 3,4-methylenedioxymethamphetamine (MDMA; ecstasy), γ-hydroxybutyrate (GHB; G, liquid ecstasy), and flunitrazepam (Rohypnol). Other drugs frequently used in clubs, raves, nightclubs, and bars are **ketamine** (special K, vitamin K), a hallucinogen; **methcathinone** (Cat, Khat), a stimulant; **LSD**, a hallucinogen; and methamphetamines, a highly addictive stimulant (Metropolitan Drug Commission [MDC], 2011).

The abuse of **prescription drugs** for nonmedical reasons is increasing rapidly (pain killers, sedatives, and stimulants). **Prescription pain killers** (such as OxyContin, Vicodin, and Percodan) are increasingly abused, especially among middle-school and high-school youth as well as adults and older adults. Nonmedical use of prescription drugs may result in dangerous addictions requiring withdrawal precautions during hospitalization, and increasingly result in overdose and death.

Anabolic-Androgenic Steroids

The abuse of **anabolic-androgenic steroids,** synthetic substances related to male hormones (e.g., testosterone), is no longer associated with just body builders and professional athletes to build muscles and boost athletic performance. Unfortunately, steroid abuse has spread to include school-age children, models, business professionals, and others.

There has been a steady increase in steroid use for both tenth and twelfth graders from 2007 through 2010 (NIDA, 2010a). The actual prevalence of steroid abuse in the United States is extremely difficult to ascertain because most studies that measure drug abuse do not include steroids.

Nicotine

Nicotine is the psychoactive drug in tobacco, and nicotine dependence is considered the most common form of chemical dependence in the United States today. Research claims that nicotine is as addictive as heroin, cocaine, or alcohol (Centers for Disease Control and Prevention [CDC], 2011a). There is evidence that cigarette smoke contains more than 7000 chemicals, and about 70 of those cause cancer (CDC, 2011a). These chemicals alter mood, appetite, and alertness in ways users find pleasant and beneficial. In 2009, 20.6% of all adults were current smokers. Tobacco use is the leading cause of preventable deaths. In the United States one in five deaths results from tobacco use. Tobacco smokers die an average of 13 to 14 years earlier than nonsmokers (CDC, 2011b).

Psychiatric Comorbidity

It seems that certain areas of the brain, like the circuits in the brain that use the neurotransmitter dopamine, can affect both drug use disorders as well as other mental illnesses. The neurotransmitter dopamine is typically affected by addictive substances and is also associated with schizophrenic depression and other psychiatric disorders (NIDA, 2010b). This in part may explain the high rate of psychiatric disorders co-occurring with chemical addictions. Comorbidity research is also studying genes that may predispose an individual, either directly or indirectly, to both an addiction and a mental disorder (NIDA, 2010b).

A large percentage of people with schizophrenia and mood disorders present with alcohol/substance dependence. Other psychiatric disorders that may be seen concurrently in people addicted to substances include acute and chronic cognitive impairment disorders, attention deficit disorder, borderline and antisocial personality disorders, anxiety disorders, and depression.

Nonchemical addictions contribute to emotional problems in young and old alike. Eating disorders and compulsive behaviors (e.g., Internet gambling, cell phone sexting, sexual addictions) are also highly associated with substance use. Nicotine addiction is high among all groups of people with substance dependence as well as those with psychiatric mental health issues.

Suicide is a high risk among individuals who abuse alcohol or drugs. The level of suicide and alcohol/drug addiction among our armed services both in war zones and after returning to the United States is rising at an alarming rate. Many of these veterans were addicted or became addicted during their tours of duty. However, even without the traumatic effects witnessed during war, the suicide rate among substance-addicted individuals is much higher than that for the general population, estimated to be three to four times higher. Substance abuse increases the risk of suicide among children, adolescents, adults, and older adults. Refer to Chapters 10 through 19 as well as Chapter 23 for more information on the relationship between substance abuse and the rates of suicide among various clinical disorders.

People with co-occurring/comorbid mental illness often experience more severe and chronic medical, social, and emotional problems. Because these individuals have two or

EXAMINING THE EVIDENCE

Gambling—A Real Addiction

I have several male college friends who drink and smoke regularly and seem to be seriously in debt because of gambling. Is this common and can gambling be considered a real addiction? Is there hope for improvement?

Sadly, this is becoming more of a problem. The top four most popular forms of gambling for college students are lottery, card games, pools, and raffles (Barnes et al., 2010). Prevalence rates for gambling are staggeringly high with about 80% of the population gambling at least once in their lifetime. Gambling is widespread across the United States with all states (except Hawaii and Utah) legalizing at least some type of gambling. A small percentage of gamblers, between 0.1% and 2.7%, develop into pathological gamblers whose behaviors parallel the symptoms of substance abuse/dependence (Beaver et al., 2009).

People usually display susceptibility to diverse addictions in sequence or simultaneously, so frequently many people smoke and drink while they are gambling. Gamblers are five times as likely as those in the general population to be dependent on alcohol and nearly seven times as likely to be dependent on nicotine (Miller, 2010). Being a college student is associated with higher levels of alcohol use and problem drinking, but being male was the strongest predictor of both problem gambling and problem drinking (Barnes et al., 2010).

Pathological gambling is now considered an "addiction" in the new *DSM-5 (Diagnostic and Statistical Manual of Mental Disorders, edition 5,* to be published in May 2013). It had previously been classified as an "impulse control disorder" in the *DSM-IV.* Many strategies for treating gambling are based on those used for substance use disorders. There is no consensus yet about which therapies are best, but two have emerged as particularly promising. Gamblers Anonymous, a 12-step program modeled on Alcoholics Anonymous, is probably the most common intervention for pathological gambling. Participants acknowledge they are powerless over their gambling behavior and try to enter into recovery with support from members and through reliance on a spiritual higher power. Another therapy is cognitive behavioral therapy (CBT) where gamblers learn to recognize distorted thinking or rationalizations about gambling and change the way they think about gambling; in addition, gamblers discover how to identify and avoid gambling triggers. Preliminary research suggests that even brief attempts at these interventions may help people reduce gambling behaviors. Much more research is needed to determine the best treatment strategies, but there is hope that by listing gambling as an "addiction" clinicians will be able to offer treatments that are most likely to help (Miller 2010).

Barnes, G.M., et al. (2010). Comparisons of gambling and alcohol use among college students and noncollege young people in the United States. *Journal of American College Health, 58*(5), 443-452.

Beaver, K., et al. (2009). Gender differences in genetic and environmental influences on gambling: results from a sample of twins from the National Longitudinal Study of Adolescent Health. *Addiction Research Report, 105,* 536-542.

Miller, M. (2010). Pathological gambling. *Harvard Mental Health Letter, 27*(2), 1-3.

more disorders, they are vulnerable to both substance-abuse relapse and worsening of the psychiatric disorder. In addition, substance-abuse relapse often leads to psychiatric decompensation and worsening of psychiatric problems often leads to substance-abuse/use relapse.

Medical Comorbidity

Although marijuana is the most common *illicit* drug of abuse, alcohol abuse is the most prevalent of the substance-abuse disorders. Therefore *alcohol*-related medical problems are the comorbidities most commonly seen in medical settings. The risk of health problems related to alcohol abuse is almost endless. Alcohol can damage the brain and most body organs. Especially vulnerable to alcohol-related damage is the cerebral cortex, responsible for higher brain functions, problem solving, and decision making. The hippocampus is also affected, which is the center of memory and learning, as well as the cerebellum, which helps coordinate our movements. Specific disorders that involve the central nervous system include Wernicke's

encephalopathy and Korsakoff's psychosis. Other disorders affect the gastrointestinal system (e.g., esophagitis, gastritis, pancreatitis, alcoholic hepatitis, and cirrhosis of the liver).

Cardiovascular risks are also significant. Alcohol can raise the levels of triglycerides in the blood. Excessive alcohol intake results in stroke, cardiomyopathy, cardiac dysrhythmia, and sudden cardiac death (American Heart Association [AHA], 2011). Also commonly associated with long-term alcohol use or abuse is tuberculosis, all types of accidents, suicide, and homicide.

Cocaine abusers may experience extreme weight loss and malnutrition, myocardial infarction, brain damage, and stroke. **Methamphetamine** abusers are likely to suffer from hypothermia, seizures, brain damage, kidney damage, stroke, and death.

Nicotine in the form of tobacco can cause chronic lung disease, coronary heart disease, chronic obstructive pulmonary disease (COPD), and stroke as well as cancer of the lungs, larynx, esophagus, mouth, and bladder (CDC, 2011c). Approximately 50% of Americans who do not smoke are exposed to secondhand smoke. A comprehensive scientific report concluded that there is no risk-free level of exposure to secondhand smoke (SHS). Secondhand smoke is responsible for heart disease and lung cancer in nonsmoking adults and is extremely harmful to infants and children (U.S. Department of Health and Human Services [USDHHS], 2006). A recent study found a significant association between exposure to SHS and major depressive disorder (MDD), general anxiety disorder (GAD), and attention deficit hyperactivity disorder (ADHD) in white participants, but only conduct disorder was linked to SHS in Mexican-American groups. There were no correlations between SHS and African-American participants (Brauser & Lie, 2011).

The effects of *anabolic-androgenic steroid (AAS)* use can be serious and permanent if an individual does not stop taking these drugs (e.g., liver damage, renal failure, heart attack, elevated cholesterol levels, and serious depression, especially in withdrawal). Some of the untoward effects of steroid use in men are shrinking of the testicles, infertility, development of breasts, and increased risk for prostate cancer. Women often show male pattern baldness, changes in menstrual cycle, growth of facial hair, and a deepening of the voice. Stunting of growth attributable to premature skeletal maturation and accelerated pubertal changes can occur in adolescents using AASs (NIDA, 2009). Research also suggests that users may experience paranoid jealousy, delusions, and violent mood swings (NIDA, 2009). The route of drug administration both influences medical complications and affects addictive potential. For example, **intravenous drug users** have a higher incidence of infections, venous sclerosis, and testing positive for HIV/AIDS. **Intranasal users** may have sinusitis and a perforated nasal septum. **Smoking a substance** increases the likelihood of respiratory tract problems. Both smoked and injected drugs enter the brain within seconds, producing a powerful rush of pleasure lasting a short period of time, necessitating taking more of the drug more often to recapture the high. Refer to Table 19-2 for a description of physical complications associated with various classes of drugs and their routes of administration.

THEORY

There is no single cause of substance abuse. Multiple factors contribute to substance use, abuse, and addiction in any individual.

Biological Theories

There are three areas of the brain that are necessary for life-sustaining functions and at the same time enhance compulsive drug use that marks addiction (NIDA, 2010c):

- **Brainstem**—controls basic functions such as heart rate, breathing, and sleeping
- **Limbic system**—contains the brain's reward circuit that links brain structures controlling feelings of pleasure, thereby motivating us to repeat behaviors causing pleasure, such as eating, viewing art, listening to music
- **Cerebral cortex**—includes areas that process information from our senses (seeing, hearing, feeling, and taste) as well as areas that power our ability to think, plan, solve problems, and make decisions

The individual variation in a person's susceptibility to become addicted supports the premise that genetic/biological variations, psychological factors, and sociocultural influences all play a role in addiction.

Genetic Theories

Genetic factors are believed to account for between 40% and 60% of a person's vulnerability to addiction (Black & Andreasen, 2011). It is generally accepted that genetic factors play an important risk factor for psychoactive drug use. For example, it is generally accepted that alcoholism is three to four times more likely to occur in children of alcoholic parents than in children of nonalcoholic parents.

It has also been demonstrated that alcohol and drugs of abuse have specific effects on selected neurotransmitters. *Dopamine* is a neurotransmitter that plays a major role in all addictions, but the concepts that apply to dopamine can relate to other neurotransmitters as well. Dopamine is the brain chemical present in regions of the brain that regulate motivation, emotion, cognition or learning, and the ability to experience pleasure and pain.

All drugs of abuse (e.g., nicotine, cocaine, marijuana, methamphetamines) directly or indirectly affect the limbic (reward) system. The reward system consists of the ventral tegmental area (VTA), the nucleus accumbens, and part of the cerebral cortex. These brain circuits allow us to feel pleasure and they increase the response to dopamine as rewards from pleasurable activities (e.g., food, music, art, sex). However, the first time an individual uses a drug of abuse neurons in the reward pathway release an unusually large amount of dopamine, resulting in exaggerated feelings of pleasure. The neurons in the reward pathway communicate through electrical signals that are passed from one neuron to another across a small gap called a synapse. Dopamine is then released into the synapse, crosses to the next neuron, and binds to that neuron's dopamine receptor (NIDA, 2010c,d). It is this binding that produces the initial unnaturally intense feelings of pleasure.

As a result of this flood of neurotransmitters (dopamine in this case), the neurons try to regulate the level of dopamine in the brain either by reducing the number of dopamine receptors or by synthesizing less dopamine. Eventually, dopamine's ability to stimulate the reward center becomes very ineffective, and the individual uses increasingly more of the drug to raise dopamine levels to normal or higher levels; this vicious cycle of taking increasing amounts of the drug to even feel "normal" begins the cycle of tolerance to the drug and eventual dependence or addiction. Other nerve cells release *γ-aminobutyric acid (GABA),* which is an inhibitory neurotransmitter that helps moderate neuronal activity and protects the receptor nerve from becoming overstimulated (NIDA, 2010c).

Opioid drugs act on opioid receptors. Alcohol and other central nervous system (CNS) depressants act on GABA receptors. This finding helps explain the addictive and cross-tolerance effects that occur when alcohol use is combined with benzodiazepine use. Cocaine and amphetamines act on the dopamine and *serotonin systems,* producing the intense rush and resulting intense lows, reinforcing compulsive use.

TABLE 19-2   PHYSICAL COMPLICATIONS RELATED TO DRUGS OF ABUSE

ROUTE	PHYSICAL COMPLICATIONS	ROUTE	PHYSICAL COMPLICATIONS
Narcotics (e.g., Heroin), PCP, Cocaine or Crack, Methamphetamines		**Marijuana**	
Intravenous*	Human immunodeficiency virus (HIV)	Smoking, ingestion	Impaired lung structure
	Acquired immunodeficiency syndrome (AIDS)		Chromosomal mutation—increased incidence of birth defects
	Hepatitis		Micronucleic white blood cells—increased risk of disease as a result of decreased resistance to infection
	Bacterial endocarditis		
	Renal failure		
	Cardiac arrest		Stroke
	Coma		Possible long-term effects on short-term memory
	Seizures		
	Respiratory arrest	**Nicotine**	
	Dermatitis	Smoking, chewing	*Heavy chronic use associated with:*
	Pulmonary emboli		Emphysema
	Tetanus		Cancer of the larynx and esophagus
	Abscesses—osteomyelitis		
	Septicemia		Lung cancer
			Peripheral vascular diseases
Cocaine, Methamphetamines			Cancer of the mouth
Intravenous, intranasal, smoking	Perforation of nasal septum (when taken intranasally)		Cardiovascular disease
			Hypertension
	Respiratory paralysis		
	Cardiovascular collapse	**Heroin**	
	Hyperpyrexia	Intravenous,* smoking	Constipation
	Intracerebral hemorrhage		Dermatitis
			Malnutrition
Caffeine			Hypoglycemia
Ingestion	Gastroesophageal reflux		Dental caries
	Peptic ulcer		Amenorrhea
	Increased intraocular pressure in unregulated glaucoma		
	Tachycardia	**Inhalants**	
	Increased plasma glucose and lipid levels	Sniffing, snorting, bagging (inhalation of fumes from a plastic bag), huffing (placing an inhalant-soaked rag in the mouth)	Tachycardia
			Dysrhythmias
			Nervous system damage
PCP			Hearing loss
Ingestion	Respiratory arrest		Bone marrow damage
			Suffocation caused by displacing oxygen in the lungs, leading to respiratory depression/arrest

*The complications listed can result from any drug taken intravenously.

Psychological Theories

Although no known addictive personality type exists, associated psychodynamic factors have been identified such as lack of tolerance for frustration and pain, lack of impulse control, lack of success in life, lack of affectionate and meaningful relationships, low self-esteem, lack of self-regard, and strong propensity for risk-taking behaviors. People who abuse two or more substances simultaneously (polysubstance abusers) are more likely to report an unstable childhood and self-medicate than are those who abuse alcohol alone. Multiple studies link personality disorders (e.g., antisocial, borderline, and narcissistic) and substance abuse.

SOCIETAL AND CULTURAL CONSIDERATIONS

Societal and family values can be strong influences on whether a person's use/abuse of alcohol or illicit drugs becomes an addiction problem. If a person's family uses/abuses drugs their children are more likely use these substances as well. If an individual's friends use drugs, peer pressure often prevails on an individual to use drugs as well. It has been found that youth and teenagers are more susceptible to peer pressure if they lack a close bond with parent(s), they spend a large amount of time away from home, and they have increased reliance on peers as opposed to parents (Black & Andreasen, 2011).

Women in general are diagnosed with substance use at lower rates than men. However, girls and young women become addicted faster and are apt to suffer the consequences of substances of abuse more rapidly than boys and young men.

In Asian cultures, the prevalence rate for alcohol abuse is believed to be relatively low. This is partly because of a deficiency of aldehyde dehydrogenase, the chemical that breaks down alcohol acetaldehyde. In approximately half of the Asian population, if the level of alcohol acetaldehyde increases in the blood severe flushing and palpitations may occur. This reaction is thought to be effective in preventing many Asians from drinking. In contrast, in Native Americans and Alaska Natives, the prevalence rate for alcohol dependence or abuse is quite high: 70% compared with 11% to 32% for their white, African-American, and Japanese American counterparts (USDHHS, 1999).

Special Populations

Pregnant Women

Alcohol use during pregnancy can have negative physical, mental, and behavioral consequences. If a pregnant woman takes a drink, the unborn child takes the same drink. Alcohol is extremely neurotoxic and interferes with the ability of the fetus to receive enough oxygen and nourishment for normal cell development in the brain as well as other organs. A study conducted at the University of California, San Diego points to a zero tolerance for alcohol during pregnancy, supporting the Surgeon General's Report for restricting alcohol during the entire pregnancy. The University of California study suggests that the total amount of alcohol throughout the entire pregnancy was the largest factor for signs of fetal alcohol syndrome, not necessarily binge drinking. The results indicated that the end of the first trimester is the most vulnerable time for the fetus (Solomon, 2012). Fetal alcohol syndrome (FAS) is the most extreme example of the effect of alcohol on fetal development. Slightly less severe are the fetal alcohol spectrum disorders (FASDs).

There are three basic criteria that need to be present in order to make the diagnosis of FAS: (1) mental retardation, (2) delayed growth and development, and (3) distinctive facial abnormalities. FAS and FASD are lifelong conditions that result in permanent physical disabilities (e.g., hearing, eyesight, facial abnormalities, organ deformities, heart and kidney defects), mental disabilities (e.g., mental retardation, learning disabilities, memory impairment, CNS handicaps), and behavioral problems (e.g., hyperactivity, poor impulse control, irritability, criminal behavior) (CDC, 2006).

According to Martin (2010), **women who smoke cigarettes prenatally** have babies that (1) are twice as likely to be low birth weight; (2) have increased risk of developmental issues (e.g., cerebral palsy, learning disabilities), congenital abnormalities, and respiratory tract problems; and have increased risk for SIDS (sudden infant death syndrome).

Secondhand smoke exposure is also thought to be a cause of SIDS, respiratory tract problems, ear infections, and asthma attacks in infants and children (USDHHS, 2006).

Mothers who take opiates during pregnancy are more likely to experience intrauterine fetal deaths and are at a higher risk for infant death. Infants born to opiate-dependent mothers are addicted at birth and experience withdrawal symptoms.

Chemically Impaired Nurses, Nursing Students, and Health Care Workers

Impairment of a health care professional is the inability or impending inability to practice according to accepted standards as a result of substance use, abuse, or dependency (Baldisseri, 2007). According to Monroe and Kenaga (2011), up to 20% of practicing nurses are addicted to substances. That would be approximately one in five nurses practicing today. Nursing students are just as vulnerable to addictions. In a review of the literature and of substance-abuse policies in the nursing profession, the conclusion was that mandating punitive action makes it more difficult for impaired nurses to seek early intervention and assistance, which makes it more likely that the public will be endangered. It also makes it more difficult for colleagues to report a fellow colleague. However, "in helping colleagues and students recover from an addictive disorder by providing a non-punitive atmosphere is a life-saving first step for nurses, students, and those in their care" (Monroe & Kenaga, 2011). Therefore the **alternative-to-discipline (ADT) programs** appear to be as effective as, if not more than, the traditional approach of reporting addicted health care professionals. Although the choices for action are varied (e.g., "alternative-to-discipline" or "peer assistance" programs), early intervention is essential, and the only choice that is wrong is for others to do nothing.

Often, the impaired nurse volunteers to work additional shifts to be nearer to the source of the drug. The nurse may leave the unit frequently or spend a lot of time in the bathroom. When the impaired nurse is on duty, more patients may complain that their pain is unrelieved by their narcotic analgesic or that they are unable to sleep, despite receiving sedative medications. Increases in inaccurate drug counts and vial breakage may occur. Examples of other behaviors may include the following (*SMART Recovery*, 2008-2011):

> A colleague may observe such signs as tendency to isolate, preference for working alone to avoid being caught, irritability with peers, dramatic changes in mood, especially after bathroom breaks, decrease in productivity as the disease progresses, lateness and tardiness for work, or arrive at work early and stay late (in order to attain drugs), odor of alcohol on breath, frequent

intoxication at social functions, isolation from social functions to drink alone, slurred speech, illegible writing charts, if handwriting was usually neat.

If indicators of impaired practice are observed, they must be reported to the nurse manager. Intervention is the responsibility of the nurse manager and other nursing administrators.

Researchers state that one of the benefits of the **alternative-to-discipline (ADT)** program is that it allows managers to remove nurses from the work environment quickly, unlike traditional disciplinary procedures that can extend for months to years. The approach of these programs provides nonjudgmental support and treatment that encourages the impaired colleague to stay in the profession (Rivers, 2011). According to Rivers (2011), the aim of these ADT programs is to help impaired nurses "recover from addiction, reduce the chance of dismissal, and return nurses to work under strict monitoring guidelines, with random substance checks, support and meetings with managers and regulators."

Clear documentation by coworkers (specific dates, times, events, consequences) is crucial. Once the nurse manager has been informed, the legal and ethical responsibilities for in-house reporting have been met. If the impaired nurse remains in the situation and no action is taken by the nurse manager, then the information must be taken to the next level in the chain of command. These measures can prevent harm to patients under the impaired nurse's care and can save a colleague's professional career or even life.

Reporting an impaired colleague is not easy, even though it is our responsibility. Often he or she has high levels of denial and is not receptive to interventions. By the same token, the colleague of an impaired nurse may deny or rationalize what is happening, thus enabling the impaired nurse to potentially endanger lives while becoming sicker and more isolated (Box 19-1 can be used as a check to discern enabling behaviors).

Rehabilitative programs, either peer assistance programs or ADT programs, are offered by most, although not all, of the state boards of nursing. Some state boards of nursing allow impaired nurses to avoid disciplinary action if they seek treatment.

CLINICAL PICTURE

Tolerance and Withdrawal

The diagnosis of substance dependence/addiction involves the concepts of tolerance and withdrawal. As mentioned previously, tolerance is a need for higher and higher doses to achieve the desired effect. Withdrawal occurs after a long period of continued use, so that stopping or reducing use results in specific physical and psychological signs and symptoms, usually drug-specific withdrawal symptoms. Information on signs and symptoms of intoxication and withdrawal from specific substances of abuse are presented later in this chapter.

Flashbacks

Flashbacks are transitory recurrences of perceptual disturbance caused by a person's earlier hallucinogenic drug use; flashbacks occur during the person's drug-free state. Visual

---

BOX 19-1   HAVE I ENABLED?

Have I:

Excused or ignored behaviors in a peer that may be suggestive of impairment and justified those behaviors as "just having a bad day" or "stress"?

Never told the supervisor about behaviors possibly indicative of impairment that I observed because I was afraid of being wrong and did not want anyone to get angry at me?

Accepted responsibility for my colleague's unfinished work and at times attempted to counsel and solve his or her problem?

Believed that nurses do not use drugs or alcohol to the point of practice impairment and that substance use can be stopped at any time unless the person is morally weak?

Liked to use drugs or alcohol myself to relax or enjoy with friends? I do not want anyone to look at me. In fact, I have used a few discontinued drugs from work myself. Doesn't everyone?

Exonerated a peer's irresponsible actions by covering for attendance or tardiness? Have I cosigned wastes I have not truly witnessed or corrected the narcotic count to account for a discrepancy?

Defended a colleague when it was suggested there may be a problem with impairment?

From Smith, L., Taylor, B. B., & Hughes, T. L. (1998). Effective peer response to impaired nursing practice. *Nursing Clinics of North America, 33*(1), 105-119.

---

distortions, time expansion, loss of ego boundaries, and intense emotions are reported. Often flashbacks are mild and perhaps pleasant, but at other times individuals experience repeated recurrences of frightening images or thoughts. Flashbacks are common in individuals who are suffering from posttraumatic stress disorder (PTSD) as well.

Codependence

Codependence is a cluster of behaviors originally identified through research involving the families of alcoholic patients. Living with a substance-abusing or alcoholic individual is a source of stress and requires family system adjustments. People who are codependent often exhibit overresponsible behavior—doing for others what others could just as well do for themselves. They have a constellation of maladaptive thoughts, feelings, behaviors, and attitudes that effectively prevent them from living full and satisfying lives. Symptomatic of codependence is valuing oneself by what one does, what one looks like, and what one has, rather than by who one is (Box 19-2).

Synergistic Effects

When some drugs are taken together, the effect of either or both of the drugs is intensified or prolonged. For example,

BOX 19-2 OVERRESPONSIBLE (CODEPENDENT) BEHAVIORS

Codependent individuals find themselves:

- Attempting to control someone else's drug use
- Spending inordinate time thinking about the addicted person
- Finding excuses for the person's substance abuse
- Covering up the person's drinking or drug taking or lying
- Feeling responsible for the person's drinking or drug use
- Feeling guilty for the addicted person's behavior
- Avoiding family and social events because of concerns or shame about the addicted member's behavior
- Making threats regarding the consequences of the alcoholic's or drug abuser's behavior and failing to follow through
- Eliciting promises for change
- Feeling like they are "walking on eggshells" on a routine basis to avoid causing problems, especially in relation to alcohol or drug use
- Allowing moods to be influenced by those of the addicted person
- Searching for, hiding, and destroying the abuser's drug or alcohol supply
- Assuming the alcoholic's or substance abuser's duties and responsibilities
- Feeling forced to increase control over the family's finances
- Often bailing the addicted person out of financial or legal problems

combinations of alcohol plus a benzodiazepine, alcohol plus an opiate, and alcohol plus a barbiturate produce syn-ergistic effects. All these drugs are CNS depressants. Taking two of these drugs together results in far greater CNS depression than the simple sum of the effects of each drug. Many unintentional deaths have resulted from lethal drug combinations.

Antagonistic Effects

Many people combine drugs to weaken or inhibit the effect of one of the drugs (i.e., for the antagonistic effect). For example, cocaine is often mixed with heroin (speedball). The heroin (CNS depressant) is meant to soften the intense let-down of withdrawal from cocaine (CNS stimulant). **Naloxone (Narcan),** an opiate antagonist, is often given to people who have overdosed on an opiate (usually heroin) to reverse respiratory and CNS depression. Because the duration of action of naloxone may be less than that of the narcotic that was taken, further monitoring and possible additional doses of naloxone may be needed.

APPLICATION OF THE NURSING PROCESS

ASSESSMENT

Assessment of chemical impairment is becoming more complex because of the increase in the simultaneous use of and dependence/addiction/on multiple substances (**polydrug abuse).** Accurate assessment becomes even more complicated in the presence of coexisting psychiatric disorders or physical illnesses, including human immunodeficiency virus (HIV) infection, acquired immunodeficiency syndrome (AIDS), dementia, and encephalopathy.

Sensitivity to multicultural and racial issues is important in interpreting symptoms, making diagnoses, providing clinical care, and designing prevention strategies. Refer to Box 19-3 for areas to be covered in overall assessment for patients who use substances.

Initial Interview Guidelines

Current alcohol or other drug problems can be detected by asking two questions that are easily integrated into a clinical interview. These two questions are:

1. In the past year, have you ever gotten drunk or used drugs more than you intended?
2. Have you felt you wanted or needed to cut down on your drinking or drug use in the past year?

From those two initial questions, the nurse can then pinpoint specific drugs depending on the particular clinical situation. The nurse should ask questions in a straightforward, nonjudgmental fashion. Specific details include name(s) of drug(s) used, route, quantity, time of last use, and usual pattern of use.

The CAGE-AID assessment is a commonly used tool in screening alcohol and substance abuse.

Responses that serve as red flags and indicate the need for further assessment are rationalizations ("You'd smoke dope, too, if..."); automatic responses, as if the question were predicted; and slow, prolonged responses, as if the person were being careful about what to say. If the person is not able to provide a drug history, the nurse should assess for indications of substance abuse, such as dilated or constricted pupils, abnormal vital signs, needle marks, tremors, and alcohol on the breath. *The nurse should also obtain history information from family and friends* when available. Clothing should be checked for drug paraphernalia, such as used syringes, crack vials, white powder, razor blades, bent spoons, and pipes.

Further Initial Assessment

There is a consistent and significant association between alcohol/drug use and injury. Intracranial hematomas, subdural hematomas, and other conditions can remain unnoticed if the symptoms of acute alcohol intoxication and withdrawal are not distinguished from the symptoms of a brain injury. Therefore neurological signs (pupil size, equality, and reaction to light) should be assessed, especially in comatose patients suspected of having traumatic injuries. In addition, questions about

BOX 19-3 OVERALL ASSESSMENT GUIDE FOR SUBSTANCE USE

History of Patient's Substance Use

1. What are the dates of first use, number of substances being taken, pattern of use, amount, frequency, periods of sobriety, time last taken?
2. Was patient treated previously for substance abuse? What was the outcome?
3. Is there a history of blackouts, delirium, or seizures?
4. Is there a history of withdrawal symptoms, overdoses, and complications from past substance use?
5. Is there a family history of drug or alcohol problems?

Medical History

1. Does the patient have any coexisting physical conditions (e.g., HIV infection)?
2. What medications does the patient presently take?
3. What is the patient's current medical status? Mental status?

Psychiatric History

1. Is there a history of comorbid psychiatric problems? Depression? Personality disorder? Conduct disorder? Schizophrenia?
2. Has the patient undergone treatment for a specific disorder? What medications were given and what was the outcome?

3. Is there a history of abuse (physical, sexual)? Family violence?
4. Is there a history of suicide? Violence toward others?
5. Is the patient having suicidal thoughts?

Psychosocial Issues

1. Does the patient have a poor work record related to substance use?
2. How has the patient's substance use affected his or her relationships with others?
   - Family
   - Friends
   - Professional relationships
   - Community involvement
3. How has the substance use affected the patient's ability to meet usual role expectations (e.g., parent, spouse, friend, employee)?
4. Is there a police or criminal record or legal problems related to substance use (e.g., vehicle accidents, driving while intoxicated, physical violence)?
5. Who does the patient identify as his or her support system? Who does the patient trust? Who cares for the patient? Who will help the patient if the patient asks for help?
6. Does the patient use coping styles that contribute to the maintenance of his or her drug or alcohol lifestyle?

alcohol or drug use should be asked as part of the assessment of any trauma. A urine toxicology screen or blood alcohol level (BAL) measurement can be useful for assessment purposes.

Assessment strategies must include collection of data pertaining to both substance dependence and psychiatric impairment. Individuals with previously established psychiatric impairment may be experiencing substance abuse or dependence if they exhibit increasing frequency of symptoms, exacerbation without obvious reason, or chronic noncompliance with treatment regimens. Self-medication or use of a substance in response to symptomatology secondary to psychiatric impairment is a common phenomenon when a person is overwhelmed or dealing with psychic pain. Substance abuse can remain undetected in those who are depressed, suicidal, or anxious unless a thorough history is taken. Similarly, the understanding and treatment of substance-dependent people are enhanced by inquiries about symptoms of depression and anxiety.

Once specific data are obtained, it is helpful to know if the person is abusing a substance or is actively dependent on the substance.

Psychological Changes

Certain psychological characteristics are associated with substance abuse, including *denial, depression, anxiety, dependency, hopelessness, low self-esteem,* and *various psychiatric disorders.* It is often

difficult to determine which comes first—psychological changes or substance abuse. People who are addicted to substances are threatened on many levels.

Addicts establish a **predictable defensive style** to protect themselves against threats, such as disruptions in their lifestyle and the consequences of withdrawal. The elements of this style include various defense mechanisms (denial, projection, rationalization), as well as characteristic thought processes (all-or-none thinking, selective attention) and behaviors (conflict minimization and avoidance, passivity, and manipulation). Refer to Chapter 11 for further discussion on defense mechanisms. The substance abuser is not able to relinquish these maladaptive coping styles until more positive and functional skills are learned.

Signs of Intoxication and Withdrawal
Central Nervous System Depressants

CNS depressant drugs include alcohol, benzodiazepines, and barbiturates. Symptoms of intoxication, overdose, and withdrawal, along with possible treatments, are presented in Table 19-3.

Withdrawal reactions to alcohol and other CNS depressants are associated with severe morbidity and mortality, unlike withdrawal from other drugs. The syndrome for alcohol withdrawal is the same as that for the entire class of CNS depressant drugs. Alcohol is used here as the prototype. The time intervals are delayed when other CNS depressants are the main drugs of

TABLE 19-3 CENTRAL NERVOUS SYSTEM DEPRESSANTS

DRUGS	INTOXICATION EFFECTS	OVERDOSE EFFECTS	POSSIBLE OVERDOSE TREATMENTS	WITHDRAWAL EFFECTS	POSSIBLE WITHDRAWAL TREATMENTS
Benzodiazepines Glutethimide Alcohol (EtOH)	*Physical:* Slurred speech Incoordination Unsteady gait Drowsiness Decreased blood pressure *Psychological-perceptual:* Disinhibition of sexual or aggressive drives Impaired judgment Impaired social or occupational function Impaired attention or memory Irritability	Cardiovascular or respiratory depression or arrest (mostly with barbiturates) Coma Shock Convulsions Death	*If awake:* Keep awake. Induce vomiting. Give activated charcoal to aid absorption of drug. Check vital signs (VS) every 15 min. *Coma:* Clear airway; insert endotracheal tube. Give intravenous (IV) fluids. Perform gastric lavage with activated charcoal. Check VS frequently for shock and cardiac arrest after patient is stable. Initiate seizure precautions Possibly perform hemodialysis or peritoneal dialysis. Administer flumazenil (Romazicon) IV.	*Cessation of prolonged heavy use:* Nausea and vomiting Tachycardia Diaphoresis Anxiety or irritability Tremors in hands, fingers, eyelids Marked insomnia Grand mal seizures *After 5 to 15 years of heavy use:* Delirium	Perform carefully titrated detoxification with similar drug. *Note:* Abrupt withdrawal can lead to death.

choice or are used in combination with alcohol. In addition, as patient's age, their symptoms of withdrawal continue for longer periods and are more severe than those in younger patients.

Multiple drug and alcohol dependencies can result in simultaneous withdrawal syndromes that present a bizarre clinical picture and may pose problems for safe withdrawal. Family and friends may help provide important information that can assist in care planning. Two alcohol withdrawal syndromes are described next: (1) alcohol withdrawal and (2) the more severe alcohol withdrawal delirium.

Alcohol withdrawal. The early signs of withdrawal develop within a few hours after cessation or reduction of alcohol (ethanol) intake; they peak after 24 to 48 hours and then rapidly and dramatically disappear, unless the withdrawal progresses to alcohol withdrawal delirium. The person may appear hyperalert, manifest jerky movements and irritability, startle easily, and experience subjective distress often described as "shaking inside." Grand mal seizures may appear 7 to 48 hours after cessation of alcohol intake, particularly in people with a history of seizures. Careful assessment followed by appropriate

medical and nursing interventions can prevent the more serious withdrawal reaction of delirium.

Consistent and frequent orientation to time and place may be necessary. Encouraging the family or close friends (one at a time) to stay with the patient in quiet surroundings can help increase orientation and minimize confusion and anxiety.

Illusions are usually terrifying for the patient. Illusions are misinterpretations of objects in the environment, usually of a threatening nature. For example, a person may think that spots on the wallpaper are blood-sucking ants. However, illusions can be clarified; this reduces the patient's terror: "See, they are not ants, they are just part of the wallpaper pattern."

Alcohol withdrawal delirium. Alcohol withdrawal delirium is considered a medical emergency and can result in death even if treated. Death is usually a result of sepsis, myocardial infarction, fat embolism, peripheral vascular collapse, electrolyte imbalance, aspiration pneumonia, or suicide. The state of delirium usually peaks 2 to 3 days (48 to 72 hours) after cessation or reduction of intake (although it can occur later) and lasts 2 to 3 days.

TABLE 19-4	**RELATIONSHIP BETWEEN BLOOD ALCOHOL LEVEL AND EFFECTS IN A NONTOLERANT DRINKER**	
BLOOD ALCOHOL LEVEL	**BLOOD ALCOHOL ACCUMULATION**	**EFFECTS**
0.05 mg %	1-2 drinks	Changes in mood and behavior; impaired judgment
0.08 mg %	5-6 drinks	**Legal level of intoxication in most states.** Clumsiness in voluntary motor activity
0.20 mg %	10-12 drinks	Depressed function of entire motor area of the brain, causing staggering and ataxia; emotional lability
0.30 mg %	15-19 drinks	Confusion, stupor
0.40 mg %	20-24 drinks	Coma
0.50 mg %	25-30 drinks	Death caused by respiratory depression

In addition to anxiety, insomnia, anorexia, and delirium, features include the following:
- Autonomic hyperactivity (e.g., tachycardia, diaphoresis, elevated blood pressure)
- Severe disturbance in sensorium (e.g., disorientation, clouding of consciousness)
- Perceptual disturbances (e.g., visual or tactile hallucinations)
- Fluctuating levels of consciousness (e.g., ranging from hyperexcitability to lethargy)
- Delusions (paranoid), agitated behaviors, and fever (temperatures of 100° to 103° F)

Immediate medical attention is warranted in alcohol withdrawal delirium (see Pharmacological, Biological, and Integrative Therapies for a full discussion of medical treatments).

Alcohol is the only drug for which objective measures of intoxication exist. The relationship between BAL and behavior in a nontolerant individual is shown in Table 19-4. Knowledge of the BAL assists the nurse in determining the level of intoxication and the level of tolerance, and in ascertaining whether the person accurately reported recent drinking during the nursing history. These factors are also assessed by means of behavioral cues. As tolerance develops, a discrepancy is seen between BAL and expected behavior. A person with tolerance to alcohol may have a high BAL but minimal signs of impairment, as indicated in the following vignette.

> **VIGNETTE**
>
> Clarence comes to the emergency department with a BAL of 0.31 mg %. He is stuporous and ataxic and has slurred speech. The fact that he is still alive indicates a high tolerance for alcohol. A nursing history conducted as Clarence sobers reveals an extensive drinking history. When the blood alcohol level is this high, assessing for withdrawal symptoms is crucial.

The nursing history, physical examination, and laboratory tests are used to gather data about drug-related physical problems. The extent of impairment depends on individual susceptibility as well as the amount of drug used and the route of administration. Each class of drugs has its own physiological signs and symptoms of intoxication, which are summarized in the tables for each substance class.

Central Nervous System Stimulants

Table 19-5 outlines the physical and psychological effects of intoxication from abuse of amphetamines and other psychostimulants, possible life-threatening results of overdose, and emergency measures for both overdose and withdrawal. All stimulants accelerate the normal functioning of the body and affect the CNS. Common signs of stimulant abuse include dilation of the pupils, dryness of the nasal cavity, and excessive motor activity.

When a person who has ingested a stimulant experiences chest pain, has an irregular pulse rate, or has a history of heart trouble, the person should be taken to an emergency department immediately.

Cocaine and crack. Cocaine is a naturally occurring stimulant extracted from the leaf of the coca bush. Crack is an inexpensive, widely available alkalinized form of cocaine. When crack is smoked, it takes effect in 4 to 6 seconds, producing a fleeting high (5 to 7 minutes) followed by a period of deep depression that reinforces addictive behavior patterns and guarantees continued use of the drug. Cocaine is classified as a schedule II substance—"high abuse potential with some recognized medical use."

Cocaine exerts two main effects on the body: anesthetic and stimulant. As an anesthetic it blocks the conduction of electrical impulses within the nerve cells that are involved in sensory transmission, primarily pain transmission. It also acts as a stimulant for both sexual arousal and violent behavior. Cocaine produces an imbalance of neurotransmitters (dopamine and norepinephrine) that are most likely responsible for many of the physical withdrawal symptoms reported by heavy chronic cocaine users: depression, paranoia, lethargy, anxiety, insomnia, nausea and vomiting, and sweating and chills—all signs of the body struggling to regain its normal chemical balance.

TABLE 19-5	CENTRAL NERVOUS SYSTEM STIMULANTS				
DRUGS	INTOXICATION EFFECTS	OVERDOSE EFFECTS	POSSIBLE OVERDOSE TREATMENTS	WITHDRAWAL EFFECTS	WITHDRAWAL TREATMENTS
Cocaine, crack (*short acting*) Note: High obtained in 3 min snorted, 30 sec injected, 4-6 sec smoked (crack) Average high lasts 15-30 min for cocaine; 5-7 min for crack	*Physical:* Tachycardia Dilated pupils Elevated blood pressure Nausea and vomiting Insomnia *Psychological-perceptual:* Assaultiveness Grandiosity Impaired judgment Impaired social and occupational functioning Euphoria	Respiratory distress Ataxia Hyperpyrexia Convulsions Coma Stroke Myocardial infarction Death	Antipsychotics *Medical and nursing management for:* Hyperpyrexia (ambient cooling) Convulsions (diazepam) Respiratory distress Cardiovascular shock Acidification of urine (ammonium chloride for amphetamine)	Fatigue Depression Agitation Apathy Anxiety Sleepiness Disorientation Lethargy Craving	Antidepressants (e.g., desipramine) Dopamine agonist (e.g., bromocriptine)
Amphetamines (*long acting*) Dextroamphetamine Methamphetamine Ice (synthesized for street use)	Increased energy Increased wakefulness, increased respirations, increased hyperthermia, and euphoria *Severe effects:* State resembling paranoid schizophrenia Paranoia with delusions* Psychosis Visual, auditory, and tactile hallucinations Severe to panic levels of anxiety Potential for violence	Same as above	Same as above	Same as above	Same as above

*Paranoia and ideas of reference may persist for months afterward.

Methamphetamine. **Methamphetamine** is a highly addictive stimulant related to amphetamines, but it has a longer lasting and more toxic effect on the CNS. Methamphetamines have neurotoxic (brain damaging) effects, destroying brain cells that contain dopamine and serotonin. Over time, as a result of reduced levels of dopamine, Parkinson-like symptoms can develop. Prolonged use results in cracked teeth, skin infections, stroke, lung disease, kidney or liver damage, birth defects, and in many cases death.

Nicotine

Nicotine is highly addictive and used worldwide. At least 20% of the U.S. population meets the criteria for nicotine dependence. A high proportion of psychiatric outpatients are nicotine dependent, which makes them even more susceptible to the medical sequelae of cigarette smoking. High among the list are lung cancer and other cancers, emphysema, and cardiovascular disease, as well as adverse pregnancy outcomes as discussed earlier.

Nicotine can act as a stimulant, depressant, or tranquilizer. Nicotine can also be chewed (in smokeless tobacco), which adds mouth cancer to the list of dangers.

Opiates

The opiate drug class includes opium, morphine, heroin, codeine, fentanyl and its analogues, methadone, and meperidine

TABLE 19-6   OPIATES*

DRUGS	INTOXICATION EFFECTS	OVERDOSE EFFECTS	POSSIBLE OVERDOSE TREATMENTS	WITHDRAWAL EFFECTS	USE IN WITHDRAWAL TREATMENTS
Opium (paregoric) Heroin Meperidine (Demerol) Morphine Codeine Methadone (Dolophine) Hydromorphone (Dilaudid) Fentanyl (Sublimaze) Fentanyl analogue	*Physical:* Constricted pupils Decreased respiration Drowsiness Decreased blood pressure Slurred speech Psychomotor retardation *Psychological-perceptual:* Initial euphoria followed by dysphoria and impairment of attention, judgment, and memory	Possible dilation of pupils as a result of anoxia Respiratory depression or arrest Cardiac arrest and death Coma Shock Convulsions Death	Narcotic antagonist (e.g., naloxone [Narcan]) to quickly reverse central nervous system depression	Yawning Insomnia Irritability Runny nose (rhinorrhea) Panic Diaphoresis Cramps Nausea and vomiting Muscle aches ("bone pain") Chills Fever Lacrimation Diarrhea	Methadone tapering Clonidine-naltrexone Vivitrol: (naltrexone for extended release injectable suspension over 1-month period) Buprenorphine: for treatment acts as substitute

*An opiate is a derivative or synthetic that affects the central nervous system and the autonomic nervous system. Medically it is used primarily as an analgesic (pain killer). Consistent use causes tolerance and distressing withdrawal symptoms.

(e.g., Demerol). Heroin has become cheaper and more potent. Novices often start by ingesting the drug nasally. Table 19-6 lists signs and symptoms of opiate intoxication, overdose, and withdrawal, as well as possible treatments.

Marijuana

Marijuana *(Cannabis sativa)* is an Indian hemp plant in which **tetrahydrocannabinol (THC)** is the active ingredient. Research has established that marijuana is addictive, and heavy use impairs the ability of young people to concentrate, learn, and retain information (Brown University Health Education, 2008) and is implicated in mental health decline. THC has mixed depressant and hallucinogenic properties. Marijuana, the leaves of the cannabis plant, is generally smoked, but it can be ingested. Desired effects include euphoria, detachment, and relaxation. Other effects include talkativeness, slowed perception of time, inappropriate hilarity, heightened sensitivity to external stimuli, and anxiety or paranoia. Overdose and withdrawal (other than craving) rarely occur.

Hallucinogens

See Table 19-7 for signs and symptoms of hallucinogen intoxication and overdose.

Lysergic acid diethylamide (LSD) and LSD-like drugs. LSD (also known as "acid"), mescaline (peyote), and psilocybin (magic mushroom) are hallucinogens. Mescaline and the mushroom *Psilocybe mexicana* (from which psilocybin is isolated) have been used for centuries in religious rites by Native Americans living in the southwestern United States and northern Mexico. The hallucinogenic experience produced by LSD results in flashbacks and persistent perception disorder as well as hallucinations.

PCP. PCP, or 1-(phenylcyclohexyl)piperidine, is also known as angel dust, horse tranquilizer, and peace pill. The signs and symptoms of PCP intoxication range from acute anxiety to acute psychosis as well as aggression, violence, and loss of coordination. The drug produces a generalized anesthesia that lessens the sensations of touch and pain and makes staff interventions difficult. Chronic use of PCP can result in long-term effects such as dulled thinking, lethargy, loss of impulse control, poor memory, and depression.

Suicidal risk is always assessed, especially in cases of toxicity or coma. Refer to Chapter 23 for more information on suicide assessment.

Inhalants

For some early teenagers (ages 13 through 17) inhalants are often the first drugs of abuse, because they are often found in the home or can easily be purchased. Inhalant use is also referred to as "huffing" or "backing." Inhalants include volatile solvents such as spray paint, glue, cigarette lighter fluid, and propellant gases used in aerosols. Types of inhalants, signs of intoxication, and side effects are listed in Table 19-8. Inhalant use may be an early marker of substance abuse and should be the focus of increased preventive efforts and early diagnosis and treatment.

TABLE 19-7 HALLUCINOGENS*

DRUGS	INTOXICATION EFFECTS	OVERDOSE EFFECTS	POSSIBLE OVERDOSE TREATMENTS
Lysergic acid diethyl-amide (LSD) Mescaline (peyote) Psilocybin	*Physical:* Pupil dilation Tachycardia Diaphoresis Palpitations Tremors Incoordination Elevated temperature, pulse, respiration *Psychological-perceptual:* Fear of going crazy Paranoid ideas Marked anxiety, depression Synesthesia (e.g., colors are heard; sounds are seen) Depersonalization Hallucinations, although sensorium is clear Grandiosity (e.g., thinking one can fly)	Psychosis Brain damage Death	Keep patient in room with low stimuli—minimal light, sound, activity. Have one person stay with patient; reassure patient, "talk down" patient. Speak slowly and clearly in low voice. Give diazepam or chloral hydrate for extreme anxiety or tension.
1-(1-Phenylcyclohexyl) piperidine (PCP)	*Physical:* Vertical or horizontal nystagmus Increased blood pressure, pulse, and temperature Ataxia Muscle rigidity Seizures Blank stare Chronic jerking Agitated, repetitive movements Belligerence, assaultiveness, impulsiveness Impaired judgment, impaired social and occupational functioning *Severe effects:* Hallucinations, paranoia Bizarre behavior (e.g., barking like a dog, grimacing, repetitive chanting speech) Regressive behavior **Violent, bizarre behaviors** Very labile behaviors	Psychosis Possible hypertensive crisis or cardiovascular accident Respiratory arrest Hyperthermia Seizures	*If alert:* *Caution:* Gastric lavage can lead to laryngeal spasms or aspiration. Acidify urine (cranberry juice, ascorbic acid); in acute stage, ammonium chloride acidifies urine to help excrete drug from body—may continue for 10-14 days. Put in room with minimal stimuli. Do not attempt to talk down patient! Speak slowly, clearly, and in a low voice. Administer diazepam. Haloperidol may be used for severe behavioral disturbance (*not* a phenothiazine). **Institute medical intervention for:** Hyperthermia High blood pressure Respiratory distress Hypertension

*A hallucinogen produces *abnormal mental phenomena* in the cognitive and perceptual spheres; for example, distortion in space and time, hallucinations, delusions (paranoid or grandiose), and synesthesia may occur.

TABLE 19-8   INHALANTS

DRUG	INTOXICATION EFFECTS	OVERDOSE EFFECTS	TREATMENT
Volatile solvents (e.g., paint thinners, glues, gasoline, dry cleaner fluid) **Gases** (e.g., butane, propane, nitrous oxide) **Nitrates** (e.g., isoamyl, isobutyl, commonly known as "poppers") **Aerosols** (e.g., spray paint, hair or deodorant sprays, fabric protector sprays, vegetable oil sprays)	Similar to alcohol: Slurred speech, lack of inhibitions, euphoria, dizziness, drunkenness, violent behavior	Liver and brain damage, heart failure, respiratory arrest, suffocation, coma, death Capable of interfering with oxygen supply to vital organs by destroying oxygen-carrying ability of red blood cells; associated with fatal cardiac rhythm **Long-term use** can lead to deterioration of myelin sheath of nerve fibers, resulting in muscle spasms and tremors, or even permanent difficulty with basic movements such as walking, bending, and talking	Support affected systems Neurological symptoms may respond to vitamin B_{12} and folate

Data from National Institute on Drug Abuse. (1998). *Research report series: inhalant use* (NIH Pub. No. 94-3819). Washington, DC: U.S. Department of Health and Human Services; National Institute on Drug Abuse. (updated 2011). Retrieved February 9, 2012, from www.drugabuse.gov/publications/infofacts/inhalants.

Rave/"Club Drugs"

Raves or techno dances are all-night dance parties attended by large numbers of adolescents (ranging from age 13 to young adults in their middle to late twenties) (MDC, 2011). Raves are known for their electric music and the liberal use of techno drugs such as ecstasy. **Ecstasy** (also called MDMA, Adam, yaba, and XTC) is a prototype of a class of substituted amphetamines that also includes MDA (methylenedioxyamphetamine, or "love") and MDE (3,4-methylenedioxy-N-ethylamphetamine, or "Eve"). These recreational drugs produce subjective effects resembling those of stimulants and hallucinogens. Club drugs are used also in nightclubs, bars, parties, and places where young people gather to dance.

MDMA primarily affects the neurons/neurotransmitters that relate to serotonin. Serotonin is a regulator of mood, aggression, sexual activity, sleep, and sensitivity to pain. MDMA acts to prolong the effects of serotonin in the brain as well as to increase the amounts of serotonin released from the neurons. It has similar effects on norepinephrine, which can cause an increase in heart rate and blood pressure. MDMA releases dopamine to a much lesser extent than the other neurotransmitters (NIDA, 2010g).

After MDMA is taken, subjective side effects include euphoria, increased energy, increased self-confidence, increased sociability, and a feeling of closeness to people. Because of their psychostimulant and psychedelic effects, ecstasy and the other drugs listed are increasingly abused. Adverse effects such as hyperthermia, heart failure, and kidney failure have occurred. Deaths from acute dehydration have been reported. Chronic heavy recreational use of ecstasy is thought to be responsible for

sleep disorders, depressed mood, persistent elevation of anxiety level, impulsiveness, and hostility as well as selective impairment of episodic memory and weakening of memory and attention.

Note: As mentioned earlier in the chapter, there are a number of chemically manufactured street drugs that contain combinations of properties. Some of these drugs can be hallucinogenic and also have stimulant or amnesic properties, among others.

Drugs Used to Perpetrate Sexual Assault

The drugs most frequently used to facilitate a sexual assault (rape) are **flunitrazepam (Rohypnol or "roofies"),** which is a fast-acting benzodiazepine, and γ-**hydroxybutyrate (GHB)** and its congeners. They are odorless, tasteless, and colorless; mix easily with drinks; and can result in unconsciousness in a matter of minutes. Perpetrators use these drugs because they rapidly produce disinhibition and relaxation of voluntary muscles; they also cause the victim to have lasting anterograde amnesia. Alcohol potentiates their effects. See Chapter 22 for more on these drugs.

ASSESSMENT GUIDELINES
Chemically Impaired Patients

1. Assess for a severe or major withdrawal syndrome.
2. Assess for an overdose to a drug or alcohol that warrants immediate medical attention.
3. Assess the patient for suicidal thoughts or other self-destructive behaviors.
4. Evaluate the patient for any physical complications related to drug abuse.

5. Explore the patient's interests in taking actions to address his or her drug or alcohol problem.
6. Assess the patient and family for knowledge of community resources for alcohol and drug treatment.

DIAGNOSIS

Nursing diagnoses for patients with psychoactive substance use disorders are many and varied because of the large range of physical and psychological effects of drug abuse or dependence on the user and his or her family. Comorbid psychiatric problems also must be addressed. Potential nursing diagnoses for people with substance use disorders are listed in Table 19-9.

OUTCOMES IDENTIFICATION

When planning care for patients with substance use problems, the patient's cultural background and values need to be reflected in the plan of care. The following are some examples of outcomes:

- Remaining free from injury while withdrawing from the substance
- Attending programs for treatment and maintenance of sobriety (e.g., Alcoholics Anonymous [AA], Cocaine Anonymous [CA], Narcotics Anonymous [NA], or group therapy, cognitive behavioral therapy, or other)
- Attending a relapse prevention program during the active course of treatment
- Verbalizing cues or situations that pose increased risk of drug use
- Having a stable group of drug-free friends and socializing with them at least three times a week by *(date)*
- Demonstrating *(1, 2, or 3)* new skills in dealing with troubling feelings (anger, loneliness, cravings, anxiety)

PLANNING

Planning care requires attention to the patient's social status, income, ethnic background, gender, age, substance use history, and current condition. It is safest to propose abstinence as a treatment goal for all addicts. Abstinence is strongly related to good work adjustment, positive health status, comfortable interpersonal relationships, and general social stability. Planning must also address the patient's major psychological, social, and medical problems as well as the substance-using behavior. Involvement of appropriate family members is essential.

Unfortunately, a person's social status and social relations often deteriorate as a result of addiction. Job demotion or job loss, with resultant reduced or nonexistent income, may occur. Meeting basic needs for food, shelter, and clothing is thereby hampered. Marriage and other close relationships deteriorate and fail, and the person is often left alone and isolated. The lack of interpersonal and social supports is a complicating factor in treatment planning for the addict.

IMPLEMENTATION

The aim of treatment is self-responsibility, not compliance. A major challenge is improving treatment effectiveness by matching subtypes of patients to specific types of treatment. Although addicts share some characteristics and dynamics, significant differences exist within the addict population with regard to physiological, psychological, and sociocultural processes. These differences influence the recovery process either positively or negatively.

Often the choice of inpatient or outpatient care depends on cost and the availability of insurance coverage. Outpatient programs work best for employed substance abusers who have an involved social support system. People who have no support and structure in their day often do better in inpatient programs when these programs are available.

In addition, neuropsychological deficits have been associated with long-term alcohol abuse as well as with other substances (e.g., methamphetamines). Impairment has been found in abstract reasoning ability, ability to use feedback in learning new concepts, attention and concentration spans, cognitive flexibility, and subtle memory functions. These deficits undoubtedly have an impact on the process of treatment.

At all levels of practice, the nurse can play an important role in the intervention process by recognizing the signs of substance abuse in both the patient and the family and by being familiar with the resources available to help with the problem.

Communication Guidelines

Communication strategies are designed to address behaviors that almost all substance abusers have in common, including dysfunctional anger, manipulation, impulsiveness, and grandiosity. The nurse's ability to develop a warm, accepting relationship with an addicted patient can help the patient feel safe enough to start looking at problems with some degree of openness and honesty. It is important to communicate in culturally appropriate ways.

A useful tool for helping the resistant addict develop a willingness to engage in treatment is known as substance-abuse intervention. The concept behind this approach is that addiction is a progressive illness and rarely goes into remission without outside help. Significant others arrange for a meeting with the addict to point out current problems and to offer treatment alternatives. The steps or elements are outlined in Box 19-4 and can be applied to all substances of abuse.

Health Teaching and Health Promotion
Relapse Prevention

Relapses are common during a person's recovery because addiction is a chronic medical illness, such as diabetes, hypertension, and asthma, and has both physiological and behavioral components (NIDA, 2010e). The goal of relapse prevention is to help individuals learn from "trigger situations" so that periods of sobriety can be lengthened over time and so that lapses and relapses are not viewed as total failure.

TABLE 19-9 POTENTIAL NURSING DIAGNOSES FOR SUBSTANCE ABUSE

SIGNS AND SYMPTOMS	NURSING DIAGNOSES*
Vomiting, diarrhea, poor nutritional and fluid intake	*Imbalanced Nutrition: Less Than Body Requirements*
	Deficient Fluid Volume
	Risk for Electrolyte Imbalance
Audiovisual hallucinations, impaired judgment, memory deficits, cognitive impairments related to substance intoxication or withdrawal (deficits in problem solving, ability to attend to tasks and grasp ideas)	*Impaired Environmental Interpretation Syndrome*
	Risk for Violence to Self or Others
	Ineffective Impulse Control
	Acute or Chronic Confusion
Changes in sleep-wake cycle, interference with stage 4 sleep, inability to sleep or long periods of sleeping related to effects of or withdrawal from substance	*Disturbed Sleep Pattern*
	Insomnia
	Sleep Deprivation
Lack of self-care (hygiene, grooming), failure to care for basic health needs	*Ineffective Health Maintenance*
	Self-Neglect
	Bathing Self-Care Deficit/
	Feeding Self-Care Deficit
	Nonadherence to Health Care Regimen
Feelings of hopelessness, inability to change, feelings of worthlessness, feeling that life has no meaning or future	*Hopelessness*
	Spiritual Distress
	Situational Low Self-Esteem
	Chronic Low Self-Esteem
	Risk for Self-Directed Violence
	Risk for Suicide
Family crises and family pain, ineffective parenting, emotional neglect of others, increased incidence of physical and sexual abuse of others, increased self-hate projected to others	*Interrupted Family Processes*
	Impaired Parenting
	Risk for Other-Directed Violence
	Dysfunctional Family Processes
	Ineffective Relationship
	Ineffective Impulse Control
Excessive substance abuse affecting all areas of a person's life: loss of friends, poor job performance, increased illness rates, proneness to accidents and overdoses	*Ineffective Coping*
	Impaired Verbal Communication
	Social Isolation
	Risk for Loneliness
	Anxiety
	Ineffective Relationship
	Risk for Suicide
Increased health problems related to substance used and route of use, as well as overdose	*Activity Intolerance*
	Ineffective Airway Clearance
	Ineffective Breathing Pattern
	Impaired Oral Mucous Membrane
	Risk for Infection
	Decreased Cardiac Output
	Sexual Dysfunction
	Risk for Impaired Liver Function
Total preoccupation with and majority of time consumed by taking and withdrawing from drug	*Risk-Prone Health Behavior*
	Ineffective Impulse Control
	Ineffective Coping
	Impaired Social Interaction
	Dysfunctional Family Processes: Substance Dependence

Nursing Diagnoses—Definitions and Classification 2012-2014. Copyright © 2012, 1994-2012 by NANDA International. Used by arrangement with Blackwell Publishing Limited, a company of John Wiley and Sons, Inc.

BOX 19-4 STEPS IN AN INTERVENTION

1. All the people concerned about and affected by the person's substance abuse are gathered together to present their case. The intervention must be rehearsed before it is actually carried out, usually with the support and guidance of a counselor.
2. Specific evidence related to the substance abuse is presented by each person, and it is written so that each person does not have to rely on memory in a tense situation.
3. Timing must be right:
   - There must be current evidence available.
   - The intervention must take place after a crisis is precipitated by substance use and *not* when the person is under the influence of the substance or in severe withdrawal.
4. The intervention requires privacy. It is held in a place where no interruptions can occur.
5. The use of defenses is anticipated. No reaction is made to them.
6. Genuine, but firm, concern is demonstrated.
7. Substance abuse is understood as a disease.
8. Treatment alternatives are presented.
9. Responses to possible outcomes are prepared. The goal is to get the affected person into treatment. If the substance abusing person agrees to accept treatment, then he or she is taken immediately to a detoxification unit, where arrangements have been made previously. If the person refuses, then family members state that his or her decision must force them to make decisions of their own because they are no longer willing to live with the addicted person's behavior.

Adapted from Johnson, V. E. (1986). *Intervention: how to help someone who doesn't want help.* Minneapolis: Johnson Institute.

APPLYING THE ART

A Person With Chemical Dependency

SCENARIO: During our previous two encounters, 34-year-old Kristen had repeatedly insisted she would "quit using and take my med." Now Kristen, a single mom, has just learned that her own mother had gained legal custody of Kristen's three preschool-aged children related to charges of child neglect. Before each of her two psychiatric hospitalizations in the past year, Kristen had chosen heroin over taking her psychotropic medication, and that decision then impaired taking care of her children.

THERAPEUTIC GOAL: By the end of this interaction, Kristen will show progress towards taking responsibility for acting-out behavior and acknowledge that choosing heroin when feeling out of control compounds her losses.

STUDENT-PATIENT INTERACTION	THOUGHTS, COMMUNICATION TECHNIQUES, AND MENTAL HEALTH NURSING CONCEPTS
Kristen: *Glances my way and motions "come on" as she rapidly paces the hallway.*	
Student's feelings: *I'm surprised Kristen did not even stop to greet me.*	
Student: "Kristen, I'm having trouble keeping up with you. You seem really upset."	I had learned in report about Kristen losing custody of her children. Initially she had cried out but her tears quickly turned to angry pacing. I *offer self* by walking with Kristen, then *reflect* feelings.
Student's feelings: *Addiction makes me angry. Kristen shows such promise and then abandons everything when heroin calls. I know that some people at school see nothing wrong with "recreational" use of drugs. I look around the addictions unit and see pain everywhere.*	
Kristen: "Yes, I'm upset. My so-called mother stole my kids! I never injured my kids. I just asked my 5-year-old whether he wanted new shoes or wanted Mommy to feel better. It's not my fault. So my mother gets upset and bought the shoes. She thinks she can buy their love."	Kristen uses *projection*, blaming her mother for the loss of her children. I remember that clients with addiction use *"stinking-thinking,"* which includes *denial* ("I'd never hurt my kids"), *rationalization* ("It wasn't me who chose heroin over shoes"), and *projection*.
Student: "Kristen, I'm concerned with what is happening with you, but I'm having trouble keeping up. Could you walk a little slower, so I can hear you clearly?"	I think Kristen may be *ambivalent*, not sure if she can tolerate me or anyone.
Student's feelings: *I really am concerned with her welfare even though I feel frustrated that she totally denies her addiction.*	

Continued

APPLYING THE ART—cont'd

A Person With Chemical Dependency

STUDENT-PATIENT INTERACTION	THOUGHTS, COMMUNICATION TECHNIQUES, AND MENTAL HEALTH NURSING CONCEPTS
Kristen: *Kicks over a chair, whirls and grabs my forearm, pulling me toward her.* "Get up here then if you care so much!"	She is escalating. I see staff on their way to help. Anxiety is communicated interpersonally. I need to talk her down.
Student's feelings: *Okay. I am okay. I need to mindfully breathe and stay calm and in charge of me. I must admit though I don't like my arm being grabbed.*	
Student: "Kristen, stop." *Louder voice, then quieter.* "You're hurting my arm." *Quietly concerned, trying to make eye contact.*	I *set limits* and *give information.*
Kristen: *Meets my eyes and loosens her grip. Sarcastically:* "Here comes the cavalry!" *Three staff approach, but wait as I speak.*	Though Kristen uses sarcasm, she nonetheless responds to the staff's arrival by loosening her grip on my arm.
Student's feelings: *I feel kind of honored that the staff trusts that I am doing well enough to wait to see if they're needed.*	
Student: "Kristen, I trust that you and I can get through this." *Pausing.* "Thank you for loosening your grip." *Concerned look.* "I know you're upset. Please let go." *She does.* "Thank you Kristen." *Staff steps back, carefully watching as Kristen slowly walks to the chair. Kristen uprights the chair she kicked over, then we both sit down.*	I *offer self* and use *reflection.* I treat Kristen with respect as well as model socially appropriate interactions by saying please and thanks to Kristen for letting go of my arm.
Student's feelings: *I made it through this with no one hurt. I feel more confident but I'm also really relieved that the staff responded so quickly. I know the staff was ready to intervene if needed.*	
Kristen: "I don't know what got into me. I never meant to hurt you."	She not only let go of me, she also fixed the chair.
Student: *I make eye contact.* "It's frightening to be grabbed. I'm okay now. How about you?"	I assess and also let Kristen know my feelings. Her choices affect others. I nonjudgmentally accept Kristen, but not the hurtful behavior.
Kristen: *Nods.* "I'm sorry. Sometimes I feel so out of control."	
Student's feelings: *Kristen tries to make things right by apologizing and fixing the chair.*	
Student: "You kicked the chair and grabbed my arm but you were also able to say 'sorry.' "	I name the observed *acting-out behavior* but also give *support* by saying, "You were able to…"
Kristen: "I meant the 'sorry.' I always mean it. Then the pressure builds and…" *Points to the needle tracks on her arms.*	She uses heroin as a dysfunctional way to cope with anxiety. Then the heroin compounds her problems.
Student: "So when you feel out of control, maybe even overwhelmed, you turn to heroin? *Kristen nods. And then…overwhelmed. I am so thankful I have other ways to cope and people who care about me.*	
Kristen: "I am gone. No more Kristen. I forget all the hassles. Then it all crashes down. I lose everything. I've screwed up everything again."	In choosing heroin she also chooses "no more Kristen." The drug erodes her self-esteem and even her sense of self.
Student's feelings: *Some days I think how far I still have to go to be a nurse. Then I think of Kristen's long, long road to reach a drug-free life.*	
Student: "Everything?"	I use *restatement,* encouraging her to go on.

APPLYING THE ART—cont'd

A Person With Chemical Dependency

STUDENT-PATIENT INTERACTION	THOUGHTS, COMMUNICATION TECHNIQUES, AND MENTAL HEALTH NURSING CONCEPTS
Kristen: "Myself, my kids." *Starts to cry.*	Kristen shows *partial insight* but so far, avoids attending *Narcotics Anonymous.*
Student: *I lean forward, waiting quietly.* **Student's feelings:** *I want to fill the silences, but I contain my anxiety.*	I use *attending* behavior.
Kristen: "I miss them so much! They deserve better than me. I need to go lie down." *She begins to turn away.*	Kristen uses *withdrawal* by physically retreating to her room.
Student's feelings: *Kristen feels exhausted by all of the emotions she's experienced.*	
Student: "Okay, I'll check with you after lunch."	I *give information* and accept Kristen's decision to leave in order to give her control and build trust.
Student's feelings: *I need to debrief in a clinical conference. I'm feeling exhausted too.*	
Kristen: *Nods, walking toward her room.*	

VIGNETTE

Bill, 20 years old and single, is transported to the emergency department in a coma. He is accompanied by his mother, with whom Bill lives in a small apartment. Bill had been in his room at home. When his mother was not able to rouse him, she dialed 911 for an ambulance. A syringe and some white powder were found next to Bill. His breathing is labored, and his pupils are constricted. Vital signs are taken: his blood pressure is 60/40 mm Hg and his pulse is 132 beats per minute. Bill's situation is determined to be life threatening.

Bill's mother is extremely distressed, but she is able to report to the staff that Bill has a substance-abuse problem and had been taking heroin for 6 months before entering a methadone maintenance program. It is decided at this point to administer a narcotic antagonist, and naloxone is given intramuscularly. After this, Bill's breathing improves, and he responds to verbal stimuli. His mother later tells staff that Bill has been in the methadone maintenance program for the past year but has not attended the program or received his methadone for the past week. At their urging, she calls the program, which arranges to send an outreach worker, Mr. Rodriguez, to talk to her and Bill. An appointment is made with Mr. Rodriguez for the following Monday. Mr. Rodriguez knows that Bill's future ultimately rests with Bill and talks to him regarding how he perceives his situation, where he wants to go, and what he thinks he needs to get there.

After talking to Bill and reviewing Bill's history, the health care team decides that a self-help, abstinence-oriented recovery program might be the most helpful treatment. Bill has not been taking drugs a long time, he has a job, and he appears motivated. Naltrexone (Trexan) will be given in conjunction with relapse prevention training, and Bill will regularly attend Narcotics Anonymous meetings.

General strategies for relapse prevention are cognitive and behavioral: recognizing and learning how to avoid or cope with threats to recovery; changing lifestyle; learning how to participate fully in society without drugs; and securing help from other people, or social support. Box 19-5 identifies relapse prevention strategies.

Awareness of Co-occurring/Comorbid Principles

The nurse needs to be aware of clinical practice guidelines that have been developed through research involving individuals with co-occurring diagnoses. The following six principles are applicable in inpatient and outpatient settings (Minkoff, 2003):

1. Expect a patient to have at least one co-occurring disorder.
2. Treatment success is increased when providers are empathic and hopeful, and work as a team.
3. Both addiction programs and mental health programs need a dual focus, which requires appropriate training for staff.
4. The substance use disorder and the psychiatric disorder are considered primary and need simultaneous treatment.
5. Recovery occurs in stages, and treatment should be matched to the patient's needs and level of motivation and engagement.
6. Outcomes must be individualized to support progress in small steps over a long period.

Psychotherapy and Therapeutic Modalities

Achieving sobriety is only the first step toward what will be a long and complex recovery. It is felt by NIDA (2010e,f) that in order to be successful the treatment program has to focus on many aspects of the person's life that have been altered because of addiction. Examples will include the individual's medical, social, vocational, legal, and psychological needs. The most

BOX 19-5   RELAPSE PREVENTION STRATEGIES

Basics

1. Keep the program simple at first; 40% to 50% of patients who abuse substances have mild to moderate cognitive problems while actively using.
2. Review instructions with health team members.
3. Use a notebook and record important information and telephone numbers.

Skills

Take advantage of cognitive behavioral therapy to increase your coping skills. Identify which important life skills are needed:

1. Which situations do you have difficulty handling?
2. Which situations are you managing more effectively?
3. For which situations would you like to develop more skills to act more effectively?

Relapse Prevention Groups

Become a member of a relapse prevention group. These groups work on:

1. Rehearsing stressful situations using a variety of techniques.
2. Finding ways to deal with current problems or ones that are likely to arise as you become drug free.
3. Providing role models to help you make necessary life changes.

Enhancement of Personal Insight

Therapy—group, individual, or family—can help you gain insight and control over a variety of psychological concerns, for example:

1. What drives your addictions?
2. What constitutes a healthy supportive relationship?
3. How can you increase your sense of self and self-worth?
4. What does your addictive substance give you that you think you need and cannot find otherwise?

Adapted from Zerbe, K.J. (1999). *Women's mental health in primary care* (pp. 94-95). Philadelphia: Saunders.

recent guiding principles for the Recovery Paradigm for addictions include (Brauser & Barclay, 2012) the following crucial components:

- Emerges from hope
- Is person-driven
- Occurs through many pathways
- Is holistic
- Is supported by peers and allies
- Is supported through relationships and social networks
- Is culturally based
- Is supported by addressing trauma
- Involves the individual, family, and community
- Is based on respect

Psychotherapy assists patients in identifying and using alternative coping mechanisms to reduce reliance on substances. Eventually, psychotherapy can assist recovering addicts to become increasingly comfortable with sobriety.

An important aspect of recovery in AA and a host of other recovery modalities is *spirituality.* Spirituality levels and spiritual practices are related to improved outcomes (Slaymaker, 2009). Higher spiritual levels often correlate with a sense of purpose, gratitude, and forgiveness, which are all aspects of spirituality (Slaymaker, 2009).

The following therapies or components of therapies have been found effective for people on the road to recovery (NIDA, 2010e,f):

- **Cognitive behavioral therapy (CBT).** CBT helps patients to recognize and avoid old triggers to using, and offers behavioral strategies to cope with situations that are most likely to induce cravings and abuse of drugs.
- Motivational incentives. Much like token therapy, positive reinforcements are provided (such as privileges) when a patient participates in counseling sessions, maintains a therapeutic drug regimen, or remains drug free, for example.
- Motivational interviewing. Provides strategies to evoke rapid and internally motivated change to stop drug use and facilitate treatment.
- **Group therapy.** Group therapy is an extremely important element of recovery for most individuals with substance use disorders.

Many critical issues arise during the first 6 months of sobriety. These include the following:

- Physical changes take place as the body adapts to functioning without substances.
- Numerous signals occur in the patient's internal and external world that previously were cues to drinking and drug use. Different responses to these cues need to be learned.
- Emotional responses (feelings that were formerly diluted by substance use) are now experienced full strength. Because they are so unfamiliar, they can produce anxiety.
- Responses of family and coworkers to the patient's new behavior must be addressed. Sobriety disrupts a system, and everyone in that system needs to adjust to the change.
- New coping skills must be developed to prevent relapse and ensure prolonged sobriety.

Whatever therapy a person chooses, it needs to be directive, open and honest, and caring. The therapeutic process involves teaching the patient to identify the physical and emotional changes that are occurring at the present time. Confidentiality must be maintained throughout therapy *except* when it conflicts with requirements for mandatory reporting in certain circumstances (e.g., child abuse, danger to self or others).

Self-Help Groups for Patient and Family

Counseling and support should be encouraged for all families with a drug-dependent member. Al-Anon and Alateen are self-help groups that offer support and guidance for adults and teenagers, respectively, in families with a chemically dependent member. Other such organizations include Adult Children of Alcoholics (ACA), Pills Anonymous (PA), Narcotics Anonymous (NA), and Cocaine Anonymous (CA), to name but a few.

Self-help groups assist family members in dealing with many common issues. Their work is based on a combination of educational and operational principles centered on acceptance of the disease model of addiction, including pragmatic methods for avoiding enabling behaviors.

Twelve-Step Programs

Alcoholics Anonymous (AA) is the prototype for all the 12-step programs that were subsequently developed for many types of addiction. These programs offer the behavioral, cognitive, and dynamic structure needed in recovery. Three basic concepts are fundamental to all 12-step programs:

1. Individuals with addictive disorders are powerless over their addiction, and their lives are unmanageable.
2. Although individuals with addictive disorders are not responsible for their disease, they are responsible for their recovery.
3. Individuals can no longer blame people, places, and things for their addiction; they must face their problems and their feelings.

Using the 12 steps is often referred to as "working the steps" and helps a person refrain from addictive behaviors as well as fostering individual change and growth. In addition to AA, other 12-step programs include PA, NA, CA, and Valium Anonymous.

SMART (Self-Management and Recovery Training): SMART is also a self-help program. SMART is rooted in "cognitive behavioral therapy"; the program emphasizes the following four key points (*Smart Recovery,* 2008-2011; Upchurch, 2011):

1. Enhancing and maintaining motivation to abstain
2. Coping with urges
3. Problem solving (managing thoughts, feelings, and behaviors)
4. Lifestyle balance (balancing momentary and enduring satisfactions) (see www.Smartrecovery.org)

Residential Programs

Residential treatment programs are best suited for individuals who have a long history of antisocial behaviors as well as addiction. The goal of treatment is to effect a change in lifestyle, including abstinence, development of social skills, and elimination of antisocial behavior. Follow-up studies suggest that patients who stay in such programs 90 days or longer exhibit a significant decrease in illicit drug use and recorded arrests and an increase in legitimate employment.

Intensive Outpatient Programs

Most treatments for substance-abusing patients take place in the community. The steps addicted people follow in an intensive outpatient program include a variety of psychotherapeutic and pharmacological interventions along with behavioral monitoring. Intensive outpatient treatment programs are becoming more popular because they are viewed as flexible, diverse, cost-effective, and responsive to the specific needs of the individual. Reduction in program length can significantly increase the number of patients completing a program without influencing clinical effectiveness (Bamford et al., 2003).

Outpatient Drug-Free Programs and Employee Assistance Programs

Outpatient drug-free programs are better suited to an individual who is simultaneously addicted to two or more drugs (polydrug abuse) and/or alcoholic abusers. These centers may offer vocational education and placement, counseling, and individual or group psychotherapy. Employee assistance programs have been developed to provide delivery of mental health services in occupational settings. Many hospitals and corporations offer their employees counseling and support as an alternative to job termination when the employee's work performance is negatively affected by his or her impairment.

Pharmacological, Biological, and Integrative Therapies

Alcohol Withdrawal Treatment

The treatment of withdrawal symptoms has the following two major goals (APA, 2006):

1. Help the person achieve detoxification as safely and comfortably as possible.
2. Enhance the person's motivation for abstinence and recovery.

Not all people who stop drinking require management of withdrawal. This decision depends on the length of time and the quantity of alcohol involved, history of withdrawal complications, and overall health status. Medication should not be given until the symptoms of withdrawal are seen. Drugs that are useful in treating alcohol withdrawal delirium are listed in Table 19-10. For an overview of pharmacotherapy for other substances of abuse, see Table 19-11.

EVALUATION

Favorable treatment outcome is judged by increased lengths of time in abstinence, decreased denial, acceptable occupational functioning, improved family relationships, and, ultimately, ability to relate normally and comfortably to other human beings. The ability to use existing supports and skills learned in treatment is important for ongoing recovery. For example, recovery is actively viable if, in response to cues to use the substance, the patient calls his or her sponsor or other recovering persons; increases attendance at 12-step meetings, aftercare, or other group meetings; or writes feelings in a log and considers alternative action. Continuous monitoring and evaluation increase the chances for prolonged recovery.

TABLE 19-10   ALCOHOL WITHDRAWAL DELIRIUM

DRUG	PURPOSE
Sedatives	
Benzodiazepines*	
Chlordiazepoxide (Librium)	Provides *safe* withdrawal and has anticonvulsant effects; chlordiazepoxide and diazepam are cross-addicting
Diazepam (Valium)	Has anticonvulsant qualities
Oxazepam (Serax)	Not metabolized in the liver
Lorazepam (Ativan)	Not metabolized in the liver
Seizure Control	
Carbamazepine (Tegretol) or valproic acid (Depakote)	Reduces the requirement (dose) of a benzodiazepine; not effective when used alone
Magnesium sulfate	Increases effectiveness of vitamin B_1 and helps reduce postwithdrawal seizures
Thiamine (vitamin B_1)	Given intramuscularly or intravenously before glucose loading to prevent Wernicke's encephalopathy
Alleviation of Autonomic Nervous System (ANS)	
Beta-blockers (propranolol) *or* alpha-blockers (clonidine)	May help reduce ANS hyperactivity (e.g., tremor, tachycardia, elevated blood pressure, diaphoresis)
Folic acid	Most effective in short time
Multivitamins	Malabsorption due to heavy long-term alcohol abuse causes deficiencies in many vitamins

*Benzodiazepines should be discontinued once detoxification is complete.

TABLE 19-11   PHARMACOTHERAPY FOR SUBSTANCE USE DISORDERS*

INDICATIONS	PRESCRIBING	ADVANTAGES	RISKS
Disulfiram (Antabuse)			
Helps prevent relapse of alcohol abuse. Ingested in combination with alcohol, it will cause nausea, vomiting, headache, and flushing.	**Induction:** 250-500 mg daily for 2 weeks **Maintenance:** 250 mg daily; range is 125-500 mg daily **Labs:** LFTs initially, then at 10-14 days, every 6 months thereafter	Useful in patients who have maintained sobriety but who have a history of relapse, current motivation, and a witnessed ingestion.	Metallic aftertaste; dermatitis; severe reaction or death could result from alcohol ingestion
Naltrexone (Revia)			
Helps with alcohol cravings, possibly by reducing the reinforcing effects of alcohol. Also used to block the effects of opiates.	**Induction for opiate dependence:** Be sure patient is opioid-free for 7-10 days; confirm by UDS Start with 25 mg. If no withdrawal reaction, increase by another 25 mg; continue at 50 mg daily.	Very useful in the acute recovery phase of alcohol dependence (first 12 weeks).	Nausea, abdominal pain; constipation; dizziness; headache; anxiety; fatigue
Vivitrol (Naltrexone for Extended-Release, Injectable Suspension)			
Vivitrol is used for alcohol abuse only (should not be used if patient has opioid dependence).	**Induction for alcohol dependence:** Start at 50 mg daily. Continue at 50 mg daily. *Vivitrol (injection in buttocks):* Be sure patient is alcohol-free for at least 1 week: 380 mg/vial **Labs:** UDS, LFTs before; 6 months thereafter	Vivitrol may be easier for patients recovering from alcohol dependency to use consistently.	Vivitrol should not be used by a patient who is also using opioids, such as heroin

TABLE 19-11	PHARMACOTHERAPY FOR SUBSTANCE USE DISORDERS*—cont'd		
INDICATIONS	**PRESCRIBING**	**ADVANTAGES**	**RISKS**
Acamprosate (Campral)			
Helps with alcohol cravings, possibly by reducing intensity of prolonged withdrawal syndrome. Benefit emerges after 30-90 days.	**Induction:** Begin two, 333-mg tablets, tid Patients with renal impairment may need dosage reduction **Maintenance:** 666 mg tid **Labs:** BUN, creatine, creatinine clearance	Reasonably safe in patients with mild to moderate hepatic impairment (excreted via the kidneys). Need to have been abstinent at least 7 or more days.	Diarrhea and decreased libido
Buprenorphine Hydrochloride (Subutex); Buprenorphine Hydrochloride and Naloxone Hydrochloride (Suboxone)			
Treatment for outpatient detoxification and maintenance by specially trained and registered physicians.	**Induction:** Begin 8 mg SL on day 1, 16 mg day 2 **Maintenance:** Continue 16 mg SL daily thereafter; range is 4-24 mg daily **Labs:** UDS at induction, and monthly thereafter; LFTs on induction, and every 6 months thereafter	Buprenorphine can prevent symptoms of withdrawal in patients addicted to opiates; is an alternative to maintenance treatment with methadone.	Dizziness; nausea; respiratory depression

*Drug doses provided here are to be used as general guidelines. Results from current research, effects of specific doses, and "risk to benefit" changes should all be considered, along with physician preference, when determining the optimal dose for each patient.
BUN, blood urea nitrogen; *LFTs,* liver function tests; *SL,* sublingual (under the tongue); *tid,* three times daily; *UDS,* urine drug screen.

KEY POINTS TO REMEMBER

- A host of designer drugs that are easy to obtain (along with prescription drugs and methamphetamines) are increasingly being used by youths and teenagers. They are extremely addicting within a short period of time. These drugs lead to damage in the brain, interfere with psychological/social growth, decrease the potential for a productive future, and terminate the life span of too many children and teenagers.
- Substance use and dependence occur on a continuum, and addiction develops over a period of time.
- The tendency to abuse a substance can be influenced by a combination of genetic, biological, sociological, and environmental factors.
- Assessment of patients with substance use disorders needs to be comprehensive, aimed at identifying common medical and psychiatric comorbidities.
- Patients with a **dual diagnosis** have more severe symptoms, experience more crises, and require longer treatment for successful outcomes.

- A person's substance use or addiction affects everybody—family, friends, coworkers, and others—and may lead them to adopt codependent behaviors to cope and minimize the behaviors of the abuser.
- Relapse is an expected complication in the recovery of addictions, and treatment includes a significant focus on teaching relapse prevention.
- Successful treatment modalities include a dual diagnosis approach, relapse prevention, self-help groups, psychotherapy, and psychopharmacotherapy.
- Nurses need to be aware of their own feelings about substance use so that they can provide empathy and hope to patients.
- Nurses themselves are at higher risk for substance use disorders and should be vigilant for signs of impairment in colleagues both to ensure the safety of patients and to safeguard effective treatment for the colleague.

APPLYING CRITICAL JUDGMENT

1. Write a paragraph describing your possible reactions to a drug-dependent patient to whom you are assigned.
   A. Would your response be different depending on the substance, for example, alcohol versus heroin, or marijuana versus cocaine? Give reasons for your answers.
   B. Would your response be different if the substance-dependent person were a professional colleague? How?

2. You have observed a fellow nursing colleague and friend using a substance of abuse on the unit, as well as exhibiting erratic behavior and using questionable judgment regarding patient care.
   A. What courses of action do you have, and what would be your responsibility if you chose to report your observations to a supervisor?
   B. Given this hypothetical example, what actions would you take if this situation actually occurred in the near future? Discuss the rationale for the answer you chose.
   C. What would be the positive aspects of getting your colleague and friend into an ADT program/peer counseling program?

3. Rosetta Seymour is a 14-year-old teenager who has started abusing oxycodone with her friends. She says that the pills are relatively easy to obtain.
   A. Briefly discuss the trend in abuse of prescription drugs among teenagers.
   B. When Ms. Seymour asks you why she needs to take increasing amounts of the drug to get "high," how would you explain to her the concept of tolerance?
   C. If she had just ingested oxycodone, what would you find on assessment of physical and behavioral-psychological signs and symptoms?
   D. If she came into the emergency department with an overdose of oxycodone, what would be the emergency care? What might be effective long-term care?

4. Tony Garmond is a 45-year-old mechanic. He has a 20-year history of heavy drinking and he says he wants to quit but needs help.
   A. Role-play with a classmate an initial assessment. Identify the kinds of information you would need to have in order to plan holistic care.
   B. Mr. Garmond tried stopping by himself but is in the emergency department with delirium tremens. What are the dangers for Mr. Garmond? What are the appropriate medical interventions?
   C. What are some possible treatment alternatives for Mr. Garmond when he is safely detoxified? How would you explain to him the usefulness and function of self-help recovery programs such as AA/SMART or others? What are some more traditional treatment options that might be successful with Mr. Garmond? Look up available referrals for Mr. Garmond that exist in your community.

CHAPTER REVIEW QUESTIONS

Choose the most appropriate answer(s).

1. When intervening with a patient who is intoxicated from alcohol, it is useful for a nurse to first:
   1. let the patient sober up.
   2. decide immediately on care goals.
   3. ask which drugs other than alcohol the patient has recently used.
   4. gain compliance by sharing personal drinking habits with the patient.

2. A patient was discharged from the hospital on Ativan 1 mg tid. After 3 months she enters the ER, shaking, sweating and crying. The patient is most likely demonstrating:
   1. tolerance to Ativan and requires an increased dose.
   2. a possible adverse reaction from mixing the Ativan with other meds and alcohol.
   3. a panic attack that will probably require another inpatient admission.
   4. withdrawal symptoms after trying to stop the drug on her own.

3. As a nurse evaluates a patient's progress, which treatment outcome would indicate a poor general prognosis for long-term recovery from substance abuse? The patient demonstrates:
   1. improved self-esteem.
   2. enhanced coping abilities.
   3. improved relationships with others.
   4. expectations for only occasional drug use in the future.

4. What statement best indicates positive progress in recovery from alcohol dependence?
   1. I understand now that my job may be the root cause of my addiction.
   2. I am powerless over the effects alcohol has on me.
   3. I will never use alcohol again.
   4. I realize that nutritious food and daily exercise is the best way to stay sober.

5. Select the patient statement that indicates a possible dual diagnosis.
   1. I am so busy all the time that I rarely get any sleep.
   2. It is difficult for me to get up every morning and face the day.
   3. I need a drink of alcohol before breakfast.
   4. Drinking alcohol helps me to function better.

REFERENCES

Abuse. (2007). *The American Heritage Dictionary*. Published by Houghton Mifflin. Retrieved February 9, 2012, from http://medicaldictionary.thefreedictionary.com/P/drug%20abuse.

Addiction. (n.d.) *The American Heritage Science Dictionary*. Retrieved February 9, 2012, from http://dictionary.reference.com/browse/addiction.

Addiction. (n.d.) *Collins English Dictionary—Complete & Unabridged, 10th ed.* Retrieved February 9, 2012, from http://dictionary.reference.com/browse/addiction.

American Heart Association. (2011). *Alcoholic beverages and cardiovascular diseases*. Retrieved April 9, 2012, from http://www.heart.org/HEARTORG/GettingHealthy/NutritionCenter?Alcoholic-Beverages-a-.

American Psychiatric Association (APA). (2006). *Practice guidelines for the treatment of patients with substance use disorders* (2nd ed.). Retrieved November 4, 2006, from www.psychiatryonline.com/content.aspx?aID=141079.

Baldisseri, M. R. (2007). Impaired healthcare professional. *Critical Care Medicine*, 35(2), 106–116.

Bamford, Z., Booth, P. G., McGuire, P. G., et al. (2003). Treatment outcome following day care for alcohol dependency: the effects of reducing program length. *Health and Social Care in the Community*, 11(5), 440–445.

Black, D. W., & Andreasen, N. C. (2011). *Introductory textbook of psychiatry* (5th ed.). Washington, DC: American Psychiatric Publishing.

Brauser, D., & Barclay, L. (2012). *Substance abuse organization releases new definition of recovery*. Retrieved February 9, 2012, from www.Medscape.org/viewarticle/756558_print.

Brauser, D., & Lie, D. (2011). *More evidence secondhand smoke bad for kid's mental health*. Retrieved April 25, 2011, from www.medscape.org/viewarticle/740832?SRC=cmemp.

Brown University Health Education. (2008). *Marijuana*. Retrieved April 2, 2008, from www.brown.edu/student_services/health_services/health-education/atod/marijuana.

Centers for Disease Control and Prevention (CDC). (Updated 2011a). *Smoking and tobacco: fact sheet: smoking cessation*. Retrieved April 21, 2011, from www.CDC.gov/tobacco/data_statistics/fact_sheets/cessation/.

Centers for Disease Control and Prevention (CDC). (Updated 2011b). Smoking and tobacco use: fast facts. Retrieved 4/21/2011 from www.CDC.gov/tobacco/data_statistics/facts_sheets/fast_facts/.

Centers for Disease Control and Prevention (CDC). (Updated 2011c). *Smoking cessation*. Retrieved April 21, 2011, from www.CDC.gov/tobacco/data_sheets/cessation/.

Centers for Disease Control and Prevention (CDC). (2006). *Fetal alcohol spectrum disorders*. Retrieved July 30, 2007, from www.Cdc.gov/ncbddd/fas/fasask.htm.

Martin, T. (2010). *Smoking during pregnancy*. Retrieved May 2, 2011, from http://quitsmoking.about.com/od/tobaccostatistics/a/SGRpregnancy.

Metropolitan Drug Commission (MDC). (2011). *Rave/drugs*. Retrieved April 27, 2011, from www.metrodrug.org/drugs/club drugs.aspx.

Minkoff, K. (2003). Dual diagnoses. In A. Tasman, J. Kay, & J. A. Lieberman (Eds.), *Psychiatry* (2nd ed., vol. 2, pp. 2333–2341). West Sussex, England: Wiley.

Monroe, T., & Kenaga, H. (2011). *Don't ask, don't tell: substance abuse and addiction among nurses*. Retrieved April 22, 2011, from http://onlinelibrary.wiley.com/doi/10.1111/J.1365–February7,2002.2010.035.

National Institute on Drug Abuse (NIDA). (2010a). *NIDA Infofacts: high school and youth trends*. Retrieved April 20, 2011, from www.nida.nih.gov/infofacts/hsyouthtrends.html.

National Institute on Drug Abuse (NIDA). (2010b). *Research report series: comorbidity: addiction and other mental illnesses*. Washington, DC: U.S. Department of Health and Human Services.

National Institute on Drug Abuse (NIDA). (2010c). *Drugs and the brain*. Retrieved April 21, 2011, from www.nida.nih.gov/scienceofaddiction/brain.html.

National Institute on Drug Abuse (NIDA). (2010d). *Drugs, brain, and behavior—the science of addiction*. Retrieved April 21, 2011, from www.nida.nih.gov/scienceofaddiction/brain.html.

National Institute on Drug Abuse (NIDA). (2010e). *Treatment and recovery*. Retrieved April 25, 2011, from www.nida.nih.gov/scienceof addiction/treatment.html.

National Institute on Drug Abuse (NIDA). (2010f). *Addiction and health*. Retrieved April 11, 2011, from http://drugabuse.gov/publications/science-addiction/drugs-brain.

National Institute on Drug Abuse (NIDA). (2010g). *InfoFacts: MDMA (ecstasy)*. Retrieved April 19, 2011, from www.drugabuse.gov.

National Institute on Drug Abuse (NIDA). (2009). *NIDA Infofacts: steroids (anabolic-androgenic)*. Retrieved April 20, 2011, from www.drugabuse.gov/infofacts/steroids.html.

Office of National Drug Control Policy (ONDCP). (2010). *Fact sheet: consequences of illicit drug use in America*. Retrieved April 19, 2011, from www.whitehousedrugpolicy.gov/publications/html1/consdru.

Rivers, K. (2011). *Support needed to help nurses tackle substance abuse*. Retrieved April 27, 2011, from http://news.Vanderbilt.edu/2011/02/help-nurses-tackle-substance.

Slaymaker, V. (2009). *The 12 steps: building the evidence base: the latest research initiative seeks insight into how spirituality affects recovery*. Retrieved April 27, 2011, from http://findarticles.com/p/articles//mi_mOQTQ/is_3_7/ai_n 320998.

SMART Recovery. (2008-2011). Retrieved April 26, 2011, from www.smartrecovery.org/intro/findimpaired nurse.

Solomon, M. (2012). *Drinking late in the first trimester may be the most hazardous*. HealthDay.com. 6 February 2012. Retrieved April 09, 2012 from http://news.yahoo.com/drinking-first-trimester-may-be-most hazardous-140610141.html.

Substance Abuse and Mental Health Services Administration (SAMHSA). (2011). *Results from the 2010 National Survey on Drug Use and Health: summary of national findings*. Retrieved April 09, 2012, from http://www.samhsa.gov.MSDUH/2k10NSDUH/2k1OReasuts.htm.

Upchurch, K. Y. (2011). *SMART way to fight addictions*. Retrieved May 1, 2011, from www.HeraldSun.com/view/full_story/12522072/article-SMA.

U.S. Department of Health and Human Services (USDHHS). (2006). *New Surgeon General's report focuses on the effects of second-hand smoke*. Retrieved June 10, 2007, from www.hhs.gov/news/press/2006pres/20060627.html.

U.S. Department of Health and Human Services. (1999). *Mental health: culture, race and ethnicity. A supplement to mental health: a report of the Surgeon General*. Retrieved February 6, 2004, from www.mentalhealth.org/cre/default.asp.

Verdejo-Garcia, A. (2011). *Novel therapies for cognitive dysfunction secondary to substance abuse*. Retrieved August 17, 2011, from www.psychiatrictimes.com/substance-related-disorders/content/article/10168/187-5588.

Volkow, N. D. (2010). *Message from the Dir. on "bath salts"—emerging and dangerous products*. Retrieved April 20, 2011, from www.nida.nih.gov/about/welcome/MessageBathSalts 211.h.

UNIT 4

Caring for Patients Experiencing Psychiatric Emergencies

Ann Wolbert Burgess, DNS, RNCS, FAAN
Pioneer in Forensic Nursing

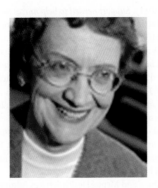

Dr. Ann Burgess is an internationally known pioneer and researcher in the rapidly expanding field of forensic nursing. She is a board-certified clinical specialist in psychiatric mental health nursing and a sexual assault nurse examiner.

She is currently Professor of Psychiatric Mental Health Nursing at Boston College, where she teaches courses in victimology, forensic science, forensic mental health (the study of offenders), case studies in forensics, and forensic science lab.

Dr. Burgess is a prolific writer, having authored 9 nursing textbooks focusing on psychiatric nursing and crisis intervention and 10 books addressing the assessment and treatment of child, adolescent and adult sexual assault victims and serial offenders. She has coauthored more than 150 articles and book chapters, including monographs for the Department of Justice on child sex rings, adolescent rape victim mentality, adolescent runaways, child molesters and abductors, juvenile prostitution, and infant abductions.

Her research with victims of abuse began in 1972 when Dr. Burgess and Lynda Lytle Holmstrom cofounded one of the first hospital-based crisis intervention programs for rape victims at Boston City Hospital. It was through their research that the diagnosis of Rape-Trauma Syndrome (a form of posttraumatic stress disorder) established validity and has been admissible in more than 300 appellate court decisions.

Since that time, her research has expanded to include the abuse of children and pornography; sexual abuse in patterns of crime scenes; children eyewitnesses in child sex abuse trials; ethics and sexual assault; sexual abuse and exploitation of children; and infant kidnapping and more. Her work continues in the study of elder abuse in nursing homes, cyber stalking, and Internet sex crimes among other areas of victimization.

Her most recent articles in 2011 reflected her current investigative interests— *Online Social Networking Patterns Among the Adolescence, Young Adults, and Sexual Offenders; Using Trauma Informed Framework to Care for Incarcerated Women; and Criminalistics and the Forensic Nursing Process.*

In conjunction with the FBI, Dr. Burgess studied serial perpetrators of sexual homicide, rape, and child sexual offenses as well as the possible relationships between child sexual abuse and exploitation, juvenile delinquency, and the eventual expression of criminal behavior. She has often provided testimony as an expert witness, sometimes in high-profile cases.

In the early days of forensic nursing, the focus was on sexual assault and abuse cases. Now forensic nurses may help with crime scene investigations, work with offenders in prison, counsel schoolchildren, conduct death investigations, and at times be summoned to provide courtroom testimony.

Dr. Burgess has been the recipient of numerous awards and appointments, including election to the Institute of Medicine (IOM), a part of the National Academy of Sciences.

CHAPTER

20

Crisis and Mass Disaster

Elizabeth M. Varcarolis

evolve WEBSITE

http://evolve.elsevier.com/Varcarolis/essentials

KEY TERMS AND CONCEPTS

adventitious crisis/crisis of
   disaster, p. 389
crisis intervention, p. 387
critical incident stress debriefing
   (CISD), p. 395
maturational crisis, p. 388
National Incident Management
   System (NIMS), p. 389

phases of crisis, p. 390
primary care, p. 394
secondary care, p. 394
situational crisis, p. 389
terrorism, p. 389
tertiary care, p. 394
triage, p. 390

OBJECTIVES

1. Discuss what is meant by a crisis and identify at least six or more principles of crisis intervention (refer to Box 20-1: Foundation for Crisis Intervention).
2. Discuss what is meant by primary, secondary, and tertiary crisis intervention. Give a clinical example of the kinds of intervention needed for each phase of crisis intervention.
3. What is a triage team, why is it needed, what are its responsibilities during an adventitious crisis/mass disaster?
4. Discuss the importance of teamwork and collaboration when identifying the initial needs of people facing an adventitious crisis/mass disaster.
5. Plan patient-centered care for a person who has experienced an adventitious crisis/mass disaster and identify the potential cognitive and emotional states likely to be present.
6. Identify the mental health safety needs that people may face if they do not obtain support during and/or after a crisis (refer to Chapter 10 for more information to answer this question).
7. When planning intervention for an individual subjected to a crisis event, name the three critical areas you would assess, and give examples of the kinds of questions you would ask to obtain the information necessary for planning effective care.
8. Provide an overview of critical incident stress debriefing (CISD), including its purpose and process.

A child is killed in a drive-by shooting; a husband announces to his wife of 30 years he wants a divorce; tornadoes rip through the Midwest, South, and Southeast, leaving devastation, death, and homelessness in their wake. What do these situations have in common? Each of these situations could be the precipitant of a crisis—an event that leaves individuals, families, or whole communities struggling to cope.

Everyone experiences crises. The experience itself is not pathological but rather represents a struggle for equilibrium and adjustment when problems seem unsolvable. A crisis presents both a danger to personality organization and a potential opportunity for personality growth. The outcome depends on how the individual, family, or community perceives and deals with the crisis and what outside supports are available at the time the crisis occurs.

Crises are acute, time-limited occurrences experienced as overwhelming emotional reactions to any of the following:
- A stressful situational event
- A developmental event
- A societal event
- A cultural event
- The perception of an event

Crisis intervention is what nurses and other health professionals do to assist those in crisis to cope. Interventions need to be broad, creative, and flexible.

PREVALENCE AND COMORBIDITY

Many factors may limit a person's ability to problem solve or cope with stressful life events or situations. Some of these factors include the presence of other stressful life events, mental illness, substance abuse, history of poor coping skills, diminished cognitive abilities, preexisting physical health problems, limited social support network, and developmental or physical challenges.

THEORY

Erich Lindemann, an early crisis theorist, conducted a classic study in the 1940s on the grief reactions of close relatives of victims who died in the Coconut Grove nightclub fire in Boston. This study formed the foundation of crisis theory and clinical intervention. Lindemann was convinced that even though acute grief is a normal reaction to a distressing situation, preventive interventions could eliminate or decrease serious personality disorganization and devastating psychological consequences from the sustained effects of severe anxiety. He believed that the same interventions that were helpful in bereavement would prove just as helpful in dealing with other types of stressful events and proposed a crisis intervention model as a major element of preventive psychiatry in the community.

In the early 1960s, **Gerald Caplan** (1964) further elaborated on crisis theory and outlined crisis intervention strategies. Since that time, our understanding of crisis and effective intervention has continued to be refined and enhanced by numerous contemporary clinicians and theorists (Behrman & Reid, 2002; Roberts, 2000).

In 1961 a report of The Joint Commission on Mental Illness and Mental Health addressed the need for community mental health centers throughout the country. This report stimulated the establishment of crisis services, which are now an important part of mental health programs in hospitals and communities.

Donna Aguilera and **Janice Mesnick** (1970) provided a framework for nurses for crisis assessment and intervention, which has grown in scope and practice. Aguilera (1998) continues to set a standard in the practice of crisis assessment and intervention.

Roberts's seven-stage model of crisis intervention (2005) is a more contemporary model useful in helping individuals who have suffered from an acute situational crisis as well as people who are diagnosed with acute stress disorder (Figure 20-1).

The devastating effects of the September 11 World Trade Center terrorist attack and the distressing lack of response to hurricane Katrina emphasized the need for crisis assessment and intervention by community mental health providers throughout the country to deal with all types of crises and the people who had been traumatized—victims, families, rescue workers, and observers (Everly, 2000; Howard & Goelitz, 2004; Lowry & Lating, 2002). Crisis theory defines specific aspects of crisis basic to crisis intervention (Box 20-1).

The ways of assessing crisis described in the following sections are derived from established crisis theory and constitute a sound knowledge base for the application of the nursing process to treatment of a patient in crisis. An understanding of three areas of crisis theory enables application of the nursing process: (1) types of crisis, (2) phases of crisis, and (3) aspects of crisis that have relevance for nurses.

CLINICAL PICTURE

Types of Crises

There are three basic types of crises: (1) maturational, (2) situational, and (3) adventitious (disasters). It is possible to experience two types of crisis situations simultaneously. For example, a 51-year-old woman may be going through a midlife crisis (maturational) when her husband dies suddenly of cancer (situational). The presence of more than one crisis further taxes the individual's coping skills. People who have preexisting mental health problems are vulnerable and prone to crisis. Psychiatric emergencies are covered in Chapters 21 through 24.

Maturational Crisis

A process of maturation occurs throughout life. Erik Erikson (1902-1994) identified eight stages of growth and development in which specific maturational tasks must be mastered. The path (stages) to adulthood is stressful and at times can be overwhelming. Erikson declared that each of these stages constitutes a crisis in personal growth and development. Each developmental stage can thus be referred to as a maturational crisis.

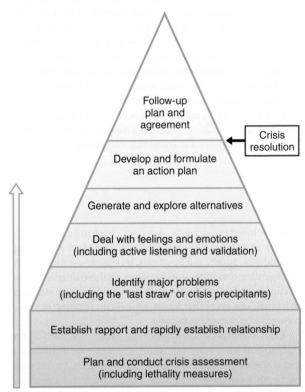

FIGURE 20-1 Roberts' seven-stage model of crisis intervention. (From Roberts, A. R. [Ed.]. [2005]. *Crisis intervention handbook* [3rd ed.]. New York: Oxford University Press.)

BOX 20-1   FOUNDATION FOR CRISIS INTERVENTION

- A crisis is self-limiting and is usually resolved within 4 to 6 weeks.
- The resolution of a crisis results in achievement of one of three different functional levels. The person will emerge at:
  - A *higher* level of functioning
  - The *same* level of functioning
  - A *lower* level of functioning
- The goal of crisis intervention is to return the individual to the precrisis level of functioning.
- The form of resolution of the crisis depends on the actions of the individual and the intervention of others.
- During a crisis people are often more open to outside intervention than they are at times of stable functioning. With intervention a person can learn different adaptive means of problem solving to correct inadequate solutions.

- A person in a crisis situation is assumed to be mentally healthy and to have functioned well in the past but is presently in a state of disequilibrium.
- Crisis intervention deals with the person's present problem and resolution of the immediate crisis only. Addressing material not directly related to the crisis can take place at a later time. Crisis intervention deals with the "here and now."
- A nurse must be willing to take an active, even directive, role in intervention; this is in direct contrast to what occurs in conventional therapeutic intervention, which stresses a more passive and nondirective role for the practitioner.
- Early intervention probably increases the chances for a good prognosis.
- A patient is encouraged to set realistic goals and plan an intervention with the nurse that is focused on the current situation.

When a person arrives at a new stage, formerly used coping styles are no longer appropriate, and new coping mechanisms have yet to be developed. For a time, the person is without effective defenses. This often leads to increased anxiety, which may manifest as variations in the person's normal behavior. Marriage, the birth of a child, and retirement are examples of maturational crises.

Alcohol and drug addiction can interrupt an individual's progression through the maturational stages. This phenomenon is too often seen among teenagers. When the addictive behavior is controlled (by the late teens), the young person's growth and development will resume at the point at which it was interrupted. A young person whose addiction is arrested at 19 years of age may have the social and problem-solving skills of a 14-year-old. Often these teenagers do not receive or accept treatment, and their adult coping skills are diminished or absent.

Successful resolution of these maturational tasks leads to development of basic human qualities. Erikson believed that the way these crises are resolved at one stage affects the ability to pass through subsequent stages because each crisis provides the starting point for moving to the next stage. If a person lacks support systems and adequate role models, successful resolution may be difficult or may not occur. Unresolved problems in the past and inadequate coping mechanisms can adversely affect what is learned in each developmental stage.

When a person is experiencing severe difficulty during a maturational crisis, professional intervention may be indicated.

> **VIGNETTE**
>
> Loretta, 41 years old, gets married for the first time to her high school sweetheart. Although he was previously married with children, the couple planned to have a child early in their marriage. When Loretta finds that she is unable to conceive because of early menopause, she becomes distraught. She is severely anxious, experiences extreme feelings of guilt, is unable to sleep, and consequently no longer is able to function as a manager of a small software company. Her concerned husband takes her to the community health center.

Situational Crisis

A situational crisis arises from an external rather than an internal source. Often the crisis is unanticipated. Examples of external situations that can precipitate a crisis include loss of a job, death of a loved one, unwanted pregnancy, a move, change of job, change in financial status, divorce, and severe physical or mental illness.

Some refer to these events as "critical life problems" because they are encountered by most people during the course of their lives. Whether these events precipitate a crisis depends on such factors as the degree of support available from caring friends and family members, a person's general emotional and physical

> **VIGNETTE**
>
> Don, 56 years old, has held a middle management position in his company for 25 years. When his company downsized and many of the middle managers were forced to retire, Don was devastated. He has been looking for another job for 9 months, but so far has no prospects. His family's health care is about to expire. His perception of himself as a competent family provider is shattered and his self-esteem has plummeted. He has been drinking heavily, staying up late, and sleeping late into the morning. He has closed himself off from family and friends.

status, social supports available in the community, and a person's ability to understand and cope with the meaning of the stressful event.

As in all crises or potential crisis situations, the stressful event involves a loss or change that threatens a person's self-concept and self-esteem. To varying degrees, successful resolution of a crisis depends on resolution of the grief associated with the loss.

Adventitious Crisis

An adventitious crisis, or crisis of disaster, is not a part of everyday life; it is unplanned and accidental. Adventitious crises may result from (1) a natural disaster (e.g., floods, fires, tornadoes, earthquakes), (2) a national disaster (e.g., war, riots, airplane crashes), or (3) a crime of violence (e.g., rape, assault, murder in the workplace or school, bombings, or spousal or child abuse). Every disaster is a unique challenge.

A distinction needs to be made between adventitious crisis and terrorism. Terrorism differs from a national disaster and other mass casualties in that a terrorist attack is meant to harm/maim/kill innocent civilians. In war zones, however, there are expectations that others are trying to intentionally inflict suffering and death. A terrorist attack occurs suddenly and "there is no warning or expectation, and there are no rules or guidelines for how to prepare and how to react" (Portelli et al., 2011). Even so, terrorism causes mass casualties.

Regardless of the cause (e.g., national, natural, terrorism), disasters result in mass casualties that affect a large number of victims who need the response of multiple organizations (Norman & Weiner, 2011). **Mass casualty incidents** (MCIs) result in excessive morbidity and mortality along with extensive damage to property, roadways, and electrical lines, limiting a region's ability to respond. These disasters can leave local governmental operations, medical systems, and local first responders overwhelmed and exhausted.

Recent mass casualty incidents (MCIs) include acts of terrorism (e.g., 9/11 Twin Towers); hurricanes (e.g., Katrina); earthquakes, some causing tsunamis (e.g., American Samoa, Indonesia, Japan); floods; and devastating tornadoes (e.g., Midwest, South and Southeast). School shootings (e.g., Virginia Tech; Columbine; DeKalb, Illinois) and other mindless shootings (such as the one in Tucson, Arizona in 2011) continue to make the headlines, leaving families, communities, and our youth changed forever. Eventually the media frenzy abates and people are left to try to put their lives together, rebuild homes and communities, mourn their dead, and recover from the long-term effects of trauma.

Statistics show that natural disasters have risen remarkably since 1990 with the biggest jump from 2000 to 2009, during which the world has witnessed some of the most devastating and destructive natural disasters in recorded history (Fraser, 2010). Presently, there is no reason to believe this trend will end.

Disaster Response

The National Incident Management System (NIMS) has been established to "provide a systematic approach to guide departments and agencies at all levels of government, nongovernmental organizations, and the private sector to work seamlessly" during disaster situations (NIMS, 2008). There is still a need for better planning in vulnerable areas and clearer lines of communication among community, state, and federal disaster agencies in order to be effective in mitigating morbidity and mortality.

Efficient response to disaster requires a triage team and an ability to distribute casualties to the most appropriate facility or holding ground for proper care. The underlying principle of triage is to separate those who need rapid medical care from those with more minor injuries, thus reducing the urgent burden on medical facilities and organizations and making the most efficient use of available resources. Triage helps responders do the greatest good for the greatest number of casualties.

The first needs during a disaster often are rescue efforts, evacuation plans and execution, food and shelter, medical attention, and physical safety. Since 2000 the Department of Homeland Security oversees a variety of agencies that focus on the safety and security of people in disasters in the United States. Providing medical disaster relief is under the jurisdiction of the National Disaster Medical System (NDMS). There are, however, nongovernmental agencies as well that take volunteer nurses and physicians to various parts of the United States and the world to help disaster victims, including the International Medical Corps (IMC). This group sends medical personnel to places such as Indonesia, for example, during the catastrophic tsunami disaster.

After immediate needs are met, people need help in reconstructing and normalizing their lives. People need housing, food, jobs, and availability of posttrauma counseling.

Common phenomena experienced following a disaster are *cognitive* (e.g., memory impairment, difficulty making decisions or problem solving, recurring or intrusive images), *behavioral* (e.g., withdrawal, relapse in chemically dependent people, under- or overeating, under- or oversleeping), or *emotional* (e.g., flood of emotions such as anxiety, fear, anger, numbness, helplessness). Common sequelae of a crisis, particularly a disaster, are posttraumatic stress disorder and depression. **The need for psychological first aid (crisis intervention) and debriefing after any crisis situation for all age-groups (children,** adolescents, adults, and older adults) **cannot be overstressed.** If concerns are not addressed or treated, individuals are vulnerable to stress-related disorders. *Critical incident stress debriefing* is discussed later in this chapter.

Disaster nursing, stemming from critical care nursing, is a new frontier, and from the preceding information one can see the great need for nurses in this area. Check out www.RedCross.org for volunteer opportunities and training programs for nurses.

Self-Care for Nurses

Nurses work with people in crisis all of the time—in the emergency department (ED); on medical, surgical, psychiatric, obstetric, and pediatric units; or with family and friends—and deal with crises in their own lives. Nurses need to constantly monitor personal feelings and thoughts when dealing with people in crisis and be aware when they need self-help. Self-monitoring and self-care should be integral to crisis intervention. This is especially true when confronted with mass casualties and natural disasters. Nurses may respond with anxiety to a patient's situation or anxiety level and try to repress such feelings to maintain personal comfort.

When nurses are unaware of personal feelings and reactions, they may unconsciously prevent the expression of the painful feelings in the patient that are precipitating the nurse's own discomfort. Thus, closing off feelings in the patient can render the nurse ineffective. There may be times when the nurse, perhaps for personal reasons, feels he or she cannot deal effectively with a patient's situation. The nurse might ask a colleague to work with a particular patient. This will give the nurse a chance to work through some uncomfortable or painful personal issues.

It is crucial in beginning crisis intervention that supervision and guidance are available as a fundamental part of the training process. The supervisor should be an experienced professional, such as a nurse counselor, nursing supervisor, or other health care expert. Nurses new to crisis intervention often face common problems that must be addressed before they become comfortable and competent in the role of crisis counselor. For example, nurses set unrealistic goals and become frustrated or have difficulty dealing with some issues, such as suicide. A number of schools of nursing now offer master's degrees in disaster nursing.

Even seasoned nurses and other health care workers working in disaster situations can become overwhelmed by witnessing catastrophic loss of human life (as in acts of terrorism, plane crashes, or school shootings) or mass destruction of people's homes and belongings (as in floods, fires, or tornadoes) that leave many families bereft of a sense of stability, well-being, and shelter. Disaster nurses need supportive ties and access to debriefing. Debriefing is an important step for staff in coming to terms with overwhelming violent or otherwise disastrous situations once they are over. It helps staff place the crisis in perspective and begin healing themselves. Debriefing is discussed in more detail later in the chapter.

Phases of Crisis

Caplan (1964) identified the following four distinct **phases of crisis:**

- *Phase 1:* A person confronted by a conflict or problem that threatens the self-concept responds with increased feelings of anxiety. The increase in anxiety stimulates the use of problem-solving techniques and defense mechanisms in an effort to solve the problem and lower anxiety.
- *Phase 2:* If the usual defensive response fails, and if the threat persists, anxiety continues to rise and produce feelings of extreme discomfort. Individual functioning becomes disorganized. Trial-and-error attempts at solving the problem and restoring a normal balance begin.
- *Phase 3:* If the trial-and-error attempts fail, anxiety can escalate to severe and panic levels, and the person mobilizes automatic relief behaviors, such as withdrawal and flight. Some form of resolution (e.g., compromising needs or redefining the situation to reach an acceptable solution) may be made in this stage.
- *Phase 4:* If the problem is not solved and new coping skills are ineffective, anxiety can overwhelm the person and lead to serious personality disorganization, depression, confusion, violence against others, or suicidal behavior (Greenstone & Leviton, 2002; Jordan, 2003; Lowry & Lating, 2002).

█ APPLICATION OF THE NURSING PROCESS

ASSESSMENT

A person's equilibrium may be adversely affected by one or more of the following: (1) an unrealistic perception of the precipitating event, (2) inadequate situational supports, and (3) inadequate coping mechanisms (Aguilera, 1998). It is crucial to assess these factors when a crisis situation is evaluated because data gained from the assessment are used as guides for both the nurse and the patient in setting realistic and meaningful goals as well as in planning possible solutions to the problem situation.

After determining whether there is a need for external controls because of suicidal or homicidal ideation or gestures, the nurse assesses three main areas: (1) the patient's perception of the precipitating event, (2) the patient's situational supports, and (3) the patient's personal coping skills.

Assessing the Patient's Perception of the Precipitating Event

Whether an event is a crisis is based on the perspective and strengths of the patient. Whereas having a physician's appointment canceled would seem to be a trivial annoyance to most people, for someone who is vulnerable from severe schizophrenia the change could instigate a crisis and lead to disorganization. Therefore it is important to view the event through the eyes of the patient. The nurse's initial task is to assess the individual's or family's perception of the problem. The more clearly the problem can be defined, the better the chance that an effective solution will be found. Sample questions that may facilitate the assessment include the following:

- Has anything particularly upsetting happened to you within the past few days or weeks?

- What was happening in your life before you started to feel this way?
- What leads you to seek help now?
- Describe how you are feeling right now.
- How does this situation affect your life?
- How do you see this event as affecting your future?
- What would need to be done to resolve this situation?

VIGNETTE

Laura, a 15-year-old girl, is brought to the emergency department (ED) after slashing her wrists. She was found by her mother, who returned home early from a date. Her mother called the police, and they rushed Laura to the hospital. After Laura is seen by the medical personnel, she is taken to the psychiatric nurse working in the ED. The nurse speaks calmly, introduces herself, and tells Laura she would like to spend some time with her. The nurse states, "It looks as if things are pretty overwhelming. Is that how you are feeling?" The nurse makes the observation that things must be very bad if Laura wants to kill herself. Laura sits slumped in a chair, her head hanging down, with tears in her eyes.

Assessing Laura's Perception of the Precipitating Event

Nurse: "Laura, tell me what has happened."

Laura: "I can't...I can't go home. No one cares. No one believes me. I can't go through it again."

Nurse: "Tell me what you can't go through again, Laura."

Laura starts to cry, shaking with sobs. The nurse sits quietly for a while, offers her some tissues, and then speaks.

Nurse: "Tell me what is so terrible. Let's look at it together."

After a while, Laura starts telling the nurse that when she was 9 years old, her mother had a boyfriend. When the mother would go to work, the boyfriend would touch her and eventually forced her to have sex, threatening to kill her if she told anyone. When she was 11, the boyfriend moved out. Two weeks ago Laura's mother told her that the old boyfriend was coming back to live with them. When Laura told her mother what had happened years ago, her mother called her a liar and said if it was a choice between Laura and the boyfriend, she would choose the boyfriend.

Assessing the Patient's Situational Supports

The patient's support systems are assessed to determine the resources available. Does the stressful event involve important people in the support system? Is the patient isolated from others, or are there family and friends who can provide the vital support? Family and friends may be asked to aid the individual by offering material or emotional support (e.g., lending money, offering services, being available to give affection and understanding). If these resources are not available, the nurse or counselor acts as a temporary support system while relationships with individuals or groups in the community are established. The following are some sample questions to ask:

- With whom do you live?
- To whom do you talk when you feel overwhelmed?
- Who can you trust?
- Who is available to help you?
- Where do you go to worship (or talk to God)? Where do you go to school or to other community-based activities?
- During difficult times in the past, who did you want most to help you?
- Who is the most helpful?

VIGNETTE
Assessing Laura's Situational Supports

Nurse: "Laura, who can you go to? Do you have any other family?"

Laura: "No, my dad left when I was little, and we are pretty much alone. My mom never allowed me to play with other kids."

Nurse: "Do you have anyone you can talk to?"

Laura: "No, I really don't have any friends. The other kids think I am stuck up. My mom always had something for me to do in the house."

Nurse: "What about teachers or a minister or rabbi?"

Laura: "My teachers are nice, but I can't tell them things like this. Besides, they wouldn't believe me either."

Assessing the Patient's Personal Coping Skills

In crisis situations it is important to evaluate the person's level of anxiety. Common coping mechanisms may be overeating, drinking, smoking, withdrawing, seeking out someone to talk to, yelling, fighting, or engaging in other physical activity (Behrman & Reid, 2002). The potential for suicide or homicide must be assessed. If the patient is suicidal, homicidal, or unable to take care of personal needs, hospitalization should be considered (Aguilera, 1998). Some sample questions to ask include the following:

- Have you thought of killing yourself or someone else? If yes, have you thought of how you would do this?
- What do you usually do to feel better?
- Did you try it this time? If so, what was different?
- What helped you through difficult times in the past?
- What do you think might happen now?

VIGNETTE

The nurse learns that Laura does very well in school. Laura explains that when she studies, she can forget her problems and get lost in other worlds. Getting good grades also has another reward: it is the only time her mother says anything nice about her.

Assessing Laura's Personal Coping Skills

Nurse: "What do you think would help your situation?"

Laura: "I don't want to die. I just don't know where to turn."

The nurse tells Laura that she wants to work with her to find a solution, and that she is concerned for Laura's safety and well-being.

ASSESSMENT GUIDELINES
Crisis

1. Identify whether the patient's response to the crisis warrants psychiatric treatment or hospitalization to minimize decompensation (suicidal behavior, psychotic thinking, and violent behavior).
2. Determine if the patient is able to identify the *precipitating event*.
3. Assess the patient's understanding of his or her present *situational supports*.
4. Identify the patient's usual *coping skills* and determine what coping mechanisms may help the present situation.
5. Determine whether there are certain religious or cultural beliefs that need to be considered in assessing and intervening in this person's crisis.
6. Assess whether this situation is one in which the patient needs primary intervention (education, environmental manipulation, or new coping skills), secondary intervention (crisis intervention), or tertiary intervention (rehabilitation).

DIAGNOSIS

A person in crisis may exhibit various behaviors that indicate a number of problems. See Table 20-1 for some signs and symptoms of people in crisis that may be used as a guide for identifying potential nursing diagnoses.

For the example in the preceding vignette, the assessment of Laura's (1) perception of the precipitating event, (2) situational supports, and (3) personal coping skills provides the nurse enough data to formulate two diagnoses and to work with Laura in setting goals and planning interventions.

VIGNETTE
Nursing Diagnoses for Laura

The nurse formulates the following nursing diagnoses for Laura:

- *Anxiety (moderate/severe)* related to fear of renewed sexual abuse and lack of protection as evidenced by ineffectual problem solving and feelings of impending doom
- *Compromised Family Coping* related to inadequate understanding by her mother's inability to listen to daughter's fears

---

OUTCOMES IDENTIFICATION

The planning of realistic patient outcomes is done in conjunction with the patient or family. Realistic outcomes are made to fit within the person's cultural and personal values. The nurse will document the outcomes as measurable goals that are

TABLE 20-1	**POTENTIAL NURSING DIAGNOSES FOR CRISIS INTERVENTION**
SIGNS AND SYMPTOMS	**NURSING DIAGNOSES***
Overwhelmed, depressed, states that has nothing in life worthwhile, self-hate and feelings of being ineffectual are assessed	*Risk for Self-Directed Violence* *Chronic Low Self-Esteem* *Spiritual Distress* *Hopelessness* *Powerlessness*
Confused, highly anxious, incoherent, crying or sobbing, shows extreme emotional pain	*Anxiety (moderate, severe, panic)* *Acute Confusion* *Sleep Deprivation*
Has difficulty with interpersonal relationships, isolated, has few or no social supports	*Social Isolation* *Risk for Loneliness* *Impaired Social Interaction*
Unable to function at work, school, or home at previous level; has difficulty concentrating or completing simple tasks	*Ineffective Coping* *Interrupted Family Processes* *Caregiver Role Strain*
Has experienced traumatic, emotionally overwhelming event or loss; unable to work through over-whelming loss or event	*Risk for Post-Trauma Syndrome* *Rape-Trauma Syndrome* *Dysfunctional Grieving* *Chronic Sorrow*

*Nursing Diagnoses—Definitions and Classification 2012-2014. Copyright © 2012, 1994-2012 by NANDA International. Used by arrangement with Blackwell Publishing Limited, a company of John Wiley and Sons, Inc.

realistic and include a time estimate (ANA, 2007). Without the patient's involvement, the outcome criteria (goals at the end of 4 to 8 weeks) may be irrelevant or unacceptable solutions to that person's crisis.

For example, a nurse new to crisis intervention who suggests that a woman leave her husband because he beats her may be surprised to find that the woman has different thoughts on what she wants as a solution. Thus outcomes are always established with the patient, and they have to be congruent with the patient's needs, values, and (in some instances) cultural expectations. The nurse evaluates the outcome for safety as well as other factors and works on contingency plans when necessary.

VIGNETTE

A social worker is called. Laura, the nurse, and the social worker meet together. All agree that Laura should not return to her mother's home if the boyfriend returns. The nurse then meets with Laura and her mother; however, her mother continues to berate Laura for lying. She says she does not care what Laura says. She has her own life to live, and if Laura does not like it she can move out.

The nurse and Laura set four goals together:
1. Laura will return to her precrisis state within 2 to 6 weeks.
2. Laura and staff will find a safe environment for her before the boyfriend moves back.
3. Laura, with the support of staff, will have at least two outside supports available within 24 hours.
4. Laura will receive continued evaluation and support until the immediate crisis is over (6 to 8 weeks).

PLANNING

Nurses are called on to plan and intervene through a variety of crisis intervention modalities, such as disaster nursing, mobile crisis units, group work, health education and crisis prevention, victim outreach programs, and telephone hotlines.

The nurse may be involved in planning and intervention for an individual (e.g., cases of physical abuse), for a group (e.g., students after a classmate's suicide event or shooting), or for a community (e.g., disaster nursing after tornadoes, shootings, and airplane crashes).

The following questions are answered (Aguilera, 1998):
- How much has this crisis affected the person's life? Can the patient still go to work? Attend school? Care for family members?
- How is the state of disequilibrium affecting significant people in the patient's life (e.g., wife, husband, children, other family members, boss, boyfriend, and girlfriend)?

Data from the answers to these two questions will guide the nurse in determining the immediate action that should be taken.

IMPLEMENTATION

Crisis intervention is considered to be a function of the basic level nurse and has two basic initial goals:
1. **Patient safety.** External controls may be applied for protection of the person in crisis if the person is suicidal or homicidal.
2. **Anxiety reduction.** Anxiety reduction techniques are used so that inner resources can be mobilized.

During the initial interview, the person in crisis first needs to gain a feeling of safety. Solutions to the crisis may be offered so that the patient is aware of other options. Feelings of support and hope will temporarily diminish anxiety. The nurse needs to play an active role by indicating that help is available. The availability of help is conveyed by the competent use of crisis intervention skills and genuine interest and support. It is not conveyed by the use of false reassurances and platitudes, such as "Everything will be all right." Crisis intervention requires a creative and flexible approach through the use of traditional and nontraditional therapeutic methods. The nurse may act as educator, adviser, and model, always keeping in mind that it is the patient who solves the problem, not the nurse. The following are important assumptions when working with a patient in crisis:
- The person is in charge of his or her own life.
- The person is able to make decisions.
- The crisis counseling relationship is one between partners.

The nurse helps the patient refocus to gain new perspectives on the situation. The nurse supports the patient during the process of finding constructive ways to solve or cope with the problem. It is important for the nurse to be mindful of how difficult it is for the patient to change his or her behavior. See Table 20-2 for crisis interventions and corresponding rationales.

> **VIGNETTE**
> After talking with the nurse and the social worker, Laura seems open to going to a foster home. She also agrees to talk to a counselor at her school. The nurse sets up an appointment at which she, Laura, and the school counselor will meet. The nurse will continue to see Laura twice a week.

Levels of Nursing Care

There are three levels of nursing care in crisis intervention. These three levels are (1) primary, (2) secondary, and (3) tertiary. Psychotherapeutic nursing interventions in crisis are directed toward these three levels of care.

Primary

Primary care promotes mental health and reduces mental illness to decrease the incidence of crisis. On this level, the nurse can:

- Work with an individual to recognize potential problems by evaluating the stressful life events the person is experiencing.
- Teach individual specific coping skills, such as decision making, problem solving, assertiveness skills, meditation, and relaxation skills, to handle stressful events.
- Assist an individual in evaluating the timing or reduction of life changes to decrease the negative effects of stress as much as possible. This may involve working with a patient to plan environmental changes, make important interpersonal decisions, and rethink changes in occupational roles.

Secondary

Secondary care establishes intervention during an acute crisis to *prevent* prolonged anxiety from diminishing personal effectiveness and personality organization. The nurse's primary focus is to ensure the safety of the patient. After safety issues are addressed, the nurse works with the patient to assess the patient's problem, support systems, and coping styles. Desired goals are explored and interventions planned. Secondary care lessens the time a person is mentally disabled during a crisis. Secondary-level care occurs in hospital units, emergency departments, clinics, or mental health centers, usually during daytime hours.

TABLE 20-2 INTERVENTIONS FOR PATIENTS IN CRISIS

INTERVENTION	RATIONALE
1. Assess for any suicidal or homicidal thoughts or plans.	1. Safety is always the first consideration.
2. Take initial steps to make patient feel safe and to lower anxiety.	2. When a person feels safe and anxiety decreases, the individual is able to problem solve solutions with the nurse.
3. Listen carefully (e.g., make eye contact, give frequent feedback to make sure you understand, summarize what patient says at the end).	3. When a person believes that someone is really listening, this can translate into the belief that someone cares about the person's situation and that help may be available. This offers hope.
4. Crisis intervention calls for directive and creative approaches. Initially the nurse may make phone calls (arrange babysitters, schedule a visiting nurse, find shelter, contact a social worker).	4. Initially a person may be so confused and frightened that performing usual tasks is not possible at that moment.
5. Assess patient's support systems. Rally existing supports (with patient's permission) if patient is overwhelmed.	5. People are often overwhelmed and nurses need to take an active role.
6. Identify needed social supports (with patient's input) and mobilize the most needed first.	6. Patient's needs for shelter help with care for children or elders, medical workup, emergency medical attention, hospitalization, food, safe housing, and a self-help group are determined.
7. Identify needed coping skills (problem solving, relaxation, assertiveness, job training, newborn care, improving self-esteem).	7. Increasing coping skills and learning new ones can help with current crisis and assist with minimizing future crises.
8. Plan with patient interventions acceptable to both counselor and patient.	8. Patient's sense of control, self-esteem, and compliance with plan are increased.
9. Plan regular follow-up to assess patient's progress (e.g., phone calls, clinic visits, home visits as appropriate).	9. Plan is evaluated to see what works and what does not work.

Tertiary

Tertiary care provides support for those who have experienced a severe crisis and are now recovering from a disabling mental state. Social and community facilities that offer tertiary intervention include rehabilitation centers, sheltered workshops, day hospitals, and outpatient clinics. Primary goals are to *facilitate optimal levels of functioning and prevent further emotional disruptions.* People with severe and persistent mental problems are often extremely susceptible to crisis, and community facilities provide the structured environment that can help prevent problem situations. See Chapter 27 for an extensive discussion on community supports for people with severe and persistent mental problems.

Critical incident stress debriefing. Critical incident stress debriefing (CISD) is an example of a tertiary intervention directed toward a group that has experienced a crisis (Everly et al., 2000). CISD consists of a seven-phase group meeting that offers individuals the opportunity to share their thoughts and feelings in a safe and controlled environment. CISD is used to debrief staff on an inpatient unit following the suicide of a patient (see Chapter 23); to debrief staff following incidents of patient violence; to debrief crisis hotline volunteers; to debrief schoolchildren and school personnel after shootings have occurred in a school; and to debrief rescue and health care workers who have responded to a natural disaster or a terrorist attack such as that on the World Trade Center (Hammond & Brooks, 2001).

The phases of CISD are the following:
1. *Introductory phase*—The purpose of the meeting is explained; an overview of the debriefing process is provided; participants are motivated; confidentiality is assured; guidelines are explained; team members are identified; and questions are answered.
2. *Fact phase*—Participants are assisted in discussing the facts of the incident; participants are asked to introduce themselves and tell how they were involved in the incident and what happened from their perspective.
3. *Thought phase*—All participants are asked to discuss their first thoughts of the incident.
4. *Reaction phase*—Participants engage in freewheeling discussion and talk about the worst thing about the incident—what they would like to forget and what was most painful.
5. *Symptom phase*—Participants describe cognitive, physical, emotional, or behavioral experiences that they had at the scene of the incident and explain any symptoms they felt following the initial experience.
6. *Teaching phase*—The normality of the symptoms that have been expressed is acknowledged and affirmed; anticipatory guidance is offered regarding future symptoms that may be experienced by participants; the group is involved in stress management techniques.
7. *Reentry phase*—Participants review old material discussed, introduce new topics they want to discuss, ask questions, and discuss how they would like to bring closure to the debriefing. Debriefing team members answer questions, inform, and reassure; provide handouts and other written material; provide information on referral sources for additional help; and summarize the debriefing experience with encouragement, support, and appreciation.

VIGNETTE

The nurse performs secondary crisis intervention and meets with Laura twice weekly during the next 4 weeks. Laura is motivated to work with the social worker and the nurse to find another place to live. The nurse suggests several times that Laura starts to see a counselor in the outpatient clinic after the crisis is over so that she can talk about some of her pain. Laura is not interested, and says she will talk to the school counselor if she needs to talk. Three weeks after the attempted suicide, foster placement is found for Laura. The couple seems interested in Laura, and Laura appears happy about the attention she is receiving.

EVALUATION

The evaluation for a person in crisis is usually performed 4 to 8 weeks after the initial interview, although it can be done earlier (e.g., by the end of the visit the anxiety level will decrease from severe to moderate). If the intervention has been successful, the person's level of anxiety and ability to function should be at precrisis levels. Appropriate questions to ask during evaluation are as follows:
- Is the patient safe?
- Has the patient developed more adaptive ways to cope with stress and anxiety?
- Does the patient have a stronger existing support system?
- Has the patient maintained an optimum level of functioning?
- Has the patient returned to the precrisis level of functioning?

Often a person chooses to seek advice on additional areas of concern and is referred to other agencies for more long-term work. Crisis intervention often serves to prepare a person for further treatment.

VIGNETTE

After 6 weeks Laura and the nurse decide that the crisis is over. Laura remains aloof and distant. The nurse evaluates Laura as being in a moderate amount of emotional pain, but Laura feels she is doing well and is beginning to feel more secure and accepted. The nurse's assessment indicates that Laura has other serious issues (e.g., the issue of her earlier sexual assaults), and the nurse strongly suggests that she could benefit from further counseling. The decision, however, is up to Laura, who says she is satisfied with the way things are and again states that if she has any problems she will talk to her school counselor.

APPLYING THE ART

A Person Needing Crisis Intervention

SCENARIO: I met 38-year-old Richard when he brought his son Lamar to the community health free clinic for his allergy shot. Richard asked if I had time to talk during Lamar's postinjection waiting period. Lamar played with other children while Richard described his gratitude that his son was able to get allergy injections despite Richard's lack of health insurance. Richard then recounted his mixed feelings about his wife being 2 months' pregnant. He saw no way to care for his expanding family on his minimum wage income.

THERAPEUTIC GOAL: By the end of this interaction, Richard will acknowledge controlled breathing as one method of limiting a panic attack and make the decision to enter psychotherapy.

STUDENT-PATIENT INTERACTION	THOUGHTS, COMMUNICATION TECHNIQUES, AND MENTAL HEALTH NURSING CONCEPTS
Richard: *After several silent moments.* "You're a nursing student right? May I ask you a question?"	
Student: "Go on." *Nodding.*	I wonder where this is going and if I will know the answer to his question. I give a *general lead* encouraging Richard to continue.
Student's feelings: *When I get anxious, I must remind myself that I don't have to know everything. My instructor is nearby.*	
Richard: "How long can a person's heart pound really hard and fast before it gives out?" *At my immediately alert expression, Richard added,* "It's not happening now."	Belatedly, I use my assessment skills. Richard is not hyperventilating; his breaths are even and slow. His face is not flushed. He does not talk or look like he is experiencing pain or vertigo.
Student's feelings: *I have to become more aware of what I show nonverbally. Hopefully, I just looked alert and not panicked.*	
Student: "You are trying to understand some symptoms you've been having?" *He nods.* "Tell me more."	I *clarify* then ask an *indirect question.* I wonder if he has ever had a full cardiac workup. Probably not, because he does not have health insurance.
Student's feelings: *Our distribution of health care dollars falls short for the Richards of the world. I feel sadness then anger. I worry about all my debt from school, but in comparison, the pressure Richard must feel seems overwhelming.*	
Richard: "A few weeks ago, out of the blue my heart starts pounding for at least 15 minutes. It always feels like my heart will pound right out of my chest!"	Richard sounds like he may be in a crisis. I will need to assess the crisis balancing factors: his perception of the events, his coping mechanisms, and situational supports.
Student: "That would be so frightening. You said 'it always feels,' so these 'heart pounding' times continue?"	I use *restatement* and ask a *direct question.* I know that physiologically such palpitations alone from a healthy heart muscle are not life threatening.
Student's feelings: *I would worry too if my heart started pounding for no reason I could figure out.*	
Richard: "Yes, my chest pounds and I start breathing fast. It feels like any minute now, I'm going to die."	If there is nothing physically wrong with Richard's heart, and his symptoms are from anxiety, then the biochemical changes from moderate to severe levels of anxiety should abate in a few minutes. However, if Richard refuels the flight-or-fight response with catastrophic thinking like, 'I'll die!" his anxiety can grow into a full-fledged panic attack.
Student's feelings: *I feel empathy for Richard. The wife's pregnancy likely set Richard up for crisis but something within the last 24 to 48 hours acted as a precipitating event. In other words, I wonder what made today the day that Richard recognized he needed help? What in the last 48 hours makes this overwhelming?*	
Student: "How do you get yourself through all of this?"	I ask an *open question.* I also imply that Richard has been able to *cope* (the second balancing factor), despite his fears.

APPLYING THE ART—cont'd

A Person Needing Crisis Intervention

STUDENT-PATIENT INTERACTION	THOUGHTS, COMMUNICATION TECHNIQUES, AND MENTAL HEALTH NURSING CONCEPTS
Richard: "The first few times I rushed to the ER, but after the second or third time they checked out my heart; they said there was nothing wrong with my heart. That made me feel stupid. The doctor said I was panicking. Like I'm a nut case." *Shakes his head.* "Maybe I am."	Richard uses *projection* when he says the ER staff made him feel stupid. Maybe he wonders that about himself. Richard re-encounters *autonomy vs. shame and doubt* with the palpitations beyond his control; he feels shame when he says words like "stupid" and "nut case."
Student's feelings: *Satisfied that there is no physical heart problem, I feel frustrated that there is such a stigma about mental illness, unlike physical illnesses.*	
Student: "Sounds like you're upset at how you were treated but maybe you're also worried something is really wrong with your heart or your head or both."	I again *attempt to translate into feelings,* which communicates empathy.
Student's feelings: *Maybe I went too far with that "really wrong" part. Sometimes it's hard to know when to allow the patient space or when to try for insight.*	
Richard: *Impatiently brushing away tears.* "What if this panic thing hits me at work? What happens to my family?"	He was able to let himself know how overwhelmed he feels, even though he quickly gets rid of the tears. In crisis intervention work, *perception* of oneself rests at the core of the patient's *perception* of the *crisis event.*
Student's feelings: *I admire how Richard cares so much for his family. I feel that way about my family, too. Sometimes, I feel guilty about all the time and money it takes for me to get through nursing school. Sometimes the demands of school take so much away from my family. I need to mindfully breathe. Right now my focus needs to be on Richard.*	
Student: "Right now you feel as though facing the problem means you will not be able to work." *He nods.* "I wonder if it's possible that knowing more about panic disorder could, on the other hand, bring a way to regain some control in your life."	I *validate* then ask an *indirect question.* I remember that the fear of having a panic attack out in public or for Richard, at work, adds to the sense of loss of control and can even contribute to agoraphobia.
Richard: *Takes a deep breath, and then begins hyperventilating with a scared look on his face.*	Richard is starting to have a panic attack!
Student's feelings: *I am breathing faster too, feeling anxious.*	
Student: "Calm down! Please calm down." *Richard starts breathing even faster.*	I gave premature advice. In essence I said, "You calm down," like a parent would say. If Richard were able to, he would have already found a way to *cope* with my nontherapeutic advice. I know that anxiety is communicated interpersonally. I need to think this through.
Student's feelings: *What's wrong with me! When someone tells me to calm down it usually makes me angry instead. It's like one more pressure on me when I'm already having trouble. I need to offer myself to work with Richard first. I need to be in charge of my actions and reactions. I will stay calm and use my listening skills to talk Richard through this. Where, oh where is my teacher?*	
Student: "Richard, could you breathe with me?" *He makes fleeting eye contact.* "Now slowly exhale all the air as I count." *I slow my pace.* "One…two… three…four…. Now breathe in slowly…one… two…three…. Again fully and slowly exhale: one… two…three…and four. Now slowly inhale counting one…two…three…. Again, exhale, always one count longer. You have the rhythm now. Keep breathing and counting as I lightly put my fingers on your pulse."	From studying about panic disorder I learned the benefits of *controlled breathing* during an attack. Counting distracts the patient from automatic catastrophic thoughts while exhaling for one count longer than the inhale combats the tendency to hyperventilate. *Asking* Richard to breathe with me and *role modeling* how to do so works a lot better than commanding him to "calm down." By breathing together, I *offer self.*
Student's feelings: *Richard seems to be responding. I'm relieved. I will have a lot to talk about in postconference.*	

Continued

APPLYING THE ART—cont'd

A Person Needing Crisis Intervention

STUDENT-PATIENT INTERACTION	THOUGHTS, COMMUNICATION TECHNIQUES, AND MENTAL HEALTH NURSING CONCEPTS
Richard: *After 4 minutes of breathing and counting,* "I can't believe it. I'm getting to be okay."	Richard's pulse rate gradually changes from 180 down to 85. I watch and breathe with him, only counting aloud as needed to remind him to breathe slowly.
Student's feelings: *I'm amazed that what I did actually helped Richard. It's really true that mental health nursing comes in handy anywhere and everywhere.*	
Student: "You were able to breathe and count and thus take some control over the panic episode."	I give *support* by saying "you were able to…"
Richard: "I don't understand. Why did that work?"	
Student: "The rapid breathing and scary thoughts that worsen the heart palpitations cannot happen when you exhale completely and keep on slowly counting each breath."	I *teach* about how mindfully controlling the breathing inhibits hyperventilation and distracts Richard away from automatic dysfunctional thoughts like, "I'm going to die."
Richard: *Sighs.* "I still don't get why this panic thing is happening, but at least now I feel some hope."	An advanced practice nurse psychotherapist could help Richard learn more about the physiology of panic as well as ways to manage stress. He could also most likely keep a record of his *dysfunctional thoughts* and learn how to do *health self-talk* instead.
Student's feelings: *Richard feels hope and that combats powerlessness. I feel hopeful for him. It almost always helps me to talk someone I trust about painful things in my own life. Finding someone to talk to would help Richard with the third balancing factor: situational support.*	
Student: "I'm guessing the panic episodes might be your body's way of letting you know you might need to take some time for you." *Nodding, Richard sighs.* "Would you be ready to talk with someone who could help?"	I do some *teaching* as I suggest a *plan of action.* With help, Richard may look deeper at the onset of his panic symptoms. They started right around the time of learning that he was going to be a father again.
Richard: *Nods.* "If I could get good at that breathing thing, I could manage the panic even if it happens at work."	Something at work in the last 48 hours may have been the trigger for Richard to ask for my help today.
Student's feelings: *I really hope Richard will find therapy that he can afford. I care about what happens to him.*	
Student: *My instructor rounds the corner.* "Let's ask about a referral."	I *offer self* by saying, "let's *together* ask…." The minimum crisis intervention goal targets Richard to return to the precrisis state with no panic attacks. The maximum goal aims for growth.
Richard: "Thank you."	

▮ KEY POINTS TO REMEMBER

- A crisis is not a pathological state but a struggle for emotional balance.
- Crises offer opportunities for emotional growth but can also lead to personality disorganization.
- There are three types of crisis: maturational, situational, and adventitious.
- Adventitious crises/crises of disaster result in mass casualty incidents causing injury, trauma, and/or destruction to large groups of people, communities, and real estate.
- The National Incident Management System (NIMS) is established to help federal, state, city, and nongovernment groups operate seamlessly during a crisis event.

- Situational and maturational crises are usually resolved within 4 to 6 weeks.
- Crisis intervention therapy is short term, from 1 to 6 weeks, and focuses on the present problem only.
- Resolution of a crisis takes three forms: a person emerges at a higher level, at the precrisis level, or at a lower level of functioning.
- Social support and intervention can promote successful resolution.
- Crisis therapists take an active and directive approach with the patient in crisis.
- The patient is an active participant in setting goals and planning possible solutions.

KEY POINTS TO REMEMBER—cont'd

- Crisis intervention is usually aimed at the mentally healthy person who generally is functioning well but is temporarily overwhelmed and unable to function.
- The crisis model can be adapted to meet the needs of people in crisis who have long-term and persistent mental problems.
- The steps in crisis intervention are consistent with the steps of the nursing process.
- Specific qualities in the nurse that can facilitate effective intervention are having a caring attitude, an ability to be flexible in planning care, an ability to listen, and an active approach.
- The basic goals of crisis intervention are to reduce the individual's anxiety level and to support the effort to return to the person's precrisis level of functioning.
- During a disaster triage helps make the most efficient use of available resources.
- Critical incident stress debriefing is a group approach that helps groups of people who have been exposed to a crisis situation.

APPLYING CRITICAL JUDGMENT

1. List the three important areas of crisis assessment once safety concerns have been identified. Give examples of two questions in each area that need to be answered before planning can take place.
2. Barbara is 21 years old and a junior in nursing school. She tells her nursing instructor that her father (age 45 years) has just lost his job. Her father has been drinking heavily for years, and Barbara is having difficulty coping. Because of her father's alcoholism and the increased stress in her family, Barbara wants to leave school. Her mother has multiple sclerosis and thinks Barbara should quit school to take care of her.
   A. How many different types of crisis are occurring in this family? Discuss the crises from the viewpoint of each family member.
   B. If this family came for crisis counseling, what areas would you assess and what kinds of questions would you ask to evaluate each member's needs and the needs of the family as a unit (perception of events, coping styles, social supports)?
   C. Formulate some tentative goals you might set in conjunction with the family.
   D. Utilizing informatics, identify by name appropriate referral agencies in your community that might be helpful to this family.
   E. If you were going to be counseling this family, how would you set up follow-up visits for the family? Would you see the family members together, alone, or in a combination during the crisis period (4 to 6 weeks)? How would you decide whether follow-up counseling was indicated?
3. Identify an adventitious crisis/crisis of disaster that happened recently in your life or one that you know about.
   A. If you are among a group of first responders, what would be the initial responsibility of your team?
   B. Identify the needs of the people that would have to be met after life-and-death decisions have been made.
   C. Discuss how you could mitigate against potential future mental health issues the disaster victims might face.

CHAPTER REVIEW QUESTIONS

Choose the appropriate answer(s).

1. Which statement about crisis theory provides a basis for nursing intervention?
   1. A crisis is an acute, time-limited phenomenon experienced as an overwhelming emotional reaction to a problem perceived as unsolvable.
   2. A person in crisis usually has had adjustment problems and has coped inadequately in his or her usual life situations.
   3. Crisis is precipitated by an event that enhances the person's self-concept and self-esteem.
   4. Nursing intervention in crisis situations rarely has the effect of ameliorating the crisis.

2. The main goal of the initial nursing assessment with a client in crisis is to:
   1. obtain a thorough medical history.
   2. arrange for a family meeting as soon as possible.
   3. determine the precrisis level of functioning.
   4. encourage the patient to return to normal activities.

3. In planning care for a person experiencing a crisis, it is important for the nurse to first:
   1. ensure that the discharge plan includes a medication appointment.
   2. encourage the patient to discuss past coping strategies.
   3. refer the patient to an outpatient therapist within his/her provider network.

    4. collaborate with the health team to determine the anticipated discharge date.

4. For a nurse working in crisis intervention, which belief would be least helpful?

    1. A person in crisis is incapable of making decisions.

    2. The crisis counseling relationship is one between partners.

    3. Crisis counseling helps the patient refocus to gain new perspectives on the situation.

    4. Anxiety reduction techniques are used so the patient's inner resources can be accessed.

5. Which of the following is not a function of critical incident stress debriefing (CISD)? To debrief:

    1. staff after incidents of patient violence.

    2. a hotline volunteer after a patient's suicide.

    3. a patient after transplant surgery.

    4. search and rescue workers after a natural disaster.

REFERENCES

Aguilera, D. C. (1998). *Crisis intervention: theory and methodology* (8th ed.). St Louis: Mosby.

Aguilera, D. C., & Mesnick, J. (1970). *Crisis intervention: theory and methodology.* St Louis: Mosby.

American Nurses Association (ANA). (2007). American Psychiatric Nurses Association, & International Society of Psychiatric–Mental Health Nurses. *Psychiatric–mental health nursing: scope and standards of practice.* Washington, DC: Nursesbooks.org.

Behrman, G., & Reid, W. J. (2002). Post-trauma intervention: basic tasks. *Brief Treatment and Crisis Intervention, 2,* 310–348.

Caplan, G. (1964). *Symptoms of preventive psychiatry.* New York: Basic Books.

Everly, G. S., Jr. (2000). Crisis management briefings (CMB): large group crisis intervention in response to terrorism, disasters and violence. *International Journal of Emergency Mental Health, 2,* 53–57.

Everly, G. S., Jr., Lating, J. M., & Mitchell, J. T. (2000). Innovations in group crisis intervention: critical incident debriefing (CISD) and critical incident stress management (CISM). In A. R. Roberts (Ed.), *Crisis interventions handbook: assessment, treatment, and research* (2nd ed., pp. 77–100). New York: Oxford University Press.

Fraser, R. (2010). *Why have natural disasters increased?* Retrieved May 3, 2011, from www.thetrumpet.com/?q=7020.5552.0.0.

Greenstone, J. L., & Leviton, S. C. (2002). *Elements of crisis intervention: crises and how to respond to them* (2nd ed.). Pacific Grove, CA: Brooks/Cole.

Hammond, J., & Brooks, J. (2001). The World Trade Center attack. Helping the helpers: the role of critical incident stress management. *Critical Care, 5*(6), 315–317.

Howard, J. M., & Goelitz, A. (2004). Psychoeducation as a response to community disaster. *Brief Treatment and Crisis Intervention, 4,* 1–10.

Jordan, K. (2003). A trauma and recovery model for victims and their families after a catastrophic school shooting: focusing on behavioral, cognitive, and psychological effects and needs. *Brief Treatment and Crisis Intervention, 3,* 397–411.

Lowry, J. L., & Lating, J. M. (2002). Reflections on the response to mass terrorist attacks: an elaboration on Everly and Mitchell's 10 commandments. *Brief Treatment and Crisis Intervention, 2,* 95–104.

National Incident Management System (NIMS). (2008). Washington, DC: U.S. Department of Homeland Security.

Norman, L. D., & Weiner, E. E. (2011). Emergency preparedness and response for today's world. In B. Cherry, & S. R. Jacob (Eds.), *Contemporary nursing: issues, trends, & management* (5th ed.). St Louis: Elsevier/Mosby.

Portelli, I., Fulmer, T., & Marr, M. C. (2011). Disaster nursing during terrorist events. In P. S. Cowen, & S. Moorhead (Eds.), *Current issues in nursing* (8th ed.). St Louis: Mosby/Elsevier.

Roberts, A. R. (2000). *Crisis intervention handbook: assessment, treatment, and research* (2nd ed.). New York: Oxford University Press. 77–100

Roberts, A. R. (2005). *Crisis intervention handbook: assessment, treatment, and research* (3rd ed.). New York: Oxford.

Child, Partner, and Elder Violence

Elizabeth M. Varcarolis

℮volve WEBSITE

http://evolve.elsevier.com/Varcarolis/essentials

KEY TERMS AND CONCEPTS

Adult Protective Services (APS),
   p. 416
child abuse, p. 403
Child Protective Services (CPS),
   p. 413
cycle of violence, p. 409
elder abuse, p. 415
emotional abuse, p. 402

intimate partner violence (IPV),
   p. 407
perpetrators, p. 403
physical abuse, p. 402
safety plan, p. 413
teen dating violence (TDV),
   p. 408
victims, p. 403

SELECTED CONCEPT: Family Violence

Family violence is prevalent among all ethnic, religious, age groups, social and socioeconomic groups. From mansions to middle-class homes in good neighborhoods, and more visibly in lower socioeconomic groups such as ghettos, projects, and all areas in between, violence and victimization exists.

Besides family abuse, abuse by trusted authority figures is part of the picture of violence in our society. Spiritual abuse (pastors, priests, faith healers) and care-giver abuse (physicians, dentists, baby-sitters, teachers) are examples of some trusted figures in our society who by their violence cause devastating and lifelong trauma to their victims.

OBJECTIVES

1. Differentiate among the three types of family abuse and give two physical and behavioral indicators for each.
2. Provide patient-centered care by demonstrating how you would communicate with (a) a parent who was suspected of child abuse and (b) a woman who is the victim of intimate partner violence (IPV).
3. Compare and contrast at least five characteristics of an abusive parent or caretaker with those of an abuser involved in intimate partner violence (IPV).
4. Discuss the assumed characteristics of the caretaker for an abused elder and other possibilities that you include in the family assessment in order to intervene effectively.

Continued

OBJECTIVES—cont'd

5. Incorporate evidence-based practice when describing the importance of obtaining and recording forensic data gathered both for a child and for an abused partner.

6. Discuss the teamwork and collaboration needed when obtaining forensic data both from a child and from an abused partner.

7. Using a clinical example, describe the factors that make an older adult more vulnerable to abuse.

8. Using informatics, summarize the concept of elder abuse and the functions of Adult Protective Services (APS) that apply in your state.

9. Prepare a handout for your classmates listing the procedures and contact numbers in your state for reporting suspected child and elder abuse (perform a computer search).

10. Using informatics find at least two referrals in your community that you could give to a victim of intimate partner violence (IPV) to find safety and group or individual therapeutic support.

Domestic violence is a huge public health and criminal justice problem throughout the world as well as in the United States. Domestic violence has enormous consequences affecting millions of women, men, and children. Physical and psychological trauma causes long-lasting and devastating damage to people's lives, children's lives, and the lives of future generations. Violence has moved from the home to schools, the workplace, neighborhoods, the road, and even the air—it touches every corner of community life. Family violence and abuse is prevalent among all ethnic, religious, social, and socioeconomic groups as well as among all age-groups. Domestic violence occurs in residences ranging from mansions and estates, to middle-class homes in "good" neighborhoods, to ghettos and building projects, and all areas in between. Aside from family abuse, abuse by trusted authority figures is part of the picture of violence in our society. Spiritual abuse (e.g., pastors, priests, faith healers) and caregiver abuse (e.g., physicians, dentists, babysitters, and teachers) exemplify how some trusted figures in our society have caused devastating and lifelong trauma to their victims.

The nurse is often the first point of contact for people experiencing family violence and is in the ideal position to contribute to prevention, detection, and effective intervention. All forms of interpersonal abuse can be devastating. Abuse can take the form of emotional, physical, or sexual abuse and neglect. **Emotional abuse** destroys the person's spirit and the ability to succeed later in life, feel deeply, or connect emotionally with others.

Physical abuse includes emotional abuse in addition to the potential for long-term physical deformity, internal damage, acute painful tissue damage, bone damage, and, in some cases, death. The consequences of being sexually abused may never be resolved if treatment is unavailable, causing behavioral and emotional difficulties throughout the person's life.

Sensitivity is required on the part of the nurse who suspects family violence. A person who feels judged or accused of wrongdoing is most likely to become defensive, and any attempts at changing coping strategies in the family will be thwarted. It is better for the nurse to ask about ways of solving disagreements or methods of disciplining children, rather than use the word abuse or violence, which appear judgmental and are therefore threatening to the family.

Some findings that should alert the nurse to the possibility of family violence are listed in Box 21-1. Lesbian, gay, bisexual, and transgender (LGBT) victimization will be discussed in Chapter 24: Anger, Aggression, and Violence.

THEORY

Most theories of intrafamily violence are related to psychology, sociology, or culture. According to researchers and authors, most conventional explanations of intrafamily violence remain partial and incomplete. These authors assert that most theories of violence are one-dimensional and separately emphasize different, yet related phenomena. They advocate for a theory of violence that provides a comprehensive explanation that incorporates an integration of interpersonal,

---

BOX 21-1 INDICATORS FOR FAMILY VIOLENCE

- Recurrent emergency department (ED) visits for injuries attributed to being "accident prone"
- Presenting problems reflecting signs of high anxiety and chronic stress:
  - Hyperventilation
  - Panic attacks
  - Gastrointestinal disturbances
  - Hypertension
  - Physical injuries
- Depression
- Stress related conditions:
  - Insomnia
  - Violent nightmares
  - Anxiety
  - Extreme fatigue
- Eczema
- Loss of hair

institutional, and structural violence. Domestic violence is extremely complex. There is no single theory that explains intrafamily violence, but rather it is most likely an interaction of societal, cultural, and psychological factors as well as neurobiological influences.

Social Learning Theory

Learning theory or the **intergenerational violence theory** of family violence relies on role modeling, identification, and human interaction (Sadock & Sadock, 2007). Learning theory proposes that a child who witnesses abuse or is abused in the family of origin learns that violence is an acceptable reaction to stress, and internalizes the violent behavior as a behavioral norm. If the violent acting-out behaviors are condoned in the family or social milieu, then the person is rewarded with a sense of power and control over others. Intergenerational abuse is considered a contributing factor in some cases of intimate partner violence (IPV), elder abuse (adults who were abused as children retaliate against their parents in later life), and child abuse.

Societal and Cultural Factors

Some correlates that exist with family abuse include the following:

- Poverty or unemployment
- Communities with inadequate resources
- Overcrowding
- Social isolation of families

The classic "frustration-aggression" hypothesis (Dollard et al., 1939) proposes that when frustration is high in response to the societal situations mentioned in the preceding text, frustration leads to aggression. Although these factors do correlate with family violence, they do not "cause" family violence. Not all frustrated individuals respond to frustration with violence. Some people respond to high levels of frustration with despair, depression, and resignation or attempt to change the situation (Sadock & Sadock, 2007).

The "patriarchal theory" (often referred to as feminist theory), which is advanced by social and behavioral scientists, holds the view that male dominance in our political and economic structure exists to enforce the differential status of men and woman. In many subcultures, women are viewed as property of or "belonging to" men, are subservient, and are kept relatively powerless. Violence against women is a major public health concern first declared by The United Nations *Declaration of the Elimination of Violence Against Women* (General Assembly United Nations, 1993) which states:

> Recognizing that violence against women is a manifestation of historically unequal power relations between men and women, which have led to domination of the discrimination against women by men and to the prevention of the full advancement of women, and that violence against women is one of the crucial social mechanisms by which women are forced into a subordinate position compared to men.

Psychological Factors

Psychological theories focus on the abuser having personality traits that "cause" abusiveness. The abuser has no control over his or her violence and, as such, is not at fault. For example, the **perpetrators** of violence have no control because they have a mental illness, or they are addicted to drugs and alcohol. It is now known that many abusers, as well as their **victims,** are considered "normal" after psychological testing. By the same token, most people who have a mental disorder do not demonstrate violent behavior.

The use of legal and illegal drugs (e.g., prescription, over-the-counter, or illicit drugs; alcohol; or solvents) may coexist with family violence, but not everyone who abuses substances is involved in family violence and not all cases of family violence include substances of abuse (National Council on Alcoholism and Drug Abuse [NCADA], 2009). However, when the two do coexist, it is a matter of genuine concern. Both family violence and substance abuse problems usually require outside assistance, and both need to be addressed together. Unfortunately, often when an abuser stops abusing a substance, family violence does not stop (NCADA, 2009).

Some abusers argue that they are physically unable to control their anger and aggression. This "loss of control" is not supported by their behavior, however. Perpetrators of family violence will most likely choose not to hit their bosses or a policeman, no matter how frustrated or angry they become. Abusers often plan where (in the home), when (no one is around), and how (leave no visible marks) they will inflict violence (Minnesota Advocates for Human Rights [MAHR], 2006). See Chapter 24 for neurobiological factors related to violence and interventions for angry and aggressive patients.

Other psychological factors include some of the following traits: low self-esteem, poor problem-solving skills, history of impulsive behavior, hypersensitivity (sees self as victim), and narcissism (centers on self, lacks compassion for others). People with aggressive traits are usually immature (although some are able to present a mature façade to the outside world).

CHILD ABUSE

A report of child abuse is made every 10 seconds, and almost five children die every day as a result of child abuse (Childhelp, 2011). **Child abuse** takes place when a child is harmed by someone else physically, psychologically, sexually, or by acts of neglect. Each state is responsible for providing its own definition of child abuse. These definitions must meet the minimum standards established by the federal government through the Child Abuse and Prevention Act (CAPA):

> Any recent act or failure to act on the part of a parent or caregiver, which results in death, serious physical harm, sexual abuse or exploitation, or act of failure to act which presents an immediate risk of serious harm.

Generally, most states recognize four different types of abuse: physical, emotional, sexual, and neglect. Table 21-1 provides definitions of different types of child abuse, some physical indicators, and some behavioral indicators.

The actual occurrences of child abuse are grossly underreported; as previously mentioned, close to five children die every day as a result of child abuse. Children younger than 4 years of age are at greatest risk of severe injury or death. In 2008 80% of deaths occurred among children younger than 4 years old and 10% among children 4 to 7 years old; and the majority of these were infants 1 year and younger (Centers for Disease Control and Prevention [CDC], 2010a; U.S. Department of Health and Human Services [USDHHS], 2009). Parents are thought to account for nearly 80% of child abuse cases (Pillado et al., 2010). Siblings can also be perpetrators of emotional, physical, and sexual abuse. Statistics concerning this common, yet unrecognized abuse are even less available. Among children confirmed by child protective agencies as being maltreated, 59% experienced neglect, with the next highest being physical abuse

TABLE 21-1   TYPES OF CHILD ABUSE AND PHYSICAL AND BEHAVIORAL INDICATORS

TYPE OF ABUSE	PHYSICAL INDICATIONS	BEHAVIORAL INDICATIONS
Physical Abuse Occurs when a caretaker allows or inflicts intentional physical injury that causes a substantial risk to the child's well-being and health.	Bruises/wounds in differing stages of healing Unexplained burns, bruises, welts, broken bones, internal injuries, bite marks, etc. Bald patches on scalp Subdural hematoma (child younger than 2 years) Retinal hemorrhage	Excessive fear of parents or constant effort to please Wary of adult contact Post-trauma syndrome (e.g., nightmares) Obvious attempts to hide bruises or injuries Withdrawn, depressed, or aggressive disruptive behavior Regressive behavior
Neglect Failure to provide for the child's basic needs.	*Physical neglect:* Malnourished Underweight, poor growth pattern Inadequately supervised Poor hygiene Unattended physical problems Inappropriate dress *Educational neglect:* School problems or failure Not enrolled in mandatory school for age of child	Soiled clothing, poor hygiene Begging, stealing food Emaciated or have distended belly Extended stay at school (early arrival–late departure) Psychosomatic complaints Delinquency Alcohol or drug abuse Abandonment Chronic truancy Special educational needs not being attended
Sexual Abuse Sexual abuse perpetrated on nonfamily member. Some types include: • Exhibitionism • Touching or manipulating the child's sexual organs • Oral, anal, or vaginal sex • Having child touch perpetrator • Masturbation in front of or with the child	Difficulty in walking or sitting Vulvovaginitis Urinary tract infections Torn, stained, or bloody underclothing Bruises or bleeding in external genitalia, vaginal or anal areas Venereal disease, especially in preteens In boys, pain on urination or penile swelling or discharge Foreign matter in rectum, vagina, or urethra	Mistrust of adults Abnormal or distorted view of sex Bizarre, sophisticated, or unusual sexual behavior or knowledge Phobias: fear of the dark, men, strangers, leaving the house Delinquent or running away Self-injury or suicidal thoughts or behaviors Mental disorders may develop (e.g., posttraumatic stress disorder, depression, multiple personality disorder, eating disorders, conduct disorders, anxiety disorder)

TABLE 21-1	TYPES OF CHILD ABUSE AND PHYSICAL AND BEHAVIORAL INDICATORS—cont'd	
TYPE OF ABUSE	**PHYSICAL INDICATIONS**	**BEHAVIORAL INDICATIONS**
Emotional or Psychological Abuse Behaviors that convey to the child that he or she is worthless, flawed, unloved, or unwanted: • Constant criticism • Insults • Harsh demands • Threats and yelling • Ignoring the child • Denying child opportunities to receive positive reinforcement	Speech disorders Lag in physical development	Difficulty in learning and living up to potential Lack of self-confidence Inappropriate adult-like behavior or infantile behavior Dramatic behavior changes (e.g., aggressiveness, compulsive seeking of affection or approval)

(USDHHS, 2009). Research conducted by the CDC (2010a) states that one in four girls and one in six boys may be sexually abused before adulthood. However, more than one type of abuse can co-occur, and emotional abuse is always part of the picture.

An interesting problem in industrialized countries—where financial resources have increased and family size has decreased—is overindulgence of children, which is considered an abuse of neglect. Although overindulgence is the farthest issue from a health care worker's mind during an assessment, it is a serious problem that results in social impairment, emotional stunting (particularly empathy), and physical problems caused by inactivity and obesity. However, during these recent years of recession, more families are slipping into lower socioeconomic brackets, which greatly increases family stress and may lead to all types of abuse, including child abuse, IPV, and also elder abuse.

Theories of the biochemistry and neuroanatomy of aggression and violence are discussed in Chapter 24: Anger, Aggression, and Violence.

APPLICATION OF THE NURSING PROCESS

ASSESSMENT

Child

Often the abused child is excessively fearful of a parent or caregiver. The child may appear disheveled and neglected and have a history of absenteeism. Guidelines for interviewing the child suspected of being abused are presented in Box 21-2.

Reassure children that they will not be punished or hurt and that they did not do anything wrong. Children should not feel pressured to talk about any topics they are unwilling or unable to discuss. The experience should be nonthreatening and supportive and not resemble a trial or inquisition. Preschoolers may be better able to express their experiences by reenacting the incident with dolls or drawings.

BOX 21-2	INTERVIEW GUIDELINES FOR ASSESSMENT OF A CHILD

Do
- Conduct the interview in private.
- Sit next to the child, not across the table or desk.
- Tell the child that the interview is confidential.
- Use language the child understands.
- Ask the child to clarify words that you do not understand.
- Tell the child if any action will be required.

Do Not
- Allow the child to feel "in trouble" or "at fault."
- Suggest answers to the child.
- Probe or press for answers the child is not willing to give.
- Display shock or disapproval of parent, child, or situation.
- Force the child to remove clothing.
- Conduct the interview with a group of interviewers.

Open-ended questions are best. Possible questions include the following:
- How did this happen to you?
- Who takes care of you?
- What do you do after school?
- Who are your friends?
- What happens when you do something wrong?

Parent or Caregiver

Abusing parents vary by degrees of intelligence and education, and come from all socioeconomic backgrounds and religious affiliations. Specific characteristics are often found

BOX 21-3   CHARACTERISTICS OF ABUSIVE PARENTS

- A history of violence, neglect, or emotional deprivation as a child
- Low self-esteem, feelings of worthlessness, depression
- Poor coping skills
- Social isolation (may be suspicious of others)
- Few or no friends, little or no involvement in social or community activities
- Involved in a crisis situation—unemployment, divorce, financial difficulties
- Rigid, unrealistic expectations of child's behavior
- Frequently uses harsh punishment
- History of severe mental illness, such as schizophrenia
- Violent temper outbursts
- Looks to child for satisfaction of needs for love, support, and reassurance
- Projects blame onto the child for his or her "troubles"
- Lack of effective parenting skills
- Inability to seek help from others
- Perceives the child as bad or evil
- History of drug or alcohol abuse
- Feels little or no control over life
- Low tolerance for frustration
- Poor impulse control

BOX 21-4   INTERVIEW GUIDELINES FOR ASSESSMENT OF A PARENT OR CAREGIVER

Do
- Conduct the interview in private.
- Be direct, honest, and professional.
- Be understanding.
- Be attentive.
- Inform the person if you must make a referral to Child Protective Services and explain the process.

Do Not
- Try to "prove" accusations or demands.
- Display horror, anger, or disapproval of parents or situation.
- Place blame on or make judgments about the parent(s) or child.

either singly or in combination among parents who abuse their children (Box 21-3). Guidelines for interviewing a parent or caregiver suspected of abusing a child are presented in Box 21-4.

Questions that are open-ended and require a descriptive response can be less threatening and elicit more relevant information than questions that can be answered yes or no. For example:

- What arrangements do you make when you have to leave your child alone?
- How do you punish your child?
- When your infant cries for a long time, how do you get him or her to stop?
- What does the child do to make you cry?
- Do you get time for yourself?
- How are things between you and your partner?

DIAGNOSES AND OUTCOMES IDENTIFICATION

The most immediate concern is to ensure the child's safety and well-being. Therefore safety, Injury, and *Risk for Injury* are primary. Other nursing diagnoses might include *Disabled Family Coping, Post-Trauma Syndrome, Anxiety, Fear, Impaired Parenting, Acute Pain, Delayed Growth and Development,* and *Imbalanced Nutrition: Less Than Body Requirements.*

The following is a list of short-term goals for the child experiencing abuse, the outcome of which should be "Physical abuse, sexual abuse, or neglect has ceased."

1. Receive medical care for injuries within an hour.
2. Notify proper state authorities to ensure continued safety for child after abuse is suspected.
3. Maintain child's safety until adequate home and family assessment can be made.

IMPLEMENTATION

When child abuse is suspected, nurses are *legally* responsible for reporting to the appropriate child protective agency designated by each state (as are social workers, medical and mental health professionals, teachers, and childcare providers). Each state mandates that a report must be filed when "suspected" abuse or neglect is encountered. Some states require all people to report suspected child abuse. Reports remain confidential. (For more on reporting child abuse and neglect go to www.childwelfare.gov/ or call 1-800-422-4453.)

The emergency department (ED) is usually where first contact is made with the abused child and family. Table 21-2 includes a list of nursing interventions to be used with the abused child and his or her family and rationales for the interventions.

The physician or nurse practitioner caring for an abused child should incorporate help from a variety of sources to ensure the long-term safety of the child, for example, social workers, home health agencies, financial counselors, local mental health facilities, alcohol and drug treatment centers, and parenting centers.

Follow-Up Care

There have been long-standing questions over whether treatment for abuse and neglect of children is valuable. A comprehensive analysis of interventions for child maltreatment (Skowron & Reineman, 2005) found that, "On average, individuals involved

TABLE 21-2   INTERVENTIONS FOR THE ABUSED CHILD AND THE CHILD'S FAMILY

INTERVENTION	RATIONALE
1. Adopt a nonthreatening, nonjudgmental relationship with parents.	1. If parents feel judged or blamed or become defensive, they may take the child and either seek help elsewhere or seek no help at all.
2. Understand that children do not want to betray their parents.	2. Even in an intolerable situation, the parents are the only security the child knows.
3. Provide (or have physician provide) a complete physical assessment of the child.	3. Allows health care worker to provide competent care and to substantiate reporting to child welfare agency, if required.
4. Use of dolls might help child tell how "accident" happened.	4. Child might not know how to articulate what happened or might be afraid of punishment. Dolls can be an easier way for the child to act out what happened.

Forensic Issues

1. **Be aware of your agency's and state's policy in reporting child abuse.** Contact supervisor or social worker to implement appropriate reporting.	1. Health care workers are mandated to report any cases of suspected or actual child abuse.
2. Ensure that proper procedures are followed, and evidence collected.	2. If child is temporarily taken to a safe environment, appropriate evidence helps protect the child's welfare.
3. Keep accurate and detailed records of incident: • Verbatim statements of who caused the injury and when it occurred • A body map to indicate size, color, shape, areas, and types of injuries with explanation • Physical evidence, when possible, of sexual abuse Use of photos can be helpful. Check hospital policy.	3. Accurate records could help ensure child's safety and court presentation.
4. Forensic examination of the sexually assaulted child should be conducted according to specific protocols: • Provided by law enforcement agencies • Follow state guidelines (www.childwelfare.gov)	4. Proper collection, handling, and storage of forensic specimens are crucial to court presentation.

Adapted from Varcarolis, E. M. (2011). *Manual of psychiatric nursing care plans: diagnoses, clinical tools, and psychopharmacology* (4th ed.). St Louis: Saunders.

in a counseling or therapeutic program were better off than 71 percent of those who did not experience treatment in terms of various psychological, cognitive and behavioral outcomes (e.g. anxiety, depression, aggressiveness, etc.)."

Primary Prevention

Many factors exist in cases of child abuse. Often, substance abuse is found in abusive families. Additional related factors are single parenthood, teen parents, or parents with mental retardation or disorders; a vulnerable child (e.g., unwanted pregnancy, low-birth-weight baby); or a child that is difficult to care for because of physical or mental handicap (e.g., hyperactivity, colic). Mothers who were abused as children or are abused by their partner are more likely to abuse their child.

Societal risk factors also play an important role. Poverty is thought to be among the most frequently and persistently noted risk factor in known cases of child abuse. Cowen and Cowen (2011) note that even at minimum wage ($6.55 an hour) parents working full-time are unable to pay for the basic necessities for their families, and this trend is spreading to more and more American families (National Center for Children in Poverty, 2009). "Families that live in lower socioeconomic neighborhoods rarely have affordable healthcare, sufficient social resources, are more at risk for violent crimes in their neighborhoods, and often lack extended family support."

Early diagnosis of actual or potential child abuse and intervention correlates with a more positive prognosis. Box 21-5 identifies common features of a successful child abuse prevention program.

INTIMATE PARTNER VIOLENCE

Intimate partner violence (IPV) is defined as "a pattern of assault and course of behaviors that may include physical injury, psychological abuse, sexual assault, progressive social isolation, stalking, deprivation, intimidation and threats" between current or former partners of an intimate relationship, regardless of gender or marital status (*Healthy People* Fact Sheet, 2010).

It has been well established that the abused as well as those who become the violent domestic partner can come from any race and religious, economic, or educational background. In

BOX 21-5   **COMMON FEATURES OF A SUCCESSFUL CHILD ABUSE PROTECTION PROGRAM**

- Strengthen and establish links with family and community support systems.
- Create opportunities for parents to feel empowered to act on their own behalf.
- Enhance coordination and integration of services needed by families.
  - Parenting skills
  - Coping skills
  - Anger management
  - Normal child development
  - Parent support group
- Provide settings where parents and children can gather, interact, support, and learn from each other.
- Enhance community awareness of the importance of healthy parenting practices.
- Provide emergency support for parents 24 hours a day.

Adapted from Bethea, L. (1999). Primary prevention of child abuse. *American Family Physician, 59*(15).

addition, both the abuser and the abused can be any age and married, single, divorced, or never married.

Although the majority of the victims of reported domestic violence are women, and domestic violence is the number one cause of ED visits by women, a growing body of research is revealing the prevalence and significance of domestic violence by women against men (American Psychological Association [APA], 2011). Actual statistics are hard to ascertain since there is drastic underreporting by women and even more so by men.

Intimate partner violence is not exclusive to heterosexual couples; IPV occurs in lesbian, gay, bisexual, and transgender (LGBT) communities as well.

Although the exact numbers of abused domestic partners are not known, it is estimated that up to 25% to 37% of all women experience battering, and of those who are battered 50% to 60% are battered during pregnancy. IPV is the leading cause of female homicides and injury-related deaths during pregnancy (*Healthy People* Fact Sheet, 2010). Birth defects and infant deaths are frequent outcomes of abuse of a woman during pregnancy. In 2007, 2340 deaths were the result of IPV, and of these deaths, 70% were females and 30% were males (CDC, 2011). IPV is the leading cause of homelessness among women.

Teen dating violence (TDV) is a disturbing trend, with approximately 25% to 33% of adolescents reporting verbal, physical, emotional, or sexual abuse from a dating partner each year (The President of United States of America, 2011; WebMD, 2008). About 1 in 11 teens reports being a victim of physical dating violence each year (CDC, 2010b). Although women are usually the victims in adult partner abuse, in teen relationships girls and boys abuse each other about equally (WebMD, 2008).

Abuse among college students remains high. Violence experienced at the hands of previous partners is estimated to be about 32% whereas violence inflicted by current partners is approximately 21%. Although it has been reported that one in five high school girls has been physically or sexually abused by a dating partner (CDC, 2010b), it is also estimated that one in four female students will experience a sexual assault over the course of her college career (The Safe Place, 2009). Teen abuse takes many forms: extreme possessiveness and jealousy, stalking (e.g., constant texting to monitor partner and partner's choice of friends), manipulation and total control of partner, demeaning partner in front of friends, threatening to commit suicide, or forced intimacy are just a few examples. Teen bullying will be discussed in Chapter 24.

Depression, posttraumatic stress disorder (PSTD), and anxiety disorders as well as suicide ideation and actual suicide attempts are potential sequelae to battering for all age-groups.

Because women are five to eight times more likely than men to be victimized by intimate partners, this discussion will use the female pronoun to denote the battered person (*Healthy People* Fact Sheet, 2010). For the same reason, the male pronoun will be used when speaking of the violent partner, with the understanding that males are also victims of IPV.

An abusive relationship is all about instilling fear and wanting to have power and control in the relationship. Anger is one way that the abuser tries to gain authority. He may also turn to physical violence (e.g., kicking, punching, grabbing, slapping, or strangulation), sexual violence (forcing sexual intercourse or performing sexual acts against the victim's will), or psychological violence (e.g., threats of death or death of a child, use of weapons). IPV has severe, long-reaching effects. Children who reside in homes where IPV occurs are vulnerable to feelings of responsibility, guilt, emotional distress, behavioral regression, somatic complaints, posttrauma disorder, PTSD, alcohol or drug abuse, and more. Children who live in an atmosphere of IPV are 30% to 60% more likely to be abused as well (Goodman, 2006).

Unfortunately, children from violent homes are more likely to model the actions they see around them in their own lives and carry the legacy of a violent home forward.

CHARACTERISTICS OF INTIMATE PARTNER VIOLENCE

The Battered Partner

Women do not ask to be beaten, nor do they enjoy being battered. The battered partner lives in terror of the next beating. Women do not usually initiate the violence, but when they are aggressive toward their violent mate, it is usually in self-defense. Approximately 93% of women who killed their mates had been battered by them (Asians Against Domestic Abuse [AADA], 2004).

The abused woman is often the subject of extreme and irrational jealousy, isolation, and verbal as well as physical abuse. Feelings of powerlessness and low self-esteem are common. After constant belittlement, insults, and degradation, the abused becomes so psychologically destroyed that she begins to believe

TABLE 21-3 **BEHAVIORAL CHARACTERISTICS OF INTIMATE PARTNER VIOLENCE**	
CHARACTERISTICS OF VIOLENT PARTNER	**CHARACTERISTICS OF BATTERED PARTNER**
Denial and Blame: Denies that abuse occurs, shifts responsibility of abuse to partner	Eventually believes that if she does or says "the right thing," the abuse will stop. If she does not do anything "wrong," then abuse will not occur
Emotional Abuse: Belittles, criticizes, insults, uses name calling, undermines	Becomes psychologically devastated and begins to believe partner's words
Control Through Isolation: Limits family or friends, controls activities and social events, tracks time or mileage on car, activities, stalks at work, takes to and from work or school, may demand permission to leave house	Gradually loses sight of personal boundaries for self, children; becomes unable to assess blame without validation from a supportive network
Control Through Intimidation: Uses behaviors to instill fear such as through vile threats, breaks things, destroys property, abuses pets, displays weapons, threatens children, and threatens homicide or suicide, increasing physical, sexual, or psychological abuse	Results in constant fear and terror that becomes cumulative and oppressive; contemplates suicide, completes suicide, contemplates homicide, occasionally completes suicide in self-defense
Control Through Economic Abuse: Controls money, makes partner account for all money spent; if partner works, calls excessively, forces partner to miss work; refuses to share money	Economic and emotional dependency may result in depression, high risk for secret drug or alcohol abuse. If works, frequently loses job from partner stalking and harassing
Control Through Power: Makes all decisions, defines role in the relationship, treats spouse like a servant, and takes charge of the home and social life	Continues to lose sense of self, becomes unsure of who she is, defines self in terms of partner, children, job, others; lacks self-power

her abuser's insults. Because of the physical or sexual abuse and threats, the abused lives in a world of terror and fear for her life and the lives of her children. These families are usually isolated, and they have few if any friends or outside influences. The violence and pain that exist inside the home remain secret. Table 21-3 lists characteristics of the abused woman and violent partner.

The Batterer

Violence is a learned behavior used by a person to control others. Frequently violent partners were raised in a home where they themselves were beaten or where they witnessed parental beatings. A batterer has a low sense of self, poor impulse control, and limited tolerance for frustration, and senses a lack of control in his life. Abusing someone less powerful or more vulnerable helps the violent partner feel more in control, powerful, and masculine (if male). Men who batter have no guilt and lack concern over their aggressiveness. Batterers may appear well adjusted from the outside, but usually have only superficial relationships with others. They are extremely possessive, are pathologically jealous, believe in male supremacy in relationships, and often have a drug or alcohol problem, which is not a cause of the abuse but often an excuse for the abuse. Batterers may be linked into types. Batterers with sociopathy (dyssocial tendencies) are thought to be more lethal than those with less psychopathology. Unfortunately, irrespective of the frequency or the lethality of the violent behavior, it is illegal and leaves lifetime scars on the victim, if not death. Unfortunately,

treatment approaches for all subtypes of batterers have thus far not proven very effective.

Cycle of Violence

Abuse toward a person in a partner relationship is not merely an exchange of blows, but rather a process that increases in intensity and escalates over time without valid provocation. The abusive relationship may start subtly. It may start by the abuser being critical of the way the partner dresses, disciplines the kids, or cares for the home. Or the abuser becomes unreasonably jealous, possessive, and watchful of the partner's activities. No matter how it begins, the process is always slowly progressive. The abuse becomes more frequent, intense, and life threatening over time. In Walker's classic study of 400 women in violent families (Walker, 1979), the cycle of violence was first operationally defined. The cycle of violence consists of three phases: (1) tension-building phase, (2) acute battering phase, and (3) honeymoon phase. Figure 21-1 shows behaviors that characterize the steps in the cycle.

The cycle of violence is a continuing cycle that is hard to break without help. It is important to recognize, however, that the cycle does not apply to many cases of IPV. In a small number of cases, the violence might not escalate to lethal levels or may cycle less frequently. Whatever pattern the violence follows, trust is broken, and shame and fear are constantly underneath the surface of the lives of the victims. Many women report that their partners never repent and that the violence is not cyclical but a constant presence in their lives.

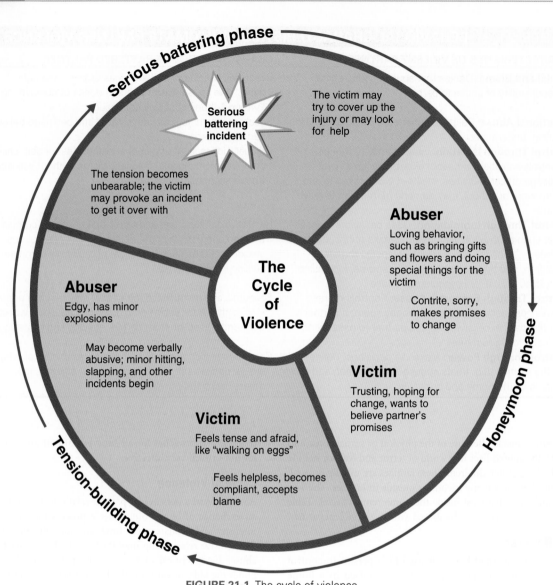

FIGURE 21-1 The cycle of violence.

Why Abused Partners Stay

There are many reasons women stay in violent domestic situations. Perhaps one of the *strongest* motives for staying is fear that the attacks will become even more violent or that the woman or her children could be murdered if they are found by the batterer. This is a very real concern, and women are at high risk of further violence or even death when they threaten to leave or if they are later found by their abuser. The following are some other reasons many women cannot leave the abusive relationship:

- They have no other means of financial support.
- They have no support system after living in isolation for long periods.
- They are afraid to be alone or think they cannot survive without the partner.
- They experience depression or loss of psychological energy necessary to leave.
- Their self-esteem is low, and they believe that the batterer is powerful and omniscient.

Some women may also have the following beliefs:

- They deserve the beatings because they did something "wrong."
- They can control the beatings by not doing anything to upset their partners.
- They need to stay for the sake of the children.
- They are still positively reinforced by the honeymoon phase of the battering cycle.

APPLYING THE ART

A Person Experiencing Partner Violence

SCENARIO: I met 28-year-old Maddie in the emergency department where she had been seen 3 weeks before for a dislocated shoulder, which she attributed to falling down the basement steps while carrying a basket of laundry. This time she complains of cramping and is in her second month of pregnancy. Her left eye showed bruising, partially masked by heavy makeup. I introduced myself and my role as Maddie rested in an exam room waiting for the nurse-midwife.

THERAPEUTIC GOAL: By the conclusion of this interaction, Maddie will verbalize the intent to access her support system, decreasing her isolation.

STUDENT-PATIENT INTERACTION	THOUGHTS, COMMUNICATION TECHNIQUES, AND MENTAL HEALTH NURSING CONCEPTS
Maddie: "I feel better now. The cramps barely hurt. I don't need that exam. I need to get home. I'm fine really." ***Student's feelings:*** *Falling down the steps plus a bruised face and now cramping. I feel deeply concerned, and I wonder if there's a connection.*	She uses *denial* that she does not need the exam, and that she is "fine really."
Student: "You say you feel better, but still you're cramping." *She shrugs her shoulders.* "You're anxious to leave, almost as though you're fearful." *She wrings her hands, looking downward.* ***Student's feelings:*** *I'm worried for her. I need to work up the courage to ask her about abuse.*	I use *restatement* then *attempt to translate into feelings*. She is moving into *moderate anxiety*. She is still able to focus her thoughts.
Maddie: "It's not worth it."	
Student: "Not worth it. The exam?" ***Student's feelings:*** *I feel concerned that she actually may see herself as "not worth it."*	I *restated* then asked a *direct question* to *clarify*. Maybe I should have stopped after "not worth it" to keep her options for answering open. Physical abuse is always emotionally damaging, too.
Maddie: *Glancing at me.* "I just need to get home before 5:30." ***Student's feelings:*** *I hope she will open up to me. I must take charge of my feelings. There's stigma attached to abuse, almost like it's the victim's fault. I want her to know whatever happens, she's okay by me.*	I need to focus on building her comfort level with me.
Student: "Maddie, I appreciate how difficult this must be. I am concerned about you." *I learn toward her and make eye contact.*	Attempting to translate into feelings facilitates empathy. My nonverbals and words need to be congruent and show nonjudgmental acceptance.
Maddie: *Silent. Bites her lip.*	
Student: "Could you share with me what happens at 5:30?"	Using the word "could" in my *question* gives her a choice, which empowers her.
Maddie: "He gets home. He can't know about the baby." *She starts to cry.* ***Student's feelings:*** *I feel sad at all she has to worry about.*	She must feel overwhelmed.
Student: "The 'he' is your husband?" *She nods.* "You seem afraid of him." *She opens her mouth then closes it again.* "I sense you've been hurt by him before."	I clarify the indefinite pronoun "he" and *attempt to translate into feelings.*
Maddie: "Before, after, and during! I used to be better at reading Steve's moods but I've been so worried about my baby. He punched my stomach when I didn't cook his eggs right this morning. He punched my stomach!" *Begins to tear up.* "Maybe he suspects." ***Student's feelings:*** *I just realized why I'm feeling so anxious. When I was young, I remember a neighbor and her kids that my family sheltered one night. She cringed describing the beating, but she also went back to her husband the very next morning.*	Like many *battered women*, Maddie describes how she anticipates her husband's needs. She may show *codependent behavior* by needing to be needed.

Continued

APPLYING THE ART—cont'd

A Person Experiencing Partner Violence

STUDENT-PATIENT INTERACTION	THOUGHTS, COMMUNICATION TECHNIQUES, AND MENTAL HEALTH NURSING CONCEPTS
Student: "Maybe he suspects?" **Student's feelings:** I'm hoping she shares some of her burden with me.	Restatement says, "go on." Sharing her pain with me decreases its intensity.
Maddie: "That I'm pregnant. He's always accusing me of running around, but I swear I never did! I never would. I love him." Sobs. "He's wonderful on his good days."	
Student: "He's wonderful on the good days, but not so wonderful on the bad days."	I verbalize the implied opposite pole, e.g., "good days" implies bad days, too. My acceptance gives her permission to talk more about the painful parts.
Maddie: Nods. "The bad days happen more often. One day he's going to kill me." Winces with another cramp. "I'll never forgive him or myself if I lose my baby."	I am remembering that people in chronically abusive relationships suffer depression and anxiety. Over time posttraumatic stress disorder can emerge.
Student: "You feel in danger for your life and now, for your baby's life, too." **Student's feelings:** Should I focus on her danger first or her not feeling able to forgive herself? She's carrying so much. What kind of man beats his wife? How can she think him wonderful, at all?	I summarize her deepest fears. Any part that is "wonderful" undoubtedly occurs during the honeymoon phase of the abuse cycle.
Maddie: Closes her eyes. Silent for 3 minutes. **Student's feelings:** It's tough for me to wait quietly. I want her to leave him but this is her life, not mine. I'll mindfully breathe to keep myself calm, yet focused. My instructor will be making rounds soon. I feel a need to debrief.	I need to think this through. I do not want to add to the stigma by judging her. I remember about learned helplessness, when battering chips away at self-esteem, initiative, and hope.
Maddie: "You're still here." Smiles and makes eye contact.	
Student: "Yes, Maddie, I'm guessing you're thinking deeply about your options. Is there anyone who can help you through this?" **Student's feelings:** I so much want to tell her to leave him but then I'm just one more person telling her what to do.	She is ambivalent. She wrestles with the pain of leaving as compared to the pain of staying. Maybe she will accept some information or at least the number for the women's shelter.
Maddie: "I think it's time I told my parents. I know they suspect something. I've lied and lied. I feel so ashamed."	
Student: "Sounds to me that, like other battered women, you made tough choices that enabled you to survive." I look at Maddie and offer my hand. **Student's feelings:** I'm taking a risk in calling her a battered woman if she's not ready.	I give information as I offer self by reaching for her hand.
Maddie: Holds my hand, looking up as the nurse-midwife comes in.	
Maddie: Nods. "I don't know what I'm going to do yet, but I'm going to call my mom." **Student's feelings:** She recognizes her loneliness. I feel so proud of her courage.	Isolation from supports fits the victimizer's agenda of ensuring dependency on the abuser alone.
Student: "You're making the decision to tell her about the abuse."	My statement acts like an indirect question.
Maddie: "Yes, I've been so lonely. Yes." **Student's feelings:** Maddie really may take this step. I feel hopeful.	

APPLICATION OF THE NURSING PROCESS

ASSESSMENT

Abused women are most often seen in the ED, but they may be seen in a physician's office or clinic. There is wide agreement that improved health care response to victims of domestic violence is needed. Many hospitals and health care systems across the country are designing and implementing screening and intervention programs to help meet this need. Following this example, a number of model middle schools and high schools are more acutely aware of the growing trend of teen violence and are committed to helping their students. In many of these schools teen counselors are working with the teachers/administration to identify and help teens in violent dating relationships.

If an injury that brings a woman to the ED does not match her explanation of the mechanism of injury or if the patient minimizes the abuse, IPV might be suspected. If IPV is suspected, a complete physical history needs to be done, including x-rays and a neurological examination. Because rape may be part of the abusive scenario, this should be evaluated as well, especially if the woman is pregnant, exposed to sexually transmitted diseases (STDs), or has any signs of infection or trauma.

Signs of abuse may include burns, bruises, scars, and other wounds in various stages of healing, particularly around the head and neck. Physical examination includes assessing for signs of internal injuries such as concussions, perforated eardrums, abdominal injuries, eye injuries, and strangulation marks on the neck. Broken or fractured bones, such as arms, pelvis, ribs, clavicle, legs, and jaw, are other signs of abuse. An examination might reveal burns from cigarettes, acids, scalding liquids, or appliances.

There are always psychological and emotional scars. The woman might present with signs of high anxiety and stress and complain of insomnia, chest pain, back pain, dizziness, stomach upset, trouble eating, or severe headache, for example. Signs of posttraumatic stress disorder (PTSD) are often present and should be part of an assessment. A brief history may reveal a series of falls, "accidents," and recent emergency department visits. A woman with any indication of IPV should always be seen alone, without her partner present.

Three questions are often sufficient to reveal current or prior IPV:

1. Have you been hit, kicked, punched, or otherwise hurt by someone within the past year? If so, by whom?
2. Do you feel safe in your current relationship?
3. Is there a partner from a previous relationship who is making you feel unsafe now?

Always ask if the children are also being hit or hurt in any way, and if suspected or confirmed, Child Protective Services need to become involved.

An assessment of the patient's support systems, suicide potential, and coping responses (e.g., learned helplessness, substance abuse, denial) should be included in the assessment. Once the history of abuse has been ascertained, careful documentation such as verbatim verbal statements and physical findings should be recorded using a body map (refer to Table 21-4). Ask the woman if she would allow photos to be taken.

DIAGNOSIS AND OUTCOMES IDENTIFICATION

IPV is a situational crisis that threatens a woman's physical and psychological health, as well as her life and possibly the lives of her children. Therefore *Risk for Violence, Risk for Injury, Acute/Chronic Pain, Risk for Trauma,* and *Risk for Self-Directed or Other-Directed Violence* are all nursing diagnoses that might need immediate focus. Others that need to be considered include *Social Isolation, Disturbed Sleep Pattern, Powerlessness, Disturbed Personal Identity, Risk for Post-Trauma Syndrome,* and *Disabled Family Coping.*

Unfortunately, women who are treated in the ED may admit to IPV but seldom return for treatment. Nurses often have strong reactions when children or women are violently treated. However, in the case of partner abuse, it is up to the abused partner to make the decision to stay in the battering situation or to leave. It is most helpful for the woman if the nurse can accept the woman's decision in a nonjudgmental way and support the woman in her decision.

Therefore the obvious outcome for health care personnel would be to see the woman opt for a safe environment for herself and her children in the form of safe houses, a caring relative, or a friend. Because that is not usually the woman's decision, the nurse can provide the woman with referrals (numbers for safe houses, hotlines, and support groups, legal counseling in verbal and written forms) as well as a safety plan. Box 21-6 contains an example of a basic IPV safety plan.

IMPLEMENTATION

Table 21-4 lists several interventions and their rationales related to the initial ED visit. It is important that the battered partner begins to understand the following facts:

- No one deserves to be beaten.
- She cannot make anyone hurt her.
- It is not her fault.

A Note on Programs for Batterers

Various types of programs across the country have been set up for men who batter their partners. Although the focus is on reducing or eliminating domestic violence, it also offers men options other than fines or incarceration. Programs vary in strategies, but usually the first priorities are to protect the victims and to stress that the behavior and attitudes of the offender are accountable for the abuse in the relationship (Hayward et al., 2007). A qualitative descriptive study, which examined eight women's perceptions of court-mandated batterer treatment programs, stated the women perceived the programs helping in some ways. For example, the women believed for the most part that communication had improved and that most of the men had developed alternate ways of

BOX 21-6 BASIC INTIMATE PARTNER VIOLENCE SAFETY PLAN

It is important, whenever possible; to work with a domestic violence advocate to develop a safety plan that fits your needs.

- Move to a room with more than one exit, avoiding rooms with potential weapons (e.g., kitchen knives).
- Know the quickest route out of your home.
- Know the quickest route out of your workplace. Determine resources employer may have to protect employees. Pack a bag beforehand with essential clothes, valuables, and documents for you and each of your children, including a calling card/cell phone/address book and at least a 1-month supply of all medications for you and your children. Keep it hidden but make it easy to grab quickly. Include the documents that apply, such as birth certificates, social security card, photo identification or passports, welfare identification, green card, marriage certificate, legal protection or restraining orders, health insurance papers and medical cards, children's school records, work permits, immigration papers, investment records/account numbers, rental agreements, lease or house deed registration, and insurance information.
- Tell your neighbors about your abuse and ask them to call the police when they hear a disturbance.
- Have a code word to use with your kids, family, and friends when you need help.
- Have a safe place selected in case you ever have to leave.
- Use your instincts.
- You have the right to protect yourself and your kids.
- Call the National Domestic Violence Hotline at 1-800-799-7233 or the National Teen Dating Abuse Helpline at 1-866-331-9474 for further information and guidance.

From Goodman, P. E. (2006). The relationship between intimate partner violence and other forms of family and societal violence. *Emergency Medical Clinics of North America, 24(4)*, 889-903; Violence Against Women: *Violence against women: safety plan list.* (2009). Retrieved May 9, 2011, from http://womanshealth.gov/violence/planning.

TABLE 21-4 INTERVENTIONS FOR INTIMATE PARTNER VIOLENCE: EMERGENCY DEPARTMENT

INTERVENTION	RATIONALE
1. Ensure that medical attention is provided to patient. Ask permission to take photos.	1. If patient wants to file charges, photos boost victim's confidence to press charges now or in the future.
2. Set up interview in private and ensure confidentiality.	2. Patient might be terrified of retribution and further attacks from partner if she reveals abuse.
3. Assess in a nonthreatening manner information concerning: • Sexual abuse • Drugs of abuse • Thoughts of suicide or homicide	3. These are all vital issues in determining appropriate interventions: • Increases risk for post-trauma syndrome. • Many victims self-medicate. • May seem the only way out of an intolerable, catastrophic situation.
4. Encourage patient to talk about the battering incident without interruptions.	4. When patients share their stories, attentive listening is essential.
5. Ask how patient is faring with the children in the home.	5. In homes in which the mother is abused, children also tend to be abused.
6. Assess if patient has a safe place to go when violence is escalating. If she does not, include a list of shelters or safe houses with other written information.	6. When abused patients are ready to leave their abusers, they will need to go quickly.
Forensic Issues	
1. Identity if patient is interested in pressing charges. If yes, give verbal and written information on: • Local attorneys who handle spousal abuse cases • Legal clinics • Battered women's advocates	1. Often the spouse or partner is afraid of retaliation, but when ready to seek legal advice, an appropriate list of lawyers well trained in this area is needed.
2. Know the requirements in your state about reporting suspected spousal abuse.	2. Many states have or are developing laws or guidelines for protecting battered women.
3. Discuss with patient an escape plan during escalation of anxiety before actual violence erupts (see Box 21-2).	3. Document escape plan and include shelter and referral numbers. This can prevent further abuse to children and patient.

TABLE 21-4	INTERVENTIONS FOR INTIMATE PARTNER VIOLENCE: EMERGENCY DEPARTMENT—cont'd
INTERVENTION	**RATIONALE**
4. Throughout work with battered spouses emphasize that the beatings are not their fault.	4. When self-esteem is eroded, victims often believe that they deserved the beatings because they did something "wrong."
5. Encourage patient to reach out to family and friends whom they might have been avoiding.	5. Old friends and relatives can make helpful allies and validate that patient does not deserve to be beaten.
6. Know the psychotherapists in the community who have experience working with battered spouses or partners.	6. Psychotherapy with victims of trauma requires special skills on the part of even an experienced therapist.
7. If patient is not ready to take action at this time, provide a list of community resources: a. Hotlines b. Shelters c. Battered women's groups d. Battered women's advocates e. Social services f. Medical assistance or Aid to Families with Dependent Children (AFDC)	7. It can take time for patients to make decisions to change their life situation. People need appropriate information.

Adapted from Varcarolis, E. M. (2011). *Manual of psychiatric nursing care plans: diagnoses, clinical tools, and psychopharmacology* (4th ed.). St Louis: Saunders.

dealing with acting out their angry, impulsive urges in physical ways. However, even when the physical violence lessened or abated, the emotional, verbal, or sexual abuse remained and may have increased (Hayward et al., 2007). In these situations, the core problem with the aggressor was that the need to exert constant and strict control remained. It is felt by many that in order to change the dynamics of abuse the aggressor needs to work at changing his perceptions of himself and the world, which can reduce the need for violent control.

ELDER ABUSE

Elder abuse is a serious and rapidly growing problem, and with the large number of aging baby boomers, in the next decade and beyond there will be an overwhelming number of adults 65 years of age or older (Institute of Medicine of the National Academies, 2008). Unfortunately, the health care system is woefully unprepared for this emerging phenomenon. A number of estimates indicate that approximately 6% of older adults are mistreated annually as reported by Fulmer and Blankenship (2011). The actual rate of elder abuse will increase proportionately to the increase in the elder population, especially if the health care system is without appropriate manpower to administer assessments and provide effective interventions to protect older Americans.

The World Health Organization (2002) states that elder abuse is "a violation of human rights and a significant cause of injury, illness, lost productivity, isolation and despair." There are three common categories of elder abuse: domestic, institutional, and self-neglect. The five common kinds of elder abuse are physical or sexual, psychological, financial abuse or exploitation, and neglect (Box 21-7).

> **BOX 21-7 FIVE KINDS OF ELDER ABUSE**
>
> 1. **Physical abuse:** The infliction of physical pain or injury (e.g., slapping, bruising, restraining) (approximately 20%).
> 2. **Psychological abuse:** The infliction of mental anguish (e.g., humiliating, intimidating, threatening) (approximately 20%).
> 3. **Financial abuse or exploitation:** The misuse of someone's property and resources by another person (approximately 20%).
> 4. **Neglect:** Failure to fulfill a caretaking obligation to provide goods and services (e.g., abandonment, denial of food or health-related services) (approximately 40%). This category may also include self-neglect.
> 5. **Sexual abuse:** Nonconsensual sexually molesting, (either by refusal or incapacity to refuse) sexual contact (percentage unknown).
>
> From International Council of Nurses Fact Sheet. *Elder abuse.* Retrieved February 10, 2007, from www.icn.ch/matters_elder.htm.

Although awareness of elder abuse emerged as a growing problem in America in the 1970s (Granny abuse), even today elder abuse has not received the major attention it needs to address the problem effectively, although many safeguards have been instituted in the last decade at the national level. Also, it is estimated that the majority of cases (from 70% to 80%) of elder abuse are never reported.

All 50 states and the District of Columbia have some form of elder abuse prevention laws and have established reporting systems. The **Adult Protective Services (APS)** division of each state receives and investigates reports of suspected elder abuse. To be eligible for APS help in most states, an older adult has to be deemed unable to care for him or herself. This leaves many older adults who are mentally and physically healthy unprotected in a situation in which they are physically or financially being exploited by family members. The result is that the definitions of elder abuse and the APS programs differ among states, resulting in a "patchwork of laws, definitions, and services throughout the country" (Quinn & Zielke, 2005, p. 451), which is still true today. These widely differing definitions and terminologies make it impossible to know the actual extent of the problem or to conduct sound research. There have been some recent movements at the national level to standardize the approach to the study of elder mistreatment.

CHARACTERISTICS OF ELDER ABUSE

The Abused Elder

The percentage of older adults (defined as 60 years or older) is growing in the United States because people are living longer and the baby boomers are aging. Seniors can be especially vulnerable to abuse as well as to other crimes. Age-related syndromes often result in frailty and functional decline, making an older adult even more at risk for abuse, neglect, and self-neglect. This frailty and decline also place older adults at greater risk for sexual abuse that, when reported, is often disbelieved. Elder abuse is most often diagnosed in older adults who have depression, alcohol or drug abuse, dementia, psychosis, loss of executive function, or other psychiatric illness, which compounds an older adult's vulnerability.

People older than 80 years of age are two to three times more likely to suffer abuse and neglect than older adults in the 60- to 80-year-old age-group, and victims of elder abuse are three times more likely to die than older adults who are not mistreated (Quinn & Zielke, 2005). Older women are more likely than men to suffer from abuse or neglect, and the majority of victims are white.

The Abuser

Early studies on elder abuse focused on the caretaker's stress and burden as a causative factor in the abuse. More recent research indicates that the characteristics of the elder abuser more closely resemble the characteristics of the abuser in partner abuse (IPV). Most often the abuser is a middle-age adult child or other family member. Often the caregiver is financially dependent on the older adult. Typically, the elder abuser will possess personality traits similar to those of the abusive person involved in child abuse or intimate partner violence. The family member inflicting the abuse may not be a cruel or insensitive person, but instead be a caring individual under extreme stress. In many cases the caregiver is grappling with a mental health issue, a substance abuse problem, or an inability to cope with the overwhelming stress of his or her daily life (Fulmer & Blankenship, 2011). It is the nurse's responsibility to carefully observe the family and determine their needs. Then the nurse

and family must explore possible interventions to lessen family tension/anxiety, or, in extreme cases, decide whether the elder needs to be removed from the home.

APPLICATION OF THE NURSING PROCESS
ASSESSMENT

Physicians, nurses, and other health care professionals are often the only outside contact an older adult may have. In most states, health care workers (nurses, nurses' aides, and physicians) are mandated to report elder abuse and neglect to APS. However, it is likely that only a very small fraction of reportable cases get referred to APS.

Victims of violence have twice as many physician and clinic visits as those not subjected to abuse. Because victims of abuse or neglect are most likely to be abused by family members, the abused is often afraid to reveal the abuse. There may be threats against disclosure, the abused may experience deep shame, or the abused may want to protect a loved one. The abused elder may also be afraid of retribution, or that he or she will be put into a nursing home. It is important, therefore, that family and friends communicate about suspected abuse. Health care workers should make a routine evaluation for signs or symptoms of abuse when older adults visit health care facilities, especially on a frequent basis.

Some of the signs of abuse are very similar to those of the victim in child abuse or IPV. Some additional red flags include the following:

- Fear of being alone with caregiver
- Obvious malnutrition
- Bedsores or skin lesions
- Begging for food
- In need of medical or dental care
- Left unattended for long periods
- Reports of abuse or neglect
- Passive, withdrawn, or emotionless behavior
- Concern over finances
- Valuables missing

When patients are referred by friends, family, police, social services, or others in situations in which the patient cannot leave the home, house calls are necessary. House calls allow the clinician to make an assessment of how the older adult functions in his or her own environment, and in that case self-neglect, abuse, or financial exploitation is easier to detect.

DIAGNOSIS AND OUTCOMES IDENTIFICATION

Nursing diagnoses for abused older adults are much the same as with other cases of abuse. *Risk for Injury, Acute or Chronic Pain, Fear, Anxiety, Risk for Self-Directed* and *Risk for Other-Directed Violence* have been discussed. However, two areas that particularly apply to an abused older adult are neglect and financial exploitation. Nursing diagnoses that may be appropriate include *Impaired Home Maintenance, Self-Care Deficit, Caregiver Role Strain, Adult Failure to Thrive,* and *Powerlessness.*

Successful long-term outcomes include the following:
1. Physical, emotional, sexual abuse has ceased.
2. Neglect or financial exploitation has ceased.
3. Plans are in place to maintain safety.
4. The elder states he or she feels more comfortable in the home.
5. Follow-up visits reveal less anxiety and tension between the caregiver and the elder.

Most hospitals and community centers have protocols that offer guidelines for nurses and other health care workers for suspected elder abuse. Immediate physical safety is always the first concern. Each state has its own protocols, but they all provide guidance to health care workers in case of suspected elder abuse. However, not all the needs of a particular older adult may be met through the protocols. Once abuse is suspected, referral to APS is appropriate.

There are a number of services that Adult Protective Services (APS) can offer to address issues of patient neglect, abuse, and other forms of mistreatment. These services are voluntary, and the patient has the right to accept or decline them. According to Dyer and colleagues (2005), APS interventions include the following:

- Arranging for housing services (e.g., emergency housing, repairs, modification for disabilities)
- Obtaining medical services
- Addressing personal needs (e.g., food delivery, food stamps, caretaker services)
- Providing service coordination (case manager, referrals to appropriate service groups)
- Serving as patient advocate
- Implementing legal interventions

Unfortunately, there is no empirical evidence that the interventions that are presently in place are effective, since most of them involve reporting and referring (Fulmer & Blankenship, 2011). Greater social supports could readily be a protective factor for elders of abuse, and further research is needed in this area to prepare for the ever-increasing needs of the elderly.

IMPLEMENTATION

Interventions include providing medical services, implementing legal interventions, and involving social services. Table 21-5 includes interventions for suspected elder abuse.

EVALUATION

Failures in interventions with abusive families often are not related to personal deficits but instead to inadequacies in the social, economic, and political systems in which we all live. A very real problem is that of the social exclusion of many disadvantaged individuals who are unable to afford helping services. Nurses can direct interventions to the social environment and can question, among other things, the acceptance of corporal punishment as a technique for guiding behavior in children, the unequal burden of caregiving responsibilities placed on women, the low priority given to education and preparation for parenthood, and the belief that one has little social value if one is older.

Evaluation of interventions (IPV, child, elder) can be based on whether the survivor acknowledges the violence, is willing to accept intervention, or is removed from the violent

TABLE 21-5	INTERVENTIONS FOR SUSPECTED ELDER ABUSE	
INTERVENTION	**RATIONALE**
1. Check your state for laws regarding elder abuse.	1. All states have adopted laws to help protect elders and support their needs for safety.
2. Involve Adult Protective Services (APS) if abuse is suspected.	2. APS can offer many sources to help guard the safety and well-being of abused elders.
3. Meet with other family members to identify stressors and problem areas.	3. Other family members may be unaware of the abuser's stress level or the lack of safety available for the abused family member.
4. If there are no other family members, notify other community agencies that might help the abuser and elder stabilize the situation; for example: • Support group for elder • Support group for abuser • Meals on Wheels • Day care for seniors • Respite services • Visiting nurse services	4. Minimizes family stress and isolation, and increases safety.
5. Encourage abuser to seek counseling.	5. Increases coping skills and social supports.
6. Suggest that family members meet on a regular basis for problem solving and support.	6. Encourages family to learn and solve problems together.

situation. With more long-term interventions, evaluation should be made by all members of the health care team on an ongoing basis. Because violence is a symptom of a family in distress, diagnosis, interventions, and evaluation should ideally

be carried out by a multidisciplinary team that includes a physician, a nurse, a social worker, an attorney, and perhaps a psychiatrist. Follow-up is crucial in helping decrease the frequency of family violence.

KEY POINTS TO REMEMBER

- Physical and emotional trauma causes long-lasting and devastating damage to people's lives, and is often passed down to future generations.
- The actual incidence of child, partner, or elder abuse is unknown, because current statistics most likely represent only a small portion of the actual victims.
- All states have mandatory guidelines for reporting child abuse and elder abuse. Victims of IPV can be given guidelines for reporting abuse and obtaining legal help, but it is ultimately the responsibility of the individual to file a report of abuse.
- Guidelines for "what to do" and "what not to do" when interviewing a child suspected of being abused are included.
- Characteristics of the parent or caregiver who abuse their child or elder are outlined.

- Characteristics of a violent partner and caregiver to an abused elder are discussed.
- Abuse never just ceases without intervention; in most cases it usually escalates over time and in intensity.
- Forensic examination procedures of children suspected of being abused and of victims involved in IPV are outlined, and the responsibility of the nurse, clinician, or physician is described.
- Nursing diagnoses and long-term outcomes are similar in all abuse cases, although each individual has unique needs.
- Guidelines for nursing interventions for child, partner, and elder abuse in each section of this chapter have been outlined.

APPLYING CRITICAL JUDGMENT

1. Six-year-old Sammy is rushed to the ED by a neighbor who found him wandering in the street in only a dirty undershirt, seemingly dazed. He is covered in what appears to be cigarette burns, is cachectic, and has bruises on his wrists and ankles. He appears fearful and confused and does not respond to questioning except to say, "I hurt. I don't feel good."
   A. What is your first priority?

   B. Write documentation following forensic nursing guidelines (draw a map and describe physical behaviors and verbatim comments).
   C. What else could you do to document his injuries?
   D. What other evidence might you and other members of the treatment team gather?
   E. Role play with a classmate what you would say when reporting Sammy's situation to Child Protective Services.

CHAPTER REVIEW QUESTIONS

Choose the most appropriate answer(s).
1. An elderly man, accompanied by his son with whom he lives, arrives in the ED with many bruises and states he has difficulty moving his left shoulder. The priority nursing action is to:
   1. discuss the injuries with the patient without his son present.
   2. call the police to report possible abuse.
   3. arrange for a social work consultation.
   4. have the patient call in another family member as a witness.
2. When treating a woman who has been trapped in an abusive marriage for many years, which statement would a nurse expect not to hear?
   1. "If I'm patient, he'll change."
   2. "I deserve to be beaten."
   3. "I'll stay for the sake of the children."
   4. "No adult has the right to control or harm another."
3. When making assessments the nurse should bear in mind that a common characteristic of an abusing parent is:
   1. being female.
   2. having poor coping skills.

   3. having realistic expectations of child behavior.
   4. abstaining from use of chemical substances of abuse.
4. During a nursing assessment, which of the following is a "red flag" for suspecting that a patient has been a victim of physical violence?
   1. Patient's explanation does not match the injury.
   2. Patient has no history of stress-related physical problems.
   3. Patient mentions having a concerned, supportive spouse.
   4. Patient is anxious but open and direct in explaining the complaint or injury.
5. An elderly woman has been emotionally and financially abused by her family for years. The nurse has difficulty understanding why she allows this abuse to recur. The best approach is to:
   1. encourage the patient to break ties with her family.
   2. avoid talking about the concept of abuse.
   3. understand that the patient may feel helpless to make change.
   4. believe that the patient is not concerned about the abuse.

REFERENCES

American Psychological Association (APA). (2011). *Male victims of 'Intimate Terrorism' can experience damaging psychological effects.* Retrieved May 9, 2011, from www.APA.org/news/press/releases/2011/04/intimate-terrorism.

Asians Against Domestic Abuse (AADA). (2004). *National statistics.* Retrieved January 28, 2007, from www.aadainc.org/Statistics.htm.

Bethea, L. (1999). Primary prevention of child abuse. *American Family Physician, 59*(6).

Centers for Disease Control and Prevention (CDC). (2011). *Understanding intimate partner violence: fact sheet.* Retrieved May 9, 2011, from www.cdc.gov/violence/prevention.

Centers for Disease Control and Prevention (CDC). (2010a). *Child maltreatment: facts at a glance.* Retrieved May 7, 2011, from www.CDC.gov/violence/prevention.

Centers for Disease Control and Prevention (CDC). (2010b). *Dating violence facts.* Retrieved May 10, 2011, from www.CDC.gov/.Choo serespect/understanding_dating__violence_facts.

Childhelp. (2011). *National child abuse statistics.* Retrieved May 7, 2011, from www.childhelp.org/pages/statistics.

Cowen, J. A., & Cowen, P. S. (2011). Child maltreatment: nursing considerations. In P. S. Cowen, & S. Morehead (Eds.), *Current issues in nursing* (8th ed.). St Louis: Mosby/Elsevier.

Dollard, J., Doob, L., Miller, N., et al. (1939). *Frustration and aggression.* New Haven, CT: Yale University Press.

Dyer, C. B., Heisler, C. J., Hill, C. A., & Kim, L. C. (2005). Community approaches to elder abuse. *Clinics in Geriatric Medicine, 21*(2), 429–447.

Family Violence, Spring 2011. *Intimate partner violence.* Retrieved May 7, 2011, from http://blogs.longwood.edu/familyviolence 2011/intimate-partner-violence/.

Fulmer, T., & Blankenship, J. L. (2011). Nursing care: victims of violence—elder mistreatment. In P. S. Cowen, & S. Moorehead (Eds.), *Current issues and nursing* (8th ed., pp. 721–725). St Louis: Mosby/Elsevier.

General Assembly United Nations. (1993). *Declaration of the elimination of violence against women (resolution 48/104).* Retrieved February 3, 2007, from http://daccessdds.un.org/doc/UNDOC/GEN/N94/095/05/PDF/N9409505.pdf.

Goodman, P. E. (2006). The relationship between intimate partner violence and other forms of family and societal violence. *Emergency Medicine Clinics of North America, 24*(4), 889–903.

Hayward, K. S., Steiner, S., & Spould, K. (2007). *Women's perceptions of the impact of a domestic violence treatment program for male perpetrators.* Retrieved May 11, 2011, from www.Medscape.com/viewarticle/561278.

Healthy People Fact Sheet. (2010). *Intimate partner violence and Healthy People 2010 fact sheet.* Washington, DC: U.S. Department of Health and Human Services.

Institute of Medicine of the National Academies. (2008, updated 2010). *Retooling for an aging America: building the healthcare workforce.* Retrieved May 5, 2011, from www.IOM.edu/Reports/2008/Retooling-for-an-Aging-America-Building-the-Health.

International Council of Nurses Fact Sheet. *Elder abuse.* Retrieved February 10, 2007, from www.icn.ch/matters_elder.htm.

MedlinePlus. (2011). *For young women, 'controlling' partner often abusive, too.* Retrieved May 9, 2011, from www.nlm.nih.gov/MEDLINEplus/news/fullstory_110752.html.

Minnesota Advocates for Human Rights (MAHR). (2006). *Stop violence against women: evolution of theories of violence.* Retrieved August 14, 2007, from www.stopvaw.org/Evolution_of_Theories_of_Violence.html.

National Center for Children in Poverty (NCCP). (2009). *Child poverty.* Retrieved May 3, 2011, from www.nccp.org/topic/child poverty.html.

National Council on Alcoholism & Drug Abuse (NCADA). (2009). *Family violence and substance abuse.* Retrieved May 1, 2011, from www.ncada-stl.org-tml.

Pillado, O., Kim, T., & Dierksing, C. B. (2010). *Fact sheet: child maltreatment.* (Spring, 2010). Southern California Academic Center of Excellence on Youth File in Prevention, Riverside: University of California. Retrieved May 1, 2011.

The President of the United States of America. (2011). *Presidential proclamation—national teen dating violence awareness and prevention month 2011.* Retrieved May 3, 2011, from www.whitehouse.gov/the-press-office/2011/01/31/presidential–proclamation-nation.

Quinn, K., & Zielke, H. (2005). Elder abuse, neglect, and exploitation: policy issues. *Clinics in Geriatric Medicine, 21*(2), 449–457.

Sadock, B. J., & Sadock, V. A. (2007). *Kaplan & Sadock's synopsis of psychiatry: behavioral sciences/clinical psychiatry* (10th ed.). Philadelphia: Lippincott Williams & Wilkins.

Skowron, E. A., & Reineman, D.H.S. (2005). Psychological interventions for child maltreatment. *Psychotherapy: Theory Research, Practice, and Training, 42,* 52–71.

The Safe Place. (2009). *Dating violence on college campuses: college dating violence.* Retrieved May 10, 2011, from www.thesafeplace.org/the basics/in-your-community/domestic-and-dating–violence.

United Nations High Commissioner For Human Rights. (1993). *Declaration on the elimination of violence against women: proclaimed by Gen. assembly resolution 48/104 of 20 December 1993.* Retrieved February 12, 2012, from www2.ohchr.org/english/law/eliminatio nvaw.htm.

U.S. Department of Health and Human Services (USDHHS). (2009). Administration on Children, Youth, and Families (ACF). *Child maltreatment 2007.* Washington, DC: U.S. Government Printing Office.

Walker, L. (1979). *The battered woman.* New York: Harper & Row.

WebMD. (2008). *Mental health: domestic violence-teen relationship abuse.* Retrieved May 10, 2011, from www.webmd.com/mental–health/tc/domestic–violence–teen–relationships–abuse.

World Health Organization. (2002). *Active ageing. A policy statement.* Geneva, Switzerland: Author.

Zolotor, A. J., Denham, A. C., & Weil, A. (2009). Intimate partner violence. *Primary Care Clinics in Office Practice, 39*(1).

Sexual Violence

Elizabeth M. Varcarolis

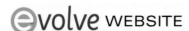 WEBSITE

http://evolve.elsevier.com/Varcarolis/essentials

KEY TERMS AND CONCEPTS

acquaintance rape, p. 421

date rape, p. 421

date rape drug, p. 427

forensic evidence, p. 422

institutional protocol, p. 426

marital partner rape, p. 421

rape, p. 421

rape kits, p. 426

rape-trauma syndrome, p. 427

sexual assault, p. 421

sexual assault nurse examiner
   (SANE), p. 426

sexual assault response team
   (SART), p. 426

survivor, p. 421

victim, p. 421

SELECTED CONCEPTS: **Survivor Versus Victim**

A **survivor** is an individual who has experienced a sexual assault and has worked through many of the issues and is going forward in their lives. The term **victim** is used for a person who has experienced a sexual assault, and can become a survivor with time, intervention, and/or counseling.

All individuals who have been the recipient of sexual violence suffer severe, deep, and emotional scars. Besides physical trauma (e.g., STDs, pregnancy) psychological consequences include depression, anxiety, difficulties with daily functioning, low self-esteem, eating disorders, self-destructive behaviors, substance abuse, and higher rates of suicide than in the general population, among others.

OBJECTIVES

1. Give examples of teamwork and collaboration by identifying the various functions and disciplines that constitute members of the sexual assault response team (SART).
2. Evaluate how sexual assault nurse examiners (SANEs) promote safety by describing the areas of expertise they provide to a victim of sexual violence.
3. Identify vulnerabilities that might be risk factors for sexual assault.
4. Summarize the characteristics of a perpetrator of sexual assault.
5. Incorporate evidence-based practice by identifying the specific data collected in the forensic component of the assessment that may be used as criminal evidence in court.
6. Promote safety by stating the guidelines, according to the Centers for Disease Control and Prevention (CDC) and

the American College of Obstetricians and Gynecologists (ACOG), for emergency treatment of a woman who has been sexually assaulted.
7. Provide patient-centered care by delineating the symptoms of rape-trauma syndrome that you would include in your teaching to a victim of sexual assault to prepare him/her for the second phase.
8. Formulate a list of community supports that can be offered to a sexually assaulted individual in your community, if a SART is not available in your area.
9. Utilizing informatics, describe the documentation of your initial assessment of a victim of sexual assault (objective and subjective data) along with a body map.
10. Differentiate between the terms survivor and victim as used in this chapter.

Sexual assault is an act of violence, power, and hate—not sex—and most often results in devastating severe and long-term trauma. It is often committed in the context of unequal power in order to demonstrate dominance and control. Sexual violence is related to teen pregnancy and the transmission of sexually transmitted diseases (STDs), including human immunodeficiency virus (HIV). Research has demonstrated that there is a long litany of other mental health issues that are more prevalent in people who have been sexually assaulted—such as depression, suicide, or use of alcohol, tobacco, and drugs. This will be discussed further in the chapter.

For our purposes here we will use the term survivor to denote someone who has experienced a sexual assault, has addressed many of the issues, and is moving on with his or her life. The term victim will be used for a person who has experienced a sexual assault and can become a survivor with time, intervention, and/or counseling. Sexual assault, sexual violence, and rape may be used interchangeably throughout this chapter.

The Centers for Disease Control and Prevention (CDC) encourages consistent definitions to monitor the incidence of sexual violence (SV). The following definitions apply to all survivors "who do not consent, or who are unable to consent or refuse to allow the act" (CDC, 2009):

- **A completed nonconsensual sexual act** is defined as contact between the penis and the vulva or the penis and the anus involving penetration, however slight; contact between the mouth and penis, vulva, or anus; or penetration of the anogenital opening of another person by a hand, finger, or other object.
- **An attempted, but not completed, sexual act**
- **Abusive sexual contact** refers to inappropriate touching and fondling; intentional touching, either directly or through the clothing, of the genitalia, anus, groin, breast, inner thigh, or buttocks of any person without his or her consent, or of a person who is unable to consent or refuse.

- **Noncontact sexual abuse** includes threatened sexual violence, exhibitionism, voyeurism, verbal or behavioral sexual harassment, taking nude photographs of another person without his or her consent or knowledge, or of a person who is unable to consent or refuse.

Sexual violence among children also includes:

- Coercing children to inappropriately touch the molester, often a trusted person
- Showing children pornographic photos and videos
- Initiating inappropriate conversations involving sexual topics

Sexual assault/sexual violence (SV) is an umbrella term encompassing the crimes of rape, date rape, acquaintance rape, gang rape (two or more perpetrators), marital/partner rape, sexual molestation, incest, statutory rape, and sexual assault of older adults.

Rape is a legal term rather than a medical diagnosis. Legal definitions of rape vary among states. For example, Ohio defines rape as (Cleveland Clinic Foundation, 2009):

…when sex is nonconsensual (not agree upon), or person forces another person to have sex against his or her will. It also occurs when the victim is intoxicated from alcohol or drugs. Rape includes intercourse in the vagina, anus, or mouth and is a felony offense, which means it is among the most serious crimes a person can commit. Rape is a crime that can happen to men, women, or children.

Date rape is a form of acquaintance rape, but in the case of date rape (Cleveland Clinic Foundation, 2009): "The victim agreed to spend time with the attacker. Perhaps the victim even went out with the attacker more than once. Date rape is still rape."

Rape should be considered a criminal act with long-term and wide-ranging medical, psychological, legal, and social sequelae (Viguera & Mian, 2004).

Presently, there is no mandated reporting for crimes of sexual assault unless they involve abuse of a minor or an elder. It is the responsibility of survivors of assault to make the decision to report the crime and it is the responsibility of health care workers to offer support, to provide information on obtaining legal counsel, and—with the patient's permission—to secure forensic evidence by a qualified person (evidence that can be used in court) for future prosecution.

PREVALENCE AND COMORBIDITY

Please note that statistics on sexual violence/assault are always approximate, are often varied, and may only refer to reported cases. It is safe to infer that the actual numbers of sexual assault are very much higher than the quoted statistics. Both rape and child sexual molestation are among the most underreported crimes. Statistics compiled by Roger Williams University (RWU, 2011a,b) and by Parents for Megan's Law (PML, 2007a) revealed that only 1% to 10% of these crimes are ever disclosed.

Children: Child Sexual Abuse/Incest

Statistics on child sexual assault/incest appear to be reaching an all-time high. Refer to Chapter 21 for further discussion on child abuse. The statistics for the sexual assault of children are appalling. For example, it is estimated that one in three girls and one in six boys are sexually molested by the time they reach 18 years old, and nearly 30% of the cases of child sexual assault reported to Child Protective Services (CPS) involved children between the ages of 4 and 7 years (PML, 2007a). The frightening statistic is that about 75% of the molestations are inflicted by family members. Abuse is likely to occur over a long-term, ongoing relationship and to escalate over time; it is estimated to last an average of 4 years (PML, 2007a). Even though strangers could be involved, the greatest percentage of molesters other than family members are persons the child trusts outside of the family, such as teachers, clergy/priests, babysitters, or family friends (Teen Breaks, 2011a).

The effects of **child sexual abuse** can last a lifetime. Sense of worth, distortion of self-concept, confusion about their place in the world, and disruption in affective capabilities are common. Unfortunately, people who were sexually assaulted as children are 4.7 times more likely to be sexually assaulted later in life. Abused children, compared to nonabused children, have higher rates for depression, substance abuse, dissociative disorders, other personality disorders, and anxiety disorders later in life (PML, 2007a). Child sexual violence that stays untreated may result in mental health issues, drug and alcohol abuse, crime, higher rates of suicide (either attempted or completed), and (not surprisingly) perpetuation of sexual abuse.

High School

The CDC (2011) states that 8% of high school students reported being forced to have sex; 11% of those were females and 5% were males. Date rape is also reported in high school students, as well as physical and emotional abuse.

Young Adults

Among college women, it is estimated that 20% to 25% will experience an attempted or completed rape by the end of their college career (CDC, 2011) and 90% will know their attackers. Perhaps the majority of sexual assaults in young adults are **acquaintance rapes/date rapes.** People ages 16 to 19 have the highest rate of sexual victimization of any age-group (PML, 2007b). Alcohol and other drugs often play a part of sexual assault, whether taken by the victim, the perpetrator, or both. Contrary to what some young men might think, intoxication by alcohol/drugs is not an excuse for sexual violence; sexual assault is still considered rape under the law. There are also drugs available to help facilitate sexual assault. Often these drugs are used for **gang rapes** (two or more sexual attackers). Although the number of rapes related to date rape drugs seems to be increasing, it is impossible to know the exact statistics. The following are some of the reasons an assaulted woman may not report her abuse:

- The woman believes it is her fault.
- The woman does not consider the incident sexual assault.
- The woman does not want to report her abuser for fear of reprisal.
- The woman does not want to get her "friend or date" in trouble.
- The woman does not want others to know about the assault.
- The woman cannot remember the incident clearly enough to feel she would be believed by others, especially if she had been drinking and/or taking other drugs.

Another consideration is that date rape drugs are cleared from the body fairly quickly, and detecting them in the emergency department or other treatment center is often difficult (RWU, 2011b). A urine sample must be obtained within a certain period of time to prove the existence of date rape drugs. The date rape drugs γ-hydroxybutyrate (GHB), flunitrazepam (Rohypnol), and Ketamine are used mostly on college campuses (e.g., fraternity houses, bars, raves, clubs, or nightclubs). Refer to Table 22-1 for more information on these drugs. Young men also must be cautious about taking a drink that contains a date rape drug. See Applying Critical Judgment at the end of this chapter for ways to minimize ingestion of a date rape drug. However, it is important to remember that the most common drug used to facilitate the crime of rape is still alcohol.

Male Victims of Sexual Assault

Sexual assault is usually committed by men against women, but it can be committed by women against men or between people of the same gender. The majority of perpetrators are male; however, women also sexually assault men. Women can force men to have sex, particularly if the male is younger and more vulnerable, and often through blackmail. Women also sexually assault other women, although the statistics are difficult to ascertain.

According to RWU (2011a), recent crisis center statistics claim that in up to 10% of sexual assaults men reported being the victim, and almost all male rape victims were raped by other men. Gay men are victims of sexual assault slightly more

TABLE 22-1   DRUGS ASSOCIATED WITH SEXUAL ASSAULT

MECHANISM OF ACTION	EFFECT	ADDITIONAL INFORMATION
GHB (γ-hydroxybutyric acid)*		
Central nervous system depressant	Onset is within 10 to 20 minutes; duration is dose related and is from 1 to 4 hours *Lower doses:* Produces euphoria, amnesia, hypotonia, and depressed respiration *Higher doses:* Can cause seizures, unconsciousness, nausea and vomiting, coma, and death	GHB needs 12 hours to be excreted from the body Used to treat narcolepsy Rapidly metabolized; difficult to detect in emergency departments and other treatment facilities
Rohypnol (flunitrazepam)†		
Potent benzodiazepine; 10 times stronger than diazepam	Impact is within 10 to 30 minutes and lasts 2 to 12 hours Becomes more potent when combined with alcohol Causes dizziness, amnesia, lack of motor coordination, confusion, nausea and vomiting, respiratory depression, and blackout episodes lasting 8 to 24 hours	Not legal in United States Detected in urine for up to 72 hours
Ketamine‡		
Anesthetic frequently used in veterinary practice; also hallucinogenic substance related to PCP (phencyclidine)	Onset is rapid, 20 minutes orally; duration is only 30 to 60 minutes Amnesia effects may last longer Usually administered as a powder that is snorted, smoked, injected, or dissolved in drinks Causes dissociative reaction with a dreamlike state leading to deep amnesia and analgesia and complete compliance of the survivor Later, survivor may be confused, paranoid, delirious, and combative with drooling and hallucinations	

*Street names include liquid ecstasy, salty water, scoop, homeboy, grievous bodily harm.
†Street names include "forget" drug, roofies, club drug, roachies, rophies, Mexican Valium.
‡Street names include special K, K, vitamin K, bump, kitkat, purple, super C.

often than heterosexual men, especially if they are the target of hate crimes. However, heterosexual men are raped in very large numbers. The vast majority of men who are sexually assaulted are assaulted by men who consider themselves heterosexual, although they may be bisexual (which is in keeping with the understanding that rape is a crime of violence and control). Although a great percentage of male rapes occur in prisons and the military, male rape can happen in cars, restrooms, colleges, universities, at work, or in the home. Jefferies (2011) states that the incidence of male on male rape may be much higher than what current statistics reveal. Jefferies quotes statistics that report that one in five women will be raped in their lives and one in seven males will be raped in their lives. The general statistics for male on male rapes often do not take into account the large number of unreported male on male rapes in prisons and in the military. The incidence of male on women rapes in the military is finally being acknowledged. Jefferies states in the April 2011 issue of a *Newsweek* article, titled "The Military Secret Shame," that male on male rapes most often

remain unreported. When the number of male on male rapes unreported in the American prison system is also considered, as revealed in the *The Economist* (2011), the extent and brutality of male on male sexual violence is revealed. Although laws addressing male on male rape have been established, they are often not acknowledged or enforced, and the culture of blaming the victim still persists.

It has been reported that more than 50% of gay men and lesbians recounted at least one incidence of coercion by a same-sex partner. Gay and lesbian sexual survivors may not come forward for fear of facing homophobia and prejudice as well as making their personal lives more public (DC Rape Crisis Center, 2007).

All individuals who have been the recipient of sexual violence suffer severe, deep, and emotional scars that may stay with them the rest of their lives. Beyond the physical trauma, such as risk of transmission of sexually transmitted diseases (STDs), human immunodeficiency virus (HIV), or pregnancy, psychological consequences can cause long-term psychological trauma. Some of the painful consequences caused by sexual assault include depression, anxiety, difficulties with daily functioning, low self-esteem, eating disorders, self-destructive behaviors, substance abuse disorders, and higher rates of suicide than in the general population. Although the risk exists for both male and female rape victims, male rape victims are more likely to commit suicide and to become infected with HIV through anal tears than are women. Timely and age-appropriate interventions can greatly help mitigate the devastating psychological sequelae and help victims become survivors; when emotional symptoms are confronted and addressed, the abused individual has a better chance of leading a full and productive life.

Cultural Considerations

Sexual violence occurs in all socioeconomic groups; it occurs in the suburbs, in rural communities, and in large cities; and it occurs in well-educated upper-class families, in middle-class families, and in poor and disadvantaged families. Sexual violence occurs across all ages to men, women, and children.

Cultural and societal factors play a part in forming attitudes, for example, cultural and societal norms that maintain women's inferiority and support male superiority and sexual entitlement. In such groups, often weak laws and policies related to gender equity and high tolerance for crimes of violence coexist. Some college fraternities reflect a societal context that could encourage violence toward women, and sexual assault on campus is thought to be increasing. More recently, even the Peace Corps has been cited as allegedly choosing to ignore male on female sexual assault.

The military is another societal group in which sexual assaults of women resulting from gender inequality along with norms that support masculine dominance have become a concern, and changes within military policy are in the process of being implemented. More recent information has revealed increasing male on male violence in the military, which again is related to positions of power. To instigate substantial change, strong, enforceable laws need to be established and rape must be recognized as a serious crime for which the perpetrator should be held responsible.

EXAMINING THE EVIDENCE

Help for Abusive Teenagers

Is there anything that can be done to help all these teen abusers we have been reading about in the news before they end up in jail? Also, is there truth to the theory about texting and electronic use possibly increasing teen aggression?

Uncontrolled adolescent anger is a significant public health concern and continues to be a contributing force in the three leading causes of adolescent death: homicide, suicide, and injuries. Unfortunately, adolescent anger does not seem to be diminishing. Violent incidents can vary in intensity and degree from bullying through psychological or physical harm to death (Pomeroy & Browning, 2010). Negative life events, perceived lack of family support, and decreased optimism are strongly linked to increased levels of anger (Puskar & Ren, 2008). A recent national survey revealed that the prevalence of adolescent depression is now close to 9%, but only 20% to 25% of youth who need mental health treatment actually receive it (Lusk & Melnyk, 2011).

Teen dating violence is an increasingly serious and underreported public health problem. One in four teenage girls in a relationship has suffered physical violence, such as being slapped by a boyfriend, whereas one in six has been pressured into having sex (Potter, 2010). Technology influences the dynamics of dating violence. Technologies redefine the boundaries of romantic relationships in ways that provide fertile ground for conflict and abuse. Participants are constantly available to one another by cell phones and other means. Electronically saved voicemails and text messages are available for scrutiny by insecure partners.

Individuals easily contact ex-partners by sending texts or posting messages on social networking sites (Draucker & Martsolf, 2010).

There are significant problems with the delivery of psychological health care services to teens—such as limited resources of time, finance, or qualified providers. In fact, there is such a shortage of providers that often the patient must wait weeks to months to be seen by a psychiatric provider, and then have only a 20-minute session (instead of the customary 50 minutes) because overworked providers have been forced to reduce session times to accommodate their increasing patient loads (Lusk & Melnyk, 2011). However, there are interventions that have proven successful in decreasing aggression. Cognitive behavioral therapy (CBT) emphasizes to the teen how particular thoughts can affect emotions (Lusk & Melnyk, 2011) and structured group therapy sessions highlight the physiological process of anger and presents techniques to promote relaxation and self-regulation (Gaines & Barry, 2008). Clinicians can also help by exploring with adolescent clients the way technology affects their dating relationship, by helping them to recognize use of aggression in technology, and by assessing if they need assistance managing electronic aggression (Draucker & Martsolf, 2010). In addition, community-based interactive theater programs for middle school students—performances with students role playing scripts that address healthy/unhealthy relationships, bullying, or sexual harassment—have also been effective (Fredland, 2010). Family therapy in which efforts toward changing family/school dynamics are the

EXAMINING THE EVIDENCE—cont'd

Help for Abusive Teenagers

focus continue to be emphasized. Family therapists must be family advocates, working in an increasingly globalized and multicultural world, respecting and understanding the need for cultural sensitivity, diversity, support, and optimism (Ungar, 2010).

Hopefully in the future, early detection of teen problems by schools and primary care providers will be enhanced and resources such as group therapy can be implemented to expedite services. In general, as the teen's self-esteem and optimism increase, anger, aggression, and abuse are decreased.

Draucker, C., & Martsolf, D. (2010). The role of electronic communication technology in adolescent dating violence. *Journal of Child and Adolescent Psychiatric Nursing, 23*(3), 133-142.

Fredland, N. (2010). Nurturing healthy relationships through a community based interactive theater program. *Journal of Community Health Nursing, 27,* 107-118.

Gaines, T., & Barry, L. (2008). The effect of a self-monitored relaxation breathing exercise on male adolescent aggressive behavior. *Adolescence, 43*(170), 292-300.

Lusk, P., & Melnyk, B. (2011). COPE for the treatment of depressed adolescents: lessons learned from implementing an evidence-based practice change. *Journal of the American Psychiatric Nurses Association, 17*(4), 297-309.

Pomeroy, E., & Browning, P. (2010). Youths in crisis. *Social Work, 55*(3), 197-201.

Potter, E. (2010). Violent teenage relationships. *British Journal of School Nursing, 5*(2), 59.

Puskar, K., & Ren, D. (2008). Anger correlated with psychosocial variables in rural youth. *Issues in Comprehensive Pediatric Nursing, 31,* 71-78.

Ungar, M. (2010). Families as navigators and negotiators: facilitating culturally and contextually specific expressions of resilience. *Family Process, 49*(3), 421-434.

Submitted by Lois Angelo.

THEORY

Vulnerable Individuals

Sexual assault occurs within all age-groups, genders, cultures, and socioeconomic backgrounds, but some groups appear more vulnerable and some situations are more conducive to sexual assault. Some of this has been previously stated; however, it all bears repeating.

- **Gender:** Women have a higher vulnerability rate than men (approximately 3 to 1). Both genders are more vulnerable if they are handicapped, have cognitive problems, or have mental disorders.
- **Age:** People ages 16 to 19 have a higher rate of sexual victimization than any other age group. Children are most vulnerable between the ages of 8 and 12. One in three girls and one in six boys are sexually abused before the age of 18, which constitutes up to 44% of sexual assaults or rape.
- **Older adults:** Domestic violence against older adults includes physical and sexual abuse; the perpetrators are most often adult children, especially sons, but can also include spouses, caregivers, health care providers, or other relatives. When an older adult is cognitively or functionally impaired, the likelihood of being sexually assaulted increases (Blackwood, 2005).
- **History of sexual violence:** Women who were raped before the age of 18 are two to three times more likely be sexually assaulted as adults.
- **Drug and alcohol use:** Use of alcohol or drugs by the perpetrator, the victim, or both is related to increased rates of victimization.
- **High-risk sexual behavior:** High-risk sexual behavior is a vulnerability that is often a consequence of childhood sexual abuse.

- **Poverty:** Poverty can make women and children more vulnerable and place them in more dangerous situations. Poor women may be at risk when they need to support themselves or their children and trade sex for food, clothing, money, or other necessary items.
- **Ethnicity or culture:** Native Americans have a one in three chance of being raped at some point in their lives. This is more than double that of non–Native American woman (Fears & Lydersen, 2007a,b) or Hispanic women.

The Perpetrator of Sexual Assault

The causes of violence toward women are multifaceted and involve biological, psychological, and social factors.

Biological Factors

From a *biological* perspective, neurophysiological factors may be a risk factor in violent behavior. Alterations in the functioning of neurotransmitters—such as serotonin, dopamine, norepinephrine, acetylcholine, and γ-aminobutyric acid—may interfere with cognition and behavior (Chapter 24).

Psychosocial Factors

From a *psychosocial* standpoint, studies have found a high incidence of psychopathology and personality disorders among sexual offenders. Antisocial personality disorder, in which people are viewed as objects, is one of the most prevalent. The act of rape involves a need for control, power, degradation, and dominance over others rather than sexual satisfaction. It is thought that some sexual offenders have difficulty finding willing sexual partners and resort to coercion or rape.

Many characteristics of a perpetrator of sexual assault are the same as those found in perpetrators of child abuse, intimate partner violence, and elder abuse (Chapter 21). Not surprisingly, most perpetrators of sexual abuse report being sexually assaulted as children. Some other characteristics include:

- Impulsive and antisocial tendencies
- Association with sexually aggressive and delinquent peers
- Preference for impersonal sex
- Hostility toward women
- Childhood history of sexual and physical abuse, or witness of family violence as a child
- Membership in a gang
- Belonging to a societal group that often refuses to acknowledge acts of sexual assault (e.g., some parts of the military, prisons, and even parts of the Peace Corps to a smaller degree)

APPLICATION OF THE NURSING PROCESS

ASSESSMENT

Sexual assault response teams (SARTs) are available across the country to help survivors of sexual violence cope with the present and aftermath of sexual violence. These teams are a collaborative effort, and include (a) mental health agencies, (b) rape crisis advocates, (c) law enforcement personnel, (d) detectives or investigators, (e) emergency departments, (f) sexual assault nurse examiners (SANEs), and (g) attorneys (Mosteller, 2010). SANEs are forensic nurses who have been certified to work with victims of sexual violence. Some of the functions of the SANE are to perform a physical examination of the survivor, collect forensic evidence, provide expert testimony regarding forensic evidence collected, support the psychobiological needs of the survivor, be part of the sexual assault response team (SART), and work closely with law enforcement agencies and the prosecutor's office.

Calling Hotlines or Other Sources

If the sexually assaulted individual calls a hotline, a sexual assault and violence prevention center, the police, or a campus medical center, there is certain information the sexually assaulted person needs to know. The assaulted person should have an advocate who can explain more about the person's options and rights (refer to Box 22-1).

Emergency Departments

When an individual who has been sexually assaulted seeks treatment, he or she is most likely seen in the emergency department (ED). People who have been sexually assaulted often go to the ED to find emotional support, help in regaining a sense of control, and reassurance regarding their safety. A sexual assault victim who arrives at the ED should not be left alone. The staff should provide privacy, and the victim should be a priority in triage.

The nature of sexual assault carries with it complex implications, and the individual requires psychological support,

---

| BOX 22-1 | INFORMATION TO HELP A RECENT VICTIM OF SEXUAL VIOLENCE IN THE AFTERMATH OF RAPE (EITHER ON THE PHONE OR IN PERSON) |

1. Go to a safe place immediately.
2. Consider reporting the rape to the police, or the campus police if it happened on campus.
3. You can report the assault and later choose not to pursue criminal proceedings.
4. If you choose not to report the assault immediately, you can do it at a later time.

Preserve evidence of the rape:

1. Do not wash your hands or face.
2. Do not shower or bathe.
3. Do not brush your teeth.
4. Do not change clothes or straighten up the area where the assault took place.

Offer information regarding the locations of a sexual assault response team (SART), a violence prevention resource center, a crisis center, or an emergency department in the area.

Explain that even if the victim chooses not to press charges, the victim can still have a forensic examination without the rape being reported to the police.

Data from UC San Diego. *What to do if you are raped.* Retrieved May 23, 2011, from www.UCSD.edu/current-students/wellness/_organizations/sarc/if-you-are-raped.html.

---

medical care, documentation of pertinent history, a thorough physical examination, and collection of specimens for use as forensic evidence. Often the physical examination and the collection of evidence are performed by a gynecologist, an ED attending physician, or a SANE. The person who collects the evidence should be knowledgeable in the collection of such data. Unfortunately, facilities differ widely in the kind of care they provide, and the ideal is not always the case—care is not always compassionate, comprehensive, or competent. Most hospitals have an institutional protocol for evidence collection and use "rape kits." Correct preservation of body fluids and swabs is essential because DNA (deoxyribonucleic acid; genetic mapping) can help identify the rapist. If a date rape drug is suspected, a urine sample should be collected.

The individual has the right to refuse legal help and medical examination. Sexual assault survivors need to know they have the right to refuse police assistance but still can choose to have forensic evidence collected. To collect evidence, a *consent form must be signed* to take photographs, perform a pelvic examination, and carry out any other procedures necessary to collect evidence and provide treatment. The individual also needs to know that all documentation is confidential—that no one can access the information without permission, unless the case goes to court. Treatment and documentation need to be accurate and meticulous (Ernoehazy et al, 2009) because the documentation constitutes legal evidence.

Caution is proposed against the use of pejorative language when documenting the history, findings, and verbatim statements. For example:

- Instead of "alleged," use *reported*
- Instead of "refused," use *declined*
- Instead of "intercourse," use *penetration*
- Instead of "in no acute distress," *describe the behavior*

After the immediate medical issues of the patient have been addressed, it is important to perform as many elements of the *forensic examination* that the individual will allow. Once the evidence is collected, it is imperative that providers maintain a "chain of custody" until it is turned over to the authorities.

ASSESSMENT GUIDELINES

Sexual Assault

1. Assess and document the circumstances of the event, including presence of threats (force, trauma, weapons, resistance, sexual acts), location of incident, and circumstances surrounding the assault. *Document in patient's own words* when possible.
2. Gather data that may be used as criminal evidence in court using the institution's protocol.
3. After consent forms have been signed, forensic evidence (debris) should be obtained from clothing, fingernail scrapings, head hair, and pubic hair; smears for sperm and/or acid phosphatase should be taken from any orifice involved. (*Note:* Elevated prostatic acid phosphatase levels are indicative of the presence of semen.) Permission for any photographs taken during the assessment also needs to be obtained. (Guidelines 3 through 8 are all considered forensic evidence and can be used in court at a later date.)
4. Assess for evidence of any physical trauma (e.g., bites, stab wounds, contusions, gunshot wounds). Use drawings and photos.
5. Perform pelvic exam to identify vaginal and cervical trauma (perform anal exam in males and sodomized females). Culture for STDs.
6. Perform psychological assessment, noting reactions to the rape event (e.g., crying, fearfulness, agitation, preoccupation). Describe all behavior in writing.
7. Perform a mental status examination.
8. Determine drug use by either assailant or survivor. Assess situation for potential involvement of date rape drug if it occurred in a large gathering (e.g., college campus, bar). A urine sample might be useful if timing is correct. Emphasize to individuals that even if they were drinking, they are *not* at fault for being assaulted. (See Table 22-1 for drugs associated with sexual assault.)
9. Identify the victim's support system (e.g., family and friends or others the person trusts), and ask for permission to involve them. Explain possible delayed reactions that might occur.

DIAGNOSIS

Rape-Trauma Syndrome

The nursing diagnosis *Rape-Trauma Syndrome* is a variant of posttraumatic stress disorder (PTSD) and is a common sequela of psychological trauma. Left untreated, psychologically traumatic events can have devastating effects. PTSD, depression, panic disorder, suicidal ideation and attempts, and substance abuse are more prevalent among survivors of sexual assault.

There are two phases of rape-trauma syndrome. The acute phase begins immediately after the crisis, followed by the long-term phase, which may occur as long as 2 weeks after the rape and may last years if untreated. *Rape-Trauma Syndrome: Compound Reaction* is also a likely diagnosis and includes both the acute phase of disorganization and the long-term recovery phase. Unfortunately, some people with PTSD (as a result of rape or other trauma) never fully resolve or recover from devastating traumatic events.

The Acute Phase

Typical reactions to crisis often reflect cognitive, affective, and behavioral disruptions. The most common responses are shock, numbness, and disbelief. A person may appear self-contained and calm. At other times, cognitive function may be impaired, and the person may have difficulty making decisions, solving problems, or concentrating. Or the person may cry, become hysterical, be restless, or even smile.

The Long-Term Phase

It is important to teach individuals what to expect during this phase so they will be prepared and not feel that they are "going crazy" or "losing their mind." It is also important to understand that all assault survivors will deal with the event in their own manner. Common symptoms of PTSD related to sexual assault include the following:

- **Re-experiencing the trauma:** Recurrent nightmares about the rape, flashbacks, or uninvited, intrusive thoughts day or night
- **Social withdrawal:** Called "psychic numbing" and involves not experiencing feelings of any kind
- **Avoidance behaviors and actions:** Avoidance of all places and activities, as well as thoughts or feelings, that could recall events about the rape
- **Increased psychological arousal characteristics:** Exaggerated startle response, hypervigilance, sleep disorders, or difficulty concentrating
- **Fears and phobias:** Fear of being alone, fear of sexual encounters, fear of the indoors or outdoors are just some examples
- **Nightmares and difficulty sleeping:** Vivid nightmares of the event waking the individual and causing terror, disturbing sleep, and preventing sleep

OUTCOMES IDENTIFICATION

Short-Term Goals

The patient will:

- Have a short-term plan for handling immediate situational needs before leaving the ED.
- Have a written list of common physical, social, and emotional reactions that may follow a sexual assault before leaving the ED.
- State the results of the physical examination completed in the ED.
- Have written access to information on obtaining competent legal counsel and community supports (individual or group) before leaving the ED.
- Have a follow-up appointment with a rape counselor or crisis counselor.
- Have support from family and friends.
- Have a list and telephone numbers of clinics or rape crisis counselors.

Long-Term Goals

The ideal outcome is that the person eventually will be able to:

- Find ongoing support to help the individual deal with the many confusing and terrifying issues and thoughts regarding the event(s).
- Return to precrisis level of functioning with minimal or no residual symptoms (survivor).

- Experience hopefulness and confidence in going ahead with life plans.
- Have comfortable and enjoyable sex (it may TAKE MANY YEARS to become a survivor for this to happen)

IMPLEMENTATION

These patients require compassionate care. **Follow the sexual assault protocol provided in your ED procedure manual. Most protocols will include the following guidelines:** treatment of all physical injuries, STD prophylaxis, pregnancy prevention (if patient agrees and your state laws allow), forensic evidence collection, and counseling.

Compassionate care involves approaching the person who has been sexually assaulted in a nonjudgmental and empathic manner. Patients need to hear and understand that the rape is *not their* fault, and confidentiality should be stressed repeatedly. It is important to help survivors and their significant others separate the issues of vulnerability from blame. Although individuals may have made choices that made them more vulnerable to assault, they are **not** to blame for the rape. See Table 22-2 for a list of interventions to be used for the victim of sexual assault.

Pharmacological, Biological, and Integrative Therapies

Emergency Department

As discussed, treatment of the sexually assaulted individuals should address physical injuries, pregnancy prophylaxis, and

TABLE 22-2 INTERVENTIONS FOR SEXUAL ASSAULT	
INTERVENTION	**RATIONALE**
1. Have someone stay with the patient (friend, neighbor, sexual assault advocate, or staff member) while he or she is waiting to be treated in the ED.	1. People in high levels of anxiety need someone with them until anxiety level is down to moderate. Never leave the patient alone.
2. **Very important:** Approach patient in a nonjudgmental manner.	2. Nurses' attitudes can have an important therapeutic effect. Displays of shock, horror, disgust, or disbelief can increase anxiety and shame.
3. **Confidentiality is crucial.**	3. The patient's situation is not to be discussed with anyone other than medical personnel involved unless patient gives consent.
4. Explain to the patient the signs and symptoms that many people experience during the long-term phase, for example: a. Nightmares b. Phobias c. Anxiety, depression d. Insomnia e. Somatic symptoms	4. Many individuals think they are going crazy and are not aware that this is a process that many people in their situation have experienced.
5. Listen and let the patient talk. **Do not** press the patient to talk.	5. When people feel understood, they feel more in control of their situation.
6. Stress that the patient did the right thing to save his or her life.	6. Victims of rape might feel guilt or shame. Reinforcing that they did what they had to do to stay alive can reduce guilt and maintain self-esteem.

TABLE 22-2 INTERVENTIONS FOR SEXUAL ASSAULT—cont'd

INTERVENTION	RATIONALE
7. **Do not** use judgmental language: • Reported *not* alleged • Declined *not* refused • Penetration *not* intercourse • Instead of reporting "no acute distress," describe the behavior	7. Pejorative terms often reflect old myths and a lack of knowledge and understanding regarding the rape victim's experience and need for immediate intervention. Words like "alleged," "refused," and "intercourse" all minimize the devastation of the event.
Forensic Examination and Issues 1. Assess the signs and symptoms of physical trauma.	1. Most common injuries are to the face, head, neck, extremities.
2. **Explain and get permission from patient to take photos and specimens.**	2. Patient's consent is needed to collect and document evidence, which may be later used in court.
3. Make a body map to identify size, color, and location of injuries. Ask permission to take photos.	3. Accurate records and photos can be used as legal evidence in the future.
4. Carefully explain all procedures before doing them (e.g., "We would like to do a vaginal [rectal] examination and do a swab. Have you had a vaginal [rectal] examination before?").	4. The individual is experiencing high levels of anxiety. Matter-of-factly explaining what you plan to do and why you are doing it can help reduce fear and anxiety.
5. Explain the forensic specimens you plan to collect; inform patient that specimens can be used for identification and prosecution of the rapist, for example: • Debris in head hair and pubic hair • Skin from underneath nails • Semen samples • Blood • Urine sample (if date rape drug is suspected)	5. Collecting body fluids and swabs is essential (DNA) for identifying the rapist.
6. Encourage patient to consider treatment and evaluation for sexually transmitted diseases before leaving the ED.	6. Many survivors are lost to follow-up after being seen in the ED or crisis center and will not otherwise get protection.
7. Offer prophylaxis to pregnancy.	7. Approximately 5% of women who are raped become pregnant.
8. All data must be carefully documented: • Verbatim statements • Detailed observations of physical trauma • Detailed observation of emotional status • Results from the physical examination • All lab tests should be noted	8. Accurate and detailed documentation is crucial legal evidence.
9. Arrange for support follow-up: • Rape counselor • Support group • Group therapy • Individual therapy • Crisis counseling	9. Many individuals can be burdened with constant emotional trauma. Depression and suicidal ideation are frequent sequelae of rape. The sooner the intervention, the less complicated the recovery may be.

sexually transmitted diseases. Common examples of physical injuries may be abrasions or contusions. More serious injuries might include broken bones, knife wounds, and injuries around the eyes, nose, and abdomen. The most common injuries are to the face, head, neck, and extremities.

According to the 2005 National Crime Victimization Survey, 5% of rapes resulted in pregnancy for a one-time unprotected sexual assault (Rape, Abuse & Incest National Network [RAINN], 2006). The American College of Obstetricians and Gynecologists (ACOG, 2004) recommends offering emergency contraception to all women who have been assaulted or are at risk of pregnancy. Even if a woman chooses not to take the medication for personal reasons, treatment should be available.

The Centers for Disease Control and Prevention (CDC) recommends prophylactic STD treatment for the most common sexually transmitted diseases (chlamydia, gonorrhea,

APPLYING THE ART

A Person Experiencing Sexual Assault

SCENARIO: A neighbor brought 40-year-old Margaret to the ED following her report of a sexual assault by a 20-something male who gained access to Margaret's home by claiming the need to make a phone call because of car trouble. The ED staff were very busy caring for many acute patients. My student status enabled me to provide continuity of care so I could stay with Margaret, never leaving her alone in the ED. I established the contact, struggling to hear Margaret, who spoke in a whisper.

THERAPEUTIC GOAL: By the close of this interaction, Margaret will allow herself to acknowledge her survival and to express her concerns.

STUDENT-PATIENT INTERACTION	THOUGHTS, COMMUNICATION TECHNIQUES, AND MENTAL HEALTH NURSING CONCEPTS
Margaret: *Voice tense.* "I don't want to be alone. Not now. Not ever." **Student's feelings**: *I would be afraid to be alone, too, if someone attacked me in my own home. But why did she trust a stranger? I struggle with countertransference. I have to be alert to not blame the victim as a way to distance myself; if I make this Margaret's fault, then rape cannot happen to me.*	Margaret started our interaction with a whisper, which makes me think she may be reacting with the *controlled style* in this *acute phase of the rape-trauma syndrome*. Yet, her tense assertion of not wanting to be alone may indicate the *expressed style*.
Student: "I am staying right here with you. You've been through a terrible ordeal."	I *offer self* and *attempt to translate* into feelings.
Margaret: "I feel so ashamed."	Earlier Margaret asked for water and I had to say no until all the evidence is collected. I am staying alert and especially careful to follow the rape crisis protocol for this ED for Margaret's sake and for any legal ramifications.
Student: "What happened was not your fault. You don't have anything to be ashamed of." **Student's feelings:** *Without thinking, I immediately reassured Margaret that she has no reason to be ashamed. Even as I speak the words, I notice Margaret pulling away. I wonder now, if I wasn't really reassuring myself.*	Reassurance seems supportive but actually discounts the patient's feelings. Margaret feels more alone now.
Margaret: "You don't understand. No one does." *Looking downward.*	
Student: "You're right. I don't understand what you went through. Margaret, I care about what happened to you and I want to understand." **Student's feelings:** *I do care about Margaret.*	I *offer self* and *give control* to Margaret, acknowledging that only she knows her experience.
Margaret: "I don't know how I will ever tell my husband." *Eyes swell with tears, which she angrily brushes away, then proceeds to rub her temples.*	
Student: "You feel worried about his reaction."	I *attempt to translate into feelings* by saying "worried." I assess Margaret's *anxiety* to be at least *moderate*. *Physical signs* arise at the *severe level* and Margaret is now rubbing her temples, as though she has a headache. Though she did not report a headache at the intake assessment, Margaret's stress and anxiety may be stimulating additional physiological responses.
Margaret: "Why would he even want to be with me—damaged goods."	

APPLYING THE ART—cont'd

A Person Experiencing Sexual Assault

STUDENT-PATIENT INTERACTION	THOUGHTS, COMMUNICATION TECHNIQUES, AND MENTAL HEALTH NURSING CONCEPTS
Student: "You feel damaged, unlovable." ***Student's feelings:*** *I feel sad that she has the added burden of dealing with the reactions of loved ones who might not be supportive.* **Margaret:** "Unlovable." *Eyes again fill with tears. Margaret presses her fists against her eyelids.*	I use *restatement* and *attempt to translate into feelings.*
Student: "Margaret, it's okay to cry." *Margaret shakes her head.*	I give permission to lend *support* and *acceptance.*
Student: "I wonder what it would mean to you to cry." **Margaret:** *Breathing deeply to suppress tears.* "That I am a weak woman, so weak I couldn't stop that monster." ***Student's feelings:*** *It's kind of scary. This could be me at another time.*	I ask an *indirect question* to assess underlying dynamics. She uses the word "monster." It must have been such a horrible violation of her personhood.
Student: "You had the strength to stay alive. You did what you had to do to survive. Your instincts acted properly to keep you alive." **Margaret:** "I am alive. Damaged, but alive." *Eyes water.*	I give *support* affirming that Margaret was, in fact, able to stay alive. She survived the assault.
Student: "You look close to tears." *She nods.* "It's okay to grieve, to let your feelings out." **Margaret:** *Sobs, accepts a tissue, and holds on to my hand.* ***Student's feelings:*** *I feel Margaret's trust that she reaches for my hand.*	I *make an observation.* Sharing the pain and allowing the *grief* decrease the intensity of the pain. Just then the rape crisis counselor and sexual assault nurse examiner arrive.

trichomoniasis, and bacterial vaginosis [BV]). The guidelines also recommend a collection of serum for immediate evaluation for HIV, hepatitis B (if not immunized), and syphilis. Any survivor with abrasions should be immunized for tetanus if 5 years have elapsed since the last immunization.

Pharmacology

Short-term treatment with a benzodiazepine may help ameliorate acute anxiety and agitation that follow a trauma. Antidepressants (selective serotonin reuptake inhibitors [SSRIs]) may be helpful for symptoms of PTSD such as hyperarousal, agitation, and insomnia and in the treatment of depression and panic attacks.

Psychotherapy

Crisis counseling should always be available to any person who has been sexually assaulted, including referrals to their family physician, community psychologist, or community rape crisis line, for example. If no SART is available, information on support groups, therapists, and attorneys who work with sexual assault survivors should be provided before the person leaves the ED. A list of safe houses should also be available for those involved with intimate partner violence (IPV). Caring for survivors is not completed in a single visit. Their emotional state and other psychological needs should be assessed within 24 to 48 hours by phone after being treated and actual resolution may take years in some cases.

Group therapy or support groups can be beneficial for survivors. Sharing experiences with others who are going through the devastating physical and emotional aftermath of rape can be healing and break through feelings of isolation, shame, and guilt.

Therapy for Rapists

Alterations in thinking and behavior need to be undertaken in order to effect change. Unfortunately, most rapists do not acknowledge the need for change. No single method or program of treatment has been found to be totally effective.

EVALUATION

Most patients will be able to eventually resume their previous lives after supportive services and crisis counseling or therapy. If survivors are relatively free of signs of PTSD and their lifestyles are close to their lifestyles before the rape, the recovery is considered successful. Too often, without counseling of some kind, various sequelae of the assault may remain for years or a lifetime.

KEY POINTS TO REMEMBER

- Sexual assault is an act of violence, control, and hate; it is a criminal offense that often results in severe long-term psychiatric trauma for the victim.
- To preserve forensic evidence, the victim should be aware of precautions to take before contacting the police, crisis center, or emergency facility.
- Contact with the sexual assault patient usually takes place in the ED. Ideally, nurses with special training (SANEs) assess the patient, collect data, and provide information and referrals (e.g., therapists, legal counsel, support groups) for patients before they leave the ED.
- Permission is necessary for collecting forensic data, performing a pelvic examination, and taking photographs. Confidentiality is stressed.
- Following the sexual assault, a forensic examination is conducted and evidence is collected. The patient should be given medications to protect against STDs, evaluated for pregnancy, offered prophylaxis, and tested for HIV and syphilis. If abrasions are noted, a tetanus shot may be indicated in accordance with the guidelines of the CDC and ACOG.

- Careful documentation of findings (diagrams and photos), observations of emotional status, and description of the events surrounding the assault are documented using verbatim statements whenever possible.
- Assessment for "date rape" drugs should be included if description of the event indicates that possibility. In such a case, a urine sample may be obtained.
- To help alleviate anxiety, explanations of all interventions or procedures are provided to the patient before they are performed.
- Before leaving the ED, sexually assaulted individuals are told what kinds of reactions are commonly experienced by sexually traumatized victims following a crisis.
- Follow-up counseling, support groups, and resources to effective legal attorneys who specialize in sexual assault should always be given before discharge from the ED.

APPLYING CRITICAL JUDGMENT

1. Sally M. is brought by a friend to the ED. She is dazed, and the friend explains that a few friends went to a bar and met some guy Sally had met at a party on campus. He bought them all drinks. Sally said that after a few drinks, "I felt funny and don't remember much except that I woke up outside the back of the bar with my underclothes off and a number of reddened marks and abrasions on my breasts and arms. I have so much pain and burning in my vagina. I feel like I'm going crazy, I am so frightened." Her friends found her semiconscious and brought her to the ED. Sally appears confused and alternates between crying uncontrollably and staring into space. She repeatedly says she wants to wash up and change clothes, but her friend wanted her to come into the ED as soon as possible.
   A. Chart the objective and subjective symptoms of Sally's physical and emotional trauma using the guidelines from this chapter including a body map.
   B. After Sally consents to the forensic examination, how would you describe to her the procedures that will be performed during the forensic and pelvic examination?
   C. Why might you ask Sally for a urine specimen at this time?
   D. Sally is afraid and does not want her parents or anyone on campus to know what happened, and especially does not want to be reported to the police. What information could you give to her that may allay some of her concerns?
   E. Describe the emergency medical treatment that should be offered to all sexually assaulted individuals.

   F. There is no SART in your area but you know that Sally may experience devastating sequelae of her sexual assault that can take years or longer to resolve. What kinds of supports and referrals should Sally be given before she leaves the ED?
   G. Use the computer to find websites that are available in your community to aid rape victims; print a handout with names, addresses, and phone numbers.
   H. Determine if there is a sexual assault response team (SART) in your community. Using the computer, secure the phone number, address, and website address and share this information with your classmates.
   I. Determine if there is a sexual assault nurse examiner (SANE) in any of your community clinics or crisis centers and share this information with your classmates.
2. A friend calls you at 3 AM and tells you that she has been raped and has run out of the man's apartment to a nearby coffeehouse, not knowing what to do. You tell her you will meet her at the coffeehouse and then take her to the emergency department. You tell her not to go home. What are some other things you would instruct your friend not to do to help preserve evidence?
3. Share among five different young people in separate situations the following guidelines for diminishing the ingestion of date rape drugs when at large parties, raves, night clubs, or rock concerts, for example (RWU, 2011a).
   1. Do not accept open drinks (i.e., alcoholic or nonalcoholic beverages from strangers or others you do not know well or trust; this includes drinks that are in a glass).

APPLYING CRITICAL JUDGMENT—cont'd

2. When in bars or clubs always get your drink directly from the bartender and do not take your eyes off the bartender when you order; do not use the waitress or let somebody else go to the bar for you. At parties only accept drinks in closed containers: bottles, cans, or Tetra Paks.

3. Never leave your drink unattended or turn your back on your table.

4. Do not drink from "resources like punch bowls, pitchers, tubbs, or community water/juice bottles."

5. Stay alert; if there is talk of date rape drugs or your friends seem "too intoxicated" for what they have taken, leave the party or club immediately and do not go back!

From U.S. Department of Health and Human Services, National Institutes of Health, National Institute on Drug Abuse, 6001 Executive Blvd., Washington, DC. Available at http://teenadvice.about.com/Box.

CHAPTER REVIEW QUESTIONS

Choose the most appropriate answer(s).

1. A 19-year-old college student, Jan, is taken to the ED by her friend. Her friend states that she was sexually assaulted at a frat party. Jan has given permission for a forensic examination (photos and specimens). Choose the nursing action you would take when working with a victim of sexual assault.
   1. Suggest she should clean up before the vaginal exam in order to feel less violated.
   2. Explain that everything will be okay, and that it usually takes a month or two to get over, in order to calm her down.
   3. Try to get her to tell you as much about the assault that she can remember, so you can put the information in your report to the police.
   4. Explain all procedures before doing them (e.g., vaginal and rectal exams, obtaining forensic specimens (e.g., semen samples, debris pubic hair, etc).

2. In the medical record of a victim of rape, which of the following types of data are inappropriate to document?
   1. Observations of the patient's physical trauma using a body map
   2. Assessment of signs and symptoms of emotional trauma
   3. Verbatim statements made by the patient
   4. Details of the patient's sexual history

3. When an ED nurse is providing care to a rape victim, which two of the following are important elements of care?
   1. Providing nonjudgmental care
   2. Conveying disgust that this would happen
   3. Aligning with her sense of blaming herself
   4. Assuring confidentiality

4. Which of the following observations, if found in the medical record of a sexual assault survivor, would indicate that "reorganization" after a rape crisis was not yet complete? The patient is:
   1. free from somatic reactions.
   2. generally positive about self.
   3. calm and relaxed during interactions.
   4. experiencing frequent nightmares.

5. A patient asks the nurse if she should leave her husband who has been sexually violent to her. The best response by the nurse would be:
   1. "It will be safer for you to divorce your husband."
   2. "Often women are in more danger during the separation period."
   3. "He will appreciate you more after you leave him."
   4. "I cannot professionally respond to your question."

REFERENCES

American College of Obstetrics and Gynecology (ACOG). (2004). *Acute care of sexual assault victims.* Retrieved July 30, 2007, from www.acog.org/departments/dept_notice.cfm?recno=17&; bulletin=1625.

Blackwood, C. L. (2005). Sexual assault. *Clinics in Family Practice, 7*(1).

Breaks, StarmanTeen (2011a). *Incest, and sexual abuse.* Retrieved May 17, 2011, from www.teenbreaks.com/sexual abuse/incestsexual abuse.cfm.

Breaks, Teen (2011b). *Rape and date rape.* Retrieved May 17, 2011, from www.teenbreaks.com/sexualabuse/rapedaterape.cfm.

Centers for Disease Control and Prevention (CDC). (2011). *Understanding sexual violence: fact sheet.* Retrieved May 16, 2011, from www.cdc.gov/violenceprevention.

Centers for Disease Control and Prevention (CDC). (2009). *Sexual violence: definitions.* Retrieved May 21, 2011, from wwwcdc.gov/Violenceprevention/sexualviolence/definition.html.

Cleveland Clinic Foundation. (2009). *Raising healthy infants, children and teens: rape and date rape.* Retrieved May 21, 2011, from http://my.clevelandclinic/healthy_living/violence/hic_rape_and_date_rape.aspx.

DC Rape Crisis Center. (2007). Retrieved February 10, 2007, from www.dcrcc.org/same-sex.htm.

Ernoehazy, W., Dyne, P. L., et al. (2009). *Sexual assault: emergency department care.* Retrieved May 21, 2011, from http://emedicine.medscape.com/article/806120-treatment.

Fears, D., & Lydersen, K. (2007a). *Native American women face high rape rate.* Retrieved August 20, 2011, from http://washingtonpost.com./wp-dyn/content/article/2007/04/25/AR 2007042502778.ht.

Fears, D., & Lydersen, K. (2007b). *Native American women phase 5 rape rates, report says*. Retrieved August 20, 2011, from www.WashingtonPost.com/wp-dyn/then/article/2007/04/25/yeah theyare200704250778.ht.

Jefferies, D. B. (2011). *The sexual rape of men*. Retrieved May 17, 2011, from www.womans radio.com/articles/The-Rape-of-Men/9507.html.

Mosteller, S. (Summer 2010). *The efficacy of SART's related rape trauma*. International Association of Forensic Nurses. Retrieved May 22, 2011, from www.iafn.org/display common.cfm?an=1&sub articlenbr=487.

National Crime Victimization Survey. (2005). *Crime and survivors statistics*. Retrieved February 8, 2007, from www.ojp.usdoj.gov/bjs/cvict.htm.

Parents for Megan's Law and Crime Victims Center (PML). (2007a). *Statistics: child sexual abuse*. Retrieved May 21, 2011, from www.parentsformeganslaw.org/public/statistics_childsexual abuse.html.

Parents for Megan's Law and Crime Victims Center (PML). (2007b). *Statistics-rate: who are the victims?* Retrieved May 22, 2011, from www.parentsformeganslaw.org/public/statistics_rape.html.

Rape, Abuse & Incest National Network (RAINN). (2006). *Pregnancies resulting from rape*. Retrieved February 8, 2007, from rainn.org/get-information/statistics/sexual-assault-victims.

Roger Williams University (RWU). (2011a). *Sexual assault: date rape drugs*. Retrieved May 22, 2011, from www.rwu.edu/studentlife/studentservices/counselingcenter/sexualassault/date rapedrug.

Roger Williams University (RWU). (2011b). *Sexual assault: rape myths and facts*. Retrieved May 22, 2011, from www.rwu.edu/studentlife/studentservices/counselingcenter/sexual assault/.

Starman, U. K. (2011). *Myths about male rape, the rape of men*. Retrieved May 21, 2011, from HCWaest.org.uk/survivors/male/myths_about_male_rape.htm.

The Economist. (May 5, 2011). Combating rape in prisons: Little and late, efforts to stop the sexual abuse of prisoners are welcomed but overdue. Retrieved May 28, 2011, from http://www.economist.com/node/18651484.

Tjaden, P., & Thoennes, N. (2006). *Extent, nature, and consequences of rape survivorization: findings from the National Violence Against Women Survey*. Washington, DC: National Institute of Justice, Report NCJ 2103346.

UC San Diego. *What to do if you are raped*. Retrieved May 23, 2011, from, www.ucsd.edu/current-students/wellness/_organizations/sart/if you are raped.html.

Viguera, A. C., & Mian, P. (2004). The patient who has been sexually assaulted. In T. A. Stern, J. B. Herman, & P. L. Salvin (Eds.), *Massachusetts General Hospital guide to primary care psychiatry* (2nd ed.). New York: McGraw-Hill.

Suicidal Thoughts and Behaviors

Elizabeth M. Varcarolis

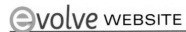 WEBSITE

http://evolve.elsevier.com/Varcarolis/essentials

KEY TERMS AND CONCEPTS

completed suicide, p. 436
Modified SAD PERSONS Scale
p. 440
physician-assisted suicide (PAS),
p. 436
postvention, p. 442

psychological postmortem
assessment, p. 446
suicidal ideation, p. 436
suicide, p. 436
suicide attempt, p. 436

SELECTED CONCEPT: Thoughts on Suicide

"Suicide in its many forms has inspired everything from condemnation to romanticism, most focusing on the morality of taking one's own life and whether it can be justified as a reasonable option."

Most people do not want to die; they just don't know how to live with their prolonged deep psychic pain.

And, what about a patient whose every moment is suffering intractable pain from a terminal illness, and wants to leave life with some dignity, and has control over when and how to say goodbye to loved ones. *(Vaughanbell, 2008)*

OBJECTIVES

1. Contrast and compare pros and cons of the "right to die" physician-assisted suicide (PAS) as outlined in the chapter.
2. Explain the role of culture, religion, and socioeconomic status as they relate to suicidal risk.
3. Provide patient-centered care by discussing the implications of the risk factors identified in the Modified SAD PERSONS Scale when determining risk for suicide potential.
4. Promote safety by discussing the kinds of safety procedures that are followed for an acutely suicidal individual who has been hospitalized.
5. Describe the need and rationale for postvention for family or friends of an individual who has completed suicide.
6. Discuss the need for a psychological postmortem assessment postvention that includes all staff involved in an inpatient suicide.

OBJECTIVES—cont'd

7. Identify the needed interventions that might provide quality improvement methods to help identify and prevent suicide for our returning war veterans.

8. Summarize the overt, covert, and behavioral clues and the steps in evaluating the lethality of a suicide plan for an individual who is contemplating suicide.

9. Utilizing informatics, make a list of community support groups within your community that might help people who are suicidal, such as support groups for veterans, suicide hotlines, crisis centers, substance use groups (e.g., AA, SMART).

10. Applying communication techniques, identify some of the most important dialogue and questions needed to promote safety.

Suicide is an act of desperation. Most individuals do not want to die; they just do not know how to go on living with their psychic and/or physical pain. Suicide is a global problem, and according to the World Health Organization (WHO), in the last 45 years suicide rates have increased by 60% worldwide (Befrienders Worldwide, 2009). WHO also found that suicidal thoughts, plans, and attempts appear to be similar across the globe (Nauret, 2008).

Suicide or completed suicide is the act of intentionally ending one's own life and opting for nonexistence. The act of purposeful self-destruction by taking one's own life arouses intense and complex emotions in others. Suicide attempt includes all willful, self-inflicted, life-threatening attempts that have not led to death. Suicidal ideation means a person is thinking about self-harm. *Always* take an individual very seriously if he or she mentions some form of suicidal ideation. *Always* ask, "Are you thinking of harming [killing] yourself?" Listen very carefully to what the person does and does not say. Appropriate nursing interventions are outlined later in this chapter.

Suicide can be understood from a variety of different perspectives: religious, philosophical, sociological, psychological, and biological.

The more recent growth of the secular philosophy—the foundation of which is respect for an individual's will and basic human rights—has influenced the perception of suicide in our society. This philosophy has led to a movement that supports the right of mentally competent adults to humanely end their own suffering. The natural extension of this perspective is the practice of physician-assisted suicide (PAS) for the terminally ill, which operates under very strict guidelines. For example, Washington state, which passed the PAS Law in 2009, states that the following conditions must exist:

- The patient must not have any neuromedical or psychiatric conditions that impair capacity to reason and process information.
- The patient must be diagnosed as having less than 6 months to live.
- The patient must make a request orally and in writing, and have the agreement for PAS approved by two different physicians.
- After a 15-day waiting period, the patient must then make the request again.

In the United States, there are presently (February, 2012) only two states that have legalized PAS: Oregon (Death with Dignity Law) and Washington. There are a couple of states that have bills pending legislation. However, it may be helpful to understand why some people are proponents of physician-assisted suicide. The following statement was made by Montana's State Justice Warren when the law first passed before it was overturned by the state legislator in 2011 (Kirkland, 2010):

…a competent, incurably ill person (who is)…going through prolonged (terminal) suffering and shows excruciating physical deterioration to hang on to the last possible moment…. The state has not come close to showing that it has any interest, much less a 'compelling' one in serving a competent, incurably ill individual's autonomous decision to contain a licensed physician's assistance in dying so that she(he) may die with the same human dignity with which she(he) was born.

At present, only a few jurisdictions legally sanction PAS, besides Oregon and Washington state, and those include the Netherlands, Belgium, and Switzerland (CBC News, 2009). The "right to die with dignity" issue is vastly controversial and complex.

PREVALENCE AND COMORBIDITY

In 2007, suicide was the eleventh leading cause of death in the United States for all age-groups (Centers for Disease Control and Prevention [CDC], 2010). The greatest number of suicides occur in younger and middle-aged adults (Conwell et al., 2011). It is the third leading cause of death for adolescents 15 to 24, as well as the fastest growing group of suicides (Black & Andreasen, 2011). Suicide is the second leading cause of death for those between 25 and 34 years old, and the third leading cause of death for those 35 to 44 years old (CDC, 2010). Among older adults, suicide is the eighth leading cause of death for the 55- to 64-year-old age group and it seems to have declined in those 65 and older (CDC, 2010, 2011).

However, this is likely to change again because the baby boomer cohort (1946 to 1964) has a higher rate of suicide than any other cohort group and the front runners of this group started reaching the age of 65 in 2011 (Conwell et al., 2011).

Epidemiological surveys have demonstrated that 90% of suicide attempters have a diagnosable psychiatric condition (Mann, 2011).

The risk of suicide in people with a major depressive disorder (MDD) is about 20 times that of the general population. Alcohol and substance abuse are often contributing factors. Patients who have schizophrenia, dementia, bipolar disorder, anxiety disorder (especially panic disorder and posttraumatic stress disorder [PTSD]), personality disorders (such as borderline, paranoid, and antisocial), and other psychiatric disorders all have higher rates of suicide than people in the general population.

The Department of Veterans Affairs has been tracking the **suicide rate among Iraq and Afghanistan veterans** since 2008. The statistics show that one in five deaths of young veterans is a result of suicide (Glantz, 2010). This does not account for the risky behavior that resulted in a disproportionate rate of veterans returning to civilian life and dying from motorcycle accidents, motor vehicle accidents, or unintentional poisonings. Psychologists speculate that these deaths are most likely related to risky behaviors common among people with PTSD (Glantz, 2010). For example, in California, more than 1000 veterans died of suicide between the years 2005 and 2008. This suicide rate was three times higher than the number of servicemen from California who were killed in the Iraq and Afghanistan conflicts over the same period (Glantz, 2010).

Traumatic brain injury (TBI) refers to any type of trauma to the head that affects brain functioning. It is estimated that between 15% and 23% of returning war veterans have experienced a TBI, which can have a severe impact on a person's functioning (Beck Institute Blog, 2010). It is believed that those who tested positive for TBI were more likely to be diagnosed with depression, anxiety disorders, PTSD, adjustment disorders, psychosis, and bipolar disorders (Tull, 2010). The most prevalent mental health problems that veterans have upon their return are PTSD, depression, extreme alcoholism, and often combinations of these three.

Physical illnesses may also play a role in increasing suicide risk. It is estimated that 5% of suicide completers had a serious medical condition at the time of their suicide (Black & Andreasen, 2011). For example, people with terminal and/or painful diseases such as acquired immunodeficiency syndrome (AIDS), cancer, chronic renal failure requiring hemodialysis, head injury, multiple sclerosis, and Parkinson's disease are at an increased risk for suicide. Intentional death, either physician-assisted or self-inflicted, may be a means of escaping from intolerable pain and extreme limitations imposed by illness. Therefore nurses may well encounter individuals with suicidal thoughts or active intent in outpatient settings, intensive care units, nursing homes, or medical-surgical units; during home visits; or even among one's own circle of family and friends.

Certain medications may also contribute to symptoms of depression, thus raising an individual's risk for suicide. Some medications commonly associated with depression are antihypertensives, benzodiazepines, calcium channel blockers, corticosteroids, hormonal medications, and medications to treat pain.

THEORY

Sigmund Freud (1856-1939) developed some of the first psychological theories of suicide in the early 1900s. Freud described suicide as a murderous attack on an ambivalently loved, internalized significant person, often referred to as murder in the 180th degree. Building on Freud's theory, **Karl Menninger** (1893-1990) suggested that all suicides experience three interrelated emotions: revenge, depression, and guilt.

Edwin Shneidman (b. 1918) proposed that victims of suicide suffer unbearable psychological pain, a sense of isolation, and the perception that death is the only solution to their situation. In essence, an individual feels that "there is no way out." Shneidman identified self-destructive behaviors (e.g., compulsive use of drugs, hyperobesity, gambling, self-harmful sexual behaviors, and medical noncompliance) as **sub-intentioned suicide.**

Herbert Hendin, medical director of the American Foundation of Suicide Prevention, states that Shneidman was the first person in the United States to call public attention to the problem of suicide. Hendin goes on to say that, "however, the biggest advances in the field of suicide prevention in the last 15 years have been in the field of biology and the pharmacology of depression and suicide; it borders on malpractice for a doctor not to prescribe medication for seriously depressed individuals" (Curwen, 2004).

Contributing Risk Factors for Suicide

Many risk factors may be involved, but there is no single theory that explains suicide. There are, however, some commonalities. Mann (2011) cites a number of clinical studies that indicate factors that are thought to contribute to an increased risk for suicide. Such factors include aggressive/impulsive traits, hopelessness or pessimistic traits, substance abuse and alcoholism, a history of physical or sexual abuse during childhood, a history of head injury or neurological disorder, and cigarette smoking. Therefore, there are many factors that influence the risk for suicide, but it is thought that acute risk is associated with anxiety, insomnia, and substance abuse.

People who attempt or complete suicide often have poor critical thinking skills, have troubled emotional lives (depression, anger, anxiety, guilt, boredom), and have a low threshold for emotional pain. Please note that a person may experience one or more risk factors and not be suicidal.

Poland (2009) cites recent assessment of markers for youth suicide that involved family and developmental background:

- Children or teens who lost a parent to suicide are three times more likely to commit suicide
- Childhood maltreatment
- Problematic family relations
- History of bullying and victimization
- Family history of suicide
- Socioeconomic problems
- Parental psychopathology
- Peer problems
- Legal and/or discipline problems

See Figure 1-1 on p. 6 for a clinical algorithm for the suspicion of suicide risk.

Neurobiological Aspects of Suicide

Serotonin (5-HT, 5-hydroxytryptamine) is an important neurotransmitter. Scientists have identified a strong association between suicide and the molecular genetics of the neurotransmitter serotonin. For example, people who attempted suicide have lower serotonin functioning; however, those who have completed suicide have the lowest levels. Studies of the brains of those who have completed suicide show abnormalities of the serotonin system in parts of the prefrontal cortex in an area of the brain called the *ventral medial prefrontal cortex* (Mann, 2011). Low levels of serotonin in cerebral spinal fluid (CSF) have long been associated with impulsive suicide-like violence (Black & Andreasen, 2011). Low levels of serotonin are known to be a significant factor in people who develop depression.

Biological responses to *stress* may also constitute a risk factor for many people. The **noradrenergic system** is a mediator of acute stress responses and overactivity of that system has been associated with both severe anxiety or agitation and higher suicidal risk, according to Mann's (2011) research of the literature. The **hypothalamic-pituitary-adrenal (HPA) axis** is another major stress response system. The HPA axis is associated with major depression and suicide victims often exhibit HPA axis abnormalities (Mann, 2011).

Genetic Factors

Suicide has long been shown to cluster in some families; therefore family history is pertinent. A striking example is the novelist Ernest Hemingway's family in which five members in four generations committed suicide (a number of Hemingway's family members suffered from mental illness or substance abuse). Several lines of research indicate both twin and adoption studies are linked to suicide behavior independent of psychiatric disorders (Black & Andreasen, 2011). For example, concordance rates are higher in monozygotic twins (same genetic makeup) than dizygotic twins (two separate genetic makeups). When identical twins (monozygotic) are adopted out to separate homes, the suicide concordance rate is significantly higher than in fraternal twins (dizygotic) who are adopted out to separate homes. To date, no specific gene has been isolated; however, research is looking at a genetic link between serotonin-related genes and suicidal behavior and impulsive aggression (Mann, 2011).

Societal Factors

Societal factors that may increase the potential for suicide include loss or lack of social supports, negative life events, and severe life stress. Therefore suicide potential is apt to be higher among individuals facing these circumstances, including those who are impoverished; are recently divorced, separated, or bereaved; are childless or homeless; live alone; have few to no supports; and are grappling with recent negative life events. Suicide also seems to be higher among the unemployed. The CDC (2011) studied suicide rates from 1928 to 2007, and for the most part found that during economic turndowns and weakened economies the suicide rate seemed to rise, and during economic expansions the suicide rate seemed to fall, especially for people in the working age-group (i.e., 25 to 64 years old).

Psychological Factors

People who are psychotic are at a high risk for suicide, especially those who experience command hallucinations telling them to kill themselves or having delusions that they must die. There is a trio of psychological-emotional factors often present when people become suicidal: hopelessness, helplessness, and feelings of worthlessness. Hopelessness refers to lack of purpose in life, helplessness refers to lack of social supports, and worthlessness refers to low self-esteem or lack of love for self. In other words, people may contemplate suicide when they feel trapped and there is "no way out." Often this type of thinking is precipitated or intensified by a negative and overwhelming event.

Suicide risk factors include:

- Presence of a plan
- Previous suicide attempt
- History of mental disorder, particularly depression or alcohol or drug abuse
- Impulsive or aggressive tendencies
- Adverse life events, recent or expected loss
- Feelings of hopelessness or isolation
- Family history of mental or substance abuse disorder
- Family history of suicide, or prior suicide attempt
- Family violence, including physical or sexual abuse
- Incarceration
- Exposure to suicidal behavior of others, including family, peers, newsworthy persons, or fiction
- Chronic physical illness, particularly if associated with chronic pain

Age

Adolescents and young adults. Suicide rates are increasing at the highest rate in the 14- to 24-year-old age group. The data seem to point to increased rates of alcohol/drug use in depression among this age cohort. American Native Americans have the highest suicide rate (National Adolescent Health Information Center [NAHIC], 2006). The strongest risk factors for youth are substance abuse, aggression, disruptive behaviors, depression, and social isolation. The following other factors are related to youth suicide:

- Frequent episodes of running away
- Frequent expressions of rage
- Family loss or instability
- Frequent problems with parents
- Withdrawal from family and friends
- Expression of suicidal thoughts or talk of death or the afterlife when sad or bored
- Difficulty dealing with sexual orientation
- Unplanned pregnancy
- Perception of school, work, or social failure

Older adults. A study by the CDC (2011) examining suicide rates from 1928 to 2007 found that two age-groups—65 to 74

EXAMINING THE EVIDENCE

But I Am Not a Psych Nurse...Dealing With Suicide in Nonpsychiatric Settings

I have noticed in my clinical rotations that there are many "psych" and suicidal patients admitted all over the hospital and not just to psychiatry. I plan to work on a medical-surgical unit, and never thought I would be dealing with these issues. How much should I know about taking care of the suicidal patient?

You definitely need to be capable of caring for suicidal patients in all kinds of health care facilities.

The Joint Commission's *Sentinel Events Alert* warns that the rate of suicide in nonpsychiatric patients has been increasing. Suicide is the eleventh leading cause of death in the United States, and in hospitals primarily occurs in emergency departments and medical-surgical inpatient units. The *Alert* urges greater attention to the risk for suicide for these patients and recommends education for health care workers about warning signs that may indicate when patients in the general hospital are contemplating harming themselves. Suicide is one of the five most serious and most frequently reported events made to The Joint Commission (Freeman, 2011). Nearly 25% of completed suicides occur in nonpsychiatric settings, and this topic remains an inadequately addressed concern (Guptill, 2011).

Because many patients do not have a psychiatric history or history of suicide attempts, assessment of risk factors can be difficult. Some risk factors for hospitalized nonpsychiatric patients are dementia, traumatic brain injury, chronic pain or intense acute pain, poor/terminal prognosis, and substance abuse (Freeman, 2011). Among the reported events, the location of the suicides included bathroom, closet, shower, and patient room (Boudreaux, 2011). It is easy to create a safety plan for the person who declares he or she is suicidal, but it is very different for people who appear calm and rational but have chronic illnesses that impact their body, lifestyle, or finances (Fiebig, 2011). The psychological well-being of persons who make serious attempts is usually minimally addressed whereas the focus is on the immediate physical concerns. Suicide and self-harm attempts are highly stigmatized and lead to shame and guilt in the attempter, and even resentment and anger from families and caregivers. Health care workers may not know how to discuss these issues with patients (Guptill, 2011).

Staff needs to be educated about suicide risk factors such as a history of suicide, recent losses, and use of antidepressants. Encouraging staff to role-play situations such as scenarios in which an actively suicidal patient wants privacy in the restroom, refuses to talk with you, or states he/she is truly "fine" has been found to decrease staff anxiety. Necessary interventions to ensure safety are to monitor the patient for "cheeking" medications for a future overdose and to remove sharps, belts, ropes, and glass objects from the patient area. Because attempts may only take a second to complete, close staff supervision is essential at all times, including monitoring toileting and bathing activities. Training materials with policies, procedures, communication techniques, and mental health resources in the hospital and community must be easily accessible on every hospital unit (Guptill, 2011). Recently, following a suicide in an ED, a "wraparound safety system" was instituted for patients identified as a suicide risk—there is a "warm handoff" of the patient from point to point, so that the patient is never left alone (Boudreaux, 2011).

Staff must feel empowered to take actions such as placing a patient on constant observation and/or contacting the mental health professional if changes occur or if there are any questions/concerns (Freeman, 2011). Screening tools for depression can be utilized on any unit, but need to be user-friendly for all those without specialized training. Staff must be alert to patients who appear calm and rational and sincerely state they will not harm themselves. Blindly trusting a suicidal patient can prove deadly (Guptill, 2011).

The challenge is that most health care providers do not want to talk about suicide in acute care (Boudreaux, 2011). The fact that two thirds of patients who commit suicide have seen a primary care provider in the month before their deaths indicates that health care professionals in general are missing opportunities to intervene. Even though there is discomfort and often fear of the topic of suicide, we need to make suicide risk a part of routine health assessments in all specialty areas in order to save lives.

Boudreaux, E. (2011). Suicides in the hospital: the liability risk nobody wants to talk about. *Healthcare Risk Management, 33*(3), 25-36.

Fiebig, W. (2011). What if patients don't volunteer info? *ED Management,* January 2011.

Freeman, G. (2011). TJC warns of ED suicide risks. *Healthcare Risk Management, 33*(1), 10-11.

Guptill, J. (2011). After an attempt: caring for the suicidal patient on the medical-surgical unit. *Medsurg Nursing, 20*(4), 163-168.
Contributed by Lois Angelo.

years and 75 years and older—exhibited decreasing rates in that time period, contrary to present thinking. However, as mentioned previously, with the influx of the baby boomer cohort, this trend toward decreasing suicide rates among older adults may well change (refer to Chapter 28).

Risk factors to be assessed among older adults include social isolation, solitary living arrangements, widowhood, lack of financial resources, poor health, and feelings of hopelessness.

Most older adults who commit suicide have visited their primary care physician in the month before the suicide, sometimes that very day. Recognition and treatment of depression in the medical setting are promising ways to prevent suicide in older adults.

CULTURAL CONSIDERATIONS

When examined as a function of age, gender, and race, the statistics for suicide identify a more complex picture. For example, the rates for both black and white women are the lowest, with white females committing more suicides than black females. Female suicide rates peak through midlife and then subsequently decline. Black males represent the next highest group of suicides, with these men experiencing two peaks—first in young adulthood and second in old age. However, the highest rates of suicide overall are for white men at every point in life. The rates for this group are dramatically higher than any other group, increasing significantly during midlife and then dramatically peaking in the oldest age group (Conwell et al., 2011).

The meaning of suicide has traditionally reflected the religious beliefs of a culture. For example, in cultures derived from a Judeo-Christian background, life is considered a gift, and to take away one's life is a sin. Cultures that derived from Catholic teachings (South America, Spain, Italy, Ireland) often have lower rates of suicide (Carroll-Ghosh et al., 2003). By the same token, people who practice the Japanese Shinto religion believe in reincarnation. Therefore death may be seen as an honorable solution to life's problems. Japan has the second highest rate of suicide among industrialized nations since the economy declined in the late 1990s, and a high percentage of suicide rates are attributed to poor job prospects (Yamaguchi, 2011). Research supports the growing concern over the suicide rates among migrant communities such as African and East Asian Americans. This trend appears to be increasing with native and indigenous populations, such as Native Americans in the United States and Alaska and the regional needs in Australia and New Zealand (Befrienders Worldwide, 2009). According to the CDC (2010) the suicide rate among American Indian/Alaskan Native adolescents and young adults age 15 to 34 are 1.8 times higher than the national average for that age group.

There are protective factors in many cultures or subcultures. Protective factors for African-American men and women as a whole include religion and the role of the extended family, both of which provide a strong social support system. Among Hispanic Americans, the Roman Catholic religion (in which suicide is a sin) and the importance given to the extended family decrease the risk for suicide. Among Asian Americans, suicide rates are noted to increase with age. Beliefs that reduce suicide include adherence to religions that tend to emphasize interdependence between the individual and society (i.e., self-destruction is seen as disrespectful to the group or selfish).

APPLICATION OF THE NURSING PROCESS

ASSESSMENT

There are a number of tools one can use to ascertain risk factors when assessing for potential suicidal behaviors. An acronym that can facilitate the health care worker's recall when in the midst of crisis situations is the Modified SAD PERSONS Scale (Box 23-1). The SAD PERSONS Scale is commonly used today in emergency departments since it is well suited to emergency department staff by helping them evaluate the urgency of the need for referrals to mental health sources/or protective care (Wyatt and colleagues, 2012).

Verbal Clues

Always take a suicide threat seriously. Whether a person makes 1 or 1000 threats, take the threat seriously. Assessing verbal clues includes the following:

Overt statements
- "I can't take it anymore."
- "Life isn't worth living anymore."
- "I wish I were dead."
- "Everyone would be better off if I died."

Covert statements
- "It's okay now. Everything will be fine."
- "Things will never work out."
- "I won't be a problem much longer."
- "Nothing feels good to me anymore, and probably never will."
- "How can I give my body to medical science?"

Behavioral Clues

Sudden behavioral changes may be noticed, for example:
- Giving away prized possessions
- Writing farewell notes
- Making out a will
- Putting personal affairs in order
- Having global insomnia
- Exhibiting a sudden and unexpected improvement in mood after being depressed or withdrawn
- Neglecting personal hygiene

Lethality of Plan

The evaluation of a plan is extremely important in determining the degree of suicide risk. The main elements in assessment should include the following:
- How detailed is the plan?
- How lethal is the proposed method?

BOX 23-1 MODIFIED SAD PERSONS SCALE*

S	Sex	1 male
A	Age	1 if <19 or >45 years, or*
D	Depression or hopelessness†	2
P	Previous attempts or psychiatric care	1
E	Excessive alcohol or drug use	1
R	Rational thinking loss (psychotic or organic illness)	1
S‡	Separated, widowed, divorced	1
O	Organized plan or serious attempt	2
N	No social support	1
S‡	Stated future intent (determined to repeat or ambivalent)	1

Guidelines for Action

POINTS	CLINICAL ACTION
0-5	May be safe to discharge (depending upon circumstances). (If sent home, have follow-up appointment arranged and discharge patient with family/friend.)
6-8	Probably requires psychiatric consultation.
>8	Probably requires hospital admission, voluntary or involuntary. (Would need agreement of two psychiatrists for involuntary admission.)

Data from Patterson, W.M., Dohn, H.H., Bird, J., et al. (1983). Evaluation of suicidal patients: the SAD PERSONS Scale. *Psychosomatics, 24,* 343-349; Wyatt, J.P., Illingworth, R.N, Graham, C.A., et al. (2012). *Oxford handbook of emergency medicine* (4th ed., p. 609). Oxford, England: Oxford University Press. There has been more than one modification to the SAD PERSONS Scale by Patterson and colleagues.
*Attempt (**A**) also in this modified scale.
†Two points are given for the combination of depression (hopelessness) and previous attempt.
‡The original SAD PERSONS Scale had **social supports lacking** for the first **S** and **sickness** for the second **S** (which is also a risk factor). In this version, the second **S** stands for **stated future intent.**

- Guns, hanging, carbon monoxide, and staging a car crash are extremely lethal.
- Slashing wrists, inhaling natural gas, and ingesting pills are lower-risk methods.
- Availability of means. Does the person have a gun? Access to a tall building? (Availability is a crucial factor when carrying out a plan.)

ASSESSMENT GUIDELINES

Suicide Risk

1. If a person appears depressed, displays any verbal or behavioral clues, or causes you to be concerned, **always ask: "Are you thinking of harming or killing yourself?"**
2. Assess precipitating event: "Is there something difficult you are facing?"
3. Assess risk factors *as well as* protective factors.
4. Assess history of suicide (e.g., in family, friends), degree of hopelessness and helplessness, and lethality of plan.
5. If there is a history of a suicide attempt, assess:
   - Intent: Is there a high probability of being discovered?
   - Lethality: Was the method used highly lethal or less lethal?
   - Injury: Did the patient suffer physical harm? (e.g., Was the patient admitted to an intensive care unit?)
6. Determine whether the patient's age, medical condition, or psychiatric diagnosis causes the patient to be at higher risk.
7. Red flags include the following:
   - The patient suddenly changes from sad or depressed to happy and peaceful. Often a decision to commit suicide gives a feeling of relief and calm.
   - The patient gives away treasured possessions.
8. If the patient is to be managed on an outpatient basis, also assess the following:
   - Social supports
   - Significant others' knowledge of the signs of potential suicidal ideation (e.g., increasing withdrawal, preoccupation, silence, and remorse)
   - Knowledge of community resources that the patient and family could use for support during the crisis

DIAGNOSIS

Risk for Suicide is the most immediately important nursing diagnosis, and self-restraint from suicide is the ideal outcome. Other nursing diagnoses include *Ineffective Coping, Hopelessness, Social Isolation, Spiritual Distress, Chronic Low Self-Esteem, Disturbed Thought Processes,* and *Post-Trauma Syndrome* among others.

OUTCOMES IDENTIFICATION AND PLANNING

Interventions during the crisis attempt to accomplish both short-term and long-term outcomes include:

Short-term outcomes
- Will have a family member/friend stay with the suicidal individual overnight
- Will have a follow-up appointment with a counselor/therapist
- Will have a list and telephone numbers of self-help groups, hotlines, organizations, therapists in the area where the individual lives

TABLE 23-1 INTERVENTIONS DURING THE CRISIS PERIOD	
INTERVENTION	**RATIONALE**
Forensic Issues	
1. **Follow institutional protocol** for suicide regarding creating a safe environment (taking away potential weapons—belts, sharp objects; checking what visitors bring into patient's room).	1. Provides safe environment during time patient is actively suicidal and impulsive; self-destructive acts are perceived as the only way out of an intolerable situation.
2. Keep accurate and thorough records of patient's behavior—both verbal and physical—as well as all nursing and physician actions.	2. These might become court documents. If patient's needs or requests are not documented, they do not exist in a court of law.
3. Put on either *suicide precaution* (one-on-one monitoring at arm's length away) or *suicide observation* (15-minute visual check of mood, behavior, and verbatim statements), depending on level of suicide potential.	3. Protection and preservation of the patient's life at all costs during crisis is part of medical and nursing staff responsibility. **Follow institutional protocol.**
4. Keep accurate and timely records and document patient's activity—usually every 15 minutes—including what patient is doing, with whom, etc. **Follow institutional protocols.**	4. Accurate documentation is vital. The chart is a legal document regarding patient's "ongoing status" and interventions taken.
5. If accepted at your institution, construct a *no-suicide contract* with the suicidal patient. Use clear, simple language. When contract expires, it is renegotiated.	5. The *no-suicide contract* helps patients know what to do when they begin to feel overwhelmed by pain (e.g., "I will speak to my nurse/counselor/support group/family member when I first begin to think of harming myself").
6. Encourage patients to talk about their feelings and problem-solve alternatives.	6. Talking about feelings and looking at alternatives can minimize suicidal acting out.

Longer-term outcomes

- Optimizes events and environmental factors to help minimize further self-destructive acts
- Is able to explore alternatives and increase problem-solving skills
- Has shown evidence of increased coping skills
- States feelings of isolation and loneliness are less and not so hurtful
- Is engaged in treatment for co-occurring mental health issues (e.g., depression, substance abuse, PTSD)

IMPLEMENTATION

Unfortunately, there seems to be a lack of evidence that supports any particular approach to suicide prevention. Although restriction of access to means, treatment of depression, assistance with problem-solving skills and other therapies, and prescription of psychotropic medications may be effective, none of these interventions has been systematically investigated.

Some interventions are considered to support a person's resilience and act as protective factors:

- Family and community support
- Effective and appropriate clinical care for mental, physical, and substance abuse disorders
- Restricted access to highly lethal methods of suicide
- Cultural and religious beliefs that discourage suicide and support self-preservation instincts
- Acquisition of learned skills for problem solving, conflict resolution, and nonviolent management of disputes
- Cognitive behavioral therapy

Nursing interventions during the crisis are outlined in Table 23-1. Nursing interventions after the crisis period are outlined in and Table 23-2.

Communication Guidelines

Nurses and other health care providers use communication skills and counseling techniques as one of their most important tools. Communication and counseling skills used by the nurse working with a suicidal person are practiced (1) in the community, (2) in the hospital, and (3) on telephone hotlines. During a suicidal crisis, the following information should be conveyed to the patient in all settings:

- The crisis is temporary.
- Unbearable pain can be survived.
- Help is available.
- You are not alone.

Psychotherapy

See Table 23-3 for interventions to be used during follow-up psychotherapy.

Postvention

Intervention for family and friends ("survivors") of a person who has committed suicide—postvention—should be

TABLE 23-2 INTERVENTIONS AFTER THE CRISIS PERIOD

INTERVENTION	RATIONALE
1. Arrange for patient to stay with family or friends. If no one is available and the person is highly suicidal, hospitalization must be considered.	1. Relieves isolation and provides safety and comfort.
2. Weapons and pills are removed by friends, relatives, or the nurse.	2. Helps ensure safety.
3. Encourage patients to talk freely about feelings (anger, disappointments) and help plan alternative ways of handling anger and frustration.	3. Gives patients alternative ways of dealing with overwhelming emotions and gaining a sense of control over their lives.
4. Encourage patient to avoid decisions during the time of crisis until alternatives can be considered.	4. During crisis situations, people are unable to think clearly or evaluate their options.
5. Contact family members; arrange for individual or family crisis counseling.	5. Re-establishes social ties and mobilizes family support to deal with precipitating event(s) or overwhelming situation.
6. Activate links to social supports in the community (e.g., self-help groups).	6. Diminishes sense of isolation and provides contact with individuals who care about the suicidal person.
7. If anxiety is extremely high or patient has not slept in days, an antianxiety or antidepressant might be prescribed. **Only a 1- to 3-day supply of medication should be given. Family member or significant other should monitor pills for safety.**	7. Relief of anxiety and restoration of sleep loss can help the patient think more clearly and might help restore some sense of well-being. Use of SSRIs is felt to be safe for a depressed adult. **Fluoxetine is the only FDA-approved antidepressant for treatment in children** (Barclay & Vega, 2006).

TABLE 23-3 INTERVENTIONS FOR FOLLOW-UP PSYCHOTHERAPY

INTERVENTION	RATIONALE
1. Identify situations that trigger suicidal thoughts (define the precipitating event).	1. Identifies targets for learning more adaptive coping skills.
2. Assess patient's strengths and positive coping skills (talking to others, creative outlets, social activities, problem-solving abilities).	2. Identifies areas to build on and draw from when planning alternatives to self-defeating behaviors.
3. Assess patient's coping behaviors that are not effective and that result in negative emotional sequelae: drinking, angry outbursts, withdrawal, denial, and procrastination.	3. Identifies areas to target for teaching and planning strategies for supplanting negative behaviors with more effective and self-enhancing behaviors.
4. Encourage patients to look into their negative thinking, and reframe negative thinking into neutral objective thinking.	4. Cognitive reframing helps people look at situations in ways that allow for alternative approaches.
5. Point out unrealistic and perfectionistic thinking.	5. Constructive interpretations of events and behavior open up more realistic and satisfying options for the future.
6. Spend time discussing patient's dreams and wishes for the future. Identify short-term goals that can be set for the future.	6. Renewing realistic dreams and hopes can give promise to the future and meaning to life.
7. Identify things that have given meaning and joy to life in the past. Discuss how these things can be reincorporated into the present lifestyle (e.g., religious or spiritual beliefs, group activities, creative endeavors).	7. Reawakens in patient abilities and experiences that tapped areas of strength and creativity. Creative activities give people intrinsic pleasure and joy, and a great deal of life satisfaction.

APPLYING THE ART

A Person With Suicidal Behaviors

SCENARIO: I met 55-year-old Raymond on the adult psychiatric unit following a suicide attempt from a self-inflicted gun-shot would. Raymond had damaged the right side of his neck, face, and part of his ear, but missed every vital vessel and somehow lived. He had shown improvement by participating more actively in group therapy and had progressed from one-to-one observation (no farther than an arm's length away) to close constant observation within continuous visual range. I was meeting with him for the third time.

THERAPEUTIC GOAL: By the conclusion of this encounter, Raymond will feel comfortable enough with me to reveal his suicide attempt.

STUDENT-PATIENT INTERACTION	THOUGHTS, COMMUNICATION TECHNIQUES, AND MENTAL HEALTH NURSING CONCEPTS
Student: "Raymond, I'm here after lunch as agreed."	I *offer self.* Being back when I said I would be builds trust.
Raymond: *Avoids eye contact.* "You can stay if you want. I don't feel like talking much." *Glances up briefly then stares at the floor.*	Although I need to *evaluate* my *nursing practice*, Raymond's behavior change most likely came from his *mood disorder. Depression* influences his perception of just about everything.
Student's feelings: *While reserved, earlier Raymond's voice had more animation. He also made eye contact. Did I do something wrong to impair the relationship?*	
Student: "I'll stay here with you." *I lean toward him with a concerned expression.*	I offer *self* with words and with attending behavior. My silence shows nonjudgmental acceptance.
Student's feelings: *I have the hardest time waiting. I keep wanting to fill the silence. I sit on the left because Raymond has hearing loss on the right from the gunshot wound.*	
Raymond: *Silent for 4 minutes.* "My wife wants a divorce."	Does this increase his suicide risk further? Such a lethal method...to shoot yourself. I remember that sometimes when a suicide fails the patient sees self once again as a failure.
Student's feelings: *Divorce. Another loss. I am beginning to pick up his feelings of hopelessness.*	
Student: "How devastating. How hurtful."	*Reflection* communicates empathy because I have to really connect to be able to discern his probable feeling.
Student's feelings: *Sometimes when I use reflection, I worry that it sounds fake. Maybe because I'm still having to think about how to ask things. Even if I'm wrong about his feelings, I hope he senses that I care, because I do.*	
Raymond: *Nods.* "She said she can't take it anymore."	
Student: "You say she can't take it anymore?"	*Restatement* helps him elaborate.
Raymond: "My depression. Doing this." *Touches the dressing on his ear, carefully shakes his head side to side, then stares downward.*	*Suicide* acts as a two-edged sword, hurting the survivors as well as the patient. I remember reading that suicide also acts as an *attempt* to *communicate*, but what?
Student's feelings: *I wonder what his marriage was like before this. When I have trouble with the people I love I often feel bad about myself too.*	
Student: "You shake your head, like you feel regret."	I *make an observation* and use *reflection.*
Raymond: "About so many things. At my age I should be able to readily name my accomplishments but all I see are my failures. I can't believe she had an affair. Then I look at how I've screwed up and no wonder. I can't even kill myself right."	At the root of all this rests low self-esteem paired with depression. Was his suicide attempt a way to punish his wife as well as himself for being as he says "a screw-up"?
Student's feelings: *Where do I start? His despair makes me feel down, too.*	His age puts him into *generativity vs. stagnation.* To feel he has no accomplishments sounds like stagnation rather than meeting the generativity task.
Student: "You're having trouble finding any reason to choose to live."	The 3-month period after an attempt remains high risk for another suicide attempt. I need to actively assess his suicide potential.
Student's feelings: *I should have checked the chart to see if he has attempted suicide before.*	
Raymond: "Some days more than others."	He feels *ambivalent.* I double-check that the staff member assigned to the close constant observation is indeed watching him.
Student's feelings: *I'm feeling worried that he may attempt again.*	

APPLYING THE ART—cont'd

A Person With Suicidal Behaviors

STUDENT-PATIENT INTERACTION	THOUGHTS, COMMUNICATION TECHNIQUES, AND MENTAL HEALTH NURSING CONCEPTS
Student: "So, sometimes you are able to find something in you worth saving." ***Student's feelings:*** *I feel hopeful that he lets himself experience "some days" when he finds a reason to choose life. I need to help him get the feelings out, both the despair and the hope.*	I give *support.* Using the words, "you are able to" reinforces his *self-esteem.*
Raymond: "I guess so, but not today. Not with divorce papers in my hand." ***Student's feelings:*** *He sounds unsure. It's painful to struggle with depression. I know what depression feels like.*	In report this morning, the nurse indicated that Raymond's antidepressant and therapies may be starting to help. I remember that as *depression lifts,* the patient may experience the energy needed to carry through the *suicide plan.*
Student: "Today you're feeling pretty hopeless." *He nods.* "So hopeless you're thinking about suicide again?" ***Student's feelings:*** *My anxiety skyrockets. Okay. I am right here in the chair next to him. He and I are both safe right now. I can do this.*	His *suicide risk* suddenly increased with the impact of the divorce papers. He does not have a weapon but he could rip out his stitches. I stay alert and watch his hands.
Raymond: *Nods.* **Student:** "Do you have a plan right now?" ***Student's feelings:*** *My heart rate is increasing but I'm keeping my voice calm.*	I ask a *direct question* to *assess suicide risk.* I need to tell staff as soon as I can. He needs to be on a one-to-one with staff only an arm's length away.
Raymond: "It'd be easier at home." ***Student's feelings:*** *He's given a lot of thought to this. I'm doing okay with connecting with Raymond.*	Raymond continues to talk and that is so much healthier than hurting himself.
Student: "So you've thought of suicide while in the hospital, too." **Raymond:** *Looks down.* ***Student's feelings:*** *Is Raymond avoiding eye contact? I don't want to lose the connection.*	The *current risk* takes precedence over thoughts of suicide at home. I *validate* with him. He uses *avoidance.* What is he hiding?
Student: "Raymond, I care about you. Have you done or are you planning to do something to yourself right now?" **Raymond:** *Mumbles.* **Student:** *Moving closer.* "Raymond, I need your help with this. Please. Did you do something?" ***Student's feelings:*** *Part of me prays he will answer me!*	I assess suicidality with a *direct question.* Communicating caring gives support. A *caring relationship* deters suicide.
Raymond: "I saved up all my pills and took them all." **Student:** "When? What? How many?" ***Student's feelings:*** *I feel frantic. Okay, self, mindfully breathe.*	Too many *questions* at once. I will overload him. I need help now.
Student: *I stop asking questions. I call and motion to staff. The nurse comes over to assess and begin emergency intervention with Raymond.* ***Student's feelings:*** *I feel relieved to get help.*	The whole *treatment team* on the psych unit works together. *Confidentiality* always includes the explanation that danger to self or others always gets reported.
Student: *As Raymond is transported off the unit, I walk alongside and I hold out my hand.* "Raymond, you were able to tell me about overdosing. That's a beginning of caring about yourself." ***Student's feelings:*** *By holding out my hand, I nonverbally ask permission to touch.*	My words and nonverbals give *support.*
Raymond: *Squeezes my hand.* ***Student's feelings:*** *I needed to know that he knows that I care.*	

initiated within 24 to 72 hours after the death. Natural feelings of denial and avoidance predominate during the first 24 hours (Thompson, 1996). Mourning the death of a loved one who has committed suicide is painful at all times. Family and friends are often faced with the process of mourning without the normal social supports—unfortunately, neighbors, acquaintances, and even family and friends are often confused and may blame the family for the death. Families with members who have committed suicide are often stigmatized and isolated.

Survivors often feel that they are "going crazy" and need to be told that these feelings are normal. Survivors also need outlets for the undercurrent of anger against the deceased, who is responsible for the trauma, confusion, and pain inflicted on them. Unfortunately, few friends or family members of a person who has committed suicide seek counseling. Pronounced feelings of anger and guilt are common reactions. Within 6 months of the suicide, 45% of the survivors report mental deterioration, with symptoms of depression or posttraumatic stress disorder. Family members of the suicide victim exhibit a higher rate of suicide—4.5 times greater than the risk found in families in which no suicide occurred.

People exposed to traumatic events, such as family/friends who have committed suicide or sudden death of a family member/friend, often manifest the following posttraumatic stress reactions: irritability, sleep disturbances, anxiety, exaggerated startle reaction, nausea, headache, difficulty concentrating, confusion, fear, guilt, withdrawal, anger, and reactive depression. The particular pattern of the emotional reaction and the type of response differ with each survivor depending on the relationship to the deceased, circumstances surrounding the death, and coping mechanisms of the survivor. The ultimate contribution of suicide or sudden loss intervention in survivor groups is to create an appropriate and meaningful opportunity to respond to suicide or sudden death. To reduce the trauma associated with the sudden loss, posttrauma loss debriefing can help initiate an adaptive grief process and prevent self-defeating behaviors.

Self-Care for Nurses

All health care members who provided care for a suicide victim are similarly traumatized by suicide, including medical staff, nursing staff, and ancillary staff. Staff may also experience symptoms of posttraumatic stress disorder with guilt, shock, anger, shame, and decreased self-esteem. Other patients on the unit who may have suicidal tendencies need to be closely monitored as well. The first 24 hours after inpatient suicide is crucial for both safety and crisis management reasons (Ballard et al., 2008).

Among the tasks for staff and administrators is a thorough **psychological postmortem assessment**. The event is carefully reviewed together by all members of the treatment team to identify the potential overlooked clues or faulty judgments, as well as to determine changes that are needed in agency protocols. Most facilities have a clear policy about interventions with families after suicide. Although some lawyers advise all health care personnel who had contact with the family to secure legal counsel, others recommend designating a spokesperson who can follow up and provide family and friends with support without discussing the details of the client's care. Referrals need to be made available to family members and friends to assist them in dealing with and addressing the many emotional reactions and problems that may easily develop, especially among children and adolescents.

With regard to *documentation,* all staff need to ensure that the record is complete and entries are completed in a timely fashion. Legal cases have shown that the client should be periodically evaluated for suicidal risk, that the treatment regimen should provide high-level security, and that staff members should be informed of the individual's treatment.

An excellent article entitled *Aftermath of Suicide in the Hospital: Institutional Response* was first published in *Psychosomatics* (Ballard et al., 2008) and can be downloaded from http://psy.psychiatryonline.org.

Self-help groups are extremely beneficial for survivors of a suicidal family member or friend. Many people join self-help groups, even if the suicide took place 25 to 30 years previously. Self-help groups for the survivors of a family member or friend who committed suicide are similar to all other self-help groups. Essentially, these groups are operated by people who have lost someone through suicide.

Box 23-2 gives some guidelines for coping with a suicide loss. Also, the American Foundation for Suicide Prevention can provide helpful information (www.afsp.org).

BOX 23-2 GUIDELINES FOR SURVIVORS OF SUICIDE

- Know you can survive. You may not think so, but you can.
- Know you may feel overwhelmed by the intensity of your feelings, but all your feelings are normal.
- Anger, guilt, confusion, and forgetfulness are common responses. You are not crazy; you are in mourning.
- Having suicidal thoughts is common. It does not mean that you will act on these thoughts.
- Find a good listener with whom to share. Call someone if you need to talk.
- Do not be afraid to cry. Tears are healing.
- Give yourself time to heal.
- Remember, the choice was not yours. No one is the sole influence in another's life.

- Give yourself permission to get help.
- Be aware of the pain of your family and friends.
- Steer clear of people who tell you what or how to feel.
- Know that there are support groups that can be helpful. If you cannot find one, ask a professional to help start one.
- Call on your personal faith to help you through.
- It is common to experience physical reactions to your grief, such as headaches, loss of appetite, inability to sleep.
- Wear out all of your questions, anger, guilt, or other feelings until you can let them go. Letting go does not mean forgetting.
- Know that you will never be the same again, but you can survive and go beyond just surviving.

Modified from Dunne, E., McIntosh, J., & Dunne-Maxim, K. (1987). *Suicide and its aftermath: understanding and counseling the survivors*. New York: Norton.

KEY POINTS TO REMEMBER

- People who attempt or complete suicide often share many risk factors, but people who have experienced the same risk factors are not always suicidal.
- Psychosis, substance abuse, poor problem-solving skills, impulsivity, and low threshold for pain place people at high risk for suicide when overwhelmed.
- Adolescents, older adults, white males, and Native Americans have the highest rates of completed suicide. Some cultures play a protective role.
- Always try to identify the precipitating event for clues to areas of intervention.
- Assessment should include verbal clues, behavioral clues, and lethality of the plan as evaluation of the risk factors.
- The Modified SAD PERSONS Scale gives a quick overview of major risk factors.

- If suicidal risk is assessed, always ask directly, "Are you thinking of killing yourself?"
- During the crisis period when a person is acutely suicidal, specific interventions can prove helpful (in or out of the hospital) and many save lives (see Table 23-1).
- After the crisis period is over, other interventions can prove helpful in increasing coping skills, enhancing problem solving, and minimizing isolation and loneliness (see Table 23-2).
- Intervention for family and friends of a person who has completed suicide is called postvention. Postvention can help lessen the guilt, anger, grief, pain, and the myriad of emotions that can stay with survivors for years.

APPLYING CRITICAL JUDGMENT

1. Sam Tee is a 62-year-old man whose wife recently died of leukemia. His only son moved to California 2 years ago with his two daughters. Sam had been caring for his wife for 3 years before her death and has become withdrawn and despondent since her death. He is now in the ED after a "fender bender" and is getting two stitches on his ear; his blood alcohol level is 0.9 He does admit to being very depressed after losing his wife, and when you are questioning him about the lethality of plan, he admits to having a gun in the house for protection. You ask Mr. Tee if he has thought about harming himself and he says, "Well, there is always a last resort, isn't there?"

   A. How many risk factors does Sam have using the Modified SAD PERSONS Scale?

   B. Do you think he needs hospitalization? If not, what should be put in place before he returns home? Explain the rationale behind your answer.

   C. What are Sam's needs? What kinds of referrals do you think would help him deal with this crisis?

   D. What do you think about the "fender bender"?

   E. Name at least three groups in your community to which you could refer Sam.

2. Have you ever known anyone who has committed suicide? Contemplated suicide? If so, looking back at the risk factors, do you think there were any options open to these individuals? If so, what might have been available for an effective intervention(s)?

CHAPTER REVIEW QUESTIONS

Choose the most appropriate answer(s).

1. Charles Brown, age 52, lost his wife in an automobile accident 4 months ago. Since then, he has been severely depressed, withdrawn from contacts with family and friends, and taken to drinking to "numb the pain." On the SAD PERSONS assessment scale, how many points does Mr. Brown have?
   a. 3
   b. 4
   c. 5
   d. 6

2. What is the most accurate rationale when planning care for suicidal patients in an inpatient setting?
   1. Suicidal attempts are not likely to occur if there is a consistent team approach.
   2. Aggressive behaviors on the unit indicate a need for staff education.
   3. A completely safe milieu eliminates the chance of suicidal behavior.
   4. There are safety risks in any plan of care that promotes responsibility and growth.

3. Which patient statement indicates that a patient may be a safety risk to self or others?
   1. I really hate being here.
   2. When do staff check patient rooms?
   3. All the rules here are ridiculous.
   4. Which staff are scheduled for tomorrow?

4. In assessing an ER patient who reports taking an overdose of aspirin (ASA), what is the best answer for the nurse to request in assessing the patient?
   1. "How long have you been depressed?"
   2. "Describe your support system."
   3. "When did you take the pills and how many?"
   4. "Are you willing to be hospitalized?"

5. Which statement is correct regarding care of the suicidal patient?
   1. The more specific the plan, the more likely the patient will attempt suicide.
   2. Teens and elderly persons rarely have suicidal ideation.
   3. Patients who survive suicide attempts rarely try again.
   4. Discussion of suicidal thoughts enhances aggressive thinking.

REFERENCES

Beck Institute Blog. (2010). *Veterans with TBI and suicidality.* Retrieved May 31, 2011, from www.beckinstituteblog.org/?category_name=suicide.

Ballard, E. D., Pao, M., Horowitz, L., et al. (2008). Retrieved August 23, 2011, from http://psychiatryonline.org. First published in (2008). *Psychosomatics,* 49(6).

Barclay, L., & Vega, C. (2006). *Antidepressants linked with attempted suicide risk in certain patients.* Retrieved January 18, 2007, from www.medscape.com/viewarticle/548961.

Befrienders Worldwide. (2009). *Suicide statistics.* Retrieved May 31, 2011, from www.befrienders.org/info/index.asp?Page URL=statistics.php.

Black, D. W., & Andreasen, N. C. (2011). *Introductory textbook of psychiatry* (5th ed.). Washington, DC: American Psychiatric Publishing.

Carroll-Ghosh, T., Victor, B. S., & Bourgeois, J. A. (2003). Suicide. In R. E. Hales, & S. C. Yudofsky (Eds.), *Textbook of clinical psychiatry* (4th ed.). Washington, DC: American Psychiatric Publishing.

CBC News. (February 9, 2009). *The fight for the right to die.* Retrieved May 27, 2011, from www.cbc.ca/news/Canada/story/2009/02/09/f-assisted-suicide.html.

Centers for Disease Control and Prevention (CDC). (2011). *Study looks at suicide rates from 1928-2007.* Retrieved May 31, 2011, from www.cdc.gov/media/release/2011/p0414_suiciderates.html.

Centers for Disease Control and Prevention (CDC). (Summer 2010). *Suicide: facts at a glance.* Retrieved May 12, 2011, from www.cdc.gov/violenceprevention.

Conwell, W., Van Orden, K., & Caine, E. D. (2011). Suicide in older adults. In G. S. Alexopoulos, & D. N. Kiosses (Eds.), *Psychiatric clinics of North America* (vol. 34, no. 2). Philadelphia: W.B. Saunders.

Curwen, T. (2004). *His work is still full of life.* Retrieved July 13, 2007, from www.cartercenter.org/news/documents/doc1755.html.

Glantz, A. (2010). *After service, veteran deaths surge: suicide: vehicle accidents, and drug overdoses take lives.* Retrieved May 28, 2011, from www.baycitizen.org/veterans/story/after- JP service-veteran-deaths-surge/.

Juhnke, G. A., Hovestadt, A. J. (1995). *Modified SAD PERSONS Scale.* Using the scale to promote superviser suicide assessment knowledge. *The Clinical Supervisor* 13:31-40.

Kirkland, M. (2010). *US Supreme Court: the right to die vs. the value of life.* Retrieved May 27, 2011, from www.upi.com/Top_News/US/2010/03/21/US-Supreme-Court.

Mann, J. J. (Modified 2011). *Neurobiological aspects of suicide. Using.* Retrieved May 28, 2011, from www.omh.state.ny.us/omhweb/savinglives/volume 2/neurobiological.html.

National Adolescent Health Information Center (NAHIC). (2006). *Suicide: adolescents & young adults: 2006 fact sheet.* Retrieved July 23, 2007, from http://nahic.ucsf.edu/downloads/Suicide.pdf.

National Survey on Drug Use and Health (NSDUH). (2009). *Suicidal thoughts and behaviors among adults.* Retrieved May 28, 2011, from www.oas.samsah.gov/2k9/165/Suicide.htm.

Nauret, R. (2008). *Suicidal risk similar worldwide.* Retrieved May 25, 2011, from http://psychocentral.com/news/2008/02/01/suicidal-risks-similar-worldwide/1865.html.

Patterson, W. M., Dohn, H. H., Bird, J., et al. (1983). Evaluation of suicidal patients: The SAD PERSONS scale. *Psychosomatics,* 24, 343–349.

Poland, S. (2009). *Youth suicide prevention: physicians can make the difference.* Retrieved May 18, 2009, from www.Medscape.com/viewarticle/588917.

Sadock, B. J., & Sadock, V. A. (2007). *Kaplan & Sadock's synopsis of psychiatry* (10th ed.). Philadelphia: Wolters Kluwer/Lippincott Williams & Wilkins.

Thompson, R. (1996). *Post-traumatic loss debriefing: providing immediate support for survivors of suicide and sudden loss*. Ann Arbor, MI: Erie Clearinghouse on Counseling and Personal Services.

Tull, M. (2010). *Posttraumatic stress disorder (PTSD): traumatic brain injuries (TBI) in veterans up mental health risk*. Retrieved May 30, 2011, from http://ptsd.about.com/od/ptsdandthemilitary/a/TBIinOEFOIFVets.htm.

Vaughanbell (2008). *The philosophy of suicide*. Retrieved 8/23/11 from http://mindhacks.com/2008/05/18/the-philosophy of suicide/.

Wyatt, J. P., Illingworth, R. N., Graham, C. A., et al. (2012). *Oxford handbook of emergency medicine* (4th ed., p. 609). Oxford, England: Oxford University Press.

Yamaguchi, M. (2011). *Japan suicide rate still among the world's highest due to low job prospects*. Retrieved May 30, 2011, from www.huffingtonpost.com/2011/03/04/japan-suicide-rate-still-_n_831430.html.

CHAPTER

24

Anger, Aggression, and Violence

Elizabeth M. Varcarolis

evolve WEBSITE

http://evolve.elsevier.com/Varcarolis/essentials

KEY TERMS AND CONCEPTS

aggression, p. 451
anger, p. 451
bullying, p. 451
catastrophic reaction, p. 463
critical incident debriefing, p. 461
comfort rooms, p. 461

de-escalation techniques, p. 456
lateral bullying, p. 451
restraint, p. 457
seclusion, p. 457
violence, p. 457

SELECTED CONCEPT

Bullying can be defined as an offensive, intimidating, malicious, condescending behavior designed to humiliate. Bullying is usually persistent, systematic, and ongoing and is an intentional display and use of *violence,* as subtle as it might appear in some instances.

The term **bullying** is often used when a person or group has power over another.

Lateral bullying refers to bullying by a person of equal status.

OBJECTIVES

1. Discuss the interplay of neurobiology, medical history, past history, and sociological/demographic issues that contribute to risks for violence.
2. Promote safety by demonstrating the physical indicators of a patient who is beginning to escalate out of control.
3. Provide patient-centered care by comparing and contrasting interventions for a patient who is angry and loud in the pre-escalation phase with those for a patient who is escalating to the aggressive phase.
4. Identify the specific safety measures you would take when engaged in de-escalating an aggressive individual.
5. Plan patient-centered nursing care for a patient who is in seclusion.
6. Incorporate evidence-based practice by describing the use of communication and procedures implemented when placing an individual in restraints.
7. Discuss how teamwork and collaboration are vital to applying seclusions or restraints to a patient who is a danger to self or others.
8. Discuss how quality improvement methods can develop from the process of critical incident debriefing.
9. Document an example of the areas for which the nurse must provide written information when violence was averted or actually occurred.
10. Incorporate evidence-based practice by discussing calming and reassuring communications with the patient with a neurocognitive disorder who is disorientated and confused.

The news media brings us daily coverage of terrorism, we watch war on TV in our living rooms, and we hear of violent acts almost every day (such as school shootings, road rage, drive-by shootings, bullying in all strata of American life). We question the effect of exposure to violent video games and the number of murders we witness on our electronic devices every day. Do all of these sources of exposure to violence make us less sensitive and more tolerant to violence?

Universal differentiation among the terms anger, aggression, and violence is difficult or almost impossible because of cultural perceptions and social backgrounds. Anger is a normal—and not always logical—human emotion, and no judgment needs to be passed on it. Anger varies in intensity from mild irritation to intense fury and rage.

Anger can be defined as "an emotional state that may range in intensity from mild irritation to intense fury and rage. Anger has physical effects including raising the heart rate and blood pressure levels of adrenaline and noradrenaline." (Medical Dictionary, 2004). Anger is an emotion like any other emotion, which is usually a response to something that is happening or has happened. Anger may arise as a response to feelings of vulnerability and uneasiness because of a frustration of desire, feelings of hurt, fear, vulnerability, a threat to one's needs (emotional or physical), or a challenge. Simply put, anger is an unplanned reaction to a stressor. Anger is a universal emotion, but not everyone responds to anger with aggression or violence. When anger is managed in a constructive manner (e.g., assertive communication, critical reasoning), anger can help keep people safe and meet needs. Anger becomes unhealthy if it gets in the way of a person's functioning, relationships, or puts others at risk. When anger is left unchecked and escalates, the results often lead to negative forms of aggression or violence. The acting out of anger may meet immediate needs, but at the expense of causing emotional or physical harm to ourselves or others.

Aggression is not the same as violence. Aggression may be appropriate or self-protective—as in protecting oneself, one's family, or a person being bullied—or aggression, defined in the more familiar manner, can be destructive. One definition of aggression includes "the act of initiating hostilities, a feeling of hostility that arouses thoughts of attack, and/or a disposition to behave aggressively" (WordNet 3.1, 2012). These behaviors reflect rage, hostility, and potential for physical assault or verbal destructiveness and can be directed at others or oneself; aggression is a hostile reaction that occurs when control over anger is lost. It is used in an attempt to regain control over the stressor or flee the situation.

Violence does not always have anger as its origin, but it does have the discrete intention of doing harm to a specific person or group and "...connotes extreme, unjustifiable aggression violating social sanctions and causing destruction to another as is its planned result" (Victoroff, 2009, p. 2671). Violence has been defined as "an unjust, unwarranted, or unlawful display of force to inflict harm upon, damage, or violate" (Collins English Dictionary, 2009). Acts of violence lead to significant physical and emotional harm to others. Bullying is an all too common form of violence in our society, workplaces, and even in cyberspace (Brooks, 2011).

BULLYING IN THE NURSING PROFESSION

Lateral violence and bullying seem to have been well documented among health care professionals (Center for American Nurses, 2008), and have been referred to by some as the "silent epidemic." A study by Rowe and Sherlock (2005) found that the most frequent source of bullying in the health care environment was among nurses (27%), followed by patient's families (25%), physicians (22%), and patients (17%). Unfortunately, bullying occurs in all professions. In her article *Bullying Among Nurses*, Dellasega (2009) states:

> Nurses are really vicious to each other.... It's not one hospital. It's not one type of nurse. It's the new nurse, it's the nurse who transferred from another floor, it's the ICU nurses feeling superior to the MedSurg nurses—it is endless.

According to Stokowski (2010), from 21% to 46% of surveyed nurses stated that they had been bullied or witnessed bullying in the hospital workplace. Bullying occurs between persons with different levels of authority (e.g., supervisor or manager bullying a staff nurse) (Center for American Nurses, 2008). Another study found that 65% of nurses had witnessed at least one episode of lateral bullying (Stokowski, 2010). Lateral bullying refers to bullying among those of equivalent status (e.g., employee to employee, nurse to nurse). Bullying or lateral bullying usually infers persistent, systematic, ongoing violence toward a person or group.

Stokowski (2010) identified a list of behaviors that represent bullying among the nursing profession according to a number of nurses who have researched this topic. A partial list includes the following:

- Providing unwanted or invalid criticism, excessively monitoring another's work
- Gossiping, spreading lies or false rumors, assigning derogatory nicknames
- Taking credit for another person's work without acknowledging his or her contribution, blocking career pathways and other work opportunities
- Publicly making derogatory comments about staff members or their work, including use of body language (eye rolling, dismissive behavior), often in front of others
- Using sarcasm or ridicule, making someone the target of practical jokes
- Blaming someone without factual justification
- Allocating unrealistic workloads and not supporting colleagues
- Being condescending or patronizing
- Using physical or verbal innuendo or abuse, using foul language, raising one's voice and shouting or humiliating someone in front of colleagues
- Breaking confidences

Dellasega (2009) identified some attributes that may make one more likely to be bullied:

- Being a new graduate or a new hire
- Receiving a promotion or honor that others feel is undeserved
- Having difficulty working well with others
- Receiving special attention from physicians
- Working under conditions of severe understaffing

All kinds of bullying behaviors create a toxic environment for **all** staff. Nurses new to the health care environment need mentors, support, and encouragement to make them feel proud of the profession they have chosen, and comfortable enough not to leave it. Health care workers who are bullied should be given alternatives and support, and policies should be established to help eliminate an atmosphere where bullying and/or violence exists. Those who are bullied are prone to negative feelings about self, humiliation, poor self-concept, and great emotional pain, and many can suffer severe reactions that may last a lifetime, such as depression, posttraumatic stress disorder (PTSD), anxiety disorders, and worse.

PREVALENCE AND COMORBIDITY

Anger, aggression, and violence are common aspects of social interaction and occur in all environments. Workplace violence in the health care system is notably higher than that found in private sector industries and is not confined to the United States. Workplace-related violence against nurses is a major international occupational health problem. Violence can occur anywhere in the hospital, but is most frequent in psychiatric units, emergency departments (EDs), waiting rooms, and geriatric units. Emergency department nurses experienced the highest rate of on-the-job violence. According to the Emergency Nurses Association (ENA), "more than half of nurses (53.4%) reported experiencing verbal abuse and more than one in 10 (12.9%) experienced physical violence" (Human Capital, 2012).

Specific **medical and neurocognitive disorders** can result in agitated, aggressive, or violent behavior. For example, certain brain tumors, Alzheimer's disease, temporal lobe epilepsy, and traumatic brain injury (TBI) to certain parts of the brain can cause changes in personality that include increased aggression/violence. Other medical conditions that may affect an individual's control of violence are infections, subdural hematomas, Tourette's syndrome, degenerative disorders, endocrine-metabolic imbalances, and intoxication.

THEORY

Environmental and Demographic Correlates of Violence

Probably the strongest predictor of adult violence is *childhood aggression*. Behaviors such as setting fires or performing acts of animal cruelty during childhood, or being diagnosed with conduct disorder, are red flags (Black & Andreasen, 2011). Many violent adults also suffered violence in childhood

(e.g., physical, sexual, emotional abuse), perpetuating the cycle of violence.

One of the strongest contributing factors to violent behavior in clinical settings is the *abuse of alcohol and other substances of abuse* (intoxication or withdrawal), such as amphetamines, cocaine, hallucinogenic drugs, sedative-hypnotics, and others.

Democratic correlates include risk factors such as male gender, young age (15 to 24 years), and family history of violence (Sadock & Sadock, 2010).

Persons of **lower socioeconomic status** are more likely to be perpetrators as well as victims of violence. Poorer populations are more apt to experience discrimination, family breakdown, alienation, and constant fight for survival (Black & Andreasen, 2011). Socially, angry reactions are learned and reinforced through the family and societal norms.

Neurobiological Factors
Brain Structure

There is no one site in the brain responsible for anger, aggression, and/or violence, although there are many areas of the brain that are believed to contribute in some way to either increasing or decreasing these emotions.

Anger biologically stimulates the *hypothalamus,* causing the body to react to the anticipation of harm. Another site known to be associated with aggression is the *limbic system,* which mediates primitive emotion and behaviors that are necessary for survival. The limbic system contains several structures that appear to have a role in regulating the behavior of aggression in humans and animals as well, judging events as either aversive or rewarding. These areas are the hippocampus, septum, cingulate, fornix, and *amygdala*. It is thought that the "amygdala is a vital nexus in the neural network supporting aggression and violence" (Victoroff, 2009, p. 2675) and that the amygdaloid cells are the cells that respond to perceived threats (e.g., emotional facial expressions).

The temporal lobe of the brain receives messages from both the limbic system and the hypothalamus. In the temporal lobe, memory is thought to be integrated; memory of previous insults is important in the cognitive appraisal of threat in the face of new stimuli. This lobe is also the source of complex partial seizures, which may lead to aggressive behavior. One theory is that the prefrontal cortex may play a role in modulating the aggressive impulses in a social context and making judgments of these impulses (Gross & Sanders, 2008). Both magnetic resolution imaging (MRI) studies and positron emission tomography (PET) in the prefrontal cortex showed changes in violent individuals. MRIs show a reduction in the volume of their prefrontal gray matter. PET scans reveal decreased prefrontal blood flow and metabolism (Gross & Sanders, 2008).

Neurotransmitters

It seems that most of the neurotransmitters have some connection or play some part in aggression and violence. However, to date the presence or absence of a single neurotransmitter has not been conclusively identified as a contributing factor for violence, although there have been studies and theories.

In numerous studies, low central *serotonin (5-HT, 5-hydroxytryptamine)* function has been correlated with impulsive aggression as well as an impulsive history of suicide, and with low levels of 5-hydroxyindoleacetic acid (5-HIAA), a metabolite of serotonin, in cerebrospinal fluid (CSF). It is unclear, however, if low levels of 5-HIAA in CSF are a marker for impulsivity or a certain kind of aggression.

As complicated as the catecholamines *(norepinephrine [NE] and epinephrine)* are, they are also thought to play a role in preparing the body for the fight-or-flight response, both on a peripheral level (preparing muscles and cardiac status for fight) and on a cognitive level. NE may enhance vigilance or help in mediating aggression and violence; the effect of NE is unclear at the present time.

EXAMINING THE EVIDENCE

Bullying: Alive and Well in Today's Workplace

I will be graduating soon and am looking forward to a career as an RN. With all the revelations about bullying in nursing, is there a way I can avoid being abused?

Unfortunately, in the nursing profession where "caring" for others is the main focus, bullying is widespread—30% of nurses indicate that they deal with aggression daily, with serious negative outcomes for RNs and their patients. Sabotage, undermining, and destruction of integrity are prevalent with both coworkers (horizontal bullying) and supervisors (bullying toward those with less power) (King-Jones, 2011).

Presently, many facilities and nurse managers condone bullying in all its forms and bullying is definitely a form of violence. It is a significant reason why many nurses leave their work setting and some choose to leave the profession of nursing. There are multiple strategies that can be utilized by both nurse managers and staff nurses to eliminate this abuse/aggression in the workplace. Since peer on peer violence (horizontal violence) is often observed by those in administration, nurse managers have a responsibility to become knowledgeable about hospital bullying in all its forms, to recognize their contributions toward its continuation/enhancement, and to implement strategies toward creating a positive work environment (Brunt, 2011).

The following steps have proven successful for administrators—name the problem and use the term horizontal violence, if appropriate; raise this issue at staff meetings (Longo & Sherman, 2007); take an anonymous survey of nurses on the unit to determine their perception of the emotional climate; distribute a handout on specific bullying behaviors (Dellasega, 2009); allow staff to tell stories of horizontal violence; engage in self-awareness activities of own leadership style to ensure that there is no support or participation in any aggressive/abusive activities; and ensure that all staff participating in horizontal violence be held accountable. One of the most effective leadership strategies is a zero tolerance policy for horizontal violence that is also supported by the facility/human resources department. It is also necessary for human resources to include the concept of horizontal violence/workplace bullying and the use of assertiveness training in orientation programs. A recent study stated that new nurses who were given structured opportunities to practice assertive response statements to abusers were successful in stopping the behaviors when they actually occurred (Longo & Sherman, 2007).

Nurse managers also need to eliminate the "shame and blame" culture common in health care where mistakes are greeted with finger pointing and accusations rather than viewed as learning experiences and opportunities for improvement. There needs to be continual awareness by management that backstabbing, gossiping, and not passing on information are all forms of sabotage that create a major dysfunction in the workplace. In addition, novice nurse workloads should be adjusted to allow opportunities for success, rather than for failure. By enhancing collegiality and collaboration, nurse managers will be helping to decrease horizontal violence and increase staff satisfaction (Weinand, 2010).

Some individual strategies for RNs to combat horizontal violence include the following: work cooperatively with each other despite feelings of personal dislike; do not be overly inquisitive about each other's lives; repay favors and compliments; do not engage in conversations about coworkers; stand up for the absent team member in a conversation where there is criticism (Brunt, 2011). If you witness a bullying situation, intervening in a positive manner can help to change the negative dynamic. Comforting a struggling colleague with a friendly word/an offer of support can be invaluable (Dellasega, 2009).

Hopefully, in the near future nurses not only can avoid the abuse but also can deal with it directly, work on its elimination, and create a workplace culture that celebrates staff achievement and values the gifts that each RN brings to the culture of nursing (Longo & Sherman, 2007).

Brunt, B. (2011). Breaking the cycle of horizontal violence. *ISNA Bulletin,* February/March/April 2011, 6-10.
Dellasega, C. (2009). Bullying among nurses. *American Journal of Nursing, 109*(1), 52-58.
King-Jones, M. (2011). Horizontal violence and the socialization of new nurses. *Creative Nursing, 17*(2), 80-86.
Longo, J., & Sherman, R. (2007). Leveling horizontal violence. *Nursing Management, 38*(3), 34-37.
Weinand, M. (2010). Horizontal violence in nursing: history, impact, and solution. *Journal of Chi Eta Phi Sorority, 54*(1), 23-26.
Contributed by Lois Angelo.

Dopamine (DA) activates the reward center of the brain. One theory regarding dopamine is that if violence is rewarded with an increase in dopamine levels in the brain, then violence is a rewarded behavior and will continue. On the other hand, if the use of aggression/violence does not increase dopamine levels, motivation for aggression is decreased (Victoroff, 2009).

Genetic Factors

Twin studies, adoption studies, studies of twins reared apart, and family and molecular genetic studies have long suggested that there is a genetic component in the etiology of violence. However, as yet there has been no specific chromosomal abnormality associated with increased risk for aggression (Gross & Sanders, 2008). Although there seem to be genetic contributions to aggression, most scientists agree that genetic characteristics alone do not account for the complexities of human behavior.

Most likely the study of the neurobehavioral aspect of violence—particularly frontal lobe dysfunction, altered serotonin metabolism, and the influence of heredity—will lead to a deeper understanding of factors in the genesis of violence. They emphasize that social and evolutionary factors also play a role.

CULTURAL CONSIDERATIONS

Violence is a complex issue. As mentioned previously, socioeconomic issues as well as medical and psychiatric issues are all contributing factors. The different rates of violent crime among societies and within subcultures emphasize the importance of social factors in the genesis of violence. For example, race **or** ethnicity may be a factor. It is estimated that an African-American male has about a 1 in 30 chance of death from homicide, whereas a white male has about a 1 in 180 chance of being murdered (Sadock & Sadock, 2010). A study in 2005 found that 92.6% of African-American victims were murdered by African-American perpetrators. However, white victims were murdered by white perpetrators 84.8% of the time, dispelling a common myth that the more advantaged population suffers violence from the disadvantaged population (Sadock & Sadock, 2010).

Males in general are far more violent than females. Individuals with the highest prevalence of violence appear to be lower-class men with substance abuse disorders or major mental disorders. A subculture that supports the use of intimidation and aggression as an acceptable way of problem solving and achieving social status can reinforce the use of violence as acceptable behavior. This is particularly true in an environment where healthy, appropriate, and effective ways of dealing with frustration, anger, and aggression are not modeled.

APPLICATION OF THE NURSING PROCESS

ASSESSMENT

Subjective Data

On admission, a comprehensive history of the patient is gathered from a variety of sources (utilize informatics to obtain the patient's history, both medical and psychological), including family, friends, and the patient when appropriate. It is important to take an accurate history of the patient's background and usual coping skills, as well as to determine the patient's perception of the issue (if possible). For example, does the patient have a history of previous violence, substance abuse, or psychotic behavior?

The patient should be asked the following questions (Black & Andreasen, 2011):

1. Have you ever thought of harming someone else?
2. Have you ever seriously injured another person?
3. What is the most violent thing you have ever done?

Objective Data

Expressions of anxiety and anger generally look similar. Both may involve increased demands, irritability, frowning, redness of the face, pacing, twisting of the hands, or clenching and unclenching of the fists. Changes in mood and behavior from quiet to talkative and loud, from talkative to silent and withdrawn, from calm to angry, or from depressed to elated also may occur. Box 24-1 identifies signs and symptoms that indicate the risk of escalating anger, which may in turn lead to aggressive behavior. Simple observation of these signs, however, does not provide the information necessary to determine the appropriate intervention.

> **VIGNETTE**
>
> A male abuser has been admitted to the unit for spousal and child abuse. He is considered at high risk for violent acting-out behaviors. Violence can be anticipated to be toward female authority figures and female staff members.

> **VIGNETTE**
>
> An intoxicated, homophobic male is admitted to the unit for detoxification. Violence can be anticipated if an all-male team is brought together to escort the patient to a quiet room.

ASSESSMENT GUIDELINES

Anger, Aggression, Violent Acting Out

1. A history of violence is the single best predictor of future violence.
2. Paranoid ideation and frank psychosis (e.g., command hallucinations) are indicators of possible aggression or violence.
3. Patients who are hyperactive, impulsive, or predisposed to irritability are at higher risk for violence.
4. Assess the patient's risk for violence:
   - Does the patient have a wish or intent to harm?
   - Does the patient have a plan?
   - Does the patient have means available to carry out the plan?
   - Does the patient have demographic risk factors, including male gender, ages 14 to 24 years, low socioeconomic status, and low support system?
5. Aggression occurs most often in the context of limit setting by the nurse.

BOX 24-1   SOME PREDICTIVE FACTORS OF VIOLENT OUTCOMES*

1. Signs and symptoms that usually *(but not always)* precede violence:†
   a. Angry, irritable affect
   b. Hyperactivity: most important predictor of imminent violence (e.g., pacing, restlessness, slamming doors)
   c. Increasing anxiety and tension: clenched jaw or fist, rigid posture, fixed or tense facial expression, mumbling to self (patient may have shortness of breath, sweating, and rapid pulse rate)
   d. Verbal abuse: profanity, argumentativeness
   e. Loud voice, change of pitch, or very soft voice forcing others to strain to hear
   f. Intense eye contact or avoidance of eye contact

2. Recent acts of violence, including property violence
3. Stone silence
4. Suspiciousness or paranoid thinking
5. Alcohol or drug intoxication (withdrawal)
6. Possession of a weapon or object that may be used as a weapon (e.g., fork, knife, rock)
7. Milieu characteristics conducive to violence:
   a. Loud
   b. Overcrowding
   c. Staff inexperience
   d. Provocative or controlling staff
   e. Poor limit setting
   f. Staff inconsistency (e.g., arbitrary revocation of privileges)

*Violent outcomes include screaming, cursing, yelling, spitting, biting, throwing objects, hitting, and punching at self or others.
†Sometimes violence may be perceived to come from "out of the blue."

---

6. Patients with a history of inability to control anger and limited coping skills, including lack of assertiveness or use of intimidation, are at higher risk of using violence.
7. Assess self for personal triggers and responses likely to escalate patient violence, including patient characteristics or situations that trigger impatience, irritation, or defensiveness.
8. Assess personal sense of competence when in any situation of potential conflict; consider asking for the assistance of another staff member.
9. Assess any personal negative thoughts or feelings you might hold toward the patient that might escalate both your anxiety and the anxiety of the patient.

DIAGNOSIS

The safety of patients and others is always the first priority. When anxiety escalates to levels at which there is a threat of harm to self or others, *Ineffective Impulse Control, Risk for Self-Directed Violence* and *Risk for Other-Directed Violence* are primary diagnoses. If a patient's anxiety is escalating and not amenable to early nursing interventions, and if de-escalating techniques are not effective, psychopharmacological means or restraints may be necessary to ensure the safety of patients and staff.

Initially, when anxiety begins to escalate and there is a potential for aggression, *Ineffective Coping* (overwhelmed or maladaptive) is a likely nursing diagnosis. Patients may have coping skills that are adequate for daily events in their lives but are overwhelmed by the stresses of illness or hospitalization. Therefore *Risk for Stress Overload* might be appropriate. A more long-term nursing diagnosis for patients who have a pattern of maladaptive coping that is marginally effective and consists of a set of coping strategies that have been developed to meet unusual or extraordinary situations (e.g., abusive families) would constitute *Ineffective Family Coping*.

Nurses can teach patients methods of coping that will decrease anxiety and distress. However, patient behavior may escalate quickly, or the patient may mask early signs of distress. Nurses may be distracted and may miss those early signs, even when they are visible. Other nursing diagnoses may include *Confusion, Disturbed Thought Processes, Disturbed Sensory Perception,* and others.

OUTCOMES IDENTIFICATION

Short-term or intermediate outcome goals may include the following:
- The patient will display nonviolent behaviors toward self and others *(by date)*.
- The patient will recognize when anger and aggressive tendencies begin to escalate and employ at least one new tension-reducing behaviors at that time (time outs, deep breathing, talking to a previously designated person, employing an exercise such as jogging) *(by date)*.
- The patient will make plans to continue with long-term therapy (individual, family, group, anger management) to work on violence-prevention strategies and increase coping skills *(by date)*.

Long-term outcome goals may include the following:
- The patient and others will remain free from injury.
- Hostile and abusive behavior toward others, property, animals, and so on will cease.
- Use of assertive and cognitive reasoning behaviors to replace aggressive behaviors is in constant evidence.
- A variety of healthy anxiety reduction techniques to keep anger in check will be used.
- Aggressive/violent impulses will be controlled.

PLANNING

Planning interventions necessitates conducting a sound assessment, including history (previous acts of violence, comorbid disorders), present coping skills, and willingness and capacity of the patient to learn alternative and nonviolent ways of handling angry feelings. However, one of the most important aspects of planning is consistency of approach among staff. A clear management approach to dealing with violent situations and individuals includes staff well-versed in unit protocols and well-trained in **de-escalation techniques.** The following questions help determine appropriate planning.

Does the patient have:
- Good coping skills but is presently overwhelmed?
- Marginal coping skills?
- A tendency to use anger or violence as a way to cover other feelings and gain a sense of mastery or control?
- A neuropsychiatric or chronic psychotic disorder?
- A tendency toward violence?
- Cognitive deficits (in the form of misinterpretation of environmental stimuli) that predispose to anger?

Does the situation call for:
- Psychotherapeutic approaches to teach the patient new skills for handling anger?
- Immediate intervention to prevent overt violence (de-escalation techniques, restraints or seclusion, or medications)?

Does the environment provide:
- A safe, therapeutic milieu?
- Privacy for the patient?
- Enough space for patients, or is there overcrowding?
- A healthy balance between structured time and quiet time?

Do the skills of the staff call for:
- Additional education in verbal de-escalation techniques?
- Counseling interventions because of punitive and arbitrary approaches to patients?
- Additional training in restraint techniques?

Planning also involves attention to the number of personnel who are available to respond to a potentially violent situation.

IMPLEMENTATION

Ensuring Safety

Promoting safety is always a first consideration. **Ensure your safety first.** You must feel safe to be able to communicate in a calm manner. Staff and other personnel should be alerted in case reinforcement is needed. The goals are that no one will become hurt and the patient will experience the least restrictive interventions. The following is a list of specific interventions for working with a potentially angry, aggressive, or violent patient:

1. All patients should be searched for contraband and dangerous objects when admitted to the unit and after visits.
2. In some cases supervised visits are advised.
3. Give the patient space. Always minimize personal risks. Stay at least one arm's length away from patient. Use more space if patient is anxious or if you want more space. *Always trust your instincts.*
4. Give adequate space for the patient and staff to ensure easy withdrawal from an escalating situation.

> ### BOX 24-2 SETTING LIMITS
>
> 1. Set limits in only those areas in which a clear need exists to protect the patient or others.
> 2. Establish realistic and enforceable consequences of exceeding limits.
> 3. Make patient aware of limits and the consequences of not adhering to the limits before incidents occur. The patient should be told in a clear, polite, and firm manner what the limits and consequences are, and should be given the opportunity to discuss any feelings or reactions to them.
> 4. All limits should be supported by the entire staff, written in the care plan, and communicated verbally to all involved.
> 5. When a decision to discontinue the limits is made by the entire staff, the decision is based on consistent desired behavior, not promises or sporadic efforts.
> 6. The staff should formulate their own plan to address their own difficulty in maintaining consistent limits.

Adapted from Chitty, K.K., & Maynard, C.K. (1986). Managing manipulation. *Journal of Psychosocial Nursing and Mental Health Services, 24*(6).

---

5. Know where panic buttons or alarms are located. Sometimes it is necessary to wear a body alarm to ensure safety.
6. Exit strategies apply to both the nurse and the patient. The nurse should be positioned between the patient and the door, but not directly in front of the patient or in front of the doorway. Facing the patient can be interpreted as confrontational, and it can also make the patient feel trapped. It is better to stand off to the side and encourage the patient to have a seat.
7. Set limits at the outset (Box 24-2).
   - Direct approach: "Violence is unacceptable." Describe the consequences (restraints, seclusion). Best for confused or psychotic patients.
   - Use the indirect approach if patient is not confused or psychotic. Give patient a choice. "You have a choice. You can take this medication and go into the interview room (or hallway, for example) and talk, or you can sit in the seclusion room until you feel less anxious."
8. When interviewing a patient whose behavior begins to escalate:
   - Provide feedback about what you observe: "You seem to be very upset." Such an observation allows exploration of the patient's feelings and may lead to de-escalation of the situation.
   - If the patient's behavior continues to escalate, end the interview and assure the patient that the staff will provide for the patient's safety (as well as everyone else's safety); then leave the patient.
9. Having enough staff is essential for a show of strength and is often enough to avert confrontation. Only one person should talk to the patient, but staff need to maintain an unobtrusive presence in case the situation escalates.

10. Give the patient the opportunity to voluntarily walk to the quiet room without assistance when team interventions seem appropriate.
11. Do not touch the patient unless the team is with you and you are ready for a possible restraint situation.
12. In the event of a restraint or seclusion situation, the team functions as a single unit, with each member assigned a limb or a function as previously practiced according to unit protocols and policy.
13. Avoid wearing dangling earrings, necklaces, or ponytails. The patient may become focused on these and grab at them, causing serious injury. This is a serious danger.

Stages of the Violence Cycle

When interventions to prevent or deal with patient violence are considered, it is important to take into account the stages of the violence. These stages include the preassaultive stage, the assaultive stage, and the postassaultive stage when the patient returns to baseline. See Chapter 11 for nursing interventions for moderate levels of anxiety that escalates to severe and panic levels.

Preassaultive Stage: De-escalation Approaches

During the preassaultive stage, the patient becomes increasingly agitated. Staff requires training in both verbal techniques of de-escalation and physical techniques to restrain without harm. The better trained the staff, the less chance that either staff or patient will be injured. Frequently verbal interventions are sufficient during this stage. Interventions at this stage are listed in Table 24-1.

Throughout these procedures, maintain the patient's self-esteem and dignity. Linehan (1993) states that respect can be maintained if the nurse operates from the following assumptions:

- Patients are doing the best they can.
- Patients want to improve.
- Patient's behaviors make sense within their worldview.

The use of empathic statements such as, "It sounds like you are in pain and confused," "You're here to get help, and we're going to try to figure out what's going on," and "Let us help you, don't be afraid" can aid in reducing anxiety and anger. These statements reinforce the feeling that the person is in a safe environment and that everyone is there to help in his or her treatment (Petit, 2005).

VIGNETTE

A 24-year-old male who was in an automobile accident is bedridden with a pelvic fracture. During his first day of admission, he yells at each nurse who walks by his room, using expletives in his demands that the nurse enter the room.

Intervention

The nurse who is assigned to the patient for the evening stops in his doorway after he yells at her. She asks in a calm, nonsarcastic manner showing mild disbelief, "Is this working for you? Do nurses really come in here when you yell at them that way?" The patient responds sullenly, justifying his behavior by complaining about his care. The nurse responds by saying, "It seems to me that you need to feel you can get care when you need it." The patient responds in a loud voice that he has been waiting 20 minutes for a bedpan and how would she like it? The nurse gets him his bedpan, and he has calmed down somewhat. The nurse's challenge has caught his attention. The nurse then goes on to suggest (i.e., teach) alternative strategies for contacting her and other nurses. The strategies are immediately put into use by the patient.

When health care personnel can teach patients alternate strategies and healthier ways to meet their needs, then patients have more choices and thus more control over their situation.

Assaultive Stage: Medication, Seclusion, Restraint

The American Psychiatric Nurses Association (APNA) (2000, rev. 2007, p. 5) *Seclusion and Restraint Standards of Practice* states:

> Any staff providing care to persons at risk for harming themselves or others and who participates in seclusion and restraint shall have received training and demonstrate current competency in all aspects of dealing with behavioral emergencies.

Be sure to know the unit/hospital protocol for seclusion and restraint in whatever part of the hospital you choose to work.

If the patient progresses to the assaultive stage, the staff must respond quickly. Generally, a team approach with at least five staff members is advisable to restrain a resistant patient, but the team may be larger if the patient requires it. One leader speaks to the patient and instructs members of the team. Only the leader will communicate with the patient. The interventions include the use of medications and seclusion or physical restraints.

Seclusion "is the involuntary confinement of a person alone in a room or an area where the person is physically prevented from leaving. It may only be used for the management of violent or self-destructive behavior" (APNA, 2007). Restraint refers to (1) "any manual method, or mechanical device, material or equipment attached or adjacent to patient's body where they cannot move their arms, legs, body, or head freely" (Health Care Financing Administration [HCFA], 1999) or (2) "a drug or medication when it is used as a restriction to manage the person's behavior or restrict the person's freedom of movement and is not a standard treatment or dosage for the person's condition" (APNA, 2007).

The least restrictive means of restraint is always tried first and seclusion/restraint is used only after alternative interventions have been attempted (e.g., medications, verbal interventions, decrease in sensory stimulation, removal of a particular problematic stimulus, presence of a significant other, frequent

TABLE 24-1   INTERVENTIONS FOR THE PREASSAULTIVE STAGE

INTERVENTION	RATIONALE
1. Pay attention to angry and aggressive behavior. Respond as early as possible (e.g., Box 24-1).	1. Minimization of angry behaviors and ineffective limit setting are the most frequent factors contributing to the escalation of violence.
2. Assess personal safety and provide for self-care.	2. Pay attention to the environment. • Leave door open or use hallway. Choose a quiet place, but one that is visible to staff. • Have a quick exit available. • If you are uncomfortable, have other staff nearby. • The more angry the patient, the more space needed to feel comfortable. • Never turn your back on an angry patient. • If *on home visit,* go with a colleague. • Leave immediately if there are signs that behavior is escalating out of control.
3. Appear calm and in control.	3. The perception that someone is in control can be comforting and calming to an individual who is beginning to lose control.
4. Do not try to speak while the aggressive person is yelling.	4. Loudly arguing with the patient will only escalate anger and violence.
5. Speak softly in a nonprovocative, nonjudgmental manner.	5. When the tone of voice is low and calm and the words are spoken slowly, anxiety levels in others may decrease.
6. Demonstrate genuineness and concern. • Do not treat the individual in a humiliating manner. • Ask "What will help now?"	6. Even the most psychotic schizophrenic individual may respond to nonprovocative interpersonal contact and expressions of concern and caring.
7. Set clear, consistent, and enforceable limits on behavior (Box 24-2) (e.g., "It's okay to be angry with Tom, but it is not okay to threaten him. If you are having trouble controlling your anger we will help you.").	7. Gives patient understanding of expectations and consequences of not adhering to those behaviors.
8. If patient is willing, both nurse and patient should sit at a 45-degree angle. Do not tower over or stare at the patient.	8. Sitting at a 45-degree angle puts you both on the same level but allows for frequent breaks in eye contact. Towering over or staring can be interpreted as threatening or controlling by paranoid individuals.
9. When patient begins to talk, listen. Use clarification.	9. Allows patient to feel heard and understood, helps build rapport, and energy can be channeled productively.
10. Acknowledge the patient's needs regardless of whether the expressed needs are rational or irrational, possible or impossible to meet.	10. Contributes to individual's perception that the nurse is trying to understand, and try to understand the cores of the aggression. Determine how some of the patient's needs can be met in a productive way.

observation, and use of a sitter who provides 24-hour one-to-one observation of the patient).

Seclusion or restraint is used in the following circumstances (APNA, 2007):

- The patient presents a clear and present danger to self.
- The patient presents a clear and present danger to others.
- The patient has been legally detained for involuntary treatment and is thought to pose an escape risk.
- The patient requests to be secluded or restrained.

Before the development of psychotropic medications, seclusion and restraint were extremely common methods of managing aggressive behavior. In the past half century their use has decreased dramatically as a result of effective medications, as well as concern that such restriction was overused, abusive, and/or dangerous. All facilities that use seclusion and restraint have strict regulatory policies that should follow state, federal, and regulatory agency guidelines. Students as well as all staff members should be familiar with their institutions' policies.

APPLYING THE ART

A Person With Anger and Aggression

SCENARIO: I'd just attended group on the forensic unit where the group leader had to set limits with 24-year-old Hector. During our initial one-to-one, Hector had been almost overly polite in contrast with his abrasiveness with some of the other patients in group. I followed Hector out of the group room.

THERAPEUTIC GOAL: By the end of this interaction, Hector will identify at least one incident where a person can demonstrate an action of kindness or caring towards another and still see self as masculine.

STUDENT-PATIENT INTERACTION	THOUGHTS, COMMUNICATION TECHNIQUES, AND MENTAL HEALTH NURSING CONCEPTS
Hector: *In harsh loud voice.* "Bunch of losers." ***Student's feelings:*** *I was taken aback and intimidated by how lightening-fast Hector's anger arose when some other guys took the seats that Hector had chosen for us during group.*	He went from being friendly with me this morning to this abrupt outburst of anger.
Student: "You're talking about what just happened in group." *I walked towards the seating area closest to the nursing station.* ***Student's feelings:*** *After Hector's bullying episode in group, I feel safer in plain view.*	I *validate* to make sure I understand his reference. I am beginning to realize that Hector's earlier politeness and charm might have to do with his *personality disorder*.
Hector: *In a loud and angry voice.* "Just because I made those guys get out of those seats. What did you think? You think that's such a big deal?"	
Student: "But why did you have to yell and scream at them? I remember some yelling and swearing." ***Student's feelings:*** *I didn't think this through with all his anger coming out. I am reacting defensively, and I'm feeling like I am in way over my head. I feel like I need a break.*	Asking a *why question* is nontherapeutic for sure. He will take it as criticism. I hope he does not get any angrier.
Student: "What were you feeling when you saw they were in the seats you wanted?" ***Student's feelings:*** *I hope he focuses on his feelings rather than my accusatory "why" question.*	I attempt to *translate* into feelings. When in doubt, always go for feelings.
Hector: "Look, I always get a raw deal. The leader likes those guys better than me."	After all this I do not think I will be going with him to *occupational therapy*. That way, I will get to consult my instructor to check if I am on the right track.
Student: "But when this happened, you were feeling… what?" ***Student's feelings:*** *It really is okay to take care of myself. Knowing I can access my teacher soon lets me refocus and attend to Hector's needs.*	I again ask him to *focus* on his feelings.
Hector: "Nothing. Never mind."	I wonder what makes Hector unable to look at his feelings at all. He refers to the leader like he is competing for attention. Almost like *sibling rivalry*. Perhaps all that macho talk hides *low self-esteem*.
Student: "I think I'd feel frustrated when directed to give the other patients their original chairs back. Maybe even a little embarrassed."	I *give information* about self but really the intent serves to *reflect* Hector's possible feelings.
Hector: *Avoids eye contact.* "My dad would've pounded the ____ out of me for letting those guys win."	
Student: "You are able to say how your dad taught lessons with his fists. I'm guessing any little boy would feel enormous pressure when interacting with others means either you win or you get pounded." ***Student's feelings:*** *I'm beginning to see how powerless Hector must feel somewhere inside all that bravado. I am beginning to feel some compassion for him.*	I give *support* by using the words "you are able to" in order to encourage Hector to recognize a link between his current responses and past abusive experiences.

Continued

APPLYING THE ART—cont'd

A Person With Anger and Aggression

STUDENT-PATIENT INTERACTION	THOUGHTS, COMMUNICATION TECHNIQUES, AND MENTAL HEALTH NURSING CONCEPTS
Hector: "He was just teaching me how to be a man."	He justifies his father pounding on him. A *history of violence* is the best *predictor of violence*. Hector defines how to be a man the same way his father did. Does he know other ways exist?
Student: "I wonder if a person can be a man in other ways besides winning or losing. This morning I saw you help when someone bumped the patient carrying breakfasts back for those who eat on the unit." ***Student's feelings:*** *My belief in my nursing self fluctuates. But I do feel some rapport exists between us.*	I use an *indirect question* and make an *observation* of his recent behavior. I know that when a person feels comfortable with you, even if one uses "nontherapeutic techniques" a person will often understand the intent behind the words.
Hector: "What a mess."	
Student: "And you helped anyway. Then when the patient apologized so much, you told him, 'It's okay. Accidents happen.'"	I *make observations* describing Hector's healthier behaviors, like spontaneously helping another.
Hector: "Others helped too."	Hector excels at generating *negative attention*. He does not know what to do with *positive feedback*.
Student: "You also spoke kindly to him."	Again I *make an observation* and give my attention to *positively reinforcing* his kind act.
Hector shrugs.	
Student: "Sometimes it seems manliness and kindness might coexist in one person."	I deliberately link Hector's kind words with his earlier idea of manhood.
Hector: *Nods slightly.* "I need a drink of water." *Goes to water fountain.*	His *intermittent explosive disorder* is most likely connected to his repeated abusive "lessons" equating any vulnerability or even a kindness as weakness.
Student's feelings: *I feel glad that he nods even slightly. I find it difficult to make even small changes, like regularly flossing my teeth. What must Hector's world be like? I have people who care about me. Who does he have for support...especially since he's an expert at pushing others away?*	Hector nods, showing *partial understanding* that demonstrating kindness is okay for a man, although it appears to make him anxious as he uses physical withdrawal (getting a drink) to protect himself (fight-or-flight response).

A patient may not be held in seclusion or restraint without a physician's order (either verbal, written, or telephone order). Sometimes this is not possible, and the decision is made by a qualified staff member to initiate seclusion or restraint because of a behavioral emergency. However, either way, the patient must be evaluated within 1 hour by a physician or licensed independent practitioner (LIP). Restraints may be preferred when staff believe that continued verbal and calming strategies would allow the patient to de-escalate and that restraints could be removed at the earliest possible time (Stokowski, 2007). Mechanical restraints are avoided in individuals who have a history of sexual abuse and trauma, and they also are contraindicated in patients who may be at risk for positional asphyxia or sudden cardiac collapse (Stokowski, 2007). Once in restraint, a patient must be protected from all sources of harm. Each team member is trained in the correct use of physical restraining maneuvers as well as the use of physical restraints. The team is organized before approaching the patient so that each team member knows

his or her individual responsibility regarding limb securing. Before approaching the patient, the team is prepared with the correct number and size of restraints and with medication, if ordered. The team leader explains to the patient in a straightforward manner exactly what the team is about to do and why. If restraints are to be used, the patient is informed at this point of the team's intent and the reason for the team's actions. Sometimes the patient is ready to cooperate and moves to the seclusion room, where either four-point or two-point restraints may be used.

Once the patient is restrained, the nurse might administer an intramuscular injection of an antipsychotic or an antihistamine, depending on the physician's order. The nurse's role is to provide an explanation to the patient for the medication and to make sure that the patient is properly restrained so that the medication can be safely administered. Throughout this time, the team leader continues to relate to the patient in a calm, steady voice, communicating decisiveness, consistency, and control.

While the patient is restrained and in seclusion, staff closely monitor the patient to determine the patient's ability to reintegrate into the unit activities. Usually every 15 minutes face-to-face observation is made through the door window. A person 14 years or younger should have constant face-to-face observation. Reintegration is gradual and is geared to the patient's ability to handle increasing amounts of stimulation. If the reintegration proves to be too much for the patient and results in increased agitation, the patient is returned to the room or to another quiet area.

Generally a structured reintegration is the best approach. For instance, reintegration can begin by reducing four-point restraints to two-point restraints. Once the patient no longer requires the locked seclusion room, the patient may be given specified time-out periods to leave the room and move slowly into the milieu of the unit. The time-out periods are gradually lengthened until the patient is able to maintain control within the unit.

> **VIGNETTE**
>
> A 19-year-old male has a 2-year history of quadriplegia. This patient also has a history of drug abuse that began in grade school, an inability to set or work toward long-term goals, and a primary coping style of anger and intimidation. The patient is admitted to an inpatient psychiatric unit because of increasing suicidal ideation. He clearly communicates to staff that his preferred means of coping with anger is to "cuss people out" and run into them with his wheelchair. However, in the hospital, the consequence of wheelchair assaults is that the patient is secluded in his room, which he finds intolerable. The patient asks the staff to help him manage his anger.
>
> **Intervention**
>
> The nurse assigned to this young man sets aside time to interview him regarding the triggers for his anger. He identifies several issues that "make him angry." These typically relate to feeling unheard and controlled by the staff. Together the nurse and patient examine alternative ways for him to deal with these situations, such as telling the staff that he does not feel that they are listening to him and letting them know that he needs to be involved in the planning of his care to increase his sense of control. The patient and nurse role play a situation in which the patient is told by a staff member that he must attend a group session. Such a situation would usually result in the patient becoming angry and aggressive, but in the role-played situation he is willing to "try out" alternative communication techniques to communicate his feelings to the staff member and thus to handle his anger. In addition, the patient is willing to enter into a behavioral contract with the nurse, stating that he will not curse at staff or assault anyone with his wheelchair. Instead, he will let the staff know when he is feeling angry and what the triggering issue is so that a nonaggressive resolution can be found.

> **Response**
>
> Because this patient is motivated to gain increased personal control, he responds positively to these suggestions. In addition, once it becomes clear that feeling unheard and out of control underlies most episodes of anger, the patient is able to target these issues for problem solving. He rapidly develops effective and appropriate ways to make himself heard and understood. He also becomes adept at communicating when he feels out of control and at finding ingenious ways of negotiating control on issues that are particularly important to him. The patient's suicidal impulses, which occur when he is frustrated, also diminish.

Potential future alternatives to reduce seclusion and restraint. Sivak (2012) points that there is no evidence that supports the therapeutic value of seclusion and restraint and reports that 150 people die a year as a real result of these practices with the mentally ill and leave others psychologically harmed, physically injured, or traumatized (SAMHSA, 2011). New approaches that focus on the recovery model are being researched and developed for the purpose of reducing the use of seclusion and restraint. One potential intervention which came out of the recovery movement is the use of **comfort rooms** in which the psychiatric facility sets aside a "comfort room" in which a person could go voluntarily to self manage anxiety and distress (Sivak, 2012).

Postassaultive Stage

Once the patient no longer requires seclusion or restraints, the staff should review the incident with the patient as well as among themselves. Discussion with the patient is an important part of the therapeutic process. Reviewing the incident allows the patient to learn from the situation, identify the stressors that precipitated the out-of-control behavior, and plan alternative ways of responding to these stressors in the future.

Critical Incident Debriefing

Staff analysis of an episode of violence, referred to as **critical incident debriefing,** is crucial for a number of reasons. *First,* a review is necessary to ensure that quality care was provided to the patient. Staff members need to critically examine their response to the patient. Questions to be answered include the following:

- Could we have done anything that would have prevented the violence?
- If yes, then what could have been done, and why was it not done in this situation?
- Did the team respond as a team? Were team members acting according to the policies and procedures of the unit? If not, why not?
- Is there a need for additional staff education regarding how to respond to violent patients?
- How do staff members feel about this patient? About this situation? Feelings of fear and anger must be discussed and handled. Otherwise, the patient may be dealt with in a punitive and nontherapeutic manner.

Second, the profound effects of workplace violence do not, unfortunately, disappear after the incident is over, and the harm is not only to the individual assaulted. Clements and colleagues (2005) state that some nurses will internalize (depression, avoidance, withdrawal) and others will externalize (anger, outbursts, fluctuating mood) emotional and behavioral responses. These are normal responses to an abnormal event. However, agencies need to provide support and debriefing to prevent long-term psychological sequelae for all types of workplace violence (Alexy & Hutchins, 2006). Employee morale, productivity, use of sick leave, transfer requests, and absenteeism are affected by patient violence, especially if a staff member has been injured. Staff members must feel supported by their peers as well as by the organizational policies and procedures established to maintain a safe environment.

Documentation of a Violent Episode

Most facilities provide standardized seclusion and restraint records. There are a number of areas in which the nurse *must* provide documentation in situations in which violence either was averted or actually occurred:

- Assessment of behaviors that occurred during the preassaultive stage *(time)*
- Nursing interventions and the patient's responses *(time)*
- Evaluation of the interventions used
- Detailed description of the patient's behaviors during the assaultive stage
- All nursing interventions used to defuse the crisis
- Patient's response to those interventions
- Name(s) of person(s) called to assess the patient and order any medications, seclusion, and/or restraints *(time)*
- Time patient put in restraints or seclusion
- Observations of and interventions performed while the patient was in restraints or seclusion (food, toileting, vital signs, verbatim statements, and general behaviors) (15 to 30 minutes depending on state law)
- Any injuries to staff or patient
- The way in which the patient was reintegrated into the unit milieu *(time and behavior)*

See Chapter 6 for more definitive legal and procedural guidelines.

Anticipating Increased Anxiety and Anger in Other Hospital Settings

Hospitals can be lonely, scary places for many people. Patients often feel that they are not being heard, and they may feel vulnerable, discounted, frightened, out of control of their situation, and tired. Some patients may have specific vulnerabilities for responding to their increasing anxiety and loss of autonomy through the use of violence. Therefore some patients with poor coping skills or mental or neurological problems may resort to anger, intimidation, or violence to obtain their short-term goals of feelings of control or mastery. For others, the anger occurs when limited or primitive attempts at coping are unsuccessful and alternatives are unknown. For these patients, anger and violence are particular risks in inpatient settings.

This is especially true for hospitalized patients with chemical or alcohol dependency who may be anxious about not having access to their substance of choice; they may have well-founded concerns that any physical pain will be inadequately addressed. Many patients with marginal coping also have personality styles that externalize blame. That is, they see the source of their discomfort and anxiety as being outside themselves; relief must therefore also come from an outside source (e.g., the nurse, medication).

Interventions begin with attempts to understand and meet the patient's needs. For instance, baseline anxiety can be moderated by the provision of comfort items before they are requested (e.g., decaffeinated coffee, deck of cards); this can build rapport and acts symbolically to reassure the patient. Anxiety also can be minimized by reducing ambiguity. This strategy includes clear and concrete communication. An interaction providing clarity about what the nurse can and cannot do is most usefully ended by offering something within the nurse's power to provide (i.e., leaving the patient with a "yes").

Interventions for anxiety might also include the use of distractions, such as magazines, action comics, and video games. Generally, distractions that are colorful and do not require sustained attention work best, although this varies according to the patient's interests and abilities. Finally, patients with a high level of baseline anxiety and limited coping skills are helped when their interactions with the treatment team are predictable; this might include speaking with the physician at a specific time each day or having the patient see a single spokesperson from the treatment team each day.

Because some patients have limited coping skills, once anxiety is moderated, nursing interventions include teaching alternative behaviors and strategies. With increased tools to deal with anxiety and frustration, patients have the opportunity to have choices and an increased sense of control over their behaviors.

Often, anger may be communicated via verbal abuse directed at the nurse. If attempts to teach alternatives have not been successful, three interventions can be used:

1. The first is to leave the room as soon as the abuse begins; the patient can be informed that the nurse will return in a specific amount of time (e.g., 20 minutes) when the situation is calmer. This is said in a straightforward manner. If the nurse is in the middle of a procedure and cannot leave immediately, the nurse can discontinue conversation and eye contact, completing the procedure quickly and efficiently before leaving the room. Note that the nurse avoids chastising, threatening, or responding punitively to the patient.
2. Withdrawal of attention to the abuse is successful only if a second intervention is also used. This step requires attending positively to, and thus reinforcing, nonabusive communication by the patient. Interventions can include discussing non–illness-related topics, responding to requests, and providing emotional support.
3. Patients who are regularly verbally abusive may respond best to the predictability of routine, such as scheduled contacts with the nurse (e.g., every 30 minutes or every

60 minutes) as long as the patient's behavior is not abusive. Such a contract works only to the extent that the nurse maintains the scheduled contacts as agreed on and other staff members must be informed of the care plan and remain consistent so that they do not inadvertently sabotage it by responding to incidental requests by the patient. If the patient's illness or injury requires nursing care outside the scheduled contact times, these visits can be carried out in a calm, brief manner. This contract is negotiated with the patient and addresses the patient's anxiety about getting needs met and being heard.

Implementing appropriate interventions can be difficult when the nurse is feeling threatened. Remaining matter-of-fact with patients who habitually use anger and intimidation can be difficult because these people are often skillful at making personal and pointed statements. It is important for the nurse to remember that patients do not know their nurses personally and thus have no basis on which they can make accurate judgments. Nurses can also vent their own responses elsewhere, with other staff or family members, or via critical incident debriefing.

Anxiety Reduction Techniques

There are a number of strategies that nurses can teach and individuals can learn to help control anxiety and minimize anxiety escalation, including relaxation training, deep breathing exercises, journaling, meditation, learning more effective critical reasoning techniques, learning to listen rather than jump impulsively, taking time out, and physical exercise. Sometimes people need more in-depth teaching, in which case a trained anger management therapist is indicated.

Interventions for Patients With Neurocognitive Deficits

Patients with cognitive deficits are particularly at risk for acting aggressively. Such deficits may result from delirium, dementia (e.g., Alzheimer's disease, multi-infarct dementia), or brain injury. Traditional approaches to disorientation and to the agitation that it can cause have relied heavily on reality orientation and medication. Reality orientation consists of providing the correct information to the patient about place, date, and current life circumstances. For some patients, orientation does not work. Because of their cognitive disorder, they can no longer "enter into our reality," and they become frightened and agitated and may become aggressive.

Sedating medication may calm agitation, but in some cases the risks may outweigh the benefits. Sedation only further clouds a patient's sensorium, which makes disorientation worse and increases the risks of falls and injuries. It is better to examine alternative interventions.

Sometimes the patient with a cognitive disorder experiences such severe agitation and aggression that it is referred to as a **catastrophic reaction.** The patient may scream, strike out, or cry because of overwhelming fear. Adopting a calm and unhurried manner is the best response. The steps for making contact with a patient experiencing a catastrophic reaction are listed in Box 24-3.

To respond effectively to episodes of agitation, it is crucial to identify the antecedents, or precursors, of the episode, and the consequences of such episodes. Once antecedents are understood, interventions are often obvious. Consequences of agitation also may be a factor if they serve to reinforce the behaviors. For example, an older man who loves ice cream and becomes calm when it is given to him becomes agitated more often when ice cream is routinely used to stop his angry behaviors.

Finally, patients who misperceive their setting or life situation may be calmed by validation therapy. Some disoriented patients believe that they are young and feel the need to return to important tasks that were a significant part of their earlier years. For example, an older woman may insist that she must go home to take care of her babies. Telling the patient that her

BOX 24-3 COGNITIVE DEFICITS AND THE CATASTROPHIC REACTION: MAKING CONTACT

Cognitive deficits result in:
- A decreased ability to interpret sensory stimuli
- A decreased ability to tolerate sensory stimuli

Striking out represents fear or the feeling that the environment is out of control.

The presence of a second agitated person (e.g., staff member) leads to increased agitation; therefore:
1. Face the patient from within 2 feet, remaining as calm and unhurried as possible.
2. Say the patient's name.
3. Gain eye contact.
4. Smile.
5. Repeat steps (2) through (4) several times if necessary, to gain and maintain eye contact.
6. Use gentle touch and keep voice soft (the person often matches this tone and lowers his or her voice also).
7. Ask the patient if there is a need to use the bathroom.
8. Help the patient regain a sense of control—ask what is needed.
9. Validate the patient's feelings: "You look upset. This can be a confusing place."
10. Use short, simple sentences. Complex explanations just represent more noise.
11. Decrease sensory stimulation.
12. Get the patient to use rhythmic sources of self-stimulation (e.g., humming, a rocking chair).

Adapted from Rader, J., Doan, J., & Schwab, M. (1985). How to decrease wandering, a form of agenda behavior. *Geriatric Nursing, 6*(4), 196-199.

babies have grown up and that she no longer has a home is not only cruel but also nontherapeutic and will result in increased agitation. It is often more helpful to reflect back to the patient the feelings behind her demand and to show understanding and concern for her worry.

Rather than attempting to reorient the patient, the nurse asks the patient to further describe the setting or situation referenced by the patient (e.g., the need to return home). During the conversation the nurse can comment on what appears to be underlying the patient's distress, thus validating it. For example, the woman who believes that she needs to return home to care for her children is asked to tell the nurse more about her children. The nurse may note that the patient misses her children and may be lonely: "Mrs. Green, you miss your children, and the hospital can be a lonely place."

As the nurse shows interest in aspects of the patient's life, the nurse establishes himself or herself as a safe, understanding person who can be trusted. In turn, the patient often becomes calmer and more open to redirection. When patients reminisce in this fashion, they often reorient themselves: "Of course, they're all grown and doing well on their own now." See Chapter 18 for a more extensive discussion on interventions for people with cognitive impairments.

VIGNETTE

An 81-year-old female with Alzheimer's disease always becomes agitated during her morning care; this comes to be a time dreaded by her caregivers. Careful observation of the antecedents to episodes of agitation reveals a natural course to the morning problems. The patient is initially calm when care begins. However, one staff person gives morning care to the patient and her roommate at the same time, moving between the two. Observation of the process reveals that the patient becomes distracted by cues being given to her roommate and often startles when the caregiver returns to her. As this process continues over several minutes, the patient becomes increasingly distressed and then agitated. When a change is made so that the patient's care is provided by one person who remains with her throughout the process, the patient's morning agitation ends.

Psychotherapy

Management of chronic aggression requires comprehensive neuropsychological testing and cognitive behavioral assessment to establish the appropriate treatment approach for each individual. Besides psychopharmacological treatment, individual therapies may include behavioral management, cognitive behavioral techniques, family interventions, and psychosocial supports (Sanders, 2004).

The cognitive behavioral assessment includes determining the psychotherapeutic approach most appropriate for a chronically aggressive patient. Data are obtained regarding the type of aggressive behavior, psychiatric diagnosis, and patient's

intellectual ability. For example, individuals with schizophrenia and those with organic brain disease (mental retardation, dementias, autism, brain injury) who experience a marginal response to medications might do well with behavioral techniques. People with personality disorders whose aggression is secondary to difficulties in regulating emotional states (people with borderline personality disorder, antisocial traits, or narcissistic patients) are often more effectively treated with cognitive behavioral techniques if motivated. It should be noted that anger treatment is *not* indicated for those who cannot control their violent behavior or whose violent behavior fits their own personal goals and is experienced in a positive or satisfactory manner by the violent individual (Quanbeck, 2006).

Behavioral interventions are based on social learning theory. This theory supports the belief that social behaviors are learned and acquired over time through two mechanisms: (1) experiencing success or failure as a result of one's own actions and (2) observing the positive and negative consequences of others' behaviors (Quanbeck, 2006). The goal of behavioral intervention is to restructure the consequences of a person's actions so that the link between aggressive behavior and its reinforcers is weakened, whereas the link between alternative, more socially acceptable behaviors is reinforced.

One such behavioral strategy is the **token economy.** In this behavioral approach, a person earns a "token" when socially acceptable behaviors are demonstrated. This token can be accumulated and traded for privileges (e.g., games, TV time, or snacks) (Quanbeck, 2006). Often social skills training is used in conjunction with behavioral programs, teaching the individual alternative and effective behaviors for getting needs met. Patients often learn assertive and self-control skills in an individual or a group setting.

Cognitive behavioral approaches are based on anger management techniques. Novaco's (1997) cognitive behavioral model of anger asserts that anger and aggression are mediated by a person's perception of threat from others and an ability to formulate strategies for managing conflict in a nonaggressive manner. A key ingredient in teaching such behaviors is to help patients find motivation for learning skills to manage their anger, and to see the benefits to their lives from implementation of these skills. Anger management skills training programs teach participants the following key components:

- Stress inoculation (imagining angry scenarios and using relaxation techniques to decrease arousal)
- Identifying and challenging cognitive distortions (misattributing the intentions of others as hostile)
- Identifying their own unique early signs of anger so they are more aware when they need to use anger management skills
- Early recognition of potentially provocative situations and implementation of nonaggressive responses (problem solving)
- Providing a person with behavioral skills for managing conflict, such as walking away

Dialectical behavior therapy (DBT) (Linehan, 1993) is effective in people with borderline personality disorders and has also been found useful to treat violence and anger in male forensic patients.

Pharmacological, Biological, and Integrative Therapies

Medications for Acute Aggression

Medications that are most frequently used in emergency violent situations are **atypical antipsychotics** (e.g., intramuscular [IM] risperidone, olanzapine, ziprasidone) or high-potency **typical neuroleptics** (e.g., IM haloperidol). They are both first-line treatments for acute aggression and psychosis-induced violence. **Benzodiazepines** (e.g., lorazepam) are often the first choice for acute aggressive episodes, especially in episodic dyscontrol and incipient rage episodes (Stokowski, 2007).

Atypical antipsychotics have fewer side effects, although most are not available in short-acting IM injectable form if the patient refuses to take oral medication. Olanzapine short-acting IM injectable has many caveats for use and should be used only if the person has shown previous dystonic or severe extrapyramidal symptoms from IM haloperidol, the person needs an antipsychotic but has preexisting stable cardiac disease, or there has been no response 1 hour after giving IM lorazepam (Gaskell, 2006).

Among the typical antipsychotics, haloperidol is usually the first choice. It is sedating, can be given in higher doses, and is less likely to cause orthostatic hypotension. However, in large doses there are risks for hypotension, oversedation, and acute dystonic reactions.

Lorazepam is often a first choice among the benzodiazepines. Violence, aggression, and suicidality associated with panic or anger attacks are responsive to benzodiazepines.

Medications for Chronic Aggression

Chronic aggression is a common problem in psychiatry, and aggression can be diminished only after a therapeutic dose of the appropriate medication is used for 4 to 8 weeks. Carbamazepine is useful for intermittent explosive disorder, borderline personality disorder, posttraumatic stress disorder, and schizophrenia. Beta-blockers (e.g., propranolol, nadolol, pindolol) and buspirone (BuSpar) are helpful in organically based violence (e.g., dementias, head injuries, stroke). Beta-blockers are useful in decreasing aggressive behavior in schizophrenia. Lithium is effective in a wide range of Axis I and Axis II disorders (e.g., bipolar disorder, borderline personality disorder, conduct disorder, and episodic dyscontrol). Anticonvulsants (e.g., phenytoin, carbamazepine) have been shown to reduce impulsive rage reactions in individuals with antisocial and borderline personality disorders, substance use disorder, attention deficit disorder, and intermittent explosive disorder.

EVALUATION

Evaluation of the care plan is essential for patients who are angry and aggressive. A well-considered plan has specific outcome criteria. Evaluation provides information about the extent to which the interventions have achieved the outcomes. If the outcomes have not been achieved, the plan must be revised. Revision focuses on all aspects of the nursing process:

- Was the assessment accurate and thorough?
- Were the nursing diagnoses applicable to the assessment data?
- Did the nursing diagnoses accurately drive nursing interventions?
- Was the plan comprehensive and individualized?
- Were interventions appropriate?
- Were interventions carried out properly?
- If restraint or seclusion was needed, was the protocol followed correctly and was safety for staff as well as patient maintained?
- Were guidelines to improve quality improvement methods found for future use?

For instance, the initial plan may have included assessment of the environmental stimuli that precede a patient's agitation. Once these are identified the plan provides interventions that are specific to those stimuli. However, the plan can work only if staff members evaluate the effectiveness of the approach by noting the extent to which agitation is decreased. Evaluation may reveal that the patient's agitation has decreased except in specific situations. The plan is then revised to include these situations.

■ KEY POINTS TO REMEMBER

- Angry emotions and aggressive actions are difficult targets for nursing intervention.
- Nurses benefit from an understanding of how the angry and aggressive patient should be approached.
- Understanding patient cues to escalating aggression, appropriate intervention goals for individuals in a variety of situations, and helpful nursing interventions is important for nurses in any setting.
- The roles of sociocultural influences and neurobiological vulnerabilities are intertwined in a person's propensity for violence.

- Cues to assess when anger is escalating (verbal and nonverbal, including facial expressions, breathing, body language, and posture) are provided.
- Assess the patient's history. A patient's past aggressive behavior is the most important indicator of future aggressive episodes.
- Many approaches are effective in helping patients de-escalate and maintain control.
- The general hierarchy of interventions for coping with aggression is verbal intervention, psychopharmacology, seclusion, and then restraint.

Continued

KEY POINTS TO REMEMBER—cont'd

- Different interventions are used depending on the patient's level of anger.
- Guidelines for de-escalation of patient behavior are given.
- Specific medications such as antipsychotics, lithium, and antianxiety medications may be useful.
- Seclusion or restraints may be needed to ensure the safety of the patient as well as the safety of other patients and the staff.

- Each unit has a clear protocol for the safe use of restraints and for the humane management of care during the time the patient is restrained, as well as clear guidelines for understanding and protecting the patient's legal rights.
- Careful documentation of any incidence of escalating violence, especially leading to seclusion or restraints, must be made according to the laws of your state.

APPLYING CRITICAL JUDGMENT

1. Mr. Arnold, a 24-year-old man, is currently in the manic phase of bipolar disorder. He is admitted to an inpatient unit. Staff note that the patient is agitated and irritable and has a history of assault. He shouts at the nurse in a loud piercing voice, yelling that she is a "slut, a mut, tut-tut." He is pacing anxiously, invading the staff's personal space, and pointing his finger at the staff.
   A. What are the appropriate nursing diagnoses for Mr. Arnold at this time?
   B. Describe how you would document his behavior at this time.
   C. What interventions would most likely be initiated by you and your colleagues at this time? Explain your rationale for your decision.
   D. Describe the kinds of objective and subjective data you would document as well as the frequency of documentation according to the protocols of your hospital.
   E. List the various aspects of interventions of patient care for someone who is in seclusion.
   F. Role play verbal techniques you could use during any other interventions being initiated at this time.

2. In the morning 2 days later, Mr. Arnold comes to the nurses' desk and asks for a pass. When told that the physician needs to write an order for his pass and the physician would not be on duty until the afternoon, Mr. Arnold becomes verbally loud, demanding that the nurse phone the physician "right this minute to get that pass."
   A. What interventions by you and your colleagues would be most appropriate to start at this time?
   B. Role play your verbal techniques.
   C. What are the personal safety measures you and your colleagues would take when treating a patient with escalating aggression?
3. Write a summary of the protocols for intervening with irate patients as found in the hospital procedure manual.
4. Describe a time in your life when you have witnessed bullying or have been bullied by others.
   A. If you were the one being bullied, describe how you felt and the long-term effects it had on you.
   B. If you were watching a coworker being bullied by a staff member in charge, how might you react today?
   C. Have you ever witnessed or been involved in a student to student, nurse to nurse, or colleague to colleague incidence of bullying? What would you do today?

CHAPTER REVIEW QUESTIONS

Choose the most appropriate answer(s).

1. Due to a patient's angry outburst, the nurse makes the determination that the patient may soon become physically violent. Select the priority nursing action.
   1. Take the client aside and speak in soft tones.
   2. Call for assistance.
   3. Tell the client to return to his room.
   4. Encourage other patients to help calm down the patient.
2. After a few days on an inpatient unit, a patient with a history of explosive outbursts states to the nurse, "I am really feeling angry now." The nurse determines that this represents:
   1. a clear threat.
   2. anti-social behavior.
   3. positive behavioral change.
   4. continued negativity.

3. To help prevent displays of anger and aggression, the nurse must understand that anger and aggression are preceded by feelings of:
   1. vulnerability.
   2. depression.
   3. elation.
   4. isolation.
4. Which of the following is most useful to the nurse planning intervention for an angry patient?
   1. Creative, individualized approaches to the patient's behavior by staff members
   2. The availability of group therapy sessions focused on cathartic expression of emotion
   3. An understanding of the patient's medical diagnosis
   4. Consistency of approach to the patient by staff members

5. After a client was sent to a quiet room following aggressive comments to several patients, the nurse explains the purpose of this intervention to the patient:

   1. This provides a means to ensure safety for you and other patients.

2. This is what happens to all patients who become too aggressive.

3. This keeps you away from the other patients.

4. This is part of your treatment plan.

REFERENCES

Alexy, E. M., & Hutchins, J. A. (2006). Workplace violence: a primer for critical care nurses. In H. J. Thompson, & E. M. Alexy (Eds.), *Violence, injury and trauma*. Philadelphia: Saunders.

American Psychiatric Nurses Association (APNA). (2000, rev. 2007). *Seclusion and restraint standards of practice*. Retrieved May 29, 2011, from www.apna.org.

American Psychological Association. (2007). *Controlling anger—before it controls you*. Retrieved March 15, 2007, from http://apa.org/topics/controlanger.html.

Black, D. W., & Andreasen, N. C. (2011). *Introductory textbook of psychiatry* (5th ed.). Washington, DC: American Psychiatric Publishing.

Brooks, B. E. ((Updated 2011). Workplace violence and bullying prevention. *Small Business Monthly*. Retrieved February 14, 2012, from http://www.sbmon.com/DesktopModules/EngagePublish/printerfriendly.aspx?itemId=148.

Center for American Nurses. (2008). *Lateral violence and bullying in the workplace* (pp. 1–12). Retrieved June 1, 2011, from www.centerforamericannurses.org.

Clements, P. T., DeRanieri, J. T., Clark, K., et al. (2005). Workplace violence and corporate policy for health care settings. *Nursing Economics, 23*(3), 119–124.

Collins English Dictionary. (Complete & Unabridged 10th Edition). 2009 © William Collins Sons & Co. Ltd. 1979, 1986. © Harper-Collins Publishers 1998, 2000, 2003, 2005, 2006, 2007, 2009.

Dellasega, C. A. (2009). Bullying among nurses. *American Journal of Nursing, 109*, 52–58.

Gaskell, C. (2006). *Guidelines for the management of acute behavioural disturbance in adult and older people in inpatient wards*. Cambridge and Peterborough Mental Health Partnership NHS Trust. A Cambridge University Teaching Trust. Retrieved July 11, 2007, from www.cambsphn.nhs.uk/documents/Clinical/Rapid_Tranquillisation_Guidelines14122005.pdf.

Gross, A. F., & Sanders, K. M. (2008). Aggression and violence. In T. A. Stern, J. F. Rosenbaum, A. Fava, J. Biederman, & S. L. Rauch (Eds.), *Massachusetts General Hospital comprehensive clinical psychiatry* (pp. 895–906). Philadelphia, Mosby/Elsevier.

Health Care Financing Administration (HCFA), Centers for Medicare & Medicaid Programs. (1999). *Hospital conditions of patient's rights: interim final rule*. Washington, DC: Author.

Human Capital. (2012). Nursing profession is life with occupational hazards. Retrieved May 14, 2012, from http://rwif.org/humancapital/product. jsp? id= 74136.

Linehan, M. (1993). *Cognitive-behavioral treatment of borderline personality disorder*. New York: Guilford Press.

Medical Dictionary. (2004). *Definition of anger*. Retrieved February 15, 2012, from http://www.medterms.com/script/main/art.asp?articlekey=33843.

Novaco, R. W. (1997). Remediating anger and aggression with violent offenders. *Legal and Criminological Psychology, 2*, 77–88.

Petit, J. R. (2005). Management of the acutely violent patient. *Psychiatric Clinics of North America, 28*(3), 701–711.

Quanbeck, C. (2006). Forensic psychiatric aspects of inpatient violence. *Psychiatric Clinics of North America, 29*(3), 743–760.

Rowe, M. M., & Sherlock, H. (2005). *Stress and verbal abuse in nursing: do burned out nurses eat their young?* Retrieved June 7, 2011, from *Journal of Nursing Mangement, 13*(3), 242–248.

Sadock, B. J., & Sadock, V. A. (2010). *Kaplan & Sadock's pocket handbook of clinical psychiatry* (5th ed.). Philadelphia: Wolters Kluwer/Lippincott Williams & Wilkins.

Sadock, B. J., & Sadock, V. A. (2007). *Kaplan & Sadock's synopsis of psychiatry* (10th ed.). Philadelphia: Lippincott Williams & Wilkins.

Substance Abuse and Mental Health Services Administration (SAMHSA). (2011). *A seclusion and restraint overview*. Retrieved February 14, 2012, from http://www.samhsa.gov/matrix2/seclusion_matrix.aspx.

Sanders, K. M. (2004). The violent patient. In T. A. Stern, J. B. Herman, & P. L. Slavin (Eds.), *Massachusetts General Hospital guide to primary care psychiatry* (2nd ed.). New York: McGraw-Hill.

Sivak, K. (2012). Implementation of comfort rooms to reduce seclusion, restraint use, and acting out behaviors. *JPN, 50*(2), 24–34.

Stokowski, L. A. (2010). *A matter of respect and dignity: bullying in the nursing profession*. Retrieved January 21, 2011, from www.Medscape.com/view article/729474.

Stokowski, L. (2007). *Alternatives to restraint and seclusion in mental health settings: questions and answers for psychiatric nurse experts*. Retrieved January 17, 2011, from www.medscape.com/view article/555686.

Victoroff, J. (2009). Human aggression. In B. J. Sadock, V. A. Sadock, & P. Ruiz (Eds.), *Kaplan and Sadock's comprehensive textbook of psychiatry* (9th ed., pp. 2671–2702). Philadelphia: Wolters Kluwer/Lippincott Williams & Wilkins.

WordNet 3.1 (2012). *Aggression*. Available at http://wordnet.princeton.edu. Retrieved February 14, 2012, from Princeton University "About WordNet." WordNet. Princeton University, 2010.

Care for the Dying and Those Who Grieve

Kathy Kramer-Howe

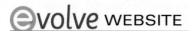 WEBSITE

http://evolve.elsevier.com/Varcarolis/essentials

KEY TERMS AND CONCEPTS

anticipatory mourning, p. 470
bereavement, p. 475
caring presence, p. 472
compassion, p. 473
disenfranchised grief, p. 475
end-of-life conversations, p. 472

Four Gifts, p. 471
Four Tasks of Mourning, p. 475
grief, p. 474
hospice and palliative care, p. 476
mourning, p. 470

SELECTED CONCEPT: Compassion

Compassion is the ability to be with someone who is suffering. Thus, compassion is a relational phenomenon. It is less like a feeling and more like a human capacity that is developed and sustained in relationship to others. It needs to be shared and passed on. In other words, even brief and fleeting expressions of compassion nourish this quality in our self and in others. Truly hearing the suffering of others puts us in touch with our own needs and vulnerabilities, and we might want to turn away to protect ourselves.

However, it's important to remember that compassion is developmental throughout life, and we can grow in our abilities (Hoisington 2007). Think of compassion as a practice, or a habit of thought and action that connects us meaningfully with others. *(Hoisington, 2007)*

OBJECTIVES

1. Identify the teamwork and collaboration involved in the care for those at the end-of-life according to the hospice movement.
2. Discuss the hospice movement in terms of (a) purpose, (b) philosophy and goals, (c) settings, (d) use of palliative treatment, and (e) various supports available to families.
3. Explain the interventions you would take to help grief-stricken caregivers in the following areas:
   a. Helping the bereaved caregivers come to terms with their feelings
   b. Helping people say goodbye
   c. Helping families maintain "hope"
   d. Establishing a presence
4. Teach a classmate some guidelines health care professionals can use to assess bereaved caregivers and their dying loved one's spiritual issues.
5. Describe and discuss the Four Tasks of Mourning as identified in this chapter.
6. Describe the importance of self-care interventions for nurses in relationship to the phenomena of *compassion* as well as *disenfranchised grief.*
7. Select at least four nursing goals at end-of-life, and discuss how you would address these issues.
8. Compare and contrast the terms *bereavement* and *mourning.*
9. Discuss and give examples of the various phenomena experienced during the normal grief process (e.g., sensations of somatic distress, changes in behavior).
10. Identify the behavioral outcomes that indicate healthy bereavement.
11. Delineate at least five symptoms of a complicated grief reaction.
12. Describe some of the short-term interventions that can be used to help a person experiencing complicated grief come to terms with his or her loss.

Health care professionals are uniquely positioned to provide leadership in our national conversation about how we care for those at end-of-life. Resources, medical options, and belief systems about end-of-life seem to be on a collision course in contemporary North American society. The capabilities of modern medicine seem to promise an inexhaustible supply of treatment options. Reuters quoted the CEO of a major pharmaceutical company as saying, "People want to have a choice, they want to know what is available, and if it's good, they want to have it… Americans have a funny approach to this—they think death is optional" (Brennan, 2006). However, the cost of current health care practices is unsustainable; it is estimated that about one third of overall health care resources are spent in the last year of life (Harding, 2010). Unlike in previous historical periods, the way most of us think about death and dying (and mourning) is no longer grounded in real human experience; instead, we have been culturally infiltrated with American values such as being strong, "never saying die," relying on technology, and staying youthful. These attitudes permeate health care as well, with the result that most nurses and physicians are ill-prepared to face the mortality of others, let alone their own impermanence. For these and other reasons, there is now a vital need for competencies in end-of-life care throughout health care professions. Those who seek expertise in this area will lead the way as we struggle towards meaningful, timely, and honest conversations about how we die.

Following the 1997 mandate of the International Council of Nurses stating that nurses have a primary responsibility to ensure a peaceful death to those at life's end, the American Association of Colleges of Nursing (2012) convened an expert panel on this topic. The expert panel developed end-of-life competency statements and suggestions for how academia could incorporate these topics into existing study areas. The competencies include expert palliative care and symptom management, bioethics, cultural sensitivity, and supporting grief and mourning. A total of 5 of the 15 competencies involve expert communication and counseling skills. In this chapter we will survey the typical conditions under which we die in America, and focus on communication skills and models that can help navigate this crucial and universal phase of life.

What do we know about dying in America? A study reported in the *Journal of the American Medical Association* asked family members of 1578 decedents about care in the setting in which death occurred. Questions centered on whether health care workers provided the desired physical and emotional comfort to the dying, supported shared decision making, treated the dying with respect, attended to the family's emotional needs, and provided coordinated care. More than 67% of deaths occurred in an institution, with the remainder occurring at home. Of these latter cases, just less than half of individuals received home hospice services. Some key findings are that one in four people who died did not receive adequate pain medication and one in two received inadequate emotional support. Families receiving home hospice care were the most satisfied on all these measures, with more than 70% of the families rating hospice care as excellent (Teno et al., 2004). The chances of dying in pain increase for people who do not speak English or who are poor, African American, Hispanic, elderly, or female (Byock, 1997). This study and others point to the need for comprehensive improvements in the care of the dying and their families.

Hospice care is a model for compassionate, holistic, and medically managed end-of-life services. After early good results shown by volunteer hospices in the 1970s, Congress enacted the Medicare hospice benefit in 1982. In 2008 there were about 4850 hospices throughout 50 states, a blend of not-for-profit, privately held for-profit, and government-owned and operated types. The National Hospice and Palliative Care Organization estimates that in 2008 38.5% of all deaths in the United States were under the care of a hospice program (approximately 1.45 million persons received hospice care). The diagnoses most commonly treated were cancer (38.3%), debility unspecified (15.3%), heart disease (11.7%), dementia (11.1%), and lung disease (7.9%). The median length of stay in 2008 was just 21.3 days. The average length of service was 69.5 days. Health care cost savings provided by hospice are calculated based on diagnosis and length of stay.

Hospice care is delivered by a multidisciplinary team of physicians, nurses, chaplains, social workers, certified nursing aides, volunteers, and bereavement counselors. All medications and supplies related to the terminal diagnosis are covered by Medicare reimbursement, and many other insurance providers mimic the Medicare benefit. Although most patients are cared for in the place they call "home," hospices provide for short-term acute inpatient care as well as respite periods for the caregivers. Patients are perceived as living fully until they die; their choices and preferences are respected and incorporated in the plan of care. The patient/family is considered the unit of care and receives counseling support around the tasks of anticipatory grief and mourning as well as spirituality and meaning-making. Research shows that hospice care extends life in many cases for days, weeks, or months.

Palliative care is a medical specialty that grew out of the hospice movement. The term was selected by Dr. Balfour Mount because the concept of "hospice" does not exist in some languages, and when it does, it is typically equated with "the end of life" (Hallenbeck, 2003). Palliation (*palliare* in Latin means to cloak or to shield) refocuses end-of-life care on symptom relief and acceptance of dying as a natural process. According to the *Standards of Practice for Hospice Programs* established by the National Hospice and Palliative Care Organization (NHPCO), "The test of palliative care lies in the agreement between the individual, physician(s), primary caregiver, and the (palliative) team that the expected outcome is relief from distressing symptoms, the easing of pain, and/or enhancing the quality of life. The individual's choices and decisions regarding care are paramount and must be followed" (NHPCO, 2004). Palliative care teams are becoming more commonplace in hospitals and other medical and home health settings, "whenever comfort, support and quality of life are significant concerns for a terminal illness" (Hutchings, 2002, p. 409). Electing hospice care is appropriate when the patient leaves the hospital or physician's office with the understanding that cure is no longer possible, but that there are many sophisticated medical and holistic interventions still available for this phase of living.

NURSING GOALS IN END-OF-LIFE CARE

Nursing the terminally ill and supporting their families require special skills, personal awareness, and ongoing self-care. Because of their daily, hands-on care and the mandate of the profession to comfort the patient, nurses have a heightened

proximity to the experiences and feelings of their patients. It is natural and helpful to be affected by the people being cared for, but witnessing the transition from active treatment to dying can be challenging, especially in the absence of relevant communication about end-of-life choices. Skills in communicating with terminally ill patients and their families are among the nine essential areas of end-of-life (EOL) care for psychiatric nurses (Durkin, 2003). The nine topics are: (1) defining/goals of communication; (2) the importance of listening; (3) barriers to communication; (4) delivering bad news/truth telling; (5) recognizing family dynamics in communication; (6) sensitivity to culture, ethnicity, values, and religion; (7) discussion of options/decisions with patient/family; (8) communication among interdisciplinary team members/collaboration; and (9) responding to requests for assisted suicide. Patients with diagnosed mental disorders require quality EOL care, just as do others, but psychiatric conditions may pose special challenges. The presence of a mood disorder or psychosis makes the assessment of end-of-life choices more complex. The psychiatric nurse can be an effective advocate for this vulnerable population. Because many academic settings seriously lag in offering coursework in EOL care, supplementary training such as the Toolkit for Nursing Excellence at End-of-Life Transition (TNEEL) can be very helpful (www.tneel.uic.edu/).

We will focus on a few of the nine essential areas of end-of-life care for nurses within the context of the challenges of anticipatory mourning (Doka, 1989). This term, though far from perfect, helps people recognize that grief is a part of the complex process of living with a terminal prognosis. From the moment of diagnosis, families begin to both experience and anticipate losses. For most people, the focus remains on treating the medical condition and coping with a lifestyle that is continually changing. Thus the presence of grief can remain muted or disguised. "Grief" is an umbrella term for a broad range of symptoms of loss—emotional, physical, cognitive, social, and spiritual. "Mourning" refers to the efforts one makes to manage grief. During anticipatory grief, caregivers have identified the primary emotions as anger (protesting that this is happening, anger at the patient for not fighting harder, anger at the medical system, displaced anger at others because of helplessness in the face of suffering, anger at God), sadness (sorrow and regret for the present and the future), hurt (pain over what the patient is enduring, the pain of being unable to protect each other, the pain of loss), fear and anxiety (a pervasive sense that something more should or could be done, dread of what is coming next, loss of control, a sense that time is running out), and bridled grief (experiencing hits or bursts of grief, but keeping it in check as long as the patient is alive) (Clukey, 2007).

Helping Bereaved Caregivers Make Sense of Their Feelings

Once a distressing symptom has been identified as grief, there are many activities of mourning that can bring some relief and improve coping. Actively mourning includes talking about feelings, journaling or writing, emoting, expressing what needs to be said, resolving and forgiving things that hurt, recognizing differences in grieving styles and abilities, using simple ritual, seeking support outside the family, and planning for a changed life. People often rehearse important events in life, such as becoming a parent, moving to a new home or job, getting married or divorced. It can also help people to rehearse life as it may be after loved ones decline further and ultimately die. One wife and mother in her thirties caring for her husband at home confessed that she frequently imagined herself at her husband's viewing and funeral. She thought this was probably an unloving and disloyal thing to do while he was living, and was relieved to find out that perhaps it was primarily a means of coping with her anticipatory grief. She visualized herself having survived the thing most feared (his death) and having a role and identity beyond (his funeral) to give herself the strength to go through what was coming.

VIGNETTE

Naming Something Gives Us Options

Julie was the wife, younger by 20 years, of a hospice patient dying of lung cancer. Julie cared for Edward in their home with help from the hospice team. During each home visit, the hospice social worker noticed that Julie seemed more drawn and fatigued. That was understandable, since Edward was getting weaker, thinner, and more confined to his room. The social worker asked Julie what was most distressing to her at this time. In tears, she said that Edward was no longer looking fondly at her or wanting to spend time together. She thought he no longer loved her, and this was deeply painful to her. The social worker described the phenomenon of anticipatory grieving, and talked about the many losses they were both experiencing. "You mean Edward is grieving?" Julie said, with amazement. "Yes," replied the social worker. "You are too. Just think of all that he will soon be forced to leave, most of all you, the love of his life. One way to deal with that is to withdraw early, to avoid some of the pain of parting." Julie's relief was obvious. She easily grasped that, while she wanted to grow closer as she anticipated his death, Edward might need to shut her out. Thereafter, she began to act on her mourning needs by being with him more, even as she supported Edward's needs by letting him know she understood how hard this was for him. Of course, Julie was grief-stricken when he died, but she had been able to express her love, reminisce about their life together, reflect the value of Edward's life back to him, and say goodbye. In addition, she had been spared needless suffering before his death due to prematurely pulling apart from each other.

Helping People Say Goodbye

It is helpful for a nurse to understand the experience of families caring for a terminally ill patient. When bereaved caregivers

were asked about their main challenges in a series of interviews (Clukey, 2007), they identified the following:

- Adjusting to caregiving demands. This challenge becomes all-consuming and includes physical, emotional, and practical stressors. With the patient getting so much attention, you can help by inquiring of caregivers how they are doing and what they are feeling. Listen and ask open-ended questions. Ask how you can help them.
- Gathering information. Most caregivers have a need to understand everything they can about the diagnosis, treatment options, and medical care for their loved ones. Anxiety usually surrounds these topics, and obtaining information may buttress a sense of control. You can help by communicating acceptance of their need to understand things. Encourage them to ask questions, as often as necessary. Slow down, repeat instructions, and check in frequently to see if they would like anything clarified.
- Finalizing the connection to the dying person. This is often done by spending time with the patient and enjoying things together. Reminiscing, looking at photographs, and visiting are all ways to show appreciation for the person's life. Barriers to this process may be the tendency to protect each other by pretending that time will never run out; loss of energy, alertness, and focus; the effects of medications; and resistance to feeling the pain of grief.

Dr. Ira Byock provides a simple structure to this process in the **Four Gifts** of resolving relationships (Byock, 2004). In essence, they invite the movement through four phases of communication:

- Forgiveness (I forgive you, please forgive me.)
- Love (I love you, I know you love me.)
- Gratitude (Thank you, and I receive your thanks.)
- Farewell (We will have an enduring connection.)

Each emotional movement opens into the next. Think of these as simple, natural, spontaneous, and creative. When they have taken place, people report a sense of peace and gratification. You can help by providing information about Byock's model, encouraging the family to express what is important to them, providing a caring presence, and understanding that successful bereavement includes a sense that one was able to say goodbye. For example, out of town family members can speak to a nonresponsive patient through a telephone held to the patient's ear; a card or letter can be read to a dying patient and placed in his or her hands on behalf of a family member who cannot be at the bedside. These simple interventions help satisfy the need to finalize the connection with the loved one.

Helping Families Maintain Hope

Families seem to need to have hope as long as the dying person is present. *Do not think of hope as a form of denial of reality.* Hopefulness can coexist with knowledge that recovery or longevity is not a realistic goal. Some include the hope that the loved one knows how important he or she is to them; the hope that the caregivers are not falling short in their efforts at providing comfort; or the hope that the dying person knows how much he or she will be missed. Many hopes center on the actual dying scene.

The plan was for John to move from the ICU to home with hospice care, have his ventilator removed at that time, and die peacefully surrounded by his family. A hospice bereavement counselor was consulted to help prepare John's four teenage grandchildren for his death. When the counselor arrived at the hospital late on the afternoon of his impending transfer home, she discovered that John was too fragile to be moved and would be extubated in the ICU instead. His wife, two adult children, and the four grandchildren were gathered in a waiting room, restless and worried. The counselor worked closely with the ICU nurse to orchestrate for the family the task of finalizing the relationship. They were invited to gather around him, touch him, tell him what he meant to them, share stories, and connect with him as each one preferred. The patient was not able to respond, but the nurse suggested that he might be able to hear them anyway. Gradually the family relaxed and expressed many things, crying, laughing, and holding hands. Then the staff asked if anyone wanted time alone with John. His wife immediately stepped forward. After her, each one requested private time. Finally, they were asked to leave the room so he could be medicated and extubated in privacy. Each step was carefully explained by the nurse and counselor. Finally, the whole family circled his bed weeping or silent as he gradually stopped breathing. The two staff members kept vigil with them in a corner of the room. His death was peaceful and quiet. So was the family, as each person gave him a final kiss before leaving the room.

The patient, if cognitively intact, often has preferences about where he or she will die, with what level of consciousness, with what people around, and with what level of comfort. Each family member will usually have a sense of how it will be at the time of the death. Some know they want to be present. Others prefer to remember the patient alive. When the hopes of the survivors are not met, people usually need to reconcile themselves with their disappointment during the period of bereavement. You can help by understanding the function of hope during the time of anticipatory mourning. You can listen carefully when hopes are being abandoned or reformulated as conditions change. Be sensitive to the fact that each member of the family, including the patient, will have differing hopes. Assess hopes by asking open-ended questions such as, "How would you like her to feel about that?" or "Ideally, how would you like this to work out?"

The Intervention of Presence

When survivors of terminally ill loved ones describe what was most helpful to them, high on the list is the presence of people who could just "be there" (Clukey, 2007). For the health care practitioner, this means that the art of presence needs to be seen as a preferred treatment intervention, and not simply as the absence of being able to "do something for them." Effective presence requires that the care provider accept the reality of suffering, helplessness, mourning, and mortality itself (Ingalls, 2007). It asks one to slow down, put other demands aside for a while, and simply be there. Watch and listen, tolerate pauses and silences, and use open-ended questions. *People going through intense life experiences report that they do not remember what others said to them, but only what the others made them feel. The intentional presence of another person makes people feel seen, valued, and important.* A hospice nurse recognized a young woman now going through nursing school, and the young woman said, "When my mother was dying a few years ago and I was fifteen, you were the nurse. The house was so chaotic, everyone was so busy. But you came and sat beside me on the stairs for a while. We didn't even speak, but that meant more to me than I can say. I think that's why I want to be nurse today, so I can do that for someone else." It seems paradoxical, but the caring presence of a health care professional in shared helplessness can bring solace and support to a dying person and the family.

Facilitating End-of-life Conversations

There are many documented barriers to having end-of-life conversations. Although awareness of the need to communicate our end-of-life choices is steadily growing in the United States, as of 2006 it was estimated that only 29% of people had executed a living will. In hospital settings, patients and families may create barriers by concealing the extent of their worry and grief, feeling confused and fearful about dying, and by cultural preconditions. Physicians may fear bearing bad news, not fully understand advance directives, view death as the enemy, have medical-legal concerns, and lack training in interpersonal relational processes. The medical system itself does not encourage or typically reimburse for end-of-life discussion, or make clear whose responsibility it is to initiate and document such dialogues (Larson & Tobin, 2000). Although training programs for physicians exist (such as Education for Physicians on End-of-Life Care [EPEC]), nurses may be well positioned to take an active role in this area. The following small research study bears this out.

Nurses in Italy devised a tool to elicit preferences about "a good death." This was a structured interview tool to be used by the physician with the patient. Certain preconditions needed to be met, however, such as the patient's awareness of the diagnosis and prognosis. Patients were considered poor candidates if they had strong psychological defenses or severe cognitive impairment. Other barriers identified in this study included lack of time for physicians to properly use the tool, or not finding the right moment to introduce it. Physicians also said that they expected strong emotional reactions from patients. Filter questions were used to allow the patient to opt out of the task at several points. Ironically, the patients who participated did not have particularly intense emotional reactions. The instrument covered topics such as how the patient wanted to be involved in medical and nursing decision making; how he or she wished to be informed about the disease process and medications; attitudes towards complementary medicine, intolerable symptoms, or procedures; preferences for delivery of care and companionship; preferences for knowing that he or she is dying; preparing for death (meaningful actions and events, key actions or passages before dying, levels of consciousness); spirituality and transpersonal issues; place and atmosphere at time of death; and religious preferences. Although many staff concerns emerged around introducing and completing the interview, those patients who elected to do it appeared to benefit, as did the care team, from expressing their personal preferences. Interestingly, it was concluded that nurses or psychologists might have better results than physicians for several reasons, such as patient perception of heightened significance when speaking with a physician, physician discomfort with emotions and relationships, and the fact that nurses and psychologists are more accustomed to communicating with patients on these issues (Borreani et al., 2008).

Assessing for Spiritual Issues

Most professional nursing associations call for nurses to assess client spirituality in all health care delivery settings. Hospices have policies and sample assessments to address this issue, and spirituality in health care is increasingly a subject of research (Millison, 1995). Clients report that they feel cared about when medical personnel are interested in their spirituality. However, they seem to prefer that such discussions occur in the context of ordinary conversation and human sharing (Hart et al., 2003). It is useful to distinguish between religion and spirituality, while acknowledging that they are aspects of the same human tendency to seek meaning and connection with something greater than self. Spirituality encompasses questions about how our lives relate to the rest of creation without requiring a specific religious affiliation, for example: What energizes our lives? What will survive our personal death, if anything? How do we explain to ourselves the things that happen in life? When do we feel most peaceful? How have we surmounted life's hardest challenges?

Imbedded in ordinary life stories you will hear spiritual themes such as how clients assign meaning and value, how they experience connections and becoming, and when they have sensed a transcendent realm or a dimension beyond the self (Stephenson et al., 2003). Spirituality goes beyond religious affiliation and practices and can be an important component of how an individual defines hope and healing. Here are some simple guidelines:

- **Start the conversation.** Allow yourself to be genuinely interested without feeling that you have to be an expert or have the answers. Ask open-ended questions and listen in a spirit of seeking to understand the patient, not to "fix" him or her.
- **This is the patient's story.** Avoid using the lens of your own belief system. This is the patient's and family's framework of values. You are there to learn and support, not to change their spirituality or faith, or lack thereof.
- **Refer to a counselor with spiritual expertise.** There will be times when a patient and/or family wishes to share with a counselor, or the medical team thinks it would be helpful. A chaplain can bring a perspective that complements that of the patient's and/or family's formal religious leader or community.

- **Seek to hear unspoken questions.** Sometimes a patient's existential issues are not communicated in words. These may be unspoken questions such as: "Do you know what I am hoping for today?" "Can you tell if I am feeling despair?" "Do you know what brings me courage and peace?" "Can you help calm my fears?" Sometimes, by listening to a patient's dreams, these unspoken emotional or spiritual states can also be explored and addressed.
- **Be empowered by the process.** This ongoing assessment may help nurses explore their own spirituality. They can grow more comfortable hearing and expressing spiritual concepts in everyday language. The plan of care will become more individualized and meaningful when influenced by spirituality.

SELF-CARE FOR NURSES

One of the hazards and challenges of becoming a professional care provider is that of practicing self-care. First, we must understand why this is so important. Then we must establish habits of good self-care. Finally, we must continually return to these habits as they are pushed into the background by the necessities of life and work. Nursing requires many skills and much knowledge, but also a great deal of compassion. **Compassion** is the ability to be with someone who is suffering. Thus, compassion is a relational phenomenon. It is less like a feeling and more like a human capacity that is developed and sustained in relationship to others. It needs to be shared and delivered. In other words, even brief and fleeting expressions of compassion nourish this quality in our self and in others. Truly hearing the suffering of others puts us in touch with our own needs and vulnerabilities, and we may feel like protecting ourselves from that vulnerability. One way to do that is to engage in our own thoughts rather than deeply listening to another's need. Many in helping professions worry that they are not as compassionate as they would like to be, and tell themselves that they are "failures." However, it is important to remember that compassion is developmental throughout life, and we can grow in our abilities (Hoisington, 2007). Think of compassion as a practice or a habit of thought and action that connects us meaningfully with others. Discover what practices keep refilling your reservoir of compassion and make them habitual.

To balance a work life that centers on others, create habits that reconnect you with your own life, your well-being, your commitment to work, and your enjoyment of the larger world. Find people you can trust at work and support each other. Accept each other's failings, successes, vulnerabilities, and intentions. Work for systemic changes at work that will enhance self-care, such as exercise programs and periodic debriefings and memorials when patients die. Review key ethical standards regularly. They express the highest and best goals of nursing care. Continue to increase your knowledge base and professional certifications. Ask your supervisor to e-mail inspiring or appreciative messages to the staff. Take a few moments to thank and appreciate each other. Use your spiritual belief system to provide a sustaining context for human suffering and human kindness.

Self-Care for Nurses and Staff

Sometimes nurses need to mourn the death of a person for whom they have provided care and developed fondness. An entire staff may need to mourn the death of a particular patient or an overload of recent deaths. After patients die, nurses may be faced with managing their own tasks of mourning, such as making sense of the death, dealing with mild to intense emotions, and realigning relationships. In one oncology unit, it was found that simply providing a support session where nurses could express their grief over the death of a beloved younger patient significantly relieved their distress. The feelings they needed to talk about included anger at the meaninglessness of a young person dying; guilt that they did not do more; sadness for the wife and children; lack of appropriate closure; and questions about mortality (Herrle, 1987). Some medical settings expose health care workers to daily suffering, grief, and death. Albert (2001) states that "in the face of overwhelming, unending death, health care workers may come to question their deepest values, the meaning of their existence, and the value of the work they do." To promote retention and self-care, it is imperative that such settings provide regular opportunities for debriefing and group support. This kind of grief is referred to as "disenfranchised" grief, and is discussed later in this chapter.

GRIEF AND LOSS

Loss is part of the human experience, and grief and mourning are the normal responses to loss. We grieve on a recurring basis as we face the commonplace losses in our lives, be they loss of a relationship (divorce, separation, death, abortion), health (a body function or part, mental or physical capacity), friendship, status, prestige, or security (occupational, financial, social, cultural). Some losses may be even more intangible such as the loss of a projected future or dreams. Normal losses include changes in circumstances, such as retirement, promotion, marriage, and aging.

It could be said that the course of our lives depends on how we adapt to losses and how we use change as a vehicle for growth. Changes that we do not adapt to—or fully mourn—may negatively affect our lives by sapping energy and impairing ability to connect (Volkan & Zintl, 1993). Understanding how to support healthy mourning in oneself and others is a vital life skill and can even be regarded as a public health issue. Unfortunately, contemporary mainstream U.S. culture perpetuates many damaging **myths about grief and mourning.** According to Dr. Alan Wolfelt (2006) the following are some of these myths:

- Grief and mourning are the same experience.
- There is a predictable and orderly stagelike progression to grieving.
- It is best to move away from grief rather than towards it.
- Following the death of someone important to you, the goal is to "get over it."
- Tears are an expression of weakness.

Grief refers to the thoughts and feelings experienced inside a person upon the death of someone loved. It is experienced emotionally, cognitively, physically, socially, and spiritually.

Normal grief reactions include depressed mood, insomnia, anxiety, poor appetite, loss of interest, guilt, dreams about the deceased, and poor concentration. Psychological states include shock, denial, anger, and yearning and searching for the deceased. Socially, grievers tend to experience isolation and disappointment as their friends and families fail to understand what they are facing. Spirituality is frequently either shaken or strengthened by the experience of profound loss. **Mourning** refers to all the ways in which a person expresses grief on the outside. Dr. Wolfelt calls this "grief gone public." This includes culturally determined practices such as wakes, funerals, sitting shiva, or decorating the gravesite. This is a key distinction because the passage of time alone does not always heal grief; it is what we do with the time that seems to help. Grief that remains private seems to simply travel with us through life. Sharing our grief with others seems to relieve some of its effects and allow us to move through it. Social media sites provide outlets for grievers to find understanding and meaningful connections with others. Attending grief support groups or seeing a counselor are also activities of mourning. Most people grieve, but many do not mourn. It is mourning that gradually releases us from the pain of loss.

Forty years after Dr. Elisabeth Kübler-Ross introduced the Five Stages of Dying (Kübler-Ross, 1969): the stages of denial, anger, bargaining, depression, and acceptance are overwhelmingly identified as the way we die as well as grieve. Academia and popular culture have embraced this model. Unfortunately, it does not reflect what people actually experience in mourning, but instead tends to steer them to doubt the normalcy of what they are going through. "Am I doing this right?" "Am I normal?" "Am I failing at this, because I am not feeling acceptance, and I keep getting stuck in denial over and over again?" In reality, each person's experience of grief is unique to that person, to the relationship he or she had with the loved one, to the way death happened, to the person's prior history with major losses, and to current life circumstances. It feels more like a wilderness with no signposts than an orderly progression through the aftermath of a death.

Grievers as well as those around them have bought into a belief that they should not surrender to mourning. Concerned adult children and physicians rush to start antidepressant medication as soon as a widow has trouble sleeping or eating. Younger widowers are pressured to start dating as soon as possible. Some of the first questions asked of a grief counselor are often, "How long does this last?" "What do I have to do to get through it as quickly as possible?" Self-control is valued and the dominant cultural and familial message is usually, "Shape up and get on with your life." In reality, mourning demands that who we are and the world we live in be reconstructed and remodeled in major ways. This requires much talking, working, engaging, writing, feeling, experimenting, and risk taking, supported by others who do not try to fix or rush the griever.

Instead of "getting over it" as soon as possible, successful mourning asks us to engage in a complex process of finding a new and durable connection to who we are now and to the person who died. J. William Worden (2009) describes this process as the **Four Tasks of Mourning:**

1. To accept the reality of the loss
2. To process the pain of grief while caring for the self
3. To adjust to a world without the deceased
4. To find an enduring connection with the deceased in the midst of embarking on a new life

These tasks indicate a natural movement that results when people actively engage in mourning, rather than fitting one's own experience into someone else's framework. When people "hang in there" with their mourning over time, they instinctively progress toward the final task. Finally, they are able to remember the loved one without so much pain. They have the energy to engage in life and be open to new relationships and activities. They sense that they now carry that departed person with them in an enduring way that no longer requires a physical presence. They are able to love again.

Bereavement is the social experience of dealing with the death of a loved one. It refers to the event of losing an important person to death and is derived from the Old English word *berafian,* meaning "to rob." Most cultures provide symbols and contexts for bereavement, such as wearing black or a black armband. Bereaved people experience themselves as being set apart from the current of ordinary life. Contemporary society has left behind the visible symbols of bereavement, with the result that those in mourning often feel isolated and alone. Historically, identifying them as being in a special state of grieving gave them special permission to be "under reconstruction" (Wolfelt, 2010). Nowadays, they look just like everybody else.

Nurses are affected by cultural myths about grief and mourning in the same way the rest of society is; when they are faced with a person who is grieving or dying, nurses may feel uncomfortable and unequipped to face the loss. They often feel acutely uncomfortable when witnessing expressions of deep grief and pain, and try to "fix it" with an intervention. Normal activities of mourning, such as weeping, protesting, or expressing anger or despair, are perceived as "melt downs" or signs of "losing it." Medical professionals commonly feel inadequate in the face of such "break downs" and either leave the griever, consider medicating the griever, or request a counselor for the griever. This reflects our societal misunderstandings about grief and mourning, but may also be a response to unmourned losses in the lives of the medical staff. Difficult memories and unresolved feelings may be awakened. Nurses may question whether it is acceptable to show their tears in the presence of death and grief. Conversely, they may feel distress at their lack of emotional response. Psychological support and education should be available to help staff better understand the grieving process. As nurses examine their own feelings and their personal experiences of loss, verbal and nonverbal clues to the needs of grieving family members of a dying patient become more apparent (Marks, 1976).

DISENFRANCHISED GRIEF

When patients and clients die, the professionals who cared for them experience disenfranchised grief. **Disenfranchised grief** is a term coined by Dr. Kenneth Doka (1989) to acknowledge losses that are not socially sanctioned, openly acknowledged, or publicly mourned. Grief may be disenfranchised because of the relationship of the griever (life partner, health care worker, defense attorney, divorced spouse), the loss (miscarriages or abortions, war heroes), the type of death (executions, homicides, suicides, human immunodeficiency virus/acquired immunodeficiency syndrome [HIV/AIDS]), or the grieving style (adolescent grieving rituals, men who emote, women who grieve instrumentally). In such situations mourners may not have the opportunity to publicly grieve the loss. Thus health care workers may experience real grief over the loss of a patient, a grief that may not be recognized or acknowledged by others. This grief may be solitary and uncomforted even within the griever (Albert, 2001) and may be difficult to resolve. Simple activities of mourning are essential to the continuing health and functioning of the staff. Once losses are recognized as disenfranchised, it becomes easier to support them within and among individuals sharing the same work experience.

THEORY

Studies of grief and loss by Parkes (1970, 1975), Caplan (1974), Engel (1964), Kübler-Ross (1969), and others postulated various phases of bereavement that proceed in orderly sequences within certain timeframes. The various frameworks for grieving and phases of grief are useful models for helping people to normalize the deeply felt and disturbing phenomena they experience when they confront profound loss. Denial and shock, anger and guilt, emotional turmoil, disorganization, panic, depression, loneliness, and, eventually, acceptance of the loss are common during bereavement. Models and frameworks help organize the experience of loss, but models do not provide the focus of care when facilitating the process of mourning. They are a road map. The work of mourning derives from the details of a person's unique experience.

Some of the most widely known early grief theorists are George Engel, Colin Parkes, Erich Lindemann, John Bowlby, and Edgar Jackson. Although each theorist uses different terminology, the process all of them outline is fundamentally the same. Each describes commonly experienced psychological and behavioral phenomena. However, we now know that these phenomena do not always follow a pattern of response. The following are common phenomena a person may experience at some point in the grief process:

1. Shock and disbelief
2. Denial
3. Sensation of somatic distress
4. Preoccupation with the image of the deceased
5. Guilt
6. Anger
7. Change in behavior (e.g., depression, disorganization, or restlessness)
8. Reorganization of behavior directed toward a new object or activity

---

EXAMINING THE EVIDENCE

End-of-Life Care—No Longer a Taboo

Death and dying is still very scary to me in general. How do nurses work with end-of-life patients?

You are definitely not alone in your apprehension, but there is hope that in the near future dealing with death and dying will not be such a scary situation for most people. It is widely acknowledged that death and dying is not a subject easily discussed by society and ongoing awareness building and education are required. Individuals need to document their wishes for care at end-of-life; health care providers need to initiate honest, timely, and culturally relevant discussions with those for whom they are caring; policy makers need to eliminate barriers that prevent access to hospice and palliative care; employers need to support staff who are living with serious illness or are caregivers; and the media need to explore ways to demystify dying and help normalize the experience to the general public (Radulovic, 2011).

In the past 30 years, there have been tremendous advances in medical care, particularly in end-of-life/palliative care. Yet far too many Americans still suffer from unnecessary pain and unaddressed needs at life's end (Radulovic, 2011). According to the Worldwide Palliative Care Alliance more than 100 million patients need palliative care annually, but fewer than 8% actually receive it. In the Quality of Death index, which measures end-of-life care services such as environment, quality of care, training availability, access to pain medications, and physician-patient transparency in 40 countries, the United States ranks ninth worldwide with the United Kingdom and other European countries rated higher (Silverberg, 2011).

There has been little focus on making staff more confident to help those who are dying (Sprinks, 2011). The first intervention in end-of-life care is for nurses to assess their own skill level and seek support from team members as necessary. The quality of patients' end-of-life care is greatly influenced by staff members' attitudes toward death. Nurses who feared death and avoided thoughts and discussions about death had poorer attitudes toward caring for dying patients (Matsui & Braun, 2010). Possessing good listening skills is cited as the most important characteristic needed by a health care worker when talking with a dying patient and his or her family. Interrupting patients before they have finished speaking is the most commonly ignored rule of communication. Also essential is sensitivity toward patient needs, including not discussing specifics of condition/prognosis if the patient is not ready for it (Charalambous, 2010).

Nursing strategies to conserve dignity include the following: maintain positive self-image and normal appearance (e.g., access to wigs, cosmetics, proper clothing); review success in patients' lives and their lasting legacy; discuss any suicidal thoughts in a nonjudgmental approach; allow time for patients to express their feelings and give them as much control over their care as possible; assist in supporting family and repairing conflicts; help to make the most of things they enjoy (e.g., visits with friends, foods/music, storytelling, living in the moment); and assist with spiritual comfort—finding solace in spiritual beliefs and achieving a peaceful death (Brown & Johnston, 2011).

Brown, H., & Johnston, B. (2011). Identifying care actions to conserve dignity in end of life care. *British Journal of Community Nursing, 16*(5), 238-245.

Charalambous, A. (2010). Good communication in end of life care. *Journal of Community Nursing, 24*(6), 12-14.

Matsui, M., & Braun, K. (2010). Nurses' and care workers' attitudes toward death and caring for dying older adults in Japan. *International Journal of Palliative Nursing, 16*(12), 593-598.

Radulovic, J. (2011). *Public awareness about end of life care is essential and must not be discouraged,* National Hospice and Palliative Care Association, March 29, 2011, press release.

Silverberg, E. (2011). Best countries for end of life care. *Canadian Nursing Home, 22*(2), 25.

Sprinks, J. (2011). Nurses lack confidence in end of life care. *Nursing Older People, 23*(2), 6-7.

Contributed by Lois Angelo.

Shock and Disbelief

The bereaved person's first response is that of **denial.** The person is emotionally unable to accept his or her painful loss. Denial functions as a buffer against intolerable pain and allows the person slowly to acknowledge the reality of death. The mourner may appear to be functioning like a robot. Often, the bereaved person feels numb. A death may be accepted intellectually during this stage—"It's just as well, she was suffering"—although the emotional responses are still repressed. Denial is a needed defense that lasts for a few hours or a few days. Denial can also be thought of as disbelief, and may recur over the early course of bereavement ("This morning I picked up the phone to call her and dialed her number before I remembered that she is gone"). However, persistent denial suggests that the mourning may be complicated, making it difficult to move through the process of mourning.

Development of Awareness

As denial fades, painful feelings begin to surface. The finality of the loved one's death becomes more of a reality. Waves of anguish and pain are experienced and may be localized in the chest or the epigastric area. **Anger** often surfaces at this time. Physicians and nurses are often the objects of blame. Awareness by staff that anger is often displaced onto people in the hospital environment may decrease defensive staff behaviors. **Guilt** is often experienced, and the bereaved blames himself or herself for taking or for failing to take specific actions. The griever may need to be supported patiently as he or she gradually comes to terms with a past that cannot be changed by hindsight. Guilt often indicates profound regret that things could not have been different than they were.

Crying is a common phenomenon during this stage. "It is during this time that the greatest degree of anguish or despair, within the limits imposed by cultural patterns, is experienced or expressed" (Engel, 1964). Crying can afford a welcome release from pent-up anguish and tension. Assessment of cultural patterns is important in making clinical judgments about the appropriateness of the bereaved's behavior. Failing to cry can be the result of cultural influences or environmental restraints. The person may cry in private. Inability to cry, however, may be the result of a high degree of ambivalence toward the deceased. A person who is unable to cry may have difficulty in successfully completing the work of mourning.

Since these pioneering scholars, other models describing how we grieve have emerged. Current research focuses on issues such as the relationship between grief and trauma; the grieving process during various developmental periods of life; the advantages of resiliency and adaptability in mourning; interventions appropriate for specific populations; definition of complicated or intractable grief and its treatment; and many more topics. The Association for Death Education and Counseling is a prominent professional organization that supports research and offers a certification in thanatology.

Stroebe and Schut (1999) describe mourning as "dual processes," both of which derive from models of stress and coping. The bereaved individual oscillates between **loss-oriented** and **restoration-oriented** tasks. The loss-oriented processes are those that deal with recognizing the loss, whereas the restoration-oriented processes aim at re-creating a new life. A person's ability to oscillate, or move between these spheres, is an indication of their coping and inner resources. One contribution of this model is that it normalizes distraction from the loss experience as an integral part of successful mourning. Mourners are encouraged to take breaks, experience positive emotions, delay or defer some of the pain of grieving, and essentially control the amount of grief they are able to bear.

Various phenomena experienced during bereavement are described in Table 25-1.

APPLICATION OF THE NURSING PROCESS

ASSESSMENT

Most bereaved people come to terms with their losses with support from family and friends. However, more than 30% may require professional support (Lloyd-Williams, 1995). As mentioned, unresolved grief reactions over a lifetime have been called the hidden disease and may account for many of the physical symptoms seen in physicians' offices and hospital units. Suicide is higher among people who have had a significant loss, especially if losses are multiple and grieving mechanisms are limited.

Often the history of an individual can alert health care personnel to signs or symptoms of potential difficulty a person may encounter during a time of mourning. The following questions identify risk factors that may complicate the successful completion of mourning:

1. Do any of the following factors relate to the bereaved?
   - Was the bereaved heavily dependent on the deceased?
   - Were there persistent, unresolved conflicts with the deceased?
   - Was the deceased a child? (Perhaps the most profound loss of all)
   - Does the bereaved have a meaningful relationship or support system?
   - Has the bereaved experienced a number of previous losses?
   - Does the bereaved have sound coping skills?
2. Was the deceased's death associated with a cultural stigma (e.g., AIDS, suicide, homicide)?
3. Has the bereaved had difficulty resolving past significant losses?
4. Does the bereaved have a history of depression, drug or alcohol abuse, or other psychiatric illness?
5. If the bereaved is young, are there indications for special interventions?
6. Was the deceased a veteran or victim of war?
7. Assessing for spiritual beliefs was discussed previously.

Acute grief can result in an exacerbation of any preexisting medical or psychiatric problems, and, of course, a history of depression, substance abuse, or posttraumatic stress disorder can complicate grief. Complicated grieving essentially means that the grief work is unresolved. Prolonged depression is the most common response to unresolved grief. Disturbances in mood are associated with biological changes in the body during stress-related depressive illness. Some examples include electrolyte disturbances, nervous system alterations, and faulty regulation of the autonomic nervous system. Always assess the potential for suicide. Someone who is having difficulty negotiating the work of mourning and is suffering can benefit from counseling, as mentioned earlier.

ASSESSMENT GUIDELINES

Grieving and Complicated Grieving

1. Identify whether the individual is at risk for complicated grieving (see assessment history).
2. Identify the bereaved person's cultural beliefs, length of typical grieving, and mourning rituals.
3. Evaluate for psychotic symptoms, agitation, increased activity, alcohol or drug abuse, and extreme vegetative symptoms (anorexia, weight loss, insomnia).
4. Do not overlook people who do not express significant grief in the context of major loss. These individuals might have an increased risk of subsequent complicated or unresolved grief reactions.

TABLE 25-1 PHENOMENA EXPERIENCED DURING BEREAVEMENT

SYMPTOMS	EXAMPLES
Sensations of Somatic Distress The bereaved may experience tightness in the throat, shortness of breath, sighing, mental pain, or exhaustion; food tastes like sand; things feel unreal. Pain or discomfort may be identical to the symptoms experienced by the deceased. Normally, symptoms are brief.	A woman whose husband died of a stroke complains of weakness and numbness on her left side.
Preoccupation With the Image of the Deceased The bereaved introduces into conversation, thinks about, and talks about numerous memories of the deceased. The memories are positive. This process continues with great sadness. The idealization of the deceased lets the bereaved relive the gratifications associated with the deceased and helps resolve any guilt the bereaved feels concerning the deceased. The bereaved may also assume many of the mannerisms of the deceased through identification. Identification serves the purpose of holding on to the deceased. Preoccupation with the deceased can continue for many months before it lessens.	A man whose wife has very recently died states, "I just can't stop thinking about my wife. Everything I see reminds me of her. We picked up this seashell on our honeymoon. I remember every wonderful moment we had together. The pain is so great, but the memories just keep coming." His friends notice that when he talks, his hand gestures and expressions are very like those of his recently deceased wife.
Guilt The bereaved reproaches himself or herself for real or imagined acts of negligence or omissions in the relationship with the deceased.	"I should have made him go to the doctor sooner." "I should have paid more attention to her, been more thoughtful."
Anger The anger the bereaved experiences may not be toward the object at its source. Often the anger is displaced onto the medical or nursing staff. Often it is directed toward the deceased. The anger is at its height during the first month but is often intermittent throughout the first year. The overflow of hostility disturbs the bereaved, resulting in the feeling that he or she is "going insane."	"The doctor didn't operate in time. If he had, Mary would be alive today." "How could he leave me like this…how could he?"
Change in Behavior: Depression, Disorganization, Restlessness A person may exhibit marked restlessness and an inability to organize his or her behavior. A depressive mood during routine activities is common, decreasing as the year passes and the intensity of the grief declines. Absence of depression is more abnormal than its presence. Loneliness and aimlessness are most pronounced 6 to 9 months after the death. Reorganization of behavior directed toward a new object or activity gradually occurs. The person renews his or her interest in people and activities. The grieving thus releases the bereaved from one interpersonal relationship, and new ones are free to take its place.	Six months after her husband died, Mrs. Faye states, "I just can't seem to function. I have a hard time doing the simplest tasks. I can't be bothered with socializing. I feel so down…so, so empty." Twenty months after her husband's death, Mrs. Faye tells a friend, "I'll be away this weekend. I am going fishing with my brother and his friend. This is the first time I've felt like doing anything since Harry died."

5. Complicated grief reactions require significant interventions. Suicidal or severely depressed people might require hospitalization. Always assess for **suicide** with signs of depression or other dysfunctional signs.

6. Assess support systems. If support systems are limited, find bereavement groups in the community.

7. When grieving is stalled or complicated, a person is at high risk for major depression or other mental illnesses. There are a variety of therapeutic approaches that have proved beneficial. Make referrals.

8. Grieving can bring with it severe spiritual anguish. Assess whether spiritual counseling or a specific counselor would be useful for the bereaved.

Table 25-2 presents a comparison between the symptoms of a "normal" mourning process and those of a complicated grief reaction.

TABLE 25-2 COMMON RESPONSES AND PATHOLOGICAL INTENSIFICATION DURING GRIEF

TYPICAL RESPONSE	PATHOLOGICAL INTENSIFICATION
Dying Emotional expression and immediate coping with the dying process	Avoidance; feeling of being overwhelmed, dazed, confused; self-punitive feelings; inappropriately hostile feelings
Death and Outcry Outcry of emotions with news of the death and turning for help to others or isolating self with self-soothing	Panic, dissociative reactions, reactive psychoses, suicidal ideation
Warding Off (Denial) Avoidance of reminders and social withdrawal, focusing elsewhere, emotional numbing, not thinking of implications to self or of certain themes	Maladaptive avoidance of confronting the implications of death through drug or alcohol abuse, promiscuity, fugue states, phobic avoidance, feeling of being dead or unreal
Reexperience (Intrusion) Intrusive experiences, including recollections of negative experiences during relationship with the deceased, bad dreams, reduced concentration, compulsive reenactments	Flooding with negative images and emotions; uncontrolled ideation, self-impairing compulsive reenactments, night terrors, recurrent nightmares, distraught feelings resulting from the intrusion of anger, anxiety, despair, shame, or guilt; physiological exhaustion resulting from hyperarousal
Working Through Recollection of the deceased and a contemplation of self with reduced intrusiveness of memories and fantasies and with increased rational acceptance, reduced numbness and avoidance, more "dosing" of recollections, and a sense of working it through	Feeling of inability to integrate the death with a sense of self and continued life; persistent warding-off themes that may manifest as anxious, depressed, enraged, shame-filled, or guilty moods; self-injurious behaviors; and psychophysiological syndromes
Resolution Reduction in emotional swings and a sense of self-coherence and readiness for new relationships; ability to experience positive states of mind	Failure to negotiate the process of mourning, which may be associated with inability to work or create, or to feel emotion or positive states of mind

From Horowitz, M.J. (1990). A model of mourning: Change in schemas of self and other. *Journal of the American Psychoanalytic Association, 38*(2), 297-303.

DIAGNOSIS

Four nursing diagnoses that apply to grief are *Grieving, Complicated Grieving, Risk for Complicated Grieving,* and *Chronic Sorrow* During the time of grief, especially if the grieving process is prolonged or symptomatic (e.g., profound depression or disorganization), other nursing diagnoses may come into play. *Ineffective Coping, Compromised Family Coping, Disturbed Sleep Pattern, Risk for Spiritual Distress, Disturbed Thought Processes, Chronic Sorrow,* and *Social Isolation* are examples.

Complicated Grieving or Risk for Complicated Grieving

Complicated grieving occurs when individuals have difficulty coming to terms with their loss and experience phenomena outside the normal grief reaction, which impairs their ability to function. The *DSM-IV*-TR (APA, 2000) identifies a number of symptoms that are not characteristic with normal mourning, some of which include:

1. Guilt about things other than actions taken or not taken by the survivor at the time of death
2. Thoughts of death other than the survivor feeling that he or she would be better off dead or should have died with the deceased person
3. Morbid preoccupation with worthlessness
4. Marked psychomotor retardation
5. Prolonged and marked functional impairment
6. Hallucinatory experiences other than thinking that he or she hears the voice of, or transiently sees the image of, the deceased person

TABLE 25-3 INTERVENTIONS FOR HELPING PEOPLE IN ACUTE GRIEF

INTERVENTION	RATIONALE
1. Use methods that can facilitate the grieving process (Robinson, 1997).	
a. Give your full presence: use appropriate eye contact, attentive listening, and appropriate touch.	a. Talking is one of the most important ways of dealing with acute grief. Listening patiently helps the bereaved express all feelings, even ones he or she feels are "negative." Appropriate eye contact helps to convey the awareness that you are there and are sharing the person's sadness. Suitable human touch can express warmth and nurture healing. Inappropriate touch can leave a person confused and uncomfortable.
b. Be patient with the bereaved in times of silence. Do not fill silence with empty chatter.	b. Sharing painful feelings during periods of silence is healing and conveys your concern.
2. Know about and share with the bereaved information about the phenomena that occur during the normal mourning process, because they may concern some people (intense anger at the deceased, guilt, symptoms the deceased had before death, unbidden floods of memories). Give the bereaved support during the occurrence of these phenomena and a written handout for reference.	2. Although the knowledge will not eliminate the emotions, it can greatly relieve a person who is thinking there is something wrong with having these feelings.
3. Encourage the support of family and friends. If no supports are available, refer the patient to a community bereavement group. (Bereavement groups are helpful even when a person has many friends or much family support.)	3. Friends can help with routine matters. For example: • Getting food into the house • Making phone calls • Driving to the mortuary • Taking care of the kids or other family members
4. Offer spiritual support and referrals when needed.	4. Dealing with an illness or catastrophic loss can cause the most profound spiritual anguish.
5. When intense emotions are in evidence, show understanding and support (see Table 25-4).	5. Empathic words that reflect acceptance of a bereaved individual's feelings are healing (Robinson, 1997).

OUTCOMES IDENTIFICATION

Ideally, successful outcomes would include the following. An individual:

- Can tolerate intense emotions.
- Reports decreased preoccupation with the deceased (loss).
- Demonstrates increased periods of stability.
- Tends to previous responsibilities.
- Takes on new roles and responsibilities.
- Has energy to invest in new endeavors.
- Expresses positive expectations about the future.
- Remembers positive as well as negative aspects of the deceased loved one.

PLANNING

Nurses constantly encounter people who are faced with loss, although that loss might not be the reason they first entered the medical or psychiatric health care system. In hospital settings, grief is expressed when there is a loss besides death, for example, loss of a limb from amputation or a breast after surgery for breast cancer. Sometimes simple active listening can go a long way in offering comfort and respite from loneliness, or perhaps a referral to a grieving support group is indicated. Still at other times, the nurse may realize that even though individuals present with a medical or emotional problem, they are also undergoing a profound loss; therefore the nurse might suggest the need for a referral for grief counseling, re-grief work, or psychotherapy. As mentioned, physical or emotional symptoms may be related to a complicated grief reaction.

IMPLEMENTATION

The nurse's focus when facilitating bereavement is on helping the bereaved deal with the most important issues emerging at a particular time. Often the nurse or other caregiver can best serve the grieving person simply by being present, listening with interest, and encouraging talking and the recounting of meaningful stories. Tables 25-3 and 25-4 provide guidelines for helping people grieve.

Psychotherapy

Grief is a process that most of us negotiate by receiving help from family and friends and by staying connected to community activities. Some people find comfort and support in

TABLE 25-4	**GUIDELINES FOR COMMUNICATING WITH A BEREAVED INDIVIDUAL**
SITUATION	**SAMPLE RESPONSE**
When you sense an overwhelming *sorrow*	"This must hurt terribly."
When you hear *anger* in the bereaved person's voice	"I hear anger in your voice. Most people go through periods of anger when their loved one dies. Are you feeling angry now?"
If you discern *guilt*	"Are you feeling guilty? This is a common reaction many people have. What are some of your thoughts about this?"
If you sense a *fear* of the future	"It must be scary to go through this."
When the bereaved seems *confused*	"This can be a confusing time."
In almost any *painful situation*	"This must be very difficult for you."

Adapted from Robinson, D. (1997). *Good intentions: the nine unconscious mistakes of nice people* (p. 9). New York: Warner Books.

grief counseling or support groups. Six to ten sessions of psychotherapy have been found to be helpful during the crisis period. At a later stage, the use of 15 sessions or more has a good outcome.

For people at risk for complicated grief reactions (history of mental illness, loss by suicide or homicide, facing multiple simultaneous losses, loss of a child), brief and time-limited psychotherapy may be indicated. According to Zisook and Zisook (2005), the following are essential components of effective short-term therapy:

1. **An educational component:** Helps people learn what to expect and how to normalize their confusing feelings and behaviors.
2. **Encouragement of full expression of emotions and affect:** May include writing letters to deceased, role playing, looking at pictures.
3. **An attempt to help bereaved come to peace with a new relationship to the deceased:** Involves the process of integrating the loss of the deceased into current reality.

More complicated or pathological patterns of grief may require special techniques, such as re-grief work. When a major depression or other mental health illness is involved, psychotherapeutic techniques geared to grief work as well as addressing the individual's mental health issues can help greatly in improving the person's quality of life. At times psychobiological interventions may be needed (e.g., antidepressants). Box 25-1 offers guidelines that can help people and their families cope with catastrophic loss.

BOX 25-1   GUIDELINES FOR DEALING WITH CATASTROPHIC LOSS

Take the time you need to grieve. The hard work of grief uses psychological energy. Resolution of the numb state that occurs after loss requires a few weeks at least. A minimum of 1 year, to cover all the birthdays, anniversaries, and other important dates without your loved one, is required before you can learn to live with your loss.

Express your feelings. Remember that anger, anxiety, loneliness, and even guilt are normal reactions and that everyone needs a safe place to express them. Tell your personal story of loss as many times as you need to—this repetition is a helpful and necessary part of the grieving process.

Establish a structure for each day and stick to it. Although it is hard to do, keeping to some semblance of structure makes the first few weeks after a loss easier. Getting through each day helps restore the confidence you need to accept the reality of loss.

Do not feel that you have to answer all the questions asked of you. Although most people try to be kind, they may be unaware of their insensitivity. Down the road you may want to read books about how others have dealt with similar circumstances. They often have helpful suggestions for a person in your situation.

As hard as it is, try to take good care of yourself. Eat well, talk with friends, get plenty of rest. Be sure to let your primary care clinician know if you are having trouble eating or sleeping. Make use of exercise. It can help you release pent-up frustrations. If you are losing weight, sleeping excessively or intermittently, or still experiencing deep depression after 3 months, be sure to seek professional assistance.

Expect the unexpected. You may begin to feel a bit better, only to have a brief emotional collapse. These are expected reactions. Moreover, you may find that you dream about, visualize, think about, or search for your loved one. This, too, is a part of the grieving process.

Give yourself time. Do not feel that you have to resume all of life's duties right away.

Make use of rituals. Those who take the time to say goodbye at a funeral or a viewing tend to find that it helps the bereavement process.

If you do not begin to feel better within a few weeks, at least for a few hours every day, be sure to tell your physician or primary care practitioner. If you had an emotional problem in the past (e.g., depression, substance abuse), be sure to get the additional support you need. Losing a loved one puts you at higher risk for a relapse of these disorders.

From Zerbe, K.J. (1999). *Women's mental health in primary care* (pp. 207-208). Philadelphia: Saunders.

EVALUATION

Evaluation should address whether these tasks have been accomplished. The work of mourning is over when the bereaved can remember realistically the pleasures and the disappointments of the relationship with the lost loved one. Brief periods of intense emotions may still occur at significant times, such as holidays and anniversaries, but the person or family members have energy to reinvest in new relationships that bring shared joys, security, satisfaction, and comfort. If, after a normal period (12 to months), a person has not been able to find pleasure, satisfaction, and comfort in his or her life, then reassessment and re-evaluation are indicated.

APPLYING THE ART

A Person Experiencing Grief

SCENARIO: I met 19-year-old Monica during her brief hospitalization to stabilize her insulin-resistant (type 1) diabetes. Under her veneer of sarcasm, I sensed depression as she talked about her pledging a sorority, too much partying, failing grades, and her diabetes raging out of control.

THERAPEUTIC GOAL: By the conclusion of this interaction, Monica will make at least one decision to break out of her self-destructive cycle and deal with the issue(s) and feelings she is pushing down.

STUDENT-PATIENT INTERACTION	THOUGHTS, COMMUNICATION TECHNIQUES, AND MENTAL HEALTH NURSING CONCEPTS
Monica: "You're back again. Couldn't find anything better to do?" ***Student's feelings***: *Monica's sarcasm tends to disconcert me until I remind myself that fear and loss fuel her anger.*	
Student: "Hi, Monica. I will be working with you again today. How are you?"	I ignored her comment, which *non-reinforces* the sarcasm. I am willing myself to not take it personally.
Monica: "Fine. The doctor just yelled because my right heel has a sore on it that I've ignored. If I fail one more class, I go on academic probation and finals start next week. Yeah, I'm doing just great."	I forgot that using a social greeting like, "How are you?" typically elicits an automatic "fine." Using a *broad opening* like "What's been happening with you since we talked yesterday?" would better let Monica know that I really want her to share.
Student: *Leaning in.* "Somehow your 'just great' doesn't sound so great." ***Student's feelings***: *I feel overwhelmed listening to her. Because I carry a heavy academic load, I identify with her struggles. Yet I feel some frustration that Monica does not seem to take charge of her life.*	I make an observation and then use *attending* body language to show empathy. Is that countertransference? Is that my own fear that I will lose control of all the pieces I juggle?
Monica: "No use worrying." *Leaning in and speaking quietly.*	
Student: "And yet somehow the worry creeps back in. Sometimes the worry looks like sadness or even anger. Sometimes it shows up as a blood sugar that refuses to stabilize." ***Student's feelings***: *I hope I'm not pushing her too much. We have some rapport and she lets herself vent with me.*	I refer to "the worry" and "a blood sugar" to depersonalize the reference, yet still allow Monica to choose insight, if possible.
Monica: *Nods.*	
Student: "You feel overwhelmed."	
Monica: "The doctor yelling about my foot! Wish I could hide in some hole where no one could ever find me or tell me what I should be doing."	In *crisis terms* the doctor "yelling" likely acted as the *precipitating event.*
Student: "I wonder what pressures you the most."	I ask Monica an indirect question to help her identify stress. Should I have instead attempted to translate into feelings? For example, "You're discouraged and having a hard time believing in yourself."
Monica: "The feeling that no matter what I do it isn't enough. It isn't good enough. I'm not good enough."	

APPLYING THE ART—cont'd

A Person Experiencing Grief

STUDENT-PATIENT INTERACTION	THOUGHTS, COMMUNICATION TECHNIQUES, AND MENTAL HEALTH NURSING CONCEPTS
Student: "You say you aren't good enough—for who?"	I am assessing a *balancing* factor in *crisis* when I help Monica talk about her *perception of the event* and most significantly, her perception of self.
Monica: "Since I was diagnosed when I was 6, my mother insisted I was the same as everybody else. 'The diabetes doesn't change anything, Monica. You can do anything!' So I pledge a sorority, go with the flow, ignoring what I should or shouldn't eat or drink. Then I stay out late and screw up my sleep and my blood sugar goes haywire. I feel bad, so I don't study."	Monica *projects* the blame for her trouble onto her Mother. *What must it be like for a person to deal with diabetes since 6 years old?*
Student: "So in trying to prove the diabetes does not matter, it ends up influencing major areas of your life. What does your mother say now?"	I *clarify* to try to understand Monica's meaning. I also *gather information.*
Monica: "Nothing. She doesn't know I'm in here."	Monica independently brought up the subject of her mother, so I will listen to see if her mother is a *situational support,* a *second balancing factor in crisis.*
Student: "She doesn't know?"	I *restate* to say, "Go on."
Monica: "I thought I could put it off until after finals, but my life is falling apart."	
Student: "Put what off, Monica?"	I still do not understand about "put off," so I ask an *indirect question.*
Student's feelings: *Did I do this the right way? I probably should have helped her talk about her life falling apart but I am also curious about what she has put off.*	
Monica: *Sobbing.* "She's dying. My mother is dying. She's survived the cancer so long that I never thought she'd actually die. She has maybe 2 months."	She has been grieving losing her mother.
Student: "Oh! I'm so sorry. You've been holding this pain inside, trying to put off…?"	
Student's feelings: *My feelings of sorrow came out without my thinking first.*	
Monica: "No one knows. My friends don't even know."	
Student's feelings: *I feel compassion for her. She must feel so alone.*	
Student: "I wonder what telling others would mean to you."	
Monica: "That I can't make it by myself. That it's real. She's going to die. I can't do my life without her." *Crying.*	I wonder if *unconsciously* Monica's noncompliance with her diabetes and even doing poorly at school has to do with *acting out* her belief that "I can't do my life without her." I know how devastated I would be to lose my mother.
Student's feelings: *I am picking up some of her feelings of aloneness and powerlessness with the impending death of her mom. I have to watch that I don't get sucked into these feelings but rather focus on Monica's feelings and thoughts.*	
Student: "Monica, what are you saying, that you don't want to live?"	Is she saying she cannot live without her mother? Is this a covert message about suicide?
Monica: "I wouldn't do anything to hurt myself, but I already feel so lonely, like she's gone already."	She describes *anticipatory grief.* However, Edwin Shneidman might refer to her behavior as subintentional suicide.
Student's feelings: *I feel relieved that she chooses to not hurt herself, though her lifestyle choices aren't healthy.*	

Continued

APPLYING THE ART—cont'd

A Person Experiencing Grief

STUDENT-PATIENT INTERACTION	THOUGHTS, COMMUNICATION TECHNIQUES, AND MENTAL HEALTH NURSING CONCEPTS
Student: "You feel lonely. You miss her already. In what ways have you been able to let your mother know what she means to you?"	I validate to be sure I understand. Again, I need to assess for countertransference and keep the pace at Monica's comfort level, not my own.
Student's feelings: *Helping Monica look at saying goodbye makes me think about telling the people I love how much they mean to me.*	
Monica: "I haven't gone home all semester. I barely talk when she calls. I guess if I go home I can't pretend that it's not happening anymore."	Monica uses the word *pretend*. The *denial* stage of grief plays a part, too.
Student: "It's natural to feel afraid. It's scary to let your-self experience this pain of saying goodbye." *She nods.* "I wonder what you think might happen."	I give *support* and ask an *indirect question*.
Student's feelings: *I feel good that Monica is working with me to think through how she will handle talking to her mother.*	
Monica: "Maybe I won't be strong. I'll break down."	
Student: "And then?"	I help Monica *problem-solve* by anticipating what will likely happen with each step, in order to decrease her *anxiety*. Being able to predict meets *safety needs*.
Monica: "My mom will cry, too."	
Student: "You will cry together." *Monica nods.*	
Monica: "I need to talk to her. Will you stay with me while I call?"	
Student: "Yes."	Our talking together highlighted the third crisis *balancing factor*, namely, *situational support*. Before we terminate today, I want to help Monica think about who can lend support as she juggles school, her diabetes, and the *grief* of losing her mother.
Student's feelings: *I feel honored that Monica is reaching out to me and has at least made a decision to be with her mom and share their losses together.*	Monica's decision to call her mother means she is *working through the denial stage* of the grief process and she is ready to go through the painful process of saying goodbye.

KEY POINTS TO REMEMBER

- There is a growing need for nurses to acquire competencies in end-of-life care, yet academic settings fail to provide curriculum. Nurses are encouraged to seek additional training and provide leadership in every health care setting.
- Hospice care is a model for multidisciplinary, holistic, palliative care at end-of-life.
- Hospice is an elective benefit under Medicare and is mirrored by most private insurance policies. While more patients choose hospice each year, less than 40% of deaths in 2008 occurred under hospice care.
- Anticipatory mourning describes the complex experience of patients and families during the period following a serious diagnosis. Health care professionals can guide families through some of the tasks of anticipatory mourning, while providing much needed normalization and therapeutic presence.
- A spiritual assessment should be part of every medical evaluation. It is crucial for health care professionals to avoid imposing their own views, faith, and beliefs on others, especially patients facing the vulnerabilities of serious illness and end-of-life.
- Compassion is a human quality and capacity that occurs and is nourished in relationships. It develops through a lifetime.
- Developing habits and practices of self-compassion is key to maintaining good self-care.

KEY POINTS TO REMEMBER—cont'd

- Grief is everything experienced inside a person in response to a loss, real or perceived, including the loss of a person, security, self-confidence, or a dream. Essentially, a loss results in a change in self-concept.
- Mourning is the social expression of grief—"grief gone public." Mourning is what enables people to move through the pain and trauma of major loss.
- Acute grief may last from 4 to 8 weeks; the complete process of mourning may take 1 or 2 years or longer.
- Common phenomena are evident during the experience of grief, and people usually show similar patterns of grief and mourning within their cultural norms. Culture greatly affects the patterns of response to death and dying in patients as well as nurses.
- Contemporary culture in the United States perpetuates several damaging myths about grief that have been internally absorbed by most people, and that are socially reinforced.
- Grief, when experienced by health care workers, can reactivate distressing feelings related to previous losses. If nurses have unresolved issues of grief and depression, their ability to help others is greatly minimized; therefore it is important

to recognize that staff members need psychological support when they work with people who are grieving.
- Many people are experts on loss but not on coping with loss. Health care workers can use a number of coping skills to help comfort the bereaved and facilitate mourning. Actively listening to a grieving person's story without offering banal or philosophical responses can assist in healing. Short-term grief counseling and support groups are often helpful.
- Indicators of the potential for complicated or unresolved grief include social isolation, extensive dependency on the deceased person, unresolved interpersonal conflicts, loss of a child, violent and senseless death, or a catastrophic loss. A history will often reveal potential risks for complicated grieving.
- Grief work is successful when the relationship to the deceased person has been restructured and energy is available for new relationships and life pursuits. The work of mourning is complete when the bereaved person or persons can remember realistically both the pleasures and the disappointments of the lost relationship. Outcomes for successful grief work have been identified.

APPLYING CRITICAL JUDGMENT

1. Mr. Hendrix's wife is now dying and she is ready to leave the hospital to go home with the aid of hospice. Mr. Hendrix asks you what hospice can do for his wife: "How can they help me care for her? Everything is so complicated and overwhelming. Who else will be there? I am so scared. I just don't know what to do."
   A. Since you know Mr. Hendrix is very anxious at this point, how would you explain to him clearly and concisely the services hospice can offer both he and his wife?
   B. Mr. Hendrix tells you he does not know what to say to his wife; he says that watching her die is too hard for him and it is very difficult to be with her, which makes him feel guilty. What guidelines can you give them in helping to say goodbye (consider the Four Gifts)?
   C. If you are the nurse on the hospice team, discuss ways in which you could implement at least three or four of the nine nursing goals identified in this chapter.

   D. If Mr. Hendrix has specific spiritual or religious beliefs that you believe might help him and his wife during this time, how could you assess these beliefs?
   E. Discuss the importance *to you* of how a person's spiritual beliefs or religious beliefs (e.g., What gives me strength? What is my purpose for being here? What brings me peace? How am I spiritually connected to other humans?) might help both the person who is dying as well as their loved ones.
2. What are some concrete ways in which you can help another to cope with a loss? Identify specific components in the following areas:
   A. How can you let the person tell his or her story?
   B. What is the potential therapeutic value of doing so?
   C. Avoiding banal advice, what are some things you might say that could offer comfort? Use the guidelines in Tables 25-3 and 25-4 to describe how you would help a person who is suffering a profound loss.

CHAPTER REVIEW QUESTIONS

Choose the most appropriate answer(s).
1. The nurse is talking to an adolescent about the death of his father 2 years ago. Which statement indicates a healthy progression in resolving this loss?
   1. "I never really had any feelings about his death."
   2. "I drive my father's old car which is nearly broken down, but I cannot give it up as it reminds me of him."

   3. "I still can barely make it through the day without sobbing."
   4. "Of course I loved my father, but he was not perfect."
2. Which statement indicates that a patient has successfully mourned a loss in his or her life?
   1. "She was so strong after her husband died. She never cried the whole time. She kept a stiff upper lip."

   2. "She was a wreck when her sister died. She cried and cried. It took her about a year before she resumed her usual activities with any zest."

   3. "You know, he still talks about his mother as if she were alive today, and she's been dead for 4 years."

   4. "He never talked about his wife after she died. He just picked up and went on life's way."

3. After having a mastectomy, a patient shows no emotion, asks no questions and smiles almost continually. The nursing priority is to focus on:

   1. identification of the patient's support system.

   2. a knowledge deficit pertaining to her illness.

   3. referral for the patient to see a psychiatrist.

   4. the meaning of the mastectomy to the patient.

4. A patient tells the nurse that his wife of 50 years died unexpectedly 6 weeks ago. The best response from the nurse would be:

   1. "It must be comforting to know you had a wonderful marriage."

   2. "It often takes 6 weeks to get over a loss such as yours."

   3. "Certain medications might be very helpful for you at this time."

   4. "This must be a difficult time for you now."

5. Which responses of a child to a father's untimely death represent an early stage of normal grieving? Select all that apply.

   1. The child lies in bed, banging his head against the mattress, shouting, "No, no, no!"

   2. The child refuses to go to school 2 weeks after his father's funeral, claiming "aches and pains all over my body."

   3. The child begins to obsessively attend to his game card collection and spends hours sorting and ordering cards for the first month after his father's death.

   4. The child repeatedly comes home from school and reports "seeing Dad" around a corner, but then "he just disappears."

REFERENCES

Albert, P. L. (2001). Grief and loss in the workplace. *Progress in Transplantation*, *11*(3), 169–173.

American Association of Colleges of Nursing. (2012). *Peaceful death: recommended competencies and curricular guidelines for end-of-life nursing care*. Retrieved from www.aacn.nche.edu/publications/deathfin.htm.

American Psychiatric Association (APA). (2000). *Diagnosis and Statistical Manual of Mental Disorders: DSM-IV-TR*. Washington, DC: Author.

Borreani, C., et al. (2008). Eliciting individual preferences about death: development of the End-of-life Preferences Interview. *Journal of Pain and Symptom Management*, *36*(4), 335–350.

Brennan, D. (2006). *Reuters report*. Retrieved from www.reuters.com/article/2006/11/09/us-summit-astrazeneca-americans-idUSN0844389820061109.

Byock, I. (2004). *Dying well: peace and possibilities at the end of life*. New York: Riverhead Books.

Caplan, G. (1974). *Support systems and community mental health. Lectures on concept development*. New York: Behavioral Publications.

Clukey, L. (2007). "Just be there": hospice caregivers' anticipatory mourning experience. *Journal of Hospice and Palliative Nursing*, *9*(3), 150–158.

Doka, K. (1989). *Disenfranchised grief: recognizing hidden sorrow*. New York: Lexington Books.

Durkin, A. (2003). Incorporating concepts of end-of-life care into a psychiatric nursing course. *Nursing Education Perspectives*, *4*, 184–185.

Engel, G. L. (1964). Grief and grieving. *American Journal of Nursing*, *64*(9), 93–98.

Hallenbeck, J. (2003). *Palliative care perspectives*. New York: Oxford University Press.

Harding, A. (2010). *End-of-life costs continue to climb upward*. Retrieved from www.reuters.com/assets/pring?aid=USTRE69C3KY20101014.

Hart, A., et al. (2003). Hospice clients' attitudes regarding spiritual discussions with their doctors. *American Journal of Hospice and Palliative Care*, *20*(2), 135–139.

Herrle, S. (1987). Helping staff cope with grief. *Nursing Management*, *18*(9), 33–34.

Hoisington, D. (2007). *An introduction to compassion*. Retrieved from www.CompassionSpace.com.

Hutchings, D. (2002). Parallels in practice: palliative nursing practice and Parse's theory of human becoming. *American Journal of Hospice and Palliative Care*, *19*(6), 408–414.

Ingalls, L. (2007). Bring your love: therapeutic and effective end-of-life discussions. *Home Health Care Management Practice*, *19*, 369–381.

Kübler-Ross, E. (1969). *On death and dying*. New York: Macmillan.

Larson, D., & Tobin, D. (2000). End-of-life conversations: evolving practice and theory. *Journal of the American Medical Association*, *284*(12), 1573–1578.

Lloyd-Williams, M. (1995). Bereavement referrals to a psychiatric service: an audit. *European Journal of Cancer Care*, *4*(1), 17–19.

Marks, M. J. B. (1976). The grieving patient and family. *American Journal of Nursing*, *76*, 1488–1491.

Millison, M. (1995). A review of the research on spiritual care and hospice. *Hospice Journal*, *10*(4), 3–19.

National Hospice and Palliative Care Organization (NHPCO). (2004). *Hospice fact sheet*. Retrieved from www.nho.org.

Parkes, C. M. (1975). *Bereavement: studies of grief in adult life*. Harmondsworth, England: Penguin.

Parkes, C. M. (1970). The first year of bereavement: a longitudinal study of the reaction of London widows to the death of their husbands. *Psychiatry*, *33*(4), 444–467.

Robinson, D. (1997). *Good intentions: the nine unconscious mistakes of nice people.* New York: Warner Books.

Stephenson, P., Draucker, C., & Martsolf, D. (2003). The experience of spirituality in the lives of hospice clients. *Journal of Hospice and Palliative Nursing, 5*(1), 51–58.

Stroebe, M., & Schut, H. (1999). The dual process model of coping with bereavement: rationale and description. *Death Studies, 23,* 197–202.

Teno, J., et al. (2004). Family perspectives on end-of-life care at the last place of care. *Journal of the American Medical Association, 291*(1), 88–93.

Volkan, V. D., & Zintl, E. (1993). *Life after loss: The lessons of grief.* New York: Simon and Schuster.

Wolfelt, A. (2010). *Exploring "complicated" mourning: sudden death, suicide grief & trauma loss.* Conference in Phoenix, Arizona, sponsored by Hospice of Arizona, November 16, 2010.

Wolfelt, A. (2006). *Death, grieving & mourning: wisdom teachings for caregivers.* Conference in Phoenix, Arizona, sponsored by the Arizona Hospice & Palliative Care Organization, October 25, 2006.

Worden, J. W. (2009). *Grief counseling and grief therapy: a handbook for the mental health practitioner* (4th ed.). New York: Springer.

Zisook, S., & Zisook, S. A. (2005). Death, dying and bereavement. In B. J. Sadock, & V. A. Sadock (Eds.), *Kaplan & Sadock's comprehensive textbook of psychiatry* (8th ed., vol. 11, pp. 2367–2392). Philadelphia: Lippincott, Williams & Wilkins.

Age-Related Mental Health Disorders

Shirley A. Smoyak, PhD, RN, FAAN

Pioneer Clinical Specialist, Writer, Distinguished Professor, Editor, and Living Legend in Psychiatric Mental Health Nursing

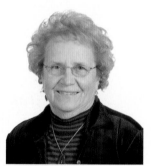

Dr. Shirley Smoyak is a baccalaureate graduate of the Rutgers University College of Nursing (1957). She was in the first class to finish the expanded 2-year master's program for psychiatric nurses developed by Hildegard E. Peplau (1959). Her doctorate, earned in 1970, is in sociology, with subspecialties in families, mental illness, and deviance.

Dr. Smoyak has been editor of the *Journal of Psychosocial Nursing and Mental Health Services (JPN)* since 1981. This is the only journal dedicated to psychiatric nurses in clinical practice. Dr. Smoyak is the author of several books, many journal articles, chapters, monographs, and videotapes. She has lectured or been a guest professor in all 50 states and in 15 foreign countries.

She is a psychiatric nurse and health care sociologist, and is a member of the Rutgers University College of Nursing. In her 51 years at Rutgers, Dr. Smoyak has taught courses in mental health and illness, psychiatric and mental health nursing, family dynamics, health care administration, culture and health, and qualitative research methods. Her current research projects are *Stalking: Criminal and Clinical Perspectives* and *Hazards of High Energy Drinks and Alcohol.* She is writing a book about the court-appointed monitoring of Greystone Park Psychiatric Hospital and the roles of monitors statewide.

Dr. Smoyak chaired the court-appointed *Doe v. Klein* Monitoring Committee, which oversaw Greystone Park Psychiatric Hospital, Morris Plains, New Jersey; she served as a monitor for 37 years. Among other efforts for better patient care, she developed a program for patients, families, and staff. In just one of the ways the citizens of New Jersey showed their appreciation for this hospital, the Rutgers–Newark Chorus performed a holiday concert in the main building chapel.

Dr. Smoyak is a Charter Member of the New Jersey Society of Certified Clinical Specialists in Psychiatric and Mental Health Nursing (1972) and a Charter Fellow of the American Academy of Nursing (1973). The American Academy of Nursing (AAN) has awarded her the distinction of Living Legend. She has served on the Board of the New Jersey State Nurses Association and as a delegate to the ANA convention many times. The NJSNA Excellence in Practice honor was awarded to her in 1990 and she was the 1995 NJSNA awardee of the Roll of Honor. In 2008 the Malta Psychiatric Nurses Association named her Distinguished Lifetime Professor. In 2009 she was awarded an Honorary Doctorate by Kingston University, London, England. In 2011 the Royal College of Nursing awarded her an Honorary Fellowship.

Children and Adolescents

Elizabeth M. Varcarolis

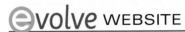

WEBSITE

http://evolve.elsevier.com/Varcarolis/essentials

KEY TERMS AND CONCEPTS

attention deficit/hyperactivity
  disorder (ADHD), p. 494
autism spectrum disorders
  (ASDs), p. 493
bibliotherapy, p. 501
conduct disorder, p. 497
dramatic play therapy, p. 501
mental status assessment, p. 491
movement and dance therapy,
  p. 501
music therapy, p. 501

oppositional defiant disorder
  (ODD), p. 497
play therapy, p. 500
recreational therapy, p. 501
resilient child/adolescent, p. 491
separation anxiety disorder, p. 499
temperament, p. 491
therapeutic drawing, p. 501
therapeutic games, p. 501
therapeutic holding, p. 501
Tourette's disorder, p. 496

SELECTED CONCEPT: Resiliency

Many children and adolescents grow up threatened by poverty, neglect, natural disasters, physical or mental illness, homelessness, abuse, or in general, are known as children at "high risk."

Children/adolescents that seem to survive with a high degree of competency have certain things in common:

1. More available resources than non-adapting children
2. Average or better intellectual skills
3. Good parenting/mentoring figure
4. Less vulnerable to stress

Studies conclude that each person has an innate capacity for resiliency provided individuals have resiliency building resources in their lives.

(Masten, 2011)

http://www.resiliency.com/htm/
whatisresiliency.htm

OBJECTIVES

1. Discuss evidence-based reasoning for having a strong background in developmental theory when performing an assessment or providing nursing care for a child or adolescent.
2. Identify the factors you would take into account in order to formulate a patient-centered care plan for a child or adolescent who is diagnosed with a mental health disorder.
3. Outline the components of a holistic assessment to determine the characteristics of mental health or mental illness in children and adolescents.
4. Identify the features with each disorder in this chapter that would qualify for a high degree of safety promotion.
5. Give examples of the kind of information you would evaluate during a developmental assessment of a child.
6. Identify the therapeutic modalities for children and adolescents that require teamwork and collaboration with other staff members and/or family members.
7. Evaluate the needs of a child with an autistic disorder and effective behavioral interventions.
8. Outline some major safety issues that parents and clinical nursing staff need to anticipate.

Children and adolescents are raised in diverse environments, and they bring with them into these environments a variety of genetic, neurobiological, and perceptual talents and temperaments. Therefore, no two children are exactly the same, and actually no one disorder is exactly the same in every child. Symptom clusters are assessed to make medical diagnoses, but nursing plans are most effective when they address the individual child or adolescent. Obviously, the promotion of *safety* is the primary priority when working with children and adolescents who have mental health problems.

For the most part, this chapter will discuss attributes and nursing measures for those disorders most frequently seen in child psychiatric clinics; however, they are not presented in order of prevalence.

Mental Retardation
Pervasive Developmental Disorders (Autistic Disorders)
Attention Deficit/Hyperactivity Disorder (ADHD)
Tic Disorders (Tourette's Disorder)
Disruptive Behavior Disorders
- Oppositional Defiant Disorder (ODD)
- Conduct Disorder (CD)

Anxiety Disorders
- Separation Anxiety Disorder. (Most of the signs and symptoms and treatment of anxiety disorders are similar for all age-groups. They are the most common disorders among children and adolescents. One exception is *Separation Anxiety Disorder*, which will be discussed in this chapter.)

PREVALENCE AND COMORBIDITY

About half of all Americans will meet the criteria for a *DSM* disorder at some time during their lives. The first onset will most likely occur in early childhood or early adolescence.

A reasonable estimate is that in the last 6 months there was nearly a 20.9% prevalence of psychiatric disorders in children ages 9 to 17 years (Bostic & Prince, 2008). Approximately one in five children and adolescents of any age in the United States suffers from a major psychiatric disorder that causes significant impairments at home, in school, and with peers (Black & Andreasen, 2011). An estimated two thirds of all young people with mental health problems are not getting the help they need. Mental illness can continue into adulthood, as evidenced by the fact that approximately 75% of 21-year-olds with mental disorders had previous mental health issues earlier in life. The federal government's recognition of these mental health problems and the efforts toward effective treatments were identified in *Mental Health: A Report of the Surgeon General* (U.S. Department of Health and Human Services [USDHHS], 1999). The following are a few of the identified barriers to assessment and treatment: (1) lack of clarity about why, when, and how children should be screened; (2) lack of coordination of multiple systems with different funding streams and eligibility requirements; (3) lack of resources; (4) lack of mental health providers; and (5) inadequate reimbursement (Children's Defense Fund, 2004).

Children with mental illness often meet the criteria for more than one diagnostic category. For example, attention deficit/hyperactivity disorder (ADHD) occurs in 60% to 90% of individuals with juvenile-onset bipolar disorder. Conduct disorders are associated with later substance use disorders, elevated rates of mood disorders, oppositional defiant disorder, and ADHD. Patients with ADHD have up to 70% comorbidity with operational defiant disorder, approximately 40% comorbidity with learning disorders, and nearly 25% comorbidity with conduct disorders (Bostic & Prince, 2008). Patients with Tourette's disorder have a high rate of comorbidity with ADHD (nearly 60% to 70%) and have 50% comorbidity with prominent obsessive-compulsive symptoms (Jummani & Coffey, 2010). Children with conduct disorder and oppositional defiant disorder are often diagnosed with a comorbid depressive disorder.

THEORY

A child's vulnerability to psychopathological conditions is the result of complex interactions between biological, psychological, genetic, and environmental variables. Younger children are harder to diagnose than older children, because the boundaries between normal and abnormal behaviors are less distinct. Intervention may be delayed until the child reaches school age to see whether a symptom is the result of a developmental lag or something more serious.

Genetic Factors

Genetic factors have been implicated in a number of childhood mental disorders, including autism, bipolar disorders, schizophrenia, ADHD, and intellectual developmental disorders (mental retardation), and some disorders have a direct genetic link, such as the intellectual impairment (mental retardation) seen in Tay-Sachs disease, phenylketonuria, and fragile X syndrome. A new research study has linked genetic mutations to autism spectrum disorder (ASD) (Nauert, 2011). Researchers using new molecular biology techniques have discovered several sporadic genetic mutations in children with autism spectrum disorders. A number of these mutated genes were located in genomes in regions that may have significant repercussions. In addition, many of these mutated genes have already been associated with schizophrenia and intellectual disability (Nauert, 2011).

Temperament, the style of behavior habitually used to cope with demands of the environment, is a constitutional factor thought to be genetically determined. It may be modified by the parent-infant relationship. In the case of the difficult-child temperament, if the caregiver is unable to respond positively to the child, there is an increased risk of insecure attachment, developmental problems, and mental disorders.

Biochemical Factors

Biochemical factors in childhood psychopathological conditions include alterations in neurotransmitters with decreases in norepinephrine and serotonin levels related to depression and suicide. In ADHD, a misfiring in the brain's executive function mediated through the prefrontal cortex is thought to lead to impaired cognitive abilities such as abstracting, structuring and organizing, and multitasking, resulting in the behavioral problems manifested in patients with this disorder (Black & Andreasen, 2011).

Environmental Factors

Environmental factors cause stress to children and adolescents and shape their development. Any type of abuse (e.g., physical, emotional, sexual) and neglect increases a child's risk for developing psychopathological conditions. Familial characteristics that correlate with child psychiatric disorders are (1) severe marital discord, (2) low socioeconomic status, (3) large families and overcrowding, (4) parental criminality, (5) maternal psychiatric disorders, and (6) foster care placement. Stressful life events are known to relate to anxiety, posttraumatic stress disorder (PTSD), conduct disorders, delinquency, impaired social and cognitive function, depression, and suicidal behaviors.

RESILIENCY

Not all vulnerable children develop mental disorders. It is assumed that constitutional resilience and a supportive environment play roles in keeping disorders from developing. Studies have shown that a resilient child/adolescent has the following characteristics:

1. A temperament that can adapt to changes in the environment
2. The ability to form nurturing relationships with other adults when a parent is not available
3. The ability to distance himself or herself from the emotional chaos of the parent or family
4. Social intelligence
5. The ability to use problem-solving skills

Studies of resilient children find that the number one important commonality is a strong relationship with a caring and competent adult. However, in the absence of that relationship, children who are resilient seek out people and environments that are good for their development, given the opportunity available to them. Other key factors in resilient children are average or better IQ scores, good attention skills, and "street-smarts" (Masten, 2011).

MENTAL HEALTH ASSESSMENT

Although much of the data gathered for a mental health assessment in children/adolescents is similar to data elicited from an adult, there are many differences as well. Important distinctions are assessment of developmental level, techniques used in the assessment, engagement of family, and presence of comorbid/co-occurring psychiatric conditions. The type of data collected to assess mental health depends on the setting, the severity of the presenting problem, and the availability of resources. The nurse is often the first health care professional to have contact with the child and completes a holistic assessment including the presenting problem, medical and developmental issues, family history, and a mental status assessment. In all cases, a physical examination is part of a complete workup.

Because developmental level is such an important part of the assessment with children and adolescents, the following questions should be included (Black & Andreasen, 2011, p. 401):

- What is the level of emotional and intellectual maturity?
- What are the patient's particular strengths?
- How do these strengths help as a protective element?
- What particular weaknesses are present?
- What stresses are affecting the child or adolescent?
- How do these stressors affect children/adolescents at this particular stage of life?
- How do gender-specific challenges affect the expression of illness and its treatment?

A mental status assessment in children and adolescents provides information about problems with thinking, feeling, and behaving (Box 26-1). This assessment is similar to that in adults except that the developmental level is considered. A developmental assessment provides information about the child's current maturational level that, when compared with the child's chronological age, identifies developmental lags and deficits. One popular assessment tool that provides this

BOX 26-1 CHILD/ADOLESCENT MENTAL STATUS ASSESSMENT

General Appearance
Size: height and weight
General health and nutrition
Dress and grooming
Distinguishing characteristics
Gestures and mannerisms
Looks or acts younger or older than chronological age

Activity Level
Hyperactivity or hypoactivity
Tics, other body movements
Autoerotic and self-comforting movements (e.g., thumb sucking, ear or hair pulling, masturbation)

Speech
Rate, rhythm, intonation
Pitch and modulation
Vocabulary and grammar appropriate to age
Mute, hesitant, talkative
Articulation problems
Other expressive problems
Unusual characteristics (pronoun reversal, echolalia, gender confusion, neologisms)

Coordination or Motor Function
Posture
Gait
Balance
Gross motor movement
Fine motor movement
Writing and drawing skills
Unusual characteristics (bizarre postures, banging, and hand biting)
Tiptoe walking, hand flapping, head shaking

Affect
Predominant emotion
Kinds of feelings expressed
Feelings appropriate to the situation
Range and stability of feelings

Intensity of feelings
Unusual characteristics (apathy, sulking, oppositional behavior)

Manner of Relating
Eye contact
Ability to separate from caregiver, be independent
Attitude toward interviewer
Behavior during interview (tolerance, impulsive, aggressive, ability to have fun or play, low frustration level)

Intellectual Functions
Fund of general information
Ability to communicate (follow directions, answer questions)
Memory
Creativity
Sense of humor
Social awareness
Learning and problem solving
Conscience (sense of right and wrong, accepts guilt and limits)

Thought Processes and Content
Orientation
Attention span
Self-concept and body image
Fantasies and dreams
Ego-defense mechanisms
Perceptual distortions (hallucinations, illusions)
Preoccupations, concerns, unusual ideas
Sex role, gender identity

Characteristics of Child's Play
Age-appropriate use of toys
Themes of play
Imagination and pretend play
Role and gender play
Age-appropriate play with peers
Relationships with peers (empathy, sharing, waiting for turns, best friends)

---

comparison is the Denver II Developmental Screening Test for infants and children up to 6 years of age.

Methods of collecting data include interviewing, screening, testing (neurological, psychological, intelligence), observing, and interacting with the child or adolescent. Histories are taken from parents, caregivers, the child (when appropriate) or adolescent, and other family members. Structured questionnaires and behavior checklists can be completed by parents and teachers.

The observation or interaction part of a mental health assessment begins with a semistructured interview in which the child or adolescent is asked about life at home with parents and siblings and life at school with teachers and peers. Because the interview is not structured, children are free to describe their current problems, even giving information about their own developmental history. Activities such as games, drawings, puppets, and free play are used for younger children who cannot respond to a direct approach. An important part of the first interview is observing the interactions between the child or adolescent, the caregiver, and siblings (if available).

COMMON DEVELOPMENTAL DISORDERS

MENTAL RETARDATION

Mental retardation is the most common of the developmental disorders.

Mental retardation is an intellectual developmental disorder that affects approximately 1% to 2% of the population (Black & Andreasen, 2011). This disorder can be mild, moderate, severe, or profound.

Causes may be a result of hereditary factors (e.g., Tay-Sachs disease, fragile X syndrome), alterations in early embryonic development (e.g., Down syndrome, fetal alcohol syndrome), pregnancy and perinatal problems (e.g., fetal malnutrition, prematurity, hypoxia, infections), and other factors such as trauma and poisoning.

Mild constitutes 85% of the individuals with intellectual developmental disorder. These children develop communication and social skills during childhood with minimal sensorimotor impairment and can be indistinguishable from children with normal IQs. They may be able to acquire up to sixth-grade academic skills and vocational skills as late teenagers. They may be capable of independent living or do better in a group home.

Moderate constitutes 10% of the individuals with mental retardation. These children develop communication and social skills during childhood but may only be able to acquire second-grade academic skills. They benefit from vocational training and can perform semiskilled work with supervision. As teenagers they have difficulty following social conventions, and this interferes with peer relationships. They do well in the community while living at home or in a supervised setting.

Severe constitutes 3% to 4% of the individuals with IDD. They acquire little or no speech during early childhood but may learn to talk and carry out basic self-care skills at a later age. They can be taught to perform simple tasks with close supervision. They can be managed living at home or in a supervised setting.

Profound mental retardation constitutes approximately 1% to 2% of individuals with IDD. These individuals usually have an identified neurological disorder causing the retardation. They have considerable sensorimotor impairments and may only develop minimal communication and self-care skills with constant supervision and highly structured settings.

The *DSM* delineates between mild, moderate, severe, or profound forms of mental retardation, by the use of specific criteria for residents within specific categories such as intellectual ability, deficits in general mental abilities, and history during the developmental period.

For example, the child with mental retardation may have impairments in communication skills, social interactions, and self-care abilities and may exhibit disruptive behaviors, depending on the severity of the intellectual and mental disruption as well as other neurological conditions or comorbidities. There is no list of specific behaviors to assess as there are for other mental disorders to categorize the individual. The nursing diagnoses will relate to the problems identified in a child/adolescent mental status assessment guide.

Nursing Diagnoses

There are several nursing diagnoses appropriate for children and adolescents with disorders that affect their intellectual development, such as mental retardation, including: *Defensive Coping, Ineffective Coping, Delayed Growth and Development, Disturbed Personal Identity, Dressing Self-Care Deficit, Impaired Verbal Communication, Risk for Impaired Parent/Child Attachment, Fear, Risk for Injury, Risk for Self-Mutilation, Ineffective Impulse Control, Risk for Self-Directed Violence, Risk for Other-Directed Violence, Impaired Social Interaction,* and *Self-Care Deficit.*

To provide child-centered care, interventions are geared toward the individual child's needs based on a sliding scale from mild to profound mental retardation.

PERVASIVE DEVELOPMENTAL DISORDERS

Pervasive Developmental Disorders such as Autistic Disorder and Asperger's Syndrome, are autistic disorders. "Autism is an abnormal self-absorption, usually affecting children, characterized by lack of response to people and actions and limited ability to communicate" (Collins English Dictionary, 2009).

These disorders are developmental disorders which cover a wide range of abilities and are essentially a group of developmental disabilities that cause problems with (Schoenstadt, 2006; CDC 2010a):
- Social skills
- Communication
- Repeated behaviors and routines
- Emotional attachment
- Other symptoms

For example, possible symptoms include (CDC, 2010a):
- **Social skills:** Avoids eye contact, avoids or resists physical contact, refers to play alone, has flat or inappropriate facial expressions, does not share interests with others, does not respond to name by 12 months of age
- **Communication:** Delayed speech and language skills, echolalia (repeats words or phrases over and over), talks in a flat, robotlike, or singsong voice, does not understand jokes, sarcasm, or teasing, gives unrelated answers to questions, uses few or no gestures
- **Repeated behaviors and routines:** Repetitive motions repeated over and over (flaps hands, rocks body, or spins self in circles, repeatedly turns light on and off), plays with toys the same way every time, gets upset by minor changes (changes furniture around, changes route going someplace familiar), has obsessive interest. When behaviors or routines are changed usually has temper tantrum, or severe frustration
- **Other symptoms:** Unusual eating habits, aggression, cause self injury, impulsive, hyperactivity, unusual reactions to the way things sound, smell, taste, look, or feel

People with autism handle information differently in their brain, and each person with a "spectrum disorder" differs greatly in the way they are affected. No two people will have the same symptoms. Autistic symptoms range from very mild to severe.

The Centers for Disease Control and Prevention (CDC, 2010b) estimates an average of 1 in 80-240 children in the United States has an autistic disorder to some degree. The incidence of autism has been increasing alarmingly in the last 10 to 15 years. There is plenty of evidence for genetic transmission of these disorders (CDC, 2010).

Although people with autistic disorders share a similar set of symptoms—impairments in social skills, communication, behaviors, routines, and other symptoms, each individual differs in terms of symptoms, severity levels, and specific needs.

Assessment

In assessing children with autism, the nurse can observe specific areas of impairment. One is impairment in communication and imaginative activity. Autism may result in delay or total absence of language, immature grammatical structure, pronoun reversal, inability to name objects, and stereotypical or repetitive use of language. Although most children like to pretend and role play, such as pretending to be a dog and barking, autistic children have a lack of spontaneous make-believe play or imaginative play and a failure to imitate.

A second characteristic of autism is impairment in social interactions. This impairment manifests itself in lack of responsiveness to and interest in others, lack of eye contact and facial responses, indifference or aversion to affection and physical contact, failure to cuddle or be comforted, and lack of friendships.

Another characteristic of autism is markedly restricted and stereotyped behaviors, interests, and activities. People with autism seem to need rigid adherence to routines and rituals, and respond catastrophically to minor changes. Stereotypical and repetitive motor mannerisms, such as rocking, are common. Autistic individuals are often preoccupied with specific objects (buttons, parts of the body, and wheels on toys) and repetitive activities.

ASSESSMENT GUIDELINES

Pervasive Developmental Disorders (Autistic Disorders)

1. Assess for developmental spurts or lags, uneven development, or loss of previously acquired abilities.
2. Assess the quality of the relationship between the child and parent or caregiver for evidence of bonding, anxiety, or tension; look for antagonism between the parent's and the child's temperaments.
3. Be aware that children with behavioral and developmental problems are at risk for abuse.
4. Assess for co-occurring conditions (e.g., intellectual developmental disorder may be present, especially with the lowest functioning individuals).
5. Assess for the child's strengths.

Diagnosis

There are several nursing diagnoses appropriate for children and adolescents with autism, including: *Ineffective Coping,* *Delayed Growth and Development, Disturbed Personal Identity, Ineffective Impulse Control, Ineffective Relationship, Impaired Verbal Communication, Impaired Social Interaction, Risk for Impaired Parent/Child Attachment, Fear, Risk for Injury, Risk for Self-Mutilation, and Dressing Self-Care Deficit.*

Implementation

Children with ASD are treated in therapeutic nursery schools, day treatment programs, and special education classes in public schools, because their education or treatment is mandated under the Children With Disabilities Act. Treatment plans include teaching parents how to modify the child's behavior and to foster the development of skills when the child is in the home setting. There are no medications to treat autism spectrum disorder. However, when needed the antipsychotic risperidone has been successfully used for symptoms of aggression, deliberate self-injury, and temper tantrums, and has shown some benefits with repetitive behaviors and hyperactivity. However, beta-blockers (e.g., propranolol) are preferred because of their lower side effect profile and increased efficacy. The selective serotonin reuptake inhibitor (SSRI) antidepressants may be used with caution in those children with autism spectrum disorders who exhibit prominent obsessive-compulsive behaviors including rigidity or compulsive rituals (Laurberg & Prince, 2010).

The ultimate *long-term outcome* is to help children with pervasive developmental disorders (autistic disorders) reach their full potential by fostering developmental competencies and coping skills. The following guidelines for nursing interventions are useful with all children in all settings:

1. Increase the child's interest in reciprocal interactions.
2. Foster the development of social skills.
3. Facilitate the expression of appropriate emotional responses, including the development of trust, empathy, shame, remorse, anger, pride, independence, joy, and enthusiasm.
4. Foster the development of reciprocal communication, especially language skills.
5. Provide for the development of psychomotor skills in play and activities of daily living (ADLs).
6. Facilitate the development of cognitive skills (attention, memory, cause and effect, reality testing, decision making, and problem solving).
7. Foster the development of self-concepts (identity, self-awareness, body image, and self-esteem).
8. Foster the development of self-control, including impulse control, tolerance of frustration, and delayed gratification.

ATTENTION DEFICIT/HYPERACTIVITY DISORDER

Attention deficit/hyperactivity disorder (ADHD) accounts for 3% to 10% of the cases of mental disorders in children or adolescents. According to Preston and colleagues (2010) most young people with ADHD will outgrow their motor restlessness/hyperactivity but will retain the core symptoms (impulsivity, impaired attention, and lack of intrinsic motivation) throughout adolescence and into adulthood. ADHD is difficult to diagnose before 4 years of age. ADHD often manifests as excessive gross motor activity that becomes less pronounced as the child matures. The disorder is most often identified when the child has difficulty adjusting to elementary school—a time when children are expected to control behavior, follow rules, and stay on task in an age-appropriate manner. The attention problems and hyperactivity contribute to low tolerance for frustration, temper outbursts, labile moods, poor academic performance, rejection by peers, low self-esteem, and disorganization. Disorganization during adolescence often is evidenced by cluttered bedrooms, disorganized lockers, and messy notebooks (Preston et al., 2010). An increased incidence of depression—up to 20%—is diagnosed in children with ADHD. Nocturnal or daytime enuresis, disruptive behavior disorders, and Tourette's disorder have been associated with ADHD.

Symptoms of ADHD include the following (Popper et al., 2002; CDC, 2009):

Inattention
- Has difficulty paying attention in tasks or play
- Does not seem to listen, follow through, or finish tasks
- Does not pay attention to details and makes careless mistakes
- Is reluctant to engage in tasks that require sustained mental effort
- Is easily distracted, loses things, and is forgetful in daily activities
- Has difficulty processing information
- Struggles to follow instructions

Hyperactivity
- Fidgets, is unable to sit still or stay seated in school
- Runs and climbs excessively in inappropriate situations
- Acts as if "driven by a motor" or constantly "on the go"
- Talks excessively
- Acts without thinking
- Finds it difficult to resist temptations or opportunities (e.g., a child may grab toys off the store shelf or play with dangerous objects; adults may commit to a relationship after only a brief acquaintance or take a job or enter into a business arrangement without due diligence)
- Has trouble sitting still during meals, school, movies

Impulsivity
- Blurts out answer before question is completed
- Has difficulty waiting his or her turn
- Interrupts, intrudes in others' conversations and games
- Is very impatient

Scientists are unsure of what causes ADHD and as yet there is no known definitive cause. However, it is thought that predisposing factors for ADHD are family history of ADHD (genes), chaotic family life (such as parental rejection, inconsistent parenting with harsh discipline, out-of-home placements, frequent shifting of parental figures, or large family size), absence of father or presence of alcoholic father (environmental factors), and adverse influences during the prenatal period (e.g., intrauterine exposure to toxic substances such as drugs, alcohol, or nicotine), perinatal period (e.g., low birth weight), and postnatal period (e.g., central nervous system insult related to trauma or infections). People with ADHD show impairment in the cortex of the frontal lobe, which is the executive center of the brain. The cortex in the frontal lobe is that region of the brain that controls our thoughts and actions (such as socialization, reason and judgment, and moral development). Brain scans of children with ADHD show underdeveloped and inactive frontal lobes as opposed to the normal child's brain, as well as changes in other areas of the brain (Greenhill & Hechtman, 2010).

ASSESSMENT GUIDELINES

Attention Deficit/Hyperactivity Disorder

1. Obtain a history detailing the nature and onset of behavioral symptoms.
2. Obtain a description of the effect of different situations on their child's behavior.
3. Observe the level of physical activity, attention span, talkativeness, and ability to follow directions and control impulses. Medication is often needed to ameliorate problems in these areas.
4. Assess difficulty in making friends and performing in school. Academic failure and poor peer relationships lead to low self-esteem, depression, and further acting-out behaviors.
5. Assess for problems with enuresis and encopresis.

Diagnosis

There are many nursing diagnoses that are appropriate for children and adolescents with attention deficit/hyperactivity disorder, including: *Impaired Social Interaction, Ineffective Impulse Control, Ineffective Relationship, Risk for Other-Directed Violence, Risk for Caregiver Role Strain, Risk for Injury, Ineffective Coping,* and *Chronic Low Self-Esteem.*

Implementation

The following are examples of nursing interventions when working with parents or caregivers of children or adolescents with ADHD:

1. Assess parent's or caregiver's knowledge of the disorder and the related behaviors and provide needed information.
2. Explore the effect of the behaviors on family life.
3. Assess the family's or caregiver's support system.
4. Discuss realistic behavioral goals and how to set them.
5. Planned activities should be geared to the abilities of the child or adolescent so that success at tasks may be realized.
6. Give positive recognition and feedback when the child is successful at a task/activity or attempts a task/activity.
7. Provide educational information about medications to both caregivers and adolescents.
8. Refer parent or caregiver to an appropriate support group.

The **interventions for ADHD** are behavior modification and pharmacological agents for the inattention and the hyperactive or impulsive behaviors, special education programs for the academic difficulties, and psychotherapy and play therapy for the emotional problems that develop as a result of the disorder. Psychostimulants are used to treat ADHD as a sluggish frontal lobe is thought to be causative of the disorder. Methylphenidate (Ritalin) is the most widely used stimulant because of its safety and simplicity of use. It is available orally and as a transdermal patch (Daytrana). Concerta is an extended-release form of Ritalin that allows once-daily dosing. Adderall is another psychostimulant (containing dextroamphetamine and amphetamine) that also calms the patient, and it is available in extended-release form. Approximately 70% to 90% of people with ADHD do fairly well when prescribed stimulants; however, because of side effects or nonresponse, up to 50% of patients may discontinue psychostimulants (Strange, 2008). Research on alternative drugs is ongoing because those children who do not respond to stimulants (almost 30% of children with ADHD) are often categorized as an "inattentive type" of ADHD that is thought by some to be a totally different kind of neurological disorder (Preston et al., 2010). Two more recently approved U.S. Food and Drug Administration (FDA) drugs that are α_2-agonist nonstimulants seem to be benefiting patients. Clonidine hydrochloride and guanfacine hydrochloride may be used as an alternative or as an adjunct with stimulants. Guanfacine seems to decrease symptoms of aggression and insomnia related to psychostimulant use, and clonidine has shown significantly improved symptoms of ADHD in children 6 to 17 years old when used in conjunction with psychostimulants. Tricyclic antidepressants or bupropion hydrochloride (i.e., Wellbutrin) may also be used (Black & Andreasen, 2011).

TIC DISORDERS

TOURETTE'S DISORDER

Transient tic disorders are common (15%) among boys between 8 and 12 years of age (e.g., excessive blinking, facial grimacing, shoulder shrugging, and head turning). Tics are stereotyped, rapid, involuntary, recurring motor movements that wax and wane over time and usually occur in response to stress, excitement, fatigue, or anxiety (Bostic & Prince, 2008; Jummani & Coffey, 2010). Tourette's disorder is the most serious of the tic disorders and involves motor and verbal tics that cause marked distress and significant impairment in social and occupational function. In Tourette's disorder (TD) a tic is a sudden, rapid, recurrent, nonrhythmic motor movement or vocalization.

Tourette's disorder may appear as early as 2 years of age, but the average age of onset is 6 to 7 years. The duration of the disorder is usually life-long, but there can be periods of remission, and the symptoms often diminish during adolescence or sometimes disappear by early adulthood. Motor tics usually involve the head but can also involve the torso or limbs, and they change in location, frequency, and severity over time. In half of the cases, the first symptom is a single tic, most often eye blinking. Other motor tics are tongue protrusion, touching, squatting, hopping, and retracing steps. Vocal tics include words and sounds (barks, grunts, yelps, clicks, snorts, sniffs, coughs). Coprolalia (uttering obscenities), although a colorful subject of films (such as *What About Bob*) and mainstream culture, is present in less than 10% of cases.

Tourette's disorder affects 4 or 5 individuals per 10,000 and is more common in males. There is a familial pattern in about 90% of cases. Vulnerability is transmitted in an autosomal dominant pattern, with 70% of females and 99% of males who have inherited the gene developing the disorder. "Nongenetic" Tourette's disorder often coexists with an autistic disorder or a seizure disorder.

Assessment

Symptoms associated with Tourette's disorder are obsessions, compulsions, hyperactivity, distractibility, and impulsivity. In addition, the child or adolescent with tics has low self-esteem from feeling ashamed, self-conscious, and rejected by peers. The fear of having tic behavior in public situations causes the individual to limit activities severely. Central nervous system (CNS) stimulants increase the severity of the tics, and therefore children with coexisting ADHD must have their medication carefully monitored.

Diagnosis

There are several nursing diagnoses appropriate for children and adolescents with Tourette's disorder, including *Anxiety, Impaired Social Interaction, Chronic Low Self-Esteem, Social Isolation, Ineffective Relationship,* and *Hopelessness.*

Implementation

The focus of treatment is on helping the child, family, and school understand and cope with the tic behaviors. This disorder is treated on an outpatient basis unless there are severe tics that severely impair the child's function at home and in school. Sometimes inpatient or day hospitalization is needed for a complete evaluation and pharmacological intervention. The drugs clonidine and guanfacine hydrochloride are currently the most effective medications for Tourette's disorder. Mild co-occurring obsessive-compulsive disorder (OCD) is responsive to cognitive therapy, and severe cases of OCD can be treated. In more severe cases of OCD an appropriate pharmacological agent should be prescribed for each symptom (Jummani & Coffey, 2010).

DISRUPTIVE BEHAVIORAL DISORDERS

OPPOSITIONAL DEFIANT DISORDER

Oppositional defiant disorder (ODD) is a persistent pattern of negativity, disobedience, defiance, and hostility directed toward authority figures (Mayo Clinic Staff, 2012).

Almost all children at some time exhibit symptoms characteristic of ODD, such as having temper tantrums, being argumentative, or refusing to obey or do chores. However, to be diagnosed with oppositional defiant disorder, these behaviors need to happen "more persistently and more frequently" than what would be considered within the range of normal behaviors.

Children with ODD exhibit persistent stubbornness, argumentativeness, testing of limits, unwillingness to concede or negotiate, and refusal to accept blame for misdeeds. This behavior is evident at home but may not be present elsewhere. These children and adolescents do not see themselves as defiant; instead, they feel they are responding to unreasonable demands or situations. According to the American Academy of Child & Adolescent Psychiatry (2011) and WebMD (2009c) symptoms may include:

- Excessive arguing with adults
- Spiteful attitude and revenge-seeking behaviors when upset
- Mean and hateful talking when upset
- Aggression toward peers
- Difficulty maintaining friendships
- Frequent temper tantrums
- Frequent anger and resentment
- Annoys other people deliberately
- Academic difficulties
- Blaming others for his or her mistakes or misbehavior

This disorder is usually evident before 8 years of age and is more common in males, until puberty when the incidence is equal. ODD often co-occurs with other disorders such as ADHD, which intensifies the challenge of effective treatment

The following are examples of nursing interventions when working with parents or caregivers of children or adolescents with ODD:

1. Assess the quality of the child/parent or caregiver relationship for evidence of bonding, anxiety, tension, or antagonism between parent's and child's temperaments, which can contribute to the development of disruptive behaviors.
2. Assess the parent's or the caregiver's understanding of growth and development, parenting skills, and handling of problematic behaviors; lack of knowledge contributes to the development of these problems.
3. Assess cognitive, psychosocial, and moral development for lags or deficits; immaturity in developmental competencies results in disruptive behaviors.

CONDUCT DISORDER

Conduct disorder is a serious behavioral and emotional disorder characterized by a persistent pattern of behavior in children and adolescents in which the rights of others and societal rules are violated. The child or adolescent acts out these patterns of behaviors in all settings and is considered a forerunner of antisocial/asocial personality disorder, since children with conduct disorder share the same symptomatology. For example (Mental Health America, 2012; WebMD, 2009):

- Aggressive behavior toward others (e.g., cruelty to animals using weapons or forcing another into sexual opportunity)
- Destructive behavior (e.g., intentional destruction such as arson, vandalism)
- Deceitfulness (e.g., conning or manipulating others, lying)
- Serious rule violations (e.g., running away from home, truancy, sexually active at a very young age)
- Other attributes of antisocial personality disorder (e.g., lack of remorse, callousness, lack of empathy for how others have been personally affected)

Childhood-onset conduct disorder can be seen as early as two years of age (irritable temperament, poor compliance, inattentiveness, impulsivity) which in later years can lead to conduct disturbance. As these children reach elementary school age aggressive tendencies with adults and peers continue to not follow social mores, and lack the ability to solve the psychosocial issues (Bernstein et al, 2011). These children are physically aggressive, have poor peer relationships with little concern for others, and lack feelings of guilt or remorse. To make matters worse, they misperceive the intentions of others as being hostile and believe their aggressive responses are justified. Although they try to project a tough image, they have low self-esteem and low tolerance for frustration, show irritability, and have temper outbursts. As time progresses their behavior includes intense anger and aggression as an emotional overreaction to perceived slights, always blame others for their own actions, and are noncompliant with demands (Bernstein et al, 2011). Early onset often indicates a poorer outcome.

Adolescent-onset conduct disorder results in less aggressive behaviors and more normal peer relationships; and these individuals are likely to have a better outcome. These pre-adults tend to act out their misconduct with their peer group (e.g., truancy, early-onset sexual behaviors, drinking, substance abuse, and risk-taking behaviors). Males are more apt to fight, steal, vandalize, and have school discipline problems, whereas girls lie, run away, and engage in prostitution. Conduct disorders lead to academic failure, failure to graduate, juvenile delinquency, and the need for the juvenile court system to assume responsibility for youths who cannot be managed by their parents. Unfortunately, interaction with other deviant peers often worsens the behaviors (Bernstein et al., 2011). Other psychiatric disorders frequently coexist with conduct disorders such as anxiety, mood disorders, learning disorders, and ADHD.

ASSESSMENT GUIDELINES

Oppositional Defiant Disorder and Conduct Disorder

1. Assess the seriousness of the disruptive behavior; determine when it started and what has been done to manage it. Hospitalization or residential placement may be necessary in addition to medication.

2. Assess the levels of anxiety, aggression, anger, and hostility toward others and the ability to control impulses.
   - Alert other team members for support in case anger/hostility escalates and interventions are needed.
   - Position yourself during the interview in a safe spot, where neither you nor the child/adolescent will feel cornered.
   - Refer to Chapter 23 for protocols and guidance for safety. Always know and follow your unit protocols.
3. Assess moral development for the ability to understand the effect of hurtful behavior on others, to empathize with others, and to feel remorse or guilt.

Diagnosis

There are several nursing diagnoses appropriate for children and adolescents with disruptive disorders, including *Ineffective Impulse Control, Defensive Coping, Delayed Growth and Development, Ineffective Relationship, Disturbed Personal Identity, Impaired Verbal Communication, Risk for Impaired Parent/Child Attachment, Risk for Impaired Attachment, Fear, Risk for Injury, Risk for Other-Directed Violence, Impaired Social Interaction,* and *Self-Care Deficit.*

Implementation

The following are guidelines for nursing interventions for children and adolescents with disruptive and conduct control disorders:

1. Protect the child or adolescent from harm and provide for biological and psychosocial needs while acting as a parental surrogate and role model.
2. Provide immediate nonthreatening feedback for unacceptable behaviors.
3. Increase the child's or adolescent's ability to trust and use interpersonal skills to maintain satisfying relationships with adults and peers.
4. Provide immediate positive feedback for acceptable behaviors.
5. Increase the child's or adolescent's ability to control impulses, tolerate frustration, and modulate the expression of affect.
6. Foster the child's or adolescent's identification with positive role models so that positive attitudes and moral values can develop that enable the youth to experience feelings of empathy, remorse, shame, and pride.
7. Use role play to help the child respond in a more acceptable manner when feeling frustrated or aggressive.
8. Foster the development of a realistic self-identity and self-esteem based on achievements and the formation of realistic goals.
9. Provide support, education, and guidance for parents or caregivers.

Overall interventions for oppositional defiant and conduct disorders focus on correcting the child's or adolescent's faulty beliefs about self and strengthening his or her ability to control impulses, which involves developing more mature and adaptive coping mechanisms. This is a gradual process not amenable to brief treatment. Conduct disorders may require inpatient hospitalization for crisis intervention, evaluation, and treatment planning, as well as transfer to therapeutic foster care or long-term residential treatment. Youths with oppositional defiant disorder are generally treated as outpatients, with much of the focus on parenting issues. Multisystemic therapy is an evidence-based model that emphasizes the home environment and the empowerment of families through several hours of treatment each week.

To control **aggressive behaviors,** a wide variety of pharmacological agents have been used, including antipsychotics, lithium carbonate, anticonvulsants, antidepressants, and β-adrenergic blockers. Cognitive behavioral therapy is used to change the pattern of misconduct by fostering the development of internal controls, both cognitive and emotional. Important components of the treatment program include learning problem-solving techniques, conflict resolution, empathy, and social interaction skills.

Families are involved in therapy and are given support in parenting skills designed to help them provide nurturance and set consistent limits. They are the key players in carrying out the treatment plan, using behavior modification techniques at home, monitoring the medication's effects, collaborating with the teacher to foster academic success, and making a home environment that promotes the achievement of normal developmental tasks. When families are abusive, drug dependent, or highly disorganized, the child may benefit from out-of-home placement.

ANXIETY DISORDERS

Anxiety becomes a problem when the child or adolescent fails to move beyond the fears associated with certain developmental stages or when anxiety interferes with normal functioning.

Anxiety disorders are the most common mental disorders of childhood and adolescence, affecting 13% of youths between the ages of 9 and 17 (Bostic & Prince, 2008; USDHHS, 1999). There may be a genetic vulnerability to anxiety disorders, which seem to occur in families. Anxiety disorders can develop in response to physical or psychosocial stressors and trauma. Cognitive theorists propose that anxiety is the result of dysfunctional efforts to make sense of life's events.

The characteristics of most anxiety disorders in children and adolescents are basically the same as those seen in adults with one exception. Anxiety in children and adolescents may be manifested in more somatic complaints such as stomachaches, headaches, or nausea and vomiting. Not infrequently, a parent may have an anxiety disorder as well. Unfortunately, many anxiety disorders seem to progress into adulthood. The one anxiety disorder specific to a child or adolescent is separation anxiety. Those anxiety disorders that can be applied to both preadults and adults are identified as agoraphobia, generalized anxiety disorder, panic disorder, specific phobia, and **social phobia.** Separation anxiety disorder as it relates to children and adolescents is discussed next.

SEPARATION ANXIETY DISORDER

Separation anxiety is very common in infants age 8 to 14 months old and toddlers clinging between 3 to 4 years of age. During this time a child might exhibit mild distressing clinging behaviors when separated from their primary caregivers, known family figures, or unfamiliar places (e.g., day care centers).

Children and adolescents with separation anxiety disorder experience extreme anxiety when they are separated or when they are anticipating separation from their familial surroundings. The anxiety-induced panic is overwhelming and excessive even for brief separations. This disorder may develop after a significant stressful event. The prevalence of the disorder in children is estimated to be about 2% to 5% with a higher incidence in females and first-degree biological relatives. Although the remission rates are high, the disorder, especially if not treated, can persist and lead to a depressed mood often accompanied by anxiety.

Some clinically significant symptoms include (Bernstein et al., 2011) (WebMD, 2009b):

- An unrealistic and lasting worry causing excessive distress when separation is imminent
- Bedwetting
- Refusal to go to sleep without being near the primary attachment figure
- Nightmares involving separation-related themes
- Physical or somatic symptoms (headaches, stomach aches, palpitations) on school days or anticipating separation primary attachment figure.
- Extreme fear of being left alone
- Repeated temper tantrums or pleading

It is believed that development of separation anxiety may be related to a traumatic separation early in the child's life such as the death of a loved one, a stay in the hospital, etc.

ASSESSMENT GUIDELINES

Anxiety Disorders

1. Assess the quality of the child/parent or caregiver relationship for evidence of anxiety, conflicts, or antagonism between the child's and the parent's temperaments.
2. Assess for recent stressors and their severity, duration, and proximity to the child.
3. Assess the parent's or the caregiver's understanding of developmental norms, parenting skills, and handling of problematic behaviors (lack of knowledge contributes to increased anxiety).
4. Assess the patient's developmental level and determine if regression has occurred.
5. Assess for physical, behavioral, and cognitive symptoms of anxiety.

Separation Anxiety Disorder

1. Assess the child's previous and current ability to separate from parent or caregiver. (The separation or individuation process may not be completed or the child may have regressed.)
2. Assess for the presence of anxiety problems in the parent or caregiver. (In addition to genetic issues, anxiety and depression can be "contagious.")
3. Assess parental response to the child's anxiety. (Increased attention reinforces behavior.)

Diagnosis

There are several nursing diagnoses appropriate for children and adolescents with separation anxiety disorders, including *Anxiety, Fear, Delayed Growth and Development, Ineffective Relationship,* and *Impaired Parenting.*

Implementation

Children and adolescents with anxiety disorders are most often treated on an outpatient basis with cognitive behavioral therapies such as environmental modifications, play therapy, counseling for the family, or school-based counseling. Therapeutic interventions are matched to the developmental level of the child. Cognitive therapy focuses on the underlying fears and concerns, and behavior modification is used to reinforce self-control behaviors. Children who refuse to start primary school are introduced gradually into the school environment with a parent or caregiver present for support for part of the day. When adolescents develop school refusals, the goal is to return them to the classroom at the earliest possible date and to give parents support in setting limits on truancy. Medications are only used if psychotherapy is unsuccessful or the anxiety levels are incapacitating. There are no medications specifically approved by the FDA for separation anxiety disorder, but the selective serotonin reuptake inhibitors (SSRIs) seem to have proven most effective.

The following are guidelines for nursing interventions for children with anxiety disorders:

1. Help the child reach full potential by fostering developmental competencies and coping skills.
2. Protect the child from panic levels of anxiety by acting as a parental surrogate and providing for biological and psychosocial needs.
3. Accept regression, but give emotional support to help the child progress again.
4. Give positive reinforcements (e.g., hugs, praise) for the small victories the child is able to accomplish. Negative reinforcements (e.g., withholding dessert, television, or computer) may increase anxiety and a sense of failure, further diminishing the child's sense of control.
5. Increase self-esteem and feelings of competence in the ability to perform, achieve, or influence the future.
6. Help the child accept and work through traumatic events or losses.

THERAPEUTIC MODALITIES FOR CHILD AND ADOLESCENT DISORDERS

Parental involvement and support is recognized as a critical factor in the supportive and educational interventions for the child or adolescent. In addition to therapy with a single family, multiple-family therapy can be used to engage families as co-therapists to help them learn to (1) like and respect others, (2) capitalize on strengths and accept shortcomings, (3) develop insight and improve judgment, (4) use new information, and (5) develop lasting and satisfying relationships.

Group therapy for younger children takes the form of play. For grade-school children, it combines playing and talking about the activity. For adolescents, it involves more talking, and focuses largely on peer relationships as well as specific problems. A challenge of using groups when working with children and adolescents lies in the contagious effect of disruptive behavior.

Groups have been used effectively to deal with specific issues in the life of a youth (e.g., bereavement, physical and sexual abuse, substance abuse, sexuality and dating, teenage pregnancy, chronic illnesses, depression, suicidal ideation).

Milieu therapy is a philosophical basis for structuring inpatient, residential, and day treatment programs. The nurse collaborates with other health care providers in structuring and maintaining a therapeutic environment that facilitates the individual's growth and positive behavioral change. The physical milieu is designed to provide a safe, comfortable place to live, play, and learn, with areas for group activity as well as private time. There may be a gym, outdoor playground, swimming pool, garden, kitchen area, or other recreational facilities, and even pets may be incorporated into the care plan. The daily schedule structures the activities (e.g., school, therapy sessions, group activities and outings, family visits).

Behavior modification is based on the principle that rewarded behavior is more likely to be repeated. Developmentally appropriate behaviors are normally rewarded with validation by a significant adult in the child's life, so modifying behavior in this manner is a standard parenting technique. To extinguish undesirable behavior, either the behavior is ignored or, if it is too disruptive or dangerous, limits that have specified consequences are set. A proactive approach to dealing with disruptive behavior includes increasing the structure of a group activity, expanding staff presence, and anticipating the contagious effects by means of "antiseptic bouncing" of a disruptive child from the activity.

One common method is the point and level system, in which points are awarded for desired behaviors and increasing levels of privileges can be earned. Points are given for behaviors such as dressing, attending school and activities on time without being disruptive, and demonstrating social skills. Each level has increasing privileges, such as leaving the unit with a staff member or having a later bedtime on weekends. At the highest level, the privilege might be to leave the unit unescorted. Earned points and level status are recorded daily. Points are collected and used to obtain specific rewards.

Removal and restraint are dangerous controversial treatment modalities for children (as well as for adults). Injuries and even death have been associated with seclusion and restraint with children. The reality is that these dangerous modalities are "loosely and erratically regulated in the United States" (Stefan, 2002). In European countries seclusion and restraint are not widely used.

Seclusion may affect superficial compliance, but has little to do with real behavioral change. The child or adolescent will usually perceive seclusion as punishment, and the experience of being overpowered by adults is terrifying, especially for one who has been abused. The use of seclusion and restraint should be used in extreme emergency. According to the American Academy of Pediatrics (1997):

> Situations that may require the short-term use of restraint in a child or adolescent include extreme, disruptive, self-injurious, or aggressive behavior as a result of drug intoxication, head injury, cerebrovascular hemorrhage, multiple trauma, or acute psychiatric disorder. Patients in status epilepticus may require short-term physical restraint to prevent injury to self or others until the seizure is controlled with antiepileptic agents. The use of the restraint, however, should not place a child or adolescent at risk of injury or deterioration of the medical condition. (p. 497)

Instead of seclusion, a unit may have an unlocked **quiet room** for a youth who needs to be removed from the situation for either self-control or control by the staff. Other approaches include the feelings room or the freedom room with objects that can be punched, kicked, and thrown. The youth is encouraged to express and work through feelings in private or with staff support.

Time-out is a common method for intervening in disruptive or inappropriate behaviors. Time-out procedures are designed so that staff can be consistent in their interventions. The child's individual behavioral goals are considered in setting limits on behavior and using time-out periods. If they are overused or used as an automatic response to a behavioral infraction, time-outs lose their effectiveness.

A youth's behavior can sometimes be so excessively destructive that physical restraint is needed. Although a mechanical restraint such as a helmet for head banging may be used, **therapeutic holding** is a long-established practice for the control of destructive behaviors. This intervention requires prompt, firm, nonretaliatory protective restraint that is gently applied and leads to a reduction in the youth's distress, greater relaxation, a return of self-control, and trust in the staff.

Cognitive behavioral therapy helps to change both cognitive processes and behaviors, thereby reducing the frequency of maladaptive responses and replacing them with new competencies. This therapy is carried out in individual or group sessions that teach youths how to cope with problems and stressors through a series of cognitive behavioral activities (e.g., cognitive rehearsal, positive affirmations, role-playing social skills and assertiveness, and relaxation techniques).

Play therapy is based on the notion that play is the work of childhood and the way a child learns to master impulses and adapt to the environment. Play is also the language of childhood and the communication medium for assessing developmental and emotional status, determining diagnosis, and instituting therapeutic interventions. There are many forms of play therapy that can be used individually or in groups. Playrooms are equipped with art supplies and a variety of toys including hand puppets, dolls, and action figures. These toys provide the child with opportunities to act out conflicts and stressful situations, to work through feelings, and with the help of the therapist to develop more adaptive ways of coping.

Dramatic play therapy is a treatment modality that uses dramatic techniques to act out emotional problems, examine subjective experience, develop new perspectives, and try out new behaviors. This modality may be used with groups of verbal children and adolescents. If they are psychotic, reality-based role plays are substituted for fantasies. Dramatic play is a form of psychodrama. Hand puppets and puppet shows are a favorite way to act out problems and solutions. Uninhibited children and adolescents enjoy acting roles in dramas that they have created spontaneously or scripted. The dramas can be videotaped for reviewing the experience and facilitating new learning.

Therapeutic games are an ideal treatment modality for children who may have difficulty talking about their feelings and problems while developing rapport with health care workers. The game might be as simple as checkers, but therapeutic games are more effective in eliciting children's fears and fantasies. A well-known game by Gardner (1986) is the *Talking, Feeling, and Doing Game* (a board game appropriate for latent and preadolescent children). The player draws a talking, feeling, or doing card, which gives instructions or asks a question, such as "All the girls in the class were invited to a birthday party except one. How did she feel?" If this game is played with a group, additional responses can be elicited.

Bibliotherapy involves using children's literature to help the child express feelings in a supportive environment, gain insight into feelings and behavior, and learn new ways to cope with difficult situations. Children unconsciously identify with the characters in the story, so the books selected should reflect the situation or feeling that is problematic for the child. It is important to assess the child's readiness for the particular topic and the child's level of understanding.

Therapeutic drawing allows children to spontaneously express themselves in artwork capturing thoughts, feelings, and tensions they may be unable to express verbally. When drawing any human figure, children leave an imprint of the inner self, revealing personality traits, strengths, weaknesses, behaviors, and interpersonal relationships including attitudes and values

of the family and cultural group. Drawings are most reliable after children are able to create objective representations of what is seen (usually between 5 and 7 years of age). Often children draw human figures, and the following characteristics are general indicators of children's emotions and are not necessarily indicative of psychopathology.

- Size of figures: very large (aggression, poor impulse control); very small (shyness, insecurity)
- Emphasis on and exaggeration of body parts: large heads (desire to be smarter), large mouths (speech problems), large arms (desire for strength and power)
- Omissions of body parts: hands (trauma, insecurity), arms (inadequacy), legs (lack of support), feet (insecure, helpless), mouth (difficulty expressing self or relating to others)
- Facial expressions: personal mood and affect
- Integration of body parts: scattered or disorganized parts indicate cognitive or psychological problems or both

Music therapy instigates changes in both the physiology of the nervous system and in social interactions. Music therapy may incorporate recorded music, songs, song writing, or use of a musical instrument. Children love to use simple noisemakers for the expression of feelings, for the development of coordination and rhythm, and as an opportunity for social interactions. Music on inpatient units is often used to create a relaxing mood for rest periods and bedtime.

Movement and dance therapy is a direct expression of the self that helps the youth become more aware of feelings and thoughts, dissipate tensions, develop greater body awareness, improve or correct a distorted body image, improve coordination, and increase social interactions. The type of movement used with children can be as simple as a game of "Follow the Leader" or it can be creative, free-form movements to the mood of the music. For older children and adolescents, more formal classes in exercise, karate, or the latest dance craze may be of interest.

Recreational therapy generally takes place off the unit and is often conducted by a recreational therapist with assistance from the nursing staff. Activities can be organized around a game that teaches psychomotor and social skills, or they can be individual activities (e.g., riding a bike, learning to swim). Special field trips and "outings" give children the opportunity to be like other children and to act appropriately in public situations. The communicated expectation is that the children's behavior will be within normal limits, and this becomes a self-fulfilling prophecy leading to increased self-control and self-esteem.

KEY POINTS TO REMEMBER

- Between 12% and 22% of children and adolescents are estimated to have emotional problems, and only a small percentage of these youths actually receive treatment.
- Risk factors known to contribute to the development of mental and emotional problems in children and adolescents include genetic, biochemical (pre- and postnatal), temperament-based, psychosocial developmental, social or environmental, and cultural factors.
- Resiliency in a preadult includes an adaptable temperament, the ability to form nurturing relationships with surrogate parental figures, the ability to distance the self from emotional chaos in parents and family, and good social intelligence and problem-solving skills.
- The most commonly diagnosed child psychiatric disorders are mood disorders, anxiety disorders, ADHD, adjustment reactions, and conduct and oppositional disorders.

- Treatment of childhood and adolescent disorders requires a multimodal approach. The ability to collaborate closely with schools, the availability of remediation services, and the incorporation of behavior modification techniques should be part of the intervention.
- Cognitive behavioral therapies, social skills groups, family therapy, parent training in behavioral techniques, and individual therapy have been found useful. Skills training may focus on a variety of areas, depending on the child's or adolescent's presenting symptoms.
- Child and adolescent psychiatric nurses are increasingly becoming aware of the need to educate the family and involve the family members in the treatment process. The family remains an integral part of the supportive and educational system for the child and adolescent.

APPLYING CRITICAL JUDGMENT

1. Thomas, a 4-year-old boy, has been diagnosed with an autism spectrum disorder.
   A. Describe the kinds of behavioral data you would find on assessment in terms of (1) communication, (2) social interactions, and (3) behaviors and activities.
   B. Name at least six realistic outcomes for Thomas.
   C. Which treatment modalities do you think would be the most effective for a child with autism spectrum disorder (ASD)? Defend your answer.
   D. What kinds of support should the family receive?
2. Nancy is a 7-year-old girl who has been diagnosed with ADHD.
   A. This child is in second grade. What clinical behaviors might she be exhibiting at home and in the classroom? Give behavioral examples for her (1) inattention, (2) hyperactivity, and (3) impulsivity.

   B. Identify at least four intervention strategies that you might suggest to be used to help her.
   C. What type of medications might help her?
3. Jeffrey is an 8-year-old boy who has been diagnosed with conduct disorder.
   A. Explain to one of Jeffrey's classmates his probable behaviors in terms of (1) aggression toward others, (2) destruction of property, (3) deceitfulness, and (4) violation of rules.
   B. What are the outcomes for this child? What is the overall prognosis for children with this disorder?
   C. What are at least seven ways you could support Jeffrey's parents?
   D. Use the computer to find locations within your community that might be the best place to refer Jeffrey's parents for support and guidance.

CHAPTER REVIEW QUESTIONS

Choose the appropriate answer(s)

1. A 6 year old diagnosed with ADHD is throwing pencils at the other children. The initial response by the nurse would be:
   1. "You might hurt others if you continue."
   2. "This is why you get into trouble."
   3. "Stop this right now."
   4. "Your doctor will have to be called."
2. The nurse working in the emergency department usually assesses adult patients, but tonight she is responsible for assessing the suicide potential of a 13-year-old adolescent. Which topic must be explored in this assessment of an adolescent that is different from such an assessment in an adult?
   1. The presence of distorted perceptions about suicide and death

2. The presence of ideas about hurting self seriously or causing death
3. Circumstances at the time suicidal thoughts are experienced
4. Identification of feelings such as depression, anger, guilt, and rejection

3. A 15-year-old boy is diagnosed with conduct disorder. He has not been attending school and states that his parents told him it was OK to stay home. The best response by the nurse would be:
   1. "Your parents are not aware of your class schedule."
   2. "Skipping classes is against the rules."
   3. "A family meeting must be arranged."
   4. "I will refer you to the principal's office."

CHAPTER REVIEW QUESTIONS—cont'd

4. Which topic would be least relevant as a focus during the assessment of a 12 year old with suspected ADHD?
   1. Effect of impulsive behavior on the child's life at home and school
   2. The child's level of physical activity and attention span
   3. The child's ability to pay attention and perform in school
   4. The child's progress with toilet training and self-care habits

5. Nurses working with children and adolescents should be focused on:
   1. avoidance of their own childhood issues.
   2. sharing aspects of their own childhood with patients' families.
   3. development of insight into their own childhood issues.
   4. teaching staff that childhood concerns can be lifelong.

REFERENCES

American Psychiatric Association (APA). (2000). *Diagnostic and statistical manual of mental disorders (DSM-IV-TR)* (4th ed, text rev.). Washington, DC: Author.

American Academy of Child & Adolescent Psychiatry (AACAP). (2011). *Children with oppositional defiant disorder.* Retrieved February 24, 2012, from http://aacap.or/page.ww?name= Children+with+ Oppositional+Defiant+Disorder& section.

American Academy of Pediatrics (AAP). (1997). *The use of physical restraint interventions for children and adolescents in acute care settings* (abstract). Retrieved February 25, 2012, from http://aappublic ations.org/content/99/3/497.full.

autism. (n.d.). *Collins English Dictionary: Complete & Unabridged 10th Edition (2009).* Retrieved June 22, 2012, from Dictionary.com website: http://dictionary.reference.com/browse/autism.

Bernstein, B. E., Pataki, C., et al. (2011). *Conduct disorder.* Retrieved February 22, 2012, from http://emedicine. Medscape.com/ article/918213-overview.

Black, D. W., & Andreasen, N. C. (2011). *Introductory textbook of psychiatry* (5th ed.). Washington, DC: American Psychiatric Publishing.

Bostic, J. Q., & Prince, J. B. (2008). Child and adolescent psychiatric disorders. In T. A. Stern, J. F. Rosenbaum, M. Fava, J. Biederman, & S. L. Rauch (Eds.), *Massachusetts General Hospital comprehensive clinical psychiatry.* Philadelphia: Mosby/Elsevier.

Centers for Disease Control and Prevention (CDC). (2010a). *Signs & symptoms, autism spectrum disorders.* Retrieved February 22, 2010, from http://www.cdc.gov/ncbddd/autism/signs.html.

Centers for Disease Control and Prevention (CDC). (2010b). *Autistic spectrum disorders.* Retrieved June 18, 2011, from www.cdc.gov/ ncbddd/autism/data.html.

Children's Defense Fund. (2004). *Newsletter from Marian Wright Edelman.* Washington, DC: Author.

Gardner, R. A. (1986). The talking, feeling, and doing game. In C. E. Schaefer, & S. E. Reid (Eds.), *Game play: therapeutic use of childhood games* (pp. 41–72). New York: John Wiley.

Greenhill, L. L., & Hechtman, L. I. (2010). Attention-deficit/ hyperactivity disorder. In B. J. Sadock, V. A. Sadock, & P. Ruiz (Eds.), *Kaplan and Sadock's comprehensive textbook of psychiatry* (9th ed., vol. 11, pp. 3560–3572). Philadelphia, PA: Wolters Kluwer/Lippincott Williams & Wilkins.

Jummani, R., & Coffey, B. J. (2010). Tic disorders. In B. J. Sadock, V. A. Sadock, & P. Ruiz (Eds.), *Kaplan and Sadock's comprehensive textbook of psychiatry* (9th ed., pp. 3609–3623). Philadelphia: Wolters Kluwer/Lippincott Williams & Wilkins.

Masten, A. S. (rev. 2011). *Resilience in children at-risk.* Retrieved June 17, 2011, from www.cchd.umn.edu/carei/reports/rpractice/ Spring 97/resilience.html.

Mental Health America. (2012). *Conduct disorder.* Retrieved January 22, 2012, from http://www.nmha.org/co-/conduct-disorder.

Mayo Clinic Staff. (2012). *Oppositional defiant disorder (ODD).* Retrieved February 22, 2012, from http://www.MayoClinic.com/ health/oppositional-defiant disorder/DS0063/DSECTION=s-.

Nauert, R. (2011). *Genetic mutations linked to autistic spectrum disorders.* Retrieved February 24, 2012, from http://psychcentral. com/news/2011/05/17/genetic-mutations-linked-to-autistic- spectrum-disorders/26248.htm.

NIMH. (2009). *Attention deficit hyperactivity disorder (ADHD).* Retrieved February 22, 2012 from http://www.nimh.gov/ publications/attention-deficit-hyperactivity-disorder/.

Preston, J. D., O'Neal, J. H., & Talaga, M. C. (2010). *Handbook of clinical psychopharmacology for therapists* (6th ed.). Oakland, CA: New Harbinger.

Schoenstadt, A. (2006). *Autism spectrum disorders symptoms.* Retrieved February 2, 2012, from http: //autism.emedtv.com/autism- spectrum-disorders/autism-spectrum-disorder-symptoms.

Stefan, S. (Summer/Fall 2002). *Legal and regulatory aspects of seclusion and restraint in mental health settings.* NETWORK, National Technical Assistance Center.

Strange, B. C. (2008). *Once-daily treatment of ADHD with guanfacine: patient implications.* Retrieved June 18, 2011 from www.ncbi.nih. gov/pmc/articles/PMC2526381/.

U.S. Department of Health and Human Services (USDHHS). (1999). *Mental health: a report of the surgeon general—executive summary.* Rockville, MD: Author.

WebMD. (2009a). *Mental health and conduct disorder.* Retrieved January 22, 2012, from http://www.webmd.com/mental- health/mental-health-conduct-disorder.

WebMD. (2009b). *Separation anxiety in children.* Retrieved February 22, 2009, from http://children.webmed.com/guide/separation-anxiety? page=2&print=true.

WebMD. (2009c). *Oppositional defiant disorder.* Retrieved February 24, 2012, from http://www.webmd.com/mental-health/opposi- tional-defiant-disorder

CHAPTER

27

Adults

Edward A. Herzog

⊖volve WEBSITE

http://evolve.elsevier.com/Varcarolis/essentials

KEY TERMS AND CONCEPTS

chemical castration, p. 518

cognitive behavioral therapy
(CBT), p. 510

community mental health centers
(CMHCs), p. 508

deinstitutionalization, p. 507

impulse control disorders, p. 511

mental health courts, p. 507

National Alliance on Mental Illness (NAMI), p. 508

outpatient commitment, p. 507

paraphilias, p. 514

programs of assertive community
treatment (PACT or ACT), p. 510

reality testing, p. 507

recidivism, p. 515

recovery model, p. 508

rehabilitation model, p. 508

severe and persistent mental illness (SPMI), p. 505

sexual disorders, p. 514

social skills training, p. 510

supported employment, p. 510

supportive psychotherapy, p. 510

teletherapy, p. 510

transinstitutionalization, p. 507

**SELECTED CONCEPT: Teletherapy and
the New Communication Technologies**
Service providers in remote locations are
using **"teletherapy,"** speaking with patients
by phone, computer-based video or closed-
circuit television when patients cannot find
transportation or travel to distant services;

   The new communication technologies
are being increasingly used to treat and
follow-up via chat messaging systems on
the healthcare website, etc. These technologies have been especially effective in
depression and anxiety disorders.
(Text) (Simon, 2011)

OBJECTIVES

1. Discuss ways in which severe mental illness affects
   society.
2. Discuss the issues and problems commonly experienced
   by those living with severe and persistent mental illness
   (SPMI). Construct a clinical picture of a man or woman
   reflecting these issues.
3. Describe evidence-based treatments for severe and persistent mental illness.
4. Role play a therapeutic interaction designed to improve
   treatment adherence for an individual with a severe and
   persistent mental illness (SPMI).
5. Describe the core behaviors and characteristics of a person
   with impulse control disorders and the implication these
   behaviors and characteristics have on society.
6. Act out in a simulation nursing interventions appropriate
   for people with impulse control disorders.
7. Describe sexual disorders and their implications for society.
8. Discuss the forms of treatment for pedophilia (pedohebe-
   philic) disorder.
9. Act out with a classmate a situation demonstrating the
   indicators/symptoms of an individual with attention defi-
   cit/hyperactivity disorder (ADHD).

This chapter focuses on mental health issues and needs affecting primarily the adult population. We will look at what it is like to have a severe and persistent mental illness (SPMI), the issues and challenges faced by those diagnosed with these illnesses, and resources and treatment programs available for illness management. Other adult mental issues examined in this chapter include disorders involving **impulse control and sexual functioning** as well as adult **attention deficit/hyperactivity disorder (ADHD)**.

UNDERSTANDING SEVERE AND PERSISTENT MENTAL ILLNESS

Categorizing mental illness according to levels of severity has tremendous implications for setting mental health policy, establishing insurance reimbursement standards, and facilitating access to appropriate care (Peck & Scheffler, 2002). In the United States each state determines how to classify mental illness for the purpose of insurance coverage.

The federal government's classifications of "serious mental illness" (SMI) and "severe and persistent mental illness" (SPMI) refer to those most deeply affected by psychiatric disorders. SMI includes 5.4% of all adults and refers to disorders that somehow interfere with social functioning. In this chapter, the focus is on SPMI, which affects about half of the people in the SMI group, or 2.6% of all adults. SPMI involves significant continuous or episodic impairment of global functioning that results in disability in 30% to 50% of cases. Disorders in this category include severe forms of depression, panic disorder, obsessive-compulsive disorder, schizophrenia, and bipolar disorder.

Individuals with SPMI usually have difficulties in multiple areas, including activities of daily living (e.g., cooking, hygiene), relationships, social interaction, task completion, communication, leisure activities, safe movement about the community, finances and budgeting, health maintenance, vocational and academic activities, and coping with stressors. Associated issues for those with SPMI include poverty, stigma, isolation, unemployment, and inadequate housing.

Extent of the Problem
Effect on the Individual

Individuals with SPMI often fall well short of their potential, experiencing significantly less academic, vocational, relational, and other forms of success than they likely would have achieved otherwise. People with SPMI often experience stigmatization and discrimination. They are more likely to be victims of crime, be medically ill, have undertreated or untreated physical illnesses, die prematurely, be homeless, be incarcerated, be unemployed or underemployed, engage in binge substance abuse, be living in poverty, and report lower quality of life than those without such illnesses (Aquila & Emanuel, 2003; Glied, 2007).

Effect on Families, Caregivers, and Significant Others

The burden on caregivers is also affected by their own coping abilities, support systems, and financial and other resources. Caregivers may not have an adequate understanding of the mental illness, they may not know how to cope with it or how to help, and they may not have access to their loved one's treatment team, leaving them feeling frustrated and powerless. Chronic caregiving demands that exceed their coping abilities can result in burnout and withdrawal from the patient, or even rejection or abuse (Hasson-Ohayon et al., 2011). Caregivers may be stigmatized by association, as if they were somehow tainted by the relationship with the SPMI person (Hasson-Ohayon et al., 2011), leading them to keep the problem a secret, thus increasing isolation.

Effect on Society

Most mental health treatment (57%) is financed with public dollars rather than private insurance, as compared with 46% for overall health care expenditures (President's New Freedom Commission on Mental Health, 2003). Untreated and inadequately treated mental illness leads to decreased productivity and other losses estimated to cost our society at least $100 billion per year (NAMI—California, 2011). Thirty-five percent

---

VIGNETTE

You are a 19-year-old nursing student working as a nursing assistant. One night, sitting alone in your dorm studying, you hear someone call your name. No one is there, and you attribute it to lack of sleep. However, over the coming weeks this happens repeatedly, and the voices begin to comment on what you are doing, criticize you, and tell you what to do. You have trouble concentrating. Your schoolwork suffers and your grades begin to drop. You feel that people know what you're thinking. You become uncomfortable being around others, begin to skip classes, avoid friends, and quit work.

Distracted by the now ever-present voices, you step into the street and are knocked off your feet by a car. A policeman comes to your aid, but you believe he wants to kill you and you try to run, only to be caught and restrained. The next few days are a confusing, frightening blur of physicians, nurses, injections, and restraints. You are on a psychiatric unit and told that you have something called a schizophreniform disorder.

Medications push the voices into the background, but you feel disconnected, like you are wrapped in layers of cotton. Just as you begin to trust some of the staff, you are discharged with an appointment to see a new physician in a mental health center far from your neighborhood. At the mental health center people look and act very strangely; some are mumbling to themselves, some get too close to you, and some pull away when you walk by. You think, "This can't be happening to me," and wonder what your future will be like.

of Supplemental Security Income (SSI) and 28% of Social Security Disability Income (SSDI) (both providing income to disabled individuals) are allocated to assist people with SMIs (NAMI, 2004).

Issues Facing Those With Severe and Persistent Mental Illness

Even with successful treatment, people with SPMI often have residual symptoms, which are milder, lingering symptoms of the disorder. Residual symptoms can lead to frustration and fear in the patient that he or she will not get better, and that the medications and treatments are not effective. In turn, the patient may decide to discontinue treatment, ironically worsening the course of the illness.

Medication side effects, particularly for the typical (standard) antipsychotic medications, can produce a wide range of distressing effects, including sedation, visual blurring, involuntary movements, weight gain, sexual dysfunction, and increased risk of medical conditions. It is important to educate patients about these side effects because some are amenable to treatment, such as extrapyramidal side effects being managed with anticholinergics. Some side effects (anticholinergic) may diminish over time whereas others can be counteracted by changes in lifestyle or behavior (e.g., learning to change position slowly to prevent dizziness from orthostatic hypotension).

One major disadvantage of the atypical antipsychotics, which have a better side effect profile but are more expensive, is metabolic syndrome (characterized by hypertension, increased insulin resistance, central obesity, and abnormal lipid levels, which increase the risk of cardiovascular disease and diabetes). Addressing side effects is essential because they may impair one's quality of life or cause (or provide a justification for) treatment nonadherence. Refer to Chapter 17 for a discussion on the typical and atypical antipsychotics and patient and family teaching plans for each of these groups of drugs.

Relapse, chronicity, and loss may occur despite adherence to medications and therapy (Ascher-Savnum et al., 2010). Disorders such as schizophrenia are usually chronic illnesses, and living with any chronic illness requires considerable effort and psychic energy and outside supports.

Depression and suicide may be the result of a profound sense of loss of preillness life and/or co-occurring major depression and/or substance abuse. For example, consider the significant disconnect between your original life trajectory and your present status if you were a successful pre-med student and 3 years later you are now unemployed and living in a group home. This loss, along with the demands and effects of chronicity on daily life, can logically lead to despair, depression, and risk of suicide (estimated that between 5% and 10% of those with SPMI commit suicide), especially if the individual has no family or outside supports.

Co-occurring medical illnesses frequently exist with SPMI, particularly hypertension (22%), obesity (24%), cardiovascular disease (21%), diabetes (12%), chronic obstructive pulmonary disease (COPD) (10%), and trauma (6%) (Miller et al., 2007). Risk of premature death (about 28 years) associated

with these disorders is 1.6 to 2.8 times greater than in the general population. People with SPMI may not provide for their own health needs and may not receive adequate care because of costs, difficulty accessing health care, or stigma or stereotyping (e.g., emergency department [ED] personnel assuming that because a person is psychotic that person's chest pain is not real). In some cases presenting complaints may be expressed in a bizarre manner, influencing the quality of health care.

Unemployment and poverty contribute to poor self-esteem and lack of identity. Eighty-five percent of people with SMIs are unemployed, and disability entitlements (received by 50% of those with SMIs) do not provide much income: On average, a person disabled by an SPMI on SSI receives income that is less than 25% of the median income (NAMI, 2008a,b). It can be difficult to find an employer open to hiring a person with a mental illness, and laws to prevent discrimination do not guarantee a job. Even if patients find a job, the income could cause them to become ineligible for health care coverage, forcing them to pay for medications out-of-pocket, in turn likely reducing medication adherence (and contributing to decreased access to health care in general) (Rosenheck et al., 2006).

Housing instability can contribute to stress for individuals with SPMIs. If patients cannot afford a car, they need to live near public transportation. To afford an inexpensive apartment they may have to live where gunshots are common occurrences—not a good situation for anyone, let alone a person overwhelmed by mental illness. An ill-timed episode of inappropriate behavior could also lead to eviction, and if the person's problems are shared among local landlords, the person could not only be refused residence but also be burdened by negative references, resulting in further rejection.

Stigma about mental illness is a significant problem. It causes others to assume that people with mental illness are less than human, dangerous, and even somehow responsible for their condition. It can leave the affected person feeling ashamed or angry, pushing him or her further away from others and reducing access to potential support systems. Stigma is perpetuated by stereotypical images or language in the media, thoughtless comments by everyday people or celebrities, and thousands of other sources. NAMI and other advocacy groups, mental health consumers and professionals, and many others are working to reduce stigma in the same way that was once necessary for developmentally disabled people. At present, many people do not yet realize that calling a mentally ill person "crazy" is equivalent to calling someone with mental retardation a "retard." Refer to Chapter 2 for more on stigma and its consequences.

Anosognosia is the inability of a person to recognize deficits from the illness due to the illness itself. With mental illness it is the brain that is sick, the same organ needed for insight and decision making. It is an extremely frustrating Catch-22, and one that is at the heart of treatment nonadherence and all its attendant problems (Amador, 2007). Would you take medicine for an illness you do not believe you have?

Social isolation and loneliness are perhaps among the most significant issues for people with chronic illnesses, not just those with SPMIs. Stigma and social stratification reduce social contact with "out" groups, such as severely mentally ill individuals. Factors such as poverty (which interferes with participation in social or recreational activities), passivity, impaired hygiene, and anxiety also reduce interaction and interfere with relationships. As a result many people with SPMIs are socially isolated and experience significant amounts of loneliness.

Medication may reduce the libido or the ability to function sexually and interfere with intimate physical relationships. Negative self-image and delusional thinking may create additional barriers to close interpersonal connections. People with SPMIs may be taken advantage of sexually or make ill-advised choices regarding sexual partners or practices, increasing the risk of sexually transmitted diseases (STDs) and unplanned pregnancies (Quinn & Browne, 2009).

Nearly half of all people with mental illnesses may be receiving inadequate therapy or medications—treatment not matching guidelines, not supported by research, or not current (NAMI, 1998). Some of the most recent medications or other treatments that are most supported by research are excluded from formularies or unapproved by third-party payers. Treatment innovations and changing standards of practice can be slow to be incorporated into practice (President's New Freedom Commission on Mental Health, 2003). Reduced public funding for health services during times of economic cutbacks can intensify problems with treatment access and quality (NAMI, 2008a,b).

Atypical antipsychotic medications can be extremely expensive, more than $20,000 per year (Becker et al., 2007). Even with Medicaid, co-pay or a spend-down (a need to exhaust one's own funds each month in order to reestablish Medicaid eligibility) may be required to obtain medications. People with insurance may find it does not cover psychiatric care or that their share of costs is prohibitively high, sometimes higher than for nonpsychiatric care.

Substance abuse has been estimated to co-occur in 50% of those with an SPMI. It may be a form of self-medication, a way of countering the dysphoria or other symptoms caused by one's illness or the sedation caused by one's medications. Nicotine use is higher in the SPMI population and is not declining as it has in the general population. Substance abuse contributes to physical health problems, reduced quality of life, incarceration, relapse, and reduced effectiveness of psychotropic treatments (Urbanoski et al., 2007).

Compared to the general population, victimization occurs more than twice as often among mentally ill people (Maniglio, 2009). Sexual victimization, such as assault or coerced sexual activity, also occurs in this vulnerable population (e.g., a patient whose boyfriend "loaned" her sexually to peers in return for drugs, compelling her to cooperate in return for housing). Factors such as impaired judgment, impaired interpersonal skills (e.g., unknowingly acting in ways that might provoke others, such as standing too close or refusing to leave), passivity, poor self-esteem, dependency, living in urban or high-crime neighborhoods, and seeming more vulnerable to criminals may contribute to this significant problem. Drug abuse and transient living conditions have been shown to be strong predictors of victimization in this population (Maniglio, 2009).

Issues Affecting Society and the Individual

Involuntary treatment involves treatment mandated by a court order and delivered without the patient's consent. Outpatient commitment was designed to provide mandatory treatment in a less restrictive setting, typically after the patient leaves the hospital or prison. Some consider it a form of assisted treatment in that it helps people who do not realize they are mentally ill to maintain the best mental health status possible (Swanson, 2010).

Criminal offenses and incarceration may be the result of desperation, impaired judgment, or impulsivity. Some patients with SPMIs cannot be persuaded to accept treatment and may not meet criteria for involuntary treatment because they are not an imminent danger to self or others. Without treatment they can become public nuisances, committing usually nonviolent crimes such as trespassing or petty theft. An example might be a man with SPMI and impaired judgment who does not dress adequately for cold weather and loiters in laundromats and libraries for warmth. When expelled, the man is at risk of hypothermia, and in such cases loved ones or police may seek the person's arrest simply to get him or her off the streets. Efforts to improve responses to people with SPMIs include educating police (e.g., through crisis intervention training programs sponsored jointly by police and mental health agencies) to identify mental illness and to distinguish it from criminal intent, and providing people with help instead of jailing them. Mental health courts are designed to assist people whose crimes are secondary to mental illness, and divert people with SPMIs to treatment instead of imprisonment.

Transinstitutionalization is the shifting of a person or population from one form of institution to another, such as from state hospitals to jails, prisons, nursing homes, or the street. Although deinstitutionalization has given the appearance of providing care in less restrictive settings and provided for financial savings to state hospitals, in a large number of cases the new setting is in fact more restrictive, and the costs have simply been transferred to another provider (Novella, 2010).

APPLICATION OF THE NURSING PROCESS

ASSESSMENT

Assessment involves observation for signs of risk to self or others, including suicidal or homicidal thinking or behaviors; depression or hopelessness; substance use/abuse, signs of relapse, especially increased impulsivity or paranoia, sleep impairment, diminished reality testing, or increased delusional thinking or command hallucinations; and inadequate attention to one's needs for proper nutrition, clothing, or medical care. Impaired judgment and psychosis increase the risk of dangerous behaviors. Such patients may start fires by leaving pots on the stove and becoming distracted or falling asleep. They may begin to respond to command hallucinations, or develop paranoid ideation that another person is a threat to them.

It is essential to observe for signs of treatment nonadherence and impending relapse. Correcting nonadherence helps prevent relapse, and early detection of relapse reduces its intensity and duration. It is also important to assess for physical health problems such as tumors or metabolic disorders, which may cause psychiatric symptoms and be mistaken for mental illness or relapse. Monitoring co-occurring illnesses ensures that self-care is satisfactory and that the patient is receiving adequate health care.

DIAGNOSIS

Nursing diagnoses for patients who have an SPMI include *Impaired Adjustment, Compromised Family Coping, Ineffective Coping, Ineffective Health Maintenance, Impaired Impulse Control, Risk for Loneliness, Noncompliance,* and *Self-neglect, Bathing Self-Care Deficit, Chronic Low Self-Esteem,* and *Chronic Sorrow.* See Table 27-1 for interventions to be used with patients who have an SPMI.

OUTCOMES IDENTIFICATION

The following are examples of potential outcome measures:
- Patient identifies "voices" as hallucinations.
- Patient demonstrates three adaptive responses when faced with hallucinations.
- Patient remains free from police involvement.
- Patient maintains stable housing.
- Patient remains free from harm.
- Patient demonstrates consistent treatment adherence.

IMPLEMENTATION

The following are interventions to be used to improve adherence with treatment:
1. Monitor side effects that encourage nonadherence and provide treatment and education to avert or minimize patient distress.
2. Simplify treatment regimens to make them more acceptable to the patient (e.g., once-per-day dosing instead of twice daily).
3. Link treatment adherence to achieving the patient's goals (not the goals of the physician or society) to increase patient motivation.
4. Emphasize and reinforce improvements, connecting them to the patient's treatment adherence.
5. Facilitate referrals for assistance with treatment costs and access to improve treatment adherence.
6. Provide psychoeducation regarding SPMI and the role of treatment in recovery to improve insight and motivation.

7. Assign consistent, committed caregivers who have (or are skilled at building) positive therapeutic bonds with the patient; trust in one's providers is essential for treatment adherence.
8. Involve the patient in support groups that have members who have greater insight and a first-hand experience with illness and treatment that the patient may be more likely to accept.
9. Provide culturally sensitive care. Cultural beliefs and practices of a patient (such as suspicious attitudes toward health care and authority figures, or valuing of self-sufficiency or privacy above health care) may be crucial in treatment adherence.
10. Consider judicious use of medication decreases or discontinuation to control side effects or improve the therapeutic alliance.
11. As indicated, and when other interventions have not been successful, use medication monitoring and long-acting forms of medication (depot injections or sustained-release formats) to maximize the benefits of medication.
12. Never reject, blame, or shame the patient when nonadherence occurs; instead, label it as simply an issue for continuing focus, often requiring numerous tries.

Pharmacological, Biological, and Integrative Therapies

State hospitals and psychiatric units in general hospitals provide inpatient care. Outpatient care for SPMI is provided by community mental health centers (CMHCs), private providers (primarily psychiatrists, psychologists, therapists, social workers, and advanced practice nurses), and private and governmental agencies. Community-based services vary with local needs and resources. It may also be difficult to "work the maze" of multiple agencies and services. See Chapter 5 for a full discussion of mental health treatment settings.

Rehabilitation Versus Recovery

Until recently the rehabilitation model has been the dominant paradigm in mental health care. It focuses on deficits, symptoms, and stability rather than on quality of life and cure. It has been criticized for emphasizing dependence on health care providers, with staff essentially functioning as parents and the patient as the dependent child. A new model of care that developed out of the consumer movement—a movement that emphasizes choices and empowerment—is called the recovery model. It is promoted by the National Alliance on Mental Illness (NAMI), a leading advocacy organization, along with many other mental health organizations and treatment providers. The *recovery model* involves a partnership between care providers and the patient, with patients having an active role in choosing and directing their treatment (Frese et al., 2009). It is a positive, hopeful, empowering strength-focused model wherein staff are in an assistive or partnership role and the consumer uses his or her strengths to achieve the highest quality of life possible (Mulligan, 2005).

TABLE 27-1 INTERVENTIONS FOR SEVERE AND PERSISTENT MENTAL ILLNESS

INTERVENTION	RATIONALE
1. Mutually develop short and long-term, patient-centered goals and interventions that will help the patient achieve the desired quality of life, rather than focus on symptom reduction.	1. Patient involvement in goal setting and treatment selection builds the therapeutic alliance, increases the patient's sense of control over his/her life, and increases the likelihood of treatment adherence and success.
2. Enhance and promote reality testing (e.g., teaching a patient, when he or she hears voices, to scan the immediate environment to see if anyone else seems to be hearing the voices; if not, encourage the patient to label it as a hallucination and to disregard it or distract self from it).	2. Impaired reality testing is common in SPMI, and contributes to hallucinations and delusional thinking. Training and encouraging the patient to verify whether experiences are real can help the patient meet his/her goals despite residual symptoms.
3. Provide psychoeducation, guidance, support, and reinforcement for actions that patients can use to manage their symptoms of SPMI (see Box 17-3 on p. 305). Include the family in psychoeducational activities as tolerated and possible.	3. Whistling or other simple auditory distractions can reduce auditory hallucinations; gaining mastery over symptoms improves function, reduces disruption, and provides one with a sense of control and confidence.
4. Reduce loneliness and isolation by interacting frequently with the patient, supporting opportunities for interaction (e.g., day programs, social and recreational events), helping the patient to manage social anxiety, helping the patient who does not want to socialize to identify and use alternative means to achieve support or comfort (e.g., pets, stuffed animals, calling support phone lines), and involving the patient in social skills training.	4. SPMIs decrease sociability and predispose individuals to isolation as a result of stigma, loss of social skills, and social discomfort. Activities that increase skill and comfort with interaction, especially with supportive people and positive role models, such as other patients who are farther along in recovery, contribute to improved functioning and a higher quality of life.
5. Encourage involvement of patients and their loved ones in NAMI support meetings and peer-based services.	5. NAMI members and peers "have been there" and can provide support, socialization, and practical suggestions for issues and problems facing patients and significant others; involvement in such groups also instills hope and empowers the patient.
6. Provide education and support regarding making sound decisions about interpersonal relations, STD prevention, and family planning.	6. People with SPMI may have impaired judgment, feel isolated, and feel vulnerable to victimization, STDs, and undesired pregnancies; patients seeking to have families may benefit from genetic counseling.
7. Connect the patient with case managers and other personnel who are likely to be able to work with him or her for extended periods and who are skilled at developing and maintaining therapeutic relationships.	7. Trusting and therapeutic relationships are key resources for achieving treatment adherence, and SPMI patients often require extended periods of working with staff to form these connections.
8. Actively promote treatment adherence by tying adherence to the patient's own goals and other motivational and educational approaches.	8. Treatment adherence reduces relapse and improves the long-term prognosis and quality of life.
9. Provide psychosocial support.	9. This aids in maintaining therapeutic rapport and helps the patient to maintain a positive self-esteem, and to cope effectively rather than maladaptively.
10. Provide regular and frequent contact with the patient, but not so much that it overstimulates the patient or contributes to paranoia.	10. Ongoing contact promotes therapeutic alliances and allows for monitoring so relapse or nonadherence can quickly be intercepted.
11. Educate, guide, support, and reinforce behaviors that prevent or control actual or potential medical comorbidities; act as an advocate as needed to ensure adequate health care for SPMI patients.	11. SPMI patients have higher burdens of physical illness, poorer hygiene and health practices, less access to effective medical treatment, and more premature mortality than the general population.
12. Involve persons with co-occurring substance abuse or addiction with Alcoholics or Narcotics Anonymous (AA or NA) and dual diagnosis (substance abuse/ mental illness [SAMI]) services.	12. Substance abuse rates are high in SPMI populations, increase relapse, and interfere with recovery; achieving sobriety is mostly associated with AA and integrated treatment programs.

Evidence-Based Treatment Approaches and Services

The following evidence-based treatment approaches are recommended for use for SPMI and available in a variety of settings in many communities.

Programs of assertive community treatment (PACT or ACT) have been shown to improve symptom management and decrease inpatient admissions, incarceration, and homelessness among people with mental illness (Coldwell & Bender, 2007). Instead of working with multiple departments or agencies, the consumer interacts with an established team of professionals who provide a comprehensive array of services all the time.

Cognitive behavioral therapy (CBT) has been effective in helping individuals with SMIs reduce and cope with symptoms such as auditory hallucinations (Penn et al., 2009). The cognitive component of CBT helps patients perceive circumstances more accurately and in a more positive light by guiding them to reconsider their perceptions and restructure their thinking to be more in line with reality. The behavioral component uses natural consequences and positive reinforcers (rewards) to shape the person's behavior in a more positive or adaptive manner.

Promotion of family support and partnerships is based on the premise that having sound support systems is one of the strongest predictors of recovery, and that treatment is enhanced when treatment providers work as empathic partners with patients and significant others (Gavois et al., 2006; NAMI, 2012). An example of this partnership is NAMI's Family-to-Family program, a psychoeducational program focusing on the skills families need to cope with their loved one's illness and to promote recovery (NAMI, 2012).

Social skills training focuses on teaching persons with SPMI a wide variety of social skills. Social deficits cause both direct and indirect functional impairment; people unable to respond assertively, for example, may instead respond aggressively or may fail to meet their needs at all. Complex interpersonal skills (such as negotiating or resolving a conflict) are broken down into subcomponents that are then taught in a stepwise fashion.

Supportive psychotherapy focuses on supporting the individual here and now, rather than on a more complex insight-oriented therapy in which change and growth are the goals. It stresses empathic understanding, improved coping, and anxiety reduction; it is informal and can be used by any member of the treatment team and in combination with other approaches; and it is suitable for use in persons benefitting from additional support (National Collaborating Centre for Mental Health, 2009).

Vocational rehabilitation and **supported employment** enhances self-esteem, improves organizational abilities, and increases socialization and income. Vocational rehabilitation has been used for many years and stresses prevocational training, employment in a sheltered setting (e.g., a consumer-managed business), and competitive employment in the general business world. Supported employment focuses on rapid employment and on-the-job training, thereby providing competitive employment from the onset, and ongoing supports (Cook et al., 2005).

Other Potentially Beneficial Approaches or Services

Although not yet evidence based to the extent of the preceding approaches, research supports potential benefits from use of the following:

- Advance directives are legal documents that give the patient the opportunity to direct how future relapses and treatment needs should be managed. Of course, an advance directive can only be considered legal if the document is signed when the patient's illness is under control and informed decisions are possible. For example, a patient can give consent to hospitalization or forced antipsychotic medications and specify when these responses may be used, minimizing the patient's loss of control over his or her treatment and avoiding the need for involuntary admission and related court involvement.

- Peer support and consumer-managed programming range from informal "clubhouses" that offer socialization, recreation, and sometimes other services to competitive businesses, such as snack bars or janitorial services that provide needed services and consumer employment while encouraging independence and building vocational skills. Certified peer specialists are specially trained consumers who are usually further along in the recovery process and who provide services to persons with SPMIs; being in recovery themselves, their guidance may be perceived as more acceptable and valid than that from staff.

- Advances in technology have the potential to reduce treatment costs, improve treatment access, and improve outcomes. Electronic records available in multiple locations via wireless technologies can assist in assessments or service delivery anywhere in the community. Service providers in remote locations are using **teletherapy**—speaking with patients by phone, computer-based video, or closed-circuit television—when patients cannot find transportation or travel to distant services; this can also save transit time for providers (Dunn et al., 2007), freeing more time available for patient care. The new communication technologies are being increasingly used to treat and follow-up patients via chat messaging systems on the health care website. These technologies have been especially useful for depression and anxiety disorders (Simon, 2011).

IMPULSE CONTROL DISORDERS

VIGNETTE

Sarah, 76, is shopping in a pharmacy when she notices the lipstick display. She rarely wears lipstick, but is drawn to the display and feels the urge to take one. She suppresses the urge, but it grows harder to resist. She ultimately snatches the lipstick and puts it in her purse. She feels a sense of relief, and an odd sort of pleasure. Over time she finds that this urge to steal things is happening repeatedly. Most of the time she cannot resist, and she sometimes takes ridiculous chances by taking things. However, later she feels ashamed and consumed with remorse and even returns the items or throws them away. Despite being caught once and threatened with jail, she continues to steal.

The problem in impulse control disorders involves a decreased ability to resist an impulse (or a drive) to perform certain acts. In most cases the pattern is one of increasing tension that builds until a particular action is taken. The actions may be impulsive (e.g., stealing) or involve considerable planning (e.g., fire setting), and range from benign or potentially harmful to self or others. The tension reduction reinforces the action and makes future resistance more difficult. Except for pathological gambling, these disorders are considered to be relatively rare.

THEORY

Biological Factors

The causes underlying impulse control disorders are not clearly established. Certain disorders or abnormalities of the brain seem to reduce one's ability to resist impulses. Violent people often show electroencephalographic variations and may have higher cerebrospinal fluid (CSF) serotonin metabolite levels (Diaz, 2010). Frontotemporal dementia or tumors (especially those affecting the right hemisphere), Parkinson's disease, and multiple sclerosis have been documented as contributing to impulsivity, as have traumatic brain injury and substance abuse, but there is not a clear link between such pathology and these disorders.

Genetic Factors

A gene associated with impulsive violence is suspected of weakening the brain's impulse control circuitry (NIMH, 2011). Although the incidence of some impulse disorders is greater within families (e.g., trichotillomania), neither this gene nor others have been linked causally to these disorders.

Psychological Factors

Theories regarding psychological causes of these disorders include an impaired ability to manage anxiety, wherein the person might be defending against (coping with) anxiety by subconsciously choosing an action that gives a sense of control over the anxiety. This theory is supported by a pattern of increased incidence of impulsive acts during periods of high stress. Some of these disorders may be a variant, or an expression, of anxiety disorders such as obsessive-compulsive disorder (OCD) or posttraumatic stress disorder (PTSD). There is also a parallel to addictive behaviors in that the patient may experience craving for the act and relief upon achieving it, supporting an addictions-based etiology (Chamberlain et al., 2007).

CLINICAL PICTURE

The *DSM-IV-TR* (APA, 2000) identifies impulse control disorders. In all cases, the diagnosis of these disorders requires elimination of all other medical and psychiatric causes—such as antisocial personality disorder or substance abuse—for the behavior in question, as well as ruling out other causations outside the arena of psychological functioning, such as seeking profit or attaining revenge. Judgment is intact and psychotic elements are absent in all six impulse control disorders. Descriptions of each disorder can be found in Table 27-2.

Effect on Individuals, Families, and Society

People with impulse control disorders are often confused and troubled by them, feeling embarrassment, shame, or guilt from their behaviors. Usually they realize that the acts are illogical or wrong, but despite their best efforts, the urge to act overwhelms them. Shame and distress accumulating from the unacceptable behaviors increase the risk of developing depression and of committing suicide (Brown et al., 2009). They may find themselves socially isolated or stigmatized.

Kleptomania is estimated to account for between 4% and 10% of all shoplifting losses (Koran et al., 2007). Gambling can cause tremendous financial losses, disrupt families, reduce job productivity, and cause loss of status, housing, possessions, jobs, and marriages. Intermittent explosive disorder and pyromania can cause injury or death to others, and can place the patient at risk of being sued or injured by the victim's defensive response. When criminal offenses are involved, society pays the costs of prosecution, incarceration, and forensic treatment, and the individual may lose civil rights (e.g., the right to vote) or private or governmental entitlements (e.g., eligibility for federal housing assistance, ability to hold a professional license or work in a particular field).

APPLICATION OF THE NURSING PROCESS

ASSESSMENT

Information suggesting the presence of an impulse control disorder is often minimized, withheld, or concealed by the patient or overlooked by staff; therefore careful assessment is important. Because the nurse's beliefs and attitudes about the behaviors in question may compromise his or her ability to perceive the disorder or remain objective about it, self-awareness is essential. For example, if the nurse believes that setting fires is simply criminal behavior and not related to a mental disorder, the nurse is not likely to identify the impulse control disorder or to pursue interventions to help the patient control these impulses.

Because actions associated with impulse control disorders may be embarrassing or even criminal in nature, building trust and conveying empathy and acceptance are key to helping the patient disclose these problems. Significant others who may be less reluctant to share information can also help identify concealed disorders. Nurses should look for patterns of recurrent

TABLE 27-2   MENTAL HEALTH DISORDERS PRIMARILY AFFECTING ADULTS

NAME	DESCRIPTION
Intermittent explosive disorder	"A mental disturbance beginning in childhood and characterized by discrete episodes of violence and aggressive behavior or destruction of property in otherwise normal individuals. The acts may occur as an overreaction to an ordinarily minor event" (Mosby's Medical Dictionary, 2009). The individual may feel depressed or remorseful afterward. They may face recrimination, arrest, civil actions, and loss of relationships and employment as a result of their actions.
Kleptomania	Kleptomania is characterized by "an abnormal, uncontrollable, and recurrent urge to steal." The objects are taken not for their monetary value, immediate need, or utility but because of the symbolic meaning usually associated with some unconscious emotional conflict, they are usually given away, returned surreptitiously, or kept and hidden (Mosby's Medical Dictionary, 2009). This behavior may begin at any age, and two thirds of the people affected are women. The behavior may occur at widely scattered intervals or be more regular and protracted. The acts are perceived as illogical and wrong.
Pyromania	Pyromania is characterized by "the recurrent compulsion to set fires. The term refers only to the setting of fires for sexual or other gratification provided by the fire itself, not to arson for profit or revenge" (Encyclopedia Britannica, 2008). Often the individual with this disorder has a fascination with fire and fire-related phenomena. These individuals are known to cause false alarms or even become firefighters for psychological gratification. This disorder may result in criminal prosecution.
Pathological gambling (gambling disorder)	Pathological gambling is characterized by the preoccupation and the inability to resist the urge to gamble despite significant disruption of one's family, finances, work, and other aspects of one's life. The individual feels aroused and positive when engaging in gambling, and experiences a relief of tension. Pathological gamblers may lie, rationalize, manipulate others, and conceal their behavior in order to maintain it. Work and social functioning may be disrupted. Most people with this disorder are men, and the incidence of this disorder is about 1% (Grant et al., 2005), but may be higher in settings where gambling opportunities are more varied and easily accessed, and in families in which other members also have the disorder (refer to Chapter 19).
Trichotillomania	Trichotillomania is a compulsion that involves pulling out one's hair in order to relieve tension. The person may pull out hair episodically for brief periods, or may engage in episodes lasting hours or longer in some cases. It tends to worsen under stress but also occurs when the person is calm, sometimes in an almost absent-minded fashion. In some cases, the hair is ingested and can produce "hairballs" similar to those seen in animals. The hair loss is often noticeable and significantly affects the individual's social comfort and causes the individual severe distress. The incidence is much higher in adult women than adult men, but about equal among boys and girls. It may be self-limited or continue for decades. Hair from any location can be involved.

Intermittent explosive disorder. (2009). *Mosby's Medical Dictionary* (8th ed.), St. Louis: Mosby Elsevier. Retrieved February 28, 2012, from http://medical-dictionary.thefreedictionary.com/intermittent explosive disorder.

Kleptomania. (2009). *Mosby's Medical Dictionary* (8th ed.). St. Louis: Mosby Elsevier. Retrieved February 28, 2012, from http://medical-dictionary.thefreedictionary.com/kleptomania.

Pyromania. (2008). © *Encyclopedia Britannica, Inc.* Retrieved February 28, 2012, from Dictionary.com, http://dictionary.reference.com/browse/pyromania.

loss of control in the patient's responses and history and should observe for signs suggesting these disorders (e.g., fascination with fire, unusual familiarity with gambling terminology, patches where hair is thin, pulling at or chewing on hair).

It is helpful to ask about circumstances that increase tension, as well as ways the patient reduces this tension. Empathic prompting can be helpful here, such as, "Sometimes people find themselves feeling tense and having urges to do different things to release the tension. Can you tell me about times when this may have happened to you?" Frank, direct questioning can set a tone for openness and prompt more candid responses; for example, "Tell me about times when you've hit someone or come close to losing control."

A patient's legal history may also suggest these disorders. Recurrent assaults or any episodes of fire setting merit further assessment. Further, the patient may be dealing with

TABLE 27-3 INTERVENTIONS FOR IMPULSE CONTROL DISORDERS

INTERVENTION	RATIONALE
1. Guide the patient to understand and practice tension reduction and stress control strategies such as stress avoidance, correction of negative self-talk, and breathing control exercises.	1. Tension usually precedes and contributes to impulsive actions; tension reduction and adaptive tension management can reduce impulsive behavior.
2. Promote the progressive substitution of alternate, less-maladaptive responses to tension, such as applying pressure to one's scalp with a thumb rather than pulling out one's hair.	2. Impulse control disorders involve maladaptive behaviors, some of which are criminal offenses; substitution of more adaptive responses can prevent negative consequences.
3. Assist the patient to explore feelings associated with the impulses, such as shame, fear, or guilt, and to manage these feelings adaptively.	3. Negative emotions contribute to stress and tension, leading to maladaptive impulsive behaviors.
4. Promote effective communication by guiding the patient to master and demonstrate assertive communication.	4. Assertiveness can improve one's ability to meet needs effectively, prevent misunderstandings, and reduce conflict and tension.
5. Assist the patient to identify the consequences of his or her actions, e.g., ask: "How do other people respond when you _____?"; "Tell me what things are like the day after you've set a fire"; or "Imagine you set the fire: what do you think will happen in the days and weeks that follow?" (anticipatory fantasy)	5. Identifying consequences can help the patient become more empathic to his/her effect on others, and increase motivation to refrain from problematic behaviors. Anticipatory fantasy guides the patient to imagine the consequences of behavior and dampen urges to act on impulses.
6. Educate the patient that drugs and alcohol may increase impulsiveness through disinhibition or impairment of judgment; educate the patient regarding the effect of "triggers," i.e., circumstances that evoke tension or impulses (e.g., going to bars).	6. Disinhibiting drugs and exposure to triggers that evoke impulsive behavior increase impulsive actions; reducing disinhibition and exposure to triggers reduces the frequency and intensity of the impulsive actions.
7. Pathological gamblers may respond well to group therapy; organizations such as Gamblers Anonymous (www.gamblersanonymous.org) provide significant assistance through support, education, and practical tips on managing gambling impulses and other concerns.	7. 12-step programs have been shown to be of significant help in reducing activities that have a compulsive or addictive component; peer support groups are effective for confronting defenses and rationalization used to support the gambling.
8. Trichotillomania patients can benefit from special hair styling, hair weaves, or other cosmetology assistance; they may require considerable support in order to access such resources, however, because of embarrassment.	8. Hair loss can create a significant cosmetic defect, resulting in impaired self-esteem and further dysfunctional coping; compensating cosmetically for such defects can enhance the person's self-image and self-esteem.

concurrent depression or be sufficiently distressed to be considering self-harm. Assessment for these risks is essential. Finally, it is always important to assess how the disorder has impacted the patient and significant others, as well as the patient's knowledge of the disorder and ways of reducing or coping with it.

DIAGNOSIS

A variety of diagnoses may apply to people with impulse control disorders, including *Impaired Impulse Control, Deficient Community Health, Impaired Adjustment, Anxiety, Compromised Family Coping, Ineffective Coping, Risk for Injury, Chronic Low Self-Esteem, Impaired Social Interaction, Ineffective Relationship,* and *Social Isolation* (NANDA-I, 2012-14).

Nursing interventions for these disorders vary with the particular disorder being addressed, but some general interventions likely to fit most related circumstances are listed in Table 27-3.

OUTCOMES IDENTIFICATION

Expected outcomes vary with the disorder but typically focus on reducing the problematic acts and substituting more adaptive means to reduce tension. Examples of desired outcomes include "Patient does not set fires," "Hair loss is reduced by 20%," "Patient substitutes corrective self-talk when experiencing impulses to act inappropriately," "Patient demonstrates use of three or more tension reduction strategies," and "Patient rates anxiety as 5 or less on a 1 to 10 scale."

IMPLEMENTATION

Pharmacological, Biological, and Integrative Therapies

Treatment strategies for impulse control disorders in most cases focus on a combination of psychotherapy and medication. Because people with these disorders usually do not manifest an imminent risk to themselves or others, or present with emergent needs, treatment is usually provided on an outpatient basis.

Psychopharmacology

Psychopharmacological interventions presently dominate in the treatment of some impulse control disorders. Selective serotonin reuptake inhibitors (SSRIs), the antidepressant bupropion (Dannon et al., 2005), and opioid antagonists (e.g., naltrexone) (Grant & Kim, 2002) are used in the treatment of kleptomania, trichotillomania, and pathological gambling. Lithium and the antipsychotic risperidone have shown to have efficacy in the treatment of conduct disorder, a child/adolescent disorder with certain similarities to intermittent explosive disorder (Ipser & Stein, 2007); lithium and SSRIs have shown possible efficacy for reducing violence.

Antidepressants and mood stabilizers have been used for this class of disorders with varying results. Opioid antagonists such as nalmefene may be of particular benefit in pathological gambling (Grant et al., 2006). Anticonvulsants, along with propranolol and similar β-adrenergic antagonists, may be useful for reducing aggression, particularly in individuals whose impulse control problems seem to stem from organic disorders such as dementia (Moeller et al., 2001).

Nonpharmacological Treatments

Nonpharmacological treatments include a variety of approaches. Hypnotherapy may be of benefit, and cognitive behavioral approaches such as habit reversal are an evidence-based practice in disorders such as trichotillomania (Bruce et al., 2005). By modifying thinking patterns and reducing thinking distortion, patients can also change their actions. Behavioral conditioning through the use of positive rewards and negative consequences is research-supported for reducing problematic habitual behaviors (Moeller et al., 2001). Group psychotherapy provides for therapeutic confrontation from peers and tends to be particularly helpful for people who have poor insight or difficulty accepting responsibility for their behavior.

SEXUAL DISORDERS

Sexual disorders involve sexual function and identity.

GENDER DYSPHORIA/GENDER IDENTITY DISORDER

Gender dysphoria/gender identity disorder is thought to be rather rare. This disorder involves persistent, strong cross-gender identification wherein a person feels he or she has a strong desire to be the opposite gender. It often first becomes apparent in childhood or adolescence, and people with this disorder may alter their dress, use hormonal medications, and even pursue surgery in order to appear as congruent as possible with their desired gender.

Gender dysphoria can be accompanied by significant embarrassment, shame, discrimination, and social isolation because many people in our society do not understand the disorder and react with repugnance.

People with this disorder experience persistent discomfort with their present gender, their gender-related roles and a strong and persistent desire to assume the characteristics (e.g., dress and mannerisms) and roles of the opposite gender. Usually the person believes that he or she was born in the wrong body, and has a strong desire to be the other gender. This experience and belief usually causes significant distress.

For those individuals who choose sexual reassignment, they engage in specific steps to ensure that this is truly what they want. The first step involves a period of counseling to assist the person in fully considering and preparing for this very involved and protracted (long-term) process. If after counseling the individual wants to proceed, they proceed to the next step. This step involves living for 1 to 2 years as a member of the opposite or desired gender (to help ensure readiness). At this time they are given hormonal therapy to suppress undesired physical characteristics and elicit desired sexual characteristics (e.g., to diminish facial hair and cause breast enlargement or to increase facial hair and alter voice). This may be the last step for many people; however, others decide to take the final step, which is surgical intervention to alter their genitalia to match those of the desired gender.

A recent book and documentary (2011) was made by Chaz Bono. Chaz Bono was born with the name of Chastity to Cher (the well-known entertainer) and Sonny Bono (was also an entertainer and later became a congressman). Chaz documented his journey throughout this process of gender change, along with the changes in his personal and social relationships and his emotions and experiences going through this process of being born female to "becoming" a male with the help of medical, hormonal, and surgical interventions.

PARAPHILIAS

Paraphilias are psychological disorders characterized by a preoccupation with sexual fantasies and related sexual urges that focus on nontraditional and socially unacceptable sexual "targets" such as children, animals, or objects. People with a paraphilia may or may not act on their urges.

As a result of divergent religious and cultural expectations, there is a degree of conflict within our society about how to define appropriate sexual behavior. For example, opinions can vary widely in terms of what is an appropriate age for the onset of sexual relations, whom one should be able to choose as a sexual partner (based on gender, age, or race, for example), and whether such relations should occur outside of marriage. The incidence of paraphilias is difficult to measure because stigma, the potential for prosecution, and other concerns cause those affected to be reluctant to disclose this information.

THEORY

Biological Factors

The cause of gender dysphoria is unknown, but theories include abnormalities in sexual hormones and related neurodevelopment in utero, or developmental aberrations in early life (Wylie, 2004). The causes underlying paraphilias have not yet been determined. As with impulse disorders, certain disorders or abnormalities of the brain seem to increase impulsiveness or reduce one's ability to resist sexual impulses, and frontotemporal dementia, tumors, and Parkinson's disease have been documented as contributing to paraphilias such as pedophilia (Rahman & Symeonides, 2008). Increased sympathetic activity and reduced serotonergic activity have been implicated in pedophilia. Traumatic brain injuries and cognitive impairment are also associated with sexual offenses (Guay, 2008), although not necessarily sexual disorders; for example, Langevin (2006) surveyed sexual offenders (not pedophiles per se) and found that 49% had suffered head trauma sufficient to cause loss of consciousness.

Psychological Factors

Theories regarding psychological causes of these disorders include failure to develop appropriate attachments in early childhood, resulting in inadequate or inappropriate attachments at later developmental stages (Sawle & Kear-Colwell, 2001). Another theory is that the disorders are learned responses to inappropriate sexual role models, causing the children to later develop an inappropriate "love map" (Fagan et al., 2002). Research also suggests that the paraphilias, particularly those associated with sexual offenses, may be caused by one's own sexual victimization; 30% to 60% of pedophiles were themselves sexually abused as children. A confounding factor limiting our understanding of these disorders is that funding entities and research institutions, perhaps because of the sometimes controversial aspects of these disorders, are sometimes reluctant to support research related to the causes and treatment of paraphilias (Arehart-Treichel, 2006).

For the most part we do not have any pathophysiological correlates for these disorders and there is no laboratory test, scan, or other widely accepted objective means of detecting them. Instead they are diagnosed on the basis of the characteristic patterns of behavior that are the symptoms of these disorders.

CLINICAL PICTURE

The *DSM* distinguishes multiple types of paraphilias, described in Table 27-4. The diagnosis of these disorders first requires eliminating all other medical and psychiatric causes of the behavior in question (e.g., criminal intent, manic episodes, dementia, substance abuse, or any disorder that causes disinhibition or impairs judgment or impulse control). Sexual disorders do not involve psychotic elements, and most have their onset during adolescence. Most people with paraphilias are male, and to be diagnosed with a paraphilia, the features must have been present for at least 6 months (i.e., occasional experiences of gratification through paraphilic-like experiences would not meet the diagnostic criteria for a paraphilia).

Although not paraphilias, sexual addiction and other forms of distress or dysfunction related to sexuality can be diagnosed as sexual disorders not otherwise specified (NOS). Other disorders related to sexuality, although not covered in this chapter or classified as sexual disorders, include those relating to chromosomal abnormalities (e.g., Klinefelter's syndrome), head trauma or other organic disorder, or compulsive use of pornography and those arising from SPMIs that affect impulse control and social and sexual interaction (e.g., schizophrenia).

Effect on Individuals, Families, and Society

The effect of paraphilias may be relatively minor and limited to the individual with the diagnosis (e.g., a person with transvestic fetishism). When people with paraphilias engage sexually with unwilling partners (e.g., frotteurism or voyeurism), victims may feel violated and experience significant and protracted psychological distress.

Pedophilic (paraphilic) offenders harm, injure, or kill their victims, and even when the victim survives or is physically uninjured, there is virtually always significant, protracted, and sometimes disabling psychological life-long damage. Survivors are at increased risk of disorders such as PTSD, depression, anxiety, and substance abuse disorders. Families, loved ones, and the general community are often traumatized and left unable to feel fully secure in the future (refer to Chapter 22).

Sexual abuse is a significant problem in our society. All pedophilics (paraphilics) are child molesters, but not all child molesters are pedophilics/paraphilics. However, only a portion of this abuse involves persons with pedophilia. Parents and caregivers commit up to 90% or more of the sexual abuse of children in the United States, and strangers are believed to account for less than 5% of child sexual offenses (refer to Chapter 21). The recidivism (repeating of a previous offense) rates for untreated child sexual offenders (both pedophilic and nonpedophilic combined) are relatively high. Up to 80% of 18- to 27-year-old offenders and up 50% for those 25- to 60-years-old reoffend within 5 years of their release from prison or hospitals, although the rate drops to almost zero for those older than 60 years (Thornton, 2006).

Patients with these disorders may be distressed by their symptoms, overwhelmed with shame or guilt. Others display more dyssocial/antisocial tendencies and are indifferent or blasé about their paraphilia, or may attempt to justify their actions through rationalization or other means. Some even lobby to decriminalize acts such as sexual relations with children. Even those who never enact their fantasies may find themselves socially isolated or stigmatized as a result of these irresistible yet unacceptable preoccupations. Disorders such as sexual addiction can contribute to guilt, marital discord, low self-esteem, and sexually transmitted diseases.

TABLE 27-4 PARAPHILIC DISORDERS

NAME	DESCRIPTION
Exhibitionism	The main characteristic of this disorder is when an individual obtains sexual arousal/pleasure by exposing their genitals to an unsuspecting stranger. An individual has strong, recurrent fantasies or acts involving exposing genitalia and has either experienced significant distress related to the fantasies or enacted these fantasies by exposing himself or herself. Exhibitionism can begin at any age but usually starts in adolescence, and the incidence seems to taper by age 40.
Fetishism	The main characteristic of fetishism is when an individual obtains sexual arousal using or thinking about an inanimate object or part of the body. The individual experiences significant distress or role impairment (e.g., as a spouse or employee), and the objects' fetish are not usual objects that can arouse sexual feelings (e.g., rubber items and shoes).
Frotteurism	Individuals with frotteurism obtain sexual arousal and gratification from rubbing their genitals against unsuspecting others in public places. These individuals experience marked distress or interpersonal difficulties as a result of the impulses or behavior.
Pedophilia	Pedophilia involves fantasized or actual sexual activity with a child who has not reached puberty. A pedophile must either have acted on the fantasies or experienced significant distress or interpersonal difficulties as a result of the fantasies. Pedophiles may focus on children of the same, opposite, or both genders, although most are heterosexually focused. They may be focused on children exclusively or may have a sexual interest in adults as well. Some people with pedophilia focus their activities on relatives (incestual form), others on non–family members, and some on both.
Sexual masochism and sexual sadism	Individuals with these disorders derive sexual gratification from having pain and/or humiliation inflicted upon themself (masochism) or creating psychological and physical pain on others (sadism). Masochism can include bondage, verbal abuse, electrical shocks, whipping, being urinated on, and being forced to humiliate oneself. Sadism includes inflicting such acts on a (usually masochistic) partner, and often involves the theme of having complete psychological and physical control over one's partner (domination). The partner may be consenting or nonconsenting.
Transvestic fetishism	Transvestic fetishism involves deriving sexual gratification by dressing as a person of the opposite gender, such as a male dressing as a female.
Voyeurism	Voyeurism involves deriving sexual gratification from observing unsuspecting persons in sexually arousing situations (e.g., undressing or engaging in sexual activity).

Societal responses to sexual offenders include educating the public, warning potential victims (via sexual offender registries and notifications of those residing nearby), and restricting access to potential victims (by prohibiting contact with children and restricting residences to areas away from schools and playgrounds). Although intended to prevent sexual offenses, these restrictions may ostracize possibly reformed offenders and create unintended consequences including isolation, unemployment, and homelessness (which may in turn make it more difficult to track and treat offenders). Information on sexual offenses and sexual offender listings can typically be found on the web pages of local law enforcement agencies.

APPLICATION OF THE NURSING PROCESS

SELF-CARE FOR NURSES

Self-care and self-assessment are essential for nurses when dealing with persons with these disorders. This is because the nurse's beliefs and attitudes about these unusual (from the nurse's perspective) or sometimes abhorrent behaviors may compromise objectivity. If the nurse is a survivor of sexual abuse, treating perpetrators can be particularly difficult and even traumatic, requiring additional support (e.g., clinical supervision to help the nurse recognize and deal with responses to the patient; counseling to help cope with reawakened memories of earlier abuse). As with impulse control disorders, actions associated with paraphilias may be embarrassing or even criminal in nature, making building trust and conveying empathy and acceptance essential. Patients often conceal or deny paraphilic thoughts and behavior, making careful assessment and validation of the patient's reports important.

ASSESSMENT

Written assessment questionnaires can elicit possibly embarrassing information without the tension of a face-to-face interview, and can form the basis of a more focused interview thereafter.

Significant others who may be less reluctant to share information can also help identify concealed issues. For example, it is not unusual for children of individuals with pedophilia to report inappropriate sexual contact during their childhood. In some cases, the patient may be dealing with concurrent depression or be sufficiently distressed to be considering self-harm, making assessment for this risk essential. This is especially true for those who recently have been accused of (or publicly exposed in reference to) sexual offenses involving children, and who face considerable shame and even hostility within their families and communities as a result; such persons are at especially high risk of suicide in the first 27 to 48 hours after incarceration. Finally, it is always important to assess how the disorder has affected the patient and significant others, as well as the patient's knowledge of the disorder and ways of reducing or coping with it.

DIAGNOSIS

A variety of diagnoses may apply to individuals with gender dysphoria disorder and paraphilias, including *Impaired* *Adjustment, Anxiety, Compromised Family Coping, Ineffective Coping, Ineffective Relationship, Risk for Injury, Chronic Low Self-Esteem, Sexual Dysfunction, Ineffective Sexuality Pattern, Risk for Other-Directed Violence,* and *Social Isolation* (NANDA, 2012-2014). Nursing interventions for these disorders vary with the disorder and its expression in a particular patient, and are affected by any comorbid mental health disorders. Some general interventions likely to fit most related circumstances are listed in Table 27-5.

OUTCOMES IDENTIFICATION

Expected outcomes vary with the disorder but typically focus on reducing the problematic acts and substituting more adaptive means to meet sexual needs. Examples of desired outcomes include "Patient reports ability to fantasize about adults as well as children," "Patient does not go to locations where children are likely to be found," "Patient does not touch any child," and "Patient rates urge to have contact with children a 5 or less on a 1 to 10 scale."

TABLE 27-5 INTERVENTIONS FOR SEXUAL DISORDERS

INTERVENTION	RATIONALE
1. Use inclusive language, set and convey a tone of acceptance, normalize disclosure pertaining to sexuality, and provide active support.	1. These actions promote free and open discussion of patient behavior and needs (Huygen, 2006).
2. Assist individuals with gender dysphoria to connect with peers and professionals who are supportive and receptive, and to access resources such as www.wpath.org and www.transgenderlaw.org, which can be good starting points for people dealing with these disorders.	2. Stigma and discrimination can cause isolation and hopelessness; connecting with others and pursuing educational resources for the patient and significant others can enhance understanding and acceptance.
3. Maintain and reinforce appropriate interpersonal boundaries with people with sexual disorders.	3. Role modeling of appropriate boundaries allows the patient to identify and adopt more effective ways of relating to others, and maintains an effective nurse-patient relationship.
4. Mutually set, track, revise, and reinforce incremental goals, along with related actions that will meet those goals.	4. Mutual goal setting increases patient "buy-in"; incremental goals are easier to attain, reducing discouragement from unmet goals and providing a series of successes that reinforce patient efforts.
5. Guide the patient to understand and practice tension reduction and stress control strategies such as avoidance of stress, correction of negative self-talk, and use of breathing control exercises.	5. High levels of stress and tension, especially when coupled with a limited or ineffective repertoire of coping strategies, increase the chance of maladaptive stress reduction behaviors.
6. Educate the patient (and, as applicable, involved support people and personnel from the criminal justice system) regarding his/her disorder: its causes, treatments, and most importantly ways to cope with and control symptoms and maladaptive behaviors.	6. Understanding the psychological and psychiatric aspects of one's disorder, as well as ways to cope with or reduce symptoms, can decrease guilt and powerlessness, instilling hope and improving the patient's sense of control.
7. Assist the patient to identify and explore feelings preceding or associated with the target behavior, such as excitement, shame, or guilt.	7. Unresolved feelings can cause desperation and lead to acting out or loss of control.

Continued

TABLE 27-5	INTERVENTIONS FOR SEXUAL DISORDERS—cont'd
INTERVENTION	**RATIONALE**
8. Assist the patient to identify the consequences of his/her actions, e.g., ask: "How do other people seem to feel about your behavior?" or "What tends to happen when you go where children play?"	8. Insight that develops from within tends to be more accepted than feedback provided externally; covert sensitization—guiding the patient to connect an undesired behavior with negative consequences—diminishes unacceptable behaviors.
9. Address comorbid disorders and mental health needs such as substance abuse or a history of sexual victimization during the patient's youth.	9. Depression and other mental disorders impair problem-solving and coping abilities, draining the patient's energy for addressing the target problems.
10. Involve the patient in group therapy with others with paraphilias; a mixture of new and recovered members is desirable.	10. Group psychotherapy allows for frank feedback and therapeutic confrontation by those who have "been there" and thus are difficult to manipulate; a mix of new and recovered members provides positive role models for the new members.

IMPLEMENTATION

Pharmacological and Therapeutic Interventions

Pedophilia/Pedohebephilic

People with sexual disorders may seek treatment when sufficiently distressed by their disorder, or when compelled to do so in order to address the concerns of spouses, significant others, or officers of the court.

People with paraphilias who commit criminal offenses may be court-ordered to submit to treatment. Except for criminal offenders with comorbid SPMIs, treatment is almost always on an outpatient basis. Although outpatient treatment has been shown to be beneficial in some cases, it has not been demonstrated to be adequately effective in preventing recidivism among pedophiles.

As a result, a movement has begun in some states to hold sexual offenders in inpatient psychiatric treatment settings (usually state forensic hospitals) for extended periods after they have completed their prison sentences (Lippke, 2008). This "preventive psychiatric incarceration" is controversial within the mental health field, because some feel it is an abuse of psychiatry to hold a person who does not require that level of clinical care (an inpatient setting), to incarcerate a person because of what he/she might do in the future, or to hold people in psychiatric settings when there may be no known (or further) psychiatric treatment available for their particular needs.

Treatment of pedophilia usually focuses on ways to decrease the patient's physical urges, since the pedophilic fantasies are remarkably persistent (Palmer, 2010). Basically, treatment involves medications and psychotherapy. The medications typically interfere with the production of the male sexual hormones, primarily testosterone. These medications are called antiandrogens and in effect produce varying degrees of chemical castration—examples include depot-leuprolide, medroxyprogesterone acetate (MPA, an analogue of progesterone), cyproterone acetate (CPA, Depo-Provera), or analogues of gonadotropin-releasing hormone. Patients receive a monthly injection, and then testosterone levels are monitored to ensure effectiveness. Group therapy is a necessary part of all modalities to help modify destructive urges.

Other Paraphilias

Other potentially helpful drugs include those that reduce compulsive or impulsive behavior (e.g., naltrexone, carbamazepine, clonazepam, and SSRIs). The following drugs are also used to treat paraphilias and sexually inappropriate behavior in other medical or psychiatric conditions, such as dementia (Light & Holroyd, 2005). They can have multiple and significant side effects, including feminization, weight gain, clotting disorders, thromboembolism, decreased fertility and sexual dysfunction, depression, and hypertension (Almeida et al., 2003; Maletzky & Field, 2003). Side effects frequently discourage use of the antiadrenergic drugs in particular, and often these are used under court order and in depot (long-acting injectable) forms to ensure adherence. In rare cases, surgical castration may be pursued by the patient in lieu of drugs.

Psychotherapeutic treatments include group and one-to-one psychotherapy and psychoeducational interventions. Cognitive behavioral therapies in particular are believed to be helpful. For people with gender dysphoria, counseling can help patients compare and choose various paths they might take, including sexual reassignment, and cope with their feelings and society's responses to this disorder.

Behavioral approaches for paraphilias can include desensitization techniques to reduce sexual responsiveness to undesired stimuli. In some cases, patients are guided to fulfill their gratification needs in non–socially-offensive ways, such as via masturbatory reconditioning and "fantasy sex." Twelve-step programs also have been effective, and treatment of comorbid disorders, particularly those that impair impulse control (e.g., substance abuse), can reduce the risk of recidivism or conversion to criminal behavior (Marshall, 2007).

ADULT ATTENTION DEFICIT/ HYPERACTIVITY DISORDER

VIGNETTE

Andrea, a 32-year-old graduate student in psychology, presents at the student health center concerned that she might have attention deficit/hyperactivity disorder (ADHD) after learning about it in class. She reports that throughout her life teachers and others told her she was extremely bright, but that somehow this was not reflected in her grades, which were B's and C's. She notes that she has difficulty maintaining concentration, often "tuning out" during lectures and having to regularly reread parts of her assignments, and that it is difficult for her to organize her work and studies.

Andrea has difficulty sitting still, frequently changing position and sometimes walking about the room. She interrupts others regularly and then apologizes but has difficulty regaining her train of thought. Distraction, worry, and irritability trouble her. She often loses track of belongings, spends much time looking for misplaced items, forgets appointments, and frequently overlooks tasks she had intended to do.

Other psychiatric and physical problems are ruled out. After treatment with methylphenidate and counseling, Andrea reports that she was able to finish a major written assignment in about one third the time and with much less stress compared with her completion of such a task before treatment. She is happy with the improvement and hopeful regarding further improvement. She says that friends have commented on the improvement, saying she seems more at ease and less scattered. She agrees to join an ADHD support group on campus and attend a 6-week follow-up appointment.

PREVALENCE AND COMORBIDITY

ADHD involves a persistent pattern of inattention, impaired ability to focus and concentrate, and hyperactivity and impulsivity that are more noticeable and more severe than would otherwise be seen at a given developmental level. It has its onset in childhood, usually peaking between the ages of 5 and 10 years (refer to Chapter 26). Although typically considered a disorder primarily of children and adolescents, the apparent decrease in prevalence of ADHD by adulthood may really be a result of the use of inadequate criteria for adult diagnosis and the enhanced ability of adults to compensate or conceal their symptoms. ADHD clearly exists in, or persists into, adulthood, albeit in many cases with a somewhat different feel or appearance compared with its expression in children (Spencer et al., 2007). New research from Norway has found that there is some overlap between ADHD and bipolar disorders with regard to rapid mood swings (Research Council of Norway, 2011). Attention deficit disorder (ADD) involves a similar presentation but without the hyperactivity.

Estimates for the incidence in children range from 3% to 10% (some research suggests up to 19%), and it is more common in males. Overall, ADHD occurs worldwide and is thought to affect 2% to 5% of the population, depending on the measurements used (Research Council of Norway, 2011). The incidence in adults has not been well established, but is likely present in nearly the same range as seen in children; however, as hyperactivity decreases over time, fewer males remain diagnosed with ADHD in adulthood, and the adult ADHD incidence is more evenly split between males and females (Greydanus et al., 2007).

ADHD contributes to a wide variety of interpersonal, social, academic, and vocational problems, and can significantly limit or disrupt a person's ability to function and negatively affect health habits and educational or socioeconomic achievement well into adulthood. It is also a controversial diagnosis in the eyes of those who believe the disorder, especially in children, is too readily and too subjectively diagnosed, and too quickly addressed through medications rather than nonpharmacological treatments.

Psychiatric comorbidity is common in ADHD, with nearly 80% of children with ADHD having at least one other diagnosis and 67% having two other diagnoses. Conduct and oppositional defiant disorders, anxiety disorders, and learning disorders are common co-occurring disorders in children; depression and antisocial personality disorder are relatively common co-occurring disorders in adults with ADHD (with antisocial elements tending to be more common in those with the combined type of ADHD), and bipolar disorder is another comorbid condition in adult ADHD patients, as mentioned previously (Spencer et al., 2007). Co-occurring physical health disorders include Tourette's disorder and other tic disorders, substance abuse, sexually transmitted diseases, traumatic brain injuries, and general traumatic injuries (Greydanus et al., 2007).

THEORY

Genetic Factors

Multiple causes and contributing factors seem to play a part in ADHD. There appears to be a strong genetic and familial component; for example, if one identical twin has the disorder, depending on the subtype involved, there is an 80% to 98% chance that the other sibling will have the disorder, and parents of children with ADHD often have features of ADHD also.

Biological Factors

Alterations in the neurotransmitters norepinephrine and dopamine have been implicated. Research suggests that the key brain areas involved in ADHD are the frontal lobe and the basal ganglia and their connections to the cerebellum; imaging studies show diminished activity (Brassett-Harknett & Butler, 2007) and relatively smaller amounts of brain matter in these areas in people with ADHD. "Biological adversity" (biological challenges) is another possible factor: fetal distress, low birth weight, prematurity, maternal bleeding, and maternal smoking and drug abuse are implicated as contributing to ADHD, as is exposure to toxins such as lead (Spencer et al., 2007). Diet may also play a role, as restrictive diets and selective food elimination have improved ADHD symptomatology in children (Pellser et al., 2009).

Psychological Factors

Theories regarding psychological causes suggest that intrafamilial conflict and distress are both causative for, and a result of, ADHD. The disorder appears to be at least aggravated by familial, social, and environmental factors. Some research suggests that the strong familial nature (increased likelihood of occurrence within a family) argues for family dysfunction being a significant contributing factor (Spencer et al., 2007).

CLINICAL PICTURE

ADHD tends to be underappreciated and underdiagnosed in adults. The diagnosis of ADHD is complicated by the complexity and varied presentation of the disorder. Because of the high percentage of patients with co-occurring mental disorders and the complexity of ADHD, a complete mental health assessment (in complicated cases, by an ADHD specialist) is highly recommended. There is no laboratory test, scan, or other objective means for detecting it. Instead, ADHD is diagnosed based on the characteristic patterns of behavior and organizational and attentional dysfunction, which are the symptoms of these disorders.

The *DSM* includes symptoms reflecting inattention and symptoms reflecting hyperactivity-impulsivity. The *DSM* does not have separate diagnostic criteria for the disorder in adults, although some experts believe separate diagnostic criteria and tools should exist (Bell, 2011). (Refer to Chapter 26 for characteristics of ADHD in children.) Individuals who have some of the diagnostic elements of ADHD but who do not meet the full criteria may be diagnosed with ADHD in partial remission (if originally diagnosed as a child) or as having ADHD NOS (e.g., if the disorder was not present before the age of 7, or if the person meets other criteria but has hypoactivity instead of hyperactivity). Some believe that childhood ADHD does not disappear as once thought, and that if properly assessed many adults who had ADHD as children would at least merit one of these lesser ADHD diagnoses.

Effect on Individuals, Families, and Society

The effect of ADHD on individuals is significant, not only while it is active (e.g., during childhood) but also even when it has diminished or resolved by adulthood. Adults diagnosed with ADHD as children tend to achieve lower socioeconomic status, complete fewer years of school, are more likely to smoke and to abuse alcohol and drugs, are more likely to have traffic incidents (e.g., road rage, accidents, speeding offenses), have more contact with police, are at greater risk of sexually transmitted diseases, change jobs more frequently, report more interpersonal and relational difficulties, and have higher rates of depression than people without ADHD (Brassett-Harknett & Butler, 2007; Spencer et al., 2007). ADHD is also significantly more prevalent in incarcerated populations, suggesting ADHD may increase the propensity toward criminal activity.

The effect on society is less well established. ADHD inhibits academic achievement at all ages, and it is believed to reduce work productivity and increase criminal justice system costs significantly, but hard data do not yet exist.

APPLICATION OF THE NURSING PROCESS

ASSESSMENT

Assessment is based on patient reports, nursing observation, and, when available, reports of employers, family members, and other third parties. Assessment should focus on behaviors supportive of the diagnosis as well as on indicators of the patient's present knowledge of and ability to cope with the disorder. Support systems play a major role in the patient achieving successful outcomes and should be assessed.

If the patient is experiencing significant distractibility or has difficulty processing complex statements, keep comments and questioning concise and clear and choose interview areas that are relatively quiet and free of distractions. If needed, prompts can help the patient organize responses and stay on track. Observe for indications of disorganization, distractibility, irritability, impulsive comments or behavior, difficulty processing information or following instructions, difficulty achieving at the expected level in social and vocational settings, and hyperactivity (excess or nonpurposeful motor activity). Substance abuse, particularly of methamphetamine and other stimulants, can mimic ADHD and should be ruled out.

DIAGNOSIS

Nursing diagnoses for ADHD include: *Impaired Social Interaction, Ineffective Impulse Control, Ineffective Relationship, Defensive Coping, Compromised Family Coping, Impaired Adjustment, Sleep Pattern Disturbance, Anxiety,* and *Personal Identity Disturbance* (NANDA, 2012-2014). Nursing interventions focus on symptom management and coping with the illness (Table 27-6). As a general rule, the interventions for adults are different from those for children.

OUTCOMES IDENTIFICATION

Examples of potential outcome measures include: "Patient demonstrates ability to stay on task by completing one task before starting another," "Patient discusses three techniques to reduce environmental distractions," and "Patient rates concentration as a 5 or greater on a 1 to 10 scale."

IMPLEMENTATION

Pharmacological, Biological, and Integrative Therapies

Medications are a well-established and researched treatment modality for ADHD. The same drugs used to treat children are also used, in most cases, to treat adults. Stimulants are the most widely used medication for ADHD, and they show a high

TABLE 27-6	**INTERVENTIONS FOR ADULT ATTENTION DEFICIT/HYPERACTIVITY DISORDER (ADHD)**
INTERVENTION	**RATIONALE**
1. Educate the patient and significant other(s) regarding ADHD: its causes, treatments, and especially ways to cope with and control its symptoms.	1. Understanding the psychological and psychiatric aspects of one's disorder, as well as ways to cope with or reduce symptoms, can decrease powerlessness, instill hope, and improve patient's sense of control.
2. Guide the patient to understand and practice stimulation reduction strategies such as environmental structuring (reducing auditory and visual distractions).	2. Environmental distractions make already impaired concentration more difficult.
3. Mutually set, track, revise, and reinforce incremental goals, along with actions that will meet those goals.	3. Mutual goal setting increases patient "buy-in"; incremental goals are easier to attain, reducing discouragement from unmet goals and providing successes that reinforce patient efforts.
4. Guide the patient to identify and use enhanced organizational skills; many techniques exist to increase organization and efficiency in completing tasks, from reminder lists to using PDAs to track appointments.	4. Enhancements in organization can improve functioning and promote a positive self-image as the patient experiences increased task success; Internet resources and print publications can be accessed for this purpose.
5. Guide the patient to identify and use enhanced time management skills (e.g., structured priority setting wherein the patient asks self, "What will happen if I do not do this task next?" and then uses those responses to determine which task to tackle next).	5. Better time management can improve functioning and reduce stress; Internet resources and published materials on this topic can be readily accessed.
6. Assist the patient to identify and explore feelings about ADHD and its effect on his/her life, and to correct any distorted self-talk pertaining to self-image.	6. ADHD may contribute to frustration or impaired self-esteem because of daily challenges and one's unmet potential; people with ADHD may be critical of themselves and use negative "self-talk" (e.g., "I am so stupid; why can't I do this? What is wrong with me!").
7. Encourage participation in ADHD support groups and vetted online support resources such as ADHD blogs.	7. Support groups and online resources can provide pragmatic "helpful hints" from peers and support from an "I've been there" perspective.
8. Address comorbid disorders and mental health needs such as substance abuse.	8. Depression and other disorders further impair problem-solving and coping abilities; substance abuse can significantly worsen impulsivity and concentration.

degree of efficacy, with 75% to 95% reporting improvement from methylphenidate (e.g., Ritalin, which is available in many different forms and formulations) and amphetamine variants (e.g., Adderall). Stimulant medications are thought to augment dopamine and/or norepinephrine neurotransmission that serves to regulate prefrontal cortex activities critical for modulation of behavior, attention, and cognition. It might seem counterintuitive for stimulants to help hyperactivity, but these medications all in some way promote enhanced dopamine and norepinephrine functioning. One concern noted in the use of such stimulants is patients sharing the medicine with others; although this is a criminal offense, such sharing has been increasing, especially among college students, and should be addressed during patient education (Diller, 2010).

Stimulants are available in short-, intermediate-, and long-acting forms, some with sustained-release technology. Longer-acting and timed-release forms allow patients to take the medicines once or twice per day before and after (rather than during) school or work, a popular feature that probably improves

adherence (inattentiveness and other features create increased adherence issues in ADHD). Concomitant use of clonidine and an antidepressant has also shown efficacy in the treatment of ADHD (Greydanus et al., 2007). Atomoxetine, a nonstimulant SSRI with antidepressant activity, enhances norepinephrine function and allows for a once-daily regimen (Scahill et al., 2004).

Psychotherapy

Psychotherapeutic treatments are of equal importance in managing ADHD. Cognitive therapy is helpful for correcting distortions in self-image and improving focus and concentration, and counseling can address co-occurring issues such as marital discord and coping with chronic illness. Psychoeducation about the disorder and its treatment and instruction in techniques for managing and coping with symptoms are essential and may be done individually or in a group setting. Support groups, helpful for addressing self-esteem and anxiety issues, can be excellent sources of helpful hints for daily management of the disorder and useful in adjusting to life with ADHD.

KEY POINTS TO REMEMBER

- Severe and persistent mental illnesses are persistent or recurrent and likely to be highly disruptive or disabling.
- Stigma and chronicity present many challenges to coping with an SPMI and contribute to a variety of other social, physical health, and mental health problems such as increases in substance abuse, poverty and unemployment, comorbid physical illnesses and premature mortality, arrest, depression, and suicide risk.
- Assertive community treatment and peer-based services (e.g., clubhouses, certified peer specialists) are evidence-based practices shown to benefit persons with SPMIs.
- Impulse control disorders involve impulsive behaviors that are disruptive and serve to relieve psychological tension. These disorders include impulsive thefts, setting fires, sudden assaults or property destruction, hair pulling, and pathological gambling.
- Impulse control disorders are treated primarily through psychotherapy and sometimes with antidepressant or anticonvulsant medications.
- Sexual disorders include gender identity dysphoria/gender identity disorders and the paraphilias. A person with gender identity/dysphoria believes his or her biological gender is incorrect, and that he or she should be the opposite gender.
- People with gender dysphoria disorders may be subject to ridicule and harassment and may experience significant distress related to their gender dissatisfaction. One intervention is gender reassignment, which involves counseling, experiencing life for 1 or 2 years as the opposite gender, using hormones, and being surgically reassigned.
- Paraphilias are disorders in which sexual gratification is obtained in atypical and often socially unacceptable ways.
- Pedophilia includes having sexual fantasies or contact with children. This disorder stirs strong feelings in staff and society.
- The causes of paraphilias are not clearly established, but neurological dysfunction may be a contributing factor.
- Psychotherapy and medications that improve neurological dysfunction or reduce sexual drive can reduce offensive sexual behavior in pedophiles.
- ADHD is associated with childhood but may continue into or first be diagnosed in adulthood. In adults it is characterized by difficulty maintaining focus and organization, and can be disruptive to task completion, employment, relationships, and other key areas of functioning.
- ADHD often goes undiagnosed in adults, who may try to compensate for its symptoms. It is treated with a combination of counseling and stimulants (or sometimes other drugs).

APPLYING CRITICAL JUDGMENT

1. You are working with a patient who has recently been diagnosed with adult ADHD. He is very impulsive and frequently makes comments to you and others that are inappropriate and rude. You find yourself avoiding him and feeling angry toward him. Describe or role play what you would say in response to help reduce such comments.
2. The parents of a 37-year-old man with an SPMI ask you for help; they are becoming frightened of their son, who is increasingly hostile in response to their efforts to get him to take showers, accept medication, and get a job. They report that they have not often been able to talk with those treating their son because of regulations restricting the sharing of private health care information. Discuss or enact how you might address both the issues of confidentiality and the conflicts experienced when they attempt to change their son's behavior.
3. Debate the pros and cons for the proposition that sexual offenders who harm children should be held indefinitely in preventive detention for the greater good of society.
4. A patient with a severe mental disorder (SMI) is about to begin outpatient services at your community mental health center after years of institutionalization in state hospitals and prisons. Discuss the major issues he will likely face, and the services that ideally would be available in your community.

CHAPTER REVIEW QUESTIONS

Choose the appropriate answer(s).

1. Federal and state categorization of mental illnesses according to levels of severity has tremendous implications for which of the following? Select all that apply.
   1. Providing a standard, nationally based medical classification to facilitate diagnosis
   2. Setting mental health policy
   3. Facilitating access to appropriate care
   4. Providing employers with the basis to understand work capacities for mentally ill employees

2. NAMI has been developed to:
   1. regulate neurotransmission along critical pathways involved in schizophrenia.
   2. provide social and employment opportunities for patients with mental health disorders through partial hospitalization programs.
   3. provide a structured, phased approach for improved management of ADHD symptoms.
   4. offer support and education for patients and families of patients with mental health disorders.

CHAPTER REVIEW QUESTIONS—cont'd

3. Which of the following are accurate statements about impulse control disorders? Select all that apply.
   1. Causes of impulse control disorders are not clearly understood.
   2. Genetic factors are not considered to contribute to impulse control disorders.
   3. Anxiety may play an important role in impulse control disorders.
   4. Impulse control disorders are frequently associated with depression.
4. Most adults with severe mental illness have economic pressures and many become homeless. The nurse needs to understand that this is due to their:
   1. lack of overall responsibility.
   2. difficulty obtaining employment.

3. neediness and often aggressive behaviors.
4. delusions and hallucinations that interfere with functioning.

5. Which of the following nursing interventions would not be considered essential when working with an adult with ADHD?
   1. Establishing a regular exercise regimen to provide physical release and daily structure
   2. Guiding the patient to identify and use enhanced organizational skills
   3. Educating the patient's significant others about causes, treatments, and ways to cope with its symptoms
   4. Guiding the patient in understanding and practicing stimulation reduction strategies

REFERENCES

Almeida, O. P., Waterreus, A., Spry, N., et al. (2003). One year follow-up study of the association between chemical castration, sex hormones, beta-amyloid, memory and depression in men. *Psychoneuroendocrinology, 29*, 1071–1081.

Amador, X. (2007). *I am not sick, I don't need help!* (2nd ed.). Peconic, NY: Vida Press.

American Psychiatric Association (APA). (2000). *Diagnostic and statistical manual of mental disorders (DSM-IV-TR)* (4th ed., text rev). Washington, DC: Author.

Aquila, R., & Emanuel, M. (2003). *Managing the long-term outlook of schizophrenia.* Retrieved July 1, 2007, from www.medscape.com/viewprogram/2680_index.

Arehart-Treichel, J. (2006). Pedophilia often in headlines, but not in research labs. *Psychiatric News, 41*(10), 37–39.

Ascher-Savnum, H., Zhu, B., Faries, D., Salkever, D., et al. (2010). The cost of relapse and the predictors of relapse in the treatment of schizophrenia. *BMC Psychiatry, 10*(1), 2–9.

Becker, M., Young, M., Ochshorn, E., & Diamond, R. (2007). The relationship of antipsychotic medication class and adherence with treatment outcomes and costs for Florida Medicaid beneficiaries with schizophrenia. *Administration and Policy in Mental Health Services Research, 34*(3), 307–314.

Bell, A. (2011). A critical review of ADHD diagnostic criteria: what to address in the *DSM-V. Journal of Attention Disorders, 15*, 3–10.

Brassett-Harknett, A., & Butler, N. (2007). Attention-deficit/hyperactivity disorder: an overview of the etiology and a review of the literature relating to the correlates and lifecourse outcomes for men and women. *Clinical Psychology Review, 27*, 188–210.

Brown, M., Linehan, M., Comtois, K., Murray, A., et al. (2009). Shame as a prospective predictor of self-inflicted injury in borderline personality disorder: a multi-modal analysis. *Behaviour Research and Therapy, 47*(10), 815–822.

Bruce, T. O., Barwick, L. W., & Wright, H. H. (2005). Diagnosis and management of trichotillomania in children and adolescents. *Pediatric Drugs, 7*(6), 365–376.

Chamberlain, S. R., Menzies, L., Sahakian, B. J., et al. (2007). Lifting the veil on trichotillomania. *American Journal of Psychiatry, 164*(4), 568–574.

Coldwell, C. M., & Bender, W. S. (2007). The effectiveness of assertive community treatment for homeless populations with severe mental illness: a meta-analysis. *American Journal of Psychiatry, 164*(3), 393–399.

Cook, J. A., Leff, H. S., Blyler, C. R., et al. (2005). Results of a multisite randomized trial of supported employment interventions for individuals with severe mental illness. *Archives of General Psychiatry, 62*, 505–512.

Dannon, P. N., Lowengrub, K., Musin, E., et al. (2005). Sustained-release bupropion versus naltrexone in the treatment of pathological gambling: a preliminary blind-rater study. *Journal of Clinical Psychopharmacology, 25*(6), 593–596.

Diaz, J. (2010). The psychobiology of aggression and violence: bioethical implications. *International Social Science Journal, 61*(200-201), 233–245.

Diller, L. (2010). ADHD in the college student: is anyone else worried? *Journal of Attention Disorders, 14*(1), 3–6.

Dunn, J. A., Arakawa, R., Greist, J. H., et al. (2007). Assessing the onset of antidepressant-induced sexual dysfunction using interactive voice response technology. *Journal of Clinical Psychiatry, 68*(4), 525–532.

Fagan, P. J., Wise, T. N., Schmidt, C. W., et al. (2002). Pedophilia. *Journal of the American Medical Association, 288*, 2458–2465.

Frese, F., Knight, E., & Saks, E. (2009). Recovery from schizophrenia: with views of psychiatrists, psychologists, and others diagnosed with this disorder. *Schizophrenia Bulletin, 35*(2), 370–380.

Gavois, H., Paulsson, G., & Fridlund, B. (2006). Mental health professional support in families with a member suffering from severe mental illness: a grounded theory model. *Scandinavian Journal of Caring Sciences, 20*(1), 102–109.

Glied, S. (2007). *Better but not well: mental health policy in the United States since 1950.* Presented at the Eighth Annual All Ohio Institute on Community Psychiatry, Beachwood, OH, March 16, 2007.

Grant, J. E., Potenza, M. N., Hollander, E., et al. (2006). Multicenter investigation of the opioid antagonist nalmefene in the treatment of pathological gambling. *American Journal of Psychiatry, 163*, 303–312.

Grant, J. E., Levine, L., Kim, D., et al. (2005). Impulse control disorders in adult psychiatric inpatients. *American Journal of Psychiatry, 162*, 2184–2188.

Grant, J. E., & Kim, S. W. (2002). Effectiveness of pharmacotherapy for pathological gambling: a chart review. *Annals of Clinical Psychiatry, 14*(3), 155–161.

Greydanus, D. E., Pratt, H. D., & Patel, D. R. (2007). Attention deficit hyperactivity disorder across the lifespan: the child, adolescent and adult. *Disease-a-Month, 53*(2), 70–131.

Guay, D. (2008). Inappropriate sexual behaviors in cognitively impaired older individuals. *American Journal of Geriatric Pharmacotherapy, 6*(5), 269–288.

Hasson-Ohayon, I., Levy, I., Kravetz, S., Vollanski-Narkis, A., et al. (2011). Insight into mental illness, self stigma, and the family burden of parents of persons with a severe mental illness. *Comprehensive Psychiatry, 52*(2), 75–80.

Huygen, C. (2006). Understanding the needs of lesbian, gay, bisexual, and transgender people living with mental illness. *Medscape General Medicine, 8*(2), 29–31.

Ipser, J., & Stein, D. J. (2007). Systematic review of pharmacology of disruptive behavior disorders in children and adolescents. *Psychopharmacology, 191*, 127–140.

Koran, L. M., Aboujaoude, E. N., & Gamel, N. N. (2007). Escitalopram treatment of kleptomania: an open-label trial followed by double-blind discontinuation. *Journal of Clinical Psychiatry, 68*(3), 422–427.

Langevin, R. (2006). Sexual offenses and traumatic brain injury. *Brain & Cognition, 60*(2), 206–207.

Light, S. A., & Holroyd, S. (2005). The use of medroxyprogesterone acetate for the treatment of sexually inappropriate behaviour in patients with dementia. *Journal of Psychiatry Neuroscience, 31*(2), 132–134.

Lippke, R. (2008). No easy way out: dangerous offenders and preventive detention. *Law and Philosophy, 27*e4, 383–1414.

Maletzky, B., & Field, G. (2003). The biological treatment of dangerous sexual offenders: a review and preliminary report of the Oregon pilot depot-Provera program. *Aggression and Violent Behavior, 8*(14), 391–412.

Maniglio, R. (2009). Severe mental illness and criminal victimization: a systematic review. *Acta Psychiatrica Scandinavica, 119*(3), 180–191.

Marshall, W. L. (2007). Diagnostic issues, multiple paraphilias, and comorbid disorders in sexual offenders: their incidence and treatment. *Aggression and Violent Behavior, 12*(1), 16–35.

Miller, B.J., Paschall, C.B., & Svendsen, D.P. (2007). *Mortality and medical comorbidity among patients with serious mental illness.* Poster presented at the Eighth Annual All Ohio Institute on Community Psychiatry, Beachwood, OH, March 16, 2007.

Moeller, F. G., Barratt, E. S., Dougherty, D. M., et al. (2001). Psychiatric aspects of impulsivity. *American Journal of Psychiatry, 158*, 1783–1793.

Mulligan, K. (2005). Recovery model seeks more than symptom relief. *Psychiatric News, 40*(18), 6.

National Alliance on Mental Illness (NAMI). (2011). News study finds NAMI family education "significantly" improves coping with mental illness. Retrieved April 18, 2012, from http://www.namisf.org/index.php?/optioncom_contents&view=article&id=83&Itemid=138.

NANDA International (NANDA-I). (2012-2014). *NANDA nursing diagnoses—definitions and classification 2012-2014*. Philadelphia: Author.

National Alliance on Mental Illness (NAMI). (2008a). *Economic crisis and mental health*. Retrieved April 30, 2011 from www.nami.org/Content/NavigationMenu/Top_Story/Economic_Crisis_and_Mental_Health.htm.

National Alliance on Mental Illness (NAMI). (2008b). *Election 2010: the 60 to 140 percent bite; state-by-state data on disability income, housing costs and people with mental illness; are candidates addressing the facts?* Retrieved April 30, 2011, from www.nami.org/Content/ContentGroups/Press_Room1/20102/October17/Election_2010_The_60_to_140_Percent_Bite;_State-by-State_Data_on_Disability_Income,_Housing_Costs_an.htm.

National Alliance on Mental Illness (NAMI). (2012). *Dual diagnosis and integrated treatment of mental illness and substance abuse disorder*. Retrieved February 19, 2012, from http://www.nami.org/Template.cfm?Section=B.

National Alliance on Mental Illness (NAMI). (2004). *Statement of Margaret Stout on behalf of NAMI before the U.S. House of Representatives, Committee on Appropriations, Subcommittee on Labor-HHS-Education and Related Agencies*. Retrieved July 2, 2007, from www.nami.org/Content/ContentGroups/Policy/Issues_Spotlights/NAMI_Presses_Congress_for_FY_2005_Funds_for_Mental_Illness_Research_and_Services.htm.

National Alliance on Mental Illness (NAMI). (1998). *Schizophrenia Patient Outcomes Research Team (PORT): call to consumers and families to take charge of system that fails to provide effective treatment and supports*. Retrieved April 30, 2011, from http://www.nami.org/Content/ContentGroups/E-News/19982/September_19982/Schizophrenia_Patient_Outcomes_Research_Team_(PORT_.htm.

National Alliance on Mental Illness—California (NAMI—California). (2011). *Time for action: the hidden cost of untreated mental illness*. Retrieved April 30, 2011, from www.namicalifornia.org/document-detail.aspx?lang=ENG&idno=4893.

National Collaborating Centre for Mental Health. (2009). *Core interventions in the treatment and management of schizophrenia in primary and secondary care (update). National Clinical Practice Guidelines, number 82*. Retrieved April 30, 2011, from www.ncbi.nln.nih.gov/books/NBK11688/.

Novella, E. (2010). Mental health care in the aftermath of deinstitutionalization: a retrospective and prospective view. *Health Care Analysis, 18*(3), 222–238.

Palmer, B. (2010). *How do doctors treat pedophiles?* Retrieved August 25, 2011, from www.slate.com/ID/2248885/.

Peck, M. C., & Scheffler, R. M. (2002). An analysis of the definitions of mental illness used in state parity laws. *Psychiatric Services, 53*, 1089–1095.

Pellser, L., Frankena, K., Toorman, J., Savelkoul, H., et al. (2009). A randomised controlled trial into the effects of food on ADHD. *European Child and Adolescent Psychiatry, 18*(1), 12–19.

Penn, D., Meyer, P., Evans, E., Wirth, R., et al. (2009). A randomized controlled trial of group cognitive-behavioral therapy vs. enhanced supportive therapy for auditory hallucinations. *Schizophrenia Research, 109*(1-3), 52–59.

President's New Freedom Commission on Mental Health. (2003). *Report of the President's New Freedom Commission on Mental Health: achieving the promise: transforming mental health in America: executive summary*. Retrieved June 28, 2007, from www.mentalhealthcommission.gov/reports/FinalReport/FullReport.htm.

Quinn, C., & Browne, G. (2009). Sexuality of people living with mental illness: a collaborative challenge for mental health nurses. *International Journal of Mental Health Nursing, 18*(3), 195–203.

Rahman, Q., & Symeonides, D. (2008). Neurodevelopmental correlates of paraphilic sexual interests in men. *Archives of Sexual Behaviour, 37*(1), 166–172.

Research Council of Norway. (2011). *New insight into ADHD.* Retrieved August 8, 2011, from www.sciencedaily.com/releases/2011/03/110301091629.htm.

Rosenheck, R., Leslie, D., Keefe, R., et al. (2006). Barriers to employment for people with schizophrenia. *American Journal of Psychiatry, 163,* 411–417.

Sawle, G. A., & Kear-Colwell, J. (2001). Adult attachment style and pedophilia: a developmental perspective. *International Journal of Offender Therapy and Comparative Criminology, 45*(1), 32–50.

Scahill, L., Carroll, D., & Burke, K. (2004). *Methylphenidate: mechanism of action and clinical update.* Retrieved June 29, 2007 from http://findarticles.com/p/articles/mi_qa3892/is_200404/ai_n9356900.

Simon. (2011). *From the couch to the computer: a new take on therapy.* Retrieved August 24, 2011, from www.nln.nih.gov/medlineplus/news/full story_115323.html.

Spencer, T. J., Biederman, J., & Mick, E. (2007). Attention-deficit/hyperactivity disorder: diagnosis, lifespan, comorbidities, and neurobiology. *Journal of Pediatric Psychology, 32*(6), 631–642.

Swanson, J. (2010). What would Mary Douglas do? A commentary on Kahan et al., cultural cognition and public policy: the case of outpatient commitment. *Law and Human Behavior, 34*(3), 176–185.

Thornton, D. (2006). Age and sexual recidivism: a variable connection. *Sexual Abuse: Journal of Research and Treatment, 18*(2), 123–135.

Urbanoski, K., Cairney, J., Adlaf, E., & Rush, B. (2007). Substance abuse and quality of life among severely mentally ill consumers: a longitudinal modeling analysis. *Social Psychiatry and Psychiatric Epidemiology, 42*(10), 810–818.

Wylie, K. (2004). Gender related disorders. *BMJ, 329,* 615–617.

e‍volve WEBSITE

http://evolve.elsevier.com/Varcarolis/essentials

KEY TERMS AND CONCEPTS

advance directives, p. 540

age discrimination, p. 528

ageism, p. 528

chemical restraints, p. 539

directive to physician, p. 541

durable power of attorney for
    health care, p. 541

elderspeak, p. 531

living will, p. 540

Omnibus Budget Reconciliation
    Act (OBRA), p. 540

Patient Self-Determination Act
    (PSDA), p. 540

physical restraints, p. 539

SELECTED CONCEPT: Ageism

Ageism is any stereotyping, prejudice, or discrimination against the older adult or in fact any age group. Ageism can be systemic, organizational, and interpersonal discrimination.

Systemic ageism is "the totality of ways in which societies foster discrimination" against older adults. *Organizational* ageism is "discriminatory policies or practices carried out by state or nonstate institutions" that are detrimental to older adults. *Interpersonal* ageism refers to "directly perceive discriminatory interactions between individuals."

(Palmore, et al., 2005, p. 333; Krieger, 1999, p. 301)

OBJECTIVES

1. Summarize the facts and myths about aging.
2. Describe the destructive and negative effects that "ageism" and "elderspeak" can have on older adults.
3. Analyze the different ways you can challenge "ageism" to change attitudes and increase the awareness of fellow students and others who care for older adults.
4. Describe the positive effects of implementing teamwork and collaboration in the various group interventions commonly used with older adults.
5. Describe the importance of a comprehensive geriatric assessment including both recommended guidelines for assessing an older adult and strategies for using the results to promote safety.

OBJECTIVES—cont'd

6. How would you apply communication strategies during your interview with any older adult?

7. Demonstrate the differences between the provision of patient-centered care for an older adult compared with that for a younger adult if the patient needs assessment and intervention for the diagnosis of depression and suicidal ideation.

8. Evaluate how you could promote safety by identifying the risk factors for elder suicide and the nursing role you would take in its prevention.

9. Demonstrate your knowledge of incorporating evidence-based care with an understanding of the physiological effects of alcohol use on an older individual compared with those on a younger adult.

10. Demonstrate your understanding of how to apply quality improvement methods in the use of physical and/or chemical restraints.

11. Discuss institutional requirements related to the Patient Self-Determination Act of 1990.

12. Use informatics to determine laws and regulations in your state for the rights of older adults who are also lesbian, gay, bisexual, or transgender (LGBT). Compare your results with the guidelines for the state of New York.

13. Contrast and compare living wills, directives to physicians, and durable powers of attorney as used in health care settings.

One of the most vulnerable populations in the United States is that of the older adult, especially as it relates to medical and mental health care access. Since this population is growing fairly rapidly, the medical and mental health access of this population is an issue that will have to be addressed by all aspects of society (e.g., socioeconomic condition, legal system, and most profoundly, our health care system). The following will address the population of the older adult as well as some of the predominant mental health concerns among this age group.

Mental Health: A Report of the Surgeon General—Executive Summary identified important considerations for promoting the mental health of the older adult (U.S. Department of Health and Human Services [USDHHS], 1999, p. 381). Three of those considerations follow:

1. Older adults can continue to learn and contribute to society in spite of physiological changes attributable to aging and increasing health problems.

2. Continued intellectual, social, and physical activity throughout the lifecycle are important for the maintenance of mental health in late life.

3. Normal aging is not characterized by mental or cognitive disorders.

However, the increasing proportion of older adults within the population has altered the socioeconomic condition in America and at the same time is transforming the practice of health care. By the year 2030, 20% of the U.S. population will consist of individuals older than 65 years of age. Among older adults, the fastest-growing subgroups are minorities, the poor, and those ages 85 years and older (Administration on Aging [AOA], 2009; President's New Freedom Commission on Mental Health, 2003).

Psychologists have divided older adults into the following age categories (Touhy & Jett, 2010):

- Young old: 65 to 74 years of age
- Middle old: 75 to 84 years of age
- Old old: 85 to 94 years of age
- Elite old: 94 years or older

On average, an older adult has three or four chronic illnesses and a nearly 20% annual risk of hospitalization (Narang & Sikka, 2006). After age 85, there is a one in three chance of developing dementia, immobility, incontinence, or another age-related disability.

Women generally outlive men an average of 7 years. Because husbands more often predecease (die before) their spouses, they benefit from the support of their wives to help with health-related issues. On the other hand, many older women lack this type of support. Women's greater longevity has significant ramifications for society at large and for the health care system in particular. Older women are more likely to be widowed, to live alone, or to be institutionalized.

There are noticeable differences between individuals in their sixties and people in their eighties. Whereas those in the younger group are relatively healthy, those in the older group are much more vulnerable, frail, and at risk for visual problems, cognitive impairment, and falls. Persons in the older age-group also have more limited economic resources and community supports and are more affected by the chronic diseases and disorders of aging (Touhy & Jett, 2010). Social Security constituted 90% or more of the income received by 35% of all Social Security beneficiaries (21% of married couples and 44% of nonmarried beneficiaries) and about 9.7% of elderly persons are living below the poverty level (AOA, 2010).

A NOTE ON PHARMACOLOGY AND THE AGING ADULT

Prescribing pharmacological agents for the elder adult is a tricky business. One major factor is that the pharmacokinetics (drug absorption, distribution, metabolism, and excretion) of any drug change as we age. Approximately 50% of accidental drug-related deaths occur in the older population (Preston et al., 2010). Other factors include noncompliance among the older adult because of complicated directions, hearing and visual impairment, cognitive and memory deficits, child-resistant packaging, and inability to afford medication (Preston et al., 2010).

A study published in the *Journal of the American Geriatrics Society* (June 24, 2011) found that anticholinergic activity, which is a side effect of many commonly used drugs (e.g., antihistamines, antidepressants), has been linked with reduced brain function and early death in elder adults (Kelland, 2011; Fox et al., 2011). Other drugs with anticholinergic effects include nifedipine, codeine, chlorpromazine, and certain tranquilizers, as well as others (Kelland, 2011). Anticholinergic properties are also found in hypertensive drugs and drugs taken for congestive heart failure. The nurse needs to review all the prescription and over-the-counter medications the patient is taking and be alert to the anticholinergic side effects. The physician needs to be notified if the patient is taking one or two medications that have this potential, since anticholinergic effects are cumulative, and physicians should avoid prescribing with multiple anticholinergic effects.

AGEISM

Ageism refers to deeply rooted negative attitudes or bias toward older people because of their age. It is a system of destructive, erroneous beliefs that stigmatize the elderly. In essence, ageism represents a dislike by the young of the old, reflecting the disparaging effects of society's attitudes toward older adults. Age prejudice is based on the notion that aging makes people increasingly unattractive, unintelligent, asexual, unemployable, and senile. Age discrimination, on the other hand, is the set of actions and/or outcomes that are perpetrated on the older adult that reflect this bias (treated on an unequal basis).

Ageism is not limited to the way the young may look at the old. It is also seen in the views of older people, who tend to be critical about themselves and their peers. Indeed, the attitudes of older adults toward their peers, particularly those with mental disabilities, are often more negative than the views held by the young (although this is not always the case). The threat of social contagion by association with the frail and infirm may simply be too strong to bear. Age proximity raises feelings of vulnerability. This may explain why older adults often do not like to be referred to as "old." By seeing themselves as "young" rather than "old," they adjust better to their advancing years.

Ageism differs from other forms of discrimination in that it cuts across gender, race, religion, sexual orientation, and national origin. In our culture, old age does not award a desirable status or membership in a prestigious club; rather, it is a social category with negative connotations. Today, a new form of ageism puts the older adult in a no-win situation: those who are wealthy are envied for their economic progress, those who are middle-class are blamed for making Social Security too costly, and those who are poor are resented for being tax burdens.

The results of ageism can be observed throughout every level of society. Even health care providers are not immune to its effects. Negative values can surface in a myriad of ways in the health care system. Financial and political support for programs for older adults is difficult to obtain; their needs are addressed only after those of younger, albeit smaller, population groups.

Ageism Among Health Care Workers

Health care personnel do not always share medical information, recommendations, and opportunities with the older adult. Studies show that older adults receive less information and sometimes less care than those who are younger. Ageism is also reflected in public policy, which leads to discrimination against older adults (Touhy & Jett, 2010).

Health care workers who deal on a daily basis with the confused, ill, and frail older adult may tend to develop a somewhat negative and biased view of them. The negative attitudes of most health care workers are often a reflection of the views of society, which again are most often characterized by negativism and stereotyping. The rendering of medical care to older adults has been burdened with pessimism, defeatism, and professional aversion. Unfortunately, such thinking can be found among professionals as well as among ancillary personnel working in nursing homes and other institutional settings.

Negative views of the older adult are frequently held by nurses. Studies have found that recruits to nursing hold ageist views, which has significant implications for practice, education, and research. Positive attitudes toward older adults and their care need to be instilled during basic nursing education. If the goal of nursing programs is to prepare students to practice in the future, then preparing students to care for older adults in a wide variety of settings is mandatory, because that *is* the future. The American Association of Colleges of Nursing (AACN) calls for nursing programs to "implement patient and family care around resolution of end-of-life and palliative care issues, such as symptom management, supportive rituals, and respect for patient and family preferences" (AACN, 2008). AACN states that this standard should be adopted in all nursing education programs (diploma, associate degree, baccalaureate programs) and beyond.

With the advance of the bulging baby boomer population that started turning 65 in 2011, there is even a greater need for increased growth of available and knowledgeable nurses and physicians within the health care system with solid background in the treatment and needs of the older adult. Even the present health care system is not prepared to care adequately for elderly persons with chronic health care needs and/or the mental health needs of people already in the system (Buckwalter et al., 2011). For over a decade there has been recognition that there is a great need within the health care system for educational programs for healthcare providers regarding older adults. Some of the suggestions that these educational programs must include the following (AACN, 2008; Lueckenotte, 2000):

- Information about the aging process
- Discussion of attitudes relating to the care of the older adult
- Sensitization of participants to their patients' needs
- Use of valid and reliable assessment tools to guide nursing practice for older adults

---

BOX 28-1 FACTS AND MYTHS ABOUT AGING

Facts

- The senses of vision, hearing, touch, taste, and smell decline with age.
- Muscular strength decreases with age. Muscle fibers atrophy and decrease in number.
- Regular sexual expressions are important to maintain sexual capacity and effective sexual performance.
- At least 50% of restorative sleep is lost as a result of the aging process.
- Older adults are major consumers of prescription drugs because of the high incidence of chronic diseases in this population.
- Older adults have a high incidence of depression.
- Many individuals experience difficulty when they retire.
- Older adults are prone to become victims of crime.
- Older widows appear to adjust better than younger ones.

Myths

- Most adults past the age of 65 years are demented.
- Sexual interest declines with age.
- Older adults are not able to learn new tasks.
- As individuals age, they become more rigid in their thinking and resistant to change.
- Older adults are financially secure and no longer impoverished.
- Most older adults are infirmed and require help with daily activities.
- Most older adults are socially isolated and lonely.
- All older adults are significantly hard of hearing and should be spoken to in a loud voice.

- Strategies in use of online guidelines to prevent and/or identify and manage geriatric syndromes
- Exploration of the dynamics of nurse-patient and staff-patient interactions
  - Grief loss and bereavement
  - Ethical and legal issues
  - Communication

Box 28-1 lists some facts and myths about aging. Simpkins (2008, p. 28), a student nurse at the time, reviewed articles on ageism and concluded:

"...nursing practice, which should be refocused to emphasize the fundamentals of nursing theory in the clinical setting. Healthcare ethics, team coordination, patient advocacy, and patient and family education would consciously shift to the forefront of the nursing process while caring for the elderly. Such evidence-based practice would ensure that patient needs are met to a greater degree, as the literature suggests that an increased awareness of ageism would result in greater patient satisfaction and improved outcomes."

ASSESSMENT AND COMMUNICATION STRATEGIES

Nurses who work with the older adult benefit from specific knowledge about normal aging, drug interactions, and chronic disease. **Geropsychiatric nurses** work with older adult patients who have mental health problems; these nurses are employed in a variety of settings, including nursing homes, assisted living facilities, community centers, inpatient units, prisons, and homeless shelters, to name a few. Geropsychiatric nurses have special skills in interviewing and assessing older adults as well as specific knowledge of effective treatment modalities, the normal aging process, and sociocultural influences on older adults and their families.

The National Institutes of Health recommends a comprehensive geriatric assessment to evaluate and manage the care and progress of all older adult patients. A comprehensive geriatric assessment includes examination of mental status, including a focus on physical health; assessment of functional, economic, and social status; and determination of environmental factors that might impinge on the older adult patient's well-being, as well as a close look at all medications the elder adult may be taking. Figure 28-1 provides an example of a comprehensive geriatric assessment. (Refer to the inside back cover for an example of a mental status exam.)

An examination and interview of an older adult conducted in unfamiliar surroundings will most likely produce anxiety. Unlike younger patients, who may be comfortable discussing personal issues such as family conflicts, feelings of sadness, sexual practices, finances, and bodily functions, older adults are part of a generation that viewed these topics as private, and as a result they may be uncomfortable discussing these personal matters. Although the more recent baby boom generation of older adults may come from a more open and so-called "sophisticated" age, it is important to respect these feelings in everyone while reviewing essential history. Older adults will guide you as to their level of comfort with personal information. The following are basic guidelines:

- Conduct the interview in a private area.
- Introduce yourself and ask the patient what he or she would like to be called. Often a younger person will address the elder by their first name, which can be perceived as demeaning and belittling to an older adult.
- Establish rapport and put the patient at ease by sitting or standing at the same level.
- Ensure that lighting is adequate and noise level is low in recognition of the fact that hearing and vision may be impaired in the older adult patient.
- Use touch to convey warmth while at the same time respecting the older adult's comfort level with personal touch.

COMPREHENSIVE GERIATRIC ASSESSMENT					

Name: Date of birth: Gender:

Physical Health

Chronic disorder

Vision	Adequate	Inadequate	Eyeglasses: Y N		Needs evaluation
Hearing	Adequate	Inadequate	Hearing aids: Y N		
Mobility	Ambulatory: Y N		Assistive device:		
	Falls: Y N				Needs evaluation
Nutrition	Albumin:	TLC:	HCT:		
	Weight:	Weight loss or gain: Y N			Needs evaluation
Incontinence	Y N	Treatment: Y N			Needs evaluation
Medications	Total number:	Reviewed & revised: Y N			
	Adverse effects/allergy:				
Screening	Cholesterol:	TSH:	B_{12}:		Folate:
	Colonoscopy: Date:		N/A		
	Mammogram: Date:		N/A		
	Osteoporosis: Date:		N/A		
	Pap smear: Date:		N/A		
	PSA: Date:		N/A		
Immunization	Influenza: Date:				
	Pneumonia: Date:				
	Tetanus: Date:		Booster:		
Counseling	Diet	Exercise	Calcium	Vitamin D	
	Smoking	Alcohol	Driving	Injury prevention	

Mental Health

Dementia	Y N	MMSE score:	Date:	Cause (if known):	
Depression	Y N	GDS score:	Date:	Treatment: Y N	

Functional Status

ADL	Bathing: I D	Dressing: I D	Toileting: I D
	Transferring: I D	Feeding: I D	Continence: Y N

FIGURE 28-1 Comprehensive geriatric assessment. *ADL,* Activities of daily living; B_{12}, vitamin B_{12}; *D,* dependent; *GDS,* Geriatric Depression Scale; *HCT,* hematocrit; *I,* independent; *MMSE,* Mini-Mental State Examination; *N,* no; *PSA,* prostate-specific antigen; *TLC,* total lymphocyte count; *TSH,* thyroid-stimulating hormone; *Y,* yes.

TABLE 28-1   COMPARISON OF DELIRIUM, DEMENTIA, AND DEPRESSION

	DELIRIUM	DEMENTIA	DEPRESSION
Onset	Sudden, over hours to days	Slowly, over months	May have been gradual with exacerbation during crisis or stress
Cause or contributing factors	Hypoglycemia, fever, dehydration, hypotension; infection, other conditions that disrupt body's homeostasis; adverse drug reaction; head injury; change in environment (e.g., hospitalization); pain; emotional stress	Alzheimer's disease, vascular disease, human immuno-deficiency virus infection, neurological disease, chronic alcoholism, head trauma	Life-long history, losses, loneliness, crises, declining health, medical conditions
Cognition	Impaired memory, judgment, calculations, attention span; can fluctuate throughout the day	Impaired memory, judgment, calculations, attention span, abstract thinking; agnosia	Difficulty concentrating, forgetfulness, inattention
Level of consciousness	Altered	Not altered	Not altered
Activity level	Can be increased or reduced; restlessness, behaviors may worsen in evening (sundowning); sleep-wake cycle may be reversed	Not altered; behaviors may worsen in evening (sundowning)	Usually decreased; lethargy, fatigue, lack of motivation; may sleep poorly and awaken in early morning
Emotional state	Rapid swings; can be fearful, anxious, suspicious, aggressive, have hallucinations and delusions	Flat; delusions	Extreme sadness, apathy, irritability, anxiety, para-noid ideation

- Summarize the interaction and invite feedback from the patient.
- Assess the cognitive, behavioral, and emotional status of the older adult—this is very important in managing the nursing care of the patient and is particularly vital for detecting delirium, dementia, and depression (Table 28-1) because their prevalence increases with age. In addition to depression, suicide and alcohol/substance abuse are major health problems among older adults.
- Evaluate any indications of abuse (physical, sexual, neglect, financial) in a discreet manner (see Chapter 21).

People talk to older adults differently. Anyone who has visited a nursing home, hospital unit with older adult patients, or even a grocery store can attest to a pernicious and condescending method of communicating with the older adult. Perhaps the worst offenders are health care workers when it comes to showing disrespect to the elderly (Leland, 2008). **Elderspeak** refers to talking to patients as if they were small children. Examples include using terms of endearment (e.g., honey, sweetie, dear), speaking in overly simple sentences and with an increased volume and pitch, and using collective pronouns (e.g., do "we" want a bath?) (Leland, 2008). This is perhaps meant to convey caring; it implies the older adult is incompetent or inferior. Studies are finding that these kinds of insults to older adults can increase their negative feelings about old age and this can have health consequences. A study conducted in 2002 by Dr. Levy and fellow researchers surveyed more than 660 people older than age 50, and found that those older adults who had a more

positive outlook on becoming older lived 7.7 years longer than elder adults with negative perceptions on aging (Leland, 2008).

Another related communication problem is when health care workers dismiss the presence of older adults in the room and speak about them rather than to them. Nursing students should consciously avoid using elderspeak. Address the older adult when asking a question, and when necessary, ask the family member or other health care worker(s) if they have anything to add. Box 28-2 provides helpful communication and interview techniques.

PSYCHIATRIC DISORDERS IN OLDER ADULTS

Not only are older adults with mental disorders less likely to be accurately diagnosed, they are also more likely to receive inappropriate or inadequate treatment compared with younger adults (Bartels & Drake, 2005; McEnany, 2011). It is important to keep in mind the presentations of mental disorders vary substantially with age. This is especially true for individuals with depression and anxiety. In this age of emerging evidence-based practice (EBP), there remains a dearth of rigorous, well-powered, randomized clinical trials to support EBP in geropsychiatric nursing (Buckwalter et al., 2011). Therefore solid evidence-based literature and studies dealing with geriatric anxiety disorder, bipolar disorders, geriatric schizophrenia, or geriatric alcohol use disorders are in short supply. Primary mental health issues affecting older adults discussed here are

---

BOX 28-2	COMMUNICATION GUIDELINES FOR INTERVIEWING THE OLDER ADULT

1. Gather preliminary data before the session and keep questionnaires relatively short.
2. Ask about often-overlooked problems, such as difficulty sleeping, incontinence, falling, depression, dizziness, or loss of energy.
3. Pace the interview to allow the patient to formulate answers; resist the tendency to interrupt prematurely.
4. Use yes-or-no or simple choice questions if the older patient has trouble coping with open-ended questions.
5. Begin with general questions such as, "How can I help you most at this visit?" or "What's been happening?"
6. Be alert for information on the patient's relationships with others, thoughts about families or coworkers, typical responses to stress, and attitudes toward aging, illness, occupation, and death.
7. Assess mental status for deficits in recent or remote memory, and determine if confusion exists.
8. Note all medications the patient is taking and assess for side effects, efficacy, and possible drug interactions.
9. Determine how fast the condition of the patient has been changing to assess the extent of the patient's concerns.
10. Include the family or significant other in the interview process for added input, clarification, support, and reinforcement.

From National Institute on Aging. (2011). *Working with your older patient: a clinician's handbook.* Bethesda, MD: Author.

depression, suicide, and alcohol and drug use. Elder abuse is also a **great** national concern. Elder abuse and *Caregiver Role Strain* are discussed in more detail in Chapter 21. Cognitive symptoms and interventions affecting the elderly adult are discussed in Chapter 18.

DEPRESSION

Depression is the most common, the most debilitating, and also the most treatable psychiatric disorder in the older adult (Byrd & Vito, 2011). Late-life depression (LLD) takes a huge toll in pain, suffering, poor quality of life, and spiritual anguish. Depression and aging can be very dangerous when the older person is also experiencing a chronic illness, loneliness, or loss of independence, and depression is the biggest risk factor for suicide (Liiades, 2010).

Health care providers frequently misinterpret clinical depression in older adults as a normal part of aging, especially if the older adult is experiencing neurological symptoms (dementia) or other physical illnesses (Byrd & Vito, 2011).

Unlike dementia, depression is treatable with medication and other interventions. In the older adult, symptoms of memory loss and other intellectual impairments or asocial or agitated behavior are generally associated with dementia but may actually be caused by depression. At times, dementia may be masked by the more frank symptoms of delirium. A careful assessment is needed to distinguish among delirium, dementia, and depression because presenting symptoms can be similar, or two or more may coincide. (See Table 28-1 for a comparison of dementia and depression.) Chapter 18 gives thorough assessment guidelines and interventions for a patient experiencing delirium or dementia.

In making an assessment, the nurse needs to be familiar with the symptoms of later-life depression. Besides the core symptoms we recognize regarding depression (see Chapter 15), sometimes depression in the elderly is expressed as physical symptoms or negative behaviors such as the following:

- Forgetfulness
- Agitation and combativeness
- Constant complaining
- Irritability
- Chronic aches and pains that do not respond to treatment
- Fatigue
- Rumination
- Easily angered
- Paranoia and suspiciousness
- Apprehension and anxiety without any cause
- Low self-esteem (feelings of insignificance or pessimism)

Often these symptoms are incorrectly assessed as a normal part of aging, which they are not. A careful evaluation of the cause of the depression is necessary. A variety of biological and psychosocial risk factors have been identified (e.g., medical illness, functional disability, social isolation, accumulation of life stressors, losses, and genetic vulnerabilities). Depression can be caused by a number of drugs (e.g., reserpine and other *Rauwolfia* derivatives, steroids, phenothiazines), by metabolic and endocrine disorders (e.g., hepatitis and adrenal and thyroid insufficiency), and by acute medical events such as cerebrovascular accident or myocardial infarction. Depression also can augment suicide potential. Thorough assessment for any medical or drug-induced side effects should be performed, as well as psychosocial and medical assessment. (See Figure 28-2 for the Geriatric Depression Scale.)

Late-life depression increases the risk for medical comorbidities, suicide, disability, and family caregiving burden. Undiagnosed late-life depression also increases the risk for unhealthy behaviors (alcohol/drug abuse, gambling) as well as the progression of other chronic illnesses (Andreescu & Reynolds, 2011; Byrd & Vito, 2011).

Late-life depression responds well to (1) *psychosocial treatments* (e.g., interventions that relieve loneliness such as group aerobic exercise sessions), (2) *talk therapies* (e.g., psychotherapy or cognitive behavioral therapy may be effective without the use of medications), and (3) *establishment of social support systems* (e.g., group meals, scheduled visitors, volunteer work)

Geriatric Depression Scale (Short Form)

		Yes	No
1.	Are you basically satisfied with your life?	○	○
2.	Have you dropped many of your activities and interests?	○	○
3.	Do you feel that your life is empty?	○	○
4.	Do you often get bored?	○	○
5.	Are you in good spirits most of the time?	○	○
6.	Are you afraid that something bad is going to happen to you?	○	○
7.	Do you feel happy most of the time?	○	○
8.	Do you often feel helpless?	○	○
9.	Do you prefer to stay at home, rather than going out and doing new things?	○	○
10.	Do you feel you have more problems with memory than most?	○	○
11.	Do you think it is wonderful to be alive now?	○	○
12.	Do you feel pretty worthless the way you are now?	○	○
13.	Do you feel full of energy?	○	○
14.	Do you feel that your situation is hopeless?	○	○
15.	Do you think that most people are better off than you are?	○	○

FIGURE 28-2 Geriatric Depression Scale (Short Form). (From Sheikh, J.I., & Yesavage, J.A. (1986). Geriatric Depression Scale (GDS): recent evidence and development of a shorter version. In T.L. Brink (Ed.), *Clinical gerontology: a guide to assessment and intervention* (pp. 165-173). New York: Haworth Press.)

(Liiades, 2010). These psychosocial and cognitive interventions can be critical in treating late-life depression since fewer than 50% of older adults on antidepressants achieve remission (Alexopoulos & Knosses, 2011).

In addition to the aforementioned therapies, antidepressants and electroconvulsive therapy (ECT) may be more appropriate for more severe depressions, especially for those persons who have suffered a life-long battle with this disorder. Elderly persons with severe depression respond similarly to middle-aged adults with depression in terms of both psychopharmacology and ECT; however, the relapse rates are higher in older adults (Andreescu & Reynolds, 2011). ECT is usually used only as a last resort in treatment-resistant elderly adults, but works well in depression with psychotic features.

Antidepressant Therapy

In choosing a drug to treat depression in the older adult, primary emphasis is placed on avoidance of possible side effects rather than on efficacy. When antidepressant therapy is initiated, low dosages (usually half the routine recommended dosage) are suggested, and the dosage is then slowly and gradually increased if needed, remembering the adage, "Start low, go slow." If the individual is at risk for suicide, then caregivers must be aware that as the depression begins to lift, there is a greater chance that the individual will complete the suicide.

The choice of which class of antidepressants to use for older adults is a complex decision. Selective serotonin reuptake inhibitors (SSRIs) have traditionally been the first-line antidepressants for older adults because of their more benign side effects and their lack of toxicity when taken in overdose. However, that view is changing. The SSRIs may also cause some problems, especially for older adults who are at greater risk for drug interactions. SSRIs need to be used with caution in older adults because it appears that SSRIs may double the risk of bone fractures and place older adults at risk for hip fractures (Liiades, 2010) and according to som reports the risk of morbidity is higher with the SSRIs than with tricyclic antidepressants. A recent study contends that SSRIs and drugs in a group

TABLE 28-2 USEFUL GROUP THERAPY MODALITIES FOR OLDER ADULT PATIENTS

REMOTIVATION THERAPY	REMINISCENCE THERAPY (LIFE REVIEW)	PSYCHOTHERAPY
Purpose of Group		
Resocialize regressed and apathetic patients	Share memories of the past	Alleviate psychiatric symptoms
Reawaken interest in the environment	Increase self-esteem	Increase ability to interact with others in a group
	Increase socialization	Increase self-esteem
	Increase awareness of the uniqueness of each participant	Increase ability to make decisions and function more independently
Format		
Groups are made up of 10 to 15 people	Groups are made up of 6 to 8 people	Group size is 6 to 12 members
Meetings are held once or twice a week	Meetings are held once or twice weekly for 1 hour	Group members should share similar:
Meetings are highly structured in a classroom-like setting	Topics include holidays, major life events, birthdays, travel, and food	• Problems
		• Mental status
Group uses props		• Needs
Each session discusses a particular topic		• Sexual integration
		Group meets at regularly scheduled times (certain number of times a week, specific duration of session) and place
Desired Outcomes		
Increase participants' sense of reality	Alleviate depression in institutionalized older adult	Decrease sense of isolation
Offer practice of health roles	Through the process of reorganization and reintegration, provide avenue by members	Facilitate development of new roles and re-establish former roles
Realize more objective self-image than older adult can		Provide information for other group
	Achieve a new sense of identity	Provide group support for effecting changes and increasing self-esteem
	Achieve a positive self-concept	

From Matteson, M.A., & McConnell, E.S. (Eds.). (1988). *Gerontologic nursing: concepts and practice* (p. 80). Philadelphia: Saunders.

of "other" antidepressants resulted in several other adverse outcomes when compared with tricyclic antidepressants (Coupland and colleagues, 2011). The risk is twofold greater from the use of SSRIs, and clinical fractures can occur from falls as well as from any stress put on the bones by even minor activity (e.g., walking or standing). Therefore a "low dose of a tricyclic (TCA) antidepressant may be more suitable in frail elderly patients at increased risk of falls and fractures" (Coupland & Hochhalter, 2011). It is also recommended that careful monitoring is needed during the first month of taking an antidepressant and after discontinuing the medication, since these are times when the risks of serious side effects are the highest (Coupland & Hochhalter, 2011).

If an SSRI is to be used, sertraline (Zoloft) is often a good choice among the SSRIs because age does not appear to affect the pharmacokinetics. Other SSRIs can cause central nervous system stimulation, resulting in increased night awakenings, insomnia, or increased plasma levels of the drug attributable to impairment of metabolism, as well as the adverse reactions mentioned previously. Low-dose TCAs may be considered, but they have been predominantly avoided in the past because of the anticholinergic effects, which remained a serious consideration. Medications are almost always used in conjunction with other types of therapy.

Psychotherapy

Clinicians may provide individual or group psychotherapy to the depressed patient. As mentioned, groups can diminish social isolation and loneliness and help the members understand that they are not alone in their situation. Group members can learn creative ways to raise their mood and increase quality of life. A number of different kinds of groups are useful for older adults (Table 28-2).

Cognitive behavioral therapy (CBT), problem-solving therapy (PST), interpersonal therapy (IPT), and supportive therapy are often used as an adjunct therapy with psychopharmacology, especially if depression in the individual has a long-term history.

SUICIDE

A study by the Centers for Disease Control and Prevention (CDC) found that two elderly age-groups (65 to 74 years and 75 years and older) experienced the most significant decline from 1928 to 2007 (CDC, 2011). The suicide rate for white males 65 and older is five times higher than that of the general population (Sadock & Sadock, 2010). Unfortunately, the baby boomer cohort (those born between 1946 and 1964) have a higher rate of suicide at any given age than any other generational cohorts. This large group with the highest rate of suicide has now entered the 65 and older age-group (a time of risk for suicide), increasing the need for evaluation and treatment of depression and suicide risk. This will be an even greater challenge for those working with older adults.

The biggest risk for suicide in the elderly person is depression. Early identification of and treatment for depression, therefore, are key measures for suicide prevention. Piechniczek-Buczek (2006) states that efforts need to be made, especially in the emergency department (ED) and primary care setting, to identify risk factors, clues, and signs of imminent threats of late-life suicide. This is feasible since perhaps as many as 70% of elderly individuals who committed suicide visited their physicians within a week to a month of their deaths (Piechniczek-Buczek, 2006).

Even though the suicide rate among older adults is high, suicides in this group are probably underreported. Suicide is often not listed on the death certificate, even if it is suspected. The numbers also do not reflect those who passively or indirectly commit suicide by abusing alcohol, starving themselves, overdosing or mixing medications, stopping life-sustaining drugs, or simply losing the will to live.

Other factors that can lead to suicide are feelings of hopelessness, uselessness, and despair. For older adults, suicide may be seen as a final gesture of control at a stage when independence is at risk or activities are limited. Severe medical illness, functional disability, alcohol abuse, history of suicide attempts, comorbid anxiety, and psychotic depression are added risk factors for suicide. For this reason, the suicide attempts of the older adult are more likely to succeed. Unlike younger people, whose suicidal gestures may be intended to draw attention to their problems, those of older adults do not signify a call for help but rather a desire to die. Financial need is another risk factor contributing to the high suicide rate. Federal reductions in programs such as Medicare, Medicaid, and food stamps, along with state-ordered cuts in medical care, cause many older Americans to worry about their future. An inverse relationship between economic conditions and suicide rate has been identified.

Assessment of Suicide Risk

The assessment of older patients must include attention to the high-risk factors that potentially contribute to suicide, such as widowhood, acute illnesses and intractable pain, status change, chronic illness, family history of suicide, chronic sleep problems, alcoholism, depression, and other losses (see Chapter 23). Losses may be personal (death of a family member or close friend), economic (loss of earnings or job), or social (loss of prestige or position). Multiple losses accompany the aging process, increasing stress at a time when the older adult may be the most vulnerable and least able to cope with stress,

thus precipitating a depressive state. Nevertheless, many older adults are able to function despite their losses. Those who concede defeat may do so because of hopelessness.

The nurse must remain vigilant for possible suicidal tendencies in patients later in life. In assessing suicide risk, the health care provider must examine previous suicidal behavior, seriousness of the intent, presence of active plans, availability of the means to commit the act, lethality of the method chosen, and the specific details of the plan. Compared to those in younger age-groups, older adults are less likely to communicate their suicidal thoughts and plans. Nurses play a vital role in the prevention of older adult suicide because of their presence in every care setting. Attention must be focused on building awareness and use of community resources in the high-risk population. Screening for depression and suicidal thinking in the older adult should be standard and can save lives.

The nurse is professionally obligated to respond and intervene with the older adult patient in crisis, especially when the patient believes that the willful destruction of life is the only option available. It is therefore very important to maintain a sensitive, compassionate, and therapeutic approach with the patient. Communication with the older adult patient must be skillful, clear, direct, and respectful of the individual's rights. For some people, these interventions may restore a sense of self and purpose so that life may be preserved (Touhy & Jett, 2010). Questions such as the following may be asked in suicide assessment:

- What kinds of thoughts do you have about a person's right to take his or her own life?
- What advantage does ending one's life offer?
- What is the most important thing you have to live for?
- Have you thought of taking your life?

Refer to Chapter 23 for the Modified SAD PERSONS Scale. Although this scale is derived from an older version, it remains an appropriate suicide assessment tool for older as well as younger adults.

Right to Die

One concern of nursing is the question of whether an older adult has the right to end his or her life by way of physician-assisted suicide (PAS) or by taking his or her own life (refer to Chapter 23). Suicide in any manner always raises spiritual and moral issues. However, there are some in society who believe that older adults with terminal illnesses and/or who suffer intractable pain should be able to control their own deaths. If an alert older adult patient is confronted with an intractable, lingering, and painful illness, with no hope of relief except through death, either by PAS or by suicide, is such an intervention justifiable?

The American Nurses Association (ANA) advises nurses not to participate in assisted suicide. It is a violation of the ANA's *Code of Ethics for Nurses* to participate in assisted suicide; however, if a patient wants their life terminated by the withdrawal of specific therapies, that does not mean withdrawal of care. ANA (1992) takes the position that nurses ethically support the provision of compassionate and dignified end-of-life care no matter what decision is made, including the withholding or withdrawing of life-sustaining treatment (Provision 1.3). This emotionally debated issue raises religious, cultural, and "right to self-determination" issues that will most likely continue as our population ages and more members of society will face painful terminal illnesses.

Although suicide is discussed in Chapter 23, specific factors that concern older adults are noted here, such as retirement-related difficulties, physical illness, economic problems, loneliness, social isolation, multiple losses, and ageism. Innovative methods to deal with these factors need to be developed for the older adult. Education of the public in general—and health care providers, in particular—is necessary to raise the level of awareness of this geriatric problem.

ALCOHOLISM AND SUBSTANCE ABUSE

The American Medical Association has termed alcohol and substance abuse among older adults a hidden epidemic sometimes referred to as the "the graying of drug users in America." This is predominantly a result of the greater lifetime rates of drug use by the baby boom generation (the Woodstock generation), gradually passing the 65-year-old threshold. Identifying alcohol and substance abuse is often difficult because personality and behavioral changes frequently are unrecognized.

Alcoholism

There are two major types of alcohol abusers: (1) an individual with early alcoholism who is now aging (longtime drinker), and (2) the late-life drinker (LLD). The aging alcoholic individual has generally had alcohol problems intermittently throughout life, with a regular pattern of alcohol abuse starting to evolve in late middle age or later. The late-life geriatric problem drinker, on the other hand, has no history of alcohol-related problems but develops an alcohol abuse pattern in response to the stresses of aging.

The stressful or reactive factors that precipitate late-onset alcohol abuse are often related to environmental conditions and may include retirement, bereavement, widowhood, and loneliness. These stressors in the older adult, who may have retired, may not drive, and may be isolated from family and friends, are often greater than the problems faced by the middle-aged adult, who has to manage a job or career and care for a family and household. Work and family responsibilities may help keep a potential alcoholic from drinking too much. Once these demands are gone and the structure of daily life is disrupted, there is little impetus to remain sober.

Alcohol and Aging

Excessive consumption of alcohol can create particular problems for older adults. They have an increased biological sensitivity to (i.e., a decreased tolerance for) the effects of alcohol. The decreased tolerance is related to a slower emptying of stomach contents and an increased sensitivity to alcohol in the brain. As people age there is also a decline in lean muscle mass and an increase in fatty tissue that can contribute to increased

blood alcohol levels (BALs) (Offsay, 2007). This diminished resistance, combined with age-related changes such as weakened manual dexterity and reduced balance and postural flexibility, can increase the likelihood of falls, burns, or other accidents.

Some drinkers, as they get older, note changes in their response to alcohol, such as the occurrence of headaches, reduction in mental abilities with memory losses or lapses, and feelings of malaise rather than well-being. These problems start to occur at lower levels of consumption than was the case in earlier years. Older adults are likely to drink more frequently but in lesser quantities than younger individuals, who tend to drink larger amounts less often. Thus the possibility of alcohol abuse in cases of only moderate ingestion by older adults often is not recognized by the friends or family of the alcohol-addicted older adult.

With aging, the body becomes less resilient; healing from injury or infection is slower, and stress is more likely to cause a loss of physiological equilibrium. As the proportion of fatty tissues to lean body mass increases with age, the individual's metabolic rate usually decreases, which increases the amount of time it takes the body to eliminate drugs.

Alcohol and Medication

The interaction of drugs and alcohol in the older adult can have serious consequences. There is a decreased functioning of the liver enzymes that metabolize alcohol, which on a short-term basis has the effect of prolonging the action of many medications, potentiating their effect. On the other hand, chronic ingestion of alcohol accelerates the metabolism of many drugs.

Older individuals can expect to reach higher blood alcohol levels than younger people with an equivalent intake of alcohol. The effects of alcohol on the brain may be one reason that alcohol abuse sometimes mimics or exacerbates normal changes of aging, because even a moderate intake of alcohol can impair the cognition and coordination skills that are already decreased with age.

Extreme care is required when treating the older alcoholic with medication. Central nervous system toxicity from psychoactive drugs increases with aging. Ingestion of antidepressants or tranquilizers can be particularly harmful because their effect is further potentiated by alcohol. The toxicity of other drugs (e.g., acetaminophen) is enhanced by alcohol-associated malnutrition and reduced stores of detoxifying substances such as glutathione.

Alcohol consumption produces a change in sleep patterns, particularly in older adults. Unlike younger individuals, older adults take longer to fall asleep and do not sleep as restfully. Although alcohol may decrease the time it takes to fall asleep, this benefit is offset by frequent awakenings during the night caused by alcohol.

Symptoms of Elder Addiction

Health practitioners need to be concerned with, and sensitive to, possible alcohol abuse among their older patients. Signs of alcohol abuse in younger individuals (e.g., alcohol-induced pancreatitis or liver disease, blackouts, major trauma) occur infrequently in older adults who are late-life drinkers (LLDs). Instead, the older alcoholic displays vague geriatric syndromes of contusions, malnutrition, self-neglect, impaired cognition, sleep disturbances, depression, and falls (Offsay, 2007). Also present may be symptoms of diarrhea, urinary incontinence, a decrease in functional status, failure to thrive, and apparent dementia. Symptoms of poor coordination or visual changes may also mimic the normal aging process but may actually be a result of excessive drinking. Although confusion and disorientation in an older patient are often associated with dementia or Alzheimer's disease, they could be caused by other factors, including alcohol abuse. Assessment of these conditions is necessary to differentiate the normal physiological changes of aging from those attributable to excessive drinking.

Whenever there is a suspicion or indication that an older adult is abusing alcohol, the health care provider should conduct a screening test. The MAST-G (Figure 28-3) is commonly used to assess alcohol problems (Menninger, 2002).

Treatment of the Older Adult Alcoholic

Because many older adults do not live in big families or have work-related contacts, they are less likely to be referred for treatment than are younger drinkers. Too often, by the time the older adult alcoholic is noticed by any treatment agencies, the patient's support systems and resources are severely decreased or depleted. Declining social, physical, and psychological performance is frequently found, which exacerbates the difficulties of loneliness, depression, monotony, accidents, social conflict, loss, and the physiological changes of aging (Wagenaar et al., 2001).

Ageism has deterred the development of treatment programs designed specifically for the older adult. Beliefs that they are too isolated, too embedded in denial of their illness, and too old to function have been detrimental to encouraging health professionals to work with chemically dependent older adults. Another factor that may play a role is that older adults often try to hide alcohol dependence because they consider such abuse sinful or feel they can handle any problems themselves (Touhy & Jett, 2010).

Treatment plans for the LLD should emphasize social therapies. Older adult alcoholics tend to be more passive than younger alcoholics and may benefit from interpersonal involvement with professional health care personnel—many respond to emotional and social support. Family therapy should be encouraged. Group therapy with other middle-aged and older alcoholics as well as self-help groups such as Alcoholics Anonymous can be effective.

The prognosis for the late-life problem drinker—a person who has lived to this point without recourse to alcohol and whose drinking is caused by losses and stress—is excellent. This individual often responds very positively to brief alcohol counseling or an alcoholic recovery program, especially if it is accompanied by environmental interventions. It is important that health care providers recognize this recovery potential. Proper education and awareness of a positive outcome for the geriatric problem drinker can increase the availability of resources; if the prognosis is good, providers and agencies should be more willing to spend resources on treatment.

For those elderly adults with long histories of alcohol use and who meet the criteria for alcohol addiction (dependence), a more rigorous treatment plan is required. This regimen needs to include detoxification, often in a 5- to 7-day inpatient unit (Offsay, 2007). Medications may also play a part in longer term treatment. Naltrexone has evidence-based efficacy and at 50 mg/day is thought to be safe for older adults when used in conjunction with periodic measurement of hepatic enzymes (Offsay, 2007).

Considering the magnitude of the problems and the likelihood that the number of older abusers will continue to increase, efforts need to be intensified to identify the causes of alcohol dependence and to develop appropriate interventions for treating it. If not, such dependence can overwhelm those charged with meeting the health and social service needs.

Substance Abuse
Illegal Drug Use

The number of older Americans seeking help from multiple substance abuse tripled from 13.7% in 1992 to 39.7% in 2008 (Substance Abuse and Mental Health Services Administration [SAMHSA], 2010). This same study by SAMHSA (2010) during the same period of time (1992 to 2008) found that the increase in marijuana abuse among the older age-group changed from 0.6% to 2.9%. Cocaine abuse nearly quadrupled from 2.9% to 11.4%, and heroin abuse doubled from 7.9% to 16%. The sheer numbers of aging baby boomers threaten to overwhelm treatment resources. Today most substance abuse treatment is geared to the young abuser; major changes will need to occur to manage a large number of older adult abusers.

Prescription and Over-the-Counter Drug Use and Abuse

Because older adult patients use both prescription and over-the-counter drugs at a higher rate than the general population, it is difficult to accurately estimate the extent to which these drugs are abused or misused. The high exposure to medications coupled with age-related physiological changes, including decreased metabolism, increased accumulation, and, in the case of long-acting benzodiazepines and anticholinergics, increased sensitivity (especially to those drugs with anticholinergic side effects), raises the likelihood of medication-related adverse events such as increased sedation, delirium, confusion, and falls, resulting in hip fractures.

SAMHSA (2010) reported that prescription drug abuse increased from 0.7% to 3.5% from 1992 to 2008. Compounding these numbers is that often the older adult will abuse two or more drugs (multidrug abuse or polydrug use), increasing the likelihood of even more severe medical, physical, and/or mental health complications.

Michigan Alcoholism Screening Testing—Geriatric Version (MAST-G)

Please answer yes or no to each question by marking the line next to the question. When you finish answering the questions, please add up how many "yes" responses you checked and put that number in the space provided at the end.

	Yes	No
1. After drinking have you ever noticed an increase in your heart rate or beating in your chest?	○	○
2. When talking to others, do you ever underestimate how much you actually drank?	○	○
3. Does alcohol make you sleepy so that you often fall asleep in your chair?	○	○
4. After a few drinks, have you sometimes not eaten or been able to skip a meal because you didn't feel hungry?	○	○
5. Does having a few drinks help you decrease your shakiness or tremors?	○	○
6. Does alcohol sometimes make it hard for you to remember parts of the day or night?	○	○
7. Do you have rules for yourself that you won't drink before a certain time of the day?	○	○
8. Have you lost interest in hobbies or activities you used to enjoy?	○	○
9. When you wake up in the morning, do you ever have trouble remembering part of the night before?	○	○
10. Does having a drink help you sleep?	○	○
11. Do you hide your alcohol bottles from family members?	○	○
12. After a social gathering, have you ever felt embarrassed because you drank too much?	○	○
13. Have you ever been concerned that drinking might be harmful to your health?	○	○
14. Do you like to end an evening with a nightcap?	○	○
15. Did you find your drinking increased after someone close to you died?	○	○
16. In general, would you prefer to have a few drinks at home rather than go out to social events?	○	○
17. Are you drinking more now than in the past?	○	○
18. Do you usually take a drink to relax or calm your nerves?	○	○
19. Do you drink to take your mind off your problems?	○	○
20. Have you ever increased your drinking after experiencing a loss in your life?	○	○
21. Do you sometimes drive when you have had too much to drink?	○	○
22. Has a doctor or nurse ever said they were worried or concerned about your drinking?	○	○
23. Have you ever made rules to manage your drinking?	○	○
24. When you feel lonely, does having a drink help?	○	○

TOTAL _____

Scoring: A score of 3 points or less is considered to indicate no alcoholism; a score of 4 points is suggestive of alcoholism; a score of 5 points or more indicates an alcohol problem.

FIGURE 28-3 Michigan Alcoholism Screening Testing—Geriatric Version (MAST-G). (© The Regents of the University of Michigan, 1991.)

ACQUIRED IMMUNODEFICIENCY SYNDROME AND AIDS-RELATED DEMENTIA

Human immunodeficiency virus (HIV) infection and AIDS remain a growing problem among the elderly (Stein, 2011).

Blood transfusions are no longer the main cause for the spread of AIDS in the older adult, unless the older adult received a blood transfusion before 1985. Research shows that older adults are sexually active and thus at risk for HIV and AIDS because of failure to practice safe sex. Men who have been treated for erectile dysfunction are also considered at risk for HIV/AIDS. With a change of demographics in this country, most HIV patients are aging as well and many are in their fifties or older (Stein, 2011). In addition, diagnosis and treatment of HIV and AIDS in the older adult are delayed because health care providers believe that this population is not sexually active. In general, lack of adequate knowledge about HIV and AIDS among older adults coupled with denial that this illness occurs in their generation increase the risk for HIV infection and AIDS in this age-group.

Older women who are sexually active are at higher risk for HIV and AIDS from an infected partner than are older men. Changes in vaginal tissue caused by the aging process can lead to tears in the vaginal mucosa during intercourse, which allow HIV to penetrate. In addition, because pregnancy is no longer a threat, use of condoms in this age-group is uncommon.

Dementia is often a sequela in people with human immunodeficiency virus (HIV) infection and AIDS. Dementia caused by AIDS and dementia caused by Alzheimer's disease can be easily confused. Therefore a careful assessment and workup are required. Health care providers must be aware that AIDS can occur in the older adult.

It is recommended that testing for HIV/AIDS be performed more regularly for older adults, even though recent studies using small sample populations did not support a need for HIV/AIDS testing in this demographic (Stein, 2011).

LEGAL AND ETHICAL ISSUES THAT AFFECT THE MENTAL HEALTH OF OLDER ADULTS

Many subjects might be included here. Among the most important for practicing nurses in any setting to be familiar with are the following:

1. Use of restraints
2. Decision making about health care
3. Elder abuse (a serious problem for the older adult addressed in Chapter 21)
4. End-of-life care (addressed in Chapter 25)

USE OF RESTRAINTS

The use of restraints is an ethical, legal, and safety concern. Restraints can be both physical and chemical. **Physical restraints** are any manual methods or mechanical devices, materials, or equipment that inhibit free movement. Examples include tightening a bedsheet to limit movement; raising side rails; applying a Posey belt; using leg, arm, and mitt restraints; or positioning a wheelchair against the wall to restrict movement. Wrist bands or devices on clothing that trigger an alarm to notify staff that an older adult is leaving a room or an area should **not** be considered restraints. **Chemical restraints** are drugs given for the very specific purpose of inhibiting a certain behavior or movement.

Physical Restraints

Whether health care providers have the right to restrain another individual physically has always been a question. Surveys undertaken by the state and federal authorities in the United States between the 1970s and 1980s revealed levels of physical restraint use as high as 75% in some facilities and levels of psychotropic drug use as high as 90% (Marchello, 2003). Physical restraints were traditionally used with hospitalized confused patients primarily to prevent disruption of medical therapies and to prevent falls. Paradoxically, they are perceived as a form of physical and psychological abuse by the patient and often the family.

Research from the mid-1980s onward has shown that restraints are more likely to cause harm than prevent it (Minnesota Department of Health [MDH], 2010). Physical restraints pose a risk of death through strangulation or asphyxiation and lead to muscle loss, incontinence, pressure sores, agitation, and bone weakness. Radziewicz and colleagues (2010) state that physical restraint of the elderly is a risk factor for:

- Severe cognitive impairment and/or physical impairment
- Fall injury risk
- Diagnosis of presence of the psychiatric disorder (e.g., alcohol withdrawal)

Restraining an elderly adult is humiliating and the immobilizing experience can lead the older adult to respond with depression, anxiety, stress-related syndromes, withdrawal, and/or agitation when minimum movement is taken away (Dharmarajan & Norman, 2003; MDH, 2010). The current standard of care is to maintain a restraint-fee policy.

More facilities are using electronic sensing systems to alert staff if a resident is about to stand up or try to get out of a bed or wheelchair. The following are examples of other alternatives to physical restraints (MDH, 2010):

- Personal strengthening and rehabilitation programs
- Increased use of hearing aids, visual aids, and mobility devices
- Safer physical environment (lower beds, adequate lighting, moving obstacles, and positioning furniture in familiar places)
- Use of door alarms for residents who may wander

Physical restraints should be used for emergency purposes only when there is a threat to the safety of the resident or others, never as a means of controlling behavior or as punishment. Physical restraints are used as a last resort; other methods used to calm the resident and prevent harm have been used and shown to be superior.

Residents in restraint-free facilities have experienced fewer injuries from falls than those in facilities using restraints. A study by Neufeld and colleagues (1999) found that serious injuries declined significantly when restraint orders were discontinued. The researchers concluded that restraint-free care is safe when a comprehensive assessment is performed and alternatives to restraints are used.

The Omnibus Budget Reconciliation Act (OBRA) of 1990 declares that each nursing home resident has the right to be free from unnecessary drugs and physical restraints. In addition, each resident must be provided with treatment to reduce dependency on chemical and physical intervention (Hogstel & Weeks, 2000). The Nursing Home Reform Amendment in OBRA details the regulatory framework governing the use of restraints in all states (Marchello, 2003).

The Joint Commission (TJC), formerly the Joint Commission on the Accreditation of Healthcare Organizations (JCAHO), developed recommendations on the use of physical restraints (JCAHO, 1999). Derived from OBRA regulations, TJC guidelines for physical restraints include the following:

1. A physician's order must be obtained.
2. Restraint application must be time limited.
3. Attempts at alternative approaches must be documented.
4. Ongoing observation and assessment of the patient must be documented.
5. Care interventions (e.g., provision of food and fluids, toileting, help with activities of daily living, and response to attempted release) must be documented.

Nurses can avoid liability by knowing the laws of their state, adhering to the policies and procedures of the institution at which they work, and using good nursing judgment. All nursing homes and hospitals should have written restraint procedures and policies available to all health care providers. If restraints are used, the nurse is responsible for the patient's safety. The patient should be restrained only for a minimal time and for a valid purpose. Use of restraints does not enhance patient care. Creative nursing skills and interventions are frequently more beneficial.

Chemical Restraints

Unfortunately, with restrictions on physical restraints and because of the lack of any FDA-approved medication, there has been an increase in off-label use of certain medications (particularly second-generation antipsychotics) as chemical restraints to control the behavior of elderly dementia patients, as well as to control the staff's working environment (Cassels, 2010). In 2008 the U.S. Food and Drug Administration (FDA) issued Black Box warnings for the off-label use of conventional or atypical antipsychotics in controlling behavioral symptoms in elderly patients with dementia, which are symptoms found in almost 50% of dementia patients (Cassels, 2010). The FDA found that the dangers included increased risk for diabetes and cerebrovascular events as well as a doubled risk for mortality. Although the warning labels have decreased the use of antipsychotics in community and hospital elderly dementia patients, they have not appeared to decrease antipsychotic use in nursing

homes across the country. A study by Chen and associates (2010) conducted a nationwide survey of nursing home use of antipsychotics and found that up to 29% of the study residents in nursing homes received at least one antipsychotic medication, and nearly 32% of the patients given antipsychotics were not psychotic and had no identified clinical indication for this therapy (Chen et al., 2010). Use of antipsychotics in the elderly population needs to be evaluated very carefully, particularly in older patients with dementia,

CONTROL OF THE DECISION-MAKING PROCESS

Patient Self-Determination Act

Since the 1960s, the public's desire to participate in decision making about health care has increased. This interest in patient advocacy was recognized when Congress passed the Patient Self-Determination Act (PSDA) in 1990, requiring that health care facilities provide clear written information for every patient regarding his or her legal rights to make health care decisions, including the right to accept or refuse treatment. The PSDA also establishes the right of a person to provide treatment directions for clinicians in the event of a serious illness. Increasing numbers of older adults are creating written directives.

An advance directive is a term used to describe living wills, durable powers of attorney for health care, and health care surrogate appointments. Health care institutions that receive federal funds are required both to provide each patient at the time of admission written information regarding his or her right to execute advance directives and to inquire if such directives have been made by the patient. The patient's admission records should state whether such directives exist. The ANA (1992) recommends that specific questions be part of every nurse's admission assessment. Box 28-3 reproduces these questions and describes the responsibilities of health care workers under the PSDA.

Such a directive indicates preferences for the types of medical care or amount of treatment desired. The directive comes into effect should physical or mental incapacitation prevent the patient from making health care decisions. These wishes can be communicated through one or more of the following: (1) a living will, (2) a directive to physician, and (3) a durable power of attorney for health care. These documents must be in writing and the patient's signature must be witnessed; depending on state and institutional provisions, notarization may be required.

Living Will

A living will is a personal statement of how and where one wishes to die. It is activated only when the person is terminally ill and incapacitated. A competent patient may alter a living will at any time. The question of whether an incompetent person can change a living will is addressed on a state-by-state basis. Executing a living will does not always guarantee its application.

BOX 28-3 NURSES' RESPONSIBILITIES AND THE PATIENT SELF-DETERMINATION ACT (1990)

Part of Nursing Admission Assessment

- Nurses should know the laws of the state in which [they] practice and should be familiar with the strengths and limitations of the various forms of advance directive.
- The ANA recommends that the following questions be part of the nursing admission assessment:
  1. Do you have basic information about advance directives, including living wills and durable power of attorney?
  2. Do you wish to initiate an advance directive?
  3. If you have already prepared an advance directive, can you provide it now?
  4. Have you discussed your end-of-life choices with your family or designated surrogate and health care workers?

Responsibilities of Health Care Workers Under the Patient Self-Determination Act of 1990

- Hospitals, skilled nursing facilities, home health agencies, hospice organizations, and health maintenance organizations serving Medicare and Medicaid patients must:
  1. Maintain written policies and procedures for providing information to their patients for whom they provide care.
  2. Give written material to patients concerning their rights under state law to make decisions about medical care, including the right to accept or refuse surgical or medical care and to formulate advance directives and provide written policies and procedures for the realization of these rights.
  3. Document in patients' records whether they have advance directives.
  4. Not discriminate in care or in other ways against patients who have or have not prepared advance directives.
  5. Make sure that policies are in place to ensure compliance with state laws governing advance directives.

Data from Schlossberg, C., & Hart, M.A. (1992). Legal perspectives. In M.M. Burke, & M.B. Walsh (Eds.), *Gerontologic nursing: care of the frail elderly* (p. 469). St Louis: Mosby; American Nurses Association. (1992). *Position statement on nursing and the Patient Self-Determination Act*. Washington, DC: Author.

Directive to Physician

In a directive to physician, a physician is appointed by the individual to serve as proxy. Many of the features of a directive to physician parallel those of a living will, such as activation only when a terminal illness is present, need for verification of the terminal illness by the physician, and requirement for patient competency at the time of signing. The directive to physician designating the physician as surrogate can be particularly useful in cases of terminal illness when an individual has no family. The physician must agree in writing to be the patient's agent and must be one of the two physicians who made the original determination that the patient is terminally ill. Unlike the living will, the directive to physician can be revoked orally at any time without regard to patient competency.

Durable Power of Attorney for Health Care

The durable power of attorney for health care differs from living wills and directives to physicians in that a person other than a physician is appointed to act as the patient's agent. The patient must be competent and of age when making the appointment and must be competent in order to revoke the power. Individuals do not have to be terminally ill or incompetent to allow the empowered individual to act on their behalf. No physician's certification is required.

Older adults who are lesbian, gay, bisexual, or transgender (LGBT) often have many conflicts within state or federal facilities such as nursing homes. Sometimes there is a cruel bias of not allowing visitation rights or power of attorney, for example, for these patients' partners. All nurses should know their state laws and should provide the same high-quality care to all patients regardless of age, gender, race, ethnicity, or sexual persuasion.

Nursing Role in the Decision-Making Process

The nurse explains the ethics and legal policies of the institution to both the patient and the family and helps them understand the concepts behind advance directives. The nurse explains that the family need not feel morally obligated to provide for all possible medical care when such care will only extend the suffering of a loved one. This is especially true when such extraordinary measures do not represent the person's values and beliefs. The nurse serves as an *advocate* and a knowledgeable resource person for the older adult patient and family. The patient is encouraged to verbalize his or her feelings and thoughts during this sensitive time of decision making. In addition, nurses are responsible for being knowledgeable about the state regulations on advance directives as well as the potential obstacles in completing the directives for the state in which they practice. Maintaining an open and continuing dialogue among patient, family, nurse, and physician is of principal importance. The nurse supports any surrogates appointed to act on the patient's behalf and seeks consultation for ethical issues the nurse feels unprepared to handle.

Every health care facility receiving federal funds is required to have written policies, procedures, and protocols in compliance with the PSDA. Nurses must prepare themselves to deal with the legal, ethical, and moral issues involved when counseling about advance directives. The law does not specify who should talk with patients about treatment decisions, but in many facilities nurses are being asked to discuss this issue with the patient. If the advance directive of a patient is not being followed, the nurse intervenes on the patient's behalf. If the problem cannot be resolved with the physician, the facility's protocol providing for notification of the appropriate supervisor is followed.

Although nurses, especially in nursing homes, may discuss options with their patients, they may not assist patients in writing advance directives because this is considered a conflict of interest. The existence of an advance directive serves as a guide to health care providers in advocating for the older adult patient's rightful wishes in this process.

KEY POINTS TO REMEMBER

- The older adult population continues to increase as the baby boomers start reaching 65 years old.
- The increase in the number of older adults poses a challenge not only to nurses but also to the entire health care system. There is much to be done to prepare and respond to the special needs of this population.
- Attitudes toward the older adult are often negative, reflecting ageism bias based solely on age.
- Ageism is found at all levels of society and even among health care providers, which affects the way we render care to our older adult patients.
- Nurses who care for older adults in various settings may function at different levels. All nurses should be knowledgeable about the process of aging and be cognizant of the differences between normal and abnormal aging changes.

- Older adults face increasing problems of alcoholism, illicit drugs, abuse and misuse of prescription and over-the-counter drugs, and suicide.
- OBRA established guidelines and a philosophy of care that mandates patients be free from unnecessary use of drugs and physical restraints.
- Nurses working with the mentally ill patient must know psychotherapeutic approaches relevant for older adults, such as remotivation and reminiscence therapy. Nurse clinicians may offer psychotherapy groups geared toward the special needs of this population.
- When it comes to dying and death, older adults' wishes and those of their families are frequently ignored. The implementation of the PSDA, passed in 1990, can afford some patients autonomy and dignity in death.

APPLYING CRITICAL JUDGMENT

1. Mr. Lopez is 70 years old and has been admitted to the intensive care unit with a diagnosis of alcohol withdrawal delirium. He is confused and combative, and threatens to strike the nurse who is trying to render care to him unless he is allowed to leave the unit. The nurse applies wrist restraints to keep Mr. Lopez from striking her and leaving the room. What are the mandates of OBRA (1990) regarding the use of restraints?
   A. How is Mr. Lopez likely to react?
   B. What are the possible legal repercussions for the nurse?
   C. Describe the physical harm that could occur to Mr. Lopez if left alone in a room while restrained.
   D. Discuss some of the safety measures that might help calm Mr. Lopez.
   E. What were the reasons that OBRA found the use of restraints dangerous for patients?
2. Mr. Lopez has received treatment for alcohol withdrawal. He appears very quiet, refuses to eat, does not sleep at night, and admits to thoughts of desperation and wishes he could die. He also confides that he attempted suicide when his wife died 5 years earlier and at that time he started drinking heavily. Which is the appropriate depression assessment

tool to use in assessing the severity of his condition? Explain your answer.
   A. What parts of the medical record of Mr. Lopez do you need to be familiar with to plan adequate nursing care? Do you need more information? Describe the information you need.
   B. If you are working with a social worker for discharge planning, what kinds of supports would you suggest be available to Mr. Lopez upon discharge?
3. Mrs. Jones comes into the hospital after a heart attack exacerbated by chemotherapy from metastasized liver cancer. Her son says that she does not want anyone to resuscitate her. Acting both as a nurse and as a patient advocate, define what is meant by advance directives and explain to both Mrs. Jones and her son the forms that need to be completed to make the patient's wishes known (e.g., living well, durable power of attorney for health care, and directive to physician).
4. Take turns with a classmate role playing "ageism" and "elderspeak" and discuss how you felt.
5. Ask an older adult (older than age 70) the changes he/she notices in his/her life (pro and con) since about age 35.

CHAPTER REVIEW QUESTIONS

Choose the most appropriate answer(s).

1. A 68-year-old man who recently retired states he is not his usual self, has a poor appetite and low energy. Physical findings were within normal limits. The priority nursing intervention is to:
   1. encourage the patient to seek diversional activities.
   2. assess the patient for depression.
   3. ask the patient if he has access to firearms.
   4. refer the patient to a dietitian for counseling.

2. Which of the following psychiatric disorders is found most frequently among older adults?
   1. Depression
   2. Dementia
   3. Anxiety
   4. Social phobia

3. Which statement regarding the use of restraints is true?
   1. Restraint-free care appreciably diminishes the overall safety of any older adult patient compared with the use of physical or chemical restraints.
   2. The nurse is responsible for patient safety during the time the patient is restrained.
   3. Chemical restraint presents less potential for patient harm than physical restraint.
   4. Restraint may be used to prevent extubation if a nursing protocol exists.

4. An elderly patient asks the nurse what contributes most to healthy aging. The best response would be: (select all that apply)
   1. regular exercise at least 90 minutes per day.
   2. a nutritious diet with plenty of fruits and vegetables.
   3. a strong support system.
   4. involvement in community activities.

5. In carrying out patients' wishes and directives as a nurse, which of the following is an unethical action for the nurse?
   1. Ignoring a "Do not resuscitate" order for an older adult patient in the intensive care unit
   2. Implementing a physician's order to withhold artificial hydration from an older adult patient in irreversible coma
   3. Adhering to the choices made for an older adult patient by the individual with durable power of attorney for health care
   4. Advocating for an older adult patient in the terminal stage of cancer who wishes to discontinue chemotherapy

REFERENCES

Administration on Aging (AOA). (2010). *A profile of older Americans: 2009*. Washington, DC: Author.

Administration on Aging (AOA). (2009). *A profile of older Americans: 2008*. Washington, DC: Author.

Alexopoulos, G. S., & Knosses, D. N. (2011). *Geriatric psychiatry: advances and directions (preface)*. Retrieved June 26, 2011, from http://www.psych.theclinics.com/article/S0193-953X(11)00031-1/fulltext.

American Association of Colleges of Nursing (AACN). (2008). *The essentials of baccalaureate education for professional nursing practice*. Washington, DC: Author. Retrieved July 5, 2011 from www.aacn.nche.edu/Education/pdf/BaccEssentials08.pdf.

American Nurses Association (ANA). (1992). *Position statement on nursing and the Patient Self-Determination Act*. Washington, DC: Author.

Andreescu, C., & Reynolds, C. F. (2011). Late-life depression: evidence-based treatment and promising new directions for research and clinical practice. In G. S. Alexopoulos, & D. N. Kiosses (Eds.), *Psychiatric Clinics of North America*. (Vol. 34, no. 2). St Louis: Elsevier.

Bartels, S. J., & Drake, R. E. (2005). Evidence-based geriatric psychiatry: an overview. *Psychiatric Clinics of North America*, *28*(4), 763–784.

Buckwalter, K. C., Beck, C., & Evens, L. K. (2011). Envisioning the future of geropsychiatric nursing. In K. D. Melillo, & S. C. Houde (Eds.), *Geropsychiatric and mental health nursing* (2nd ed., pp. 465–475). Sudbury, MA: Jones and Bartlett Learning.

Byrd, E. H., & Vito, N. A. (2011). Nursing assessment and treatment of depressive disorders of late life. In K. D. Melillo & S. C. Houde (Eds.), *Geropsychiatric and mental health nursing* (2nd ed.). Sudbury, MA: Jones and Bartlett Learning.

Cassels, C. (2010). *Inappropriate use of antipsychotics in the elderly continued use despite FDA warnings*. Retrieved July 1, 2011, from www.medscape.com/viewarticle/715257_print.

Centers for Disease Control and Prevention (CDC). (2011). *Study looks at suicide rates from 1928-2007*. Retrieved June 25, 2011, from www.cdc.gov/media/release/2011/p. 0414_suicide rates.html.

Charney, D. S., Reynolds, C. F., Lewis, L., et al. (2003). Depression and bipolar support alliance consensus statement on the unmet needs in diagnosis and treatment of mood disorders in late life. *Archives of General Psychiatry*, *60*(7), 664–672.

Chen, W., Briesacher, B. A., Field, T. S., Tjia, J., et al. (2010). *Unexplained variation across U.S. nursing homes in antipsychotic prescribing rates*. Retrieved July 2, 2011, from http://archinte.ama-assn.org/cgi/content/abstract/170/1/89.

Cole, M. G. (2005). Evidence-based review of risk factors for geriatric depression and brief preventive interventions. *Psychiatric Clinics of North America*, *28*(4), 785–803.

Coupland, C., Dhiman, P., Morriss, R., et al. (2011). *Antidepressant use and risk of adverse outcomes in older people*. Retrieved February 19, 2012, from http://www.medscape.com/viewarticle/748441.

Coupland, C., & Hochhalter, A. (2011). *Popular antidepressants not always best choice for seniors*. Retrieved August 26, 2011, from www.nlm.nih.gov/medlineplus/news/full story_114940.html.

Dharmarajan, T. S., & Norman, R. A. (Eds.), (2003). *Clinical geriatrics*. New York: Parthenon.

Fox, C., Richardson, K., Maidment, I. D., et al. (2011). Retrieved February 22, 2011, from http://www.ncbi.nln.nih.gov/pubmed/21707557.

Hogstel, M. Oh., & Weeks, S. M. (2000). Mental health. In A. G. Lueckenotte (Ed.), *Gynecological nursing* (2nd ed.). St Louis: Mosby.

Joint Commission on Accreditation of Healthcare Organizations (JCAHO). (1999). *Standards for behavioral health care.* Oakbrook, IL: Author.

Kelland, K. (2011). *Anti-cholinergic drug effects boosts elderly death risk.* Retrieved July 4, 2011 from www.medscape.com/viewarticle/745256_print.

Krieger, N. (1999). Embodying inequality: a review of concepts measures, and methods for studying health consequences of discrimination. *International Journal of Health Services, 29*(2), 295–352.

Leland, J. (2008). *And "sweetie" and "dear," a hurt for the elderly.* Retrieved June 28, 2011, from www.nttimes.com/2008/10/07/us/07aginghtml?.

Liiades, C. (2010). *Treating depression in the elderly.* Retrieved June 28, 2011, from www.everydayhealth.com/depression/understanding/treating-depression-in-elderly.

Lueckenotte, A. G. (2000). Gerontologic assessment. In A. G. Lueckenotte (Ed.), *Gerontologic nursing* (2nd ed.). St Louis: Mosby.

Marchello, V. (2003). Long-term care. In T. S. Dharmarajan, & R. A. Norman (Eds.), *Clinical geriatrics.* New York: Parthenon.

McEnany, J. P. (2011). Psychopharmacology. In K. D. Melillo, & S. C. Houde (Eds.), *Geropsychiatric and mental health nursing* (2nd ed.). Sudbury, MA: Jones and Bartlett Learning.

Minnesota Department of Health (MDH). (2010). *Minnesota Department of Health safety without restraints: a new practice standard for safe care.* Retrieved July 1, 2011, from www.health.state.mn.us/divs/fpc/safety.htm.

Menninger, J. A. (2002). Assessment and treatment of alcoholism and substance-related disorders in the elderly. *Bulletin of the Menninger Clinic, 66*(2), 166–183.

Narang, A. T., & Sikka, R. (2006). Resuscitation of the elderly. *Emergency Medicine Clinics of North America, 24*(2), 261–272.

Neufeld, R. R., Libow, L. S., Foley, W. J., et al. (1999). Restraint reduction reduces serious injuries among nursing home residents. *Journal of the American Geriatrics Society, 47*, 1202–1207.

Offsay, J. (2007). Treatment of alcohol-related problems in the elderly. *Annals of Long-Term Care, 15*(7), 39–44.

Palmore, E. B., Branch, L. G., and Harris, Deep. K. (2005). *Encyclopedia of ageism.* Binghamton, N. Y.: Haworth Pastoral Press.

Piechniczek-Buczek, J. (2006). Psychiatric emergencies in the elderly population. *Emergency Medicine Clinics of North America, 24*(2), 467–490.

President's New Freedom Commission on Mental Health. (2003). *Achieving the promise: transforming mental health care in America. Final report.* Rockville, MD: USDHHS (Pub. No. SMA-03-3832).

Preston, J. D., O'Neal, J. H., & Talaga, M. C. (2010). *Handbook of clinical psychopharmacology for therapists* (6th ed.). Oakland, CA: New Harbinger Publications.

Radziewicz, R. M., Amoto, S., & Bradas, C. (2010). *Use of physical restraints with elderly patients.* Retrieved February 21, 2012, from http://www.gerin.org/topics/physicalrestraints/want_toknow more__.

Richards, J. B., Papaioannou, A., Adachi, J. D., et al. (2007). Effect of selective serotonin reuptake inhibitors on the risk of fracture. *Archives of Internal Medicine, 167*(2), 188–194.

Sadock, B. J., & Sadock, V. A. (2010). *Kaplan and Sadock's pocket handbook of clinical psychiatry* (5th ed.). Philadelphia: Wolters-Kluwer/Lippincott Williams & Wilkins.

Sheikh, J. I., & Yesavage, J. A. (1986). Geriatric Depression Scale (GDS): recent evidence and development of a shorter version. In T. L. Brink (Ed.), *Clinical gerontology: a guide to assessment and intervention.* New York: Haworth Press.

Simpkins, C. L. (2008). Ageism's influence on healthcare delivery and nursing practice. *Journal of Nursing Student Research, 1*(1), 24–28.

Stein, J. (2011). *High-risk older patients are not screened for HIV.* Retrieved June 29, 2011, from www.medscape.com/viewarticle/743632.

Substance Abuse and Mental Health Services Administration (SAMHSA), Office of Applied Studies. (June 17, 2010). *The TEDS report: changing substance abuse patterns among older admissions: 1992 and 2008.* Rockville, MD: Author.

Touhy, T. A., & Jett, K. (2010). *Ebersole and Hess' gerontological nursing & healthy aging.* St Louis: Mosby/Elsevier.

U.S. Department of Health and Human Services. (1999). *Mental health: a report of the Surgeon General—executive summary.* Rockville, MD: Author.

U.S. Food and Drug Administration (FDA). (2008 update). Antipsychotics are not indicated for the treatment of dementia-related psychoses. Retrieved February 20, 2012, from http://www.fda.gov/drugs/drugsafety/postmarketdrugsafetyinformationforpatients andprovider.

Wagenaar, D. B., Mickus, M. A., & Wilson, J. (2001). Alcoholism in late life: challenges and complexities. *Psychiatric Annals, 31*(11), 665–672.

DSM-IV-TR Diagnostic Criteria for Mental Disorders

DSM-IV-TR CLASSIFICATION

NOS: not otherwise specified

An *x* appearing in a diagnostic code indicates that a specific code number is required.

An ellipsis (…) is used in the names of certain disorders to indicate that the name of a specific mental disorder or general medical condition should be inserted when recording the name (e.g., 293.0 Delirium Due to … Hypothyroidism).

If criteria are currently met, one of the following severity specifiers may be noted after the diagnosis:

Mild

Moderate

Severe

If criteria are no longer met, one of the following specifiers may be noted:

In Partial Remission

In Full Remission

Prior History

DISORDERS USUALLY FIRST DIAGNOSED IN INFANCY, CHILDHOOD, OR ADOLESCENCE

Mental Retardation

Note: These are coded on Axis II.

317	Mild Mental Retardation
318.0	Moderate Mental Retardation
318.1	Severe Mental Retardation
318.2	Profound Mental Retardation
319	Mental Retardation, Severity Unspecified

From American Psychiatric Association: *Diagnostic and statistical manual of mental disorders*, ed 4, text revision, Washington, DC, 2000, The Association.

Learning Disorders

315.00	Reading Disorder
315.1	Mathematics Disorder
315.2	Disorder of Written Expression
315.9	Learning Disorder NOS

Motor Skills Disorder

315.4	Developmental Coordination Disorder

Communication Disorders

315.31	Expressive Language Disorder
315.32	Mixed Receptive-Expressive Language Disorder
315.39	Phonologic Disorder
307.0	Stuttering
307.9	Communication Disorder NOS

Pervasive Developmental Disorders

299.00	Autistic Disorder
299.80	Rett's Disorder
299.10	Childhood Disintegrative Disorder
299.80	Asperger's Disorder
299.80	Pervasive Developmental Disorder NOS

Attention-Deficit and Disruptive Behavior Disorders

314.xx	Attention-Deficit/Hyperactivity Disorder
.01	Combined Type
.00	Predominantly Inattentive Type
.01	Predominantly Hyperactive-Impulsive Type
314.9	Attention-Deficit/Hyperactivity Disorder NOS
312.xx	Conduct Disorder
.81	Childhood-Onset Type
.82	Adolescent-Onset Type
.89	Unspecified Onset
313.81	Oppositional Defiant Disorder
312.9	Disruptive Behavior Disorder NOS

Feeding and Eating Disorders of Infancy or Early Childhood

307.52	Pica
307.53	Rumination Disorder
307.59	Feeding Disorder of Infancy or Early Childhood

Tic Disorders

307.23	Tourette's Disorder
307.22	Chronic Motor or Vocal Tic Disorder
307.21	Transient Tic Disorder
	Specify if Single Episode/Recurrent
307.20	Tic Disorder NOS

Elimination Disorders

—.—	Encopresis
787.6	With Constipation and Overflow Incontinence
307.7	Without Constipation and Overflow Incontinence
307.6	Enuresis (Not Due to a General Medical Condition)
	Specify type: Nocturnal Only/Diurnal Only/Nocturnal and Diurnal

Other Disorders of Infancy, Childhood, or Adolescence

309.21	Separation Anxiety Disorder
	Specify if Early Onset
313.23	Selective Mutism
313.89	Reactive Attachment Disorder of Infancy or Early Childhood
	Specify type: Inhibited Type/Disinhibited Type
307.3	Stereotypic Movement Disorder
	Specify if With Self-Injurious Behavior
313.9	Disorder of Infancy, Childhood, or Adolescence NOS

DELIRIUM, DEMENTIA, AND AMNESTIC AND OTHER COGNITIVE DISORDERS

Delirium

293.0	Delirium Due to ... [Indicate the General Medical Condition]
—.—	Substance Intoxication Delirium (refer to Substance-Related Disorders for substance-specific codes)
—.—	Substance Withdrawal Delirium (refer to Substance-Related Disorders for substance-specific codes)
—.—	Delirium Due to Multiple Etiologies (code each of the specific etiologies)
780.09	Delirium NOS

Dementia

294.xx	Dementia of the Alzheimer's Type, With Early Onset (*also code 331.0 Alzheimer's disease on Axis III*)

.10	Without Behavioral Disturbance
.11	With Behavioral Disturbance
294.xx	Dementia of the Alzheimer's Type, With Late Onset (*also code 331.0 Alzheimer's disease on Axis III*)
.10	Without Behavioral Disturbance
.11	With Behavioral Disturbance
290.xx	Vascular Dementia
.40	Uncomplicated
.41	With Delirium
.42	With Delusions
.43	With Depressed Mood
	Specify if With Behavioral Disturbance

Code presence or absence of a behavioral disturbance in the fifth digit for Dementia Due to a General Medical Condition:
0 = Without Behavioral Disturbance
1 = With Behavioral Disturbance

294.1x	Dementia Due to HIV Disease (*also code 042 HIV on Axis III*)
294.1x	Dementia Due to Head Trauma (*also code 854.00 head injury on Axis III*)
294.1x	Dementia Due to Parkinson's Disease (*also code 332.0 Parkinson's disease on Axis III*)
294.1x	Dementia Due to Huntington's Disease (*also code 333.4 Huntington's disease on Axis III*)
294.1x	Dementia Due to Pick's Disease (*also code 331.1 Pick's disease on Axis III*)
294.1x	Dementia Due to Creutzfeldt-Jakob Disease (*also code 046.1 Creutzfeldt-Jakob disease on Axis III*)
294.1x	Dementia Due to ... [Indicate the General Medical Condition not listed above] (*also code the general medical condition on Axis III*)
—.—	Substance-Induced Persisting Dementia (*refer to Substance-Related Disorders for substance-specific codes*)
—.—	Dementia Due to Multiple Etiologies (*code each of the specific etiologies*)
294.8	Dementia NOS

Amnestic Disorders

294.0	Amnestic Disorder Due to ... [Indicate the General Medical Condition]
	Specify if Transient/Chronic
—.—	Substance-Induced Persisting Amnestic Disorder (*refer to Substance-Related Disorders for substance-specific codes*)
294.8	Amnestic Disorder NOS

Other Cognitive Disorders

294.9	Cognitive Disorder NOS
	Mental Disorders Due to a General Medical Condition Not Elsewhere Classified
293.89	Catatonic Disorder Due to ... [Indicate the General Medical Condition]
310.1	Personality Change Due to ... [Indicate the General Medical Condition]

Specify type: Labile Type/Disinhibited Type/ Aggressive Type/Apathetic Type/Paranoid Type/Other Type/Combined Type/Unspecified Type

293.9 Mental Disorder NOS Due to ... *[Indicate the General Medical Condition]*

SUBSTANCE-RELATED DISORDERS

The following specifiers may be applied to Substance Dependence as noted:

[a]With Physiological Dependence/Without Physiological Dependence

[b]Early Full Remission/Early Partial Remission/Sustained Full Remission/Sustained Partial Remission

[c]In a Controlled Environment

[d]On Agonist Therapy

The following specifiers apply to Substance-Induced Disorders as noted:

[I]With Onset During Intoxication

[W]With Onset During Withdrawal

Alcohol-Related Disorders
Alcohol Use Disorders

303.90	Alcohol Dependence[a,b,c]
305.00	Alcohol Abuse

Alcohol-Induced Disorders

303.00	Alcohol Intoxication
291.81	Alcohol Withdrawal
	Specify if With Perceptual Disturbances
291.0	Alcohol Intoxication Delirium
291.0	Alcohol Withdrawal Delirium
291.2	Alcohol-Induced Persisting Dementia
291.1	Alcohol-Induced Persisting Amnestic Disorder
291.x	Alcohol-Induced Psychotic Disorder
.5	With Delusions[I,W]
.3	With Hallucinations[I,W]
291.89	Alcohol-Induced Mood Disorder[I,W]
291.89	Alcohol-Induced Anxiety Disorder[I,W]
291.89	Alcohol-Induced Sexual Dysfunction[I]
291.89	Alcohol-Induced Sleep Disorder[I,W]
291.9	Alcohol-Related Disorder NOS

Amphetamine- (or Amphetamine-like-) Related Disorders
Amphetamine Use Disorders

304.40	Amphetamine Dependence[a,b,c]
305.70	Amphetamine Abuse

Amphetamine-Induced Disorders

292.89	Amphetamine Intoxication
	Specify if With Perceptual Disturbances
292.0	Amphetamine Withdrawal
292.81	Amphetamine Intoxication Delirium
292.xx	Amphetamine-Induced Psychotic Disorder

.11	With Delusions[I]
.12	With Hallucinations[I]
292.84	Amphetamine-Induced Mood Disorder[I,W]
292.89	Amphetamine-Induced Anxiety Disorder[I]
292.89	Amphetamine-Induced Sexual Dysfunction[I]
292.89	Amphetamine-Induced Sleep Disorder[I,W]
292.9	Amphetamine-Related Disorder NOS

Caffeine-Related Disorders
Caffeine-Induced Disorders

305.90	Caffeine Intoxication
292.89	Caffeine-Induced Anxiety Disorder[I]
292.89	Caffeine-Induced Sleep Disorder[I]
292.9	Caffeine-Related Disorder NOS

Cannabis-Related Disorders
Cannabis Use Disorders

304.30	Cannabis Dependence[a,b,c]
305.20	Cannabis Abuse

Cannabis-Induced Disorders

292.89	Cannabis Intoxication
	Specify if With Perceptual Disturbances
292.81	Cannabis Intoxication Delirium
292.xx	Cannabis-Induced Psychotic Disorder
.11	With Delusions[I]
.12	With Hallucinations[I]
292.89	Cannabis-Induced Anxiety Disorder[I]
292.9	Cannabis-Related Disorder NOS

Cocaine-Related Disorders
Cocaine Use Disorders

304.20	Cocaine Dependence[a,b,c]
305.60	Cocaine Abuse

Cocaine-Induced Disorders

292.89	Cocaine Intoxication
	Specify if With Perceptual Disturbances
292.0	Cocaine Withdrawal
292.81	Cocaine Intoxication Delirium
292.xx	Cocaine-Induced Psychotic Disorder
.11	With Delusions[I]
.12	With Hallucinations[I]
292.84	Cocaine-Induced Mood Disorder[I,W]
292.89	Cocaine-Induced Anxiety Disorder[I,W]
292.89	Cocaine-Induced Sexual Dysfunction[I]
292.89	Cocaine-Induced Sleep Disorder[I,W]
292.9	Cocaine-Related Disorder NOS

Hallucinogen-Related Disorders
Hallucinogen Use Disorders

304.50	Hallucinogen Dependence[b,c]
305.30	Hallucinogen Abuse

Hallucinogen-Induced Disorders

292.89	Hallucinogen Intoxication

292.89	Hallucinogen Persisting Perception Disorder (Flashbacks)
292.81	Hallucinogen Intoxication Delirium
292.xx	Hallucinogen-Induced Psychotic Disorder
.11	With Delusions[I]
.12	With Hallucinations[I]
292.84	Hallucinogen-Induced Mood Disorder[I]
292.89	Hallucinogen-Induced Anxiety Disorder[I]
292.9	Hallucinogen-Related Disorder NOS

Inhalant-Related Disorders
Inhalant Use Disorders
304.60	Inhalant Dependence[b,c]
305.90	Inhalant Abuse

Inhalant-Induced Disorders
292.89	Inhalant Intoxication
292.81	Inhalant Intoxication Delirium
292.82	Inhalant-Induced Persisting Dementia
292.xx	Inhalant-Induced Psychotic Disorder
.11	With Delusions[I]
.12	With Hallucinations[I]
292.84	Inhalant-Induced Mood Disorder[I]
292.89	Inhalant-Induced Anxiety Disorder[I]
292.9	Inhalant-Related Disorder NOS

Nicotine-Related Disorders
Nicotine Use Disorder
305.1	Nicotine Dependence[a,b]

Nicotine-Induced Disorder
292.0	Nicotine Withdrawal
292.9	Nicotine-Related Disorder NOS

Opioid-Related Disorders
Opioid Use Disorders
304.00	Opioid Dependence[a,b,c,d]
305.50	Opioid Abuse

Opioid-Induced Disorders
292.89	Opioid Intoxication
	Specify if With Perceptual Disturbances
292.0	Opioid Withdrawal
292.81	Opioid Intoxication Delirium
292.xx	Opioid-Induced Psychotic Disorder
.11	With Delusions[I]
.12	With Hallucinations[I]
292.84	Opioid-Induced Mood Disorder[I]
292.89	Opioid-Induced Sexual Dysfunction[I]
292.89	Opioid-Induced Sleep Disorder[I,W]
292.9	Opioid-Related Disorder NOS

Phencyclidine-Related or Phencyclidine-like Disorders
Phencyclidine Use Disorders
304.60	Phencyclidine Dependence[b,c]
305.90	Phencyclidine Abuse

Phencyclidine-Induced Disorders
292.89	Phencyclidine Intoxication
	Specify if With Perceptual Disturbances
292.81	Phencyclidine Intoxication Delirium
292.xx	Phencyclidine-Induced Psychotic Disorder
.11	With Delusions[I]
.12	With Hallucinations[I]
292.84	Phencyclidine-Induced Mood Disorder[I]
292.89	Phencyclidine-Induced Anxiety Disorder[I]
292.9	Phencyclidine-Related Disorder NOS

Sedative-, Hypnotic-, or Anxiolytic-Related Disorders
Sedative, Hypnotic, or Anxiolytic Use Disorders
304.10	Sedative, Hypnotic, or Anxiolytic Dependence[a,b,c]
305.40	Sedative, Hypnotic, or Anxiolytic Abuse

Sedative-, Hypnotic-, or Anxiolytic-Induced Disorders
292.89	Sedative, Hypnotic, or Anxiolytic Intoxication
292.0	Sedative, Hypnotic, or Anxiolytic Withdrawal
	Specify if With Perceptual Disturbances
292.81	Sedative, Hypnotic, or Anxiolytic Intoxication Delirium
292.81	Sedative, Hypnotic, or Anxiolytic Withdrawal Delirium
292.82	Sedative-, Hypnotic-, or Anxiolytic-Induced Persisting Dementia
292.83	Sedative-, Hypnotic-, or Anxiolytic-Induced Persisting Amnestic Disorder
292.xx	Sedative-, Hypnotic-, or Anxiolytic-Induced Psychotic Disorder
.11	With Delusions[I,W]
.12	With Hallucinations[I,W]
292.84	Sedative-, Hypnotic-, or Anxiolytic-Induced Mood Disorder[I,W]
292.89	Sedative-, Hypnotic-, or Anxiolytic-Induced Anxiety Disorder[W]
292.89	Sedative-, Hypnotic-, or Anxiolytic-Induced Sexual Dysfunction[I]
292.89	Sedative-, Hypnotic-, or Anxiolytic-Induced Sleep Disorder[I,W]
292.9	Sedative-, Hypnotic-, or Anxiolytic-Related Disorder NOS

Polysubstance-Related Disorder
304.80	Polysubstance Dependence[a,b,c,d]

Other (or Unknown) Substance-Related Disorders
Other (or Unknown) Substance Use Disorders
304.90	Other (or Unknown) Substance Dependence[a,b,c,d]
305.90	Other (or Unknown) Substance Abuse

Other (or Unknown) Substance-Induced Disorders
292.89	Other (or Unknown) Substance Intoxication
	Specify if With Perceptual Disturbances
292.0	Other (or Unknown) Substance Withdrawal
	Specify if With Perceptual Disturbances

292.81	Other (or Unknown) Substance–Induced Delirium
292.82	Other (or Unknown) Substance–Induced Persisting Dementia
292.83	Other (or Unknown) Substance–Induced Persisting Amnestic Disorder
292.xx	Other (or Unknown) Substance–Induced Psychotic Disorder
.11	With Delusions[I,W]
.12	With Hallucinations[I,W]
292.84	Other (or Unknown) Substance–Induced Mood Disorder[I,W]
292.89	Other (or Unknown) Substance–Induced Anxiety Disorder[I,W]
292.89	Other (or Unknown) Substance–Induced Sexual Dysfunction[I]
292.89	Other (or Unknown) Substance–Induced Sleep Disorder[I,W]
292.9	Other (or Unknown) Substance–Related Disorder NOS

SCHIZOPHRENIA AND OTHER PSYCHOTIC DISORDERS

295.xx	Schizophrenia

The following Classification of Longitudinal Course applies to all subtypes of Schizophrenia:

Episodic With Interepisode Residual Symptoms (*specify if* With Prominent Negative Symptoms)/Episodic With No Interepisode Residual Symptoms

Continuous (*specify if* With Prominent Negative Symptoms)

Single Episode in Partial Remission (*specify if* With Prominent Negative Symptoms)/Single Episode In Full Remission

Other or Unspecified Pattern

.30	Paranoid Type
.10	Disorganized Type
.20	Catatonic Type
.90	Undifferentiated Type
.60	Residual Type
295.40	Schizophreniform Disorder
	Specify if Without Good Prognostic Features/ With Good Prognostic Features
295.70	Schizoaffective Disorder
	Specify type: Bipolar Type/Depressive Type
297.1	Delusional Disorder
	Specify type: Erotomanic Type/Grandiose Type/Jealous Type/Persecutory Type/Somatic Type/Mixed Type/Unspecified Type
298.8	Brief Psychotic Disorder
	Specify if With Marked Stressor(s)/Without Marked Stressor(s)/With Postpartum Onset
297.3	Shared Psychotic Disorder
293.xx	Psychotic Disorder Due to ... *[Indicate the General Medical Condition]*
.81	With Delusions
.82	With Hallucinations

—.—	Substance-Induced Psychotic Disorder *(refer to Substance-Related Disorders for substance-specific codes)*
	Specify if With Onset During Intoxication/ With Onset During Withdrawal
298.9	Psychotic Disorder NOS

MOOD DISORDERS

Code current state of Major Depressive Disorder or Bipolar I Disorder in fifth digit:

1 = Mild
2 = Moderate
3 = Severe Without Psychotic Features
4 = Severe With Psychotic Features
    Specify: Mood-Congruent Psychotic Features/Mood-Incongruent Psychotic Features
5 = In Partial Remission
6 = In Full Remission
0 = Unspecified

The following specifiers apply (for current or most recent episode) to Mood Disorders as noted:

[a]Severity/Psychotic/Remission Specifiers
[b]Chronic
[c]With Catatonic Features
[d]With Melancholic Features
[e]With Atypical Features
[f]With Postpartum Onset

The following specifiers apply to Mood Disorders as noted:

[g]With or Without Full Interepisode Recovery
[h]With Seasonal Pattern
[i]With Rapid Cycling

Depressive Disorders

296.xx	Major Depressive Disorder
.2x	Single Episode[a,b,c,d,e,f]
.3x	Recurrent[a,b,c,d,e,f,g,h]
300.4	Dysthymic Disorder
	Specify if Early Onset/Late Onset
	Specify: With Atypical Features
311	Depressive Disorder NOS

Bipolar Disorders

296.xx	Bipolar I Disorder
.0x	Single Manic Episode[a,c,f]
	Specify if Mixed
.40	Most Recent Episode Hypomanic[g,h,i]
.4x	Most Recent Episode Manic[a,c,f,g,h,i]
.6x	Most Recent Episode Mixed[a,c,f,g,h,i]
.5x	Most Recent Episode Depressed[a,b,c,d,e,f,g,h,i]
.7	Most Recent Episode Unspecified[g,h,i]
296.89	Bipolar II Disorder[a,b,c,d,e,f,g,h,i]
	Specify *(current or most recent episode)*: Hypomanic/Depressed
301.13	Cyclothymic Disorder
296.80	Bipolar Disorder NOS

293.83	Mood Disorder Due to … *[Indicate the General Medical Condition]* *Specify type:* With Depressive Features/With Major Depressive-Like Episode/With Manic Features/With Mixed Features
—.—	Substance-Induced Mood Disorder *(refer to Substance-Related Disorders for substance-specific codes)* *Specify type:* With Depressive Features/With Manic Features/With Mixed Features *Specify if* With Onset During Intoxication/With Onset During Withdrawal
296.90	Mood Disorder NOS

ANXIETY DISORDERS

300.01	Panic Disorder Without Agoraphobia
300.21	Panic Disorder With Agoraphobia
300.22	Agoraphobia Without History of Panic Disorder
300.29	Specific Phobia *Specify type:* Animal Type/Natural Environment Type/Blood-Injection-Injury Type/Situational Type/Other Type
300.23	Social Phobia *Specify if* Generalized
300.3	Obsessive-Compulsive Disorder *Specify if* With Poor Insight
309.81	Posttraumatic Stress Disorder *Specify if* Acute/Chronic *Specify if* With Delayed Onset
308.3	Acute Stress Disorder
300.02	Generalized Anxiety Disorder
293.84	Anxiety Disorder Due to … *[Indicate the General Medical Condition]* *Specify if* With Generalized Anxiety/With Panic Attacks/With Obsessive-Compulsive Symptoms
—.—	Substance-Induced Anxiety Disorder *(refer to Substance-Related Disorders for substance-specific codes)* *Specify if* With Generalized Anxiety/With Panic Attacks/With Obsessive-Compulsive Symptoms/With Phobic Symptoms *Specify if* With Onset During Intoxication/With Onset During Withdrawal
300.00	Anxiety Disorder NOS

SOMATOFORM DISORDERS

300.81	Somatization Disorder
300.82	Undifferentiated Somatoform Disorder
300.11	Conversion Disorder *Specify type:* With Motor Symptom or Deficit/With Sensory Symptom or Deficit/With Seizures or Convulsions/With Mixed Presentation
307.xx	Pain Disorder
.80	Associated With Psychological Factors
.89	Associated With Both Psychological Factors and a General Medical Condition *Specify if* Acute/Chronic
300.7	Hypochondriasis *Specify if* With Poor Insight
300.7	Body Dysmorphic Disorder
300.82	Somatoform Disorder NOS

FACTITIOUS DISORDERS

300.xx	Factitious Disorder
.16	With Predominantly Psychological Signs and Symptoms
.19	With Predominantly Physical Signs and Symptoms
.19	With Combined Psychological and Physical Signs and Symptoms
300.19	Factitious Disorder NOS

DISSOCIATIVE DISORDERS

300.12	Dissociative Amnesia
300.13	Dissociative Fugue
300.14	Dissociative Identity Disorder
300.6	Depersonalization Disorder
300.15	Dissociative Disorder NOS

SEXUAL AND GENDER IDENTITY DISORDERS

Sexual Dysfunctions

The following specifiers apply to all primary Sexual Dysfunctions:
Lifelong Type/Acquired Type
Generalized Type/Situational Type
Due to Psychological Factors/Due to Combined Factors

Sexual Desire Disorders

| 302.71 | Hypoactive Sexual Desire Disorder |
| 302.79 | Sexual Aversion Disorder |

Sexual Arousal Disorders

| 302.72 | Female Sexual Arousal Disorder |
| 302.72 | Male Erectile Disorder |

Orgasmic Disorders

302.73	Female Orgasmic Disorder
302.74	Male Orgasmic Disorder
302.75	Premature Ejaculation

Sexual Pain Disorders

| 302.76 | Dyspareunia (Not Due to a General Medical Condition) |
| 306.51 | Vaginismus (Not Due to a General Medical Condition) |

Sexual Dysfunction Due to a General Medical Condition

625.8	Female Hypoactive Sexual Desire Disorder Due to … *[Indicate the General Medical Condition]*
608.89	Male Hypoactive Sexual Desire Disorder Due to … *[Indicate the General Medical Condition]*
607.84	Male Erectile Disorder Due to … *[Indicate the General Medical Condition]*
625.0	Female Dyspareunia Due to … *[Indicate the General Medical Condition]*
608.89	Male Dyspareunia Due to … *[Indicate the General Medical Condition]*
625.8	Other Female Sexual Dysfunction Due to … *[Indicate the General Medical Condition]*
608.89	Other Male Sexual Dysfunction Due to … *[Indicate the General Medical Condition]*
—.—	Substance-Induced Sexual Dysfunction *(refer to Substance-Related Disorders for substance-specific codes)* *Specify if* With Impaired Desire/With Impaired Arousal/With Impaired Orgasm/With Sexual Pain *Specify if* With Onset During Intoxication
302.70	Sexual Dysfunction NOS

Paraphilias

302.4	Exhibitionism
302.81	Fetishism
302.89	Frotteurism
302.2	Pedophilia *Specify if* Sexually Attracted to Males/Sexually Attracted to Females/Sexually Attracted to Both *Specify if* Limited to Incest *Specify type:* Exclusive Type/Nonexclusive Type
302.83	Sexual Masochism
302.84	Sexual Sadism
302.3	Transvestic Fetishism *Specify if* With Gender Dysphoria
302.82	Voyeurism
302.9	Paraphilia NOS

Gender Identity Disorders

302.xx	Gender Identity Disorder
.6	In Children
.85	In Adolescents or Adults *Specify if* Sexually Attracted to Males/Sexually Attracted to Females/Sexually Attracted to Both/Sexually Attracted to Neither
302.6	Gender Identity Disorder NOS
302.9	Sexual Disorder NOS

EATING DISORDERS

307.1	Anorexia Nervosa *Specify type:* Restricting Type; Binge-Eating/Purging Type
307.51	Bulimia Nervosa *Specify type:* Purging Type/Nonpurging Type
307.50	Eating Disorder NOS

SLEEP DISORDERS

Primary Sleep Disorders

Dyssomnias

307.42	Primary Insomnia
307.44	Primary Hypersomnia *Specify if* Recurrent
347	Narcolepsy
780.59	Breathing-Related Sleep Disorder
307.45	Circadian Rhythm Sleep Disorder *Specify type:* Delayed Sleep Phase Type/Jet Lag Type/Shift Work Type/Unspecified Type
307.47	Dyssomnia NOS

Parasomnias

307.47	Nightmare Disorder
307.46	Sleep Terror Disorder
307.46	Sleepwalking Disorder
307.47	Parasomnia NOS

Sleep Disorders Related to Another Mental Disorder

307.42	Insomnia Related to … *[Indicate the Axis I or Axis II Disorder]*
307.44	Hypersomnia Related to … *[Indicate the Axis I or Axis II Disorder]*

Other Sleep Disorders

780.xx	Sleep Disorder Due to … [Indicate the General Medical Condition]
.52	Insomnia Type
.54	Hypersomnia Type
.59	Parasomnia Type
.59	Mixed Type
—.—	Substance-Induced Sleep Disorder (refer to Substance-Related Disorders for substance-specific codes) Specify type: Insomnia Type/Hypersomnia Type/Parasomnia Type/Mixed Type Specify if With Onset During Intoxication/With Onset During Withdrawal

IMPULSE-CONTROL DISORDERS NOT ELSEWHERE CLASSIFIED

312.34	Intermittent Explosive Disorder
312.32	Kleptomania
312.33	Pyromania
312.31	Pathologic Gambling
312.39	Trichotillomania
312.30	Impulse-Control Disorder NOS

ADJUSTMENT DISORDERS

309.xx	Adjustment Disorder
.0	With Depressed Mood
.24	With Anxiety
.28	With Mixed Anxiety and Depressed Mood
.3	With Disturbance of Conduct
.4	With Mixed Disturbance of Emotions and Conduct
.9	Unspecified
	Specify if Acute/Chronic

PERSONALITY DISORDERS

Note: These are coded on Axis II.

301.0	Paranoid Personality Disorder
301.20	Schizoid Personality Disorder
301.22	Schizotypal Personality Disorder
301.7	Antisocial Personality Disorder
301.83	Borderline Personality Disorder
301.50	Histrionic Personality Disorder
301.81	Narcissistic Personality Disorder
301.82	Avoidant Personality Disorder
301.6	Dependent Personality Disorder
301.4	Obsessive-Compulsive Personality Disorder
301.9	Personality Disorder NOS

OTHER CONDITIONS THAT MAY BE A FOCUS OF CLINICAL ATTENTION

Psychological Factors Affecting Medical Condition

316	… *[Specified Psychological Factor]* Affecting … *[Indicate the General Medical Condition]* Choose name based on nature of factors: Mental Disorder Affecting Medical Condition Psychological Symptoms Affecting Medical Condition Personality Traits or Coping Style Affecting Medical Condition Maladaptive Health Behaviors Affecting Medical Condition Stress-Related Physiological Response Affecting Medical Condition Other or Unspecified Psychological Factors Affecting Medical Condition

Medication-Induced Movement Disorders

332.1	Neuroleptic-Induced Parkinsonism
333.92	Neuroleptic Malignant Syndrome
333.7	Neuroleptic-Induced Acute Dystonia
333.99	Neuroleptic-Induced Acute Akathisia
333.82	Neuroleptic-Induced Tardive Dyskinesia
333.1	Medication-Induced Postural Tremor
333.90	Medication-Induced Movement Disorder NOS

Other Medication-Induced Disorder

995.2	Adverse Effects of Medication NOS

Relational Problems

V61.9	Relational Problem Related to a Mental Disorder or General Medical Condition
V61.20	Parent-Child Relational Problem
V61.10	Partner Relational Problem
V61.8	Sibling Relational Problem
V62.81	Relational Problem NOS

Problems Related to Abuse or Neglect

V61.21	Physical Abuse of Child *(code 995.5 if focus of attention is on victim)*
V61.21	Sexual Abuse of Child *(code 995.5 if focus of attention is on victim)*
V61.21	Neglect of Child *(code 995.5 if focus of attention is on victim)*
—.—	Physical Abuse of Adult
V61.12	(if by partner)
V62.83	(if by person other than partner) *(code 995.81 if focus of attention is on victim)*
—.—	Sexual Abuse of Adult
V61.12	(if by partner)
V62.83	(if by person other than partner) *(code 995.83 if focus of attention is on victim)*

Additional Conditions That May Be a Focus of Clinical Attention

V15.81	Noncompliance With Treatment
V65.2	Malingering
V71.01	Adult Antisocial Behavior
V71.02	Child or Adolescent Antisocial Behavior
V62.89	Borderline Intellectual Functioning *Note: This is coded on Axis II.*
780.9	Age-Related Cognitive Decline
V62.82	Bereavement
V62.3	Academic Problem
V62.2	Occupational Problem
313.82	Identity Problem
V62.89	Religious or Spiritual Problem
V62.4	Acculturation Problem
V62.89	Phase of Life Problem

ADDITIONAL CODES

300.9	Unspecified Mental Disorder (nonpsychotic)
V71.09	No Diagnosis or Condition on Axis I
799.9	Diagnosis or Condition Deferred on Axis I
V71.09	No Diagnosis on Axis II
799.9	Diagnosis Deferred on Axis II

AXIS II: PERSONALITY DISORDERS

301.0	Paranoid Personality Disorder
301.20	Schizoid Personality Disorder

301.22	Schizotypal Personality Disorder
301.7	Antisocial Personality Disorder
301.83	Borderline Personality Disorder
301.50	Histrionic Personality Disorder
301.81	Narcissistic Personality Disorder
301.82	Avoidant Personality Disorder
301.6	Dependent Personality Disorder
301.4	Obsessive-Compulsive Personality Disorder
301.9	Personality Disorder NOS

AXIS III: ICD-9-CM GENERAL MEDICAL CONDITIONS

Infectious and Parasitic Diseases (001-139)

Neoplasms (140-239)

Endocrine, Nutritional, and Metabolic Diseases and Immunity Disorders (240-279)

Diseases of the Blood and Blood-Forming Organs (280-289)

Diseases of the Nervous and Sense Organs (320-389)

Diseases of the Circulatory System (390-459)

Diseases of the Respiratory System (460-519)

Diseases of the Digestive System (520-579)

Diseases of the Genitourinary System (580-629)

Complications of Pregnancy, Childbirth, and the Puerperium (630-676)

Diseases of the Skin and Subcutaneous Tissue (680-709)

Diseases of the Musculoskeletal System and Connective Tissue (710-739)

Congenital Anomalies (740-759)

Certain Conditions Originating in the Perinatal Period (760-779)

Symptoms, Signs, and Ill-Defined Conditions (780-799)

Injury and Poisoning (800-999)

AXIS IV: PSYCHOSOCIAL AND ENVIRONMENTAL PROBLEMS

Problems with Primary Support Group (Childhood [V61.9], Adult [V61.9], Parent-Child [V61.2]), such as death of a family member; health problems in family; disruption of family by separation, divorce, or estrangement; removal from the home; remarriage of parent; sexual or physical abuse; parental overprotection; neglect of child; inadequate discipline; discord with siblings; birth of sibling

Problems Related to the Social Environment (V62.4), such as death or loss of friend, inadequate social support, living alone, difficulty with acculturation, discrimination, adjustment to life cycle transition (such as retirement)

Educational Problems (V62.3), such as illiteracy, academic problems, discord with teachers or classmates, inadequate school environment

Occupational Problems (V62.2), such as unemployment, threat of job loss, stressful work schedule, difficult work conditions, job dissatisfaction, job change, discord with boss or co-workers

Housing Problems (V60.9), such as homelessness, inadequate housing, unsafe neighborhood, discord with neighbors or landlord

Economic Problems (V60.9), such as extreme poverty, inadequate finances, insufficient welfare support

Problems with Access to Health Care Services (V63.9), such as inadequate health care services, transportation to health care facilities unavailable, inadequate health insurance

Problems Related to Interaction with the Legal System/Crime (V62.5), such as arrest, incarceration, litigation, victim of crime

Other Psychosocial and Environmental Problems (V62.9), such as exposure to disasters, war, other hostilities; discord with non-family caregivers such as counselor, social worker, or physician; unavailability of social service agencies

AXIS V: GLOBAL ASSESSMENT OF FUNCTIONING (GAF) SCALE*

Consider psychological, social, and occupational functioning on a hypothetical continuum of mental health-illness. Do not include impairment in functioning due to physical or environmental limitations. (*Note:* Use intermediate codes when appropriate, such as 45, 68, 72.)

Code

100	Superior functioning in a wide range of activities, life's problems never seem to get out of hand, is sought out by others because of his many positive qualities. No symptoms.
91	
90	Absent or minimal symptoms (e.g., mild anxiety before an examination), good functioning in all areas, interested and involved in a wide range of activities, socially effective, generally satisfied with life, no more than everyday problems or concerns (e.g., an occasional argument with family members).
81	
80	If symptoms are present, they are transient and expectable reactions to psychosocial stressors (e.g., difficulty concentrating after family argument); no more than slight impairment in social, occupational, or school functioning (e.g., temporarily falling behind in schoolwork).
71	
70	Some mild symptoms (e.g., depressed mood and mild insomnia) OR some difficulty in social, occupational, or school functioning (e.g., occasional truancy, or theft within the

*The rating of overall psychological functioning on a scale of 0-100 was operationalized by Luborsky in the Health-Sickness Rating Scale (Luborsky L: Clinicians' judgments of mental health, *Arch Gen Psychiatry* 7:407-417, 1962). Spitzer and colleagues developed a revision of the Health-Sickness Rating Scale called the Global Assessment Scale (GAS) (Endicott J et al: The global assessment scale: a procedure for measuring overall severity of psychiatric disturbance, *Arch Gen Psychiatry* 33:766-771, 1976). A modified version of the GAS was included in DSM-III-R as the Global Assessment of Functioning (GAF) Scale.

household), but generally functioning pretty well, has some meaningful interpersonal relationships.

61

60 Moderate symptoms (e.g., flat affect and circumstantial speech, occasional panic attacks) OR moderate difficulty in social, occupational, or school functioning (e.g, few friends, conflicts with peers or co-workers).

51

50 Serious symptoms (e.g., suicidal ideation, severe obsessional rituals, frequent shoplifting) OR any serious impairment in social, occupational, or school functioning (e.g., no friends, unable to keep a job).

41

40 Some impairment in reality testing or communication (e.g., speech is at times illogical, obscure, or irrelevant) OR major impairment in several areas, such as work or school, family relations, judgment, thinking, or mood (e.g., depressed man avoids friends, neglects family, and is unable to work; child frequently beats up younger children, is defiant at home, and is failing at school).

31

30 Behavior is considerably influenced by delusions or hallucinations OR serious impairment in communication or judgment (e.g., sometimes incoherent, acts grossly inappropriately, suicidal preoccupation) OR inability to function in almost all areas (e.g., stays in bed all day; no job, home, or friends).

21

20 Some danger of hurting self or others (e.g., suicide attempts without clear expectation of death, frequently violent, manic excitement) OR occasionally fails to maintain minimal personal hygiene (e.g., smears feces) OR gross impairment in communication (e.g., largely incoherent or mute).

11

10 Persistent danger of severely hurting self or others (e.g., recurrent violence) OR persistent inability to maintain personal hygiene OR serious suicidal act with clear expectation of death.

1

0 Inadequate information.

Outline for Cultural Formulation

The following outline for cultural formulation is meant to supplement the multiaxial diagnostic assessment and to address difficulties that may be encountered in applying *DSM-IV-TR* criteria in a multicultural environment. The cultural formulation provides a systematic review of the individual's cultural background, the role of the cultural context in the expression and evaluation of symptoms and dysfunction, and the effect and cultural differences they may have on the relationship between the individual and the clinician.

The clinician must take into account the individual's ethnic and cultural context in the evaluation of each of the *DSM-IV-TR* axes. The suggested cultural formulation provides an opportunity to describe systematically the individual's cultural and social reference group and ways in which the cultural context is relevant to clinical care. The clinician may provide a narrative summary for each of the following categories:

Cultural identity of the individual. Note the individual's ethnic or cultural reference groups. For immigrants and ethnic minorities, note separately the degree of involvement with both the culture of origin and the host culture (where applicable). Also note language abilities, use, and preference (including multilingualism).

Cultural explanations of the individual's illness. The following may be identified: the predominant idioms of distress through which symptoms or the need for social support are communicated (e.g., "nerves," possessing spirits, somatic complaints, inexplicable misfortune), the meaning and perceived severity of the individual's symptoms in relation to norms of the cultural reference group, any local illness category used by the individual's family and community to identify the condition, the perceived causes or explanatory models that the individual and the reference group use to explain the illness, and current preferences for and past experiences with professional and popular sources of care.

Cultural factors related to psychosocial environment and levels of functioning. Note culturally relevant interpretations of social stressors, available social supports, and levels of functioning and disability. This includes stresses in the local social environment and the role of religion and kin networks in providing emotional, instrumental, and informational support.

Cultural elements of the relationship between the individual and the clinician. Indicate differences in culture and social status between the individual and the clinician and problems that these differences may cause in diagnosis and treatment (e.g., difficulty in communicating in the individual's first language, in eliciting symptoms or understanding their cultural significance, in negotiating an appropriate relationship or level of intimacy, in determining whether a behavior is normative or pathological).

Overall cultural assessment for diagnosis and care. The formulation concludes with a discussion of how cultural considerations specifically influence comprehensive diagnosis and care.

NANDA-I Nursing Diagnoses 2012-2014

Domain 1: Health Promotion

Class 1: Health Awareness
Deficient Diversional Activity (00097)
Sedentary Lifestyle (00168)
Class 2: Health Management 153
Deficient Community Health (00215)
Risk-Prone Health Behavior (00188)
Ineffective Health Maintenance (00099)
Readiness for Enhanced Immunization Status (00186)
Ineffective Protection (00043)
Ineffective Self-Health Management (00078)
Readiness for Enhanced Self-Health Management (00162)
Ineffective Family Therapeutic Regimen Management (00080)

Domain 2: Nutrition

Class 1: Ingestion
Insufficient Breast Milk (00216)
Ineffective Infant Feeding Pattern (00107)
Imbalanced Nutrition: Less Than Body Requirements (00002)
Imbalanced Nutrition: More Than Body Requirements (00001)
Readiness for Enhanced Nutrition (00163)
Risk for Imbalanced Nutrition: More Than Body Requirements (00003)
Impaired Swallowing (00103)

Class 2: Digestion
Class 3: Absorption
Class 4: Metabolism
Risk for Unstable Blood Glucose Level (00179)
Neonatal Jaundice (00194)
Risk for Neonatal Jaundice (00230)
Risk for Impaired Liver Function (00178)
Class 5: Hydration
Risk for Electrolyte Imbalance (00195)
Readiness for Enhanced Fluid Balance (00160)
Deficient Fluid Volume (00027)
Excess Fluid Volume (00026)
Risk for Deficient Fluid Volume (00028)
Risk for Imbalanced Fluid Volume (00025)

Domain 3: Elimination and Exchange

Class 1: Urinary Function
Functional Urinary Incontinence (00020)
Overflow Urinary Incontinence (00176)
Reflex Urinary Incontinence (00018)
Stress Urinary Incontinence (00017)
Urge Urinary Incontinence (00019)
Risk for Urge Urinary Incontinence (00022)
Impaired Urinary Elimination (00016)
Readiness for Enhanced Urinary Elimination (00166)
Urinary Retention (00023)
Class 2: Gastrointestinal Function
Constipation (00011)
Perceived Constipation (00012)
Risk for Constipation (00015)
Diarrhea (00013)
Dysfunctional Gastrointestinal Motility (00196)
Risk For Dysfunctional Gastrointestinal Motility (00197)
Bowel Incontinence (00014)
Class 3: Integumentary Function

Class 4: Respiratory Function
Impaired Gas Exchange (00030)

Domain 4: Activity/Rest

Class 1: Sleep/Rest
Insomnia (00095)
Sleep Deprivation (00096)
Readiness for Enhanced Sleep (00165)
Disturbed Sleep Pattern (00198)
Class 2: Activity/Exercise
Risk for Disuse Syndrome (00040)
Impaired Bed Mobility (00091)
Impaired Physical Mobility (00085)
Impaired Wheelchair Mobility (00089)
Impaired Transfer Ability (00090)
Impaired Walking (00088)
Class 3: Energy Balance
Disturbed Energy Field (00050)
Fatigue (00093)
Wandering (00154)
Class 4: Cardiovascular/Pulmonary Responses
Activity Intolerance (00092)
Risk for Activity Intolerance (00094)
Ineffective Breathing Pattern (00032)
Decreased Cardiac Output (00029)
Risk for Ineffective Gastrointestinal Perfusion (00202)
Risk for Ineffective Renal Perfusion (00203)
Impaired Spontaneous Ventilation (00033)
Ineffective Peripheral Tissue Perfusion (00204)
Risk for Decreased Cardiac Tissue Perfusion (00200)
Risk for Ineffective Cerebral Tissue Perfusion (00201)
Risk for Ineffective Peripheral Tissue Perfusion (00228)
Dysfunctional Ventilatory Weaning Response (00034)
Class 5: Self-Care
Impaired Home Maintenance (00098)
Readiness for Enhanced Self-Care (00182)
Bathing Self-Care Deficit (00108)
Dressing Self-Care Deficit (00109)
Feeding Self-Care Deficit (00102)
Toileting Self-Care Deficit (00110)
Self-Neglect (00193)

Domain 5: Perception/Cognition

Class 1: Attention
Unilateral Neglect (00123)
Class 2: Orientation
Impaired Environmental Interpretation Syndrome (00127)
Class 3: Sensation/Perception
Class 4: Cognition
Acute Confusion (00128)
Chronic Confusion (00129)
Risk for Acute Confusion (00173)
Ineffective Impulse Control (00222)
Deficient Knowledge (00126)
Readiness for Enhanced Knowledge (00161)
Impaired Memory (00131)

Class 5: Communication
Readiness for Enhanced Communication (00157)
Impaired Verbal Communication (00051)

Domain 6: Self-Perception

Class 1: Self-Concept
Hopelessness (00124)
Risk for Compromised Human Dignity (00174)
Risk for Loneliness (00054)
Disturbed Personal Identity (00121)
Risk for Disturbed Personal Identity (00225)
Readiness for Enhanced Self-Concept (00167)
Class 2: Self-Esteem
Chronic Low Self-Esteem (00119)
Situational Low Self-Esteem (00120)
Risk for Chronic Low Self-Esteem (00224)
Risk for Situational Low Self-Esteem (00153)
Class 3: Body Image
Disturbed Body Image (00118)

Domain 7: Role Relationships

Class 1: Caregiving Roles
Ineffective Breastfeeding (00104)
Interrupted Breastfeeding (00105)
Readiness for Enhanced Breastfeeding (00106)
Caregiver Role Strain (00061)
Risk for Caregiver Role Strain (00062)
Impaired Parenting (00056)
Readiness for Enhanced Parenting (00164)
Risk for Impaired Parenting (00057)
Class 2: Family Relationships
Risk for Impaired Attachment (00058)
Dysfunctional Family Processes (00063)
Interrupted Family Processes (00060)
Readiness for Enhanced Family Processes (00159)
Class 3: Role Performance
Ineffective Relationship (00223)
Readiness for Enhanced Relationship (00207)
Risk for Ineffective Relationship (00229)
Parental Role Conflict (00064)
Ineffective Role Performance (00055)
Impaired Social Interaction (00052)

Domain 8: Sexuality

Class 1: Sexual Identity
Class 2: Sexual Function
Sexual Dysfunction (00059)
Ineffective Sexuality Pattern (00065)
Class 3: Reproduction
Ineffective Childbearing Process (00221)
Readiness for Enhanced Childbearing Process (00208)
Risk for Ineffective Childbearing Process (00227)
Risk for Disturbed Maternal–Fetal Dyad (00209)

Domain 9: Coping/Stress Tolerance

Class 1: Post-Trauma Responses

Post-Trauma Syndrome (00141)
Risk for Post-Trauma Syndrome (00145)
Rape-Trauma Syndrome (00142)
Relocation Stress Syndrome (00114)
Risk for Relocation Stress Syndrome (00149)
Class 2: Coping Responses
Ineffective Activity Planning (00199)
Risk for Ineffective Activity Planning (00226)
Anxiety (00146)
Defensive Coping (00071)
Ineffective Coping (00069)
Readiness for Enhanced Coping (00158)
Ineffective Community Coping (00077)
Readiness for Enhanced Community Coping (00076)
Compromised Family Coping (00074)
Disabled Family Coping (00073)
Readiness for Enhanced Family Coping (00075)
Death Anxiety (00147)
Ineffective Denial (00072)
Adult Failure to Thrive (00101)
Fear (00148)
Grieving (00136)
Complicated Grieving (00135)
Risk for Complicated Grieving (00172)
Readiness for Enhanced Power (00187)
Powerlessness (00125)
Risk for Powerlessness (00152)
Impaired Individual Resilience (00210)
Readiness for Enhanced Resilience (00212)
Risk for Compromised Resilience (00211)
Chronic Sorrow (00137)
Stress Overload (00177)
Class 3: Neurobehavioral Stress
Autonomic Dysreflexia (00009)
Risk for Autonomic Dysreflexia (00010)
Disorganized Infant Behavior (00116)
Readiness for Enhanced Organized Infant Behavior (00117)
Risk for Disorganized Infant Behavior (00115)
Decreased Intracranial Adaptive Capacity (00049)

Domain 10: Life Principles

Class 1: Values
Readiness for Enhanced Hope (00185)
Class 2: Beliefs
Readiness for Enhanced Spiritual Well-Being (00068)
Class 3: Value/Belief/Action Congruence
Readiness for Enhanced Decision-Making (00184)
Decisional Conflict (00083)
Moral Distress (00175)
Noncompliance (00079)
Impaired Religiosity (00169)
Readiness for Enhanced Religiosity (00171)
Risk for Impaired Religiosity (00170)
Spiritual Distress (00066)
Risk for Spiritual Distress (00067)

Domain 11: Safety/Protection 415

Class 1: Infection 417
Risk for Infection (00004)
Class 2: Physical Injury 421
Ineffective Airway Clearance (00031)
Risk for Aspiration (00039)
Risk for Bleeding (00206)
Impaired Dentition (00048)
Risk for Dry Eye (00219)
Risk for Falls (00155)
Risk for Injury (00035)
Impaired Oral Mucous Membrane (00045)
Risk for Perioperative Positioning Injury (00087)
Risk for Peripheral Neurovascular Dysfunction (00086)
Risk for Shock (00205)
Impaired Skin Integrity (00046)
Risk for Impaired Skin Integrity (00047)
Risk for Sudden Infant Death Syndrome (00156)
Risk for Suffocation (00036)
Delayed Surgical Recovery (00100)
Risk for Thermal Injury (00220)
Impaired Tissue Integrity (00044)
Risk for Trauma (00038)
Risk for Vascular Trauma (00213)
Class 3: Violence 447
Risk for Other-Directed Violence (00138)
Risk for Self-Directed Violence (00140)
Self-Mutilation (00151)
Risk for Self-Mutilation (00139)
Risk for Suicide (00150)
Class 4: Environmental Hazards 454
Contamination (00181)
Risk for Contamination (00180)
Risk for Poisoning (00037)
Class 5: Defensive Processes 461
Risk for Adverse Reaction to Iodinated Contrast Media (000218)
Latex Allergy Response (00041)
Risk for Allergy Response (00217)
Risk for Latex Allergy Response (00042)
Class 6: Thermoregulation 467
Risk for Imbalanced Body Temperature (00005)
Hyperthermia (00007)
Hypothermia (00006)
Ineffective Thermoregulation (00008)

Domain 12: Comfort

Class 1: Physical Comfort
Class 2: Environmental Comfort
Class 3: Social Comfort
Impaired Comfort (00214)
Readiness for Enhanced Comfort (00183)
Nausea (00134)
Acute Pain (00132)
Chronic Pain (00133)
Social Isolation (00053)

Domain 13: Growth/Development

Class 1: Growth
    Risk for Disproportionate Growth (00113)
Class 2: Development
    Delayed Growth and Development (00111)
    Risk for Delayed Development (00112)

Nursing Diagnoses Retired from the NANDA-I Taxonomy 2009-2014:

Health-seeking Behaviors (00084) Retired 2009-2011

Disturbed Sensory Perception (Specify: Visual, Auditory, Kinesthetic, Gustatory, Tactile, Olfactory) (00122) Retired 2012-2014

Page numbers followed by *f* indicate figures; *t*, tables; *b*, boxes.

559